Novak's
Gynecology

Novak's
Gynecology

Twelfth Edition

Editor

Jonathan S. Berek, MD, MMSC

Professor and Vice Chair
Chief of Gynecology and Gynecologic Oncology
Department of Obstetrics and Gynecology
UCLA School of Medicine
Director, UCLA Women's Reproductive Cancer Program
Jonsson Comprehensive Cancer Center
Los Angeles, California

Associate Editors

Eli Y. Adashi, MD

Professor and Director
Division of Reproductive Endocrinology and Infertility
Departments of Obstetrics and Gynecology, and Physiology
University of Maryland School of Medicine
Baltimore, Maryland

Paula A. Hillard, MD

Associate Professor
Departments of Obstetrics and Gynecology, and Pediatrics
University of Cincinnati College of Medicine
Cincinnati, Ohio

Illustration and Graphic Design

Timothy C. Hengst, CMI, FAMI

Editorial Assistance

Rebecca D. Rinehart

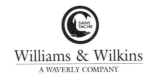

Williams & Wilkins
A WAVERLY COMPANY
BALTIMORE • PHILADELPHIA • LONDON • PARIS • BANGKOK
BUENOS AIRES • HONG KONG • MUNICH • SYDNEY • TOKYO • WROCLAW

Editor: Charles W. Mitchell
Managing Editor: Marjorie Kidd Keating
Production Coordinator: Anne Stewart Seitz
Copy Editor: Denise Wilson
Designer: Norman W. Och
Illustration Planner: Lorraine Wrzosek
Cover Designer: Wilma Rosenberger
Typesetter: Peirce Graphic Services, Inc.
Manufacturer: Metropole

ISBN 0-683-00593-6

Copyright © 1996 Williams & Wilkins
351 West Camden Street
Baltimore, Maryland 21201-2436 USA

Rose Tree Corporate Center
1400 North Providence Road
Building II, Suite 5025
Media, Pennsylvania 19063-2043 USA

Printed in Canada

Eleventh Edition, 1988

Library of Congress Cataloging-in-Publication Data

Novak's gynecology, — 12th ed. / editor, Jonathan S. Berek : associate editors,
  Eli Y. Adashi, Paula A. Hillard.
      p.   cm.
  Rev. ed. of: Novak's textbook of gynecology / Howard W. Jones III,
Anne Colston Wentz, Lonnie S. Burnett. 11thed. ©1988.
    Previous edition has main entry under Novak, Emil, 1883–1857.
    Includes bibliographical references and index.
    ISBN 0-683-00593-6 (alk. paper)
    1. Gynecology.   I. Berek, Jonathan S.   II. Adashi, E. Y.
III. Hillard, Paula Adams.   IV. Jones, Howard W. (Howard Wilbur),
1942–   Novak's textbook of gynecology.
    [DNLM: 1. Genital Diseases, Female.   2. Pregnancy Complications.
3. Gynecology—methods.   WP 100 N9351 1996]
RG101.N69   1996
618.1—dc20
DNLM/DLC   96–16316
for Library of Congress   CIP

To purchase additional copies of this book, call our customer service department at (800) 638-0672 or fax orders to (800) 447-8438. For other book services, including chapter reprints and large quantity sales, ask for the Special Sales department.

Canadian customer should call (800) 268-4178, or fax (905) 470-6780. For all other calls originating outside of the United States, please call (410) 528-4223 or fax us at (410) 528-8550.

Visit Williams & Wilkins on the Internet: http://www.wwilkins.com or contact our customer service department at custserv@wwilkins.com. Williams & Wilkins customer service representatives are available from 8:30 am to 6:00 pm, EST, Monday through Friday, for telephone access.

98 99
4 5 6 7 8 9 10

Dedication
We dedicate this book to our families—our spouses,
Deborah Berek, Toni Adashi, and Randy Hillard;
and our children, Jonathan Micah, James, and Jessica Berek;
Judah Adashi; Elena, Ian, and Nat Hillard.

Foreword

In 1940, Emil Novak published the first edition of what has been known as "Novak's Textbook." Dr. Novak was a mentor and exemplar to so many of those of us who studied gynecology and gynecologic pathology. He clearly saw the importance of this study and this field of medicine, and he provided each of us who have followed in his footsteps with a wonderful example. To us, Emil Novak was the ultimate doctor, a man who saw the study of medicine as a way to provide aid to those who suffered illness. We are indebted to him for having begun this work, taught so many who have worked in this specialty, and provided the means by which his textbook could carry on his work.

It is a pleasure and a privilege to have been asked to pen this foreword, as it has been my pleasure and privilege to have worked on this textbook and to have as colleagues in this endeavor so many superb physicians. Dr. Novak would endorse and be thankful that the text is being updated for your use. He knew, as we do, that the pursuit of academic medicine is imperative to the development of medicine in general and our field in particular. In order to provide you with the same superb resource that Emil Novak began 55 years ago, *Novak's Textbook of Gynecology* must be updated, and a new generation of men and women must accept his challenge.

Medicine as a profession has changed and will continue to change, but the basic message that Emil Novak presented in the first textbook is the same: doctors must be concerned with the welfare of patients, and in order to accomplish this task, they must have access to the latest and best information and training. Jonathan Berek and his colleagues are well schooled in the legacy of Emil Novak and all of those who have worked on this book. It is with confidence in the quality of their work that I endorse this 12th edition of *Novak's Gynecology.*

J. Donald Woodruff, MD
Richard W. TeLinde Professor Emeritus
Johns Hopkins University School of Medicine
Baltimore, Maryland

Preface to the Twelfth Edition

After a hiatus of 8 years, *Novak's Gynecology* has returned, now in its 12th iteration. The textbook has been completely revised and reorganized, but its essence is still the same—a comprehensive general textbook in gynecology. The substance reflects the wealth of information that has evolved during the 55 years since the inception of *Novak's Textbook of Gynecology.* It is an honor to have been asked to shepherd such an important book in our specialty and one that we hope will inform and educate our colleagues for many years.

We are mindful of our past and of our heritage. The textbook, originated by the faculty of the Johns Hopkins University School of Medicine, continues to reflect the contributions of that great institution. The textbook was inaugurated by Dr. Emil Novak, a gynecologist and pathologist, a pioneer in the specialty. After the fifth edition and subsequent death of Dr. Novak in 1957, many physicians of Johns Hopkins and subsequently the Vanderbilt faculty have helped carry the torch—Dr. Edmund R. Novak through the ninth edition in 1979; Drs. Howard W. Jones, Jr. and Georgeanna Seegar Jones through the tenth edition in 1981; and Drs. Howard W. Jones, III, Lonnie S. Burnett, and Anne Colston Wentz through the 11th edition in 1988. These editors, assisted by many contributors who have been faculty at Johns Hopkins, especially Drs. J. Donald Woodruff and Conrad G. Julian, have helped define the specialty of gynecology over the latter half of the 20th century. These authors gave birth to much of gynecology as we know it today—its surgical and medical therapies, reproductive endocrinology, assisted reproductive technologies, gynecologic oncology, urogynecology, and infectious diseases—which has been shaped and directed by the ideas enunciated by these physicians. The new editor is a graduate of Johns Hopkins University School of Medicine, and one of the associate editors is a former fellow in that department. We are proud to be part of that rich tradition.

This edition incorporates a new format. The design of the book was established by Dr. Leon Speroff and his colleagues in the textbook *Clinical Gynecologic Endocrinology and Infertility* and was adapted for the book *Practical Gynecologic Oncology.* By using this presentation style, this book should facilitate the study of gynecology for the student as well as the specialist.

Novak's Gynecology, 12th edition, is presented in six sections. The first, "Principles of Practice," includes the initial assessment of the gynecologic patient, the history and physical examination, and communication skills. This section addresses ethical principles of patient care, quality assessment and improvement, and the epidemiology of gynecologic conditions. The second section, "Basic Sciences," summarizes the scientific basis for the specialty—anatomy and embryology, molecular biology and genetics, and reproductive physiology. The third section, "Preventive and Primary Care," is new to *Novak's Gynecology* and reflects the importance of primary health care for women, which has evolved to address preventive care, screening, family planning, sexuality, and common psychiatric problems. The fourth section, "General Gynecology," reviews benign diseases of the female reproductive tract, the evaluation of pelvic infections, pain, intraepithelial diseases, the management of early pregnancy loss and ectopic pregnancy, the evaluation of benign breast disease, and the operative management of benign gynecologic conditions. The fifth section, "Reproductive Endocrinology," summarizes the major disorders affecting the growth, development, and function of women from puberty through menopause. The sixth section, "Gynecologic Oncology," covers malignant diseases of the female reproductive tract, breast cancer, palliative care, and pain management.

We have purposely presented a limited historical perspective on the development of the specialty. Space limitations have required a shift in emphasis from the past to the present. Our respect for the rich heritage provided by our predecessors is demonstrated by our commitment to the future of gynecologic practice and scholarship.

The editors are grateful to the many individuals who helped to create this book. Rebecca Rinehart provided superb editorial assistance, manuscript review, and revision. Tim Hengst, our outstanding medical illustrator, designed and created the original artwork. At our publishers, Williams & Wilkins, Mr. Charley Mitchell has guided the editorial process with great skill and enthusiasm. Working with him, Anne Stewart Seitz, Margie Keating, Lorraine Wrzosek, Brian Smith, Deborah K. Tourtlotte, and their team have produced the manuscript with finesse. Expert secretarial support has been provided by Tery Schooler, Sherry Weber, Rhonda McMillan, Nicole Jones, Karen Kannmacher, and Nancy Timmons. We are grateful to Drs. Yao Shi Fu, Roberta K. Nieberg, and Nagesh Ragavendra, who provided photography.

We wish to acknowledge our mentors—Dean Sherman Mellinkoff, Drs. J. Donald Woodruff, J. George Moore, and William J. Dignam (J.S.B.); George W. Mitchell, Jr., Howard W. Jones, Jr., Georgeanna Seegar Jones, Samuel S. C. Yen, and M. Carlyle Crenshaw, Jr. (E.Y.A.); and Luther Talbert (P.A.H.). We also ackowledge our colleagues—Drs. Gautum Chaudhuri, Neville F. Hacker, Robin Farias-Eisner, and Roy M. Pitkin (J.S.B.); Howard D. McClamrock (E.Y.A.); and Clarence McLain, Robert Rebar, and Margery Gass (P.A.H.). Each of these physicians and scholars provided us with guidance, wisdom, and support over the years at our respective university medical schools.

The editor is grateful to Nicole Kidman, the chair of the advisory board of the UCLA Women's Reproductive Cancer Treatment and Research Program, and Tom Cruise—whose creativity, energy, and friendship have helped stimulate this project.

We hope that this book will be a useful resource for our colleagues and for the students of the specialty of gynecology. We are proud to be members of that specialty and we look forward to its continued strength and evolution as a major force in the delivery of health care for women. We dedicate our work to the enhancement of medical services to women throughout the world.

Jonathan S. Berek

Eli Y. Adashi

Paula A. Hillard

Preface to the First Edition

Since the plan and scope of this book represent something of a departure from those followed in other textbooks of gynecology, the author feels impelled to state the ideas which furnished the incentive for the preparation of this work, and which dictated its character and scope.

First of all, no especial apology seems necessary for the combined title. While gynecology was formerly often spoken of as a branch of surgery, this is certainly not its present status. Only a small proportion of gynecological patients require surgical treatment. On the other hand, the biological aspects of gynecology have assumed vast importance, chiefly because of the amazing developments in the field of reproductive physiology and endocrinology. Many of these advances find daily application in the interpretation and management of functional disorders in women. In other words, female endocrinology is now an integral and important part of gynecology and it is so considered in this book.

Second, it has always seemed to me that the great majority of readers of textbooks on gynecology must be not at all interested in the details of operative technique, to the consideration of which most authors have devoted many pages. Certainly this applies to the general practitioner, while medical educators are now generally agreed that the medical student should not be burdened with such details in his undergraduate years. Since this book is designed for these two groups primarily, the indication seemed clear to omit the consideration of operative details. The plan followed is to carry the patient up to the point of operation, and to discuss the indications, scope and purpose of the latter, without going into descriptions of the technique itself.

Diagnosis and treatment have been accented throughout the book, as I believe most readers would wish. The traditional chapters on anatomy, history-taking, and methods of examination have been boiled down to the essentials. On the other hand, functional disorders, including especially the large group of gynecological endocrinopathies, have been treated rather elaborately, in keeping with the avowed plan of covering the combined fields of gynecology and female endocrinology. The list of references appended to each chapter makes no pretense of exhaustiveness, and preference has been given to publications most worth while, those most recent, and those written in English. The pathological aspects of gynecological disease, so fundamental to a proper understanding of the whole subject, have received adequate but not disproportionate consideration.

In the consideration of various endocrine disorders a disturbing problem presented itself. In the discussion of endocrine preparations which might be indicated in treatment, there is no doubt that the mention of various products by their commercial names would have had some advantages. On the other hand, these have appeared to be definitely outweighed by the disadvantages of such a plan, apart from its questionable delicacy. These proprietary preparations are constantly multiplying, and their commercial names are being changed from day to day. For example, there are now well over forty estrogenic preparations on the market. It would be almost impossible, in any enumeration of such therapeutic products, to avoid omission of some of them, and this might be very unfair to products perhaps just as effective as those which might be included. A complete list published today is quite likely to be very incomplete within a few months.

The sensible plan seemed to be to rely on the intelligence and initiative of the reader, who should have no difficulty in ascertaining good commercial preparations of estrogen, progesterone, chorionic hormone or any other hormone principle to which reference is made in the treatment of various disorders.

It will be noted that the work is devoted to "straight" gynecology and male endocrinology and that it does not include a consideration of disorders in allied fields which concededly obtrude themselves frequently into the practice of the gynecologist. For example, many gynecologists include female urology in their practices, while anorectal and abdominal surgical problems are often encountered, as may be problems in almost any field of medicine. For textbook purposes, however, the line must be drawn fairly sharply, and the reader will naturally expect to go to the proper sources for information in any of these allied fields.

In short, the purpose of this book is to present to the reader as much information as is possible in as practical a fashion as possible on the subjects of gynecology and female endocrinology. Whether right or wrong, the ideas behind the book represent the crystallization of many years of teaching and practice in gynecology. The author's goal has been to produce a book which would not only be suited to the needs of the medical student, but which could be carried with him into the practice of his profession.

It is a pleasant obligation to express my indebtedness to those who have been helpful to me in the preparation of this book. To a number of my friends, especially Dr. R.B. Greenblatt, of Augusta, Georgia, I am grateful for the loan of illustrations; to Dr. E.L. Krieg, for the excellent colored illustrations as well as for other photographic work; to Mr. Chester Reather, for most of the photomicrographs; to Miss Eva Hildebrandt, technician in the Laboratory of Gynecological Pathology at The Johns Hopkins Hospital and to Sister Mary Lucy, technician at Bon Secours Hospital for help in the preparation of sections for microscopic illustration; to my artist, Miss Frances Shultz, for many of the illustrations; and to my faithful secretary, Miss Helen L. Clayton, for much help throughout the project. For permission to use illustrations which have appeared in previously published articles of my own I am indebted to the publishers of the *Journal of the American Medical Association;* the *American Journal of Obstetrics and Gynecology; Surgery, Gynecology and Obstetrics;* and the *Bulletin of The Johns Hopkins Hospital.*

Certain illustrations which appeared in one of my previous books, *Gynecological and Obstetrical Pathology,* do not have a credit line in the caption. For permission to use these I wish to thank WB Saunders Company, the publishers.

Finally, it is a genuine pleasure to acknowledge the efficient and wholehearted cooperation of the publishers, Little, Brown and Co., throughout the preparation of this work.

EMIL NOVAK
Baltimore

Contributors

Jean R. Anderson, MD

Associate Professor
Department of Gynecology and Obstetrics
Johns Hopkins University School of Medicine
Baltimore, Maryland

Vicki V. Baker, MD

George W. Morley Professor of Obstetrics and Gynecology
Chief, Division of Gynecologic Oncology
Department of Obstetrics and Gynecology
University of Michigan School of Medicine
Ann Arbor, Michigan

David A. Baram, MD

Associate Professor
Departments of Obstetrics and Gynecology, and Psychiatry
University of Rochester School of Medicine and Dentistry
Rochester, New York

Ross S. Berkowitz, MD

William H. Baker Professor of Gynecology
Director of Gynecologic Oncology
Department of Obstetrics, Gynecology, and Reproductive Biology
Co-Director, New England Trophoblastic Disease Center
Harvard Medical School
Brigham and Women's Hospital and Dana Farber Cancer Institute
Boston, Massachusetts

Matthew P. Boente, MD

Associate Member
Division of Gynecologic Oncology
Department of Surgical Oncology
Fox Chase Cancer Center
Philadelphia, Pennsylvania

Joanna M. Cain, MD

Professor and Chair
Department of Obstetrics and Gynecology
Hershey Medical Center
Pennsylvania State University School of Medicine
Hershey, Pennsylvania

Daniel L. Clarke-Pearson, MD

James M. Ingram Professor and Director
Division of Gynecologic Oncology
Department of Obstetrics and Gynecology
Duke University Medical Center
Durham, North Carolina

Daniel W. Cramer, MD, ScD

Associate Professor
Department of Obstetrics, Gynecology, and Reproductive Biology
Harvard Medical School
Brigham and Women's Hospital
Boston, Massachusetts

Thomas M. D'Hooghe, MD, PhD

Assistant Professor
Department of Obstetrics, Gynecology, and Reproductive Biology
Harvard Medical School
Brigham and Women's Hospital
Boston, Massachusetts

Yao S. Fu, MD

Senior Pathologist
Department of Pathology
Saint Joseph Medical Center
Burbank, California

Joseph C. Gambone, DO

Associate Professor
Department of Obstetrics and Gynecology
UCLA School of Medicine
Los Angeles, California

Rene Genadry, MD

Associate Professor
Department of Gynecology and Obstetrics
Johns Hopkins Medical Institutions
Baltimore, Maryland

Armando E. Giuliano, MD

Clinical Professor of Surgery
Department of Surgery
UCLA School of Medicine
Los Angeles, California
Director, Joyce Eisenberg Keefer Breast Center
John Wayne Cancer Institute
Saint John's Hospital and Health Center
Santa Monica, California

Donald P. Goldstein, MD

Associate Professor
Department of Obstetrics, Gynecology, and Reproductive Biology
Director, New England's Trophoblastic Disease Center
Harvard Medical School
Brigham and Women's Hospital
Boston, Massachusetts

Neville F. Hacker, MD

Director of Gynaecologic Oncology
Royal Hospital for Women
Associate Professor of Obstetrics and Gynaecology
University of New South Wales
Sydney, Australia

Kenneth D. Hatch, MD

Professor and Head
Department of Obstetrics and Gynecology
University of Arizona Medical Center
Tucson, Arizona

Avner Hershlag, MD

Associate Professor of Obstetrics and Gynecology
Department of Obstetrics and Gynecology
Cornell University Medical College
North Shore University Hospital
Manhasset, New York

Joseph A. Hill, MD

Associate Professor
Chief of Reproductive Medicine
Department of Obstetrics, Gynecology, and Reproductive Biology
Harvard Medical School
Brigham and Women's Hospital
Boston, Massachusetts

Mark D. Hornstein, MD

Assistant Professor and Director
In Vitro Fertilization Program
Department of Obstetrics, Gynecology, and Reproductive Biology
Harvard Medical School
Brigham and Women's Hospital
Boston, Massachusetts

William W. Hurd, MD

Associate Professor
Department of Obstetrics and Gynecology
Indiana University
Indianapolis, Indiana

J. Norelle Lickiss, MD

Associate Professor and Director
Palliative Care Service
Royal Prince Alfred Hospital
Prince of Wales Hospital
Royal Hospital for Women
New South Wales, Australia

John R. Lurain III, MD

John and Ruth Brewer Professor of Gynecology and Cancer Research
Section Head, Gynecologic Oncology
Department of Obstetrics and Gynecology
Northwestern University Medical School
Chicago, Illinois

Howard D. McClamrock, MD

Associate Professor
Department of Obstetrics and Gynecology
Division of Reproductive Endocrinology
University of Maryland School of Medicine
Baltimore, Maryland

Marian L. McCord, MD

Assistant Professor
Division of Gynecology
Department of Obstetrics and Gynecology
University of Tennessee College of Medicine
Memphis, Tennessee

Otoniel Martínez-Maza, PhD

Associate Professor
Departments of Obstetrics and Gynecology, and
Microbiology and Immunology
UCLA School of Medicine
Los Angeles, California

Malcolm G. Munro, MD

Professor of Clinical Obstetrics and Gynecology
Department of Obstetrics and Gynecology
UCLA School of Medicine
Los Angeles, California

Thomas E. Nolan, MD

Associate Professor
Departments of Obstetrics and Gynecology, and Internal Medicine
Chief, General Obstetrics and Gynecology and Critical Care Obstetrics
Louisiana State University Medical Center
New Orleans, Louisiana

David L. Olive, MD

Associate Professor and Chief
Division of Reproductive Endocrinology
Department of Obstetrics and Gynecology
Yale University School of Medicine
New Haven, Connecticut

George J. Olt, MD

Assistant Professor
Division of Gynecologic Oncology
Department of Obstetrics and Gynecology
Hershey Medical Center
Pennsylvania State University School of Medicine
Hershey, Pennsylvania

Steven F. Palter, MD

Instructor
Division of Reproductive Endocrinology
Department of Obstetrics and Gynecology
Yale University School of Medicine
New Haven, Connecticut

C. Matthew Peterson, MD

Associate Professor
Division of Reproductive Endocrinology
Department of Obstetrics and Gynecology
University of Utah Medical Center
Director of Reproductive Endocrinology
LDS Hospital
Salt Lake City, Utah

Andrea J. Rapkin, MD

Associate Professor
Department of Obstetrics and Gynecology
UCLA School of Medicine
Los Angeles, California

Robert W. Rebar, MD

Professor and Director
Department of Obstetrics and Gynecology
University of Cincinnati Medical Center
Cincinnati, Ohio

Robert C. Reiter, MD

Associate Professor and Director
General Women's Health Division
Department of Obstetrics and Gynecology
University of Iowa Hospital and Clinics
Iowa City, Iowa

Gustavo C. Rodgriguez, MD

Assistant Professor
Department of Obstetrics and Gynecology
Duke University Medical Center
Durham, North Carolina

Wendy J. Scherzer, MD

Assistant Professor
Department of Obstetrics, Gynecology, and Reproductive Sciences
Temple University
Philadelphia, Pennsylvania

Daniel J. Schust, MD

Clinical Fellow
Department of Obstetrics, Gynecology, and Reproductive Biology
Harvard Medical School
Brigham and Women's Hospital
Boston, Massachusetts

David E. Soper, MD

Professor
Departments of Obstetrics and Gynecology, and Medicine
Division of Infectious Diseases
Medical University of South Carolina
Charleston, South Carolina

Nada L. Stotland, MD

Associate Professor
Departments of Psychiatry, and Obstetrics and Gynecology
University of Chicago
Medical Coordinator
Division of Mental Health
Illinois Department of Mental Health and Developmental Disabilities
Chicago, Illinois

Thomas G. Stovall, MD

Associate Professor and Head
Section of Gynecology
Department of Obstetrics and Gynecology
Bowman Gray School of Medicine
Wake Forest University
Winston-Salem, North Carolina

Phillip G. Stubblefield, MD

Professor and Chair
Department of Obstetrics and Gynecology
Boston University School of Medicine
Boston, Massachusetts

Gillian M. Thomas, MD

Professor and Head
Department of Radiation Oncology
Toronto-Sunnybrook Regional Cancer Centre
Departments of Radiation Oncology, and Obstetrics and Gynecology
University of Toronto
Toronto, Ontario, Canada

L. Lewis Wall, MD, DPhil

Associate Professor
Director of Urogynecology
Department of Obstetrics and Gynecology
Louisiana State University Medical Center
Adjunct Associate Professor of Tropical Medicine
School of Public Health and Tropical Medicine
Tulane University
New Orleans, Louisiana

Jennifer Wiltshire, MB, BcH

Director of Community Consultative Service
Central Sydney Palliative Care Service
Institute of Palliative Medicine
Royal Prince Alfred Hospital
Sydney, Australia

Robert C. Young, MD

President
Fox Chase Cancer Center
Philadelphia, Pennsylvania

Contents

PRINCIPLES
OF PRACTICE

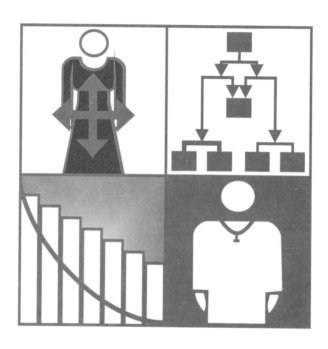

1

Initial Assessment and Communication

Jonathan S. Berek
Paula A. Hillard

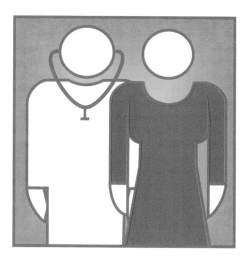

The practice of gynecology requires many skills. In addition to medical knowledge, the gynecologist should develop interpersonal and communication skills that promote patient-doctor interaction and trust. The assessment must be of the "whole patient," not only her general medical status. It should include any apparent medical condition that she has as well as the psychologic, social, and family aspects related to her situation. Environmental and cultural issues that affect the patient must be taken into account to view her in the appropriate context. Such an approach is of value in routine assessments, providing opportunities for preventive care and counseling on a continuing basis, as well as in the assessment of medical conditions.

Communication

Good communication is essential to patient assessment and treatment. The patient-physician relationship is based on communication that must be conducted in an open, honest, and careful manner so the patient's situation and problems can be accurately understood and effective solutions can be determined. Good communication requires patience, dedication, and practice.

The foundation of communication is based on key skills: empathy, attentive listening capabilities, expert knowledge, and rapport. These skills can be learned and refined (1). After establishing the initial relationship with the patient, the physician must vigilantly pursue interviewing techniques that create opportunities to foster an understanding of the patient's concerns (2). Trust is the fundamental element that encourages the patient to openly communicate her feelings, concerns, and thoughts without risk of her withholding information.

Although there are many styles of interacting with patients and each physician must determine the best way that he or she can relate to patients, physicians must convey that they are able and willing to listen and that they receive the information with utmost confidentiality (3). The Hippocratic oath demands that physicians be circumspect with all patient-related information.

Variables that Affect Patient Status

Many external variables exert an influence on the patient and on the care she receives. Some of these factors include the patient's "significant others"—her family and friends and her relationships (Table 1.1). These external variables also include psychologic, genetic, biologic, and social and economic issues. Factors that affect an individual's perception of disease and pain and the means by which they have been taught to cope with illness include one's education, attitudes, understanding of human reproduction and sexuality, family history of disease, and in some cases the need for attention (3–5). Cultural factors, socioeconomic status, religion, ethnicity, and sexual preference are important considerations in understanding the patient's response to her care in both illness and health.

We are all products of our environment, our background, and our culture. The importance of ascertaining the patient's general, social, and familial situation cannot be overemphasized (1). The context of the family can and should be ascertained directly. The family history, including a careful analysis of those who have had significant illnesses such as cancer, must be obtained. The psychological and sexual practices of the patient should be understood, and her functional level of satisfaction in these areas should be determined. **The physician must avoid being judgmental, particularly with respect to questions about sexual practices and preferences** (see Chapters 11 and 12).

Communication Skills

It is essential for the physician to communicate with a patient in a manner that allows her to continue to seek appropriate medical attention. Not only the words used, but also the patterns of speech, the manner in which the words are delivered, even "body language" and eye contact, are important aspects of the patient-physician interaction. The traditional role of the physician has been rather paternalistic, with the physician being expected to deliver direct commands and specific guidance on all matters (1). Patients are now demanding more balanced communication with their physicians and, although they do not in most cases command an understanding of medicine, they do expect to be treated with appropriate deference, respect for their intellect, and more equal stature with the physician (6). There is some evidence that giving the patient more control in the relationship with her doctor can lead to better health outcomes (3, 7, 8).

Table 1.1   Variables that Influence the Status of the Patient

Patient	Age
	History of illness
	Attitudes and perceptions
	Sexual preference
	Habits (e.g., use of drugs, smoking)
Family	Patient's status (e.g., married, separated, divorced)
	Siblings (e.g., number, ages)
	History (e.g., disease)
Environment	Socioeconomic environment
	Religion
	Culture and ethnic background

Physician-Patient Interaction

The pattern of the physician's speech can influence interactions with the patient. Some important components of effective communication between patients and physicians are presented in Table 1.2. In order for this communication to be effective, the patient must feel that she is able to discuss her problems fully. In addition, if the patient perceives that she participates in the decision and that she is given as much information as possible, she will react to the proposed treatment with lower levels of anxiety and depression. There is ample evidence that patient communication, understanding, and outcome are improved when discussions with physicians are more "dialogue" than lecture. In addition, when patients feel they have some room for "negotiation," they tend to retain more information regarding health care plans (9).

The notion of "collaborative" planning between patients and physicians has developed (9). This means that the patient becomes more vested in the process of determining health care choices. For example, if the patient is informed about the risks and benefits of hormone replacement therapy and she clearly understands them, she may be more likely to comply with the plan once it has been set jointly by her and her physician.

Studies suggest that when patients are heard, understood, more vocal, and more inquisitive, their health improves (2). **Good communication is essential for the maintenance of a relationship between the patient and physician that fosters ongoing care.** Health maintenance, therefore, can be linked directly to the influence of positive, genial interactions. Patients who are comfortable with their physician may be more likely to raise issues or concerns or convey information about potential health risks. This degree of rapport may promote the effectiveness of early interactions, including behavior modification. It will also help ensure that patients return for regular care because they feel the physician is genuinely interested in their welfare.

Table 1.2   Important Components of Communication Between the Patient and Physician: The Physician's Role

The physician is:
A good listener
Empathetic
Honest
Genuine
The physician uses:
Understandable language
Appropriate body language
A collaborative approach
Open dialogue
Appropriate emotional content
Humor and warmth
The physician is not:
Confrontational
Combative
Condescending
Overbearing
Judgmental

When patients are ill, they feel vulnerable, physically and psychologically exposed, and powerless. Because the physician has power by virtue of knowledge and status, this relationship can be intimidating. Therefore, it is essential that the physician be aware of this disparity so the balance of "power" does not shift too far away from the patient. Shifting it back from the physician to the patient may help improve outcomes (3, 7, 8).

In assessing the effects of the patient-physician interaction on the outcome of chronic illness, Kaplan identified three characteristics that are associated with better health care outcomes (8):

1. Empathetic physician and more patient control of the interview.

2. Expression of emotion by both patient and physician.

3. Provision of information by the physician in response to the patient's inquiries.

These findings related to the control of diastolic blood pressure and the reduction of hemoglobin A_{1c} in patients with diabetes, who experienced improved function and subjective evaluation of health in the presence of these characteristics. The best responses were achieved when an empathetic physician provided as much information and clarification as possible, responded to the patients' questions openly and honestly, and expressed a full range of emotions, including humor, and when the relationship was not entirely dominated by the physician (8).

In studies of gender and language, men tend to talk more than women, successfully interrupt women, and control the topics of the conversation (10). As a result, male physicians may tend to take control and be more assertive than female physicians. Men's speech tends to be characterized by interruptions, command, and lectures, and women's speech is characterized by silence, questions, and proposals (11, 12). Some patients may simply feel more reticent in the presence of a male physician, whereas others may be more forthcoming with a male than a female physician (13). While these generalizations clearly do not apply to all physicians, they can raise awareness about the various styles of communication. These patterns indicate the need for all physicians, regardless of their gender, to be attentive to their style of speech because it may affect their ability to elicit open and free responses from their patients (14, 15). Women tend to speak openly in order to express their feelings and to have them validated and shared in an attempt to gain understanding of their concerns (9–11).

With regard to communication relating to gynecologic issues, it is important to understand that different styles of communication may affect the physician's ability to perceive the patient's status and to achieve the ultimate goal of optimal assessment and compliance with medical and surgical therapies. The intimate and highly personal nature of many gynecologic conditions requires particular sensitivity to evoke an honest response.

Style

In general, the art of communication and persuasion is based on mutual respect and development of the patient's understanding of the circumstances of her health (2). Insight is best achieved when the patient is encouraged to query her physician and when she is not pressured to make decisions (3, 9). Patients who feel "backed into a corner" have the lowest compliance with recommended treatments (7).

The following are techniques to help achieve rapport with patients:

1. Use positive language, e.g., agreement, approval, and humor.

2. Build a partnership, e.g., acknowledgment of understanding, asking for opinions, paraphrasing, and interpreting the patient's words.

3. Ask rephrased questions.

4. Give complete responses to the patient's questions.

The manner in which a physician guides a discussion with a patient will determine her level of understanding and her compliance. For example, in providing a prescription, if a "command" is given to take the medication without a discussion of the rationale for it, patients may not comply, particularly if they become confused about the instructions (9). It is obviously inappropriate to prescribe hormone replacement therapy with a statement of simply "Just take one of these pills every night before you go to bed" without a discussion of the risks and benefits of taking estrogen and progesterone.

The style of the presentation of information is important to its effectiveness. The physician should avoid "speaking down" to patients, both figuratively and literally. The latter occurs when discussions take place with the patient in the supine or the lithotomy position. Such a position creates a vulnerable situation in which the patient does not feel she is an equal partner in the relationship. Serious discussions about diagnosis and management strategies should be conducted when the patient is fully clothed and face-to-face with a doctor in a private room with or without an intervening desk.

Body language also is important in interactions with patients. The physician should avoid an overly casual stance, which can communicate a lack of caring or lack of compassion. The patient should be viewed directly and spoken to with eye contact so that the physician is not perceived as "looking off into the distance" (2).

Laughter and Humor

Humor is an essential component that promotes open communication. It can be either appropriate or inappropriate. Appropriate humor allows the patient to diffuse anxiety and understand that (even in difficult situations) laughter can be healthy (16). Inappropriate humor would horrify, disgust, or offend a patient or generally make her uncomfortable or seem disrespectful of her. Laughter can be used as an appropriate means of relaxing the patient and making her feel better.

Laughter is a "metaphor for the full range of the positive emotions" (16). It is the response of human beings to incongruities and one of the highest manifestations of the cerebral process. It helps to facilitate the full range of positive emotions—love, hope, faith, the will to live, festivity, purpose, and determination (16). Laughter is a physiologic response, a release that helps us all feel better and allows us to accommodate the collision of logic and absurdity. Illness, or the prospect of illness, heightens our awareness of the incongruity between our existence and our ability to control the events that shape our lives and our outcomes. We use it to combat stress, and stress reduction is an essential mechanism used to cope with illness.

Strategies for Improving Communication

The art of communication during the medical interview is something that all physicians should understand. It is essential that interactions with patients are professional, honorable, and honest. Issues that are important to physicians regarding patient-physician interactions are presented in Table 1.3. Some general guidelines that can help to improve communication are as follows:

1. Listen more and talk less.

2. Encourage the pursuit of topics introduced by and important to patients.

3. Minimize controlling speech habits such as interrupting, issuing commands, and lecturing.

Table 1.3   Importance Attached to the Patient–Physician Relationship*

Rank	Physicians' Support Services	Always or Often	Rarely or Never
1	Answering the patient's questions about the disease and its treatment, side effects, and possible outcomes	99%	1%
2	Making sure that the patient clearly understands the explanation of the medical treatment procedures	99%	1%
3	Encouraging the patient to develop an attitude of hope and optimism concerning treatment outcome	95%	5%
4	Adjusting treatment plans to enhance compliance when the patient exhibits noncompliance	88%	12%
5	Directly counseling family members	87%	13%
6	Continuing to serve as primary physician when the patient receives supplementary treatment at another facility	85%	15%
7	Providing referral to social support groups	83%	17%
8	Providing the patient with educational materials	81%	19%
9	Helping the patient develop methods to improve the quality of his or her life	74%	26%
10	Assisting the patient in determining which of his or her coping mechanisms are most productive and helping to activate them	62%	38%
11	Providing referral to psychological counseling services	57%	43%

*Results of a physician survey of 649 oncologists in regard to patient-physician communication.
Modified from **Cousins N.** *Head First: The Biology of Hope and the Healing Power of the Human Spirit.*
New York:Penguin Books, 1989:220.

4. Seek out questions and provide full and understandable answers.

5. Become aware of discomfort in an interview, recognize when it originates in an attempt by the physician to take control, and redirect that attempt.

6. Assure patients that they have the opportunity to fully discuss their problem.

7. Recognize when patients may be seeking empathy and validation of their feelings rather than a solution. Sometimes all that is necessary is to be there as a compassionate human being.

In conducting interviews with patients, it is important for the physician to understand the patients' concerns. In studies of interviewing techniques, Branch and Malik have shown that although clinicians employ many divergent styles, the successful ones tend to look for "windows of opportunity" (i.e., careful, attentive listening with replies or questions at opportune times) (2). This skill of communication is particularly effective in exploring psychologic and social issues during brief interviews. The chief skill essential to allowing the physician to perceive problems is the ability to listen attentively.

An interview that permits maximum transmission of information to the physician is best achieved by the following approach (2):

1. Begin with an "open" question.

2. As the patient begins to speak, pay attention not only to her answers but also to her emotions and general body language.

3. Extend a second question or comment, encouraging the patient to talk.

4. Allow the patient to respond without interrupting, perhaps by employing silence, nods, or small facilitative comments, encouraging the patient to talk while the physician is listening.

5. Summarize and express empathy and understanding at the completion of the interview.

Attentiveness, rapport, and collaboration characterize good medical interviewing techniques. Open-ended questions are generally desirable, particularly coupled with good listening skills.

Premature closure of an interview and inability to get the complete information to the patient may occur for several reasons (2). It may arise from a lack of recognition of the patient's particular concern, from not providing appropriate opportunity for discussion, from the physician's becoming uncomfortable in sharing the patient's emotion, or perhaps from the physician's lack of confidence that he or she can deal with the patient's concern. One of the principal factors determining the success of the interview is lack of time. However, skilled physicians can facilitate considerable interaction even in a short time by encouraging open communication.

Many patients lack accurate information about their illness. Lack of full understanding of an illness can produce dissatisfaction with medical care, increased anxiety, distress, coping difficulties, noncompliance with treatment, and poor treatment response (17). As patients increasingly request more information about their illnesses and more involvement in decisions about their treatment, and as physicians attempt to provide more open negotiation, communication problems become more significant. Poor patient understanding stems from poor communication techniques, lack of consultation time, patient anxiety, patient denial, and in some cases, the withholding of information considered detrimental to patient welfare (17).

If clinical findings or confirmatory testing strongly suggest a serious condition, e.g., malignancy, the gravity and urgency of this situation must be conveyed in a manner that does not unduly alarm or frighten the individual. Honest answers should be provided to any specific questions the patient may want to discuss.

Allowing time for questions is important, and scheduling a follow-up visit to discuss treatment options after the patient has had an opportunity to consider the options and recommendations may be valuable. The patient should be encouraged to bring a partner or family member with her to provide moral support and to assist with questions. The patient should also be encouraged to write down any concerns she may have and bring them with her because important issues may not come to mind easily during an office visit. If the patient desires a second opinion or if a second opinion is mandated by her insurance coverage, it should be facilitated.

Valuable information can be provided by direct interview, by ancillary supporting staff providing pamphlets and other materials produced for patient education. Some studies have demonstrated that the use of pamphlets is highly effective in promoting an understanding of the condition and treatment options. Others have shown that the use of audio and videotapes have a positive impact on knowledge and can decrease anxiety (17).

The relationship between the patient and her physician is changing, as is true of all features of social interchange. The state of our health is dynamic. Many of us are fortunate to be "healthy" and in a "good state of health" for much of our lives, but some are not so fortunate. The goal of open communication between patient and physician is to achieve maximum effectiveness in diagnosis, treatment, and compliance for all patients.

Talk to the heart, speak to the soul.

Look to the being and embrace the figure's form.
Reach deeply, with hands outstretched.
Talk intently, to the seat of wisdom,
as life resembles grace.

Achieve peace within a fragile countenance.
Seek the comfort of the placid hour.
Through joyous and free reflection
know the other side of the flesh's frame.

JSB

History and Physical Examination

After a dialogue has been established, the patient assessment proceeds with obtaining a complete history and performing a physical examination. Both of these aspects of the assessment rely on good doctor-patient interchange and attention to details. During the history and physical examination, the identification of risk factors that may require special attention should be sought. These factors should be reviewed with the patient in developing a plan for her future care (see Chapter 8).

History

Following the ascertainment of the chief complaint and characteristics of the present illness, the history of the patient should be obtained. It should include her complete medical and surgical history, her reproductive history (including menstrual history), and a thorough family and social history.

A technique for obtaining information about the present illness is presented in Table 1.4. The physician should determine what other consultations may be in order to complete the evaluation. In some cases, referral to a social worker, psychologist, psychiatrist, or sexual counselor would be helpful. These issues are covered in Section III, Primary and Preventative Care (Chapters 8 through 12). Laboratory testing for routine care and high-risk factors are presented in Chapter 8.

Table 1.4   Technique of Taking the History of the Present Illness

---

The technique used in taking the history of the present illness varies with the patient, the patient's problem, and the physician.

---

1. *Allow the patient to talk about her chief complaint.* Although this complaint may or may not represent the real problem (depending on subsequent evaluation), it is usually uppermost in the patient's mind and most often constitutes the basis for the visit to the physician.

   During the phase of the interview, establish the temporal relation of the chief complaint to the total duration of the illness. Questions such as "Then up to the time of this complaint, you felt perfectly well?" may elicit other symptoms that may antedate the chief complaint by days, months, or years. In this manner, the patient may recall the date of the first appearance of illness.

   Encourage the patient to talk freely and spontaneously about her illness from the established date of onset. Do not interrupt the patient's account, except for minor promptings such as "When did it begin?" and "How did it begin?" which will help in developing chronologic order in the patient's story.

   After the patient has furnished her spontaneous account (and before the next phase of the interview), it is useful to employ questions such as "What other problems have you noticed since you became ill?" The response to this question may reveal other symptoms not yet brought forth in the interview.

Table 1.4—*continued*

Thus, in the first phase of the interview, the physician obtains an account of the symptoms as the patient experiences them, without any bias being introduced by the examiner's direct questions. Information about the importance of the symptoms to the patient and the patient's emotional reaction to her symptoms are also revealed.

2. *Because all available data regarding the symptoms are usually not elicited by the aforementioned techniques, the initial phase of the interview should be followed by a series of direct and detailed questions concerning the symptoms described by the patient.* Place each symptom in its proper chronologic order and then evaluate each in accordance with the directions for analyzing a symptom.

   In asking direct questions about the details of a symptom, take care not to suggest the nature of the answer. This particularly refers to questions that may be answered "yes" or "no." If a leading question should be submitted to the patient, the answer must be assessed with great care. Subject the patient to repeated cross-examination until you are completely satisfied that the answer is not given just to oblige you.

   Finally, before dismissing the symptom under study, inquire about other symptoms that might reasonably be expected under the clinical circumstances of the case. Symptoms specifically sought but denied are known as negative symptoms. These negative symptoms may confirm or rule out diagnostic possibilities suggested by the positive symptoms.

3. *The data secured by the techniques described in the first two phases of the interview should now suggest several diagnostic possibilities.* Test these possibilities further by inquiring about other symptoms or events that may form part of the natural history of the suspected disease or group of diseases.

4. *These techniques may still fail to reveal all symptoms of importance to the present illness, especially if they are remote in time and seemingly unrelated to the present problem.* The review of systems may then be of considerable help in bringing forth these data. A positive response from the patient on any item in any of the systems should lead immediately to further detailed questioning.

5. *Throughout that part of the interview concerning the present illness, consider the following factors:*
   a. The probable cause of each symptom or illness, i.e., emotional stress, infection, neoplasm.

      Do not disregard the patient's statements of causative factors. Consider each statement carefully, and use it as a basis for further investigation. When the symptoms point to a specific infection, direct inquiry to: water, milk, and foods eaten; exposure to communicable diseases, animals, or pets; sources of sexually transmitted disease; residence or travel in the tropics or other regions where infections are known to exist. In each of the above instances, ascertain, if possible, the date of exposure, incubation period, and symptoms of invasion (prodromal symptoms).
   b. The severity of the patient's illness, as judged either by the presence of systemic symptoms such as weakness, fatigue, loss of weight, or by a change in personal habits. The latter includes changes in sleep, eating, fluid intake, bowel movements, social activities, exercise, or work.

      Note the dates the patient discontinued her work or took to bed. Is she continuously confined to bed?
   c. Determine the patient's psychologic reaction to her illness (anxiety, depression, irritability, fear) by observing how she relates her story as well as her nonverbal behavior. The response to a question such as "Have you any particular theories about or fear of what may be the matter with you?" may yield important clues relative to the patient's understanding and feeling about her illness. The reply may help in the management of the patient's problem and allow the physician to give advice according to the patient's understanding of her ailment.

Modified with permission from **Hochstein E, Rubin AL.** *Physical Diagnosis.* New York:McGraw-Hill, 1964:9–11.

Physical Examination

A thorough general physical examination should be performed during each patient assessment (Table 1.5). In addition to the evaluation of the vital signs, examination of the breast, abdomen, and pelvis is an essential part of the gynecologic examination.

Table 1.5   Method of the Female Pelvic Examination

The patient is instructed to empty her bladder. She is placed in the lithotomy position (Fig. 1.1) and draped properly. The examiner's right or left hand is gloved, depending on his or her preference. The pelvic area is illuminated well and the examiner faces the patient. The following order of procedure is suggested for the pelvic examination:

A. External genitalia

1. *Inspect the mons pubis, labia majora, labia minora, perineal body, and anal region for characteristics of the skin, distribution of the hair, contour, and swelling.* Palpate any abnormality.

2. *Separate the labia majora with the index and middle fingers of the gloved hand and inspect the epidermal and mucosal characteristics and anatomic configuration of the following structures in the order indicated below:*

a. Labia minora

b. Clitoris

c. Urethral orifice

d. Vaginal outlet (introitus)

e. Hymen

f. Perineal body

g. Anus

3. *If disease of Skene's glands is suspected, palpate the gland for abnormal excretions by milking the undersurface of the urethra through the anterior vaginal wall.* Examine the expressed excretions by microscopy and cultures.

If there is a history of labial swelling, palpate for a diseased Bartholin gland with the thumb on the posterior part of the labia majora and the index finger in the vaginal orifice. In addition, sebaceous cysts, if present, can be felt in the labia minora.

B. Introitus

With the labia still separated by the middle and index fingers, instruct the patient to bear down. Note the presence of the anterior wall of the vagina when a cystocele is present or bulging of the posterior wall when a rectocele or enterocele is present. Bulging of both may accompany a complete prolapse of the uterus.

The supporting structure of the pelvic outlet is evaluated further when the bimanual pelvic examination is done.

C. Vagina and cervix

Inspection of the vagina and cervix using a speculum should always precede palpation.

The instrument should be warmed with tap water—not lubricated—if vaginal or cervical smears are to be obtained for the test or if cultures are to be performed.

Select the proper sized speculum (Fig. 1.2), warmed and lubricated (unless contraindicated). Introduce the instrument into the vaginal orifice with the blades oblique, closed, and pressed against the perineum. Carry the speculum along the posterior vaginal wall, and after it is fully inserted, rotate the blades into a horizontal position and open them. Maneuver the speculum until the cervix is exposed between the blades. Gently rotate the speculum around its long axis until all surfaces of the vagina and cervix are visualized.

1. *Inspect the vagina for the following:*

a. The presence of blood.

b. Discharge. This should be studied to detect trichomoniasis, monilia, and clue cells, and to obtain cultures, primarily for gonococci, and chlamydia.

c. Mucosal characteristics (i.e., color, lesions, superficial vascularity, and edema).

The lesion may be:

1) Inflammatory—redness, swelling, exudates, ulcers, vesicles

2) Neoplastic

Table 1.5—*continued*

3) Vascular

4) Pigmented: bluish discoloration of pregnancy (Chadwick's sign)

5) Miscellaneous—e.g., endometriosis, traumatic lesions, and cysts

d. Structural abnormalities (congenital and acquired).

2. *Inspect the cervix for the same factors listed above for the vagina.*
Note the following comments relative to the inspection of the cervix:

a. Unusual bleeding from the cervical canal, except during menstruation, merits an evaluation for cervical or uterine neoplasia.

b. Inflammatory lesions are characterized by a mucopurulent discharge from the os and redness, swelling, and superficial ulcerations of the surface.

c. Polyps may arise either from the surface of the cervix projecting into the vagina or from the cervical canal. Polyps may be inflammatory or neoplastic.

d. Carcinoma of the cervix may not dramatically change the appearance of the cervix or may appear as lesions similar in appearance to an inflammation. Therefore, a biopsy should be performed if there is suspicion of neoplasia.

D. Bimanual palpation

The pelvic organs can be outlined by bimanual palpation; the examiner places one hand on the lower abdominal wall and the fingers (usually two) (Fig. 1.3) of the other hand in the vagina (or vagina and rectum in the rectovaginal examination) (Fig. 1.4). Either the right or left hand may be used for vaginal palpation.

1. *Introduce the well-lubricated index and middle finger into the vagina at its posterior aspect near the perineum.* Test the strength of the perineum by pressing downward on the perineum and asking the patient to bear down. This procedure may disclose a previously concealed cystocele or rectocele and descensus of the uterus.
Advance the fingers along the posterior wall until the cervix is encountered. Note any abnormalities of structure or tenderness in the vagina or cervix.

2. *Press the abdominal hand, which is resting on the infraumbilical area, very gently downward, sweeping the pelvic structures toward the palpating vaginal fingers.*
Coordinate the activity of the two hands to evaluate the body of the uterus for:

a. Position

b. Architecture, size, shape, symmetry, tumor

c. Consistency

d. Tenderness

e. Mobility

Tumors, if found, are evaluated for location, architecture, consistency, tenderness, mobility, and number.

3. *Continue the bimanual palpation and evaluate the cervix for position, architecture, consistency, and tenderness, especially on mobility of the cervix.* Rebound tenderness should be noted at this time. The intravaginal fingers should then explore the anterior, posterior, and lateral fornices.

4. *Place the "vaginal" fingers in the right lateral fornix and the "abdominal" hand on the right lower quadrant. Manipulate the abdominal hand gently downward toward the vaginal fingers to outline the adnexa.*
A normal tube is not palpable. A normal ovary (about $4 \times 2 \times 3$ cm in size, sensitive, firm, and freely movable) is often not palpable. If an adnexal mass is found, evaluate its location relative to the uterus and cervix, architecture, consistency, tenderness, and mobility.

5. *Palpate the left adnexal region, repeating the technique described above, but place the vaginal fingers in the left fornix and the abdominal hand on the left lower quadrant.*

6. *Follow the bimanual examination with a rectovaginal-abdominal examination.*
Insert the index finger into the vagina and the middle finger into the rectum very

Table 1.5—*continued*

gently. Place the other hand on the infraumbilical region. The use of this technique makes possible higher exploration of the pelvis, since the cul-de-sac does not limit the depth of the examining finger.

7. In virgins who have an intact hymen, examine the pelvic organs by the rectal-abdominal technique.

E. Rectal examination

1. *Inspect the perianal and anal area, the pilonidal (sacrococcygeal) region, and the perineum for the following aspects:*

a. Color of the region
Note that the perianal skin is more pigmented than the surrounding skin of the buttocks and is frequently thrown into radiating folds.

b. Lesions

1) The perianal and perineal regions are common sites for itching. Pruritus ani is usually indicated by thickening, excoriations, and eczema of the perianal region and adjacent areas.

2) The anal opening is often the site of fissures, fistulae, and external hemorrhoids.

3) The pilonidal area may present a dimple, a sinus, or an inflamed pilonidal cyst.

2. *Instruct the patient to "strain down" and note whether this technique brings into view previously concealed internal hemorrhoids, polyps, or a prolapsed rectal mucosa.*

3. *Palpate the pilonidal area, the ischiorectal fossa, the perineum, and the perianal region before inserting the gloved finger into the anal canal.*
Note the presence of any concealed induration or tenderness in any of these areas.

4. *Palpate the anal canal and rectum with a well-lubricated, gloved index finger.* Lay the pulp of the index finger against the anal orifice and instruct the subject to strain downward. Concomitant with the patient's downward straining (which tends to relax the external sphincter muscle), exert upward pressure until the sphincter is felt to yield. Then, with a slight rotary movement, insinuate the finger past the anal canal into the rectum. The palpating finger should systematically examine the anal canal before exploring the rectum.

5. *Evaluate the anal canal*

a. Tonus of the external sphincter muscle and the anorectal ring at the anorectal junction.

b. Tenderness (a tight sphincter, an anal fissure, or painful hemorrhoids are the usual causes).

c. Tumor or irregularities, especially at the pectinate line.

d. Superior aspect: Reach as far as you can. Mild straining by the patient may cause some lesions, which are out of reach of the finger, to descend sufficiently low to be detected by palpation.
Examine the finger after it is withdrawn for evidence of gross blood, pus, or other alterations in color or consistency. Smear the stool to test for occult blood (guaiac).

e. Test for occult blood: Examine the finger after it is withdrawn for evidence of gross blood, pus, or other alterations in color or consistency. Smear the stool to test for occult blood (guaiac).

6. *Evaluate the rectum*

a. Anterior wall

1) Cervix: size, shape, symmetry, consistency, and tenderness especially on manipulation

14

Table 1.5—*continued*

---

2) Uterine or adnexal masses

---

3) Rectouterine fossa for tenderness or implants
   In virgins with an intact hymen, the examination of the anterior wall of the rectum is the usual method of examining the pelvic organs.

---

b. Right lateral wall, left lateral wall, posterior wall, superior aspect and test for occult blood

---

Modified with permission from **Hochstein E, Rubin AL.** *Physical Diagnosis.* New York: McGraw-Hill, 1964:342–53.

Abdominal Examination

With the patient in the supine position, an attempt should be made to have the patient relax as much as possible. Her head should be leaned back and supported gently by a pillow so the patient does not tense her abdominal muscles.

The abdomen should be inspected for signs of an intra-abdominal mass, organomegaly, or distention that would, for example, suggest ascites or intestinal obstruction. Initial palpation of the abdomen is performed to evaluate the size and configuration of the liver, spleen, and other abdominal contents. Evidence of "fullness" or mass effect should be noted. This is particularly important in patients who may have a pelvic mass and in determining the extent of omental involvement, for example, with metastatic ovarian cancer. A fullness in the upper abdomen could be consistent with an "omental cake." All four quadrants should be carefully palpated for any evidence of mass, firmness, irregularity, or distention. A systematic approach should be used, e.g., clockwise starting in the right upper quadrant. Percussion should be used to measure the dimensions of the liver. The patient should be asked to inhale and exhale during palpation of the edge of the liver.

Auscultation should be performed to ascertain the nature of the bowel sounds. The frequency of intestinal sounds and their quality should be noted. In a patient with intestinal obstruction, "rushes" as well as the occasional high-pitched sound can be heard. Bowel sounds associated with an "ileus" may be less frequent but at the same pitch as normal bowel sounds.

Pelvic Examination

The pelvic examination is typically performed with the patient in the dorsal lithotomy position (Fig. 1.1). The patient's feet should rest comfortably in stirrups with the edge of the buttocks at the lower end of the table so that the vulva can be readily inspected and the speculum can be inserted in the vagina without obstruction from the table.

The vulva and perineal area should be carefully inspected. Evidence of any lesions, erythema, pigmentation, masses, or irregularity should be noted. The skin quality should be noted as well as any signs of trauma such as excoriations or ecchymosis. The presence of any visible lesions should be quantitated and carefully described with regard to their full appearance and characteristics on palpation, i.e., mobility, tenderness, consistency. Ulcerative or purulent lesions of the vulva should be cultured as outlined in subsequent chapters, and biopsy should be performed on any lesions.

Following thorough visualization and palpation of the external genitalia, including the mons pubis and the perianal area, a speculum is inserted in the vagina. In a normal adult who is sexually active, a Pederson or Graves speculum is used. The types of specula that are used in gynecology are presented in Figure 1.2. In general, the smallest speculum necessary to produce adequate visualization should be used. The speculum should be warmed before it is inserted into the vagina, and warm water generally will provide sufficient lubrication for this procedure. The patient should be alerted to the fact that the speculum will

Figure 1.1   The lithotomy position for the pelvic examination.

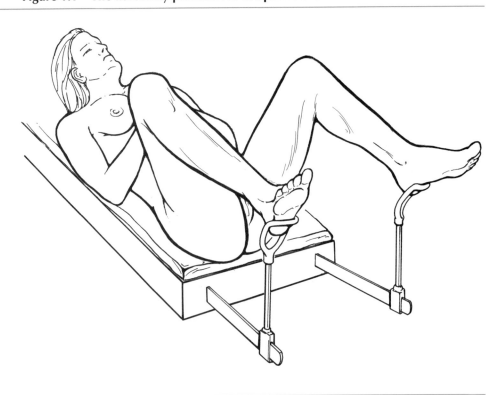

Figure 1.2   Vaginal speculae 1. Grave's extra-long, 2. Grave's regular, 3. Pederson extra-long, 4. Pederson regular, 5. Huffman "virginal," 6. Pediatric regular, and 7. Pediatric narrow.

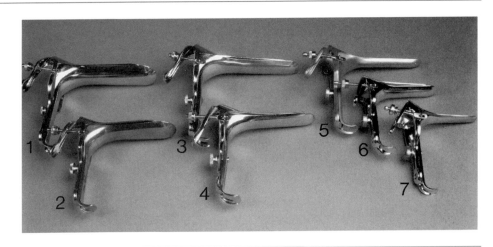

be inserted so she is not surprised by its placement. Following insertion, the cervix and all aspects of the vagina should be carefully inspected. Particular attention should also be paid to the vaginal fornices because lesions (e.g., warts) may be present in those areas and are not readily visualized unless care is taken to do so.

The appropriate technique for a Papanicolaou (Pap) test is presented in Chapter 16. Any obvious lesions on the cervix or in the vagina need to be biopsied. An endometrial biopsy is usually performed with a flexible cannula or a Novak curette as discussed in Chapter 13. Any purulence in the vagina or cervix should be cultured (see Chapter 15).

After the speculum is removed and pelvis is palpated, the first and second fingers are inserted gently into the vagina after adequate lubrication has been applied to the examination glove. In general, in right-handed physicians, the right hand is inserted into the vagina and the left hand is used on the abdomen to provide counter pressure as the pelvic viscera are moved (Fig. 1.3). The vagina, its fornices, as well as the cervix, are palpated carefully for any masses or irregularities. The fingers are placed gently into the posterior fornice so that the uterus can be moved. With the abdominal hand in place, the uterus can usually be palpated just above the surface pubis. In this manner, the size, shape, mobility, contour, consistency, and position of the uterus are documented.

The adnexa are also then palpated gently on both sides, paying particular attention to any enlargements. Again, the size, shape, mobility, and consistency of any adnexal structures should be carefully noted.

A rectal examination is performed routinely in postmenopausal women and in all premenopausal women in whom there is any difficulty ascertaining the adnexal structures (Fig 1.4). **Rectovaginal examination should also be performed in women in their forties to exclude the possibility of concurrent rectal disease** (18). In postmenopausal women who undergo rectal examination, a stool guaiac test can be performed. During rectal examination, the quality of the sphincter muscles, support of the pelvis, and evidence of masses such as hemorrhoids or lesions intrinsic of the rectum should be noted.

Figure 1.3   The bimanual examination.

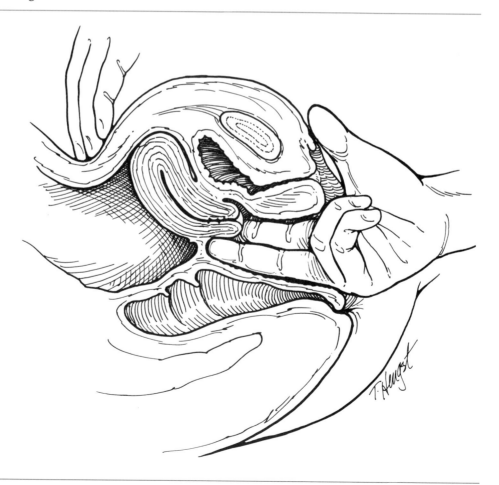

Figure 1.4   The rectovaginal examination.

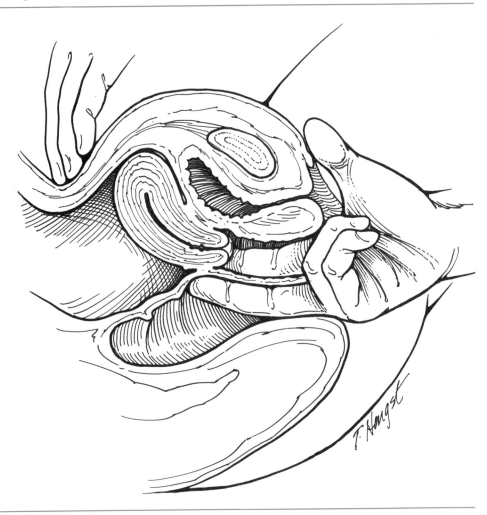

At the completion of the physical examination, the patient should be informed about the findings. When the results of the examination are normal, the patient can be reassured accordingly. When there is a possible abnormality, the patient should be informed immediately. A plan to evaluate the findings should be outlined briefly and in understandable language. The implications of any proposed procedure (e.g., biopsy) should be discussed, and the patient should be informed when the results of any tests will be available.

Examination of Pediatric Patient

A careful examination is indicated when a child presents with genital complaints. The examiner should be familiar with the normal appearance of the prepubital genitalia. The normal unestrogenized hymenal ring and vestibule can appear mildly erythematous. The technique of examination is different from that used for examining an adult and may need to be tailored to the individual child based on her age, size, and comfort with the examiner. A young child can usually be examined best in a "frog-leg" position on the examining table. Some very young girls (toddlers or infants) do best when held in their mother's arms. Sometimes the mother can be positioned, clothed, on the exam table (feet in stirrups, head of table elevated) with the child on her lap, the child's legs straddling her mother's. The knee-chest position may also be helpful for the examination (19). The child who is relaxed and warned about touching will usually tolerate the examination satisfactorily. Some children who have been abused, who have had particularly traumatic previous examinations, or who are unable to allow an examination may need to be examined with the use of anesthesia, although a gentle office exam should almost always be attempted first. If no obvious case of bleeding

18

is visible externally or within the distal vagina, an examination under anesthesia may be indicated to visualize the vagina and cervix completely. A hysteroscope, cytoscope, or other endoscopic instrument can be used to provide magnification and light source.

Examination of Adolescent Patient

A pelvic examination may be less revealing in an adolescent than in an older woman, particularly if it is the patient's first examination or if it takes place on an emergency basis. Although other diagnostic techniques (such as pelvic ultrasound) can supplement an inadequate or poorly revealing examination, an examination should usually be attempted. The keys to a successful examination lie in earning the patient's trust, explaining the components of her examination, performing only the essential components, and using a very careful and gentle technique. It is important to ascertain whether the patient has had a previous pelvic examination.

An adolescent should have a pelvic examination if she has had intercourse, if the results of a pregnancy test are positive, if she has abdominal pain, if she is markedly anemic, or if she is bleeding heavily enough to compromise hemodynamic stability. The pelvic examination occasionally may be deferred in young teenagers who have a classic history of irregular cycles soon after menarche, who have normal hematocrit levels, who deny sexual activity, and who will reliably return for follow-up.

Before a first pelvic examination is performed, a brief explanation of the planned examination (which may or may not need to include a speculum), instruction in relaxation techniques, and the use of lidocaine jelly as a lubricant can be helpful. The patient should be encouraged to participate in the examination through voluntary relaxation of the introital muscles or by using a mirror if she wishes. If significant trauma is suspected or the patient finds the examination too painful and is truly unable to cooperate, an examination under anesthesia may occasionally be necessary. The risks of general anesthesia must be weighed against the value of information that would be obtained by the examination.

Confidentiality is an important issue in adolescent health care. A number of medical organizations, including the American Medical Association, the American Academy of Pediatrics, and the American College of Obstetrics and Gynecologists, have endorsed adolescents' rights to confidential medical care. Particularly with regard to issues as sensitive as sexual activity, it is critical that the adolescent be interviewed alone, without a parent in the room. The patient should be asked if she has engaged in sexual intercourse, if she used any method of contraception, and if she feels there is any possibility of pregnancy.

Follow-Up

Arrangements should be made for the ongoing care of patients, regardless of their health status. Patients with no evidence of disease should be counseled regarding health behaviors and the need for routine care. For those with signs and symptoms of a medical disorder, further assessments and a treatment plan should be discussed. The physician must determine whether he or she is equipped to treat a particular problem or if the patient should be directed to another health professional either in obstetrics and gynecology or another specialty. If the physician feels it is necessary to refer the patient for care elsewhere, the patient should be reassured that this measure is being undertaken in her best interests and that continuity of care will be ensured.

Summary

The management of patients' gynecologic symptoms as well as abnormal findings and signs detected during examination requires the full use of a physician's skills and knowledge and poses challenges to practice the art of medicine in a manner that leads to effective alliances between physicians and their patients. Physicians must listen carefully to what patients are saying about the nature and severity of their symptoms. The art of medical history-taking must not be minimized. Physicians also must listen carefully for what patients may not be saying: their fears, anxieties, and personal experiences that lead them to react in a certain manner when faced with what is often, to them, a crisis (the diagnosis of an abnormality on examination, laboratory testing, or pelvic imaging).

Physicians must use their knowledge of gynecology gained through formal education, personal experience, teachers and mentors, and textbooks, always striving to have the latest information about a given problem. Patients often present a unique set of circumstances, medical issues, or combination of diseases. Today, the use of a textbook chapter is only a beginning. Computers have made the world of information management accessible. Physicians must learn to practice "evidence-based" medicine based on the very latest of what is known—not just impressions, recollections, or advice of colleagues. Physicians need to search the medical literature to help discover what they do not know. Patients are searching the medical literature, using computer on-line services to gain access to medical subject talk-groups, research reports, and the same literature read by physicians. Knowledge derived from an evidence base must be applied, using the art of medicine, to interact with patients to maintain health, alleviate suffering, and manage and cure disease.

References

1. **Lipkin M Jr.** The medical interview and related skills. In: **Branch WT,** ed. *Office Practice of Medicine.* Philadelphia: WB Saunders, 1987:1287–306.

2. **Branch WT, Malik TK.** Using windows of opportunities in brief interviews to understand patients' concerns. *JAMA* 1993;269:1667–8.

3. **Simpson M, Buckman R, Stewart M, Maguire P.** Doctor-patient communication: the Toronto consensus statement. *BMJ* 1991;303:1385–7.

4. **Ley P.** *Communicating With Patients.* London: Croom Helm, 1988.

5. **Butt HR.** A method for better physician-patient communication. *Ann Intern Med* 1977;86:478–80.

6. **Mishler EG, Clark JA, Ingelfinger J, Simon MP.** The language of attentive patient care: a comparison of two medical interviews. *J Gen Intern Med* 1989;4:325–35.

7. **The Headache Study Group of the University of Western Ontario.** Predictors of outcome on headache patients presenting to family physicians–a one year perspective study. *Headache* 1986;26:285–4.

8. **Kaplan SH, Greenfield S, Ware JE Jr.** Assessing the effects of physician-patient interactions on the outcomes of chronic disease. *Med Care* 1989;27:S110–27.

9. **Fallowfield LJ, Hall A, Macguire GP, Baum M.** Psychological outcomes of different treatment policies in women with early breast cancer outside a clinical trial. *BMJ* 1990;301:575–80.

10. **Spender D.** *Man Made Language.* 2nd ed. New York: Routledge & Kegan Paul Ltd., 1985.

11. **Tannen D.** *You Just Don't Understand: Women and Men In Conversation.* New York: Ballentine, 1990.

12. **West C.** Reconceptualizing gender in physician-patient relationships. *Soc Sci Med* 1993;36:57–66.

13. **Todd AD, Fisher S.** *The Social Organization of Doctor-Patient Communication.* 2nd ed. Norwood, NJ: Ablex Publishing, 1993:243–65.

14. **Roter D, Lipkin M Jr, Korsgaard A.** Sex differences in patients' and physicians' communication during primary medical care visits. *Med Care* 1991;29:1083–93.

15. **Lurie N, Slater J, McGovern P, Ekstrum J, Quam L, Margolis K.** Preventive care for women. Does the sex of the physician matter? *N Engl J Med* 1993;329:478–82.

16. **Cousins N.** The laughter connection. In: **Cousins N,** ed. *Head First. The Biology of Hope and the Healing Power of the Human Spirit.* New York: Penguin Books, 1989:125–53.

17. **Dunn SM, Butow PN, Tattersall MHN, Jones QJ, Sheldon JS, Taylor JJ, et al.** General information tapes inhibit recall of the cancer consultation. *J Clin Oncol* 1993;11:2279–85.

18. **Hochstein E, Rubin AL.** *Physical Diagnosis.* New York: McGraw-Hill, 1964.

19. **Emans SJ, Goldstein P.** The gynecologic examination of the prepubital child with vulvovaginitis: use of the knee-chest position. *Pediatrics* 1980;65:758–60.

2 Principles of Patient Care

Joanna M. Cain

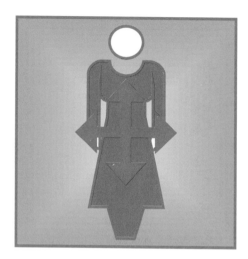

The practice of gynecology, as with all aspects of medicine, is based on ethical principles that guide patient care. These principles and concepts create a framework for ethical decision-making that applies to all aspects of practice:

- *Autonomy:* A person's right to self-rule, to establish personal norms of conduct, and to choose a course of action based on a set of personal values and principles derived from them.
- *Beneficence:* The obligation to promote the well-being of others.
- *Confidentiality:* A person's right to decide how and to whom personal medical information will be communicated.
- *Covenant:* A binding agreement between two or more parties for the performance of some action.
- *Fiduciary Relationship:* A relationship founded on faith and trust.
- *Informed Consent:* The patient's acceptance of a medical intervention after adequate disclosure of the nature of the procedure, its risks and benefits, and alternatives.
- *Justice:* The right of individuals to claim what is due them based on certain personal properties or characteristics.
- *Maleficence:* The act of committing harm (nonmaleficence obliges one to avoid doing harm).

Patient and Physician

Health care givers fulfill a basic need—to preserve and advance the health of human beings. Despite the challenges imposed by the commercial aspects of the current medical environment, for most physicians the practice of medicine remains very much a "calling," a giving of oneself to the greater good. Although much of medicine is contractual in nature, it cannot be understood in only those terms: *"The kind of minimalism that a contractualist understanding of the professional relationship encourages produces a professional too grudging, too calculating, too lacking in spontaneity, too quickly exhausted to go the second mile with his patients along the road of their distress"* (1). There is a relationship be-

21

tween physician and patient that extends beyond a contract and assumes the elements of a fiduciary relationship—a covenant between parties. The physician, having knowledge about the elements of health care, assumes a trust relationship with the patient whereby her interests are held paramount. Both the patient and the physician have rights and responsibilities in this relationship, and both are rewarded when those rights and responsibilities are upheld. **Confidentiality and informed consent are two expressions of that trust or covenantal relationship.**

Confidentiality

The patient seeking assistance from a health professional has the right to be assured that the information exchanged during that interaction is private. Privacy is essential to the trust relationship between doctor and patient. Discussions are privileged information. The right to privacy prohibits a physician from revealing information regarding the patient unless the patient waives that privilege. Privileged information belongs to the patient except when it impinges on the legal and ethical rights of institutions and society at large, regardless of the setting. In a court situation, for example, physicians cannot reveal information about their patients unless that privilege is waived by the patient. If privilege is waived, the physician may not withhold such testimony.

The privilege of privacy must be maintained even when it does not seem intrinsically obvious. A patient's family, friend, or spiritual guide, for example, has no right to medical information regarding the patient unless the patient specifically releases it. This may seem obvious but often can be overlooked, such as when a health care giver receives a call from a concerned parent, spouse, or relative inquiring about the status of a patient. The response may be a natural attempt to reassure and inform a caring individual about the patient's status. However, for her own reasons, the patient may not want certain individuals informed of her medical condition. Thus, confidentiality has been breached. **It is wise to ask patients who may be involved in decision-making and who may be informed about their status.** If a care giver is unclear of the patient's wishes regarding the person requesting information, the reply should indicate that the patient's permission is necessary before discussing her status. Finally, when trying to contact individual patients for follow-up of medical findings, it is never appropriate to reveal the reason to an individual other than the patient.

Record Keeping

Health care professionals are part of a record keeping organization. Those records are used for multiple purposes in medicine and are a valuable tool in patient care. Unfortunately, there is an increasing tendency for organizations to collect, maintain, and disclose information about individuals to whom they have no direct connection (2). Given the present lack of universal and nondiscriminatory access to health insurance in the U.S., physicians must be aware of this practice and its ramifications. Patients sign a document, often without understanding its meaning, upon registering with a health care institution or insurance plan. That document gives access to the medical record (the patient waives her privilege) to insurers and often other health care givers who request the record. The consequences of such disclosure for patients can be significant in terms of insurance coverage and potential job discrimination (3). This concern must be weighed against the need for all health care givers involved with an individual to be informed about past or present diseases or activities that may interfere with or complicate management. The use of illegal drugs, a positive human immunodeficiency virus (HIV) test result, and even a history of cancer or psychiatric illness are all exceptionally important to health care givers in evaluating individual patients. When revealed to outside institutions, however, these factors may affect the patient's ability to obtain and keep medical coverage, insurance, or even credit. **Everything that is written in a patient's record should be important to the medical care of that patient and extrinsic information should be avoided. Furthermore, it is appropriate for physicians to discuss with patients the nature of medical records and their release to other parties so patients can make an informed choice about such release.**

Legal Issues

The privilege of patients to keep their records or medical information private can be superseded by the needs of society. The classic legal decision quoted for the needs of others superseding individual patient rights is that of *Tarasoff v. Regents of the University of California* (4). That decision establishes that the special relationship between a patient and doctor may support affirmative duties for the benefit of third persons. It requires disclosure if *"necessary to avert danger to others"* but still in a fashion *"that would preserve the privacy of the patient to the fullest extent compatible with the prevention of the threatened danger."* This principle is also compatible with the various codes of ethics that allow physicians to reveal information in order to protect the welfare of the individual or the community. In other words, *"the protective privilege ends where the public peril begins"* (4).

Legislative law can also override individual privilege. The most frequent example is the recording of births and deaths, which is the responsibility of physicians. Various diseases are required to be reported depending on state law (for example, HIV status may or may not be reportable in individual states, whereas AIDS is reportable in all states). Reporting injuries caused by lethal weapons, rapes, and battering (e.g., elder and child abuse) is mandatory in some states and not others. The regulations for the reporting of these conditions is codified by law and can be obtained from the state health department. These laws are designed to protect the individual's privacy as much as possible while still serving the public interest. Particularly in the realm of abuse, physicians have a complex ethical role regardless of the law. Victims of abuse, for example, must feel supported and assured that the violent act they have survived will not make a difference in how they are treated as people. Their sense of vulnerability and actual vulnerability may be so great that reporting an incident may increase their risk of medical harm. Despite the laws, physicians also have an ethical responsibility to see to the patient's best interest, and weighing that ethical responsibility can be difficult.

Informed Consent

Informed consent is a process that involves an exchange of information directed toward reaching mutual understanding and informed decision-making. Ideally, informed consent should be the practical manifestation of respect for patient preferences (autonomy) (5, 6). Unfortunately, an act of informed consent is often misunderstood as procurement of a signature on a document. Furthermore, the intent of the consenting often is the protection of the physician from liability. Nothing could be further from either the legal or ethical meaning of this concept.

Informed consent is a conversation between physician and patient that teaches the patient about the medical condition, explores her values, and informs her about the reasonable medical alternatives. Informed consent is an interactive discussion in which one participant has greater knowledge about medical information and the other participant has greater knowledge about that individual's value system and circumstances affected by the information. This process does not require an arduous lecture on the medical condition or extensive examination of the patient's psyche. It does require adjustment of the information to the educational level of the patient and respectful elicitation of concerns and questions. It also requires acknowledgement of the various fears and concerns of both parties. Fear that the information may frighten patients, fear of the information by the patient, lack of ability to decode technical information, and inability to express lack of comprehension are among the many barriers facing physicians and patients engaging in this conversation. Communication skills are part of the art of medicine and observation of good role models, practice, and good intent can help to instill this ability in physicians (7).

Autonomy

Informed consent arises from the concept of autonomy. Pellegrino (8) defines an autonomous person as *"one who, in his thoughts, work, and actions, is able to follow those norms he chooses as his own without external constraints or coercion by others."* This definition contains the essence of what health care givers must consider as informed consent. **The choice to receive or refuse medical care must be in concert with the patient's values and freely chosen, and the options must be considered in light of the patient's values.**

Autonomy is not respect for a patient's wishes against good medical judgment. Consider the example of a patient with inoperable, advanced stage cervical cancer who demands surgery and refuses radiation therapy. The physician's ethical obligation is to seek the best for the patient's survival (beneficence) and avoid the harm (maleficence) of surgery, even though that is what the patient wishes. Physicians, then, are not obligated to offer treatment that is of no benefit to patients. The patient does, however, have the right to refuse treatment if it does not fit into her values. Thus, this patient could refuse treatment for her cervical cancer, but she does not have the right to be given any treatment she wishes.

Surrogate Decision-Makers

If the ability to make choices is diminished by extreme youth, mental processing difficulties, extreme medical illness, or loss of awareness, surrogate decision-making may be required. In all circumstances, the surrogate must make every attempt to act as the patient would have acted (9). The hierarchy of surrogate decision-makers is specified by statutory law in each state and differs slightly from state to state. For adults, the first surrogate decision-maker is a court-appointed guardian and second is a durable power of attorney, followed by relatives by degree of presumed familiarity (e.g., spouse, adult children, parents).

For children, parents are the surrogate decision-makers, except in circumstances in which the decision is life-threatening and might not be the choice a child would make later, when adult beliefs and values are formed. The classic example of this is the Jehovah's Witness parents who refuse life-saving transfusions for their child (10). Although this case is the extreme, it illustrates that the basic principle outlined for surrogate decision-making should also apply to parents. Bias that influences decision-making (in protection of parental social status, income, or systems of beliefs) needs to be considered by physicians, because the potential conflict may lead parents to decisions that are not in the best interest of the child. If there is a conflicting bias that does not allow decisions to be made in the best interest of the child or that involves a medical threat to a child, legal action to establish guardianship (normally through a child protective agency) may be necessary. This action can destroy not only the patient (child)/physician relationship but also the parent/physician relationship and may affect the long-term health and well-being of the child, who must return to the care of the parents. Such decisions should be made only after all attempts to educate, clarify, and find alternatives have been tried.

The legal age at which adolescents may make their own decisions varies by state (11). However, there is a growing trend to increase the participation of adolescents who are capable of decision-making in decisions about their health care. Because minors often have developed a value system and the capacity to make informed choices, their ability to be involved in decisions should be assessed individually rather than relying solely on the age criteria of the law and their parents' views.

Beneficence and Nonmaleficence

The principles of beneficence and nonmaleficence are the basis of medical care—the *"to do good and no harm"* of Hippocrates. However, these issues are often clouded by other decision-makers, consultants, family pressures, and sometimes financial constraints or conflicts of interests. Of all the principles of good medical care, benefit is the one that continually must be reassessed. Simple questions often have no answers. What is the medical indication? How does the proposed therapy address this issue? How much will this treatment benefit the patient? How much will it extend the patient's life? Furthermore, when confronted with multiple medical problems and consultants, physicians should ask how much treatment will be of benefit given all the patient's problems (e.g., failing kidneys, progressive cardiomyopathy, HIV-positive status, and respiratory failure) rather than necessarily attempting intubation and respiratory support to treat the immediate problem.

The benefit or futility of the treatment, along with quality-of-life considerations, should be considered in all aspects of patient care. It is best to weigh all of the relevant issues in a systematic fashion. Some systematic approaches depend on a sequential gathering of all the pertinent information in four domains—**medical indications (benefit and harm), patient preferences (autonomy), quality of life, and contextual issues (justice)** (5). Other approaches identify decision-makers, followed by facts, and then ethical principles. It is important for physicians to select an ethical model with which to practice so that, when faced with troubling and complex decisions, a system is available to help clarify the issues.

Medical Futility

The essence of good medical care is to attempt to be as clear as possible about the outcomes of the proposed interventions. If the proposed intervention (continued respiratory support or initiating support) has a very low or highly unlikely chance of success, intervention might be considered futile. Physicians have no obligation to continue or initiate therapies of no benefit (12). The decision to withdraw or withhold care, however, is one that must be accompanied by an effort to ensure that the patient or her surrogate decision-maker is educated about the decision and agrees with it. Other issues such as family concerns can, and should, modify decisions if the overall well-being of the patient and the family are best served. For example, waiting (within reason) to withdraw life support may be appropriate to allow a family to reach consensus or a distant family member to see the patient for a last time.

Quality of Life

Quality of life is a much used, often unclear term. **In the care of patients, quality of life is the effect of therapy on the patient's experience of living based on her perspective. It is perilous and wholly speculative to assume that physicians know what "quality of life" represents for a particular patient judging from a personal reaction.** It is instructive, however, to attempt to guess what it means and then seek the patient's perspective. The results may be surprising. For example, when offered a new drug for ovarian cancer, a patient might prefer to decline the treatment because the side effects may not be acceptable even when there may be a reasonable chance that her life may be slightly prolonged. In some instances, the physician may not believe that further treatment is justified but the patient finds joy and fulfillment in preserving her existence as long as possible.

Controversy exists regarding whether currently available quality-of-life measurement systems will provide information to help patients make decisions (13). Information from quality-of-life studies might be judged by criteria that include whether the measured aspects of the patient's life were based on the patient's views or the physician's clinical experience (14). Informing patients of others' experiences with alternative treatments may help in their decision-making, but it is never a substitute for the individual patients' decisions.

Professional Relations

Conflict of Interest

All professionals have multiple "interests" that affect their decisions. Contractual and covenantal relationships between physician and patient are intertwined and complicated by health care payors and colleagues, which creates considerable pressure. The conflict with financial considerations directly influences how patients lives are affected, often without their consent. Drummond and Rennie (15) described that pressure eloquently: *"Instead of receiving more respect (for more responsibility), physicians feel they are being increasingly questioned, challenged, and sued. Looking after a patient seems less and less a com-*

pact between two people and more a match in which increasing numbers of spectators claim the right to interfere and referee." An honest response to this environment is for the physician to attempt to protect his or her efforts by assuming that the physician-patient relationship is contractual, and only contractual, in nature. This allocation of responsibility and authority for the "contract" precludes the need for the covenant between the physician and patient. For example, a contract, insurance, or managed care plan may discourage referral to a more knowledgeable specialist, removing the physician's responsibility. Thus, the contract establishes the extent of the physician-patient relationship. All health care givers must decide whether they will practice within a covenantal or contractual relationship and whether the relationship they develop remains true to this decision. In either setting, a reasonable perception of that relationship is "one that allows clients as much freedom as possible to determine how their lives are affected as is reasonably warranted on the basis of their ability to make decisions" (16).

Health Care Payors

An insurance coverage plan may demand that physicians assume the role of gatekeeper and administrator. Patients can be penalized for a lack of knowledge about their future desires or needs and the lack of alternatives to address the changes in those needs. Patients are equally penalized when they develop costly medical conditions that would not be covered if they moved from plan to plan. These situations often place the physician in the position of being the arbiter of patients' coverage rather than acting as an advocate and adviser. It is an untenable position for physicians because they often cannot change the conditions of the plan but are made to be the administrators without an ability to change the structures.

In an effort to improve physician compliance with and interest in decreasing costs, intense financial conflicts of interest are brought to bear on physicians by managed care plans. If a physician's profile on costs or referral is too high, he or she might be excluded from the plan, thus decreasing the ability to earn a living or to provide care to certain patients with whom a relationship has developed. Conversely, a physician may receive a greater salary or bonus if the plan makes more money. The ability to earn a living and to see patients in the future is dependent on maintaining relationships with various plans and other physicians. These are compelling loyalties and conflicts that cannot be ignored (17–19).

These conflicts are substantially different from those of fee-for-service plans, although the ultimate effect on the patient can be the same. In fee-for-service plans, financial gain may result in failure to refer a patient, or referral is restricted to those cases in which the financial gain is derived by return referral of other patients (20). Patients may be unaware of these underlying conflicts, which elevates conflict of interest to an ethical problem. A patient has a right to know what her plan covers, to whom she is being referred and why, and the credentials of those to whom she is referred. **The reality is that health care givers make many decisions under the pressure of multiple conflicts of interest. Physicians are continually caught between self-interest and professional integrity.** Whether it is the more blatant lying about indications for a procedure in order to receive reimbursement or a more subtle persuasion to sign up for a certain protocol because of points earned for a group, the outcome for individual and society's relationship with health care givers is damaged by failure to recognize and specifically address conflicts of interest that impede decision-making (21). Focusing clearly on meeting the patient's best interest and responsibly rejecting choices that compromise the patient's needs are ethical requirements.

Institutions, third-party payors, and legislatures have avoided accountability for revealing conflicts of interest to those to whom they offer services. The restrictions of health care plans are never placed in as equally a prominent a position as the coverage. The coverage choices can be quite arbitrary, and there is no system for challenging them. The social and financial conflicts of interest of these payors can directly affect the setting and nature of the relationship between physician and patient. To deal with ambiguous and sometimes cious decision-making, revelation of the conflicts of interest and accountability for choices should be demanded by physician and patient (22).

Legal Problems

Abuses of the system (e.g., referral for financial gain) have led to proposals and legislation affecting physicians' ability to send patients to local laboratories and facilities in which they have a potential for financial gain. Although there have been clearly documented abuses, the same legislation would affect rural clinics and laboratories in which the only capital available is obtained through the rural physicians. States vary on the statutory legislation regarding this issue. Regardless of laws, however, it is ethically required that financial conflicts of interest be revealed to patients (23–26).

Another abuse of the physician-patient relationship caused by financial conflicts of interest is fraudulent Medicare and Medicaid billings. This activity resulted in the *Fraud and Abuse Act of 1987 (42. U.S.C. at 1320 a–7b)*, which prohibits any individual or entity making false claims or soliciting or receiving any "remuneration" in cash or any kind, directly or indirectly, overtly or covertly, to induce a referral. Indictment under these laws are felonies with steep fines and jail sentences and loss of the license to practice medicine. Physicians should be aware of the legal ramifications of their referral and billing practices (21, 27).

Harassment

The goal of medicine is excellence in the care of patients and, often, research and education that will advance the practice of medicine. It is ethically axiomatic that everyone involved in the process should be able to attend to that common goal on equal footing and without unwelcome harassment that interferes with employees' or colleagues' ability to work or be equally promoted in that environment. Every office and institution must have written policies on discrimination and sexual harassment that detail inappropriate behavior and state specific steps to be taken to correct an inappropriate situation. The legal sanction for this right is encoded in both statutory law through the *Civil Rights Act of 1964 (42 U.S.C.A. at 2000e–2000e–17 [West 1981 and Supp. 1988])* and reinforced with judicial action (case or precedential law) by state and U. S. Supreme Court decisions. In particular, charges of sexual harassment can be raised as a result of unwelcome sexual conduct or a hostile workplace (such as areas of medicine that have been known for antifeminist attitudes in the past). As stated in one legal case, "a female does not assume the risk of harassment by voluntarily entering an abusive, antifemale environment" (*Barbetta v. Chemlawn Service Co., 669 F, Supp. 569, WDNY, 1989*). The environment must change rather than expect the men or women to adapt because "they knew what it would be like." The tension in the legal debate regarding harassment (sexual, racial, disability) always hinges on the weight of protection of free speech and the right of the individual to equality and a nonhostile work environment.

Stress Management

There is little doubt that the day-to-day stress of practicing medicine is significant. Besides the acknowledged stress of the time pressures and responsibility of medicine, the current health care environment has had a detrimental impact on job security, with concurrent health risks (28). Stress takes a toll not only on cardiac function (29) but on practicing medicine and functioning in a life outside of medicine (30).

Responding to stress through drug or alcohol abuse increases overall health and marital problems and decreases effectiveness in practice. In a long-term prospective study of medical students, individuals with high-risk temperaments have been shown to have a high rate of premature death (particularly before 55 years of age) (31). Adequate sleep, reasonable working hours, exercise, and nutritional balance have been shown to be directly related to decreases in psychological distress (32). Simple relaxation training has been shown to decrease gastroesophageal reflux in response to stress (33).

27

The pace that physicians maintain has a seductive quality that can easily mask the need for stress reduction by means of good health practices, exercise, and relaxation training. The answer to increased stress is not to work harder and extract the time to work harder from the relaxing and enjoyable pursuits that exist outside medicine. The outcome (in terms of psychological and physical optimal functioning) of that strategy is in neither the physician's nor patient's best interest. **Both the welfare of the patient and the welfare of the physician are enhanced by a planned strategy of good health practices and relaxation. Furthermore, such a strategy is important to all members of the health care team. By providing such leadership, physicians can contribute to a better work and health care environment for everyone.**

Society and Medicine

Justice

Some of the ethical and legal problems in the practice of gynecology relate to the fair and equitable distribution of burdens and benefits. How benefits are distributed is a matter of great debate. There are various methods of proposed distribution:

1. *Equal shares* (everyone has the same number of health care dollars per year).

2. *Need* (only those people who need health care get the dollars).

3. *Queuing* (the first in line for a transplant gets it).

4. *Merit* (those with more serious illnesses receive special benefits).

5. *Contribution* (those who have paid more into their health care fund get more health care).

Each of these principles could be appropriate as a measure of allocation of just health care dollars, but each will affect individual patients in different ways. Only recently has just distribution become a major issue in health care. The principles of justice apply only when the resource is desired or beneficial and to some extent scarce (34).

The traditional approach to medicine has been for practitioners to accept the intense focus on the individual patient. However, the current changes in medicine will alter the focus from the patient to a population (35)—*"in the emerging medicine, the presenting patient, more than ever before, will be a representative of a class, and the science that makes possible the care of the patient will refer prominently to the population from which that patient comes."* Physicians are increasingly bound by accumulating outcomes data (population statistics) to modify the treatment of an individual in view of the larger population statistics. If, for example, the outcome of liver transplantation is only 20% successful in a patient with a certain set of medical problems, that transplant may instead be offered to someone in the population of people who has an 85% chance of success. Theoretically, the former individual might have a successful transplant and the procedure might fail in the latter, but population statistics have been used to allocate this scarce resource. The benefit has been measured by statistics not justice by need, queuing, merit, or contribution. This approach represents a major change in the traditional dedication of health care to the benefits of individual patients. With scarce resources, the overall benefits for all patients are considered in conjunction with the individual benefits for one patient.

There has always been an inequity in the distribution of health care access and resources. This inequity has not been seen by many health care givers who do not care for those patients who are unable to gain access, such as those who lack transportation or live in rural areas or where limits are imposed by lack of health care providers, time, and financial resources. Social discrimination sometimes leads to inequity of distribution of health care. Minorities are less likely to see private physicians or specialists, regardless of their income or source of health care funding (36–38). Thus, health care is rationed by default.

Health care providers must shift the paradigm from the absolute "do everything possible for this patient" to the proportionate "do everything reasonable for all patients" (5). To reform the health care system requires not just judicial, legislative, or business mandates but also attention to the other social components that can pose obstacles to efforts to expand health care beyond a focus on individual patients.

Health Care Reform

The tension between understanding health as an inherently individual matter (in which the receipt of health care is critical to individual well-being) versus health as a communal resource (in which distribution of well-being throughout society is the goal) underpins much of the political and social debate surrounding health care reform (39). The questions of health care reform are: what is the proper balance between individual and collective good, and who will pay for basic health care? Because much of health care reform requires a balancing of competing goals, legislation should specifically address how this balance can be achieved. The role of government would be the following:

1. Regulating access of individuals to health care.

2. Regulating potential harms to the public health (smoking, pollution, drug use).

3. Promoting health practices of benefit to large populations (immunization, fluoridation of water).

Decisions regarding both the amount and distribution of resources are often made by health care payors, not individual providers. The health insurance industry determines what are "reasonable and customary" charges and what will be covered. The government decides (often with intense special interest pressure) what will be covered by Medicare and Medicaid (40, 41). These decisions directly affect patient care. For that reason, health care givers cannot ethically remain silent when the health and well-being of their individual patients and their communities are adversely affected by health care reform decisions. Health care givers should assess proposed reforms in light of their value to the community and to individual patients and then formulate their own criteria for judging proposals for health care reform (42–45). Furthermore, initiation and support of research focused on the outcomes of care delivered by gynecologists (financial aspects, quality-of-life measures, survival, morbidity and mortality) will allow the discipline to have a real voice in determining what choices are made for health care for women.

References

1. **May WF.** Code and covenant or philanthropy and contract. *Hastings Cent Rep* 1975;5:29–38.

2. **Privacy Protection Study Commission.** *Personal Privacy in an Information Society.* Washington, DC: U.S. Government Printing Office, 1977.

3. **Cain J.** Confidentiality. In: APGO Task Force on Medical Ethics. *Exploring Medical-Legal Issues in Obstetrics and Gynecology.* Washington, DC: APGO, 1994:43–5.

4. **Justice Matthew O. Tobriner.** Majority Opinion, California Supreme Court, 1 July 1976. *California Reporter,* West Publishing Company, 1976:14–33.

5. **Jonsen AR, Siegler M, Winslade WJ.** *Clinical Ethics.* New York: McGraw-Hill, 1992:5–61.

6. **American College of Obstetricians and Gynecologists.** *Ethical Dimensions of Informed Consent.* Committee Opinion, No. 108. Washington, DC: ACOG, 1992.

7. **Katz J.** Informed consent—must it remain a fairy tale? *J Contemp Health Law Policy* 1994; 10:69–91.

8. **Pellegrino ED.** Patient and physician autonomy: conflicting rights and obligations in the physician-patient relationship. *J Contemp Health Law Policy* 1994;10:47–68.

9. **Buchanan AE, Brock DW.** *Deciding for Others: The Ethics of Surrogate Decision Making.* New York: Cambridge University Press, 1989.

10. **Ackerman T.** The limits of beneficence: Jehovah's Witnesses and childhood cancer. *Hastings Cent Rep* 1980;10:13–6.

11. **Nocon JJ.** Selected minor consent laws for reproductive health care. In: APGO Task Force on Medical Ethics. *Exploring Medical-Legal Issues in Obstetrics and Gynecology.* Washington, DC: APGO, 1994:129–36.

12. **Jecker NS, Schneiderman LJ.** Medical futility: the duty not to treat. *Camb Q Healthc Ethics* 1993;2:151–9.

13. **Gill TM, Feinstein AR.** A critical appraisal of the quality of quality of life measurements. *JAMA* 1994;262:619–26.

14. **Guyatt GH, Cook DJ.** Health status, quality of life and the individual. *JAMA* 1994;272:630–1.

15. **Rennie D.** Let us focus your worries! Health care policy: a clinical approach. *JAMA* 1994;272:631–2.

16. **Bailees MD.** The professional-client relationship. In: *Professional Ethics.* Belmont, CA: Wadsworth Publishing Co., 1981.

17. **Ellsbury K.** Can the family physician avoid conflict of interest in the gatekeeper role? An affirmative view. *J Fam Pract* 1989;28:698–701.

18. **Stephens GG.** Can the family physician avoid conflict of interest in the gatekeeper role? An opposing view. *J Fam Pract* 1989;28:701–4.

19. **Miles C.** Resource allocation in the National Health Service. In: **Byrne P,** ed. *Ethics and the Law in Health Care and Research.* New York: John Wiley and Sons, 1990.

20. **Cain JM, Jonsen AR.** Specialists and generalists in obstetrics and gynecology: conflicts of interest in referral and an ethical alternative. *Womens Health Issues* 1992;2:137–45.

21. **American College of Obstetricians and Gynecologists.** *Committee Opinion. Deception.* No. 87. Washington, DC: ACOG, 1990.

22. **Wrenn K.** No insurance, no admission. *N Engl J Med* 1985;392:373–4.

23. **Hyman D, Williamson JV.** Fraud and abuse: setting the limits on physicians' entrepreneurship. *N Engl J Med* 1989;320:1275.

24. **McDowell TN Jr.** Physician self referral arrangements: legitimate business or unethical entrepreneurialism. *Am J Law Med* 1989;15:61–109.

25. **Stark F.** Ethics in patient referrals. *Acad Med* 1989;64:146–7.

26. **Green RM.** Medical joint-venturing: an ethical perspective. *Hastings Cent Rep* 1990;20:22–6.

27. **Nocon JJ.** Fraud and abuse: employment kickbacks and physician recruitment. In: APGO Task Force on Medical Ethics. *Exploring Medical-Legal Issues in Obstetrics and Gynecology.* Washington, DC: APGO, 1994:69–74.

28. **Heaney CA, Isreal BA, House JS.** Chronic job insecurity among automobile workers: effects on job satisfaction and health. *Soc Sci Med* 1994;38:1431–7.

29. **Sloan RP, Shapiro PA, Bagiella E, Boni SM.** Effect of mental stress throughout the day on cardiac autonomic control. *Biol Psychol* 1994;37:89–99.

30. **Serry N, Bloch S, Ball R, Anderson K.** Drug and alcohol abuse by doctors. *Med J Aust* 1994;60:402–7.

31. **Graves PL, Mead LA, Wang NY, Liang KY, Klag MJ.** Temperament as a potential predictor of mortality: evidence from a 41 year prospective study. *J Behav Med* 1994;17:111–26.

32. **Ezoe S, Morimoto K.** Behavioral lifestyle and mental health status of Japanese workers. *Prev Med* 1994;23:98–105.

33. **McDonald HJ, Bradley LA, Bailey MA, Schan CA, Richter JE.** Relaxation training reduces symptom reports and acid exposure in patients with gastroesophageal reflux disease. *Gastroenterology* 1994;107:61–9.

34. **Daniels N.** *Just Health Care*. Cambridge: Cambridge University Press, 1985.

35. **Jonsen AR.** *The New Medicine and the Old Ethics*. Boston: Harvard University Press, 1990.

36. **Watson SD.** Minority access and health reform: a civil right to health care. *J Law Med Ethics* 1994;22:127–37.

37. **Watson SD.** Health care in the inner city: asking the right question. *N C Law Rev* 1993;71: 1661–3.

38. **Freeman HE, Blendon RJ, Aiken LH, Sudman S, Mullinix CF, Corey CR.** Americans report on their access to health care. *Health Aff (Millwood)* 1987;6:6–8.

39. **Burris S.** Thoughts on the law and the public's health. *J Law Med Ethics* 1994;22:141–6.

40. **Evans RW.** Health care technology and the inevitability of resource allocation and rationing decisions: part 2. *JAMA* 1983;249:2208–10.

41. **President's Commission for the Study of Ethical Problems in Medicine and Biomedical and Behavioral Research.** *Securing Access to Health Care: The Ethical Implications of Differences in Availability of Health Services*. Washington, DC: Government Printing Office, 1983:1–3.

42. **Eddy DM.** What care is essential? *JAMA* 1991;265:786–8.

43. **Sultz H.** Health policy: if you don't know where you're going, any road will take you. *Am J Public Health* 1991;81:418–20.

44. **Agich GJ.** Medicine as business and profession. *Theor Med* 1990;2:311–24.

45. **Daniels N.** Is the Oregon rationing plan fair? *JAMA* 1991;265:2232–5.

Quality Assessment and Improvement

Joseph C. Gambone
Robert C. Reiter

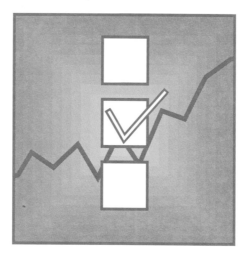

The need to measure and manage the quality of health care is essential because of its rising cost. In constant dollars, the annual per capita expense of health care in the U.S. has risen steadily from $950 in 1970 to an estimated $3400 in 1994. Much of this increase has been shifted from the individual to state and federal government and to employers (Fig. 3.1). The U.S. spends more on health care (14% of gross domestic product) than on education and defense combined. Expenditures for health care are greater than for food (1). Despite this enormous outlay of resources, there is concern about the overall quality of health care in the U.S. (2). The health status of U.S. citizens (in terms of life expectancy, neonatal mortality, and rates of illness and disability) is poorer than that of people living in most European and Scandinavian countries, the United Kingdom, Japan, and Canada, although these countries spend less per capita on health care. Quality improvement programs in other industries have shown that management methods can increase quality and reduce costs. Patients as well as private and public third-party payers are demanding ongoing quality assessment and improvement programs in health care delivery systems.

Quality Assurance

The medical profession has traditionally focused its efforts on assessing and improving the quality of health services through internal, self-imposed, *retrospective peer review*. Examples of such mechanisms are morbidity and mortality (M&M) conferences, medical society-sponsored and state-legislated peer-review programs, surgical case reviews (tissue committees), and the specialty board certification processes. These programs review adverse occurrences ("indicators") retrospectively, e.g., assessment of medical and surgical complications and review of misdiagnoses. **Although useful, these programs are not aimed at prevention of errors and they are not designed to assess and improve the effectiveness of health care services and procedures.**

The history of modern quality management in industry has its roots in the post-World War II era. Initially, the U.S. business community was not responsive to the concept that post-production inspection to detect errors and poor quality was not as efficient as producing

Figure 3.1   Sources of spending in U.S. health care, 1960–1990. Note that third-party payment has steadily replaced direct payment during this interval. (Data from U.S. Congressional Budget Office, 1992).

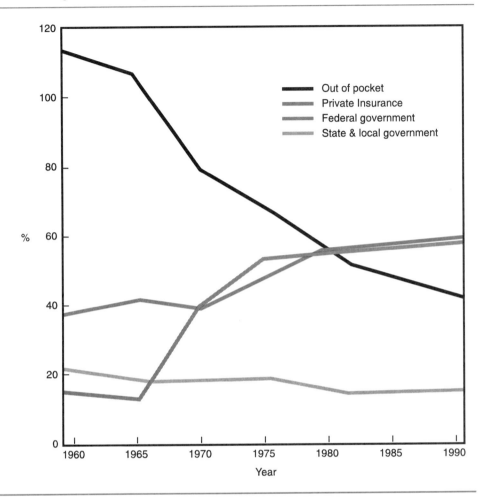

quality work and delivering a consistent level of services. Unlike their U.S. counterparts, the Japanese incorporated these newer principles of quality management into their business culture, thus transforming their reputation from one of producing low cost but inferior products. Recently, U.S. industry, government, and health care organizations are incorporating these principles into health care evaluation and practice.

Some traditional quality assurance (QA) programs have attempted to standardize quality indicators and reduce inappropriate variation in utilization of selected health services such as major surgical procedures. Examples of QA programs are the "clinical indicators" and criteria sets developed by the American College of Obstetricians and Gynecologists (ACOG). A criteria set is a consensus-derived guideline listing prerequisites (findings or prior treatments) that should be documented prior to undertaking a recommended medical or surgical procedure (Table 3.1). When used prospectively, this technique may help prevent the unnecessary procedures (e.g., hysterectomies and cesarean deliveries). Most QA initiatives are applied retrospectively, which can be an effective way to identify areas for future improvement. However, continuous and prospective "decision support" models appear to be the best way to bring about meaningful behavioral changes and make lasting improvements in health care (3).

The differences between traditional QA programs and newer quality improvement and management programs, such as continuous quality improvement (CQI) or total quality

Table 3.1   An Example of an American College of Obstetricians and Gynecologists (ACOG) Criteria-Set

Procedure

Gonadotropin-releasing hormone agonists for preoperative treatment of leiomyomata.

Indication

Leiomyomata (ICD-9-CM Codes 218.0–218.9).

Confirmation of Indication (Presence of 1 and 3 *or* 2 and 3 *or* 3)

1. Asymptomatic leiomyomata of such size that they are palpable abdominally and are a concern to the patient.

2. Excessive uterine bleeding evidenced by *either* of the following:

a. Profuse bleeding with clots or repetitive periods lasting more than 8 days.

b. Anemia due to acute or chronic blood loss.

3. Treatment prior to hysterectomy or myomectomy for large leiomyomata to facilitate surgery.

Actions Prior to Treatment

1. Eliminate anovulation and other causes of abnormal bleeding.

2. Rule out other causes of pelvic mass (e.g., pregnancy, ovarian tumor, or nongynecologic neoplasm.

3. Rule out cervical carcinoma or cytology.

4. Document that the patient was counseled regarding risks, benefits, costs, and alternatives.

Treatment

Maximum duration of preoperative treatment is 3 months.

Contraindication

1. Rapid uterine enlargement over 3–6 months prior to treatment.

2. Progressive enlargement during therapy.

Unless otherwise stated, each numbered and lettered item (except contraindications) must be present.

management (TQM), are presented in Figure 3.2. Assuming that all health care services are "normally" distributed, QA programs are designed to identify and eliminate the small percentage of substandard care represented on the left side of the normal curve (the "bad apple" approach). The majority of "standard" care occurs in the middle of the curve, however, and is the "target" of programs like CQI. Such programs are designed to prospectively study the processes of care based on need and to improve outcomes by the reduction of unintended variation (4). The right side of the curve represents "state of the art" practice usually performed under protocols at university and other large centers that are monitored by institutional review boards and national research groups such as the National Cancer Institute (NCI) and the Gynecologic Oncology Group (GOG). As more emphasis is placed on quality management programs in health care, innovations will come from traditional research and quality improvement efforts.

Quality management programs such as CQI, TQM, and performance improvement (PI) each have three essential elements (5):

1. To understand the customer and to link that knowledge to the activities of the organization.

2. To mold the culture of the organization through the deeds of leaders; to foster pride, enjoyment, collaboration, and scientific thinking.

3. To continuously increase knowledge and to control variation by scientific methods.

Figure 3.2   The hypothetical relationship between quality assurance and quality improvement.

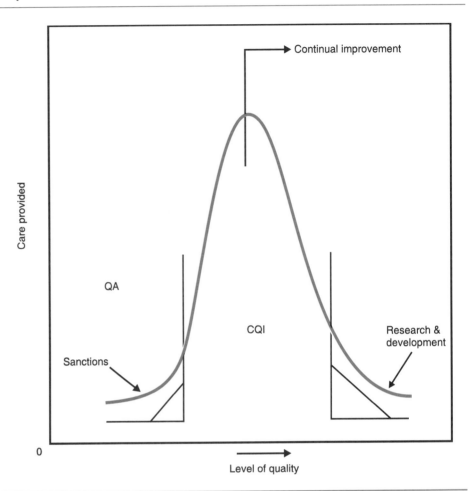

Health care professionals often do not like to refer to health care services as *products* and patients as *customers* or consumers. The older, paternalistic attitude (i.e., patients passively agreeing to health care procedures that were determined by health care providers) is being replaced by a more egalitarian view of patients as intelligent and informed consumers who participate in their care (6). The consumerism movement in health care is predicated on the belief that health care services should conform to acceptable standards of quality, efficiency, and safety (7). This newer model of improved communication and shared decision-making may alter the wasteful practice of "defensive medicine," which significantly increases health care costs (8, 9).

Principles of Quality Assessment

Quality means different things in different situations. The concept of quality in products (e.g., consumer goods and state-of-the-art machinery) is different than that of complex services (e.g., health care delivery to people). However, many of the principles of quality assessment and improvement that have been shown to improve consumer goods and services can also be applied to the evaluation and improvement of health services. There are certain principles of quality assessment that should be considered when attempting to measure and improve health care quality.

Efficacy, Effectiveness, and Efficiency

Efficacy and *effectiveness* are similar terms that are often used interchangeably to describe evaluations of outcomes of health care services and procedures. As defined by the Institute of Medicine, *efficacy* refers to what an intervention or procedure can accomplish under ideal conditions and when applied to appropriate patients (10). *Effectiveness* **refers to the actual performance in customary practice of an intervention or procedure.** An example of this difference is the theoretical success rate (efficacy) of oral contraception used for one year (99% successful at preventing pregnancy) versus the actual or "use-rate" effectiveness, usually reported to be 93–97%. Most health care decisions have been based on efficacy rates obtained from controlled clinical trials rather than actual effectiveness. One of the major challenges for quality assessment and management programs is to develop and use measurements that reflect the actual or "real-life" success rates of treatment options so that "evidence-based" decision-making can replace "authority-based" decision-making. Also, strategies need to be developed to improve patient compliance rates to increase the likelihood that the actual *effectiveness* is as close as possible to theoretical *efficacy* (11).

Efficiency **describes the relative "waste" or resource use (complications and costs) of alternative effective interventions.** To realize meaningful improvements in health services, health professionals and organizations must develop more efficient interventions (e.g., medical therapy or expectant management versus surgical treatment for abnormal bleeding) when appropriate. The goal of health care quality improvement is optimal value. *Value* **is defined as quality divided by the cost or as the quotient of outcomes (benefits) divided by resources used:**

$$\text{Value} = \frac{\text{Outcomes}}{\text{Resource Use}}$$

Optimal Versus Maximal Care

The assessment of the quality of health care depends on whether the goal of the system is to provide maximally effective or optimally effective care (12). Figure 3.3 shows a theoretical representation of the difference between maximally effective health care (Point B), in which every conceivable intervention is offered regardless of cost to those who can afford it, and optimally effective health care (Point A), in which resources are utilized in a manner that will provide the most good for as many people as possible. Maximized health care emphasizes individual intervention, whereas optimized care emphasizes public health care and prevention. If optimal health care becomes the goal of a health care system, conflicting individual and societal needs must be resolved.

When the effectiveness of health care interventions are being assessed, another variable is the course of "self-limiting" disease over time with and without treatment. Often the effectiveness of health care procedures does not consider the natural course of disease or what would happen without treatment or "watchful waiting."

Assessing Outcomes

A widely accepted system for assessing the quality of health care is based on the measurement of indicators of *structure, process,* **and** *outcome* **(13).** *Structure* **includes the resources, equipment, and people who provide health care.** *Process* **is the method by which a procedure or course of action is executed.** *Outcome* **includes the complications, adverse events, and short-term results of interventions, as well as the patient's health status and health-related quality of life after treatment, which reflects the effectiveness of the intervention.**

Evaluation of health care structure involves the assessment of the stable and tangible resources needed to provide care, such as safe and adequately sized operating rooms and properly functioning equipment. Other examples of structural elements include the aspects of the medical staff's qualifications, such as school accreditation, licensure, continuing medical education credits, and specialty board certification. Although these elements form the foundation of a health care organization or system, there is a weak correlation between structural assessment and other measures of the quality of care such as clinical outcomes (14). Therefore, many health services researchers believe that organizations need to di-

Figure 3.3   The "optimal" versus the "maximal" benefits and costs of medical treatments. *On the top panel,* the benefits to health and the costs of care are plotted. *On the bottom panel,* the cost is subtracted from the benefits, illustrating that after a certain point, additions of care may detract from the benefits. (Reproduced with permission from **Donabedian A.** The quality of care: How can it be assessed. *JAMA* 1988;260:1743–8.

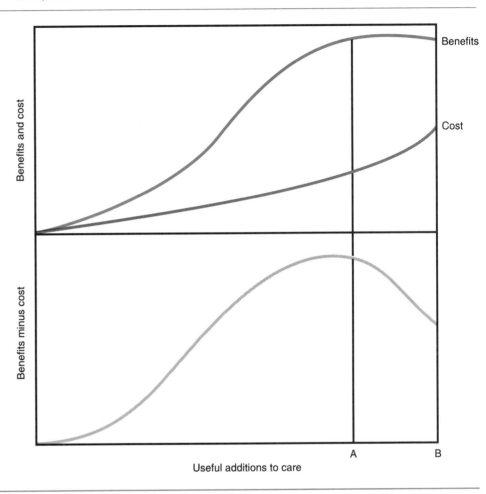

rectly measure clinical outcomes (including not only death and short-term morbidity but also disability and health-related quality of life issues) if they hope to improve both the *effectiveness* and *efficiency* of health care delivery. Ultimately, longevity and quality-of-life factors may be the only relevant outcomes of health care.

Outcomes Research

The Agency for Health Care Policy and Research (AHCPR) and its Medical Treatment Effectiveness Program was established by the U.S. Congress in the mid-1980s. Under this program, the AHCPR conducts and supports research on the outcomes of available treatments, especially those that are common or costly and are associated with substantial patient risk or burden and those for which there are treatment options. Unlike that of the National Institutes of Health (NIH), AHCPR research does not emphasize the underlying causes of disease but rather stresses the evaluation of available strategies for treating disease with particular emphasis on the outcomes that are important to, and experienced by, typical patients (15). This research also emphasizes measurement of clinical or health outcomes that are defined as those that patients can experience and value without the interpretation of the health care provider. Examples of clinical or health outcomes and their corresponding intermediate or surrogate end points are presented in Table 3.2.

Table 3.2   Clinical and Health Outcomes and Their Corresponding Intermediate or Surrogate Endpoints: Some Examples

Clinical or Health Outcomes	Intermediate or Surrogate Endpoints
Longevity	Dilated coronary arteries
Quality of life	5-year survival
Take baby home	Pregnancy
Pain relief	Fewer adhesions
No transfusion	Less blood loss

Another AHCPR initiative designed to assess outcomes to measure the quality of care is the Patient Outcomes Research Team (PORT). The 11th of 14 original PORT projects is a study of the methods of management and outcomes of childbirth. This was the first PORT that did not primarily involve Medicare and Medicaid patients and was the first in women's health care.

Quality-of-Life Measurement

Medical outcomes research has tended to focus on the assessment of short-term risks and the confirmation of pathologic diagnoses. This effort has been usually limited to quantification of mortality and major morbidity—such as infection, blood transfusion, and reoperation—occurring while the patient was hospitalized and verified by tissue diagnosis. Most standardized lists of clinical quality assurance indicators are from the *medical model* of outcomes assessment. Although the importance of these kinds of indicators seems obvious, these indicators may have little or no relevance to the more fundamental question of actual *effectiveness* of a procedure in terms of preserving or enhancing quality of life. For example, if a patient with pelvic pain undergoes a hysterectomy for leiomyomata, experiences no short-term complications, and has a diagnosis that is confirmed histologically, the procedure may be considered successful from the standpoint of surgical risk management, short-term outcome, and histologic verification. However, if the patient continues to experience pain and has no improvement in the quality of her life, the surgery has been, in reality, unsuccessful. Short-term risk indicators often have little or no bearing on whether the procedure actually works.

Behavioral Model of Health Outcomes

Efforts to measure the success or the effectiveness of health care procedures in the U.S. are based on the traditional medical model in which a patient is evaluated for a symptom, diagnosed as having a condition, and treated for that diagnosis. A procedure is usually considered successful if the diagnosis is confirmed.

Medicine has traditionally relied on short-term risk indicators and histologic confirmation because these measurements seem more objective and quantifiable. Death and infection rates, blood loss, and rates of histologic verification can all be measured and expressed numerically. Crucial to the application of a more predictive behavioral model in clinical outcomes research are several statistically valid and reliable methods to measure health-related quality of life. Many measures have been developed and validated, but few are used in clinical practice (16).

Utilizing the *behavioral model* of effectiveness, the concept of *quality-adjusted life-years* (*QALY*) has been proposed to measure the benefit, in both quantity and quality of life, of a health care procedure (17). The number of *QALY*s is determined by combining the extra years of life that a procedure offers with a validated measure of eight categories of disability and four measures of distress. The use of this methodology allows standardized comparison of the cost of entirely different health care procedures. Despite its inadequacies, the *medical model* has been the standard, but the *behavioral model* of outcomes is now becoming incorporated into health care evaluation and research (18). Scales of health-related quality-of-life issues, called the SF-36 and the SF-12 (short-form 36 and 12), have been developed (19).

Quality Improvement

Most methods for the assessment of the quality of health care have been based on the premise that quality is the sole responsibility of the health care professional. Because the practitioner's technical skills, knowledge, and interpersonal interactions are the basis for quality of patient care, many regulatory agencies (e.g., the Joint Commission on the Accreditation of Health Care Organizations [JCAHO]) and hospitals have created QA models that focus mostly on the practitioner. However, quality of care is determined by many interacting forces, and the practitioner clearly does not deliver care in isolation. The delivery of health care requires the integration and management of many processes. The practitioners' ability to deliver care is influenced by the environment, the ability and skill of support staff, policies and procedures, facilities, governing processes, methods of work, and equipment and materials available, as well as innumerable patient variables such as severity of illness, concurrent illness (comorbidity), and social support. Historically, QA efforts attempted to monitor these processes to document bad outcomes. However, this approach has not proved to be adequate in improving the quality of care (20). Regulatory agencies and hospitals are now focusing on the overall performance of health care organizations in terms of clinical or health outcomes.

Improvements in health care have been based on knowledge that physicians and other health care professionals acquired in medical and other professional schools. Improvements have been brought about by clinicians applying knowledge developed by discipline-specific experts (21). The recent national emphasis on health care reform is an indication that the past rate of improvements is not sufficient to meet the financial needs and expectations of society. Improvements in efficiency must be made at a faster pace because consumers are seeking greater value for and access to health care services. A theoretical basis for organizational change that promotes continuous improvement includes knowledge of a system, knowledge of variation, and the theory of knowledge (3, 22–24).

Knowledge of a System   The first component of continuous improvement is *knowledge of a system*. A *system* is defined as a network of interdependent components that work together to accomplish its aim. A system does not exist without an aim and is only capable of improving if there is a connection between the aim, the means of production, and the means of improving. An "open system" is one that permits continued access from *outside* the system. Because health care organizations are accountable to patients and to the community as a whole, they are considered open systems. The aim of an organization involves the integration of the knowledge of the social needs and the needs of patients.

Knowledge of a system includes the following aspects:

1. *Customer knowledge*—This is the basis of an organization's aim. The aim is derived by identifying the organization's customers and by understanding the measures used to judge quality. Meeting patient expectations is one of the most accurate ways to define quality.

2. *How the organization provides its services*—This is the means of producing a service, which involves knowledge of what is delivered, the processes or steps taken to deliver the services, the information and materials used to provide services, and the suppliers.

3. *How the organization improves what it delivers*—This involves knowledge of the aim and identification of areas for improvement that are likely to have the greatest impact.

Understanding the interrelationships between the aim, the customers, the primary areas for improvement, and the specific processes that can be improved is known as "systems thinking." If a health care organization is focused on providing as many services as possible and does not understand the needs of the community and their customers, it will eventually fail to deliver quality services.

Knowledge of Variation

Another element of continuous improvement is *knowledge of variation. Variation* is present in every aspect of our lives. There is variation in everyone's behavior, learning styles, and ways of performing a task. Although the presence of variation or "uniqueness" can be considered a kind of quality, most services are judged on the basis of predictability and a low level of variation. When a service is thought to be of high quality, we expect it to be "exactly" the same each time, and if there is to be any variation, it must be "better."

To continually improve health products and services, it is necessary to know the customers, their needs, and how they judge the quality of health services. The processes by which health services are delivered must be understood and unintended variations reduced. If an organization is to improve and be innovative, it must plan changes that are based on knowledge of what can be better. Two types of variation found in production processes are those that occur by chance (common cause) and those due to "assignable" causes (special causes) (25). The ability to differentiate between these two types of variation is essential to making improvements in health care.

Clinicians regularly make decisions in their practices based on variation. For example, a physician making frequent rounds may note a change in a patient's temperature and may decide to treat or to observe the patient based on the temperature change and on experience (i.e., judgment). If the temperature variation is seen as "special cause" (i.e., infection), a decision may be made to add an antibiotic. However, if the change or variation is interpreted as "common cause" variation in temperature due to short-term "normal" changes or "chance," it may be ignored. If this happens often, the physician may alter the frequency of observation, thereby making an improvement to the monitoring process. Frequently, however, common cause variation is not recognized in health care, and the variation is acted on prematurely, resulting in the over-utilization of resources and a lower quality of care (5). If the approach is to "measure and change," too many costly changes might be made.

Learning how to respond appropriately to variation in health care processes is a major challenge. Understanding and controlling variation in health care services should be the main emphasis of quality management. The notion of controlling variation, however, causes concern and skepticism in many health care professionals. Physicians who fear any effort to control variation are worried about the loss of options and about restrictions on their judgment. As Berwick points out (5), however, "The (problem) is not *considered, intentional variation,* but rather *unintended* or *misinterpreted* variation in the work of health care. Unintended variation is stealing health care blind today. In controlling it, the health care system could potentially recover a bounty in wasted resources that would dwarf the puny rewards of cost-containment to date."

Variation in Utilization

One of the earliest and most compelling influences on "modern" health care quality assessment in the U.S. was a series of investigations that demonstrated a wide variation in the use of health care procedures (26). Although previous investigations had documented two- to fourfold differences in the rates of selected procedures both within the U.S. and between the U.S. and other industrialized countries, these variations usually were disregarded as secondary to population differences. However, a "small-area analysis" documented similar or even greater magnitudes of variation within small (25–50 miles) geographic regions that could not be explained by differences in patient characteristics or appropriate differences in "standards of care" (27).

Variations in utilization have now been analyzed for virtually all major surgical procedures, including hysterectomy and cesarean delivery (28, 29). Also, variation in the performance of medical procedures, such as those used in the management of acute myocardial infarction and sepsis, have been identified (30). On the basis of these analyses, significant variation has been documented in utilization and in important outcomes such as complications, cost, and derived benefit (31). This type of analysis does not usually allow accurate assessment of which rate of utilization or outcome is appropriate. However, it can help to focus attention on the quality of health services and the complexities of using statistically valid methods to measure health care quality.

Variation in utilization of health care services can be categorized as follows:

1. Necessary and intended variation due to well-recognized patient differences such as severity of illness, comorbidity, and legitimate patient preferences.

2. Acceptable but reducible variation because of uncertainty and lack of accurate information about outcomes.

3. Unacceptable variation because of nonclinical factors such as habitual differences in practice style that are not grounded in knowledge or reason.

Most of the differences in utilization rates of many health care procedures result from the last two categories.

Variation in Women's Health Care

Overall, the rate of inpatient surgery for females aged 15–44 years is more than three times that of males, excluding vaginal deliveries (31). The most commonly performed major surgical procedure in the U.S. is cesarean delivery, with approximately 950,000 procedures performed annually in the U.S. Rates of cesarean delivery vary by region, state, and small geographical areas. The rates are 12–40%, and the national mean is 24%. Comparative rates for the United Kingdom are 6–12%.

Hysterectomy is the second most frequent inpatient surgical procedure in the U.S. The total annual occurrence of hysterectomy for all ages, all indications, and all institutions (federal and nonfederal) in the U.S. is approximately 600,000, which is about twice the annual occurrence of coronary artery bypass grafting and intervertebral disk repair in men and women combined (31, 32). Hysterectomy rates in the southern and western U.S. are 50% higher than those in the midwest and twice the rate in New England. A two- to fivefold variation in utilization rates has been documented within states and small geographical areas within the U.S. (28, 33). National rates in the U.S. are twice those in the United Kingdom and more than three times the rates in Sweden and Norway (34).

Hysterectomy utilization in the U.S. varies by both provider and patient characteristics. Studies of utilization patterns have demonstrated that older physicians are more likely to recommend hysterectomy than are younger physicians, and (when controlled for age) gender does not appear to influence hysterectomy decision-making (35). With respect to patient variables, although hysterectomy utilization is similar among African-American women and white women (32, 36), low income and low educational level are risk factors for hysterectomy (36, 37). By age 65, the prevalence of hysterectomy is 40% for women with a high school education and 20% for women with a college education.

Short-term outcomes of hysterectomy vary significantly by race. African-American women have substantially higher relative risks (RR) for morbidity and in-hospital mortality (RR=3.1) compared to age- and condition-matched white women (38). The reasons for this variation are not known. Quality management techniques are being applied to study and reduce these wasteful variations.

The Theory of Knowledge

The final component of knowledge for improvement is *the theory of knowledge*. The theory of knowledge refers to the need for the application of a scientific method for making improvements. One model for testing small-scale change is called the **P**lan, **D**o, **S**tudy, **A**ct (**PDSA**) method (23). Unlike the "ideal" scientific method recommended for clinical trials, the **PDSA** method does not include a control group. Although randomized controlled trials have been considered to be the best way to determine the value of health care interventions they have two distinct disadvantages. They are expensive and tend to define the *efficacy* of an intervention such as a drug or a surgical procedure. Because efficacy is the way an intervention works under ideal conditions, compared with effectiveness, which is the way an intervention works in everyday practice (10), health services researchers now recognize that it may not be possible to generalize about an intervention's effectiveness based on its efficacy as measured in a randomized trial. Also, it is too expensive to perform randomized trials in all situations in which the effectiveness of health care services need to be improved.

The **PDSA** cycle has been modified as the **F**ind a process, **O**rganize a team, **C**larify the process, **U**nderstand the variation, and **S**elect an improvement (**FOCUS**)-**PDCA** cycle and tested for health care improvements (23). In this model, the **"P"** represents the need to **"plan"** an improvement by first identifying a change that might lead to improvement and then testing the change on a small scale. During this phase, the details of who will do what, when the change will occur, and how the change will be communicated to those who will be affected are detailed. The **"D"** stands for **"doing"** or implementing the plan (change to the process) and collecting the data. The **"C"** stands for **"checking"** the data to determine if the change to the process represents an improvement, and the **"A"** stands for **"acting"** or incorporating the change into the process if it is found to be an improvement. A new cycle with another change is started if an improvement was not recognized.

Health care organizations are seeking efficient ways to optimize the way that they deliver and improve health care services. The notion that high-quality health care automatically means high cost is no longer accepted without question. At a time when many businesses have transformed themselves by using newer methods of quality management, enabling them to deliver high-quality goods and services at reasonable costs, health care professionals and organizations are beginning to test these improvement methods in medical and surgical practice.

Informed Consent and Medical Decision-Making

Available research suggests that the most efficient means of improving outcomes and quality of care is to involve the patient (customer) in the process of health care decision-making. Only occasionally (emergency care) should it be considered appropriate to exclude the patient from active participation in the process of making diagnostic or treatment choices. Because most health care decisions are elective (i.e., there is at least one other reasonable alternative for diagnosis or treatment), a process of informed collaborative choice should nearly always occur (39).

The process of informed consent evolved in the U.S. because of medical-legal liability that arose secondary to the failure to properly inform patients before treatment. Informed consent has remained unchanged over the years despite research showing that it is not adequate as the sole means of allowing a patient to make an informed decision. In one study (40), the essential elements of informed consent were discussed in only a percentage of encounters: rationale (43%), benefits (34%), risks (14%), and alternatives (12%). Other important categories of information for decision-making, such as *preferences* and *expense,* were not included or studied.

Typically, patients undergo the informed consent process in a hurried fashion that is usually not "informed" or truly "consensual" after the decision is made to proceed with a procedure. Physicians sometimes complain about the amount of time required to give adequate "informed consent" and provide informed consent nominally to comply with "risk-management" protocols. Most health care professionals, health services researchers, and consumer groups have urged fundamental changes in the way that patients are informed about elective diagnostic and treatment alternatives available to them. Including the patient in the decision-making process can improve compliance, satisfaction, and even clinical outcomes (41–43).

Recent research has indicated that patients are frequently reluctant to assert themselves in a health care setting. Although a variety of explanations has been provided for this observation, current behavioral research suggests that it is usually either because of a lack of accurate information about choices and effectiveness or a belief that they do not have the ability to choose. Accurate information regarding therapeutic options and effectiveness is also referred to as *outcome expectations;* a patient's belief about his or her ability to choose appropriately is called decision-making *self-efficacy.* In a theoretical representation of patient status in health care decision-making, a few patients are characterized as having complete autonomy (Fig. 3.4). These patients take a lead role in discussions, asking questions, introducing topics, expressing opinions, and determining clinical decisions; they can be characterized as having very high self-efficacy. At the other extreme are patients who abdicate their role in decision-making. These patients are often passive and, therefore, may be reluctant to ask questions or even express opinions and would be characterized as having low decision-making self-efficacy. Also, they may be susceptible to a phenomenon known as *demand effect,* which is the desire of the patient to conform to the perceived wishes of the physician. In health care decision-making, when there is total patient abdication, the provider does most of the talking, asks most of the questions, chooses the topics for discussion, and frequently interrupts. Patient abdication is occasionally appropriate, as when emergency treatment is needed or when treatment alternatives do not exist. In most cases that involve elective choices, however, excluding the patient from the process may lead to resentment and anger, particularly if there is a bad outcome.

In the center of this ideal model of physician-patient communication and decision-making is collaboration. The provider and patient work together to reach an appropriate decision. This kind of communication and interaction can only occur when the health care provider establishes the proper atmosphere, including sufficient time, noncoercive and open-ended discussion, and mutual respect and participation. The use of lay terminology instead of

Figure 3.4   A health care decision-making continuum. Current U.S. practice is weighted toward physician control and patient abdication. (Modified with permission from **Ballard-Reisch DS.** A model for participative decision making for physician-patient interaction. *Health Commun* 1990;2:91.)

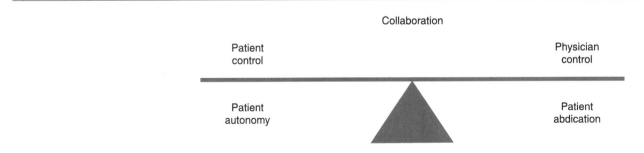

medical jargon is recommended, and the patient cannot be made to feel rushed, inferior, or intimidated. Meaningful quality improvement efforts to establish patient-centered informed consent and medical decision-making must begin with a conscious, noncynical commitment on the part of the provider to share decision-making (44). When the decision has been made collaboratively, patients are much less likely to "blame" the provider for an unpreventable poor outcome.

One approach to both quality assessment and improvement and medical decision-making that has been recommended (the **PREPARED** system) uses a checklist to analyze the *value* of a health care procedure before it is performed (7, 45). The purpose is to sequentially review the critical data categories of information, each represented by a letter in the word **PREPARED,** that should be used to determine the most appropriate course of action or choice (46):

Procedure:	The course of action being considered
Reason:	The indication or rationale
Expectation:	The chances of benefit and failure
Preferences:	Patient-centered priorities (utilities) affecting choice
Alternatives:	Other reasonable options
Risks:	The potential for harm from procedures
Expenses:	All direct and indirect costs
Decision:	Fully informed collaborative choice

Standardized procedural analysis using this sequenced checklist has been shown to improve health care decision-making by increasing patient satisfaction and self-efficacy and thereby facilitating patient choice (47). It has the potential to improve the assessment of the quality and appropriateness of both provider and patient decision-making.

Newer Methods

Health services researchers and clinicians are beginning to develop and validate newer methods for the measurement and improvement of health care quality. For example, there is a need to make valid comparisons of quality between divergent populations and to correlate clinical performance with measurable processes of care. The goal of a new branch of investigation called "clinical outcomes sciences" is to obtain valid measures of relevant outcomes that are correlated with measurable processes of care so that changes in process can be identified and initiated, thereby improving outcomes. This discipline incorporates methodologies from divergent areas such as epidemiology, clinical research, management, engineering, economics, and behavioral sciences. The methods and analytical models used in clinical outcomes investigation vary widely but share a common paradigm (Fig. 3.5).

Statistical adjustments are used to allow clinically dissimilar populations such as high-risk and low-risk patients and those with complicated and uncomplicated conditions to be compared. This procedure is called "case-mix adjustment" and controls for severity of illness and comorbidity (48, 49). Outcomes that are assessed include traditional (medical model) measures such as complications and adverse occurrences, as well as newer, well-validated measures of satisfaction, health, and functional status.

Concurrently, the processes of care are assessed. This would include measurement of resources used during an episode of care (e.g., supplies, medications, specialized personnel) and practice parameters (e.g., physician orders and nursing practices).

Measurement of the processes and outcomes of health care can be prohibitively expensive if this measurement is not integrated into the daily clinical care. For this reason, another goal of clinical quality outcomes research is to develop and incorporate methods of quality assessment into routine practice. This mechanism could be accomplished, for example, by using the SF-36 (the health-status tool derived from the RAND Medical Outcomes Survey) as a standard nursing intake form at the time of admission.

Figure 3.5 Process/outcomes analysis: Diagrammatic representation of an outcomes analysis plan. (From *Health Care Works*, Del Mar, CA, 1995.)

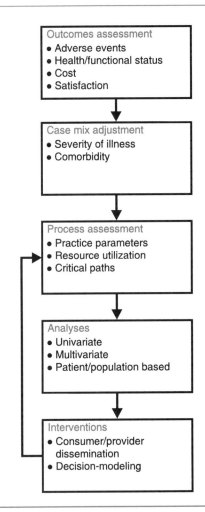

Analytical methods in clinical outcomes science rely heavily on multivariate statistics and iterative outcomes databases to provide valid correlations between measurable (and changeable) processes and outcomes. However, the mere identification of process changes that would improve outcomes does not ensure that they will, in fact, be used. For this reason, process/outcomes data must be linked to methods that will allow this information to be incorporated into clinical and operational decision-making if they are to change behavior and improve outcomes. These analyses must be readily available both geographically and temporally at the point of care (the place and time that the decision is made) if they are to improve outcomes.

Outcomes-Derived Clinical Guidelines

In the past, clinical practice guidelines or parameters have been largely derived by expert opinion and consensus. A major goal of clinical outcomes science is to allow for the development of guidelines based on *actual measured outcomes* that could "self-adjust" based on performance and newer methods of diagnosis and treatment. One such process for incorporating outcomes data into clinical practice is the "critical pathway–case management" method (45). In this method, consensus practice parameters for a given condition (e.g., management of preterm labor) are initially developed by a multidisciplinary team consisting of all professional, allied, and support services involved in the care of the target population. This list of parameters is called a "critical path" or "clinical map." The critical path details all laboratory, dietary, consultative, medical, teaching, and nursing activities that are thought to be necessary to obtain specific clinical outcomes. Outcomes of care, as well as variations from the "path," are monitored and collected continuously.

Positive and negative outcomes are then analyzed and correlated with variances from the critical pathway. These data are then returned to the multidisciplinary team, which recommends changes in the entire path based on the outcomes and variance analyses.

In one pilot study of a critical pathway method for cesarean delivery, length of stay and cost were reduced by 13% and 14%, respectively. Additionally, five of seven measurements of satisfaction, including quality of care, were improved and health status was unchanged (50).

Managed Care

Efforts to measure and improve health care quality have received progressively greater support and validation. Health care reform efforts and rapidly changing reimbursement patterns are moving away from fee-for-service toward managed care and capitation-based contracting, and this trend has led to a rapid application of modern quality management techniques in health care. The need to maintain or increase quality while decreasing costs has stimulated quality improvement initiatives. Managed care contracts are currently being awarded on the basis of both clinical outcomes and cost.

Many states and federal agencies have enacted legislation that requires health care providers to collect and disseminate comparative outcomes data in their practices. If these data are collected and analyzed appropriately, these initiatives could improve health care quality and reduce costs by facilitating rational decision-making by consumers, providers, and third-party payers. If done hastily or inappropriately, efforts to use outcomes data, although well-intended, could undermine these goals. For these reasons, standardized and validated methods for measuring the processes and outcomes of health care must be developed and integrated into everyday clinical and operational practice (51).

References

1. **Kaplan RM**. Behavior as a central outcome in health care. *Am Psychol* 1990;45:1211–20.

2. **Fuchs VR.** The best health care system in the world? *JAMA* 1992;268(7):916–7.

3. **Morris M, Gambone JC.** Making continual improvements to health care. *Clin Obstet Gynecol* 1994;37(1):137–48.

4. **Berwick DM.** Continuous improvement as an ideal in health care. *N Engl J Med* 1989;310:53–6.

5. **Berwick DM.** Controlling variation in health care: a consultation from Walter Shewhart. *Med Care* 1991;29(12):1212–25.

6. **DiMatteo MR.** The physician-patient relationship: effects on the quality of health care. *Clin Obstet Gynecol* 1994;37(1):149–61.

7. **Reiter RC, Lench JB, Gambone JC.** Consumer advocacy, elective surgery, and the "golden era of medicine." *Obstet Gynecol* 1989;74:815–17.

8. **Hickson GB, Clayton EW, Entman SS, Miller CS, Githens PB, Whitten-Goldstein K, et al.** Obstetricians' prior malpractice experience and patients' satisfaction with care. *JAMA* 1994;272:1583–7.

9. **Entman SS, Glass CA, Hickson GB, Githens PB, Whetten-Goldstein K, Sloan FA.** The relationship between malpractice claims history and subsequent obstetric care. *JAMA* 1994;272:1588–91.

10. **DeFreise GH.** Measuring the effectiveness of medical interventions: new expectations of health services research. *Health Serv Res* 1990;25:691–5.

11. **DiMatteo RM, Reiter RC, Gambone JC.** Enhancing medication adherence through communication and informed collaborative choice. *Health Commun* 1994;6(4):253–65.

12. **Donabedian A.** The quality of care: How can it be assessed? *JAMA* 1988;260:1743–8.

13. **Donabedian A.** *The Methods and Findings of Quality Assessment and Monitoring.* Ann Arbor: Health Administration Press, 1985:3.

14. **Kaplan RM, Anderson JP.** The general health policy model: an integrated approach. In: Spilker B, ed. *Quality of Life Assessment in Clinical Trials.* New York: Raven Press, 1990:131–49.

15. **Salive ME, Mayfield JA, Weissman NW.** Patient outcomes research teams and the agency for health care policy and research. *Health Serv Res* 1990;25:697–708.

16. **Deyo RA, Patrick DL.** Barriers to the use of health status measures in clinical investigation, patient care, and policy research. *Med Care* 1989;27:S254–68.

17. **Maynard A.** Developing the health care market. *Economic Journal* 1991;101:1277–87.

18. **Ware JE Jr, Kosinski M, Bayliss MS, McHorney CA, Rogers WH, Raczek A.** Comparison of methods for the scoring and statistics of SF-36 health profile and summary measure: summary of outcomes study. *Med Care* 1995;33(Suppl 4):AS264–79.

19. **Kaplan RM.** An outcomes-based model for directing decisions in women's health care. *Clin Obstet Gynecol* 1994;37(1):192–206.

20. **Batalden PB, Buchanan DB.** Patient care process improvement. In: Batalden PB, Buchanan DB, eds. *A Course, Hospital Wide Quality: Focus on Continuous Improvement.* Nashville: Hospital Corp. of America (QRG), 1990:12.

21. **Batalden PB, Nolen TW.** Knowledge for the leadership of continual improvement in healthcare. In: Taylor RJ, ed. *Manual of Health Services Management.* Gaithersburg: Aspen, 1993:1–21.

22. **Deming WE.** *The New Economics for Industry, Government and Education.* Cambridge: Massachusetts Institute of Technology, 1993.

23. **Bataldin PB, Stoltz PK.** A framework for the continual improvement of health care: building and applying professional and improvement knowledge to test changes in daily work. *Joint Comm J Qual Impr* 1993;19(10):424–52.

24. **Deming WE.** *Out of the Crisis.* Cambridge: MIT Center for Applied Engineering Studies, 1986.

25. **Shewhart WA.** *Statistical Method from the Viewpoint of Quality Control.* Washington, DC: Department of Agriculture, 1993.

26. **Wennberg JE, Gittelsohn A.** Variations in medical care among small areas. *Sci Am* 1982;246:120–34.

27. **Wennberg JE, Freeman JL, Culp WJ.** Are hospital services rationed in New Haven or overutilized in Boston? *Lancet* 1987;1:1185–9.

28. **Roos NP.** Hysterectomy: Variations in rates across small areas and across physicians' practices. *Am J Public Health* 1984;74(4):327–35.

29. **Center for Disease Control and Prevention.** Rates of cesarean delivery—United States. *MMWR* 1993;42:285–9.

30. **The Cardiology Working Group:** Cardiology and the quality of medical practice. *JAMA* 1991;265:482–5.

31. **Bickell NA, Earp JA, Garrett JM, Evans AT.** Gynecologists' sex, clinical beliefs, and hysterectomy rates. *Am J Public Health* 1994;84:1649–52.

32. **Carlson KJ, Nichols DH, Schiff I.** Indications for hysterectomy. *N Engl J Med* 1993;328:856–60.

33. **Coulter A, Peto V, Doll H.** Patients' preferences and general practitioners' decisions in the treatment of menstrual disorders. *Fam Pract* 1994;11(1):67–74.

34. **Graves EJ.** *Summary: National Hospital Discharge Survey.* Advance Data From Vital and Health Statistics: No. 199. Hyattsville: National Center for Health Statistics, 1989.

35. **Haas S, Acker D, Donahue C, Katz ME.** Variation in hysterectomy rates across small geographic areas of Massachusetts. *Am J Obstet Gynecol* 1993;169:150–4.

36. **Kjerulff K, Langenberg P, Guzinski G.** The socioeconomic correlates of hysterectomies in the United States. *Am J Public Health* 1993;83(5):106–8.

37. **Kjerulff KH, Guzinski GM, Langenberg PW, Stolley PD, Moye NE, Kazandjian VA.** Hysterectomy and race. *Obstet Gynecol* 1993;82:757–64.

38. **Wilcox LS, Koonin LM, Pokras R, Strauss LT, Xia Z, Peterson HB.** Hysterectomy in the United States, 1988-1990. *Obstet Gynecol* 1994;83(4):549–55.

39. **Gambone JC, Reiter RC, DiMatteo MR.** *The Prepared Provider: A Guide for Improved Patient Care.* Beaverton: Mosby/Great Performance, 1994:1–16.

40. **Wu WC, Pearlman RA.** Consent in medical decision-making. The role of communication. *J Gen Intern Med* 1988;3:9–14.

41. **Roter DL.** Patient participation in the patient-provider interaction: The effects of patient question asking on the quality of interaction, satisfaction and compliance. *Health Education Monogr* 1977;5:281–315.

42. **Kaplan SH, Greenfield S, Ware JE Jr.** Assessing the effects of physician patient interactions on the outcomes of chronic disease. *Med Care* 1989;27:S110–27.

43. **Greenfield S, Kaplan S, Ware JE Jr.** Expanding patient involvement in care: effects on patient outcomes. *Ann Intern Med* 1985;102:520–8.

44. **Gambone JC, Reiter RC.** Quality improvement in women's health care. In: **Moore T, Reiter RC, Rebar R, Baker V,** eds. *Gynecology and Obstetrics: A Longitudinal Approach.* New York: Churchill Livingstone, 1993:27–36.

45. **Gambone JC, Reiter RC.** Quality improvement in health care. *Curr Prob Obstet Gynecol Fertil* 1991;15(5):170–5.

46. **Gambone JC, Reiter RC.** Promising innovation or needless intervention? *J Gynecol Techniques* 1995;1:59.

47. **Gambone JC, Reiter RC, DiMatteo MR.** *The PREPARED Checklist: Putting Risk into Perspective by a Process of Informed Collaborative Choice. Communicating Risk to Patients.* Proceedings of United States Pharmacopeial Convention, September 20–21, 1994:67–9.

48. **Boyle T.** Developing severity-adjusted critical paths using medisgroups reporting. *Am J Medical Quality* 1991;4:1–12.

49. **Zander K.** Nursing care management: strategic management of cost and quality outcomes. *J Nurs Adm* 1988;18:23–30.

50. **Blegen MA, Reiter RC, Goode C, Murphy R.** Outcomes of hospital based managed care: a multivariate analysis of cost and quality. *Obstet Gynecol* 1995;86:809–14.

51. **Loegering L, Reiter RC, Gambone JC.** Measuring the quality of health care. *Clin Obstet Gynecol* 1994;37(1):122–36.

4

Epidemiology for the Gynecologist

Daniel W. Cramer

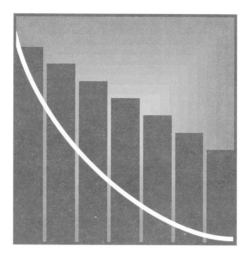

Epidemiology is the study of the occurrence of health events in human populations. Epidemiologic studies may have a variety of designs. They may encompass broad topics such as birth or death rates and how they vary among people of different nationalities or narrow topics such as the risk for a specific disease and how it changes after a specific exposure. Epidemiologic studies depend on the relationship between "exposure" (or treatment) and "disease" (Fig. 4.1). The design, strengths, and weaknesses of the principal types of epidemiologic studies and the issues that affect the validity of such studies are presented (1–6).

Study Designs

In evaluating a medical study, one should first distinguish whether it is primarily *descriptive* or *analytic* (i.e., designed to test an hypothesis about an association).

Descriptive Studies

A description of medical illnesses (or "cases") is the most common type of study. Although these reports do not "prove" associations, they often serve as the catalyst for larger prospective trials and clinical "experiments" that permit us to appropriately study these observations. **The two principal types of descriptive studies are *case series* and *cross-sectional studies*.**

Case Series or Reports

One of the most common and simplest type of study is the case report or case series. Although no epidemiologic analysis is required to prepare a case series, it should be evaluated in the spectrum of epidemiologic studies. A case series is the first step of a case-control study, which is an analytic study describing the characteristics of individuals with a particular disease and including a comparison or control group. Therefore, the manner of selection of cases in a case series (e.g., incident or prevalent cases, record-based or personal contact of patients) can affect the validity of a case-control study that is developed from a case series.

Case series often form the basis for future epidemiologic studies or can lead to public health action. Hypotheses about disease etiology or treatment are frequently developed from case

51

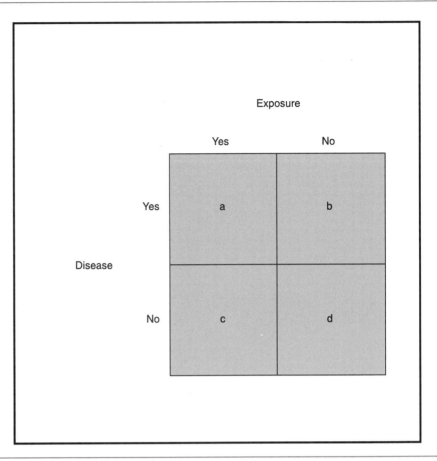

Figure 4.1   The essential design of an epidemiologic study showing the relationship between "exposure" (or treatment) and "disease."

series and then explored in analytic studies. For example, a link between oral contraceptives and thromboembolism was first suggested by case reports (7) and later confirmed in a case-control study (8). Occasionally, when case series describe the co-occurrence of "rare" exposures and "rare" diseases, they are compelling enough on their own to suggest cause and effect. Links between thalidomide and fetal limb reduction (9), the Dalkon shield and septic abortion (10), and sequential oral contraceptives and premenopausal endometrial cancer (11) emerged through case series that were persuasive enough to initiate public health action without the performance of formal epidemiologic studies. **In general, however, just because a high number of members of a case series share a particular characteristic, one cannot assume that there is a cause-and-effect relationship, because a number of selection factors could have contributed to the observation.**

A case series does not usually yield any formal epidemiologic measure other than estimates of the frequency of a particular characteristic among members of the case series. Clinicians sometimes refer to this as the "incidence" of a particular characteristic among cases, but "prevalence" is the more appropriate term.

Cross-Sectional Studies

Design

Cross-sectional studies are much larger in scope than case series and generally do not focus on a particular disease. Populations are surveyed to provide a "snapshot" of health

52

events in the population at a particular time. The Census Bureau counts the U.S. population by categories of age, sex, and ethnicity. The National Center for Health Statistics compiles a wide variety of data on the health of the U.S. population, such as occurrence of hospitalization for various conditions. State health departments are required to count the number of births and deaths annually in their population, and some maintain registries to count the number of individuals who have cancer.

Yield

Incidence Rate   **Incidence is the rate of occurrence of new cases of diseases or conditions over a specific time interval.** Cross-sectional studies often yield incidence rates in which births, new disease cases, or deaths are counted annually for a specified census region and divided by the population size to yield events per population per year. The rate is usually multiplied by a base (1000, 10,000, or 100,000) to give numbers that can more easily be tabulated. The concept of incidence provides more information regarding the occurrence of disease than does prevalence.

Age-specific incidence **refers to the number of new events occurring in 5- or 10-year age groups per year. Because of marked differences by age for most illnesses, age-specific incidence rates are the best way to describe event occurrence in a population. If the incidence rate is not specified with regard to age, it is described as "crude."**

Prevalence   **Prevalence, or frequency, is the existing number of cases at a specific point in time. Stated another way, prevalence is the frequency with which a disease or condition occurs at a particular time divided by the population size.** Prevalence is another measure frequently developed from cross-sectional studies. For example, in 1988 the Family Growth Survey Branch of the National Center for Health Statistics interviewed a sample of married couples and found the prevalence of infertility among married women younger than 45 years of age in the U.S. to be about 8.0% (12). Because prevalence measures disease status in a population rather than events occurring over time, prevalence is a proportion.

Although cross-sectional studies are primarily descriptive, they may contribute information on the etiology of disease by showing how disease varies by age, sex, race, or geography. In "ecologic" studies, disease rates in various populations are correlated with other population characteristics (e.g., endometrial cancer rates worldwide are positively correlated with per capita fat consumption and negatively correlated with cereal and grain consumption) (13). Such observations are valuable in suggesting topics for analytic studies or supporting the consistency of an association.

Analytic Studies

The purpose of an analytic epidemiologic study is to test a hypothesis about and to measure an association between exposure (or treatment) and disease occurrence (or prevention). Analytic studies may be subdivided as nonexperimental or experimental. *Nonexperimental analytic studies* include cohort and case-control studies and take advantage of "natural experiments" in which individuals do or do not have a particular disease and have or have not had an exposure of potential interest. *Experimental studies,* such as clinical trials, should meet more rigid criteria than nonexperimental studies, including randomization (in which participants are randomly assigned to exposures) and measures to ensure unbiased assessment of outcome.

Nonexperimental Studies

Cohort Studies

Design   A cohort is a group of people who have some factor in common. In the context of a survival analysis, the cohort begins with a population that is 100% well at a particular time and is followed over time to calculate the percentage of the cohort still well at later times. Survival analysis describes mortality after disease (i.e., cancer patients who died within 5 years) but can be adapted to other events (e.g., the percentage of women who continue to menstruate after 50 years of age or the percentage of infertile women who conceive after therapy).

A cohort is defined by subsets of a population who are, have been, or may in the future be exposed or not exposed to factors hypothesized to influence the occurrence of a given disease (Fig. 4.2). The exposed and nonexposed subjects are observed long enough to generate "person-years" as the denominator for incidence or mortality rates in exposed and nonexposed subsets.

Cohort studies are also called *follow-up,* longitudinal, or *prospective* studies. Although these terms suggest that the exposure is identified prior to outcome, a *retrospective cohort study,* in which the exposure and outcome have already occurred when the study is begun, is possible. For example, studies of radiation and subsequent cancer are based on records of patients irradiated many years previously. Medical records and death certificates are used to determine whether a second cancer occurred after the radiation.

Yield   Cohort studies often yield two measures of an association between exposure and illness: an attributable risk and a relative risk.

Figure 4.2   The format and calculations for a cohort study design.

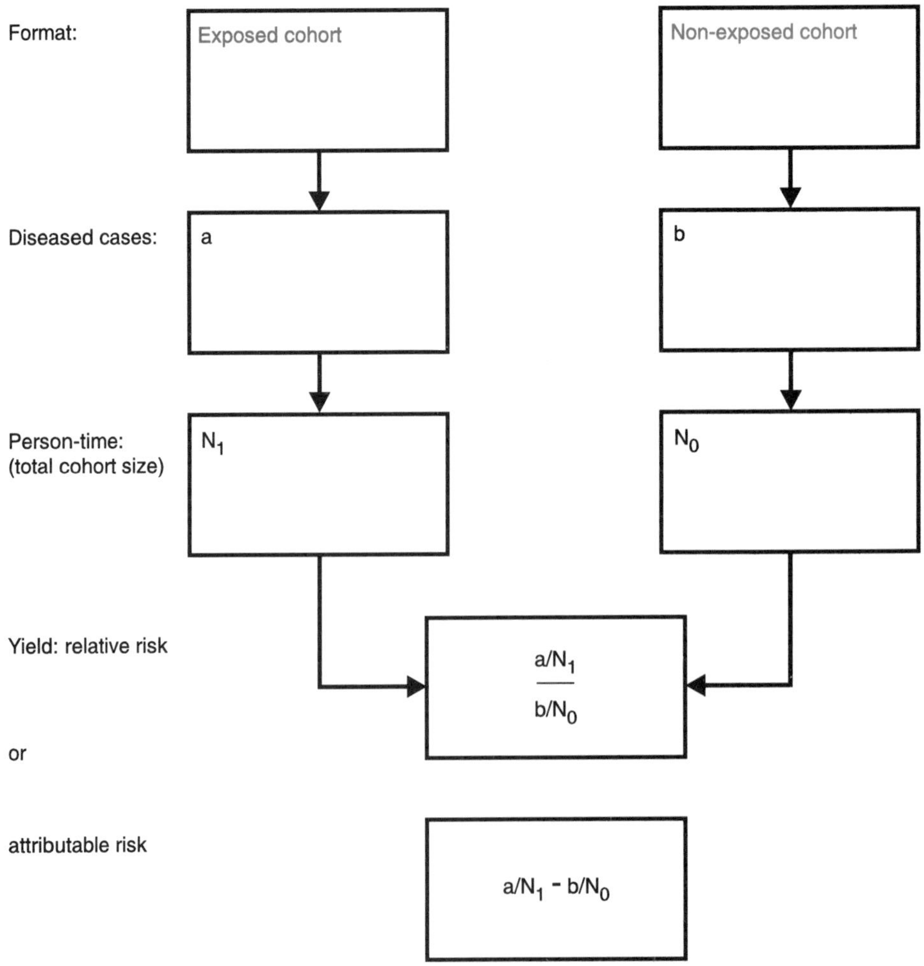

Attributable risk **is the difference between the occurrence measure in the exposed and the unexposed cohort.** The null value is zero—a positive number indicates how many cases of disease may be caused by the exposure, and a negative number indicates how many cases of disease may be prevented by the exposure.

Relative risk **divides occurrence in the exposed cohort by occurrence in the nonexposed cohort. The null value for the relative risk is 1. A value greater than 1 indicates that exposure may increase risk for the disease** (i.e., a relative risk of 1.5 indicates that exposed individuals had 1.5 times the risk for disease as unexposed individuals). **A value less than 1 indicates that exposure may decrease risk for disease** (i.e., a relative risk of 0.5 indicates that the rate in exposed individuals was one-half that of the rate in the nonexposed individuals).

Strengths and Weaknesses   The ability to obtain both attributable and relative risks is a strength of cohort studies. In addition, cohort studies are less susceptible to selection and recall bias. However, misclassification of exposure and confounding variables can occur. Disadvantages of a cohort study generally include higher cost and longer time for completion. Cohort studies are most useful for examining the occurrence of common diseases after a rare exposure. For rare exposures, an investigator may use the general population as the unexposed group. **In this type of study, the observed number of cases in the exposed cohort is divided by the number of cases expected if general population rates had prevailed in the exposed cohort. This comparison is called the** *standardized morbidity or mortality ratio (SMR)* **and is equivalent to relative risk.**

Case-Control Studies

Design   A case-control study starts with the identification of individuals with a disease or outcome of interest and a suitable control population without the disease or outcome of interest. The relationship of a particular attribute or exposure to the disease is studied by comparing how the cases and controls differed in that exposure. An alternate term frequently used to describe a case-control study is "retrospective," because the exposures are assessed after the disease has occurred.

Yield   **The yield of a case-control study is the exposure odds ratio (or simply "odds ratio") and is the ratio of exposed cases to unexposed cases divided by the ratio of exposed to unexposed controls.** If an entire population could be characterized by its exposure and disease status, the exposure odds ratio would be identical to the relative risk obtainable from a cohort study of the same population. Although it is not feasible to survey the entire population, as long as the sampling of cases or controls from the population was not influenced by their exposure status, the exposure odds ratio will approximate the relative risk. Attributable risk is not directly obtainable in a case-control study (Fig. 4.3).

Strengths and Weaknesses   The advantages of case-control studies are that they are generally lower in cost and easier to conduct than other analytic studies. Case-control studies are most feasible for examining the association between a relatively common exposure and a relatively rare disease. Disadvantages include greater potential for selection bias, information bias, and confounding variables.

Experimental Studies   Because an investigator must assign exposures according to a strict protocol, human experimental studies are limited to the study of measures that will prevent disease or the consequences of disease. Examples of experimental studies are clinical trials and field and community intervention trials.

55

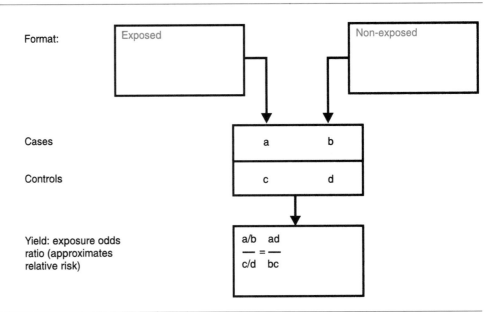

Format:

Exposed

Non-exposed

Cases

	a	b

Controls

	c	d

Yield: exposure odds
ratio (approximates
relative risk)

$$\frac{a/b}{c/d} = \frac{ad}{bc}$$

Figure 4.3   The case-control study design.

Clinical Trials

Clinical trials evaluate treatments for disease in humans. Randomization is the cornerstone of a good clinical trial because it minimizes bias, which can result from confounding variables or preferential assignment of treatment based on patient characteristics. Evidence must be provided that factors that might influence outcome, such as stage of disease, were similar in patients assigned to the study protocol compared with patients assigned to placebo or traditional treatment. Criteria for successful treatment must be clearly defined. Blinding the subject and clinician to the treatment modality may help ensure unbiased assessment of the outcome. A properly designed clinical trial will have a sufficient number of subjects enrolled to ensure that a "negative" study is powerful enough to rule out a treatment effect.

Field and Community Intervention Trials

Field and community intervention trials evaluate measures that may prevent disease, such as vaccines, dietary interventions, or screening procedures. In a field trial, the intervention is applied to individuals. In a community intervention trial, the intervention (e.g., water fluoridation) is applied on a community-wide basis rather than to individual persons. Both types of studies deal with subjects who do not yet have disease and may require large numbers of participants, especially for studies of screening procedures to prevent cancer. In the latter context, issues related to the validity of screening tests (i.e., sensitivity, specificity, and predictive value) are quite important (Table 4.1).

The *sensitivity* of a test is the proportion of persons with a true positive screening result out of all those who have the disease.

The *specificity* of a test is the proportion of persons with a true negative screening result out of all those who do not have the disease.

The *predictive value of a positive test* is defined as the number of true positive results out of all those screened with positive results.

Table 4.1 Measures of Validity for a Screening Procedure

Status Determined by Screening	True Disease Status		
	Positive	*Negative*	*Total*
Positive	a (true positives)	b (false-positives)	a + b (all screened positive)
Negative	c (false-negatives)	d (true negatives)	c + d (all screened negative)
Total	a + c (all diseased)	b + d (all nondiseased)	N (all subjects)

Measure	*Definition*	*Formula*
Sensitivity	$\dfrac{\text{True positives}}{\text{All diseased}}$	$\dfrac{a}{a + c}$
Specificity	$\dfrac{\text{True negatives}}{\text{All nondiseased}}$	$\dfrac{d}{b + d}$
Predictive value of a positive screen	$\dfrac{\text{True positives}}{\text{All screened positive}}$	$\dfrac{a}{a + b}$

Reproduced from **Cramer DW.** Epidemiology and biostatistics. In: **Berek JS, Hacker NF,** eds. *Gynecologic Oncology.* 2nd ed. Baltimore: Williams & Wilkins, 1994: 193.

The *predictive value of a negative test* is the number of true negative results out of all those screened with negative results.

The Validity of Analytic Studies

Features of an analytic study that are considered in judging its scientific validity include statistical significance, biases, dose response, consistency, and biologic credibility.

Statistical Significance

Statistical significance is determined by application of a statistical method to test the null hypothesis (i.e., the hypothesis that two factors are not associated). The degree of significance is summarized by the "P value." The P value indicates the relative likelihood that an observation is due to chance. Typically, a P value <0.05 is used to determine statistical significance. In other words, a result differing from the null hypothesis that would have been observed by chance less than 1 in 20 times is considered statistically significant.

Confidence Interval Confidence interval (CI) is a method of significance testing in which an estimation is used to determine an interval in which the "true" measure of the association is expected to occur. A 95% CI means, for example, that if a study were to be repeated many times and a 95% CI were calculated in each study, then 95% of these measurements would contain the association being studied. Confidence intervals of 95% for an odds ratio that includes the null value 1 would not be statistically significant.

Bias

A bias is a systematic error in the design, conduct, or analysis of a study that results in a mistaken conclusion.

Information Bias

Information bias occurs when subjects are classified incorrectly with respect to exposure or disease. This may occur if records are incomplete or if the criteria for exposure or outcome were poorly defined, leading to misclassification.

Recall bias is another type of information bias that may occur if cases are more likely to remember or to reveal their past exposures compared with controls. In addition to adequate criteria and complete records, blindness of observation may reduce information bias if interviewers are unaware of the status of the subjects or the purpose of the study.

Selection Bias

Selection bias may occur when correlates of the exposure or outcome influence sampling from the larger population of potentially eligible subjects. An example of selection bias that may arise in a hospital-based case-control study occurs when the combination of the disease under study and a particular exposure are more likely to lead to hospital admission (14). Using incident cases from more than one hospital, obtaining high participation rates, and attempting to describe nonparticipants are several ways to reduce or at least estimate the potential for selection bias.

Confounding Variables

A third source of potential bias is *confounding variables*. **A confounder is an extraneous variable that accounts for the apparent effect of the study variable or masks the true association.** When a factor is associated with both the study exposure and the study outcome and differs between cases and controls or cohort members, a distortion of the true association between the exposure and the disease may be produced. Age, race, and socioeconomic status are likely confounders and must be adjusted for by statistical techniques including stratification or multivariate analysis. After an analysis to control for confounding variables, the investigator will present the adjusted risk ratio that presumably reflects an association free of such variables.

Stratification means examining the association of interest only within groups that are similar with respect to a potential confounder. *Multivariate analysis* is a statistical technique used during analysis that controls a number of confounders simultaneously and is commonly used in epidemiological studies.

Dose Response

Dose response means that a change in the amount, intensity, or duration of an exposure is associated with either a consistent increase or decrease in risk for a specified disease or outcome. *Trend tests* are used to determine whether a dose response exists.

Consistency and Meta-Analysis

Consistency between findings in different populations, at different times, and by different methods or investigators is an important criterion used to judge whether there is likely to be a causal relationship. A formal method for studying consistency and pooling results from different studies is meta-analysis. **Meta-analysis is the process of combining results from several independent studies examining the same exposure (or treatment) and same outcome in order to conduct a more powerful test of the null hypothesis. A meta-analysis is conducted by assembling measures of the association from different studies, like relative risks, weighting them by the variance of the measure, and taking an overall average.** In the weighting process, the studies with the largest sample size will contribute the greatest information. A properly performed meta-analysis will also have a qualitative component that establishes criteria for acceptance of a study; e.g., only randomized studies might be chosen for a meta-analysis of the effect of a particular treatment.

Biologic Credibility

***Biologic credibility* means that an association is plausible, taking into consideration all aspects of what is known about the natural history or demographics of a disease or**

what has been observed in relevant experimental models. Whereas an imaginative epidemiologist can find an explanation for any single association, a key issue is whether a model can be proposed that accounts for a variety of exposures as well as experimental data and cross-sectional observations.

Exposures and Illnesses

The relationship between an exposure and a disease can best be determined by studying individuals who are "exposed" or "not exposed" to the item of interest (e.g., a drug or substance) and relating the groups to those who do or do not have the disease in question.

Exposures

"Exposures" that are important to women's health are either "gynecologic" exposures that affect common diseases or common exposures that affect gynecologic diseases.

Reproductive Events

The age when women begin their menstrual periods, the characteristics of their menstrual cycle, the number of times they have been pregnant, and when they cease having periods are important reproductive information that may have broad impact on many diseases, including endometriosis (15), fibroids (16), heart disease (17), osteoporosis (18), and cancers of the breast, endometrium, or ovary (19–21). Gynecologists should maintain careful records of reproductive landmarks, both for their potential usefulness in advising patients and for their relevance to clinical research.

Contraception and Sterilization

Barrier Contraception   A protective effect of barrier contraception against pelvic inflammatory disease (PID) (22), tubal infertility (23), ectopic pregnancy (24), and cervical cancer (25) has been consistently observed.

Intrauterine Devices   Current or past use of an intrauterine device (IUD) has been linked with risk for PID (26), ectopic pregnancy (27), and tubal infertility (28). It is likely that these risks could be reduced by recommending IUDs only to women at low risk for genital infections (e.g., parous women in a monogamous relationship).

Oral Contraceptives   Early epidemiologic literature on oral contraceptives (OCs) focused on adverse events including thromboembolism (particularly with high-dose formulations) (29), hypertension (30), myocardial infarction (especially in women older than 40 years of age who also smoked) (31), and liver adenomas (32). Protective effects of OCs have more recently been appreciated, including lower risk for benign breast disease (33), ovarian cysts (34), ovarian cancer (35), and PID (36). Controversy exists concerning the relationship between OC use and cervical and breast cancer. Progression of intraepithelial cervical lesions may be more frequent among OC users (37). A large case-control study of breast cancer in England suggested use of preparations containing 50 μg or more of estrogen may increase the risk for breast cancer (38). However, the possible increased risk associated with past OC use for developing breast cancer at an early age may be more than offset by a decreased risk for developing breast cancer at an older age (39).

Sterilization   Concerns that sterilization might induce early menopause (40) have not been proven. An unexpected protective effect of female sterilization has been suggested for ovarian cancer (41). This protection may derive from the reduction of uterine growth factors that reach the ovary as a result of the interruption of the utero-ovarian circulation—a hypotheses compatible with the observation that hysterectomy (even without removal of ovaries) also protects against ovarian cancer (42).

59

Menopausal Hormones

Similar to early studies of OCs, studies of menopausal hormones focused on adverse events, including endometrial cancer associated with unopposed estrogen use (43). This association has likely been obviated by the use of combined estrogen-progesterone regimens (44). More recent studies suggest protective effects on heart disease (45), osteoporosis (46), and even Alzheimer's disease (47). The association between menopausal hormones and breast cancer continues to be debated. However, a recent meta-analysis of studies of menopausal hormone use and breast cancer provided reassurance that the effect of such agents on breast cancer risk is modest (48).

Sexually Transmitted Diseases

Worldwide, sexually transmitted diseases are possibly the most important preventable cause of morbidity in women. This morbidity includes not only PID from gonorrhea and chlamydia but also chronic disease from syphilis and genitally transmitted viruses including hepatitis, human papillomavirus, and human immunodeficiency virus (HIV). The importance of public health measures to prevent the spread of sexually transmitted diseases, especially the use of barrier contraception, cannot be overemphasized, because the morbidity from these infections may carry over to the offspring.

Lifestyle

Smoking   Adverse effects of smoking on the lungs and heart are well known; however, it is less widely appreciated that smoking may be linked to tubal infertility (49), ectopic pregnancy (50), cervical cancer (51), and early menopause (52).

Alcohol   Alcohol use, in moderation, is associated with decreased risk for cardiovascular disease (53), which may come at the expense of an increased risk for breast cancer (54). It is possible that both of these effects are mediated by the ability of alcohol to retard the metabolism of estrogen, thereby leading to higher circulating levels of estrogen (55).

Exercise and Nutrition   Although aspects of exercise and nutrition cannot be fairly summarized in a single paragraph, it can be stated that gynecologic problems can occur at either extreme. The lean athlete in training who becomes amenorrheic may lose bone mass because of a lack of estrogen, as might the patient with anorexia (18). In obese women, menstrual difficulties may occur that are related to higher estrogen levels, which may, in the longer term, be associated with a higher risk for endometrial cancer (56).

Talc Use   Use of talc in genital hygiene is an exposure emphasized as a potential risk factor for ovarian cancer (57). Because there are no benefits of genital talc use, other than aesthetic, this practice should be discouraged.

Illnesses

Many gynecologists are primary care providers for women and more may assume this role in the future. Therefore, it is important for gynecologists to have an overview of the major causes of mortality in women. Reliable incidence data for gynecologic cancers and benign gynecologic problems are sometimes difficult to find, but statistics are available to guide clinical interventions.

All Causes of Mortality

Table 4.2 shows the 10 leading causes of death in 1990 for females in the U.S. by age from the National Center for Health Statistics data (58). Heart disease remains the major cause of death in women over all, but there is considerable age variation; accidents, homicides, and suicides are most important at ages 15–34 years and cancer is most important at ages 35–74 years.

Table 4.2   Mortality, 10 Leading Causes of Death by Age Group, United States, 1995

All Ages	Ages 1–14	Ages 15–34	Ages 35–54	Ages 55–74	Ages 75 +
Heart diseases 361,048	Accidents 2266	Accidents 6944	Cancer 29,302	Cancer 111,419	Heart diseases 263,041
Cancer 242,277	Cancer 694	Cancer 3434	Heart diseases 11,026	Heart diseases 84,865	Cancer 97,388
Cerebro-vascular diseases 86,767	Congenital anomalies 626	Homicide 2838	Accidents 4695	Cerebro-vascular diseases 16,889	Cerebro-vascular diseases 65,870
Pneumonia, influenza 41,646	Homicide 375	Suicide 1831	Cerebro-vascular diseases 3321	Chronic obstructive lung disease 17,049	Pneumonia, influenza 33,971
Chronic obstructive lung diseases 40,165	Heart diseases 284	Heart diseases 1491	Cirrhosis of liver 2274	Diabetes 10,995	Chronic obstructive lung diseases 21,272
Accidents 29,617	Pneumonia, influenza 148	HIV infection 1440	Suicide 2296	Pneumonia, influenza 5699	Diabetes 14,485
Diabetes 27,855	Cerebral palsy 139	Cerebro-vascular diseases 540	Diabetes 2009	Accidents 5221	Atherosclerosis 9566
Atherosclerosis 10,784	HIV infection 122	Congenital anomalies 408	Chronic obstructive lung disease 1502	Cirrhosis of liver 4442	Accidents 10,073
Nephritis 10,942	Benign neoplasms 66	Pneumonia, influenza 375	Homicide 1498	Diseases of arteries 3104	Alzheimer's disease 7908
Septicemia 11,081	Viral diseases 69	Diabetes 342	HIV infection 1615	Nephritis 2812	Septicemia 7622
All causes 1,047,853	All causes 6376	All causes 24,822	All causes 72,218	All causes 299,422	All causes 629,118

From **Wingo PA, Tong T, Bolden S.** Cancer statistics 1995. *CA Cancer J Clin* 1995; 45:7–30.

Mortality Caused by Cancer

Table 4.3 shows the five leading causes of cancer mortality in women by various ages. In women, lung cancer now accounts for more deaths than breast cancer. Colon and rectal cancers are third over all, although these cancers are the leading cause of death from cancer in women older than 75 years of age, highlighting the importance of colon cancer screening in postmenopausal patients. Pancreatic and ovarian cancers occur with about equal frequency and both remain elusive to screening.

Incidence of the Gynecologic Cancers

Figure 4.4 illustrates the age-specific incidence of genital malignancies in all females in the U.S. around 1991 (59). The incidence of invasive cervical cancer remains steady across all ages, whereas ovarian and endometrial cancer increase markedly during the perimenopausal years and dominate the picture after 50 years of age. The sharp increase

Table 4.3   Mortality for the Five Leading Cancer Sites for Females by Age Group, United States, 1995

All Ages	Ages 1–14	Ages 15–34	Ages 35–54	Ages 55–74	Ages 75 +
Lung 52,068	Leukemia 260	Breast 660	Breast 9188	Lung 30,154	Colon and rectum 15,727
Breast 43,583	Brain and CNS 220	Leukemia 432	Lung 5372	Breast 19,900	Lung 16,400
Colon and rectum 29,017	Endocrine 69	Uterus 343	Uterus 1978	Colon and rectum 11,117	Breast 13,834
Pancreas 13,161	Connective tissue 33	Brain and CNS 328	Colon and rectum 1999	Ovary 6720	Pancreas 6637
Ovary 13,247	Bone 28	Non-Hodgkin's lymphoma 209	Ovary 1779	Pancreas 5669	Ovary 4601

CNS, central nervous system.
From **Wingo PA, Tong T, Bolden S.** Cancer statistics 1995. *CA Cancer J Clin* 1995; 45:7–30.

in endometrial and ovarian cancer rates around the time of menopause may reflect anovulatory cycles associated with unopposed estrogen and increased levels of gonadotropins. Although ovarian cancer appears to rank second to endometrial cancer in terms of incidence, mortality from ovarian cancer currently exceeds the combined mortality of endometrial and cervical cancer (58).

Incidence of Benign Gynecologic Conditions

The estimated number of hospital admissions listing various benign gynecologic conditions as a discharge diagnoses shown in Table 4.4 are based on data collected by the National Hospital Discharge Survey for 1988–1990 and by the Division of Reproductive Health of the Centers for Disease Control and Prevention (60). It should be noted these data pertain to women ages 15–45 years and are based on discharges from nonmilitary hospitals. PID is the most frequent discharge diagnosis, with nearly 300,000 women hospitalized annually. Of almost equal frequency are hospitalizations for benign ovarian cysts, endometriosis, and fibroids, each of which account for the hospitalization of almost 200,000 women annually.

The estimated age-specific incidence of these conditions are shown for PID, ovarian cysts, fibroids, and endometriosis in Figure 4.5. Notable are the higher incidence of PID in the twenties and the increasing incidence of endometriosis and fibroids into the forties. The high frequency of the latter two conditions, combined with a lack of information on their etiology, suggests that these conditions should be the target for more epidemiologic research.

In 1989, there were approximately 88,400 ectopic pregnancies in the U.S., with a rate of about 16.0 per 1000 reported pregnancies compared to 4.5 per 1000 in 1970 (61). In 1970, however, the case-fatality rate was 35.5 per 10,000 ectopic pregnancies compared with 3.8 per 10,000 ectopic pregnancies in 1989, which accounted for approximately 13% of all maternal deaths that year. Ectopic pregnancy continues to contribute to maternal mortality, particularly among nonwhite populations.

Gynecologic "exposures" and gynecologic "diseases" have always been a major focus for epidemiologic research. However, gynecologists have been infrequently involved in the

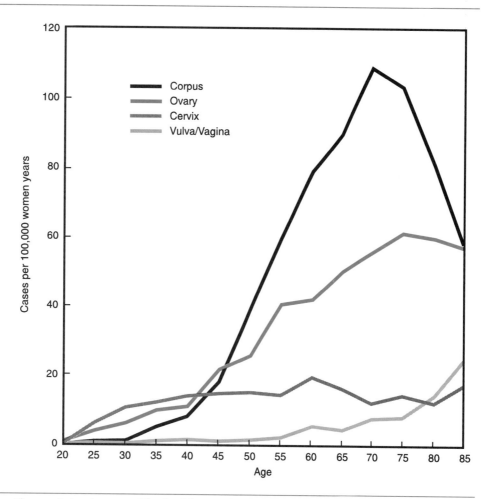

Figure 4.4   Age-specific incidence for gynecologic cancers, all U.S. females (1991). (From **Ries LAG, Miller BA, Hankey BF, Kosary CL, Harras A, Edwards BK.** *SEER Cancer Statistics Review, 1973-1991, Tables and Graphs.* Bethesda, MD: Surveillance Program, Division of Cancer Prevention and Control, National Cancer Institute, NIH Pub No. 94–2789, 1994.)

Table 4.4   Estimated number of annual hospitalizations among women of reproductive age in the United States

Group of Diagnosis	*Hospitalizations**
Pelvic inflammatory disease	287,343
Benign cysts of the ovary	190,548
Endometriosis	188,805
Menstrual disorders	182,988
Uterine leiomyomas	177,082
Prolapse/stress incontinence	101,907
Cervical intraepithelial neoplasia	60,320

*Based on discharge diagnoses for women 15 through 45 years of age in nonmilitary hospitals averaged for the period 1988–1990.
From **Velebil P, Wingo PA, Xia A, Wilcox LS, Peterson HB.** Rate of hospitalization for gynecologic disorders among reproductive-age women in the United States. *Obstet Gynecol* 1995;86:764–9.

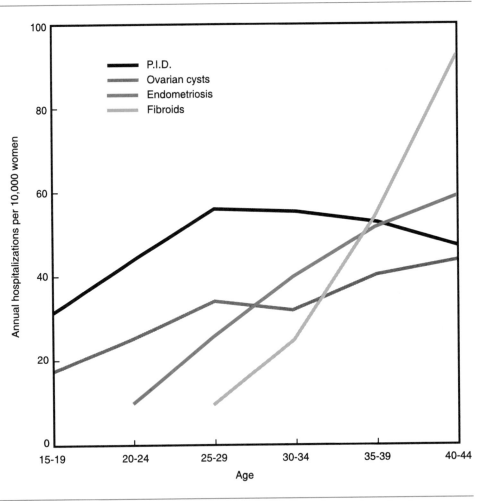

**Figure 4.5   Age-specific incidence of hospitalization for various benign gyneco-
logic conditions around 1990.** (From **Velebil P, Wingo PA, Xia A, Wilcox LS, Peterson HB.** Rate of hospitalization for gynecologic disorders among reproductive-age
women in the United States. *Obstet Gynecol* 1995;86:764–9.)

design and interpretation of such studies, and therefore, the physiologic and clinical relevance of various associations often have been inadequately discussed. Even if the gynecologist does not actually perform epidemiologic research, an understanding of epidemiologic principles will allow a more critical reading of the medical literature and sharpen the
practice of preventive medicine in gynecology.

References

1. **Dawson-Saunders B, Trapp RG.** *Basic and Clinical Biostatistics.* Norwalk: Appleton &
   Lange, 1990.

2. **Last JM.** *A Dictionary of Epidemiology.* 2nd ed. New York: Oxford University Press, 1988.

3. **Peterson HB, Kleinbaum DG.** Interpreting the literature in obstetrics and gynecology. I: Key
   concepts in epidemiology and biostatistics. *Obstet Gynecol* 1991;78:710–7.

4. **Peterson HG, Kleinbaum DG.** Interpreting the literature in obstetrics and gynecology. II: Logistic regression and related issues. *Obstet Gynecol* 1991;78:717–20.

5. **Rothman KJ.** *Modern Epidemiology.* Boston: Little, Brown, 1986.

6. **Schlesselman JJ.** *Case-Control Studies: Design, Conduct, Analysis.* New York: Oxford University Press, 1982.

7. **Tyler ET.** Oral contraceptives and thromboembolism. *JAMA* 1963;185:131–2.

8. **Research Advisory Service of the Royal College of General Practitioners.** Oral contraception and thromboembolic disease. *J R Coll Gen Pract* 1967;13:267–79.

9. **McBride WG.** Thalidomide and congenital abnormalities. *Lancet* 1961;ii:1358.

10. **Christian CD.** Maternal deaths associated with an intrauterine device. *Am J Obstet Gynecol* 1974;119:441–4.

11. **Silverberg SG, Makowski EL.** Endometrial carcinoma in young women taking oral contraceptive agents. *Obstet Gynecol* 1975;46:503–6.

12. **Chandra A, Mosher WD.** The demography of infertility and use of medical care for infertility in study designs and statistics for infertility research. In: **Cramer DW, Goldman MB,** eds. *Infertility and Reproductive Medicine Clinics of North America.* Vol. 5. Philadelphia: WB Saunders Co., 1994:283–96.

13. **Armstrong B, Doll R.** Environmental factors and cancer incidence and mortality in different countries with special reference to dietary practices. *Int J Cancer* 1975;15:617–31.

14. **Berkson J.** Limitations of the application of fourfold table analysis to hospital data. *Biometrics Bull* 1946;2:47–53.

15. **Cramer DW, Wilson E, Stillman RJ, Berger MJ, Belisle S, Schiff I, et al.** The relation of endometriosis to menstrual characteristics, smoking, and exercise. *JAMA* 1986;255:1904–8.

16. **Ross RK, Pike MC, Vessey MP, Bull D, Yeates D, Casagrande JT, et al.** Risk factors for uterine fibroids: Reduced risk associated with oral contraceptives. *BMJ* 1986;293:359–62.

17. **Matthews KA, Meilahn E, Kuller L, Kelsey JF, Caggiula AW, Wing RR.** Menopause and risk factors for coronary artery disease. *N Engl J Med* 1989;321:641–6.

18. **Jones KP, Ravnikar VA, Tulchinsky D, Schiff I.** Comparison of bone density in amenorrheic women due to athletics, weight loss, and premature menopause. *Obstet Gynecol* 1985;66:5–8.

19. **MacMahon B, Cole P.** Etiology of human breast cancer: a review. *J Natl Cancer Inst* 1973;50:21–42.

20. **MacMahon B.** Risk factors for endometrial cancer. *Gynecol Oncol* 1974;2:122–9.

21. **Cramer DW, Hutchinson GB, Welch WR, Scully RE, Ryan KJ.** Determinants of ovarian cancer risk I. Reproductive experiences and family history. *J Natl Cancer Inst* 1983;72:711–6.

22. **Kelaghan J, Rubin GL, Ory HW, Layde PM.** Barrier-method contraceptives and pelvic inflammatory disease. *JAMA* 1982;248:184–7.

23. **Cramer DW, Goldman MB, Schiff I, Belisle S, Albrecht B, Stadel B, et al.** The relationship of tubal infertility to barrier method and oral contraceptive use. *JAMA* 1987;257:2446–50.

24. **Kalandidi A, Doulgerakis M, Tzonou A, Hsieh CC, Aravandinos D, Trichopoulos D.** Induced abortions, contraceptive practices, and tobacco smoking as risk factors for ectopic pregnancy in Athens, Greece. *Br J Obstet Gynaecol* 1991;98:207–13.

25. **Aitken-Swan J, Baird D.** Cancer of the uterine cervix in Aberdeenshire. Aetiologic aspects. *Br J Cancer* 1966;20:642–59

26. **Faulkner WL, Ory HW.** Intrauterine devices and acute pelvic inflammatory disease. *JAMA* 1976;235:1851–3.

27. **Chow WH, Daling JR, Cates W Jr, Greenberg RS.** Epidemiology of ectopic pregnancy. *Epidemiol Rev* 1987;9:70–94.

28. **Cramer DW, Schiff I, Schoenbaum SC, Gibson M, Belisle S, Albrecht B, et al.** Tubal infertility and the intrauterine device. *N Engl J Med* 1985;312:941–7.

29. **Inman WHW, Vessey MP, Westerholm B, Engelund A.** Thromboembolic disease and the steroidal content of oral contraceptives. *BMJ* 1970;2:203–9.

30. **Fisch IR, Frank J.** Oral contraceptives and blood pressure. *JAMA* 1977;237:2499–503.

31. **Incidence of arterial disease among oral contraceptive users. Royal College of General Practitioners' Oral Contraceptive Study.** *J R Coll Gen Pract* 1983;33:75–82.

32. **Rooks JB, Ory HW, Ishak KG, Strauss LT, Greenspan JR, Hill AP, Tyler CW.** Epidemiology of hepatocellular adenoma and the role of oral contraceptive use. *JAMA* 1977;237:2499–503.

33. **Ory H, Cole P, MacMahon B, Hoover R.** Oral contraceptives and reduced risk of benign breast diseases. *N Engl J Med* 1976;294:419–22.

34. **Ory HW.** Functional ovarian cysts and oral contraceptives. *JAMA* 1974;228:68–9.

35. **Gross TP, Schlesselman JJ.** The estimated effect of oral contraceptive use on the cumulative risk of epithelial ovarian cancer. *Obstet Gynecol* 1994;83:419–24.

36. **Rubin GL, Ory HW, Layde PM.** Oral contraceptives and pelvic inflammatory disease. *Am J Obstet Gynecol* 1980;144:630–5.

37. **Swan SH, Brown WL.** Oral contraceptive use, sexual activity, and cervical carcinoma. *Am J Obstet Gynecol* 1981;139:52–7.

38. **UK National Case Control Study Group.** Oral contraceptive use and breast cancer risk in young women. *Lancet* 1989;1:973–82.

39. **Stadel BV, Schlesselman JJ, Murray PA.** Oral contraceptives and breast cancer. *Lancet* 1989;1:1257–9.

40. **Cattanach J.** Oestrogen deficiency after tubal ligation. *Lancet* 1985;1:847–9.

41. **Hankinson SE, Hunter DJ, Colditz GA, Willett WC, Stampfer MJ, Rosner B, et al.** Tubal ligation, hysterectomy, and risk of ovarian cancer. *JAMA* 1993;270:2813–8.

42. **Cramer DW, Xu H.** Epidemiologic evidence for uterine growth factors in the pathogenesis of ovarian cancer. *Ann Epidemiol* 1995;5:310–4.

43. **Shapiro S, Kaufman DW, Slone D, Rosenberg L, Miettinen OS, Stolley PD, et al.** Recent and past use of conjugated estrogens in relation to adenocarcinoma of the endometrium. *N Engl J Med* 1980;303:485–9.

44. **Key TJ, Pike MC.** The dose-relationship between "unopposed" oestrogens and endometrial mitotic rate; its central role in explaining the predicting endometrial cancer risk. *Br J Cancer* 1988;57:205–12.

45. **Stampfer MJ, Colditz GA, Willett WC, Manson JE, Rosner B, Speizer FE, et al.** Postmenopausal estrogen therapy and cardiovascular disease. Ten-year follow-up from the nurses' health study. *N Engl J Med* 1991;325:756–62.

46. **Lindsay R, Aitken JM, Anderson JD, MacDonald EB, Anderson JB, Clarke AC, et al.** Long-term prevention of postmenopausal osteoporosis by oestrogen. *Lancet* 1976;i:1038–41.

47. **Henderson VW, Paganini-Hill A, Emanuel CK, Dunn ME, Buckwalter JG.** Estrogen replacement therapy in older women. Comparisons between Alzheimer's disease cases and non-demented control subjects. *Arch Neurol* 1994;51:896–900.

48. **Dupont WD, Page DL.** Menopause estrogen replacement therapy and breast cancer. *Arch Intern Med* 1991;151:67–72.

49. **Phipps WR, Cramer DW, Schiff I, Belisle S, Stillman R, Albrecht B, et al.** The association between smoking and female infertility as influenced by cause of the infertility. *Fertil Steril* 1987;48:377–82.

50. **Handler A, Davis F, Ferre C, Yeko T.** The relationship of smoking and ectopic pregnancy. *Am J Public Health* 1989;79:1239–42.

51. **Brinton LA, Schairer C, Haenszel W, Stolley P, Lehman HF, Levine R, et al.** Cigarette smoking and invasive cervical cancer. *JAMA* 1986;255:3265–9.

52. **McKinlay SM, Bifano NL, McKinlay JB.** Smoking and age at menopause in women. *Ann Intern Med* 1985;103:350–6.

53. **Klatsky AL, Armstrong MA, Friedman GD.** Risk of cardiovascular mortality in alcohol drinkers, ex-drinkers and nondrinkers. *Am J Cardiol* 1990;66:1237–42.

54. **Willett WC, Stampfer MJ, Colditz GA, Rosner BA, Hennekens CH, Speizer FE.** Moderate alcohol consumption and the risk of breast cancer. *N Engl J Med* 1987;316:1174–80.

55. **Cronholm T, Rudquist V.** Effects of ethanol metabolism on oxidoreduction at C-17 in vivo in the rat. *Biochem Biophys Acta* 1982;711:159–65.

56. **Elwood JM, Cole PH, Rothman KJ, Kaplan SD.** Epidemiology of endometrial cancer. *J Natl Cancer Inst* 1977;59:1055–60.

57. **Harlow BL, Cramer DW, Bell DA, Welch WR.** Perineal exposure to talc and ovarian cancer risk. *Obstet Gynecol* 1992;80:19–26.

58. **Wingo PA, Tong T, Bolden S.** Cancer statistics 1995. *CA Cancer J Clin* 1995;45:8–30.

59. **Ries LAG, Miller BA, Hankey BF, Kosary CL, Harras A, Edwards BK.** *SEER Cancer Statistics Review, 1973-1991, Tables and Graphs.* Bethesda, MD: Surveillance Program, Division of Cancer Prevention and Control, National Cancer Institute, NIH Pub. No. 94–2789, 1994.

60. **Velebil P, Wingo PA, Xia A, Wilcox LS, Peterson HB.** Rate of hospitalization for gynecologic disorders among reproductive-age women in the United States. *Obstet Gynecol* 1995; 86:764–9.

61. **Goldner TE, Lawson HW, Xia Z, Atrash HK.** Surveillance for ectopic pregnancy—United States 1970–1989. *MMWR* 1993;42:73–85.

BASIC SCIENCE

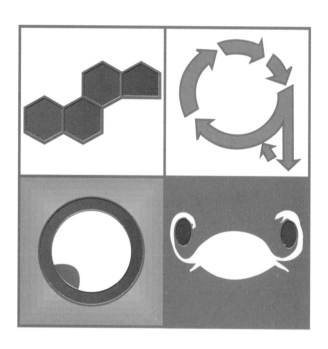

5 Anatomy and Embryology

Jean R. Anderson
Rene Genadry

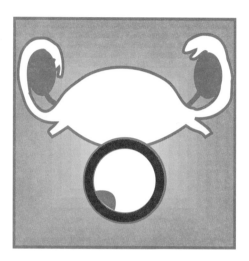

Nothing is more fundamental to the knowledge base of the practicing gynecologist than an understanding of the anatomy of the female pelvis. Although the basic facts of anatomy and their relevance to gynecologic practice do not change with time, our understanding of specific anatomic relationships and the development of new clinical and surgical correlations continue to evolve.

The anatomy of the fundamental supporting structures of the pelvis and the genital, urinary, and gastrointestinal viscera are presented in this chapter. Because significant variation has developed in the names of many common anatomic structures, the terms used here reflect current standard nomenclature according to the *Nomina Anatomica* (1); however, other commonly accepted terms are included in parentheses.

Pelvic Structure

Bony Pelvis

The skeleton of the pelvis is formed by the sacrum and coccyx and the paired hip bones (coxal, innominate), which fuse anteriorly to form the symphysis pubis. Figure 5.1 illustrates the bony pelvis, as well as its ligaments and foramina.

Sacrum and Coccyx

The sacrum and coccyx are an extension of the vertebral column resulting from the five fused sacral vertebrae and the four fused coccygeal vertebrae joined by a symphyseal articulation (sacrococcygeal joint), which allows some movement.

The essential features of the sacrum and coccyx are as follows:

1. *Sacral promontory*—the most prominent and anterior projection of the sacrum, this is an important landmark during laparoscopic insertion. It is located at the level of bifurcation of the common iliac arteries.

2. *Four paired anterior and posterior sacral foramina*—exit sites for the anterior and posterior rami of the corresponding sacral nerves; anterior foramina are also traversed by the lateral sacral vessels.

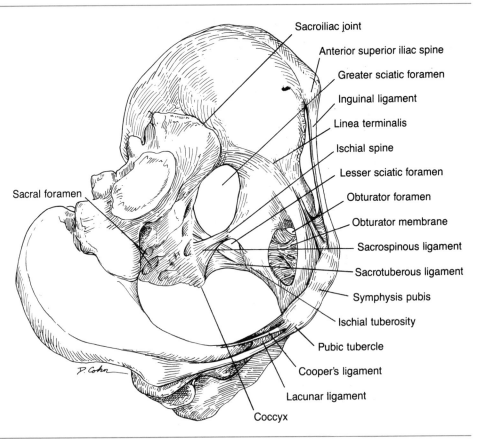

Figure 5.1   **The female pelvis.** The pelvic bones (the innominate bone, sacrum, and coccyx) and their joints, ligaments, and foramina.

3. *Sacral hiatus*—results from incomplete fusion of the posterior lamina of the fifth sacral vertebra, offering access to the sacral canal, which is clinically important for caudal anesthesia.

Laterally, the alae ("wings") of the sacrum offer auricular surfaces that articulate with the hip bones to form synovial sacroiliac joints.

Os Coxae

The paired *os coxae* or hip bones have three components: the ilium, the ischium, and the pubis. These components meet to form the acetabulum, a cup-shaped cavity that accommodates the femoral head.

Ilium

1. *Iliac crest*—provides attachments to the iliac fascia, abdominal muscles, and fascia lata.

2. *Anterior superior and inferior spine*—superior spine provides the point of fixation of the inguinal ligament.

3. *Posterior superior and inferior spine*—superior spine is the point of attachment for the sacrotuberous ligament and the posterior sacral iliac ligament.

4. *Arcuate line*—marks the pelvic brim and lies between the first two segments of the sacrum.

5. *Iliopectineal eminence (linea terminalis)*—the line of junction of the ilium and the pubis.

6. *Iliac fossa*—the smooth anterior concavity of the ilium, covered by the iliacus muscle.

Ischium

1. *Ischial spine*—delineates the greater and lesser sciatic notch above and below it. It is the point of fixation for the sacrospinous ligament; the ischial spine represents an important landmark in the performance of pudendal nerve block and sacrospinous ligament vaginal suspension; vaginal palpation during labor allows detection of progressive fetal descent.

2. *Ischial ramus*—joins that of the pubis to encircle the obturator foramen; provides the attachment for the inferior fascia of the urogenital diaphragm and the perineal musculofascial attachments.

3. *Ischial tuberosity*—the rounded bony prominence upon which the body rests in the sitting position.

Pubis

1. *Body*—formed by the midline fusion of the superior and inferior pubic rami.

2. *Symphysis pubis*—a fibrocartilaginous symphyseal joint where the bodies of the pubis meet in the midline; allows for some resilience and flexibility, which is critical during parturition.

3. *Superior and inferior pubic rami*—join the ischial rami to encircle the obturator foramen; provide the origin for the muscles of the thigh and leg; provide the attachment for the inferior layer of the urogenital diaphragm.

4. *Pubic tubercle*—a lateral projection from the superior pubic ramus, to which the inguinal ligament, rectus abdominis, and pyramidalis attach.

Pelvic Bone Articulations   The pelvic bones are joined by four articulations:

1. *Two cartilaginous symphyseal joints—the sacrococcygeal joint and the symphysis pubis*—these joints are surrounded by strong ligaments anteriorly and posteriorly, which are responsive to the effect of relaxin and facilitate parturition.

2. *Two synovial joints—sacroiliac joints*—these are stabilized by the sacroiliac ligaments, the iliolumbar ligament, the lateral lumbosacral ligament, the sacrotuberous ligament, and the sacrospinous ligament.

The pelvis is divided into the *greater* and *lesser pelvis* by an oblique plane passing through the sacral promontory, the *linea terminalis (arcuate line of the ilium)*, the pectineal line of the pubis, the pubic crest, and the upper margin of the symphysis pubis. This plane lies at the level of the superior pelvic aperture (pelvic inlet) or pelvic brim. The inferior pelvic aperture or pelvic outlet is irregularly bound by the tip of the coccyx, the symphysis pubis, and the ischial tuberosities. The dimensions of the superior and inferior pelvic apertures have important obstetric implications.

Ligaments and Foramina

In addition to the ligaments that hold together and stabilize the bony pelvis, two other ligaments—the inguinal ligament and Cooper's ligament—are of importance to the gynecologic surgeon.

Inguinal Ligament

The inguinal ligament is important surgically in the repair of inguinal hernia. The inguinal ligament is:

1. Formed by the lower border of the aponeurosis of the external oblique muscle folded back upon itself.

2. Fused laterally to the iliacus fascia and inferiorly to the fascia lata.

3. Flattens medially into the lacunar ligament, which forms the medial border of the femoral ring.

Cooper's Ligament

Cooper's ligament is used frequently in bladder suspension procedures. Cooper's ligament is:

1. A strong ridge of fibrous tissue extending along the pectineal line—also known as the pectineal ligament.

2. Merged laterally with the iliopectineal ligament and medially with the lacunar ligament.

The bony pelvis and its ligaments delineate three important foramina that allow the passage of the various muscles, nerves, and vessels to the lower extremity.

Greater Sciatic Foramen

The greater sciatic foramen transmits the following structures: the piriformis muscle, the superior gluteal nerves and vessels, the sciatic nerve along with the nerves of the quadratus femoris, the inferior gluteal nerves and vessels, the posterior cutaneous nerve of the thigh, the nerves of the obturator internus, and the internal pudendal nerves and vessels.

Lesser Sciatic Foramen

The lesser sciatic foramen transmits the tendon of the obturator internus to its insertion on the greater trochanter of the femur. The nerve of the obturator internus and the pudendal vessels and nerves reenter the pelvis through it.

Obturator Foramen

The obturator foramen transmits the obturator nerves and vessels.

Muscles

The muscles of the pelvis include those of the lateral wall and those of the pelvic floor (Fig. 5.2; Table 5.1).

Muscles of the Lateral Wall

The muscles of the lateral pelvic wall pass into the gluteal region to assist in thigh rotation and adduction. They include the pyriformis, the obturator internus, and the iliopsoas.

Muscles of the Pelvic Floor	### Pelvic Diaphragm

Pelvic Diaphragm

The pelvic diaphragm is a funnel-shaped fibromuscular partition that forms the primary supporting structure for the pelvic contents (Fig. 5.3). It is composed of the levator ani and the coccygeus muscles, along with their superior and inferior fasciae (Table 5.1). It forms the ceiling of the ischiorectal fossa.

Levator Ani

The levator ani is composed of the pubococcygeus (including the pubovaginalis, puborectalis, puborectalis, and iliococcygeus.) It is a broad, curved sheet of muscle stretching from the pubis anteriorly and the coccyx posteriorly and from one side of the pelvis to the other. It is perforated by the urethra, vagina, and anal canal. Its origin is from the tendinous arch extending from the body of the pubis to the ischial spine. It is inserted into the central tendon of the perineum, the wall of the anal canal, the anococcygeal ligament, the coccyx, and the vaginal wall.

The levator ani assists the anterior abdominal wall muscles in containing the abdominal and pelvic contents. It supports the posterior wall of the vagina, facilitates defecation, and aids in fecal continence. During parturition, the levator ani supports the fetal head during cervical dilation. The levator ani is innervated by S3–4, the inferior rectal nerve.

Urogenital Diaphragm

The muscles of the urogenital diaphragm reinforce the pelvic diaphragm anteriorly and are intimately related to the vagina and the urethra. They are enclosed between the inferior and superior fascia of the urogenital diaphragm. The muscles include the deep transverse perineal and sphincter urethrae (Table 5.1).

Blood Vessels

The pelvic blood vessels supply not only genital structures but also the following: lower urinary and gastrointestinal tracts; muscles of the abdominal wall, pelvic floor and perineum, buttocks, and upper thighs; fasciae, other connective tissue, and bones; and skin and other superficial structures. Classically, vessels supplying organs are known as visceral vessels and those supplying supporting structures are called parietal vessels.

The Major Blood Vessels

The course of the major vessels supplying the pelvis is illustrated in Figure 5.4; their origin, course, branches, and venous drainage presented in Table 5.2. In general, the venous system draining the pelvis closely follows the arterial supply and is named accordingly. Not infrequently, a vein draining a particular area may form a plexus with multiple channels. Venous systems, which are paired, mirror each other in their drainage patterns, with the notable exception of the ovarian veins. Unusual features of venous drainage are also listed in Table 5.2.

General Principles of Pelvic Blood Vessel Anatomy

"Control of the blood supply" and "meticulous hemostasis" are two of the most common exhortations to young surgeons. In developing familiarity with the pattern of blood flow in the pelvis, several unique characteristics of this vasculature should be understood and may have implications for surgical practice:

1. *The pelvic vessels play an important role in pelvic support.* They provide condensations of endopelvic fascia that act to reinforce the normal position of pelvic organs (2).

75

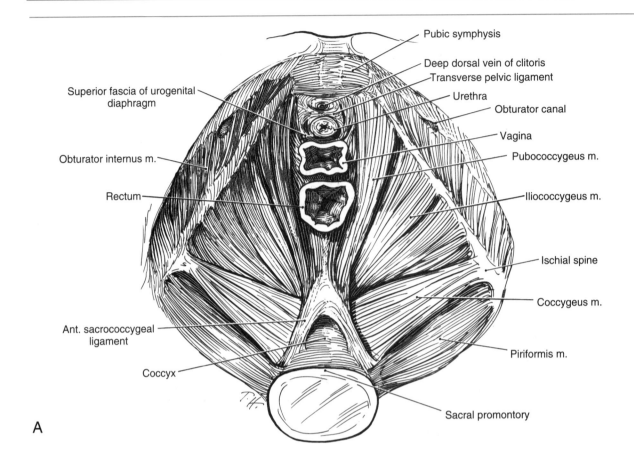

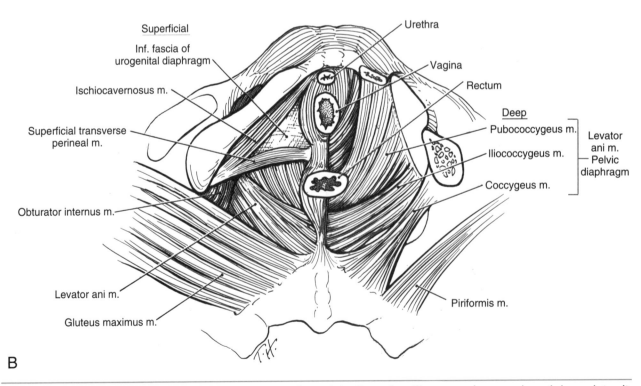

Figure 5.2   The pelvic diaphragm. *A,* A view into the pelvic floor that illustrates the muscles of the pelvic diaphragm and their attachments to the bony pelvis. *B,* A view from outside the pelvic diaphragm illustrating the divisions of the levator ani muscles. *C,* A lateral, sagittal view of the pelvic diaphragm.

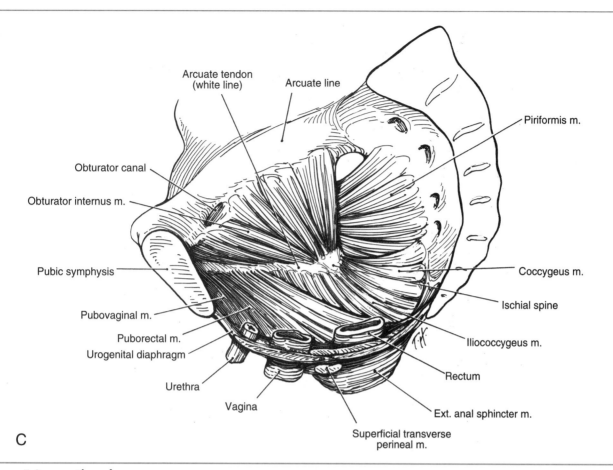

Arcuate tendon (white line)

Arcuate line

Piriformis m.

Obturator canal

Obturator internus m.

Pubic symphysis

Coccygeus m.

Ischial spine

Pubovaginal m.

Puborectal m.

Urogenital diaphragm

Iliococcygeus m.

Urethra

Rectum

Vagina

Ext. anal sphincter m.

Superficial transverse perineal m.

C

Figure 5.2—*continued*

2. *There is significant anatomic variation between individuals in the branching pattern of the internal iliac vessels.* There is no constant order in which branches divide from the parent vessel; some branches may arise as common trunks or may spring from other branches rather than from the internal iliac. Occasionally, a branch may arise from another vessel entirely (e.g., the obturator artery may arise from the external iliac or inferior epigastric artery). This variation may also be found in the branches of other major vessels; the ovarian arteries have been reported to arise from the renal arteries or as a common trunk from the front of the aorta on occasion. Patterns of blood flow may be asymmetrical from side to side, and structures supplied by anastomoses of different vessels may show variation from person to person in proportion of vascular support provided by the vessels involved. The pelvic surgeon must be prepared for deviations from "textbook" vascular patterns.

3. *The pelvic vasculature is a high-volume, high-flow system with enormous expansive capabilities throughout reproductive life.* Blood flow through the uterine arteries increases to approximately 500 ml/min in late pregnancy. In nonpregnant women, certain conditions such as uterine fibroids or malignant neoplasms may be associated with neovascularization and hypertrophy of existing vessels and a corresponding increase in pelvic blood flow. Understanding of the volume and flow characteristics of the pelvic vasculature in different clinical situations will enable the surgeon to anticipate problems and take appropriate preoperative and intraoperative measures (including blood and blood product availability) to prevent or manage hemorrhage.

Table 5.1   Muscles of the Pelvic Floor

	Origin	Insertion	Action	Innervation
Lateral Pelvic Wall				
Piriformis	Anterior aspect of S2–S4 and sacrotuberous ligament	Greater trochanter of the femur	Lateral rotation, abduction of thigh in flexion; holds head of femur in acetabulum	S1-S2; forms a muscular bed for the sacral plexus
Obturator internus	Superior and inferior pubic rami	Greater trochanter of the femur	Lateral rotation of thigh in flexion; assists in holding head of femur in acetabulum	(L5, S1) Obturator internus nerve
Iliopsoas	Psoas from the lateral margin of the lumbar vertebrae; iliacus from the iliac fossa	Lesser trochanter of the femur	Flexes thigh and stabilizes trunk on thigh; flexes vertebral column or bends it unilaterally	(L1–3) Psoas-ventral rami of lumbar nerve (L2–L3) Iliacus-femoral nerve contains the lumbar plexus within its muscle body
Pelvic Floor				
Pelvic Diaphragm				
Levator Ani Pubococcygeus Pubovaginalis Puborectalis	From the tendinous arch, extending from the body of the pubis to the ischial spine	Central tendon of the perineum; wall of the anal canal; anococcygeal ligament; coccyx; vaginal wall	Assists the anterior abdominal wall muscles in containing the abdominal and pelvic contents; supports the posterior wall of the vagina; facilitates defecation; aids in fecal continence; and during parturition, it supports the fetal head during cervical dialation	S3–S4; the inferior rectal nerve.
Coccygeus	Ischial spine and sacrospinous ligament	Lateral margin of the fifth sacral vertebra and coccyx	Supports the coccyx and pulls it anteriorly	S4–S5
Urogenital Diaphragm				
Deep transverse perineal	Medial aspect of the ischiopubic rami	Lower part of the vaginal wall; anterior fibers blend with those of the sphincter urethrae	Steadies the central perineal tendon	S2–S4; perineal nerve
Sphincter urethrae	Medial aspect of the ischiopubic rami	Urethra and vagina	Compresses the urethra	S2–S4; perineal nerve

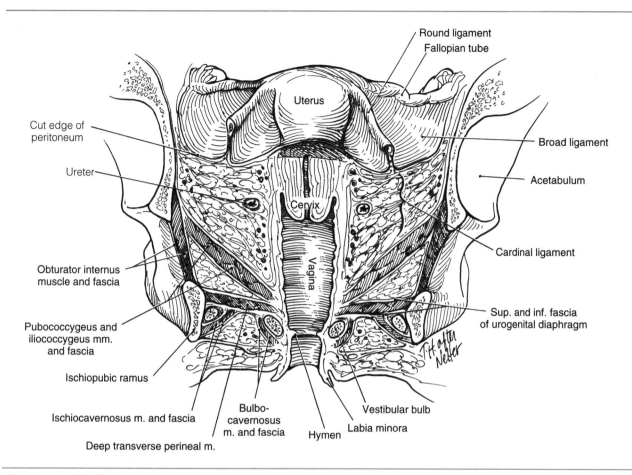

Figure 5.3   The ligaments and fascial support of the pelvic viscera.

4. *The pelvic vasculature is supplied with an extensive network of collateral connections* (Fig. 5.5) that provides rich anastomotic communication between different major vessel systems. This degree of redundancy is important to ensure adequate supply of oxygen and nutrients in the event of major trauma or other vascular compromise. Hypogastric artery ligation continues to be used as a strategy for management of massive pelvic hemorrhage when other measures have failed. Bilateral hypogastric artery ligation dramatically reduces pulse pressure in the pelvis, converting flow characteristics from that of an arterial system to a venous system and allowing use of collateral channels of circulation to continue blood supply to pelvic structures. The significance of collateral blood flow is demonstrated by reports of successful pregnancies occurring after bilateral ligation of both hypogastric and ovarian arteries (3). Table 5.3 lists the collateral channels of circulation in the pelvis.

Lymphatics

The pelvic lymph nodes are generally arranged in groups or chains and follow the course of the larger pelvic vessels, for which they are usually named. Smaller nodes that lie close to the visceral structures are usually named for those organs. Lymph nodes in the pelvis receive afferent lymphatic vessels from pelvic and perineal visceral and parietal structures and send efferent lymphatics to more proximal nodal groups. The number of lymph nodes and their exact location is variable; however, certain nodes tend to be relatively constant:

1. Obturator node in the obturator foramen, close to the obturator vessels and nerve

2. Nodes at the junction of the internal and external iliac veins

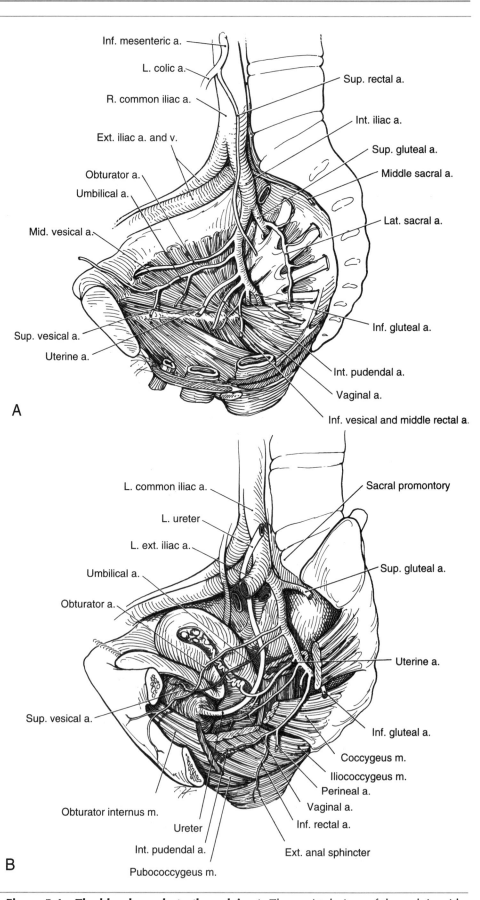

Figure 5.4   The blood supply to the pelvis. *A,* The sagittal view of the pelvis without the viscera. *B,* The blood supply to one pelvic viscera.

Table 5.2   The Major Blood Vessels of the Pelvis

Artery	Origin	Course	Branches	Venous Drainage
Ovarian	Arises from ventral surface of aorta just below the origin of the renal vessels	Crosses over common iliac vessels; in proximity to ureter over much of its course, crosses over ureter while superficial to the psoas muscle and runs just lateral to the ureter when entering the pelvis as part of the infundibulopelvic ligament	To ovaries, fallopian tubes, broad ligament; often small branches to ureter	Right side drains into the inferior vena cava; left drains into the left renal vein
Inferior mesenteric artery (IMA)	Unpaired left-sided retroperitoneal artery arising from the aorta 2–5 cm proximal to its bifurcation	IMA and its branches pass over the left psoas muscle and common iliac vessels; IMA courses anterior to the ureter and ovarian vessels above the pelvic brim	1. *Left colic*—originates above pelvic brim; supplies left transverse colon, splenic flexure, descending colon 2. *Sigmoid*—several branches; supply sigmoid colon 3. *Superior rectal (hemorrhoidal)*—divides into two terminal branches to supply rectum	Inferior mesenteric vein empties into the splenic vein
Common iliac artery	Terminal division of the aorta at fourth lumbar vertebra	Oblique and lateral course, approximately 5 cm in length	1. External iliac 2. Internal iliac	Lie posterior and slightly medial to arteries; drains into inferior vena cava
External iliac femoral artery	Lateral bifurcation of common iliac, begins opposite the lumbo-sacral joint	Along the medial border of the psoas muscle and lateral pelvic side wall; becomes femoral artery after passing under the inguinal ligament to supply lower extremity	1. *Superficial epigastric*—supplies skin and subcutaneous tissue of lower anterior abdominal wall 2. *External pudendal*—supplies skin and subcutanious tissue of mons pubis and anterior vulva 3. *Superficial circumflex iliac*—supplies skin/subcutaneous tissues of the flank 4. *Inferior epigastric*—supplies musculo-fascial layer of lower anterior abdominal wall 5. *Deep circumflex iliac*—supplies musculofascial layer of lower abdominal wall	Lie posterior and then medial to the artery as it enters the anterior thigh; drain into common iliac veins

Table 5.2—continued

Artery	Origin	Course	Branches	Venous Drainage
Internal iliac hypogastric artery	Medial bifurcation of common iliac artery, begins opposite the lumbosacral joint. The major blood supply to the pelvis.	Descends sharply into the pelvis; divides into an anterior and posterior division 3–4 cm after origin	*Posterior division:* 1. *Iliolumbar*—anastomoses with lumbar and deep circumflex iliac arteries; helps supply lower abdominal wall, iliac fossa 2. *Lateral sacral*—supplies contents of sacral canal, piriformis muscle 3. *Superior gluteal*—supplies gluteal muscles *Anterior division:* 1. *Obturator*—supplies iliac fossa, posterior pubis, obturator internus muscle 2. *Internal pudendal* 3. *Umbilical*—remnant of fetal umbilical artery; after giving off branches, as the medial umbilical ligament 4. *Superior, middle, inferior vesical*—supply bladder and one or more branches to the ureter 5. *Middle rectal (hemorrhoidal)*—supplies rectum, branches to mid vagina 6. *Uterine*—supplies uterine corpus and cervix, with branches to upper vagina, tube, round ligament, and ovary 7. *Vaginal*—supplies vagina 8. *Inferior gluteal*—supplies gluteal muscles, muscles of posterior thigh	Deep to arteries, from complex plexus and drain into common iliac veins

Table 5.2—*continued*

Artery	Origin	Course	Branches	Venous Drainage
Internal pudendal artery	Internal iliac artery; it provides the major blood supply to the perineum	Leaves the pelvis through the greater sciatic foramen, courses around the ischial spine, and enters the ischio-rectal fossa through the lesser sciatic foramen. In its path to the perineum, lies with the pudendal nerve within Alcock's canal, a fascial tunnel over the obturator internus muscle	1. *Inferior rectal (hemorrhoids)*—supplies anal canal, external anal sphincter, perianal skin, with branches to levator ani 2. *Perineal*—supplies perineal skin, muscles of superficial perineal compartment (bulbocavernosus, ischiocavernosus, superficial transverse perineal) 3. *Clitoral*—supplies clitoris, vestibular bulb, Bartholin gland, and urethra	Drain into internal iliac veins
Middle sacral artery	Midline unpaired vessel arising from posterior terminal aorta	Courses over lower lumbar vertebrae, sacrum, and coccyx Supplies bony and muscular structures of posterior pelvic wall Paired middle sacral veins usually drain into left common iliac vein		
Lumbar arteries	Segmental branches arising at each lumbar level from posterior aorta	Supplies abdominal wall muscu-lature (external/internal oblique, transversus abdominis) veins into inferior vena cava		

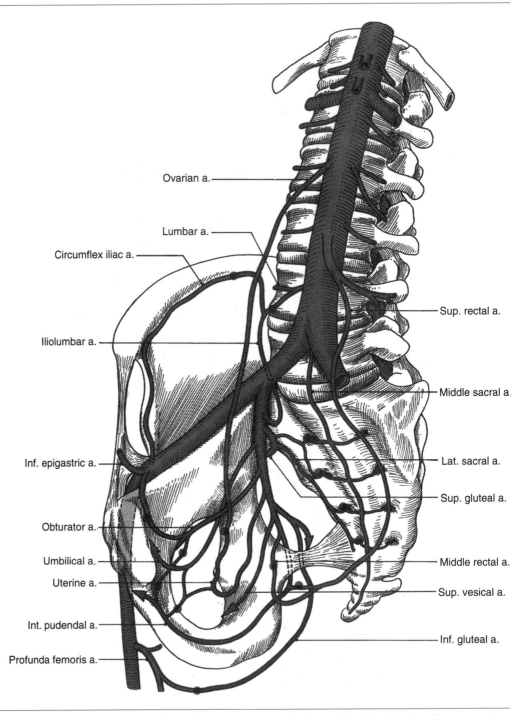

Figure 5.5   The collateral blood vessels of the pelvis. Modified with permission from **Kamina P.** *Anatomie Gynécologique et Obstétricale.* Paris: Maloine Sa Éditeur, 1984:125.

3. Ureteral node in the broad ligament near the cervix, where the uterine artery crosses the ureter

4. Cloquet's or Rosenmüller's node—the highest of the deep inguinal nodes that lies within the opening of the femoral canal.

Figure 5.6 illustrates the pelvic lymphatic system. Table 5.4 outlines the major lymphatic chains of relevance to the pelvis and their primary afferent connections from major pelvic

Table 5.3   Collateral Arterial Circulation of the Pelvis

Primary Artery	*Collateral Arteries*
Aorta	
Ovarian artery	Uterine artery
Superior rectal artery (IMA)	Middle rectal artery
	Inferior rectal artery (internal pudendal)
Lumbar arteries	Iliolumbar artery
Vertebral arteries	Iliolumbar artery
Middle sacral artery	Lateral sacral artery
External Iliac	
Deep iliac circumflex artery	Iliolumbar artery
	Superior gluteal artery
Inferior epigastric artery	Obturator artery
Femoral	
Medial femoral circumflex artery	Obturator artery
	Inferior gluteal artery
Lateral femoral circumflex artery	Superior gluteal artery
	Iliolumbar artery

and perineal structures. There are extensive interconnections between lymph vessels and nodes; more than one lymphatic pathway is usually available for drainage of each pelvic site. Bilateral and crossed extension of lymphatic flow may occur, and entire groups of nodes may be bypassed to reach more proximal chains.

The natural history of most genital tract malignancies directly reflects the lymphatic drainage of those structures, although the various interconnections, different lymphatic paths, and individual variability make the spread of malignancy somewhat unpredictable. Regional lymph node metastasis is one of the most important factors in formulation of treatment plans and prediction of eventual outcome.

Nerves

The pelvis is innervated by both the autonomic and somatic nervous systems. The autonomic nerves include both *sympathetic* (adrenergic) and *parasympathetic* (cholinergic) fibers and provide the primary innervation for genital, urinary, and gastrointestinal visceral structures and blood vessels.

Somatic Innervation

The *lumbosacral plexus* (Fig. 5.7) and its branches provide motor and sensory somatic innervation to the lower abdominal wall, the pelvic and urogenital diaphragms, the perineum, and the hip and lower extremity. The nerves originating from the muscles, the lumbosacral trunk, the anterior divisions of the upper four sacral nerves (*sacral plexus*), and the anterior division of the coccygeal nerve and fibers from the fourth and fifth sacral nerves (*coccygeal plexus*) are found on the anterior surface of the piriformis muscle and lateral to the coccyx, respectively, deep in the posterior pelvis. Table 5.5 lists each major branch by spinal segment and structures innervated. In addition to these branches, the lumbosacral plexus includes nerves that innervate muscles of the lateral pelvic wall (obturator internus, piriformis), posterior hip muscles, and the pelvic diaphragm. A visceral component, the pelvic splanchnic nerve, is also included.

Nerves supplying the cutaneous aspects of the anterior, medial, and lateral lower extremities, as well as the deep muscles of the anterior thigh, primarily leave the pelvis by passing beneath the inguinal ligament. Nerves supporting the posterior cutaneous and deep structures of the hip, thigh, and leg lie deep in the pelvis and should not be vulnerable to injury during pelvic surgery. The obturator nerve travels along the lateral pelvic wall to pass through the obturator foramen into the upper thigh, and it may be encountered in more radical dissections involving the lateral pelvic wall and in paravaginal repairs.

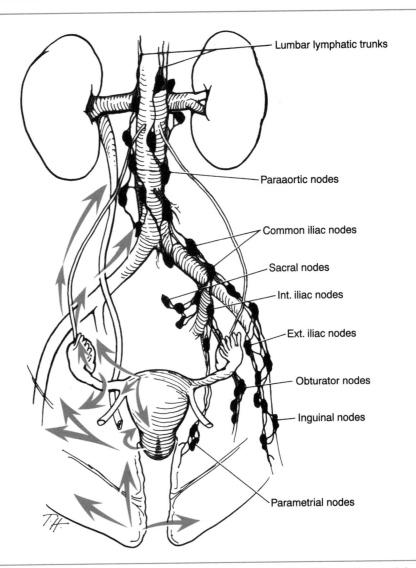

Lumbar lymphatic trunks

Paraaortic nodes

Common iliac nodes

Sacral nodes

Int. iliac nodes

Ext. iliac nodes

Obturator nodes

Inguinal nodes

Parametrial nodes

Figure 5.6 The lymphatic drainage of the female pelvis. The vulva and lower vagina drain to the superficial and deep inguinal nodes, sometimes directly to the iliac nodes (along the dorsal vein of the clitoris) and to the other side. The cervix and upper vagina drain laterally to the parametrial, obturator, and external iliac nodes and posteriorly along the uterosacral ligaments to the sacral nodes. Drainage from these primary lymph node groups is upward along the infundibulopelvic ligament, similarly to drainage of the ovary and fallopian tubes to the para-aortic nodes. The lower uterine body drains in the same manner as the cervix. Rarely, drainage occurs along the round ligament to the inguinal nodes.

The pudendal nerve crosses over the piriformis to travel with the internal pudendal vessels into the ischiorectal fossa, where it divides into its three terminal branches to provide the primary innervation to the perineum. Other nerves contribute to the cutaneous innervation of the perineum:

1. The *anterior labial nerve branches of the ilioinguinal nerve*—these nerves emerge from within the inguinal canal and through the superficial inguinal ring to the mons and upper labia majora.

2. The *genital branch of the genitofemoral nerve*—this branch enters the inguinal canal with the round ligament and passes through the superficial inguinal ring to the anterior vulva.

Table 5.4   Primary Lymph Node Groups Providing Drainage to Genital Structures

Nodes	Primary Afferent Connections
Aortic/para-aortic	Ovary, fallopian tube, uterine corpus (upper); drainage from common iliac nodes
Common iliac	Drainage from external and internal iliac nodes
External iliac	Upper vagina, cervix, uterine corpus (upper); drainage from inguinal nodes
Internal iliac Lateral sacral Superior gluteal Inferior gluteal Obturator Vesical Rectal Parauterine	Upper vagina, cervix, uterine corpus (lower)
Inguinal Superficial Deep	Vulva, lower vagina; (rare: uterus, tube, ovary)

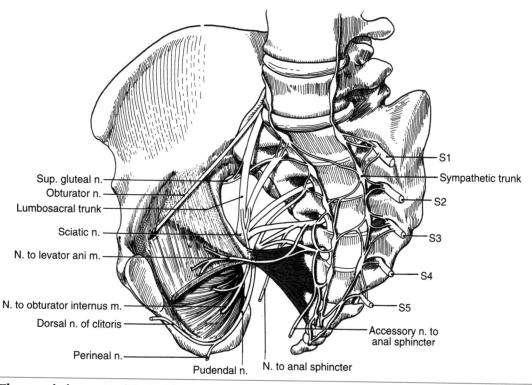

Figure 5.7   The sacral plexus. Modified with permission from **Kamina P.** *Anatomie Gynécologique et Obstétricale.* Paris: Maloine Sa Éditeur, 1984:90.

3. The *perineal branches of the posterior femoral cutaneous nerve*—after leaving the pelvis through the greater sciatic foramen, these branches run in front of the ischial tuberosity to the lateral perineum and labia majora.

4. *Perforating cutaneous branches of the second and third sacral nerves*—these branches perforate the sacrotuberous ligament to supply the buttocks and contiguous perineum.

Table 5.5   Lumbosacral Plexus

Nerve	Spinal Segment	Innervation
Iliohypogastric	T12, L1	Sensory—skin near iliac crest, just above symphysis pubis
Ilioinguinal	L1	Sensory—upper medial thigh, mons, labia majora
Lateral femoral cutaneous	L2, L3,	Sensory—lateral thigh to level of knee
Femoral	L2, L3, L4	Sensory—anterior and medial thigh, medial leg and foot, hip and knee joints Motor—iliacus, anterior thigh muscles
Genitofemoral	L1, L2	Sensory—anterior vulva (genital branch) middle/upper anterior thigh (femoral branch)
Obturator	L2, L3, L4	Sensory—medial thigh and leg, hip and knee joints Motor—adductor muscles of thigh
Superior gluteal	L4, L5, S1	Motor—gluteal muscles
Inferior gluteal	L4, L5, S1, S2	Motor—gluteal muscles
Posterior femoral cutaneous	S2, 3	Sensory—vulva, perineum
Sciatic	L4, L5, S1, S2, S3	Sensory—much of leg, foot, lower extremity joints Motor—posterior thigh muscle, leg and foot muscles
Pudendal	S2, S3, S4	Sensory—perianal skin, vulva and perineum, clitoris, urethra, vaginal vestibule Motor—external anal sphincter, perineal muscles, urogenital diaphragm

5. The *anococcygeal nerves*—these nerves arise from S4–5 and also perforate the sacrotuberous ligament to supply the skin overlying the coccyx.

Autonomic Innervation

Functionally, the innervation of the pelvic viscera may be divided into an afferent or sensory component and an efferent component; in reality, however, afferent and efferent fibers are closely associated in a complex interlacing network and cannot be separated anatomically.

Efferent Innervation

Efferent fibers of the autonomic nervous system, unlike motor fibers in the somatic system, involve one synapse outside the central nervous system, with two neurons required to carry each impulse. In the *sympathetic (thoracolumbar) division*, this synapse is generally at some distance from the organ being innervated; on the other hand, the synapse is on or near the organ of innervation in the *parasympathetic (craniosacral) division*.

Axons from preganglionic neurons emerge from the spinal cord to make contact with peripheral neurons arranged in aggregates known as autonomic ganglia. Some of these ganglia, along with interconnecting nerve fibers, form a pair of longitudinal cords called the *sympathetic trunks*. Located lateral to the spinal column from the base of the cranium to the coccyx, the sympathetic trunks lie along the medial border of the psoas muscle from T12 to the sacral prominence and then pass behind the common iliac vessels to continue into the pelvis on the anterior surface of the sacrum. On the anterolateral surface of the aorta, the *aortic plexus* forms a lacy network of nerve fibers with interspersed ganglia. Rami arising from or traversing the sympathetic trunks join this plexus and its subsidiaries.

The ovaries and part of the fallopian tubes and broad ligament are innervated by the *ovarian plexus,* a network of nerve fibers accompanying the ovarian vessels and derived from the aortic and renal plexuses. The *inferior mesenteric plexus* is a subsidiary of the *celiac plexus* and *aortic plexus* and is located along the inferior mesenteric artery and its branches, providing innervation to the left colon, sigmoid, and rectum.

The *superior hypogastric plexus (presacral nerve)* (Fig. 5.8) is the continuation of the aortic plexus beneath the peritoneum in front of the terminal aorta, the fifth lumbar vertebra, and the sacral promontory, medial to the ureters. Embedded in loose areolar tissue, the plexus overlies the middle sacral vessels and is usually composed of two or three incompletely fused trunks. It contains preganglionic fibers from lumbar nerves, postganglionic fibers from higher sympathetic ganglia and from the sacral sympathetic trunks, and visceral afferent fibers.

Just below the sacral promontory, the superior hypogastric plexus divides into two loosely arranged nerve trunks, the *hypogastric nerves.* These nerves course inferiorly and laterally to connect with the *inferior hypogastric plexuses (pelvic plexuses)* (Fig. 5.8), which are a dense network of nerves and ganglia that lie along the lateral pelvic sidewall overlying branches of the internal iliac vessels.

The inferior hypogastric plexus includes efferent sympathetic fibers, afferent (sensory) fibers, and parasympathetic fibers arising from the pelvic splanchnic nerves (S2–4) (nervi erigentes).

Figure 5.8   The presacral nerves.

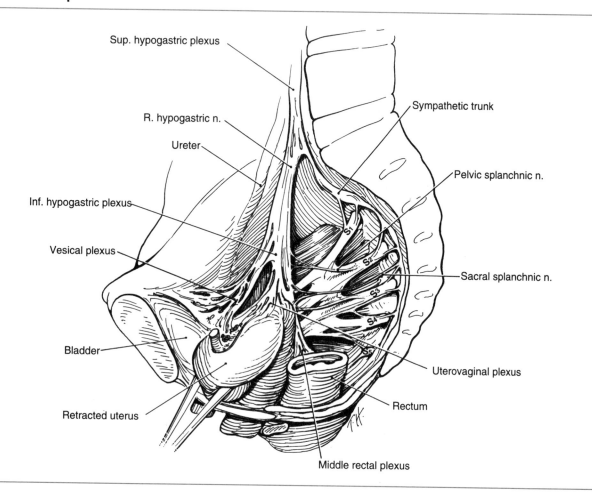

This paired plexus is the final common pathway of the pelvic visceral nervous system and is divided into three portions, representing distribution of innervation to the viscera:

1. *Vesical plexus*
   - innervation: bladder and urethra
   - course: along vesical vessels

2. *Middle rectal plexus (hemorrhoidal)*
   - innervation: rectum
   - course: along middle rectal vessels

3. *Uterovaginal plexus (Frankenhauser's ganglion)*
   - innervation: uterus, vagina, clitoris, vestibular bulbs
   - course: along uterine vessels and through cardinal and uterosacral ligaments; sympathetic and sensory fibers derive from T10, L1; parasympathetic fibers derive from S2–4.

Afferent Innervation

Afferent fibers from the pelvic viscera and blood vessels traverse the same pathways to provide sensory input to the central nervous system. They are also involved in reflex arcs needed for bladder, bowel, and genital tract function. The afferent fibers reach the central nervous system to have their first synapse within posterior spinal nerve ganglia.

Presacral neurectomy, in which a segment of the superior hypogastric plexus is divided and resected in order to interrupt sensory fibers from the uterus and cervix, has been associated with relief of dysmenorrhea secondary to endometriosis in approximately 50–75% of cases in which it has been employed (4, 5). Because efferent fibers from the adnexa travel with the ovarian plexus, pain originating from the ovary or tube is not relieved by resection of the presacral nerve. Because this plexus also contains efferent sympathetic and parasympathetic nerve fibers intermixed with afferent fibers, disturbance in bowel or bladder function may result. An alternative surgical procedure advocated in recent years is resection of a portion of the uterosacral ligaments; because they contain numerous nerve fibers with more specific innervation to the uterus, it is postulated that bladder and rectal function is less vulnerable to compromise.

An anesthetic block of the pudendal nerve is performed most often for pain relief with uncomplicated vaginal deliveries but may also provide useful anesthesia for minor perineal surgical procedures. This nerve block may be accomplished transvaginally or through the perineum. A needle is inserted toward the ischial spine with the tip directed slightly posteriorly and through the sacrospinous ligament. As anesthetic agent is injected, frequent aspiration is required to avoid injection into the pudendal vessels, which travel with the nerve.

Pelvic Viscera

Embryologic Development

The female urinary and genital tracts are closely related not only anatomically but also embryologically. Both are derived largely from primitive mesoderm and endoderm, and there is evidence that the embryologic urinary system has an important inductive influence on the developing genital system. **Approximately 10% of infants are born with some abnormality of the genitourinary system and anomalies in one system are often mirrored by anomalies in another system** (6).

It is important for the practicing gynecologist to have a basic understanding of embryology, because developmental defects may play a significant role in the differential diagnosis of certain clinical presentations and have special implications in pelvic surgery (6–10).

The following presents the urinary system, internal reproductive organs, and the external genitalia separately in order of their initial appearance, although much of their development proceeds concurrently. The development of each of these three regions precedes synchronously at an early embryologic age (Table 5.6).

Urinary System

Kidneys, Renal Collecting System, Ureters   The kidneys, renal collecting system, and ureters derive from the longitudinal mass of mesoderm (known as the nephrogenic cord) found on each side of the primitive aorta. This process gives rise to three successive sets of increasingly advanced urinary structures, each developing more caudal to its predecessor.

The *pronephros* or "first kidney" is rudimentary and nonfunctional; it is succeeded by the "middle kidney" or *mesonephros,* which is believed to function briefly before regressing. Although the mesonephros is transitory as an excretory organ, its duct, the *mesonephric (wolffian) duct,* is of singular importance for the following reasons:

1. It grows caudally in the developing embryo to open, for the first time, an excretory channel into the primitive cloaca and the "outside world."

2. It serves as the starting point for development of the metanephros, which becomes the definitive kidney.

3. It ultimately differentiates into the sexual duct system in the male.

Table 5.6   Development of Genital and Urinary Tracts by Embryologic Age

Weeks of Gestation	Genital Development	Urinary Development
4–6	Urorectal septum	Pronephros
	Formation of cloacal folds, genital tubercle	Mesonephros/mesonephric duct
		Ureteric buds, metanephros
	Genital ridges	Exstrophy of mesonephric ducts and ureters into bladder wall
6–7	End of indifferent phase of genital development	Major, minor calyces form
	Development of primitive sex cords	Kidneys begin to ascend
	Formation of paramesonephric ducts	
	Labioscrotal swellings	
8–11	Distal paramesonephric ducts begin to fuse	Kidney becomes functional
	Formation of sinuvaginal bulbs	
12	Development of clitoris and vaginal vestibule	
20	Canalization of vaginal plate	
32		Renal collecting duct system complete

4. Although regressing in female fetuses, there is evidence that the mesonephric duct may have an inductive role in development of the paramesonephric or müllerian duct (7).

Development of the *metanephros* is initiated by the ureteric buds, which sprout from the distal mesonephric ducts; these buds extend cranially and penetrate the portion of the nephrogenic cord known as the *metanephric blastema*. The ureteric buds begin to branch sequentially, with each growing tip covered by metanephric blastema. The metanephric blastema ultimately form the renal functional units (the nephrons), whereas the ureteric buds become the collecting duct system of the kidneys (collecting tubules, minor and major calyces, renal pelvis) and the ureters. Although these primitive tissues differentiate along separate paths, they are interdependent on inductive influences from each other—neither can develop alone.

The kidneys initially lie in the pelvis but subsequently ascend to their permanent location, rotating almost 90° in the process as the more caudal part of the embryo in effect grows away from them. Their blood supply, which first arises as branches of the middle sacral and common iliac arteries, comes from progressively higher branches of the aorta until the definitive renal arteries form; previous vessels then regress.

Bladder and Urethra

The *cloaca* forms as the result of dilation of the opening to the fetal exterior. The cloaca subsequently partitioned by the mesenchymal urorectal septum into an anterior urogenital sinus and a posterior rectum. The bladder and urethra form from the most superior portion of the urogenital sinus, with surrounding mesenchyme contributing to their muscular and serosal layers. The remaining inferior urogenital sinus is known as the phallic or definitive urogenital sinus.

Concurrently, the distal mesonephric ducts and attached ureteric buds are incorporated into the posterior bladder wall in the area that will become the bladder trigone. As a result of the absorption process, the mesonephric duct ultimately opens independently into the urogenital sinus below the bladder neck.

The *allantois,* which is a vestigial diverticulum of the hindgut that extends into the umbilicus and is continuous with the bladder, loses its lumen and becomes the fibrous band known as the *urachus* or *median umbilical ligament.* In rare instances, the urachal lumen remains partially patent, with formation of urachal cysts, or completely patent, with the formation of a urinary fistula to the umbilicus.

Genital System

Although genetic sex is determined at fertilization, the early genital system is indistinguishable between the two sexes. This is known as the "indifferent stage" of genital development, during which both male and female fetuses have gonads with prominent cortical and medullary regions, dual sets of genital ducts, and external genitalia that appear similar. Clinically, **gender is not apparent until approximately the 12th week of embryonic life and depends on the elaboration of** *testis-determining factor (TDY)* **and, subsequently, androgens by the male gonad.** Female development has been called the basic developmental path of the human embryo, requiring not estrogen but the absence of testosterone.

Internal Reproductive Organs

The *primordial germ cells* migrate from the yolk sac via the mesentery of the hindgut to the posterior body wall mesenchyme at approximately the 10th thoracic level, which is the initial site of the future ovary (Figs. 5.9 and 5.10). Once the germ cells reach this area, they induce proliferation of cells in the adjacent mesonephros and celomic epithelium to form a pair of *genital ridges* medial to the mesonephros. The development of the gonad is absolutely de-

92

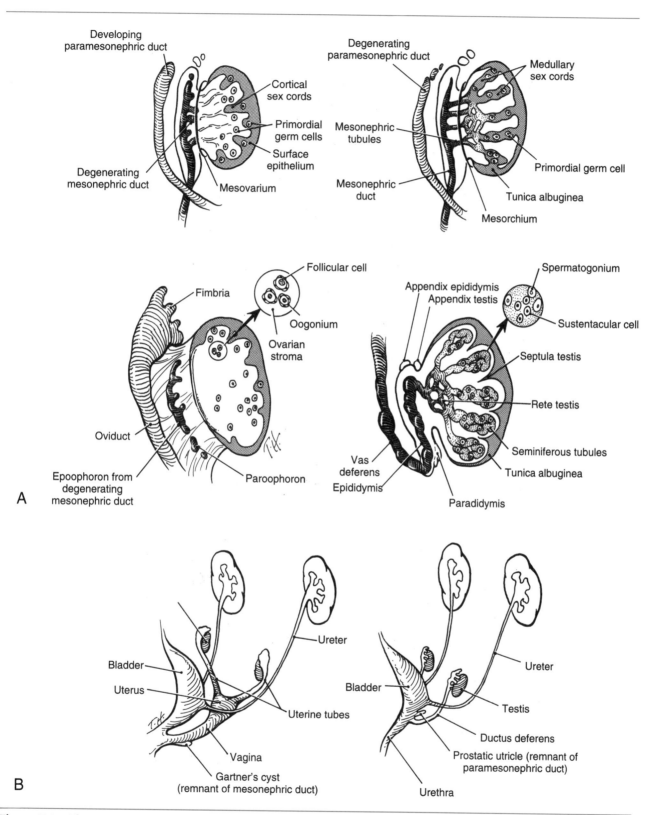

Figure 5.9   **The comparative changes of the female and male during early embryolic development.**

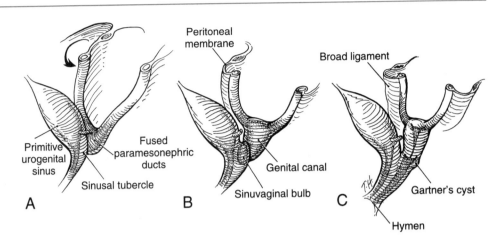

Figure 5.10   The embryonic development of the female genital tract. The formation of the uterus and vagina. *A,* The uterus and superior end of the vagina begin to form as the paramesonephric ducts fuse together near their attachment to the posterior wall of the primitive urogenital sinus. *B and C,* The ducts then zipper together in a superior direction between the third and fifth months. As the paramesonephric ducts are pulled away from the posterior body wall, they drag a fold of peritoneal membrane with them, forming the broad ligaments of the uterus. *A–C,* The inferior end of the vagina forms from the sinovaginal bulbs on the posterior wall of the primitive urogenital sinus.

pendent on this proliferation, because these cells form a supporting aggregate of cells (the primitive sex cords) that invest the germ cells and without which the gonad would degenerate.

Müllerian Ducts   The *paramesonephric* or *müllerian ducts* then form lateral to the mesonephric ducts; they grow caudally and then medially to fuse in the midline. They contact the urogenital sinus in the region of the posterior urethra at a slight thickening known as the *sinusal tubercle*. Subsequent sexual development is controlled by the presence or absence of TDY, encoded on the Y chromosome and elaborated by the somatic sex cord cells. TDY results in the degeneration of the gonadal cortex and differentiation of the medullary region of the gonad into Sertoli cells.

The Sertoli cells secrete a glycoprotein known as *anti-müllerian hormone (AMH),* which causes regression of the paramesonephric duct system in the male embryo and is the likely signal for differentiation of Leydig cells from the surrounding mesenchyme. The Leydig cells produce testosterone and, with the converting enzyme 5α-reductase, dihydrotestosterone. Testosterone is responsible for evolution of the mesonephric duct system into the vas deferens, epididymis, ejaculatory ducts, and seminal vesicle; at puberty, testosterone leads to spermatogenesis and changes in primary and secondary sex characteristics. Dihydrotestosterone results in development of the male external genitalia, prostate, and bulbourethral glands. In the absence of TDY, the medulla regresses, and the cortical sex cords break up into isolated cell clusters (the primordial follicles).

The germ cells differentiate into oogonia and enter the first meiotic division as primary oocytes, at which point development is arrested until puberty. In the absence of AMH, the mesonephric duct system degenerates, although in at least one-fourth of adult women (8) remnants may be found in the mesovarium *(epoophoron, paroophoron)* or along the lateral wall of the uterus or vagina *(Gartner's duct cyst).*

The paramesonephric duct system then develops. The inferior fused portion becomes the *uterovaginal canal,* which later becomes the epithelium and glands of the uterus and the upper vagina. The endometrial stroma and myometrium differentiate from surrounding mesenchyme. The cranial unfused portions of the paramesonephric ducts open into the celomic (future peritoneal) cavity and become the *fallopian tubes.*

The fusion of the paramesonephric ducts brings together two folds of peritoneum, which become the *broad ligament* and divide the pelvic cavity into a posterior rectouterine and anterior vesicouterine pouch or cul-de-sac. Between the leaves of the broad ligament, mesenchyme proliferates and differentiates into loose areolar connective tissue and smooth muscle.

Vagina   The *vagina* forms in the third month of embryonic life. While the uterovaginal canal is forming, the endodermal tissue of the sinusal tubercle begins to proliferate, forming a pair of *sinovaginal bulbs,* which become the inferior 20% of the vagina. The most inferior portion of the uterovaginal canal becomes occluded by a solid core of tissue (the *vaginal plate*), the origin of which is unclear. This tissue elongates over the subsequent 2 months and canalizes by a process of central desquamation, and the peripheral cells become the vaginal epithelium. The fibromuscular wall of the vagina originates from the mesoderm of the uterovaginal canal.

Accessory Genital Glands   The female accessory genital glands develop as outgrowths from the urethra (*paraurethral* or *Skene*) and the definitive urogenital sinus (*greater vestibular* or *Bartholin*). Although the ovaries first develop in the thoracic region, they ultimately arrive in the pelvis by a complicated process of descent. This descent is under the control of a ligamentous cord called the *gubernaculum,* which is attached to the ovary superiorly and to the fascia in the region of the future labia majora inferiorly. The gubernaculum becomes attached to the paramesonephric ducts at their point of superior fusion so that it becomes divided into two separate structures. As the ovary and its mesentery (the mesovarium) are brought into the superior portion of the broad ligament, the more proximal part of the gubernaculum becomes the *ovarian ligament* and the distal gubernaculum becomes the *round ligament.*

External Genitalia

Early in the fifth week of embryonic life, folds of tissue form on each side of the cloaca and meet anteriorly in the midline to form the genital tubercle (Fig. 5.11). With the division of the cloaca by the urorectal septum and consequent formation of the perineum, these cloacal folds are known anteriorly as the urogenital folds and posteriorly as the anal folds. The genital tubercle begins to enlarge, but in the female embryo, its growth gradually slows to become the clitoris and the urogenital folds form the labia minora. In the male, the genital tubercle continues to grow to form the penis, and the urogenital folds are believed to fuse to enclose the penile urethra. Lateral to the urogenital folds, another pair of swellings develops, known in the indifferent stage as labioscrotal swellings. In the absence of androgens, they remain largely unfused to become the labia majora. The definitive urogenital sinus gives rise to the vaginal vestibule, into which open the urethra, vagina, and greater vestibular glands.

Clinical Correlations   Developmental abnormalities of the urinary and genital systems can be explained and understood by a consideration of female and male embryologic development. Because of the intertwined development of these two systems, it is easy to understand how abnormalities in one may be associated with abnormalities in the other (9).

Urinary System

Urinary tract anomalies arise from defects in the ureteric bud, the metanephric blastema, or their inductive interaction with each other.

Renal Agenesis   Renal agenesis occurs when one or both ureteric buds fail to form or degenerate and the metanephric blastema is therefore not induced to differentiate into

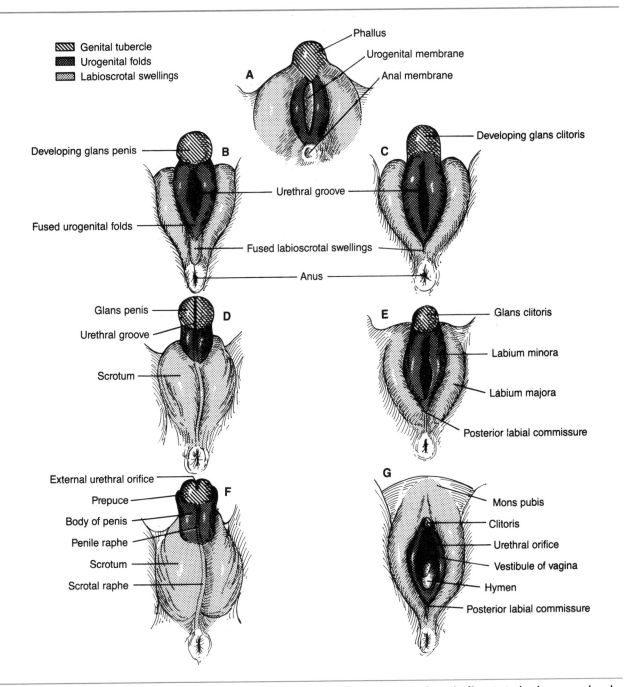

Figure 5.11   The comparative development of the female and male external genitalia. *A,* In both sexes, the development follows a uniform pattern through the seventh week and thereafter begins to differentiate. *B,* The male external genitalia. *C,* The female external genitalia.

nephrons. Bilateral renal agenesis is incompatible with postnatal survival, but infants with only one kidney usually survive and the single kidney undergoes compensatory hypertrophy. Unilateral renal agenesis is often associated with absence or abnormality of fallopian tubes, uterus, or vagina—the paramesonephric duct derivatives.

Abnormalities of Renal Position   Abnormalities of renal position result from disturbance in the normal ascent of the kidneys. A malrotated pelvic kidney is the most common result; a horseshoe kidney, in which the kidneys are fused across the midline, occurs in about one in 600 individuals and also has a final position lower than usual because its normal ascent is prevented by the root of the inferior mesenteric artery.

Duplication of the Upper Ureter and Renal Pelvis Duplication of the upper ureter and renal pelvis are relatively common and result from premature bifurcation of the ureteric bud. If two ureteric buds develop, there will be complete duplication of the collecting system. In this situation, one ureteric bud will open normally into the posterior bladder wall while the second bud will be carried more distally within the mesonephric duct to form an ectopic ureteral orifice into the urethra, vagina, or vaginal vestibule; incontinence is the primary presenting symptom. Most of the aforementioned urinary abnormalities remain asymptomatic unless obstruction or infection supervene. In that case, anomalous embryologic development must be included in the differential diagnosis.

Genital System

Because the early development of the genital system is similar in both sexes, congenital defects in sexual development, usually arising from a variety of chromosomal abnormalities, tend to present clinically with ambiguous external genitalia. These conditions are known as intersex conditions or hermaphroditism and are classified according to the histologic appearance of the gonads (see Chapter 24).

True Hermaphroditism **Individuals with true hermaphroditism have both ovarian and testicular tissue, most commonly as composite ovotestes but occasionally with an ovary on one side and a testis on the other.** In the latter case, a fallopian tube and single uterine horn may develop on the side with the ovary because of the absence of local AMH. True hermaphroditism is an extremely rare condition associated with chromosomal mosaicism, mutation, or abnormal cleavage involving the X and Y chromosomes.

Pseudohermaphroditism **In individuals with pseudohermaphroditism, the genetic sex indicates one gender and the external genitalia has characteristics of the other gender.** Males with pseudohermaphroditism are genetic males with feminized external genitalia, most commonly manifesting as hypospadias (urethral opening on the ventral surface of the penis) or incomplete fusion of the urogenital or labioscrotal folds. Females with pseudohermaphroditism are genetic females with virilized external genitalia, including clitoral hypertrophy and some degree of fusion of the urogenital or labioscrotal folds. Both types of pseudohermaphroditism are caused either by abnormal levels of sex hormones or abnormalities in the sex hormone receptors.

Another major category of genital tract abnormalities involves various types of uterovaginal malformations (Fig. 5.12), which occur in 0.16% of women (11). These malformations are believed to result from one or more of the following situations:

1. Improper fusion of the paramesonephric ducts

2. Incomplete development of one paramesonephric duct

3. Failure of part of the paramesonephric duct on one or both sides to develop

4. Absent or incomplete canalization of the vaginal plate.

Genital Structures

A sagittal section of the female pelvis is presented in Fig. 5.13.

Vagina

The vagina is a hollow fibromuscular tube extending from the vulvar vestibule to the uterus. In the dorsal lithotomy position, the vagina is directed posteriorly toward the sacrum, but its axis is almost horizontal in the upright position. It is attached at its upper end to the uterus just above the cervix. The spaces between the cervix and vagina are known as the anterior, posterior, and lateral vaginal fornices. Because the vagina is at-

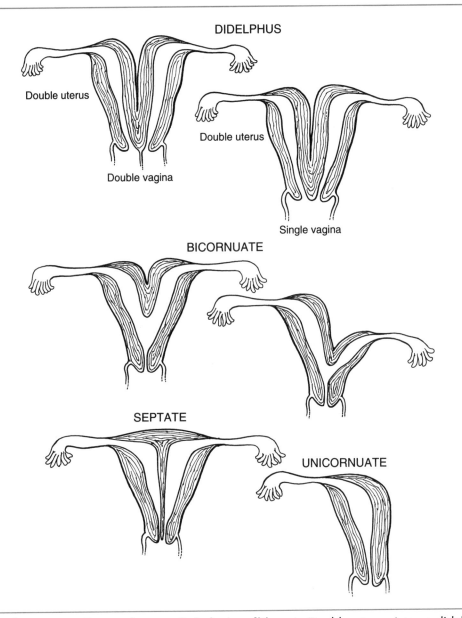

Figure 5.12 Types of congenital abnormalities. *A,* Double uterus (uterus didelphys) and double vagina. *B,* Double uterus with single vagina. *C,* Bicornuate uterus. *D,* Bicornuate uterus with a rudimentary left horn. *E,* Septate uterus. *F,* Unicornuate uterus.

tached at a higher point posteriorly than anteriorly, the posterior vaginal wall is approximately 3 cm longer than the anterior wall.

The posterior vaginal fornix is separated from the posterior cul-de-sac and peritoneal cavity by the vaginal wall and peritoneum. This proximity is clinically useful, both diagnostically and therapeutically. *Culdocentesis,* a technique in which a needle is inserted just posterior to the cervix through the vaginal wall into the peritoneal cavity, has been used to evaluate intraperitoneal hemorrhage (e.g., ruptured ectopic pregnancy, hemorrhagic corpus luteum, other intra-abdominal bleeding), pus (e.g., pelvic inflammatory disease, ruptured intra-abdominal abscess), or other intra-abdominal fluid (e.g., ascites). Incision into the peritoneal cavity from this location in the vagina, known as a *posterior colpotomy,* is experiencing a renaissance as an adjunct to laparoscopic excision of adnexal masses, with removal of the mass intact through the posterior vagina.

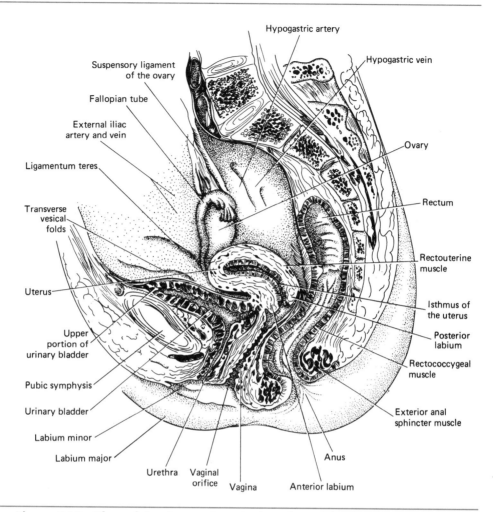

Figure 5.13   The pelvic viscera. A sagittal section of the female pelvis with the pelvic viscera and their relationships.

The vagina is attached to the lateral pelvic wall with endopelvic fascial connections to the *arcus tendineus (white line)*, which extends from the pubic bone to the ischial spine. This connection converts the vaginal lumen into a transverse slit with the anterior and posterior walls in apposition; the lateral space where the two walls meet is the vaginal sulcus. Lateral detachments of the vagina are recognized in some cystocele formation.

The opening of the vagina may be covered by a membrane or surrounded by a fold of connective tissue called the *hymen*. This tissue is usually replaced by irregular tissue tags later in life as sexual activity and childbirth occur. The lower vagina is somewhat constricted as it passes through the urogenital hiatus in the pelvic diaphragm; the upper vagina is more spacious. However, the entire vagina is characterized by its distensibility, which is most evident during childbirth.

The vagina is closely applied anteriorly to the urethra, bladder neck and trigonal region, and posterior bladder; posteriorly, the vagina lies in association with the perineal body, anal canal, lower rectum, and posterior cul-de-sac. It is separated from both the lower urinary and gastrointestinal tracts by their investing layers of endopelvic fascia.

The vagina is composed of three layers:

1. *Mucosa*—nonkeratinized stratified squamous epithelium, without glands. Vaginal lubrication occurs by transudation primarily, with contributions from cervical and Bartholin's gland secretions. The mucosa has a characteristic pattern of transverse ridges and furrows, known as rugae. It is hormonally sensitive, responding to stimulation by estrogen with proliferation and maturation. The mucosa is colonized by mixed bacterial flora with lactobacillus predominant; normal pH is 3.5–4.5.

2. *Muscularis*—contains connective tissue and smooth muscle, loosely arranged in inner circular and outer longitudinal layers.

3. *Adventitia*—consists of endopelvic fascia, adherent to the underlying muscularis.

Blood Supply   The blood supply of the vagina includes the vaginal artery and branches from the uterine, middle rectal, and internal pudendal arteries.

Innervation   The innervation of the vagina is as follows: the upper vagina—uterovaginal plexus; the distal vagina—pudendal nerve.

Uterus

The uterus is a fibromuscular organ usually divided into a lower cervix and an upper corpus or uterine body (Fig. 5.14).

Cervix

The portion of cervix exposed to the vagina is the exocervix or portio vaginalis. It has a convex round surface with a circular or slit-like opening (the external os) into the endocervical canal. The endocervical canal is approximately 2–3 cm in length and opens proximally into the endometrial cavity at the internal os.

The cervical mucosa generally contains both stratified squamous epithelium, characteristic of the exocervix, and mucous-secreting columnar epithelium, characteristic of the en-

Figure 5.14   The uterus, fallopian tubes, and ovaries.

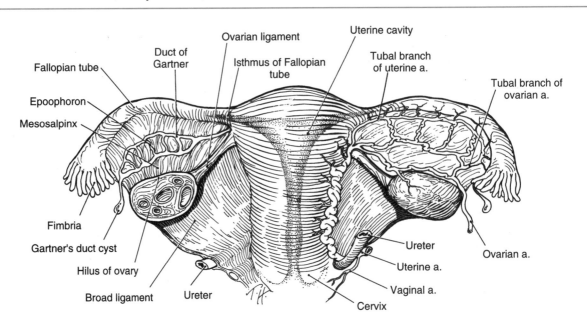

docervical canal. However, the intersection where these two epithelia meet—the squamo-columnar junction—is geographically variable and dependent on hormonal stimulation. It is this dynamic interface, the transformation zone, that is most vulnerable to the development of squamous neoplasia.

In early childhood, during pregnancy, or with oral contraceptive use, columnar epithelium may extend from the endocervical canal onto the exocervix, a condition known as eversion or ectopy. After menopause, the transformation zone usually recedes entirely into the endocervical canal.

Cervical mucus production is under hormonal influence. It varies from profuse, clear, and thin mucus around the time of ovulation to scant and thick mucus in the postovulatory phase of the cycle. Deep in the mucosa and submucosa, the cervix is composed of fibrous connective tissue and a small amount of smooth muscle in a circular arrangement.

Corpus

The body of the uterus varies in size and shape, depending on hormonal and childbearing status. **At birth, the cervix and corpus are approximately equal in size; in the adult woman, the corpus has grown to 2–3 times the size of the cervix.** The position of the uterus in relation to other pelvic structures is also variable and is generally described in terms of positioning—anterior, midposition, or posterior; flexion; and version. *Flexion* **is the angle between the long axis of the uterine corpus and the cervix, whereas** *version* **is the angle of the junction of the uterus with the upper vagina.** Occasionally, abnormal positioning may occur secondary to associated pelvic pathology, such as endometriosis or adhesions.

The uterine corpus is divided into several different regions. The area where the endocervical canal opens into the endometrial cavity is known as the isthmus or lower uterine segment. On each side of the upper uterine body, a funnel-shaped area receives the insertion of the fallopian tubes and is called the uterine cornu; the uterus above this area is the fundus.

The endometrial cavity is triangular in shape and represents the mucosal surface of the uterine corpus. The epithelium is columnar and gland-forming with a specialized stroma. It undergoes cyclic structural and functional change during the reproductive years, with regular shedding of the superficial endometrium and regeneration from the basal layer.

The muscular layer of the uterus, the myometrium, consists of interlacing smooth muscle fibers and ranges in thickness from 1.5 to 2.5 cm. Some outer fibers are continuous with those of the tube and round ligament.

Peritoneum covers most of the corpus of the uterus and the posterior cervix and is known as the serosa. Laterally, the broad ligament, a double layer of peritoneum covering the neurovascular supply to the uterus, inserts into the cervix and corpus. Anteriorly, the bladder lies over the isthmic and cervical region of the uterus.

Blood Supply   The blood supply to the uterus is the uterine artery, which anastomoses with the ovarian and vaginal arteries.

Innervation   The nerve supply to the uterus is the uterovaginal plexus.

Fallopian Tubes

The fallopian tubes and ovaries collectively are referred to as the adnexa. The fallopian tubes are paired hollow structures representing the proximal unfused ends of the müllerian duct. They vary in length from 7 to 12 cm and their function includes ovum pickup, provision of physical environment for conception, and transport and nourishment of the fertilized ovum.

The tubes are divided into several regions:

1. *Interstitial*—narrowest portion of the tube, lies within the uterine wall and forms the tubal ostia at the endometrial cavity

2. *Isthmus*—narrow segment closest to the uterine wall

3. *Ampulla*—larger diameter segment lateral to the isthmus

4. *Fimbria (infundibulum)*—funnel-shaped abdominal ostia of the tubes, opening into the peritoneal cavity; this opening is fringed with numerous finger-like processes that which provide a wide surface for ovum pickup. The fimbria ovarica is a connection between the end of the tube and ovary, bringing the two closer.

The tubal mucosa is ciliated columnar epithelium, which becomes progressively more architecturally complex as the fimbriated end is approached. The muscularis consists of an inner circular and outer longitudinal layer of smooth muscle. The tube is covered by peritoneum and, through its mesentery (*mesosalpinx*), which is situated dorsal to the round ligament, is connected to the upper margin of the broad ligament.

Blood Supply   The vascular supply to the fallopian tubes is the uterine and ovarian arteries.

Innervation   The innervation to the fallopian tubes is the uterovaginal plexus and the ovarian plexus.

Ovaries

The ovaries are paired gonadal structures that lie suspended between the pelvic wall and the uterus by the infundibulopelvic ligament laterally and the utero-ovarian ligament medially. Inferiorly, the hilar surface of each ovary is attached to the broad ligament by its mesentery (mesovarium), which is dorsal to the mesosalpinx and fallopian tube. Primary neurovascular structures reach the ovary through the infundibulopelvic ligament and enter via the mesovarium. **The normal ovary varies in size, with measurements up to 5 × 3 × 3 cm.** Variation in dimension results from endogenous hormonal production, which varies with age and with each menstrual cycle. Exogenous substances, including oral contraceptives, gonadotropin-releasing hormone agonists, or ovulation-inducing medication, may either stimulate or suppress ovarian activity and, therefore, affect size.

Each ovary consists of a cortex and medulla and is covered by a single layer of flattened cuboidal to low columnar epithelium that is continuous with the peritoneum at the mesovarium. The cortex is composed of a specialized stroma and follicles in various stages of development or attrition. The medulla occupies a small portion of the ovary in its hilar region and is composed primarily of fibromuscular tissue and blood vessels.

Blood Supply   The blood supply to the ovary is the ovarian artery, which anastomoses with the uterine artery.

Innervation   The innervation to the ovary is the ovarian plexus and the uterovaginal plexus.

Lower Urinary Tract

Ureters

The ureter is the urinary conduit leading from the kidney to the bladder; it measures approximately 25 cm in total length and is totally retroperitoneal in location.

The lower one-half of each ureter traverses the pelvis after crossing the common iliac vessels at their bifurcation, just medial to the ovarian vessels. It descends into the pelvis adherent to the peritoneum of the lateral pelvic wall and the medial leaf of the broad ligament and enters the bladder base anterior to the upper vagina, traveling obliquely through the bladder wall to terminate in the bladder trigone.

The ureteral mucosa is a transitional epithelium. The muscularis consists of an inner longitudinal and outer circular layer of smooth muscle. A protective connective tissue sheath, which is adherent to the peritoneum, encloses the ureter.

Blood Supply   This is variable with contributions from the renal, ovarian, common iliac, internal iliac, uterine, and vesical arteries.

Innervation   The innervation is through the ovarian plexus and the vesical plexus.

Bladder and Urethra

Bladder

The bladder is a hollow organ, spherically shaped when full, that stores urine. Its size varies with urine volume, normally reaching a maximum volume of ≥ 500 ml. The bladder is often divided into two areas, which are of physiologic significance:

1. The *base of the bladder* consists of the urinary trigone posteriorly and a thickened area of detrusor anteriorly. The three corners of the trigone are formed by the two ureteral orifices and the opening of the urethra into the bladder. The bladder base receives α-adrenergic sympathetic innervation and is the area responsible for maintaining continence.

2. The *dome of the bladder* is the remaining bladder area above the bladder base. It has parasympathetic innervation and is responsible for micturition.

The bladder is positioned posterior to the pubis and lower abdominal wall and anterior to the cervix, upper vagina, and part of the cardinal ligament. Laterally, it is bounded by the pelvic diaphragm and obturator internus muscle.

The bladder mucosa is transitional cell epithelium and the muscle wall *(detrusor),* rather than being arranged in layers, is composed of intermeshing muscle fibers.

Blood Supply   The blood supply to the bladder is from the superior, middle, and inferior vesical arteries with contribution from the uterine and vaginal vessels.

Innervation   The innervation to the bladder is from the vesical plexus, with a contribution from the uterovaginal plexus.

Urethra

The vesical neck is the region of the bladder that receives and incorporates the urethral lumen. The female urethra is approximately 3–4 cm in length and extends from the bladder to the vestibule, traveling just anterior to the vagina.

The urethra is lined by nonkeratinized squamous epithelium that is responsive to estrogen stimulation. Within the submucosa on the dorsal surface of the urethra are the paraurethral or Skene's glands, which empty via ducts into the urethral lumen. Distally, these glands empty into the vestibule on either side of the external urethral orifice. Chronic infection of Skene's glands, with obstruction of their ducts and cystic dilation, is believed to be an inciting factor in the development of suburethral diverticula.

The urethra contains an inner longitudinal layer of smooth muscle and outer circularly oriented smooth muscle fibers. The inferior fascia of the urogenital diaphragm or perineal membrane begins at the junction of the middle and distal thirds of the urethra. Proximal to the middle and distal parts of the urethra, voluntary muscle fibers derived from the urogenital diaphragm intermix with the outer layer of smooth muscle, increasing urethral resistance and contributing to continence. At the level of the urogenital diaphragm, the skeletal muscle fibers leave the wall of the urethra to form the sphincter urethrae and deep transverse perineal muscles.

Blood Supply   The vascular supply to the urethra is from the vesical and vaginal arteries and the internal pudendal branches.

Innervation   The innervation to the urethra is from the vesical plexus and the pudendal nerve.

The lower urinary and genital tracts are intimately connected anatomically and functionally. In the midline, the bladder and proximal urethra can be dissected easily from the underlying lower uterine segment, cervix, and vagina through a loose avascular plane. The distal urethra is essentially inseparable from the vagina. Of surgical significance is the location of the bladder trigone immediately over the middle third of the vagina. Unrecognized injury to the bladder during pelvic surgery may result in development of a vesicovaginal fistula.

Fortunately, dissection to the level of the trigone is rarely required and damage to this critical area is unusual. If dissection is carried too far laterally away from the midline, attachments between the bladder and cervix or vagina become much more denser and vascularized, resulting in increased blood loss and technical difficulty.

Lower Gastrointestinal Tract

Sigmoid Colon

The sigmoid colon begins its characteristic S-shaped curve as it enters the pelvis at the left pelvic brim (Fig. 5.15). The columnar mucosa and richly vascularized submucosa are surrounded by an inner circular layer of smooth muscle and three overlying longitudinal bands of muscle called tenia coli. A mesentery of varying length attaches the sigmoid to the posterior abdominal wall.

Blood Supply   The blood supply to the sigmoid colon is from the sigmoid arteries.

Innervation   The nerves to the sigmoid colon are derived from the inferior mesenteric plexus.

Rectum

The sigmoid colon loses its mesentery in the midsacral region and becomes the rectum approximately 15–20 cm above the anal opening. The rectum follows the curve of the lower sacrum and coccyx and becomes entirely retroperitoneal at the level of the rectouterine pouch or posterior cul-de-sac. It continues along the pelvic curve just posterior to the vagina until the level of the anal hiatus of the pelvic diaphragm, at which point it takes a sharp 90° turn posteriorly and becomes the anal canal, separated from the vagina by the perineal body.

104

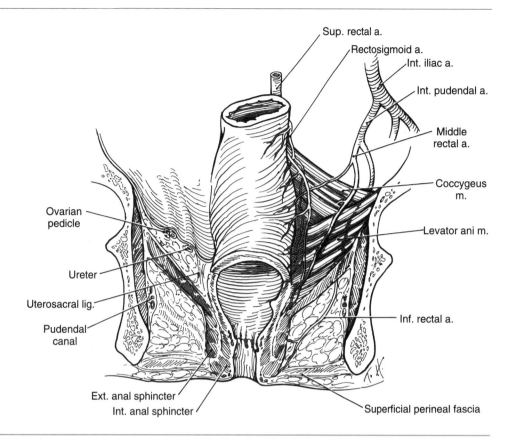

Figure 5.15   The rectosigmoid colon, its vascular supply, and muscular support.

The rectal mucosa is columnar epithelium characterized by three transverse folds that contain mucosa, submucosa, and the inner circular layer of smooth muscle. The tenia of the sigmoid wall broaden and fuse over the rectum to form a continuous longitudinal external layer of smooth muscle to the level of the anal canal.

Anal Canal

The anal canal begins at the level of the sharp turn in the direction of the distal colon and is 2–3 cm in length. At the anorectal junction, the mucosa changes to stratified squamous epithelium (the pectinate line), which continues until the termination of the anus at the anal verge, where there is a transition to perianal skin with typical skin appendages. It is surrounded by a thickened ring of circular muscle fibers that is a continuation of the circular muscle of the rectum, the internal anal sphincter. Its lower part is surrounded by bundles of striated muscle fibers, the external anal sphincter (11).

Fecal continence is primarily provided by the puborectalis muscle and the internal and external anal sphincter. The puborectalis surrounds the anal hiatus in the pelvic diaphragm and interdigitates posterior to the rectum to form a rectal sling. The external anal sphincter surrounds the terminal anal canal below the level of the levator ani.

The practicing gynecologist must be familiar with the lower gastrointestinal tract because of its anatomical proximity to the lower genital tract. This is particularly important during surgery of the vulva and vagina. Lack of attention to this proximity during repair of vaginal lacerations or episiotomies can lead to damage of the rectum and resulting fistula formation or injury to the external anal sphincter with development of fecal incontinence. Because of the avascular nature of the rectovaginal space, it is relatively easy to dissect the rectum from the vagina in the midline, which is routinely done in the repair of rectoceles.

Blood Supply   The vascular supply to the rectum and anal canal is from the superior, middle, and inferior rectal arteries. The venous drainage is a complex submucosal plexus of vessels that, under conditions of increased intra-abdominal pressure (pregnancy, pelvic mass, ascites), may dilate and become symptomatic with rectal bleeding or pain as hemorrhoids.

Innervation   The nerve supply to the anal canal is from the middle rectal plexus, the inferior mesenteric plexus, and the pudendal nerve.

The Genital Tract and its Relations

The genital tract is situated at the bottom of the intra-abdominal cavity and is related to the intraperitoneal cavity and its contents, the retroperitoneal spaces, and the pelvic floor. Its access through the abdominal wall or the perineum requires a thorough knowledge of the anatomy of these areas and their relationships.

The Abdominal Wall

The anterior abdominal wall is bound superiorly by the xiphoid process and the costal cartilage of the 7th–10th ribs and inferiorly by the iliac crest, anterior superior iliac spine, inguinal ligament, and pubic bone. It consists of the following structures.

Skin/Subcutaneous Tissue

The lower abdominal skin may exhibit striae or "stretch marks" and increased pigmentation in the midline in parous women. The subcutaneous tissue contains a variable amount of fat.

Muscles

Five muscles and their aponeuroses contribute to the structure and strength of the anterolateral abdominal wall (Fig. 5.16; Table 5.7).

Fascia

Superficial Fascia

The superficial fascia consists of two layers:

1. *Camper's fascia*—the most superficial layer, which contains a variable amount of fat and is continuous with the superficial fatty layer of the perineum

2. *Scarpa's fascia*—a deeper membranous layer continuous in the perineum with Colles' fascia (superficial perineal fascia) and with the deep fascia of the thigh (fascia lata).

Rectus Sheath

The aponeuroses of the external and internal oblique and the transversus abdominis combine to form a sheath for the rectus abdominis and pyramidalis, fusing medially in the midline at the linea alba and laterally at the semilunar line (Fig. 5.17). Above the arcuate line, the aponeurosis of the internal oblique muscle splits into anterior and posterior lamella (Fig. 5.17*A*). Below this line, all three layers are anterior to the body of the rectus muscle (Fig. 5.17*B*). The rectus is then covered posteriorly by the transversalis fascia, providing access to the muscle for the inferior epigastric vessels.

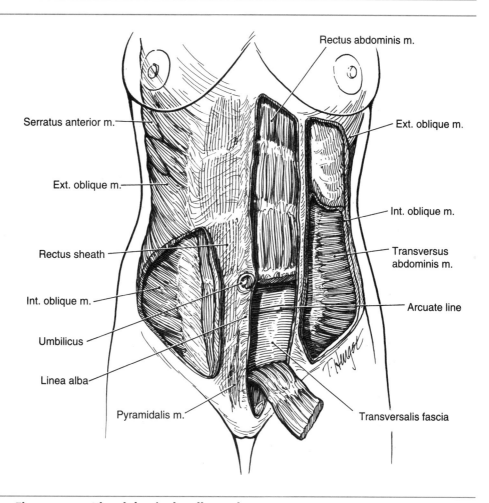

Figure 5.16   The abdominal wall muscles.

Transversalis Fascia

The transversalis fascia is a firm membranous sheet on the internal surface of the transversus abdominis muscle that extends beyond the muscle and forms a fascia lining the entire abdominopelvic cavity. Like the peritoneum, it is divided into a parietal and a visceral component. It is continuous from side to side across the linea alba and covers the posterior aspect of the rectus abdominis muscle below the arcuate line. Superiorly, it becomes the inferior fascia of the diaphragm. Inferiorly, it is attached to the iliac crest, covers the iliac fascia and the obturator internus fascia, and extends downward and medially to form the superior fascia of the pelvic diaphragm.

Characteristically, the transversalis fascia continues along blood vessels and other structures leaving and entering the abdominopelvic cavity and contributes to the formation of the visceral (*endopelvic*) pelvic fascia (12), thereby playing a critical role in the support of the pelvic organs. In the inguinal region, the fascial relationships result in the development of the inguinal canal, through which the round ligament exits into the perineum. The fascia is separated from the peritoneum by a layer of preperitoneal fat. Areas of fascial weaknesses or congenital or post-traumatic and surgical injuries result in herniation of the underlying structures through a defective abdominal wall. The incisions least likely to result in damage to the integrity and innervation of the abdominal wall muscles include a midline incision through the linea alba and a transverse incision through the recti muscle fibers that respects the integrity of its innervation (13).

Table 5.7

Muscle	Origin	Insertion	Action
External oblique	Fleshy digitations from the outer surfaces of ribs 5–12	Fibers radiate inferiorly, anteriorly, and medially, in most cases ending in the aponeurosis of the external muscle and inserting into the anterior half of the iliac crest, the pubic tubercle, and the linea alba. The superficial inguinal ring is located above and lateral to the pubic tubercle at the end of a triangular cleft in the external oblique muscle, bordered by strong fibrous bands that transmit the round ligament	Compresses and supports abdominal viscera; flexes and rotates vertebral column
Internal oblique	Posterior layer of the thoracolumbar fascia, the anterior two-thirds of the iliac crest, adn the lateral two-thirds of the inguinal ligament	Inferior border of ribs 10–12. The superior fibers of the aponeurosis split to enclose the rectus abdominus muscle and join at the linea alba above the arcuate line. The most inferior fibers join with those of the transverse abdonimis muscle to insert into the pubic crest and pecten pubis via the conjoint tendon	Compresses and supports abdominal viscera
Transversus abdominus	Inner aspect of the inferior six costal cartilages, the thoracolumbar fascia, the iliac crest, and the lateral one-third of the inguinal ligament	Linea alba with the aponeurosis of the internal oblique, the pubic crest and the pecten pubis via the conjoint tendon	Compresses and supports abdominal viscera
Rectus abdominus	Superior pubic ramus and the ligaments of the symphysis pubis	Anterior surface of the xiphoid process and the cartilage of ribs 5–7	Tenses anterior abdominal wall and flexes trunk
Pyramidalis	Small triangular muscle contained within the rectus sheath, anterior to the lower part of the rectus muscle	On the linea alba, easily recognizable shape, used to locate the midline, particularly in a patient with previous abdominal surgery and scarring of the abdominal wall	Tenses the linea alba, insignificant in terms of function and is frequently absent

Nerves and Vessels

The tissues of the abdominal wall are innervated by the continuation of the *inferior intercostal nerves* T4 to T11 and the *subcostal nerve* T12. The inferior part of the abdominal wall is supplied by the *first lumbar nerve* via the iliohypogastric and the ilioinguinal nerves. The primary blood supply to the anterior lateral abdominal wall includes the following:

1. The *inferior epigastric* and *deep circumflex iliac arteries*, branches of the external iliac artery

2. The *superior epigastric artery*, a terminal branch of the internal thoracic artery.

The inferior epigastric artery runs superiorly in the transverse fascia to reach the arcuate line, where it enters the rectus sheath. It is vulnerable to damage with abdominal incisions in which the rectus muscle is completely or partially transected or with excessive lateral

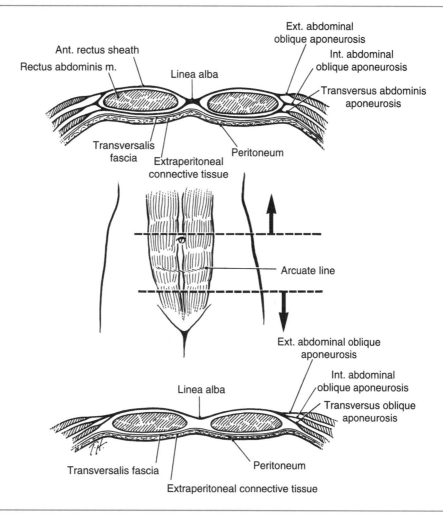

Figure 5.17   A transverse section of the rectus abdominus. The aponeurosis of the external and internal oblique and the transversus abdominus from the rectus abdominus. *A,* Above the arcuate line. *B,* Below the arcuate line.

traction on the rectus. The deep circumflex artery runs on the deep aspect of the anterior abdominal wall parallel to the inguinal ligament and along the iliac crest between the transverse abdominis muscle and the internal oblique muscle. The superior epigastric vessels enter the rectus sheath superiorly just below the seventh costal cartilage.

The venous system drains into the saphenous vein, and the lymphatics drain to the axillary chain above the umbilicus and to the inguinal nodes below it. The subcutaneous tissues drain to the lumbar chain.

Perineum

The perineum is situated at the lower end of the trunk between the buttocks. Its bony boundaries include the lower margin of the pubic symphysis anteriorly, the tip of the coccyx posteriorly, and the ischial tuberosities laterally. These landmarks correspond to the boundaries of the pelvic outlet. The diamond shape of the perineum is customarily divided by an imaginary line joining the ischial tuberosities immediately in front of the anus, at the level of the perineal body, into an anterior urogenital and a posterior anal triangle (Fig. 5.18).

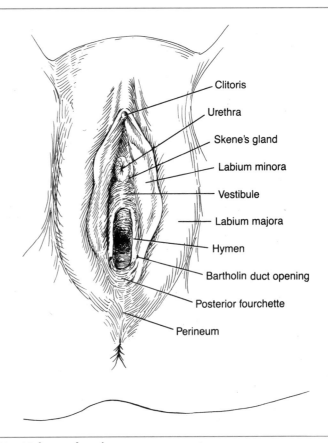

Clitoris
Urethra
Skene's gland
Labium minora
Vestibule
Labium majora
Hymen
Bartholin duct opening
Posterior fourchette
Perineum

Figure 5.18   Vulva and perineum.

Urogenital Triangle

The urogenital triangle includes the external genital structures and the urethral opening (Fig. 5.18). These external structures cover the superficial and deep perineal compartments (Figs. 5.19 and 5.20) and are known as the vulva.

Vulva

Mons Pubis

The mons pubis is a triangular eminence in front of the pubic bones that consists of adipose tissue covered by hair-bearing skin up to its junction with the abdominal wall.

Labia Majora

The labia majora are a pair of fibroadipose folds of skin that extend from the mons pubis downward and backward to meet in the midline in front of the anus at the posterior fourchette. They include the terminal extension of the round ligament and occasionally a peritoneal diverticulum, the *canal of Nuck*. They are covered by skin with scattered hairs laterally and are rich in sebaceous, apocrine, and eccrine glands.

Labia Minora

The labia minora lie between the labia majora, with which they merge posteriorly and are separated into two folds as they approach the clitoris anteriorly. The anterior folds unite to form the prepuce or hood of the clitoris. The posterior folds form the frenulum of the clitoris as they attach to its inferior surface. The labia minora are covered by hairless skin overlying a fibroelastic stroma rich in neural and vascular elements. The area between the posterior labia minora forms the vestibule of the vagina.

110

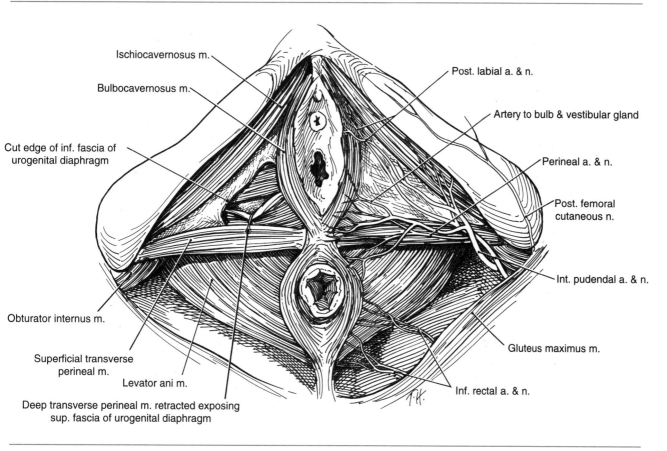

Figure 5.19   Superficial perineal compartment.

Clitoris

The clitoris is an erectile organ that is 2–3 cm in length. It consists of two crura and two corpora cavernosa and is covered by a sensitive rounded tubercle (the glans).

Vaginal Orifice

The vaginal orifice is surrounded by the hymen, a variable crescentic mucous membrane that is replaced by rounded caruncles after its rupture. The opening of the duct of the *greater vestibular glands (Bartholin)* is located on each side of the vestibule. Numerous lesser vestibular glands are also scattered posteriorly and between the urethral and vaginal orifices.

Urethral Orifice

The urethral orifice is immediately anterior to the vaginal orifice about 2–3 cm beneath the clitoris. The *Skene's gland (paraurethral)* duct presents an opening on its posterior surface.

Superficial Perineal Compartment

The superficial perineal compartment lies between the superficial perineal fascia and the inferior fascia of the urogenital diaphragm (perineal membrane) (Fig. 5.19). The superficial perineal fascia has a superficial and deep component. The *superficial* layer is relatively thin and fatty and is continuous superiorly with the superficial fatty layer of the lower abdominal wall (*Camper's fascia*). It continues laterally as the fatty layer of the thighs. The *deep* layer of the superficial perineal fascia or *Colles' fascia* is continuous superiorly with

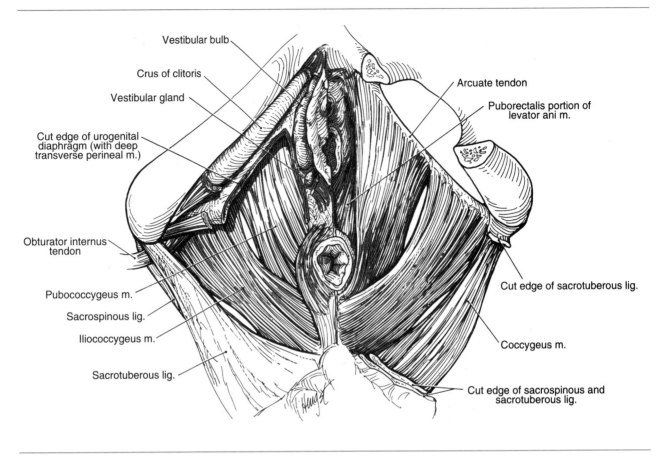

Figure 5.20   Deep perineal compartment.

the deep layer of the superficial abdominal fascia (*Scarpa's fascia*), which attaches firmly to the ischiopubic rami and ischial tuberosities. The superficial perineal compartment is continuous superiorly with the superficial fascial spaces of the anterior abdominal wall, allowing spread of blood or infection along that route. Such spread is limited laterally by the ischiopubic rami, anteriorly by the transverse ligament of the perineum, and posteriorly by the superficial transverse perineal muscle. The superficial perineal compartment includes the following.

Erectile bodies

The vestibular bulbs are 3-cm, highly vascular structures surrounding the vestibule and located under the bulbocavernosus muscle. The body of the clitoris is attached by two crura to the internal aspect of the ischiopubic rami. They are covered by the ischiocavernosus muscle.

Muscles

The muscles of the vulva are the ischiocavernosus, the bulbocavernosus, and superficial transverse perineal.

Ischiocavernosus

- Origin—ischial tuberosity
- Insertion—ischiopubic bone
- Action—compresses the crura and lowers the clitoris.

112

Bulbocavernosus

- Origin—perineal body
- Insertion—posterior aspect of the clitoris; some fibers pass above the dorsal vein of the clitoris in a sling-like fashion
- Action—compresses the vestibular bulb and dorsal vein of the clitoris.

Superficial Transverse Perineal

- Origin—ischial tuberosity
- Insertion—central perineal tendon
- Action—fixes the perineal body.

Vestibular Glands

The vestibular glands are situated on either side of the vestibule under the posterior end of the vestibular bulb. They drain between the hymen and the labia minora. Their mucus secretion helps maintain adequate lubrication. Infection in these glands can result in an abscess.

Deep Perineal Compartment

The deep perineal compartment is a fascial space bound inferiorly by the perineal membrane and superiorly by a deep fascial layer that separates the urogenital diaphragm from the anterior recess of the ischiorectal fossa (Fig. 5.20). It is stretched across the anterior half of the pelvic outlet between the ischiopubic rami. Recently, Oelrich (14) suggested that the deep compartment may be directly continuous with the pelvic cavity superiorly. Indeed, the posterior pubourethral ligaments, functioning as wing-like elevations of the fascia ascending from the pelvic floor to the posterior aspect of the symphysis pubis, provide a point of fixation to the urethra and support the concept of the continuity of the deep perineal compartment with the pelvic cavity.

According to Milley and Nichols (15), the anterior pubourethral ligaments represent a similar elevation of the inferior fascia of the urogenital diaphragm and are joined by the intermediate pubourethral ligament, with the junction between the two fascial structures arcing under the pubic symphysis. The urogenital diaphragm includes the *sphincter urethrae (urogenital sphincter)* and the *deep transverse perineal (transversus vaginae)* muscle.

The sphincter urethrae (Fig. 5.21) is a continuous muscle fanning out as it develops proximally and distally, including the following:

1. The *external urethral sphincter,* which surrounds the middle third of the urethra

2. The *compressor urethrae,* arcing across the ventral side of the urethra

3. The *urethrovaginal sphincter,* which surrounds the ventral aspect of the urethra and terminates in the lateral vaginal wall.

The deep transverse perineal muscle originates at the internal aspect of the ischial bone, parallels the muscle compressor urethrae, and attaches to the lateral vaginal wall along the perineal membrane to which it intimately attaches.

There is a common reliance of the urinary and genital tracts on several interdependent structures for support. The vagina is well anchored in its inferior portion by the urogenital diaphragm and perineal body. The uterosacral/cardinal ligamentous complex, including its vascular pedicles, secure its fixation over the levator plate, and the endopelvic fascia contribute to its lateral connections to the arcus tendineus.

Anteriorly, the pubourethral ligaments and pubovesical fascia and ligaments provide fixation and stabilization for the urethra and bladder. Posteriorly, they rely on the vagina and

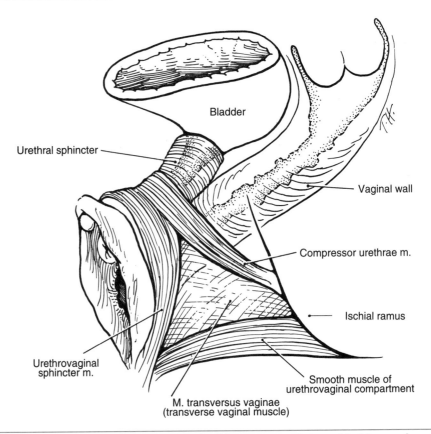

Figure 5.21   The complete urogenital sphincter musculature, bladder, and vagina.

lower uterus for support. Partial resection or relaxation of the uterosacral ligaments often leads to relaxation of the genitourinary complex, resulting in the formation of a cystocele. Various types and degrees of genital tract prolapse or relaxation are almost always associated with similar findings in the bladder or urethra or both.

Blood Supply   The blood supply to the vulva is from the superficial and deep perineal compartments as follows:

    1. External pudendal artery (from femoral artery), internal pudendal artery

    2. Venous drainage—internal pudendal veins.

The blood supply to the superficial and deep perineal compartments is as follows:

    1. Internal pudendal artery, dorsal artery of the clitoris

    2. Venous drainage—internal pudendal veins, which are richly anastomotic

    3. Lymphatic drainage—internal iliac chain.

Innervation   The innervation to the vulva and the superficial and deep perineal compartments are as follows:

    • *Vulva*—branches of the:

    1. Ilioinguinal nerve

2. Genitofemoral nerve (genital branch)

3. Lateral femoral cutaneous nerve of the thigh (perineal branch)

4. Perineal nerve (branch of pudendal)

• *Superficial and deep perineal compartments* — the perineal nerve.

Perineal Body

The perineal body or central perineal tendon is critical to the posterior support of the lower aspect of the anterior vaginal wall. It is a triangle-shaped structure separating the distal portion of the anal and vaginal canals that is formed by the convergence of the tendinous attachments of the bulbocavernosus, the external anal sphincter, and the superficial transverse perinei muscle. Its superior border represents the point of insertion of the *rectovaginal (Denonvilliers') fascia,* which extends to the underside of the peritoneum covering the cul-de-sac of Douglas, separating the anorectal from the urogenital compartment (16). The perineal body also plays an important anchoring role in the musculofascial support of the pelvic floor. It represents the central connection between the two layers of support of the pelvic floor—the pelvic and urogenital diaphragm. It also provides a posterior connection to the anococcygeal raphe. Thus, it is central to the definition of the bileveled support of the floor of the pelvis.

Anal Triangle

The anal triangle includes the lower end of the anal canal. The external anal sphincter surrounds the anal triangle, and the ischiorectal fossa is on each side.

Posteriorly, the *anococcygeal body* lies between the anus and the tip of the coccyx and consists of thick fibromuscular tissue (of levator ani and external anal sphincter origin) giving support to the lower part of the rectum and the anal canal.

The *external anal sphincter* forms a thick band of muscular fibers arranged in three layers running from the perineal body to the anococcygeal ligament. The subcutaneous fibers are thin and surround the anus and, without bony attachment, decussate in front of it. The superficial fibers sweep forward from the anococcygeal ligament, and the tip of the coccyx around the anus inserts into the perineal body. The deep fibers arise from the perineal body to encircle the lower half of the anal canal to form a true sphincter muscle, which fuses with the puborectalis portion of the levator ani.

The *ischiorectal fossa* is mainly occupied by fat and separates the ischium laterally from the median structures of the anal triangle. It is a fascia-lined space located between the perineal skin inferiorly and the pelvic diaphragm superiorly; it communicates with the contralateral ischiorectal fossa over the anococcygeal ligament. Superiorly, its apex is at the origin of the levator ani muscle from the obturator fascia. It is bound medially by the levator ani and the external sphincter with their fascial covering, laterally by the obturator internus muscle with its fascia, posteriorly by the sacrotuberous ligament and the lower border of the gluteus maximus muscle, and anteriorly by the base of the urogenital diaphragm. It is widest and deepest posteriorly and weakest medially. Thus, an ischiorectal abscess should be drained without delay or it will extend into the anal canal. The cavity is filled with fat that cushions the anal canal and is traversed by many fibrous bands, vessels, and nerves, including the pudendal and the inferior rectal nerves. The perforating branch of S2 and S3 and the perineal branch of S4 also run through this space.

The *pudendal (Alcock's) canal* is a tunnel formed by a splitting of the inferior portion of the obturator fascia running anteromedially from the ischial spine to the posterior edge of the urogenital diaphragm. It contains the pudendal artery, vein, and nerve in their traverse from the peritoneal cavity to the perineum.

115

Blood Supply   The blood supply to the anal triangle is from the inferior rectal (hemorrhoidal) artery and vein.

Innervation   The innervation to the anal triangle is from the perineal branch of the fourth sacral nerve and the inferior rectal (hemorrhoidal) nerve.

Retroperitoneum and Retroperitoneal Spaces

The subperitoneal area of the true pelvis is partitioned into potential spaces by the various organs and their respective fascial coverings and by the selective thickenings of the endopelvic fascia into ligaments and septa (Fig. 5.22). It is imperative that surgeons operating in the pelvis be familiar with these spaces, which include the following:

Prevesical Space (Retzius' Space)

The prevesical space (Retzius' space) is a fat-filled potential space bound anteriorly by the pubic bone, covered by the transversalis fascia, and extending to the umbilicus between the medial umbilical ligaments (obliterated umbilical arteries); posteriorly, the space extends to the anterior wall of the bladder. It is separated from the paravesical space by the ascending bladder septum (bladder pillars).

Figure 5.22   Schematic sectional drawing of the pelvis shows the firm connective tissue covering. The bladder, cervix, and rectum are surrounded by a connective tissue covering. The Mackenrodt ligament extends from the lateral cervix to the lateral abdominal pelvic wall. The vesicouterine ligament originating from the anterior edge of the Mackenrodt ligament leads to the covering of the bladder on the posterior side. The sagittal rectum column spreads both to the connective tissue of the rectum and the sacral vertebrae closely nestled against the back of the Mackenrodt ligament and lateral pelvic wall. Between the firm connective tissue bundles is loose connective tissue (paraspaces). (Reproduced with permission from **Von Peham H, Amreich JA.** *Gynaekologische Operationslehre.* Berlin: S Karger, 1930.)

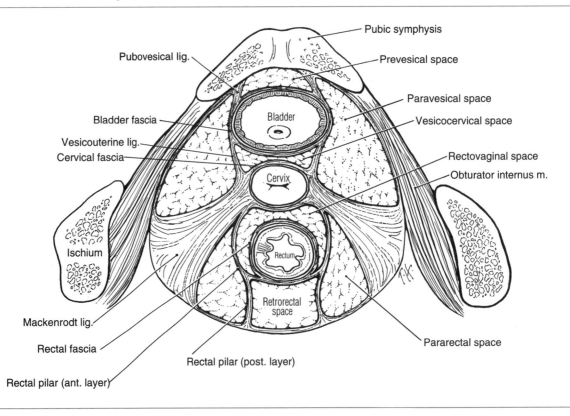

Upon entering the prevesical space, the pubourethral ligaments may be seen inserting the posterior aspect of the symphysis pubis as a thickened prolongation of the arcus tendineus fascia. Combined abdominal and vaginal bladder neck suspensory procedures usually enter the Retzius' space between the arcus tendineus and the pubourethral ligaments.

Paravesical Space

The paravesical spaces are fat filled and limited by the fascia of the obturator internus muscle and the pelvic diaphragm laterally, the bladder pillar medially, the endopelvic fascia inferiorly, and the lateral umbilical ligament superiorly.

Vesicovaginal Space

The vesicovaginal space is separated from the Retzius' space by the endopelvic fascia. This space is limited anteriorly by the bladder wall (from the proximal urethra to the upper vagina), posteriorly by the anterior vaginal wall, and laterally by the bladder septa (selective thickenings of the endopelvic fascia inserting laterally into the arcus tendineus). A tear in these fascial investments and thickenings medially, transversely, or laterally allow herniation and development of a cystocele.

Rectovaginal Space

The rectovaginal space extends between the vagina and the rectum from the superior border of the perineal body to the underside of the rectouterine Douglas' pouch. It is bound anteriorly by the rectovaginal septum (firmly adherent to the posterior aspect of the vagina), posteriorly by the anterior rectal wall, and laterally by the descending rectal septa separating the rectovaginal space from the pararectal space on each side. The rectovaginal septum represents a firm membranous transverse septum dividing the pelvis into rectal and urogenital compartments, allowing the independent function of the vagina and rectum. An anterior rectocele often results from a defect or an avulsion of the septum from the perineal body. Reconstruction of the perineum is critical for the restoration of this important compartmental separation as well as for the support of the anterior vaginal wall (17).

Pararectal Space

The pararectal space is bound laterally by the levator ani, medially by the rectal pillars, and posteriorly above the ischial spine by the anterolateral aspect of the sacrum. It is separated from the retrorectal space by the posterior extension of the descending rectal septa.

Retrorectal Space

The retrorectal space is limited by the rectum anteriorly and the anterior aspect of the sacrum posteriorly. It communicates with the pararectal spaces laterally above the uterosacral ligaments and extends superiorly into the presacral space.

Presacral Space

The presacral space is the superior extension of the retrorectal space and is limited by the deep parietal peritoneum anteriorly and the anterior aspect of the sacrum posteriorly. It harbors the middle sacral vessels and the hypogastric plexi between the bifurcation of the aorta invested by loose areolar tissue. Presacral neurectomy requires a good familiarity and working knowledge of this space.

Peritoneal Cavity

The female pelvic organs lie at the bottom of the abdominopelvic cavity covered superiorly and posteriorly by the small and large bowel. Anteriorly, the uterine wall is in contact with the posterior-superior aspect of the bladder. The uterus is held in position by the following structures:

1. The *round ligaments* coursing inferolaterally toward the internal inguinal ring

2. The *uterosacral ligaments*

3. The *cardinal ligaments,* which provide support to the cervix and upper vagina and contribute to the support of the bladder.

Anteriorly, the uterus is separated from the bladder by the vesicouterine pouch and from the rectum posteriorly by the rectouterine pouch or Douglas' cul-de-sac. Laterally, the bilateral broad ligaments carry the neurovascular pedicles and their respective fascial coverings, attaching the uterus to the lateral pelvic side wall.

The broad ligament is in contact inferiorly with the paravesical space, the obturator fossa, and the pelvic extension of the iliac fossa, to which it provides a peritoneal covering, and the uterosacral ligament. Superiorly, it extends into the infundibulopelvic ligament.

Ureter

In its pelvic path, in the retroperitoneum, several relationships are of significance and identify areas of greatest vulnerability to injury of the ureter (Fig. 5.23):

1. The ovarian vessels cross over the ureter as it approaches the pelvic brim and lie in proximity just medial to the ureter as it enters the pelvis.

2. As the ureter descends into the pelvis, it runs within the broad ligament just lateral to the uterosacral ligament, separating the uterosacral ligament from the mesosalpinx, mesovarium, and ovarian fossa.

Figure 5.23   The course of the ureter and its relationship to the sites of greatest vulnerability.

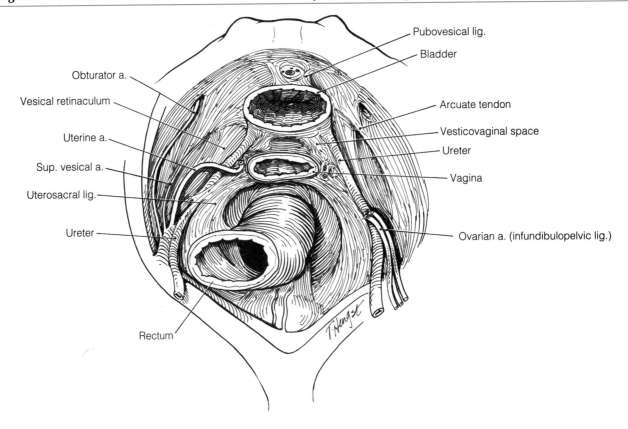

3. At approximately the level of the ischial spine, the ureter crosses under the uterine artery in its course through the cardinal ligament; the ureter divides this area into the supraureteric parametrium surrounding the uterine vessels and the infraureteric paracervix molded around the vaginal vessels and extending posteriorly into the uterosacral ligament. In this location, the ureter lies 2–3 cm lateral to the cervix.

4. The ureter then turns medially to cross the anterior upper vagina as it traverses the bladder wall.

Approximately 75% of all iatrogenic injuries to the ureter result from gynecologic procedures, most commonly abdominal hysterectomy (18). Distortions of pelvic anatomy, including adnexal masses, endometriosis, other pelvic adhesive disease, or fibroids, may increase susceptibility to injury by displacement or alteration of usual anatomy. **Despite the severity of intraperitoneal disease, however, the ureter can always be identified by using a retroperitoneal approach and remembering fundamental landmarks and relationships.**

Pelvic Floor

The pelvic floor includes all of the structures closing the pelvic outlet from the skin inferiorly to the peritoneum superiorly. It is commonly divided by the pelvic diaphragm into a pelvic and a perineal portion. The pelvic diaphragm is spread transversely in a hammock-like fashion across the true pelvis, with a central hiatus for the urethra, vagina, and rectum. Anatomically and physiologically, the pelvic diaphragm can be divided into two components—the internal and external components.

The external component originates from the arcus tendineus, extending from the pubic bone to the ischial spine, which gives rise to fibers of differing directions, including the *pubococcygeus,* the *iliococcygeus,* and the *coccygeus.*

The internal component originates from the pubic bone above and medial to the origins of the pubococcygeus and is smaller but thicker and stronger (19). Its fibers run in a sagittal direction and are divided into the following two portions.

Pubovaginalis   The fibers of the pubovaginalis run in a perpendicular direction to the urethra, crossing the lateral vaginal wall at the junction of its lower one-third and upper two-thirds to insert into the perineal body. The intervening anterior interlevator space is covered by the urogenital diaphragm.

Puborectalis   The superior fibers of the puborectalis sling around the rectum to the symphysis pubis; its inferior fibers insert into the lateral rectal wall between the internal and external sphincter.

The pelvic diaphragm is covered superiorly by fascia, which includes a parietal and a visceral component and is a continuation of the transversalis fascia (Fig. 5.24). The parietal fascia has areas of thickening (ligaments, septa) that provide reinforcement and fixation for the pelvic floor. The visceral fascia extends medially to invest the pelvic viscera, resulting in a fascial covering to the bladder, vagina, uterus, and rectum. It becomes attenuated where the peritoneal covering is well defined and continues laterally with the pelvic cellular tissue and neurovascular pedicles.

Musculofascial elements (the hypogastric sheath) extend along the vessels originating from the internal iliac artery. Following these vessels to their respective organs, the hypogastric sheath extends perivascular investments that contribute to the formation of the endopelvic fascia so critical for the support of the pelvic organs.

Thus, the parietal fascia anchors the visceral fascia, which defines the relationship of the various viscera and provides them with significant fixation (uterosacral and cardinal ligaments), septation (vesicovaginal and rectovaginal), and definition of pelvic spaces (pre-

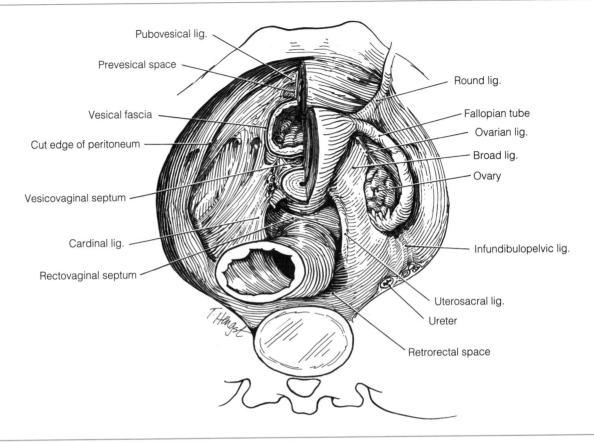

Figure 5.24   **The fascial components of the pelvic diaphragm.**

ments), septation (vesicovaginal and rectovaginal), and definition of pelvic spaces (prevesical, vesicovaginal, rectovaginal, paravesical, pararectal, and retrorectal).

For its support, the pelvic floor relies on the complementary role of the pelvic diaphragm and its fascia resting on the perineal fibromuscular complex, composed of the perineal membrane and urogenital diaphragm anteriorly, and the perineal body joined to the anococcygeal raphe by the external anal sphincter posteriorly. This double-layered arrangement, when intact, provides optimal support for the pelvic organs and counterbalances the forces pushing them downward with gravity and any increase in intra-abdominal pressure (Fig. 5.25).

Summary

Continuing review and education in anatomy are important for every pelvic surgeon. New surgical approaches are being developed to solve old problems and often require surgeons to revisit familiar anatomy from an unfamiliar perspective (e.g., through a laparoscope) or with a different understanding of complex anatomic relationships. Anatomic alterations secondary to disease, congenital variation, or intraoperative complications may make even familiar surgical territory suddenly seem foreign. All of these situations require surgeons to be perpetual students of anatomy, regardless of breadth or depth of experience.

Several strategies for continuing education in anatomy are suggested:

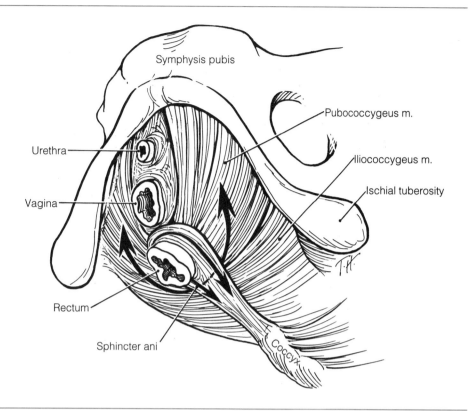

Figure 5.25   The double-layered muscular support of the pelvic diaphragm.

1. Review relevant anatomy prior to each surgical procedure.

2. Study the gynecologic literature on an ongoing basis—numerous publications over the past several years document the evolution of newer concepts regarding anatomic issues such as pelvic support.

3. Operate with more experienced pelvic surgeons, particularly when incorporating new surgical procedures into practice.

4. Periodically dissect fresh or fixed cadaveric specimens; this practice can generally be arranged through local or regional anatomy boards or medical schools or by special arrangement at the time of autopsy.

References

1. **International Anatomical Nomenclature Committee.** *Nomina Anatomica.* 6th ed. Edinburgh: Churchill Livingstone, 1989.

2. **Uhlenhuth E, Day EC, Smith RD, Middleton EB.** The visceral endopelvic fascia and the hypogastric sheath. *Surg Gynecol Obstet* 1948;86:9–28.

3. **Thompson JD, Rock WA, Wiskind A.** Control of pelvic hemorrhage: blood component therapy and hemorrhagic shock. In: **Thompson JD, Rock JA,** eds. *TeLinde's Operative Gynecology.* 7th ed. Philadelphia: JB Lippincott Co., 1991:151.

4. **Lee RB, Stone K, Magelssen D, Belts RP, Benson WL.** Presacral neurectomy for chronic pelvic pain. *Obstet Gynecol* 1986;68:517–21.

5. **Polan ML, DeCherney A.** Presacral neurectomy for pelvic pain in infertility. *Fertil Steril* 1980;34:557–60.

6. **Vaughan ED Jr, Middleton GW.** Pertinent genitourinary embryology. Review for the practicing urologist. *Urology* 1975;6:139–49.

7. **Byskov AG, Hoyer PE.** Embryology of mammalian gonads and ducts. In: **Knobil E, Neill JD,** eds. *The Physiology of Reproduction.* 2nd ed. New York: Raven Press Ltd, 1994:487.

8. **Arey LB.** The genital system. In: *Developmental Anatomy.* 7th ed. Philadelphia: WB Saunders Co., 1974:315.

9. **Moore KL.** The urogenital system. In: *The Developing Human—Clinically Oriented Embyrology.* 3rd ed. Philadelphia: WB Saunders Co., 1982:255.

10. **Semmens JP.** Congenital anomalies of female genital tract. Functional classification based on review of 56 personal cases and 500 reported cases. *Obstet Gynecol* 1962;19:328–50.

11. **Lawson JO.** Pelvic anatomy II. Anal canal and associated sphincters. *Ann R Coll Surg Engl* 1974;54:288–300.

12. **Curtis AH.** *A Textbook of Gynecology.* 4th ed. Philadelphia: WB Saunders Co., 1943.

13. **Moore KL.** *Clinically Oriented Anatomy.* 2nd ed. Baltimore: Williams & Wilkins, 1985.

14. **Oelrich TM.** The striated urogenital sphincter muscle in the female. *Anat Rec* 1983;205:223–32.

15. **Milley PS, Nichols DH.** The relationship between the pubo-urethral ligaments and the urogenital diaphragm in the human female. *Anat Rec* 1971;170:281.

16. **Uhlenhuth E, Wolfe WM, Smith EM, Middleton EB.** The rectovaginal septum. *Surg Gynecol Obstet* 1948;86:148–63.

17. **Nichols DH, Randall CL.** Clinical pelvic anatomy of the living. In: *Vaginal Surgery.* Baltimore: Williams & Wilkins, 1976:1.

18. **Symmonds RE.** Urologic injuries: ureter. In: **Schaefer G, Graber EA,** eds. *Complications in Obstetric and Gynecologic Surgery.* Philadelphia: Harper & Row, 1981:412.

19. **Lawson JO.** Pevic anatomy I. Pelvic floor muscles. *Ann R Coll Surg Engl* 1974;54:244–52.

6 Molecular Biology and Genetics

Vicki V. Baker
Otoniel Martínez-Maza
Jonathan S. Berek

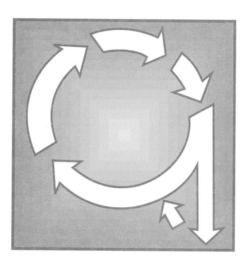

Normal cells are characterized by discrete metabolic, biochemical, and physiologic functions and responses. The observed functions and responses are influenced by the specific cell type and its genetic complement (Fig. 6.1). To orchestrate a coordinated and appropriate response, an external stimulus must be converted to an intracellular signal that is reliably transduced to the nucleus and is then converted to specific genetic messages. Through these steps, extracellular signals prompt changes in cellular function, differentiation, and proliferation. Although specific cell types and tissues by definition exhibit unique functions and characteristics, there are also many aspects of cell biology and genetics that are common to all eukaryotic cells. The general concepts of cell biology and genetics interpreted in the context of the female reproductive system are presented.

Cell Cycle

Normal Cell Cycle

The cell cycle and the factors that influence it are key to cell biology. Control of the cell cycle is the result of multiple levels of complex molecular regulation, the majority of which are poorly understood. **Progression through the cell cycle occurs through four distinct phases; G_1, S, G_2, and M (Fig. 6.2). The duration of the cell cycle (e.g., the *generation time*) may be quite variable, although most human cells complete the cell cycle in approximately 24 hours. Variations in cell cycle time reflect different durations of the G_1 phase.** With respect to the cell cycle, there are three subpopulations of cells—those that are:

1. *Terminally differentiated* and cannot reenter the cell cycle

2. *Quiescent (G_0)* but can enter the cell cycle if appropriately stimulated

3. *Dividing* (e.g., in the cell cycle)

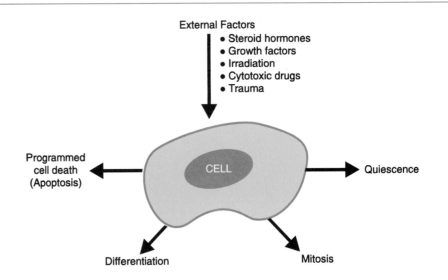

Figure 6.1 External stimuli affect the cell, which has a specific coordinated response.

Figure 6.2 The cell cycle.

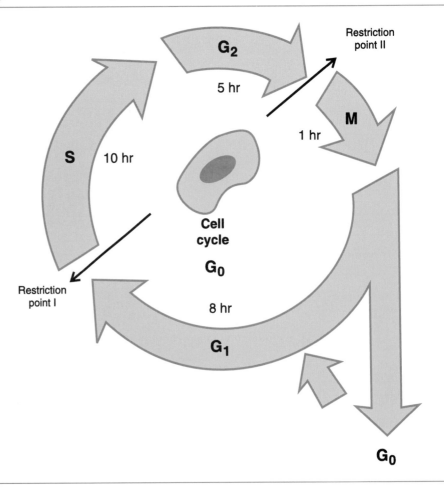

Red blood cells, striated muscle cells, uterine smooth muscle cells, and nerve cells are terminally differentiated. Other cells, such as fibroblasts, exist in the G_0 phase and are considered to be out of the cell cycle. These cells are stimulated to enter the cell cycle following exposure to specific stimuli, such as growth factors and steroid hormones. Dividing cells are found in the gastrointestinal tract, the skin, and the cervix.

G_1

In response to specific external stimuli, cells enter the cell cycle by moving from the G_0 phase into the G_1 phase. The G_1 phase of the cell cycle is characterized by diverse biosynthetic activities. The synthesis of enzymes and regulatory proteins necessary for DNA synthesis occurs during this phase of the cell cycle. **Variation in the duration of the G1 phase of the cell cycle, ranging from less than 8 hours to longer than 100 hours, accounts for the different generation times exhibited by different types of cells.**

S

The nuclear DNA content of the cell is copied during the S phase of the cell cycle. It is not known what actually triggers the initiation of DNA synthesis, but once it begins, it proceeds as an "all-or-none" phenomenon. Upon completion of this phase, the DNA content of the cell is doubled.

G_2

RNA and protein synthesis occurs during the G_2 phase of the cell cycle. The burst of biosynthetic activity provides the metabolic substrates and enzymes to meet the metabolic requirements of the two daughter cells. Another important event that occurs during the G_2 phase of the cell cycle is repair of errors of DNA replication that may have occurred during the S phase. Failure to detect and correct these genetic errors can result in a broad spectrum of adverse consequences for the organism as well as the individual cell (1). Defects in the DNA repair mechanism can be associated with an increased incidence of cancer (2).

M

During mitosis, or the M phase of the cell cycle, nuclear division occurs. During this phase, cellular DNA is equally distributed to each of the daughter cells. Mitosis provides a diploid (2n) DNA complement to each somatic daughter cell. Following mitosis, eukaryotic mammalian cells normally contain diploid (2n) DNA reflecting a karyotype that includes 44 somatic chromosomes and an XX or XY sex chromosome complement. Exceptions to the diploid cellular content include hepatocytes (4n) and the functional syncytium of the placenta.

Ploidy

Germ cells contain a haploid (1n) genetic complement after meiosis. After fertilization, a 46XX or 46XY diploid DNA complement is restored. Restoration of the normal cellular DNA content is crucial to normal function. Abnormalities of cellular DNA content cause distinct phenotypic abnormalities as exemplified by hydatidiform molar pregnancy (see Chapter 35). With complete hydatidiform mole, an oocyte without any nuclear genetic material (e.g., an empty ovum) is fertilized by one sperm. The haploid (1n) genetic content of the fertilized ovum is then duplicated and the diploid cellular DNA content is restored, resulting in a homozygous 46XX gamete. Less often, a complete hydatidiform mole results from the fertilization of an empty ovum by two sperm, resulting in a heterozygous 46XX or 46XY gamete. In complete molar pregnancies, the nuclear DNA is paternally derived, embryonic structures do not develop, and trophoblast hyperplasia occurs. A partial hydatiform mole follows the fertilization of a haploid (1n) ovum by two sperm, resulting in a 69XXX, 69XXY, or 69XYY karyotype. A partial mole contains paternal and maternal DNA, and both embryonic and placental development occur.

Both the 69YYY karyotype and the 46YY karyotype are incompatible with embryonic and placental development. These observations indicate the importance of the maternal genetic contribution, in general, and the X chromosome, in particular, to normal embryonic and placental development.

In addition to total cellular DNA content, the chromosome number is another important determinant of cellular function. Abnormalities of chromosome number, which are often the result of nondisjunction during meiosis, result in well-characterized clinical syndromes such as trisomy 21 (Down's syndrome), trisomy 18, and trisomy 13.

Nuclear division and the allocation of replicated DNA to the daughter cells is closely followed by cytoplasmic division (e.g., *cytokinesis*). Exceptions are hepatocytes and syncytiotrophoblasts, in which several nuclei exist in a common cytoplasm. After mitosis and completion of cellular division, the daughter cells continue in G_1, enter the G_0 phase, or undergo programmed cell death. The option that is pursued by the daughter cell has important implications for the integrity of the tissue and the organ.

Genetic Control of the Cell Cycle

Cellular proliferation must occur to balance cell loss and maintain tissue and organ integrity. This process requires the coordinated expression of many genes at discrete times during the cell cycle (3). To successfully complete the cell cycle, a number of *cell-division-cycle (cdc) genes* are activated. In addition, the cell must traverse two checkpoints, one at the G_1/S boundary and one at the G_2/M boundary (4, 5). **The G_1/S boundary marks the point at which a cell commits to proliferation and the G_2/M boundary marks the point at which repair of any DNA damage must be completed** (6, 7).

Cell Division Cycle Genes

Among the factors that regulate the cell cycle checkpoints, proteins encoded by the *cdc2* family of genes and the cyclin proteins appear to play particularly important roles (8, 9). **The accumulation and degradation of cyclins regulate the checkpoint at the G_1/S boundary.** It has been hypothesized that these proteins bind to specific chromosomal sites. When the chromosomal sites are fully occupied, a critical threshold is exceeded, the free intracellular concentration of cyclins increases, and the cell enters the S-phase of the cycle. By an unknown mechanism, cyclins can also inhibit progression through the cell cycle in the presence of DNA damage.

The *p53* tumor suppressor gene also appears to participate in delay of the cell cycle in order for DNA repair to be completed. As an example, cells exposed to α radiation therapy exhibit an S-phase arrest that is accompanied by increased expression of *p53*. This delay permits the repair of radiation induced DNA damage. When the *p53* gene is mutated, the S-phase arrest that normally follows radiation therapy does not occur (10, 11). A normal *p53* gene that is not mutated can be inactivated when human papillomavirus 16 E6 protein is present, and the S-phase arrest in response to ultraviolet-induced DNA damage does not occur (12).

Mitosis is initiated by activation of the *cdc2* gene at the G_2/M checkpoint (13, 14). The *p34 cdc2* protein and specific cyclins form a complex heterodimer referred to as *mitosis-promoting factor (MPF)*, which catalyzes protein phosphorylation and drives the cell into mitosis. Once the G_2/M checkpoint has been passed, the cell undergoes mitosis. In the presence of abnormally replicated chromosomes, progression past the G_2/M checkpoint does not occur.

Following cytoplasmic division, the daughter cells exit the cell cycle (e.g., enter the G_0 phase), continue in the G_1 phase of the cell cycle, or undergo programmed cell death. Failure of the progeny cells to respond to the signals that regulate cellular proliferation at this point in the cell cycle is a fundamental characteristic of the neoplastic phenotype.

Programmed Cell Death (Apoptosis)

The regulation and maintenance of normal tissue mass requires a balance between cell proliferation and programmed cell death, or *apoptosis.* When proliferation exceeds programmed cell death, the result is hyperplasia. When programmed cell death exceeds proliferation, the result is atrophy. Programmed cell death is a crucial concomitant of normal embryologic development. This mechanism accounts for deletion of the interdigital webs (15), palatal fusion (16), and development of the intestinal mucosa (17). Programmed cell death is also an important phenomenon in normal physiology (18). The reduction in the number of endometrial cells following alterations in steroid hormone levels during the menstrual cycle is, in part, a consequence of programmed cell death (19, 20). Granulosa cells also undergo programmed cell death (e.g. follicular atresia) in response to androgens (21).

Programmed cell death is an energy-dependent, active process that is initiated by the expression of specific genes. It is a process distinct from cell necrosis, although both mechanisms result in a reduction in total cell number. In programmed cell death, cells shrink and undergo phagocytosis and it affects isolated cells. Apoptosis is an energy-dependent process that results from the expression of specific genes. Conversely, in cell necrosis, groups of cells expand and lyse, and it is an energy-independent process that results from noxious stimuli. Programmed cell death is triggered by a variety of factors, including intracellular signals and exogenous stimuli such as radiation exposure, chemotherapy, and hormones. Cells undergoing programmed cell death may be identified on the basis of histologic, biochemical, and molecular biologic changes. Histologically, apoptotic cells exhibit cellular condensation and fragmentation of the nucleus. Biochemical correlates of impending programmed cell death include an increase in transglutaminase expression and fluxes in intracellular calcium concentration. The molecular mechanisms of programmed cell death are the subject of intense investigation (22, 23). The regulation of programmed cell death requires complex interactions between the *bcl-2, c-myc, p53,* and *ced-9* genes, among others.

Programmed cell death has recently emerged as an important factor in the growth of neoplasms. Historically, neoplastic growth has been characterized by uncontrolled cellular proliferation that resulted in a progressive increase in tumor burden. It is now recognized that the increase in tumor burden associated with progressive disease reflects an imbalance between cell proliferation and cell death. Cancer cells not only fail to respond to the normal signals to stop proliferating but they may also fail to recognize the physiologic signals that trigger programmed cell death.

Modulation of Cell Growth and Function

The normal cell exhibits an orchestrated response to the changing extracellular environment. The three groups of substances that signal these extracellular changes are steroid hormones, growth factors, and cytokines. The capability to respond to these stimuli requires a cell surface recognition system, an intracellular signal transduction system, and a means to elicit the expression of specific genes in a coordinated fashion to affect changes in cell structure and function.

Oncogenes and Tumor Suppressor Genes

Among the genes that participate in cell growth and function, *proto-oncogenes* **and** *tumor suppressor genes* **are particularly important** (24–26). *Proto-oncogenes* encode growth factors, membrane and cytoplasmic receptors, proteins that play key roles in the intracellular signal transduction cascade, and nuclear DNA binding proteins (Table 6.1). As a group, proto-oncogenes exert positive effects upon cellular proliferation. More than 50 proto-oncogene products that contribute to growth regulation have been identified. In contradistinction, *tumor suppressor genes* exert inhibitory regulatory effects on cellular proliferation (Table 6.2).

Table 6.1   Proto-oncogenes

Proto-oncogenes	Gene Product/Function
	Growth factors
	Fibroblast growth factor
fgf-5	
sis	Platelet-derived growth factor beta
hst, int-2	
	Transmembrane receptors
erbB	Epidermal-growth-factor (EGF) receptor
HER-2/neu	EGF-related receptor
fms	Colony-stimulating-factor (CSF) receptor
kit	Stem-cell receptor
trk	Nerve-growth-factor receptor
	Inner-membrane receptor
bcl-2	
Ha-ras, N-ras, N-ras	
fgr, lck, src, yes	
	Cytoplasmic messengers
crk	
cot, plm-1, mos, raf/mil	
	Nuclear DNA binding proteins
erbB-1	
jun, ets-1, ets-2, fos, gil 1, rel, ski, vav,	
lyl-1, maf, myb, myc, L-myc, N-myc, evi-1	

Table 6.2   Tumor suppressor genes

p53	Mutated in as many as 50% of solid tumors
Rb	Deletions and mutations predispose retinoblastoma
WT1	Mutations are correlated with Wilms' tumor
NF1	Neurofibromatosis gene
APC	Associated with colon cancer development in patients with familial adenomatous polyposis

Steroid Hormones

Steroid hormones play crucial roles in reproductive biology in addition to general physiology. To mention only a few of their roles, steroid hormones influence pregnancy, phenotype, cardiovascular function, bone metabolism, and an individual's sense of general well-being.

Steroid hormone action reflects the intracellular and genetic mechanisms that are necessary for the transduction of an extracellular signal to the nucleus to affect a physiologic response. Estrogen diffuses through the cell membrane and binds to estrogen receptors that are located in the nucleus. The receptor-steroid complex then binds to the DNA at specific sequences designated as estrogen-response elements (EREs). These steroid-responsive elements are located near the promoter regions of genes that are regulated by estrogen (27). In the uterus, these interactions result in discrete changes in gene expression, protein synthesis, and cellular and tissue function (28).

In any estrogen-responsive tissue, the estrogen receptor plays a pivotal role. The estrogen receptor has been characterized in terms of its molecular biology, structure, function, and tissue distribution. As is the case for all hormone receptors, specificity of action is conferred by the ligand-binding and the DNA-binding domains. Mutations of hormone receptors and their functional consequences illustrate their contributions to normal physiology. As an example, absence of the estrogen receptor in a male human has been reported (29). The clinical sequelae attributed to this mutation include incomplete epiphyseal closure, increased bone turnover, tall stature, and impaired glucose tolerance. The androgen-insensitivity syndrome is caused by mutations of the androgen receptor (30). Mutations of the receptors for growth hormone and thyroid-stimulating hormone have also been identified. A spectrum of phenotypic alterations are associated with these mutations. Mutations of hormone receptors also may contribute to the progression of neoplastic disease. One theory is that variants of the estrogen receptor may contribute to *tamoxifen* resistance in breast cancer, although this hypothesis is not widely accepted (31, 32).

Growth Factors

Growth factors are polypeptides that are produced by a variety of cell types and exhibit a wide range of overlapping biochemical actions (23). Growth factors bind to high-affinity cell membrane receptors and trigger complex positive and negative signaling pathways that regulate cell proliferation and differentiation (34). **In general, growth factors exert positive or negative effects upon the cell cycle by influencing gene expression related to events that occur at the G_1/S cell cycle boundary** (24).

Because of their short half-life in the extracellular space, growth factors generally act over limited distances through autocrine or paracrine mechanisms. The autocrine mechanism of growth control involves the elaboration of a growth factor that acts on the cell that produced it. The paracrine mechanism of growth control involves the elaboration of a growth factor acts on another cell in proximity.

More than 40 growth factors have been described. Those that appear to play important roles in female reproductive physiology are listed in Table 6.3. The biological response of a cell to a specific growth factor depends on the cell type and the other stimuli that are concomitantly acting on the cell. Two growth factors acting in concert may produce a very dif-

Table 6.3   Growth factors that play important roles in female reproductive physiology

Growth Factor	Sources	Targets	Actions
Platelet-derived growth factor (PDGF)	Placenta, platelets, preimplantation embryo, endothelial cells	Endothelial cells Trophoblast	Mitogen
Epidermal growth factor (EGF)	Submaxillary gland, theca cells	Granulosa cells Endometrium, cervix	Mitogen
Transforming growth factor-alpha (TGF-alpha)	Embryo, placenta, theca cell, ovarian stromal cell	Placenta Granulosa cell	Mitogen
Transforming growth factor-beta (TGF-beta)	Embryo, theca cells	Endometrium Granulosa cells Theca cells	Mitogen
Insulin-like growth factor 1 (IGF-1)	Granulosa cell	Theca cell Granulosa cell	Mediates growth hormone activity
Insulin-like growth factor 2 (IGF-2)	Theca cell	Theca cell	Insulin-like effects
Fibroblast growth factor (FGF)	Granulosa cell	Granulosa cell	Angiogenic activity Mitogen

comitantly acting on the cell. Two growth factors acting in concert may produce a very different effect from either factor independently.

The regulation of ovarian function occurs through *autocrine*, *paracrine*, and *endocrine* mechanisms (35–41). The growth and differentiation of ovarian cells is significantly influenced by the *insulin-like growth factors (IGFs)* (Fig. 6.3). The IGFs amplify the actions of gonadotropin hormones on autocrine and paracrine growth factors found in the ovary. As an example, IGF-1 acts on granulosa cells to cause an increase in cyclic adenosine monophosphate (cAMP), progesterone, oxytocin, proteoglycans, and inhibin. IGF-1 acts on theca cells to cause an increase in androgen production. The theca cell in turn produces *tumor necrosis factor-α* (TNF-α) and *epidermal growth factor (EGF),* both of which are also regulated by follicle-stimulating hormone (FSH). EGF acts on granulosa cells to stimulate mitogenesis. IGF-2 is the principal growth factor found in follicular fluid although other factors, including IGF-1, TNF-α, TNF-β, and EGF, also play important roles. Disruption of the autocrine and paracrine intraovarian pathways may be the basis of polycystic ovarian disease and disorders of ovulation.

TGF-β activates intracytoplasmic serine-threonine kinases and inhibits cells in the late G_1 phase of the cell cycle (41). It appears to play an important role in embryonic remodeling. Müllerian Inhibiting Substance (MIS), which is responsible for regression of the müllerian

Figure 6.3 The regulation of ovarian function occurs through autocrine, paracrine, and endocrine mechanisms.

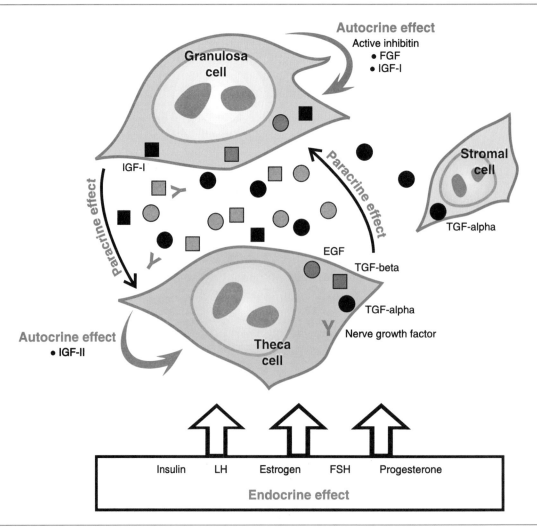

Müllerian Inhibiting Substance (MIS), which is responsible for regression of the müllerian duct, is structurally and functionally related to TGF-β (42).

TGF-α is an EGF homologue that binds to the EGF receptor and acts as an autocrine factor in normal cells. Like EGF, TGF-α promotes entry of G_0 cells into the G_1 phase of the cell cycle.

The role of growth factors in endometrial growth and function has also been the subject of several reviews (36–41). Similar to the ovary, autocrine, paracrine, and endocrine mechanisms of growth and function regulation also occur in endometrial tissue.

Cytokines are soluble medications of immune function that play important roles in normal cell biology in general and reproductive function in particular. They influence ovulation, luteinization, implantation, embryonic development, and healing following surgery. Cytokines may act in concert with growth factors to alter cell growth and differentiation.

Intracellular Signal Transduction

Growth factors trigger intracellular biochemical signals by binding to cell membrane receptors. In general, these membrane-bound receptors are *protein kinases* that convert an extracellular signal into an intracellular signal. The interaction between growth factor ligand and its receptor results in receptor dimerization, autophosphorylation, and *tyrosine kinase activation*. Activated receptors in turn phosphorylate substrates in the cytoplasm and trigger the intracellular signal transduction system (Fig. 6.4). The intracellular signal transduction system relies on serine-threonine kinases, *src*-related kinases, and G-proteins. Intracellular signals in turn activate nuclear effectors that regulate gene expression. **Many of the proteins that participate in the intracellular signal transduction system are encoded by *proto-oncogenes* that are conveniently divided into subgroups based on their cellular location or enzymatic function** (Fig. 6.5).

The *raf* and *mos* proto-oncogenes encode proteins with *serine-threonine kinase* activity. These kinases integrate signals originating at the cell membrane with those that are forwarded to the nucleus (45, 46). *Protein kinase C (PKC)* is an important component of the second messenger system that exhibits serine-threonine kinase activity. This enzyme plays a central role in phosphorylation, which is a general mechanism for activating and deactivating proteins. It also plays an important role in cell metabolism and division (47).

The SCR family of tyrosine kinases is related to PKC and includes protein products encoded by the *scr, yes, fgr, hck, lyn, fyn, lck, alt,* and *fps/fes* proto-oncogenes. These proteins bind to the inner cell membrane surface.

G-proteins   The *G-proteins* are guanyl nucleotide-binding proteins. The heterotrimeric or large G-proteins link receptor activation with effector proteins such as adenyl cyclase, which activates the cAMP-dependent, kinase-signaling cascade (48, 49). The monomeric or small G-proteins, encoded by the ras proto-oncogene family, are designated *p21* and are particularly important regulators of mitogenic signals (50). The *p21 ras* protein exhibits guanyl triphosphate (GTP) binding/GTPase activity. Hydrolysis of GTP to guanyldiphosphate (GDP) terminates *p21 ras* activity. The *p21 ras* protein influences the production of deoxyguanosine (dG) and inositol phosphate (IP)3, arachidonic acid production, and inositol phosphate turnover.

Gene Expression

Regulation of genetic transcription and replication is crucial to the normal function of the daughter cells as well as the tissues and ultimately the organism. Transmission of external signals to the nucleus by way of the intracellular signal transduction cascade culminates in the transcription and translation of specific genes that ultimately affect the structure, function, and proliferation of the cell. Cells of different lineages can be distinguished by their gene product profile.

131

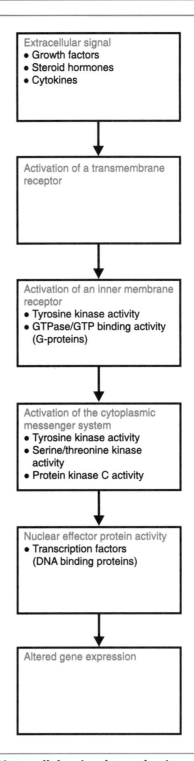

Figure 6.4   Pathways of intracellular signal transduction.

Gene replication, transcription, and translation are imperfect processes and the fidelity is less than 100% (51). Genetic errors may result in abnormal structure and function. Genomic alterations have been identified in premalignant, malignant, and benign neoplasms of the female genital tract (52–54).

In view of the critical roles that oncogenes and tumor suppressor genes play in the regulation of normal cell growth, it is understandable that mutations of these genes may causally

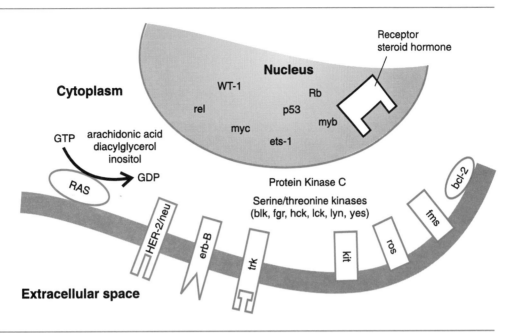

Figure 6.5   Proto-oncogenes are divided into subgroups based on their cellular location or enzymatic function.

contribute to the neoplastic phenotype. By convention, mutated proto-oncogenes are referred to as *c-oncogenes*. Mutations may occur by one of several mechanisms (Fig. 6.6).

***Amplification*   Amplification refers to an increase in the copy number of a gene.** Amplification results in enhanced gene expression by increasing the amount of template DNA that is available for transcription. Proto-oncogene amplification is a relatively common event in malignancies of the female genital tract.

Point Mutations   Point mutations of a gene, in which the codon sequence is altered, may result in altered gene action by qualitatively altering the gene product. The *ras* gene family is perhaps the best example of oncogene-encoded proteins that disrupt the intracellular signal transduction system following mutation. Transforming ras proteins contain point mutations in critical codons, i.e., 11, 12, 59, 61, that reduce GTPase activity so that *ras* is constitutively active in the GTP bound form.

Point mutations of the *p53* gene are the most common genetic mutation described in solid tumors. These mutations occur at preferential "hot spots" that coincide with the most highly conserved regions of the gene. Loss of normal *p53* gene activity removes one of the inhibitors of cell proliferation and also increases the likelihood that DNA damage may be successfully passed to daughter cells.

Deletions and Rearrangements   Deletions and rearrangements reflect gross changes in the DNA template that may result in the synthesis of a markedly altered protein product. As an example, deletion mutations of the EGF receptor affect tyrosine kinase activity. The mutated receptor is activated constitutively and transmits a signal to the cytoplasm for cellular proliferation in the absence of a bound ligand.

Summary   Genetic abnormalities, such as amplification, point mutations, and deletions or rearrangements, are progressive in successive generations. One error tends to permit additional aberrations. A variety of genetic abnormalities has been associated with the neoplastic phenotype. The end result of the genetic abnormalities found in transformed cells is defective control of the cell cycle. Proliferation may be abnormally increased with in-

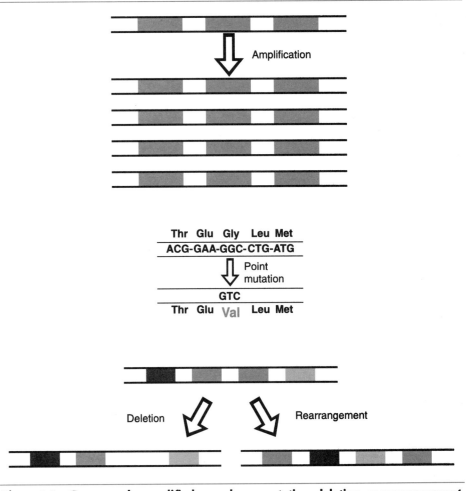

Figure 6.6   Genes can be amplified or undergo mutation, deletion, or rearrangement.

operative normal constraints on cell growth, programmed cell death may fail to occur, or some combination of the two processes may exist.

A single genetic mutation that causes cancer has not been identified. In fact, specific genetic mutations may not be as important as the accumulation of a critical number of mutations. Available data suggest that cancer results from the accumulation of mutations over time in a number of genes (55). From this perspective, exposure to factors that increase the likelihood of genetic mutations over time assumes importance in assessing cancer risk.

Immunology

The immune system plays an essential part in host defense and can respond to host cells that have undergone transformation to become neoplastic cells. These responses, whether natural or induced, can, in some cases, lead to tumor regression. As more is learned about the regulation of immune responses, new opportunities for novel immunotherapeutic approaches develop. Immunodiagnostic procedures using antitumor marker antibodies also show great promise as diagnostic and prognostic tools.

Immunologic Mechanisms

The human immune system has the potential to respond to abnormal or tumor cells in various ways. Some of these immune responses occur in an innate or antigen-nonspecific manner, whereas others are adaptive or antigen specific. Adaptive responses are specific a given antigen and also establish a memory, allowing a more rapid and vigorous response to the same antigen in future encounters (55). Various innate and adaptive immune mechanisms are involved in responses to tumors, including cytotoxicity directed to tumor cells mediated by cytotoxic T cells, natural killer (NK) cells, macrophages, and antibody-dependent cytotoxicity mediated by complementation activation (56).

Adaptive or specific immune responses are made up of humoral and cellular responses. *Humoral immune responses* refer to the production of antibodies that are antigen-reactive, soluble, bifunctional molecules composed of specific antigen-binding sites that react with foreign antigens. They are associated with a constant region that directs the biological activities of the antibody, such as the binding of antibody molecules to cells, including phagocytic cells, or the activation of complement. *Cellular immune responses* are antigen-specific immune responses mediated directly by activated immune cells rather than by the production of antibodies. The distinction between humoral and cellular responses is historical and originates from the experimental observation that humoral immune function can be transferred by serum, whereas cellular immune function requires the transfer of cells. Most immune responses include both humoral and cellular components.

Several types of cells, including cells from both the myeloid and lymphoid lineages, make up the immune system. Specific humoral and cellular immune responses to foreign antigens involve the coordinated action of populations of lymphocytes operating in concert with each other and with phagocytic cells (macrophages). These cellular interactions include both direct cognate interactions involving cell-cell contact and cellular interactions involving the secretion of and response to cytokines or lymphokines. Lymphoid cells are found in lymphoid tissues, such as lymph nodes or spleen, or in the peripheral circulation. The cells that make up the immune system originate from stem cells in the bone marrow.

B Cells, Humoral Immunity, and Monoclonal Antibodies

The cells that synthesize and secrete antibodies are B lymphocytes (56). Mature, antigen-responsive B cells develop from pre-B cells (committed B-cell progenitors) and differentiate to become plasma cells, which produce large quantities of antibodies. Pre-B cells originate from bone marrow stem cells in adults, after the rearrangement of immunoglobin genes from their germ-cell configuration to that seen in B cells. Mature B cells express cell surface immunoglobulin molecules, which these cells use as their receptors for antigen.

On interaction with antigen, and in the presence of appropriate cell–cell stimulatory signals and cytokines, mature B cells respond to become antibody-producing cells. Although the generation of antibodies directed to tumor cells is generally not thought to have a central role in antitumor immune responses, the production of monoclonal antibodies to tumor cell antigens has shown great potential for immunotherapy and tumor detection.

Kohler and Milstein developed monoclonal antibody technology more than 10 years ago, and there has been considerable interest in the use of monoclonal antibodies for detection and monitoring of tumors and for treatment (57). Monoclonal antibodies that react with tumor-associated antigens may provide new therapeutic agents for cancer. Immunotoxin-conjugated monoclonal antibodies directed to human ovarian adenocarcinoma antigens can induce tumor cell killing and can prolong survival in mice implanted with a human ovarian cancer cell line (58). However, many obstacles limit the clinical use of monoclonal antibodies, including tumor cell antigenic heterogeneity, modulation of tumor-associated antigens, and cross-reactivity of normal host and tumor-associated antigens. No unique tumor-specific antigens have been identified; all tumor antigens that have been identified to date are tumor-related antigens, which have been seen to be expressed to some extent in nonmalignant tissues. Because most monoclonal antibodies are murine, the host's immune system can also recognize and respond to these foreign mouse proteins. The use of the genetically engineered monoclonal antibodies composed of human-constant regions with specific antigen-reactive murine variable regions should result in reduced antigenicity to the host (58). This may help eliminate many of the problems associated with using murine monoclonal antibodies.

T Lymphocytes and Cellular Immunity

T lymphocytes have a central role in the generation of immune responses by acting as helper cells in both humoral and cellular immune responses and by acting as effector cells in cellular responses (55). T-cell precursors originate in bone marrow and move to the thymus, where they mature into functional T cells. During their thymic maturation, T cells learn to recognize antigen in the context of the *major histocompatibility complex (MHC)* type of the individual person. It also seems that self-responding T cells are removed during development in the thymus (54–56).

T cells can be distinguished from other types of lymphocytes by their cell surface phenotype, the pattern of expression of various molecules on the cell surface, as well as by differences in their biological functions. All mature T cells express certain cell surface molecules such as the cluster determinant (CD)3 molecular complex and the T-cell antigen receptor, which is found in close association with the CD3 complex. The expression of cell surface molecules can be quantified using monoclonal antibodies specific for these molecules. The availability of monoclonal antibody reagents specific for such markers has led to great progress in understanding the organization of the immune system in recent years. Certainly, such monoclonal antibodies are of great value in monitoring the effects on the human immune system of experimental treatment with biological response modifiers or cytokines.

T cells recognize antigen through the cell-surface T-cell antigen receptor. The structure and molecular organization of this molecule are similar to those of antibody molecules, which are the B-cell receptor for antigen. The T-cell receptor gene undergoes similar gene arrangements during T-cell development to those seen in B cells, but there are important differences between the antigen receptors on B cells and T cells. The T-cell receptor is not secreted, and its structure is somewhat different from that of antibody molecules. The way in which the B-cell and T-cell receptors interact with antigens is also quite different. T cells can respond to antigens only when these antigens are presented in association with MHC molecules on antigen-presenting cells. Effective antigen presentation involves the processing of antigen into small fragments of peptid within the antigen-presenting cell and the subsequent presentation of these fragments of antigen in association with MHC molecules expressed on the surface of the antigen-presenting cell. T cells can respond to antigen only when presented in this manner, unlike B cells, which can bind antigen directly, without processing and presentation by antigen-presenting cells (56).

There are two major subsets of mature T cells that are phenotypically and functionally distinct: *T helper/inducer cells*, **which express the CD4 cell surface marker, and the** *T suppressor/cytotoxic cells*, **which express the CD8 marker.** The expression of these markers is acquired during the passage of T cells through the thymus. CD4 T cells can provide help to B cells, resulting in the production of antibodies by B cells, and interact with antigen presented by antigen-presenting cells in association with MHC class II molecules. CD4 T cells can also act as helper cells for other T cells. CD8 T cells include cells that are cytotoxic (cells that can kill target cells bearing appropriate antigens), and they interact with antigen presented on target cells in association with MHC class I molecules. The CD8 T-cell subset also contains suppressor T cells. Suppressor T cells are cells that can inhibit the biological functions of B cells or other T cells (56).

Although the primary biological role of cytotoxic T cells seems to be lysis of virus-infected autologous cells, cytotoxic immune T cells can mediate the lysis of tumor cells directly. Presumably, cytotoxic T cells recognize antigens associated with MHC class I molecules on tumor cells through their antigen-specific T-cell receptor, setting off a series of events that ultimately results in the lysis of the target cell.

136

Monocytes and Macrophages

Monocytes and macrophages, which are myeloid cells, have important roles in both innate and adaptive immune responses; macrophages play a key part in the generation of immune receptors. T cells do not respond to foreign antigens unless those antigens are processed and presented by antigen-presenting cells. **Macrophages (and B cells) express MHC class II molecules and are effective antigen-presenting cells for CD4 T cells** (55). Helper/inducer (CD4) T cells that bear a T-cell receptor of appropriate antigen and self-specificity are activated by this antigen-presenting cell to provide help (various factors—lymphokines—that induce the activation of other lymphocytes).

In addition to their role as antigen-presenting cells, macrophages play an important part in innate responses by ingesting and killing microorganisms. Activated macrophages, in addition to their many other functional capabilities, can act as cytotoxic, antitumor killer cells.

Natural Killer Cells

A third major population of lymphocytes includes NK cells (55). These do not consistently bear cell surface markers that are characteristic of T or B cells, although they can share certain cell surface molecules with other types of lymphocytes. Characteristically, NK cells have a large granular lymphocyte morphology (59).

NK cells are effector cells in an innate type of immune response: the nonspecific killing of tumor cells and virus-infected cells. Therefore, **NK activity represents an innate form of immunity that does not require an adaptive, memory response for optimal biological function, but the anti-tumor activity can be increased by exposure to several agents, particularly cytokines such as interleukin-2 (IL-2).**

Although NK cells can express certain cell surface receptors, particularly a receptor for the crystallizable fragment (Fc) portion of antibodies and other NK-associated markers, it seems that cells with NK function are phenotypically heterogeneous, at least when compared with T or B cells. The cells that can carry out antibody-dependent cellular cytotoxicity, or antibody-targeted cytotoxicity, seem to be NK-like cells. Antibody-dependent cellular cytotoxicity by NK-like cells has been shown to result in the lysis of tumor cells *in vitro*. The mechanisms of this tumor-cell killing are not clearly understood, although close cellular contact between the effector cell and the target cell seems to be required.

Biological Response Modifiers

Most immunotherapeutic agents used in the treatment of cancer have been nonspecific agents that, when introduced into the human system, elicit a generalized inflammatory reaction and immune response, probably mediated by the secretion of a range of cytokines by many different types of cells. These agents have diverse and broad biological effects and are often referred to as immunomodulators or biological response modifiers.

The response of a given patient to treatment with biological response modifiers depends on the ability to react to treatment with a generalized immune response. It is possible that some elements of the immune response elicited by immunotherapeutic agents or biological response modifiers may be counterproductive, possibly causing immune suppression, inducing the production of cytokines that enhance tumor growth, or inducing an unfavorable or inappropriate immune response.

Bacille Calmette-Guerin (BCG) vaccine has been widely used in many tumor systems, either systemically, by injection into the lesion, or by scarification (60). Occasionally, it has been mixed with whole irradiated tumor cells and injected into the patient as a vaccine. In a large series, intracutaneous injection of melanoma lesions with BCG resulted in some tumor regression in patients with cutaneous recurrence (61), but visceral or parenchymal metastatic disease is resistant to this treatment. Although there have been some preliminary observations about the use of BCG as an adjuvant in children with acute lymphocytic

137

leukemia and with stage II melanoma, randomized studies have not shown any appreciable responses.

Cytokines, Lymphokines, and Immune Mediators

Many events in the generation of immune responses (as well as during the effector phase of immune responses) require or are enhanced by cytokines, which are soluble mediator molecules (Table 6.4) (62–82). Cytokines are pleiotropic, in that they have multiple biological functions that depend on the type of target cell or its maturational state. Cytokines are also heterogeneous, whereas some cytokines seem to be related, in the sense that they share structural features and evolution from a common ancestral precursor, most cytokines share little structural or amino acid homology. *Cytokines* (also called "*monokines*" if they

Table 6.4   Sources, target cells, and biological activities of cytokines involved in immune responses

Cytokine	Cellular source	Target cells	Biological effects
IL-1	Monocytes and macrophages Tumor cells	T cells, B cells Neurons Endothelial cells	Costimulator Pyrogen activation
IL-2	T cells (TH1)	T cells B cells NK cells	Growth Activation and antibody production Activation and growth
IL-3	T cells	Immature hemopoietic stem cells	Growth and differentiation
IL-4	T cells (TH2)	B cells T cells	Activation and growth; isotype switch to IgE; increased MHC II expression Growth
IL-6	Monocytes and macrophages T cells, B cells Ovarian cancer cells Other tumors	B cells T cells Hepatocytes Stem cells Tumor cells	Differentiation, antibody production Costimulator Induction of acute-phase response Growth and differentiation Autocrine/paracrine growth and viability-enhancing factor
IL-10	T cells (TH2) Monocytes and macrophages	T cells (TH1) Monocytes and macrophages B cells	Inhibition of cytokine synthesis Inhibition of Ag presentation and cytokine production Activation
IL-12	Monocytes	NK cells, T cells (TH1)	Induction
IFN gamma	T cells (TH1) NK cells	Monocytes/macrophages NK cells, T cells, B cells	Activation Activation Activation Enhances responses
TNFα	Monocytes and macrophages T cells	Monocytes/macrophages T cells, B cells Neurons (hypothalamus) Endothelial cells Muscle and fat cells	Monokine production Costimulator Pyrogen Activation, inflammation Catabolism/cachexia

Reproduced with permission from **Berek JS, Martínez-Maza O.** Immunology and immunotherapy. In: **Lawton FG, Neijt JP, Swenerton KD.** *Epithelial Cancer of the Ovary.* London: BMJ, 1995:224.

are derived from monocytes, "*lymphokines*" if they are derived from lymphocytes, "*inter-leukins*" if they exert their actions on leukocytes, or "*interferons*" (IFNs) if they have antiviral effects) are produced by a wide variety of cell types and seem to have important roles in many biological responses outside the immune response, such as hematopoiesis. They may also be involved in the pathophysiology of a wide range of diseases and show great potential as therapeutic agents in immunotherapy to cancer.

Although cytokines are a heterogeneous group of proteins, they share some characteristics. For instance, most cytokines are low- to intermediate-molecular-weight (10–60 kDa) glycosylated secreted proteins. They are also involved in immunity and inflammation, are produced transiently and locally (they do not generally act in an endocrine manner), are extremely potent in small concentrations, and interact with high-affinity cellular receptors that are specific for each cytokine. The cell surface binding of cytokines by specific receptors results in signal transduction followed by changes in gene expression and, ultimately, by changes in cellular proliferation or altered cell behavior, or both. Their biological actions overlap, and exposure of responsive cells to multiple cytokines can result in synergistic or antagonistic biological effects.

Interleukins

Many different cytokines are involved in immune responses, particularly the inter-leukins (IL-1, IL-2, IL-3, IL-4, IL-6, IL-7, IL-10, IL-11, and IL-12) (Table 6.4). The interleukins are heterogeneous and do not constitute a family of growth-related molecules.

Interleukin-1   *IL-1* has a wide range of biological activities, including direct effects on several cells involved in immune responses (62–82). It is involved in fever and inflammatory responses and may be involved in the pathogenesis of several diseases, such as rheumatoid arthritis. There are two defined forms of IL-1, IL-1α and IL-1β, which have similar biological activities. IL-1 can be released as a soluble form or can be found as a cell-associated molecule on the cell surface of macrophages. The primary sources of IL-1 are macrophages, the phagocytic cells of the liver and spleen, some B cells, epithelial cells, certain brain cells, and the cells lining the synovial spaces. IL-1 has a broad range of target cells and biological activities, as do most lymphokines.

Interleukin-2   *IL-2* is a lymphokine that was originally called "T-cell growth factor," which indicates one of the major biological activities of this molecule. Failure of T cells to produce IL-2 results in the absence of a T-cell-immune response and a diminution of the antibody response. Natural human IL-2 is a 15 kDa glycoprotein and is produced primarily by activated T cells. For IL-2 to exert its proliferation-inducing effects, it has to interact with a specific receptor for IL-2 on the surface of the target cell. The high-affinity receptor for IL-2 consists of two polypeptides, the α (75 kDa) and β (55 kDA) chains. After activation, T cells express greatly increased numbers of this high-affinity receptor for IL-2.

A principal role of IL-1 is in the initiation of early events in immune responses (62, 68). It functions by inducing antigen-responsive T cells to express the gene for IL-2; these T cells will then express the IL-2 receptor and will respond to IL-2 with increased proliferation. Stimulation of resting T cells with antigen presented in the context of self (antigen associated with an MHC molecule on the surface of an antigen-presenting cell) and with IL-1 therefore induces synthesis and secretion of IL-2. During this activation process, responding T cells undergo a change of alteration in their cell-surface receptors, including the expression of cell-surface receptors for IL-2. Continuing exposure to IL-2 leads to the proliferation of T cells bearing the IL-2 receptor, thereby serving as an activation and response-amplification stage in the generation of immune responses. Activated T cells not only respond to IL-2 but also produce IL-2. IL-2 can therefore act in an autocrine manner (the cells producing the lymphokine then respond to it) or in a paracrine fashion (the IL-2 produced by a T cell is taken up and responded to by neighboring cells).

139

IL-1 has other direct effects on cells of the immune system (62, 68). For instance, it can act as a B-cell activation-inducing factor and can also induce the production of other lymphokines that are involved in immune responses, such as IL-6. Since its original description as a T-cell growth hormone, IL-2 has been shown to have various other immune functions, including the promotion of B-cell activation and maturation and activation of monocytes and NK cells. Interleukin-2 can also lead directly or indirectly to the stimulation of the production of interferon and other cytokines.

Interleukin-3 *IL-3,* a factor that can increase the early differentiation of hematopoietic cells (82), may find a role in immunotherapy because of its ability to induce hematopoietic differentiation in people undergoing aggressive chemotherapeutic treatment or bone marrow transplantation. TNF-α is a cytokine that can be directly cytotoxic for tumor cells, can increase immune-cell-mediated cellular cytoxicity, and can activate macrophages and induce secretion of monokines. Other biological activities of TNF-α include the induction of cachexia, inflammation, and fever; it is an important mediator of endotoxic shock.

Interleukin-4, Interleukin-5, and Interleukin-6 B-lymphocyte activation and differentiation to immunoglobulin-secreting plasma cells is increased by cytokines produced by helper T lymphocytes or monocytes (Table 6.4) (55, 56). Several cytokines originally described as B-cell stimulating factors (*IL-4, IL-5, and IL-6*) have additional biological activities. For instance, IL-6 (a factor that can induce B-lymphocyte differentiation to immunoglobulin-secreting cells) is a pleiotropic cytokine with biological activities that include the induction of cytotoxic T-lymphocyte differentiation, the induction of acute-phase reactant production by hepatocytes, and activity as a colony-stimulating factor for hematopoietic stem cell (63). Interleukin-6 is produced primarily by activated monocyte/macrophages and T lymphocytes. Interestingly, several types of tumor cells produce IL-6, and it has been proposed as an autocrine/paracrine growth factor for different types of neoplasms (64–69). It may prove to be an effective antitumor agent by virtue of its ability to enhance antitumor T-cell-mediated immune responsiveness (69, 70).

Interleukin-8 and Interleukin-10 *IL-10,* a 35–40 kDA cytokine, also called "cytokine synthesis inhibitory factor" because of its activity as an inhibitor of cytokine production, is produced by a subset of CD4 cells, *"type 2" (TH2) cells,* and inhibits the cytokine production by another CD4 cell subset, *"type 1" (TH1) cells* (71). **TH1 and TH2 are two T-helper-cell subpopulations that control the nature of an immune response by secreting a characteristic and mutually antagonistic set of cytokines: TH1 clones produce IL-2, IFN-2, and IFN-α, while TH2 clones produce IL-4, IL-5, IL-6, and IL-10** (72). A similar dichotomy between TH1- and TH2-type responses has been reported in humans (73, 74). Human IL-10 inhibits the production of IFN-α and other cytokines by human peripheral blood mononuclear cells (75) and by suppressing the release of cytokines (IL-1, IL-6, *IL-8,* and IL-α) by activated monocytes (76–78). IL-10 also downregulates class II MHC expression on monocytes, resulting in a strong reduction in the antigen-presenting capacity of these cells (78). Together, these observations support the concept that IL-10 has an important role as an immune-inhibitory cytokine.

Because epithelial cancers of the ovary usually remain confined to the peritoneal cavity, even in the advanced stages of the disease, it has been suggested that the growth of ovarian cancer intraperitoneally could be related to a local deficiency of antitumor immune effector mechanisms (79). Studies have shown that ascitic fluid from patients with ovarian cancer contained increased concentrations of IL-10 (80). Various other cytokines are also seen in ascites obtained from women with ovarian cancer; concentrations of IL-6, IL-10, TNF-α, *granulocyte colony stimulating factor (G-CSF),* and *granulocyte macrophage colony stimulating factor (GM-CSF)* were raised appreciably (81). A similar pattern was seen in serum samples from women with ovarian cancer; IL-6 and IL-10 were often detected. Preliminary results have indicated that ovarian cancer cells do not produce IL-10, so high concentrations of IL-10 could certainly result in a peritoneal environment characterized by immune unresponsiveness and promotion of tumor growth.

Interferons

There are three types of interferons: IFN-α, IFN-β, and IFN-γ (54, 55, 83). They can interfere with viral production in infected cells and have various effects on the immune system as well as direct antitumor effects. For instance, IFN-α (a cytokine produced by T lymphocytes) can affect immune function by increasing the induction of MHC molecule expression, increasing the activity of antigen-presenting cells and thereby increasing T lymphocyte activation.

Cytokines in Cancer Therapy

Cytokines are extraordinarily pleiotropic with a bewildering array of biological activities, including some outside the immune system (54, 55, 63, 69). Because some cytokines have direct or indirect antitumor and immune-enhancing effects, several of these factors have been used in the experimental treatment of cancer.

The precise roles of cytokines in antitumor responses have not been completely described. Cytokines could exert antitumor effects by many different direct or indirect activities. It is possible that a single cytokine could increase tumor growth directly by acting as a growth factor, while at the same time increasing immune responses directed to the tumor. The potential of cytokines to increase antitumor immune responses has been tested in experimental adoptive immunotherapy by exposing the patient's peripheral blood cells or tumor-infiltrating lymphocytes to cytokines such as IL-2 *in vitro*, thus generating activated cells with antitumor effects that can be given back to the patient (84–86). Some cytokines can also exert direct antitumor effects: TNF can induce cell death in sensitive tumor cells.

The effects of cytokines on patients with cancer might be modulated by soluble receptors or blocking factors. For instance, blocking factors for TNF and for lymphotoxin were found in ascites from patients with ovarian cancer (87). Such factors could inhibit the cytolytic effects of TNF or lymphotoxin and should be taken into account in the design of clinical trials of intraperitoneal infusion of these cytokines.

Cytokines have growth-increasing effects on tumor cells in addition to inducing antitumor effects: they can act as autocrine or paracrine growth factors for human tumor cells, including those of nonlymphoid origin. For instance, IL-6 (which is produced by various types of human tumor cells) can act as a growth factor for human myeloma, Kaposi's sarcoma, renal carcinoma, and epithelial ovarian cancer cells (63–69).

Clearly, cytokines are of great potential value in the treatment of cancer, but because of their multiple, even conflicting biological effects, a thorough understanding of cytokine biology is essential for their successful use in the treatment of cancer (83–91).

Adoptive Immunotherapy   Recently, the *ex vivo* enhancement of antitumor immune cell responses, including the generation of lymphokine-activated killer (LAK) cells or the activation of tumor-infiltrating lymphocytes, has provided new immune system-based approaches for antitumor responses. In particular, adoptive immunotherapy with IL-2 can produce regression of tumor in various animal and human tumors, such as melanoma and renal cell carcinoma, when used in conjunction with the adoptive transfer of autologous LAK cells (84, 85).

Exposure of peripheral blood monoclonal cells to cytokines *in vitro* (particularly IL-2) leads to the generation of cytotoxic effect cells called "LAK cells" (85). These cells are cytotoxic for various tumor cells, including those that are resistant to NK-cell- or T-cell-mediated lysis. The treatment of patients with such *ex vivo* activated autologous cells, together with IL-2, simultaneously forms the basis of adoptive immunotherapy, a form of experimental antitumor immunotherapy.

Experimental treatment of human subjects with autologous *ex vivo* generated LAK cells and IL-2 has yielded tumor regression in some cases (84–88). This sort of treatment has resulted in some complete responses (86); the combined response rate was 27% in 146 patients with cancer who were treated in two separate studies (88–90). The overall response rate to LAK treatment is low, however, and this type of adoptive immunotherapy causes high morbidity (90). It is also costly and impractical in most medical settings.

Much current experimental work is aimed at developing more efficient and practical applications of adoptive immunotherapy (91–97). One approach involves the *ex vivo* generation of immune effector cells from tumor-infiltrating lymphocytes, which are lymphocytes that are isolated from tumors and activated and expanded *in vitro* by exposure to IL-2. They are then given concurrently with IL-2 (91, 92). This approach is hampered by the need to expand a limited number of tumor-infiltrating lymphocytes *in vitro* to generate enough effector cells for treatment. Much attention has also been directed toward the development of new methods for the generation of LAK cells or tumor-infiltrating lymphocytes, including methods that use cytokines other than IL-2 to stimulate these cells.

Another promising approach that has been explored in animal studies involves the targeting of activated T lymphocytes with a bifunctional monoclonal antibody that binds to the CD3/T-cell receptor complex (on the target tumor cell) (93). This approach has the potential advantage of allowing a large number of the activated lymphocytes to target their effects directly on tumor cells, thereby reducing the need to amplify a large number of effector cells from tumor-infiltrating lymphocytes. It also has the potential to reduce some of the side effects associated with LAK treatment, which is a more nonspecific form of adoptive immunotherapy. Adoptive immunotherapy is an active area of study and may eventually lead to effective forms of antitumor treatment.

Factors that Trigger Neoplasia

Cell biology is characterized by considerable redundancy and functional overlap so that a defect in one mechanism does not invariably jeopardize the function of the cell. However, with a sufficient number of abnormalities in structure and function, normal cell function is jeopardized and uncontrolled cell growth or cell death results. Either end point may result from accumulated genetic mutations over time. Factors have been identified that enhance the likelihood of genetic mutations, jeopardize normal cell biology, and may increase the risk of cancer.

Advanced Age

Increasing age is considered the single most important risk factor for the development of cancer (98). Cancer is diagnosed in as many as 50% of the population by 75 years of age (99). It has been suggested that the increasing risk of cancer with age reflects the accumulation of critical genetic mutations over time that ultimately culminate in neoplastic transformation. The basic premise of the multistep somatic mutation theory of carcinogenesis is that genetic or epigenetic alterations of numerous independent genes results in cancer. Factors that have been associated with an increased likelihood of cancer include exposure to exogenous mutagens, altered host immune function, and certain inherited genetic syndromes and disorders.

Environmental Factors

A number of environmental pollutants act as mutagens when tested *in vitro*. A mutagen is a compound that results in a genetic mutation. Environmental mutagens usually produce specific types of mutations that can be differentiated from spontaneous mutations. As an example, activated hydrocarbons tend to produce G-T transversions (100). A carcinogen

142

is a compound that can produce cancer. It is important to recognize that all carcinogens are not mutagens and that all mutagens are not necessarily carcinogens.

Smoking

Cigarette smoking is perhaps the best known example of mutagen exposure that is associated with the development of lung cancer when the exposure is of sufficient duration and quantity in a susceptible individual. An association between cigarette smoking and cervical cancer has been recognized for decades. More recently, it has been determined that the mutagens in cigarette smoke are selectively concentrated in cervical mucus (52). It has been hypothesized that exposure of the proliferating epithelial cells of the transformation zone to cigarette smoke mutagens may increase the likelihood of DNA damage and subsequent cellular transformation.

Radiation

Radiation exposure can also be considered an environmental mutagen that increases the risk of cancer. This statement does not apply to exposure secondary to diagnostic radiology studies, which is not associated with an increased risk of cancer. Interestingly, the overall risk of radiation-induced cancer is approximately 10% greater in women than in men (101). This difference has been attributed to gender-specific cancers, including breast cancer. With respect to gynecology, radiation therapy of cervical cancer is associated with a small increase in the risk of colon cancer and thyroid cancer.

Radiation-induced cancer may be the result of sublethal DNA damage that is not repaired (101). Normally, radiation damage prompts an S-phase arrest so that DNA damage is repaired. This requires normal *p53* gene function. If DNA repair does not occur for some reason, the damaged DNA is propagated to daughter cells following mitosis. If a sufficient number of critical genes are mutated, cellular transformation may result.

Immune Function

Systemic immune dysfunction has been recognized as a risk factor for cancer for decades. The immunosuppressed renal transplant patient may have a 40-fold increased risk of cervical cancer (52). More recently, patients infected with human immunodeficiency virus (HIV) who have a depressed CD4 cell count have been reported to be at increased risk of cervical dysplasia and invasive disease (96). Both of these examples illustrate the importance of immune function in host surveillance for transformed cells.

Another interesting example of altered immune function that may be related to the development of cervical dysplasia is the alteration in mucosal immune function that occurs in women who smoke cigarettes (52). The Langerhans cell population of the cervix is decreased in women who smoke. Langerhans cells are responsible for antigen processing. It is postulated that a reduction in these cells increases the likelihood of successful human papillomavirus infection of the cervix.

Diet

The role of diet in disease prevention and predisposition is widely recognized but poorly understood (96, 99). Dietary fat intake has been correlated with the risk of colon and breast cancer. Fiber is considered protective against colon cancer. With respect to the female reproductive system, epidemiologic studies provide conflicting results. Deficiencies of folic acid and vitamins A and C have been associated with the development of cervical dysplasia and cervical cancer. Considerable research must be performed to clarify the impact of diet on cancer prevention and development.

References

1. **Taylor AM, McConville CM, Byrd PJ.** Cancer and DNA processing disorders. *Br Med Bull* 1994;50:708–17.

2. **Kraemer KH, Levy DD, Parris CN, Gozukara EM, Moriwaki S, Adelberg S, et al.** Xeroderma pigmentosum and related disorders: examining the linkage between defective DNA repair and cancer. *J Invest Dermatol* 1994;103(Suppl 5):96S–101S.

3. **Jacobs T.** Control of the cell cycle. *Dev Biol* 1992;153:1–15.

4. **Weinert T, Lydall D.** Cell cycle checkpoints, genetic instability and cancer. *Can Biol* 1993;4:129–40.

5. **Fridovich-Keil JL, Hansen LJ, Keyomarsi K, Pardee AB.** Progression through the cell cycle: an overview. *Am Rev Respir Dis* 1990;142:53–6.

6. **Reddy GP.** Cell cycle: regulatory events in $G_1 - S$ transition of mammalian cells. *J Cell Biochem* 1994;54:379–86.

7. **Hartwell LH, Weinert TA.** Checkpoints: controls that ensure the order of cell cycle events. *Science* 1989;246:629–34.

8. **Murray AW, Kirschner MW.** Dominoes and clocks: the union of two views of the cell cycle. *Science* 1989;246:614–21.

9. **Lee MG, Norbury CJ, Spurr NK, Nurse P.** Regulated expression and phosphorylation of a possible mammalian cell-cycle control protein. *Nature* 1988;333:257–67.

10. **Kastan MB, Onyekwere O, Sidransky D, Vogelstein B, Craig RW.** Participation of p53 protein in the cellular response to DNA damage. *Cancer Res* 1991;51:6304–11.

11. **Kuerbitz SJ, Plunkett BS, Walsh WV, Kastan MB.** Wild type p53 is a cell cycle checkpoint determinant following irradiation. *Proc Natl Acad Sci U S A* 1992;89:7491–5.

12. **Gu Z, Pim D, Labrecque S, Banks L, Matlashewski G.** DNA damage induced p53 mediated transcription in inhibited by human papillomavirus type 18 E6. *Oncogene* 1994;9:629–33.

13. **Morena S, Nurse P.** Substrates for p34cdc2: in vivo veritas? *Cell* 1990;61:549–51.

14. **Lewin B.** Driving the cell cycle: M-phase kinase, its partners, and substrates. *Cell* 1990;61:743–52.

15. **Hammar SP, Mottet NK.** Tetrazolium salt and electron microscopic studies of cellular degeneration and necrosis in the interdigital areas of the developing chick limb. *J Cell Sci* 1971;8:229.

16. **Farbman AI.** Electron microscopic study of palate fusion in mouse embryos. *Dev Biol* 1968;18:93.

17. **Harmonn B, Bell L, Williams L.** An ultrasound study on the meconium corpuscles in rat foetal epithelium with particular reference to apoptosis. *Anat Embryol* 1984;169:119.

18. **Cotter TG, Lennon SV, Glynn JG, Martin SJ.** Cell death via apoptosis and its relationship to growth, development, and differentiation of both tumor and normal cells. *Anticancer Res* 1990;10:1153–60.

19. **Pollard JW, Pacey J, Cheng SUY, Jordan EG.** Estrogens and cell death in murine uterine luminal epithelium. *Cell Tissue Res* 1987;249:533–40.

20. **Nawaz S, Lynch MP, Galand P, Gershenson LE.** Hormonal regulation of cell death in rabbit uterine epithelium. *Am J Pathol* 1987;127:51–9.

21. **Billig H, Furuta I, Hsueh AJW.** Estrogens inhibit and androgens enhance ovarian granulosa cell apoptosis. *Endocrinology* 1993;33:2204–12.

22. **Williams GT, Smith CA.** Molecular regulation of apoptosis: genetic controls on cell death. *Cell* 1993;74:777–9.

23. **Vaux DL.** Toward an understanding of the molecular mechanisms of physiological cell death. *Proc Natl Acad Sci U S A* 1993;90:786–9.

24. **Baserga R, Porcu P, Sell C.** Oncogenes, growth factors, and control of the cell cycle. *Cancer Surv* 1993;16:201–13.

25. **Smith MR, Matthews NT, Jones KA, Kung H-F.** Biological actions of oncogenes. *Pharmacol Ther* 1993;58:211–36.

26. **Studzinski GP.** Oncogenes, growth and the cell cycle: an overview. *Cell Tissue Kinet* 1989;22:405–24.

27. **Landers JP, Spelsberg TC.** New concepts in steroid hormone action: transcription factors, proto-oncogenes and the cascade model for steroid regulation of gene expression. *Crit Rev Eukaryot Gene Expr* 1993;2:19–63.

28. **Stancel GM, Baker VV, Hyder SM, Kirkland JL, Loose-Mitchell DS.** Oncogenes and uterine function. In: **Milligan SR,** ed. *Oxf Rev Reprod Biol* 1993:1–42.

29. **Smith EP, Boyd J, Frank GR, Takahashi H, Cohen RM, Specker B, et al.** Estrogen resistance caused by a mutation of the estrogen receptor gene in a man. *N Engl J Med* 1994; 331:1056–61.

30. **De Bellis A, Quigley CA, Marschke KB, el-Awady MK, Lane MV, Smith EP, et al.** Characterization of mutant androgen receptors causing partial androgen insensitivity syndrome. *J Clin Endocrinol Metab* 1994;78:513–22.

31. **Fuqua SA.** Estrogen receptor mutagenesis and hormone resistance. *Cancer* 1994;74:1026–9.

32. **Osborne CK, Fuqua SA.** Mechanisms of tamoxifen resistance. *Breast Cancer Res Treat* 1994;32:49–55.

33. **Pusztal L, Lewis CE, Lorenzen J, McGee JOD.** Growth factors: regulation of normal and neoplastic growth. *J Pathol* 1993;169:191–201.

34. **Aaronson SA, Rubin JS, Finch PW, Wong J, Marchese C, Falco J, et al.** Growth factor regulated pathways in epithelial cell proliferation. *Am Rev Respir Dis* 1990;142:S7-10.

35. **Giordano G, Barreca A, Minuto F.** Growth factors in the ovary. *J Endocrinol Invest* 1992; 15:689–707.

36. **Baldi E, Bonaccorsi L, Finetti G, Luconi M, Muratori M, Susini T, et al.** Platelet activating factor in human endometrium. *J Steroid Biochem Mol Biol* 1994;49:359–63.

37. **Gold LI, Saxena B, Mittal KR, Marmor M, Goswami S, Nactigal L, et al.** Increased expression of transforming growth factor B isoforms and basic fibroblast growth factor in complex hyperplasia and adenocarcinoma of the endometrium: evidence for paracrine and autocrine action. *Cancer Res* 1994;54:2347–58.

38. **Leake R, Carr L, Rinaldi F.** Autocrine and paracrine effects in the endometrium. *Ann N Y Acad Sci* 1991;622:145–8.

39. **Giudice LC.** Growth factors and growth modulators in human uterine endometrium: their potential relevance to reproductive medicine. *Fertil Steril* 1994;61:1–17.

40. **Murphy LJ.** Growth factors and steroid hormone action in endometrial cancer. *J Steroid Biochem Mol Biol* 1994;48:419–23.

41. **Laiho M, DeCaprio JA, Ludlow JW, Livingston DM, Massaque J.** Growth inhibition by TGF-beta linked to suppression of retinoblastoma protein phosphorylation. *Cell* 1990;62: 175–85.

42. **Cate RL, Donahoe PK, MacLaughlin DT.** Müllerian-inhibiting substance. In: **Sporn MB, Roberts AB,** eds. *Peptide Growth Factors and Their Receptors.* Vol II. Berlin: Springer-Verlag, 1990:179–210.

43. **Bates SE, Valverius EM, Ennis BW, Bronzert DA, Sheridan JP, Stampfer MR, et al.** Expression of the transforming growth factor alpha/epidermal growth factor receptor pathway in normal human breast epithelial cells. *Endocrinology* 1990;126:596–607.

44. **Hunter T.** Protein kinase classification. *Methods Enzymol* 1991;200:3–37.

45. **Ralph RK, Darkin-Rattray S, Schofield P.** Growth-related protein kinases. *Bioessays* 1990;12:121–3.

46. **Simon MI, Strathmann MP, Gautam N.** Diversity of G-proteins in signal transduction. *Science* 1991;252:802–8.

47. **Speigel AM.** G-proteins in cellular control. *Curr Opin Cell Biol* 1992;4:203–11.

48. **Hall A.** The cellular function of small GTP-binding proteins. *Science* 1990;249:635–40.

49. **Mendelsohn ML.** The somatic mutational component of human carcinogenesis. In: **Moolgavkar SH,** ed. *Scientific Issues in Quantitative Cancer Risk Assessment.* New York: Birkhaeuser, Boston, Inc., 1990:22–31.

50. **Baker VV.** The molecular biology of endometrial cancer. *Clin Consult Obstet Gynecol* 1993; 5:95–9.

51. **Baker VV.** The molecular genetics of epithelial ovarian cancer. *Clin Obstet Gynecol* 1994; 21:25–40.

52. **Baker VV.** Update on the molecular carcinogenesis of cervix cancer. *Clin Consult Obstet Gynecol* 1995;7:86–93.

53. **Barrett JC.** Genetic and epigenetic mechanisms in carcinogenesis. In: **Barrett JD**, ed. *Mechanisms of Environmental Carcinogenesis.* Vol 1. Role of Genetic and Epigenetic Changes. Boca Raton: CRC Press, 1987:1–15.

54. **Abbas AK, Lictman AH, Pober JS.** *Cellular and Molecular Immunology.* Philadelphia: WB Saunders, 1991.

55. **Roitt I, Brostoff J, Male D.** *Immunology.* 2nd ed. London: Gower Medical Publishing, 1989.

56. **Boyer CM, Knapp RC, Bast RC Jr.** Biology and immunology. In: **Berek JS, Hacker NF,** eds. *Practical Gynecologic Oncology.* 2nd ed. Baltimore: Williams & Wilkins, 1994:75–115.

57. **Kohler G, Milstein C.** Continuous cultures of fused cells secreting antibody of predefined specificity. *Nature* 1978;256:495–7.

58. **Ettenson D, Sheldon K, Marks A, Houston LL, Baumal R.** Comparison of growth inhibition of a human ovarian adenocarcinoma cell line by free monoclonal antibodies and their corresponding antibody-recombinant ricin A chain immunotoxins. *Anticancer Res* 1988;8:833–8.

59. **Ortaldo JR, Herberman RB.** Heterogeneity of natural killer cells. *Ann Rev Immunol* 1984;2:359.

60. **Bast RC, Zbar B, Borsos T, Rapp RJ.** BCG and cancer. *N Engl J Med* 1974;290:1413–58.

61. **Borstein RS, Mastrangelo MJ, Sulit H.** Immunotherapy of melanoma with intralesional BCG. *Natl Cancer Inst Monogr* 1973;39:213–20.

62. **Di Giovine FS, Duff GW.** Interleukin 1: the first interleukin. *Immunol Today* 1990;11:13–20.

63. **Hirano T, Akira S, Taga T, Kishimoto T.** Biological and clinical aspects of interleukin 6. *Immunol Today* 1990;11:443–9.

64. **Watson JM, Sensintaffar JL, Berek JS, Martínez-Maza O.** Epithelial ovarian cancer cells constitutively produce interleukin-6 (IL-6). *Cancer Res* 1990;50:6959–65.

65. **Berek JS, Chang C, Kaldi K, Watson JM, Knox RM, Martínez-Maza O.** Serum interleukin-6 levels correlate with disease status in patients with epithelial ovarian cancer. *Am J Obstet Gynecol* 1991;164:1038–43.

66. **Miles SA, Rezai AR, Salazar-Gonzalez JF, Vander Meyden M, Stevens RH, Logan DM, et al.** AIDS Kaposi's sarcoma-derived cells produce and respond to interleukin-6. *Proc Natl Acad Sci U S A* 1990;87:4068–72.

67. **Miki S, Iwano M, Miki Y, Yamamoto M, Tang B, Yokokawa K, et al.** Interleukin-6 (IL-6) functions as an in vitro autocrine growth factor in renal cell carcinomas. *FEBS Lett* 1989;250:607–10.

68. **Wu S, Rodabaugh K, Martínez-Maza O, Watson JM, Silberstein DS, Boyer CM, et al.** Stimulation of ovarian tumor cell proliferation with monocyte products including interleukin-1, interleukin-6 and tumor necrosis factor-α. *Am J Obstet Gynecol* 1992;166:997–1007.

69. **Martínez-Maza O, Berek JS.** Interkeukin 6 and cancer therapy. *In Vivo* 911;5:583.

70. **Mule JJ, McIntosh JK, Jablons DM, Rosenberg SA.** Antitumor activity of recombinant interleukin 6 in mice. *J Exp Med* 1990;171:629–36.

71. **Fiorentino DF, Bond MW, Mosmann TR.** Two types of mouse helper T cells. IV. Th2 clones secrete a factor that inhibits cytokine production by Th1 clones. *J Exp Med* 1989;170:2081–95.

72. **Mosmann TR, Moore KW.** The role IL-10 in crossregulation of TH1 and TH2 responses. *Immunol Today* 1991;12:A49.

73. **Del Prete GF, De Carli M, Ricci M, Romagnant S.** Helper activity for immunoglobulin synthesis of T helper type 1 (TH1) and TH2 human T cell clones: the help of TH1 clones is limited by their cytolytic capacity. *J Exp Med* 1991;174:809–13.

74. **Romagnani S.** Human TH1 and TH2 subsets: doubt no more. *Immunol Today* 1991;12:256–7.

75. **Zlotnik A, Moore KW.** Interleukin 10. *Cytokine* 1991;3:366–71.

76. **Fiorentino DF, Zlotnik A, Mosmann TR, Howard M, O'Garra A.** IL-10 inhibits cytokine production by activated macrophages. *J Immunol* 1991;147:3815–22.

77. **Bogdan C, Vodovotz Y, Nathan C.** Macrophage deactivation by IL-10. *J Exp Med* 1991;174:1549–55.

146

78. **de Waal Malefyt R, Abrams J, Bennett B, Figador CG, de Vries JE.** Interleukin-10 (IL-10) inhibits cytokine synthesis by human monocytes: an autoregulatory role of IL-10 produced by monocytes. *J Exp Med* 1991;174:1209–20.

79. **Berek JS.** Epithelial ovarian cancer. In: **Berek JS, Hacker NF,** eds. *Practical Gynecologic Oncology.* 2nd ed. Baltimore: Williams & Wilkins, 1994:327–75.

80. **Gotlieb WH, Abrams JS, Watson JM, Velu T, Berek JS, Martínez-Maza O.** Presence of IL-10 in the ascites of patients with ovarian and other intraabdominal cancers. *Cytokine* 1992;4: 385–90.

81. **Watson JM, Gotlieb WH, Abrams JH, Kaldi K, Martínez-Maza O, Berek JS.** Cytokine profiles in ascitic fluid from patients with ovarian cancer: relationship to levels of acute phase proteins and immunoglobulins, immunosuppression and tumor classification. *Proc Soc Gynecol Invest* 1993;186:8.

82. **Shrader JW.** The panspecific hemopoietin of activated T lymphocytes (interleukin-3). *Annu Rev Immunol* 1986;4:205–30.

83. **Golub SH.** Immunological and therapeutic effects of interferon treatment of cancer patients. *Clin Immunol Allergy* 1984;4:377–41.

84. **Rosenberg SA.** Immunotherapy of cancer by systemic administration of lymphoid cells plus interleukin-2. *J Biol Resp Mod* 1984;3:501–11.

85. **Rosenberg SA, Lotze MT.** Cancer immunotherapy using interleukin-2 and interleukin-2 activated lymphocytes. *Annu Rev Immunol* 1986;4:681–709.

86. **Rosenberg SA, Lotze MT, Muul LM, Leitman S, Chang AE, Ettinghausen SE, et al.** Observations on the systemic administration of autologous lymphokine-activated killer cells and recombinant interleukin-2 to patients with metastatic cancer. *N Engl J Med* 1985;313:1485–92.

87. **Cappuccini F, Yamamoto RS, DiSaia PJ, Grosen EA, Gatanaga M, Lucci JA, et al.** Identification of tumor necrosis factor and lymphotoxin blocking factor(s) in the ascites of patients with advanced and recurrent ovarian cancer. *Lymphokine Cytokine Res* 1991;10:225–9.

88. **Rosenberg SA, Lotze MT, Muul LM, Chang AE, Avis FP, Leitman S, et al.** A progress report on the treatment of 157 patients with advanced cancer using lymphokine-activated killer cells and interleukin-2 or high-dose interleukin-2 alone. *N Engl J Med* 1987;316:889–97.

89. **West WH, Tauer KW, Yannelli JR, Marshall GD, Orr DW, Thurman GB, et al.** Constant-infusion recombinant interleukin-2 in adoptive immunotherapy of advanced cancer. *N Engl J Med* 1987;316:898–905.

90. **Berek JS.** Intraperitoneal adoptive immunotherapy for peritoneal cancer. *J Clin Oncol* 1990;8:1610–12.

91. **Topalian SL, Solomon D, Avis FP, Chang AE, Freerksen DL, Linehan WM, et al.** Immunotherapy of patients with advanced cancer using tumor infiltrating lymphocytes and recombinant interleukin-2: a pilot study. *J Clin Oncol* 1988;6:839–53.

92. **Lotzova E.** Role of human circulating and tumor-infiltrating lymphocytes in cancer defense and treatment. *Nat Immun* 1990;9:253–64.

93. **Garrido MA, Valdayo MJ, Winkler DF, Titus JA, Hecht TT, Perez P, et al.** Targeting human T-lymphocytes with bispecific antibodies to react against human ovarian carcinoma cells growing in nu/nu mice. *Cancer Res* 1990;50:4227–32.

94. **Bookman MA, Berek JS.** Biologic and immunologic therapy of ovarian cancer. *Hematol Oncol Clin North Am* 1992;6:941–65.

95. **Zighelboim J, Nio Y, Berek JS, Bonavida B.** Immunologic control of ovarian cancer. *Natural Immun* 1988;7:216–25.

96. **Berek JS, Martínez-Maza O, Montz FJ.** The immune system and gynecologic cancer. In: **Coppelson M, Tattersall M, Morrow CP,** eds. *Gynecologic Oncology.* Edinburgh: Churchill Livingstone, 1992:119.

97. **Berek JS, Lichtenstein AK, Knox RM, Jung TS, Rose TP, Cantrell JL, et al.** Synergistic effects of combination sequential immunotherapies in a murine ovarian cancer model. *Cancer Res* 1985;45:4215–8.

98. **Newell GR, Spitz MR, Sider JG.** Cancer and age. *Semin Oncol* 1989;16:3–9.

99. **Yancik R.** *Perspectives on Prevention and Treatment of Cancer in the Elderly.* New York: Raven Press, 1983.

100. **Maher VM, Yang JL, Mah MC, McCormick JJ.** Comparing the frequency of and spectra of mutations induced when an SV-40 based shuttle vector containing covalently bound residues of structurally-related carcinogens replicates in human cells. *Mutat Res* 1989;220: 83–92.

101. **National Research Council.** *Health Effects of Exposure to Low Levels of Ionizing Radiation (BEIR V).* Washington, DC: National Academy Press, 1990.

Portions reproduced with permission from **Berek JS, Martínez-Maza O.** Immunology and immunotherapy of ovarian cancer. In: **Lawton FG, Neijt JP, Swenerton KD.** *Epithelial Cancer of the Ovary.* London: BMJ, 1995:220–47.

7

Reproductive Physiology

Steven F. Palter
David L. Olive

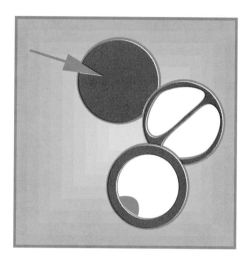

Neuroendocrinology

Neuroendocrinology represents facets of two traditional fields of medicine: endocrinology, which is the study of hormones (i.e., substances secreted into the bloodstream that have diverse actions at sites remote from the point of secretion), and neuroscience, which is the study of the action of neurons. The discovery of neurons that transmit impulses and secrete their products into the vascular system to function as hormones themselves, a process known as neurosecretion, demonstrates that the two systems are intimately linked. For instance, the regulation of the menstrual cycle is through the feedback of hormones on the neural tissue of the central nervous system (CNS).

Anatomy

Hypothalamus

The hypothalamus is a small neural structure situated at the base of the brain above the optic chiasm and below the third ventricle (Fig. 7.1). It is connected directly to the pituitary gland and is the part of the brain that is the source of many pituitary secretions. Anatomically, the hypothalamus is divided into three zones: *periventricular* (adjacent to the third ventricle), *medial* (primarily cell bodies), and *lateral* (primarily axonal). Each zone is further subdivided into structures known as nuclei, which represent locations of concentrations of similar types of neuronal cell bodies (Fig. 7.2).

Hypothalamic Interconnection: Input and Output

The hypothalamus is not an isolated structure within the CNS; instead, it has multiple interconnections with other regions in the brain. In addition to the well-known pathways of hypothalamic output to the pituitary, there are numerous less well-characterized pathways of output to diverse regions of the brain, including the limbic system (amygdala and hippocampus), the thalamus, and the pons (1). Many of these pathways form feedback loops to areas supplying neural input to the hypothalamus.

149

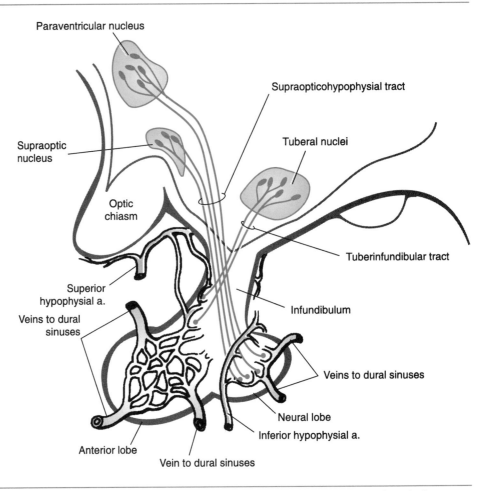

Paraventricular nucleus

Supraopticohypophysial tract

Supraoptic nucleus

Tuberal nuclei

Optic chiasm

Tuberinfundibular tract

Superior hypophysial a.

Infundibulum

Veins to dural sinuses

Veins to dural sinuses

Neural lobe

Inferior hypophysial a.

Anterior lobe

Vein to dural sinuses

Figure 7.1   The hypothalamus and its neurologic connections to the pituitary.

Several levels of feedback to the hypothalamus exist and are known as the long, short, and ultra short feedback loops. The *long feedback loop* is composed of endocrine input from circulating hormones, just as feedback of androgens and estrogens onto steroid receptors are present in the hypothalamus (2, 3). Similarly, pituitary hormones may feed back to the hypothalamus and serve important regulatory functions in *short-loop feedback*. Finally, hypothalamic secretions may directly feed back to the hypothalamus itself in an *ultra-short feedback loop*.

The major secretory products of the hypothalamus are the pituitary releasing factors (Fig. 7.3):

1. *Gonadotropin-releasing hormone (GnRH),* which controls the secretion of *luteinizing hormone (LH)* and *follicle-stimulating hormone (FSH)*

2. *Corticotropin-releasing factor (CRF),* which controls the release of *adrenocorticotrophic hormone (ACTH)*

3. *Growth hormone-releasing hormone (GHRH),* which regulates the release of *growth hormone (GH)*

4. *Thyrotropin-releasing hormone (TRH),* which regulates the secretion of *thyroid-stimulating hormone (TSH)*.

The hypothalamus is the source of all neurohypophyseal hormone production. The neural posterior pituitary can be viewed as a direct extension of the hypothalamus connected by

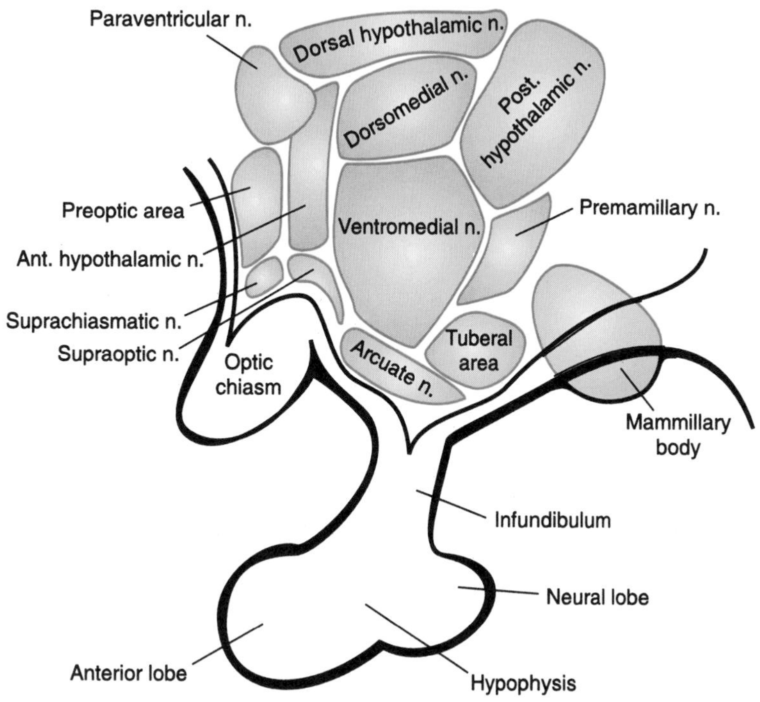

Figure 7.2   The neuronal cell bodies of the hypothalamus.

the finger-like infundibular stalk. The discovery that the capillaries in the median eminence differ from those in other regions of the brain was a major one. Unlike the usual tight junctions that exist between adjacent capillary endothelial lining cells, the capillaries in this region are fenestrated in the same manner as capillaries outside the CNS. As a result, there is no blood-brain barrier in the median eminence.

Pituitary

The pituitary is divided into three regions or lobes: *anterior, intermediate,* and *posterior.* The anterior pituitary (adenohypophysis) structurally is quite different from the posterior neural pituitary (neurohypophysis), which is a direct physical extension of the hypothalamus. The adenohypophysis is derived embryologically from epidermal ectoderm from an infolding of Rathke's pouch. Therefore, it is not composed of neural tissue, as is the posterior pituitary, and does not have direct neural connections to the hypothalamus. Instead, a unique anatomic relationship exists that combines elements of neural production and endocrine secretion. The adenohypophysis itself has no direct arterial blood supply. Its major source of blood flow is also its source of hypothalamic input—the portal vessels. Blood flow in these portal vessels is primarily from the hypothalamus to the pituitary. Blood is supplied to the posterior pituitary via the superior, middle, and inferior hypophyseal arteries. In contrast, the anterior pituitary has no direct arterial blood supply. Instead, it receives blood via a rich capillary plexus of the portal vessels that originate in the median eminence of the hypothalamus and descend along the pituitary stalk. This is not absolute, however, and retrograde blood flow has been demonstrated (4). This blood flow, combined with the location of the median eminence outside the blood-brain barrier, permits bidirectional feedback control between the two structures.

The specific secretory cells of the anterior pituitary have been classified based on their hematoxylin- and eosin-staining patterns. Acidophilic-staining cells primarily secrete GH and prolactin and, to a variable degree, ACTH (5). The gonadotropins are secreted by basophilic cells, and TSH is secreted by the neutral-staining chromophobes.

151

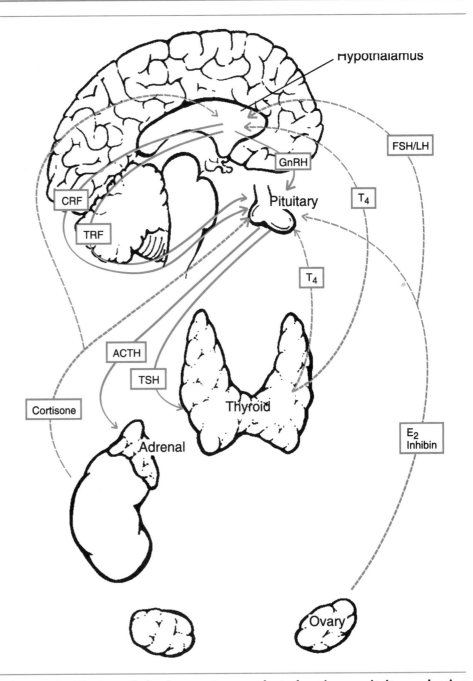

Figure 7.3 **The hypothalamic secretory products function as pituitary releasing factors that control the endocrine function of the ovaries, the thyroid, and the adrenal glands.**

Reproductive Hormones

The Hypothalamus

Gonadotropin-Releasing Hormone (GnRH)

GnRH (also called *luteinizing hormone-releasing hormone,* or *LHRH*) is the controlling factor for gonadotropin secretion (6). It is a decapeptide produced by neurons with cell bodies primarily in the arcuate nucleus of the hypothalamus (7–9) (Fig. 7.4). Embryologically, these neurons originate in the olfactory pit and then migrate to their adult locations (10). These GnRH-secreting neurons project axons that terminate on the portal vessels at the median em-

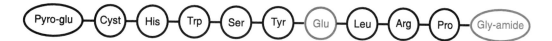

Figure 7.4   Gonadotropin-releasing hormone (GnRH) is a decapeptide.

inence where GnRH is secreted for delivery to the anterior pituitary. Less clear in function are multiple other secondary projections of GnRH neurons to locations within the CNS.

Pulsatile Secretion

GnRH is unique among releasing hormones in that it simultaneously regulates the secretion of two hormones—FSH and LH. It is also unique among the body's hormones because it must be secreted in a pulsatile fashion to be effective, and the pulsatile release of GnRH influences the release of the two gonadotropins (11–13). Using animals that have undergone electrical destruction of the arcuate nucleus and have no detectable levels of gonadotropins, a series of experiments were performed with varying dosages and intervals of GnRH infusion (13–14). Continual infusions did not result in gonadotropin secretion, whereas a pulsatile pattern led to physiologic secretion patterns and follicular growth. Continual exposure of the pituitary gonadotroph to GnRH results in a phenomenon called "down-regulation," through which the number of gonadotroph cell surface GnRH receptors is decreased (15). Similarly, intermittent exposure to GnRH will "up-regulate" or "auto-prime" the gonadotroph to increase its number of GnRH receptors (16). This allows the cell to have a greater response to subsequent GnRH exposure. Similar to the intrinsic electrical pacemaker cells of the heart, this action most likely represents an intrinsic property of the GnRH-secreting neuron, although it is subject to modulation by various neuronal and hormonal inputs to the hypothalamus.

The continual pulsatile secretion of GnRH is necessary because GnRH has an extremely short half-life (only 2–4 minutes) as a result of rapid proteolytic cleavage. The pulsatile secretion of GnRH varies in both frequency and amplitude throughout the menstrual cycle and is tightly regulated (17, 18) (Fig. 7.5). The follicular phase is characterized by frequent small amplitude pulses of GnRH secretion. In the late follicular phase, there is an increase in both frequency and amplitude of pulses. During the luteal phase, however, there is a progressive lengthening of the interval between pulses as well as a decrease in the amplitude. This variation in pulse amplitude and frequency is directly responsible for the magnitude and relative proportions of gonadotropin secretion from the pituitary, although additional hormonal influences on the pituitary will modulate the GnRH effect.

GnRH Agonists

Mechanism of Action   Used clinically, GnRH agonists are modifications of the native molecule to either increase receptor affinity or decrease degradation (19). Their use, therefore, leads to a persistent activation of GnRH receptors, as if continuous GnRH exposure existed. As would be predicted by the constant GnRH infusion experiments, this leads to suppression of gonadotropin secretion. An initial release of gonadotropins followed by a profound suppression of secretion is observed. The initial release of gonadotropins represents the secretion of pituitary stores in response to receptor binding and activation. With continued activation of the gonadotroph GnRH receptor, however, there is a down-regulation effect and a decrease in the concentration of GnRH receptors. As a result, gonadotropin secretion decreases and sex steroid production falls to castrate levels (20).

Structure—Agonists and Antagonists   As a peptide hormone, GnRH is degraded by enzymatic cleavage of bonds between its amino acids. Pharmacologic alterations of the structure of GnRH have led to the creation of agonists and antagonists (Fig. 7.4). The primary sites of enzymatic cleavage are between amino acids 5 and 6, 6 and 7, and 9 and 10. Substitution of

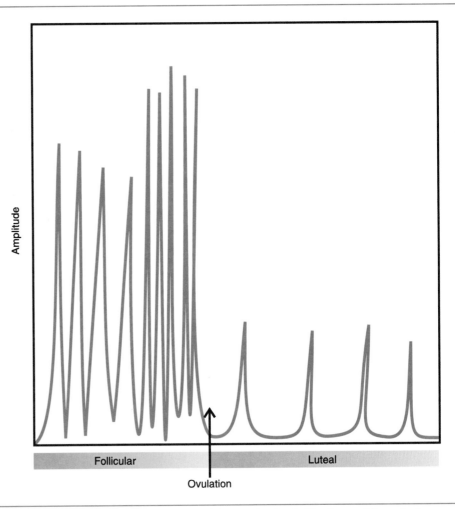

Figure 7.5   The pulsatile secretion of GnRH in the follicular and luteal phases of the cycle.

the position 6 amino acid glycine with large bulky amino acid analogues makes degradation more difficult and creates a form of GnRH with a relatively long half-life. Substitution at the carboxyl terminus produces a form of GnRH with increased receptor affinity. The resulting high affinity and slow degradation produces a molecule that mimics continuous exposure to native GnRH (19). Thus, as with constant GnRH exposure, down-regulation occurs. GnRH agonists are now widely used to treat disorders that are dependent on ovarian hormones (20). GnRH is used to control ovulation induction cycles and to treat precocious puberty, ovarian hyperandrogenism, leiomyomas, and hormonally dependent cancers. Potentially, they can be used to treat pelvic pain and premenstrual syndrome and for contraception.

The development of pure antagonists has allowed down-regulation of the pituitary-ovarian axis without the initial agonist burst (21). These antagonists differ slightly in structure from native GnRH and binding to the receptor without activation. It is expected that these antagonists will soon be available clinically.

Endogenous Opioids and Effects on GnRH   The endogenous opioids are three related families of naturally occurring substances produced in the CNS that represent the natural ligands for the opioid receptors (22–24). There are three major classes of endogenous opioids, each derived from precursor molecules:

1. *Endorphins* are named for their endogenous morphine-like activity. These substances are produced in the hypothalamus from the precursor pro-opiome-

lanocortin (POMC) and have diverse activities, including regulation of temperature, appetite, mood, and behavior (25).

2. *Enkephalins* function primarily in regulation of the autonomic nervous system. Proenkephalin A is the precursor for the two enkephalins of primary importance: met-enkephalin and leu-enkephalin.

3. *Dynorphins* are endogenous opioids produced from the precursor proenkephalin B and serve a function similar to that of the endorphins.

The endogenous opioids play a significant role in the regulation of hypothalamic-pituitary function. Endorphins appear to inhibit GnRH release within the hypothalamus, resulting in inhibition of gonadotropin secretion (26). Ovarian sex steroids can increase the secretion of central endorphins, further depressing gonadotropin levels (27).

Endorphin levels vary significantly throughout the menstrual cycle, with peak levels in the luteal phase and a nadir during menses (28). This inherent variability, although helping to regulate gonadotropin levels, may contribute to cycle-specific symptoms experienced by ovulatory women. For example, the dysphoria experienced by some women in the premenstrual phase of the cycle may be related to a withdrawal of endogenous opiates (29).

Pituitary Hormone Secretion

Anterior Pituitary

The anterior pituitary is responsible for the secretion of the major hormone-releasing factors: FSH, LH, TSH, and ACTH, as well as GH and prolactin. Each hormone is released by a specific pituitary cell type. The gonadotropins that arise from the anterior pituitary are as follows:

1. FSH and LH regulate ovarian sex steroid secretion.

2. TSH and ACTH regulate adrenal cortex glucocorticoid secretion.

3. GH and prolactin are produced by the adenohypophysis.

The Gonadotropins

The gonadotropins FSH and LH are produced by the anterior pituitary gonadotroph cells and are responsible for ovarian follicular stimulation. Structurally, there is great similarity between FSH and LH (Fig. 7.6). They are both glycoproteins that share identical alpha subunits and differ only in the structure of their beta subunits, which confer receptor specificity (30, 31). The synthesis of the beta subunits is the rate-regulating step in gonadotropin biosynthesis (32). TSH and placental chorionic gonadotropin also share identical alpha subunits with the gonadotropins. There are several forms of each gonadotropin, which differ in carbohydrate content as a result of post-translation modification. The degree of modification varies with steroid levels and is an important regulator of gonadotropin bioactivity.

Prolactin

Prolactin, a 198-amino-acid polypeptide secreted by the anterior pituitary lactotroph, is the primary trophic factor responsible for the synthesis of milk by the breast (33). Several forms of this hormone, which are named according to their size and bioactivity, are normally secreted (34). **Prolactin production is under tonic inhibitory control by the hypothalamic secretion of prolactin inhibiting factor (PIF), which most likely is dopamine (35). Therefore, disease states characterized by decreased dopamine secretion or any con-**

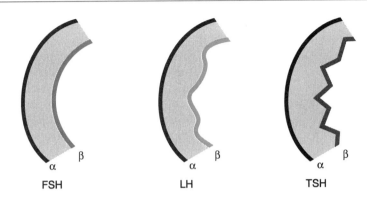

Figure 7.6   The structural similarity between FSH, LH, and TSH. The α subunits are identical and the β subunits differ.

dition that interrupts transport of PIF down the infundibular stalk to the pituitary gland will result in increased synthesis of prolactin. In this respect, prolactin is unique in comparison to all other pituitary hormones: it is predominantly under tonic inhibition, and release of control produces an increase in secretion. **Clinically, increased prolactin levels are associated with amenorrhea and galactorrhea, and hyperprolactinemia should be suspected in any individual with symptoms of either of these conditions.**

Although prolactin appears to be primarily under inhibitory control, many stimuli can elicit its release, including breast manipulation, drugs, stress, exercise, and certain foods. The existence of a releasing factor or factors for prolactin has been long hypothesized. Whereas such a factor has been identified in a variety of animal species, no physiologically significant releasing factor has been definitively identified in humans, although TRH appears to play this role to a large extent (36). Other hormones that may stimulate prolactin release include vasopressin, gamma-aminobutyric acid (GABA), dopamine, β-endorphin, vasoactive intestinal peptide (VIP), and angiotensin II (37, 38). The relative contributions of these substances under normal conditions remain to be determined.

Thyroid-Stimulating Hormone (TSH), Adrenocorticotropic Hormone (ACTH), and Growth Hormone (GH)

The other hormones produced by the anterior pituitary are TSH, ACTH, and GH. TSH is secreted by the pituitary thyrotrophs in response to TRH. Like GnRH, TRH is synthesized primarily in the arcuate nucleus of the hypothalamus and is then secreted into the portal circulation for transport to the pituitary. In addition to stimulating TSH release, TRH is also a major stimulus for the release of prolactin. TSH stimulates release of thyroid glands T_3 and T_4, which in turn negatively feeds back on pituitary TSH secretion. Abnormalities of thyroid secretion (both hyper- and hypothyroidism) are frequently associated with ovulatory dysfunction, due to diverse actions on the hypothalamic-pituitary-ovarian axis (39).

ACTH is secreted by the anterior pituitary in response to another hypothalamic releasing factor (corticotropin-releasing factor, CRH) and stimulates the release of adrenal glucocorticoids. Unlike the other anterior pituitary products, ACTH secretion has a diurnal variation with an early morning peak and a late evening nadir. Like the other pituitary hormones, ACTH secretion is negatively regulated by feedback from its primary end product, which in this case is cortisol.

GH is the anterior pituitary hormone that is secreted in the greatest absolute amount. It is secreted in response to the hypothalamic releasing factor, GHRH, as well as by thyroid hormone and glucocorticoids. This hormone is also secreted in a pulsatile fashion but with peak release during sleep. In addition to its vital role in the stimulation of linear growth, GH appears to have a role in the regulation of ovarian function, although the degree to which it serves this role in normal physiology is unclear (40).

Posterior Pituitary	**Structure and Function**

The posterior pituitary (neurohypophysis) is composed exclusively of neural tissue and is a direct extension of the hypothalamus. It lies directly adjacent to the adenohypophysis but is embryologically distinct, derived from an invagination of neuroectodermal tissue in the third ventricle. Axons in the posterior pituitary originate from neurons with cell bodies in two distinct regions of the hypothalamus, the supraoptic and paraventricular nuclei, named for their anatomic relationship to the optic chiasm and the third ventricle. Together, these two nuclei comprise the hypothalamic magnocellular system. These neurons can secrete their synthetic products directly from axonal boutons into the general circulation to act as hormones. This is the mechanism of secretion of the hormones of the posterior pituitary, oxytocin and arginine vasopressin (AVP). Although this is the primary mode of release of these hormones, numerous other secondary pathways have been identified, including secretion into the portal circulation, intrahypothalamic secretion, and secretion into other regions of the CNS (41).

In addition to the established functions of oxytocin and vasopressin, several other diverse roles have been suggested in animal models. These include modulation of sexual activity and appetite, learning and memory consolidation, temperature regulation, and regulation of maternal behaviors (42). It remains to be seen which, if any, of these functions also exist in humans.

Oxytocin   Oxytocin is a nine-amino-acid peptide primarily produced by the paraventricular nucleus of the hypothalamus (Fig. 7.7). The primary function of this hormone in humans is the stimulation of two specific types of muscular contractions (Fig. 7.8). The first type, uterine muscular contraction, occurs during parturition. The second type of muscular contraction regulated by oxytocin is breast lactiferous duct myoepithelial contractions during the milk letdown reflex. Oxytocin release may be stimulated by suckling, triggered by a signal from nipple stimulation transmitted via thoracic nerves to the spinal cord and then to the hypothalamus, where oxytocin is released in an episodic fashion (43). Oxytocin release may also be triggered by olfactory, auditory, and visual clues as well as part of a conditioned reflex in nursing animals. There is a significant release of oxytocin with stimulation of the cervix and vagina that may trigger reflex ovulation (the Ferguson reflex) in some species, although it is unclear to what extent this effect exists in humans.

Arginine-Vasopressin (AVP)   AVP (also known as *antidiuretic hormone*, or ADH) is the second major secretory product of the posterior pituitary (Fig. 7.7). It is synthesized primarily by neurons with cell bodies in the supraoptic nuclei (Fig. 7.8). Its major function is the regulation of circulating blood volume, pressure, and osmolality (43). Specific receptors throughout the body can trigger the release of AVP. Osmoreceptors located in the hypothalamus sense changes in blood osmolality from a mean of 285 mOsm/kg. Baroceptors sense changes in blood pressure caused by alterations in blood volume and are peripherally located

Figure 7.7   Oxytocin and arginine-vasopressin (AVP) are nine amino acid peptides produced by the hypothalamus. They differ only in two amino acids.

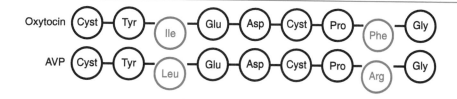

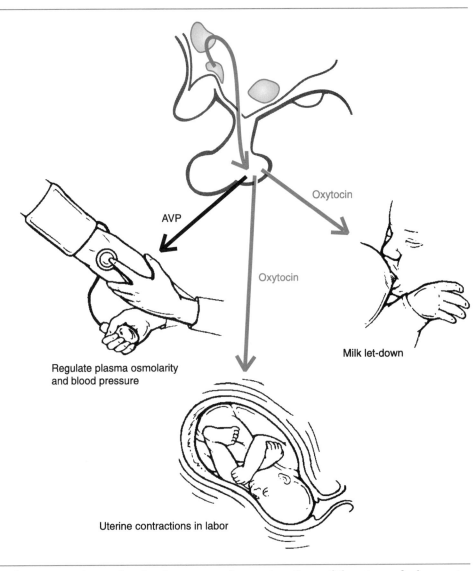

Figure 7.8 *Oxytocin* **stimulates muscular contractions of the uterus during parturition and the breast lactiferous duct during the milk letdown reflex.** *Arginine-vasopressin (AVP) regulates circulating blood volume, pressure, and osmolality.*

in the walls of the left atrium, carotid sinus, and aortic arch (44). These receptors can respond to changes in blood volume of more than 10%. In response to decreases in blood pressure or volume, AVP is released and causes arteriolar vasoconstriction and renal free water conservation. This in turn leads to a decrease in blood osmolarity and an increase in blood pressure. Activation of the renal renin-angiotensin system can also activate AVP release.

Menstrual Cycle Physiology

In the normal menstrual cycle, there is an orderly cyclical hormone production and parallel proliferation of the uterine lining in preparation for implantation of the embryo. Disorders of the menstrual cycle and, likewise, disorders of menstrual physiology may lead to various pathologic states, including infertility, recurrent miscarriage, and malignancy.

Menstruation disorder is one of the most frequent reasons women seek medical care (Table 7.1). Although helpful in formulating a diagnostic or therapeutic plan, the specific abnormalities of menstrual flow are not directly related to unique causes.

Table 7.1   Definitions of Menstrual Cycle Irregularities

Oligomenorrhea	Infrequent, irregularly timed episodes of bleeding usually occurring at intervals of more than 35 days
Polymenorrhea	Frequent but regularly timed episodes of bleeding usually occurring at intervals of 21 days or less
Menorrhagia	Regularly timed episodes of bleeding that are excessive in amount (<80 ml) and duration of flow (>5 days)
Metrorrhagia	Irregularly timed bleeding
Menometrorrhagia	Excessive, prolonged bleeding that occurs at irregularly timed, frequent intervals
Hypomenorrhea	Regularly timed bleeding that is decreased in amount
Intermenstrual bleeding	Bleeding (usually not of an excessive amount) that occurs between otherwise normal menstrual cycles

Normal Menstrual Cycle

The normal human menstrual cycle can be divided into two segments: the ovarian cycle and the uterine cycle, based on the organ under examination. The ovarian cycle may be further divided into follicular and luteal phases, whereas the uterine cycle is divided into corresponding proliferative and secretory phases (Fig. 7.9). The phases of the ovarian cycle are characterized as follows:

1. *Follicular phase*—the hormonal feedback promotes the orderly development of a single dominant follicle, which should be mature at midcycle and prepared for ovulation. The average length of the human follicular phase ranges from 10 to 14 days, and variability in this length is responsible for most variations in total cycle length.

2. *Luteal phase*—the time from ovulation to the onset of menses, with an average length of 14 days.

A normal menstrual cycle lasts from 21 to 35 days with 2 to 6 days of flow and an average blood loss of 20–60 ml. However, studies of large numbers of normally cycling women have shown that only approximately two-thirds of adult women have cycles lasting 21–35 days (45). The extremes of reproductive life (after menarche and perimenopausally) are characterized by a higher percentage of anovulatory or irregularly timed cycles (46, 47).

Hormonal Variations

The relative pattern of ovarian, uterine, and hormonal variation along the normal menstrual cycle is shown in Figure 7.9.

1. At the beginning of each monthly menstrual cycle, levels of gonadal steroids are low and have been decreasing since the end of the luteal phase of the previous cycle.

2. With the demise of the corpus luteum, FSH levels begin to rise and a cohort of growing follicles is recruited. These follicles each secrete increasing levels of estrogen as they grow in the follicular phase. This, in turn, is the stimulus for uterine endometrial proliferation.

3. Rising estrogen levels provide negative feedback on pituitary FSH secretion, which begins to wane by the midpoint of the follicular phase. Conversely, LH is at first stimulated by the secretion of estrogen throughout the follicular phase.

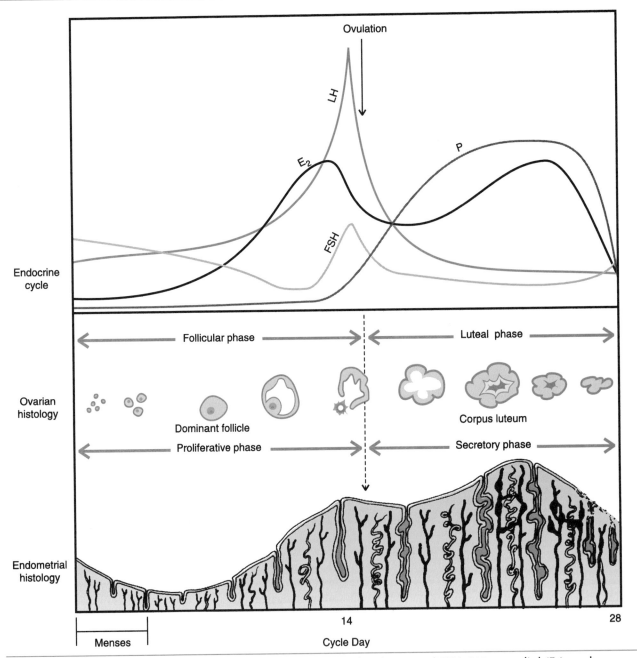

Figure 7.9   The menstrual cycle. The top panel shows the cyclic changes of FSH, LH, estradiol (E_2), and progesterone (P) relative to the time of ovulation. The bottom panel correlates the ovarian cycle in the follicular and luteal phases and the endometrial cycle in the proliferative and secretory phases.

4. At the end of the follicular phase (just prior to ovulation), FSH-induced LH receptors are present on granulosa cells and, with LH stimulation, modulate the secretion of progesterone.

5. After a sufficient degree of estrogenic stimulation, the pituitary LH surge is triggered, which is the proximate cause of ovulation that occurs 24–36 hours later. Ovulation heralds the transition to the luteal/secretory phase.

6. The estrogen level decreases through the early luteal phase in a continuation of a process that begins just before ovulation and continues until the midluteal phase, when it begins to rise again as a result of corpus luteum secretion.

7. Progesterone levels rise precipitously after ovulation and can be used as a presumptive sign that ovulation has occurred.

8. Both estrogen and progesterone levels remain elevated through the life span of the corpus luteum and then wane with its demise, thereby setting the stage for the next cycle.

Uterus

Cyclical Changes of the Endometrium

The cyclic histologic changes in the adult human endometrium were described by Noyes, Hertig, and Rock in 1950 (48) (Fig. 7.10). These changes proceed in an orderly fashion in response to cyclic hormonal production by the ovaries (Fig. 7.9). Histologic cycling of the endometrium can best be viewed in two parts: the endometrial glands and the surrounding stroma. The superficial two-thirds of the endometrium is the zone that proliferates and is ultimately shed with each cycle if pregnancy does not occur. This cycling portion of the endometrium is known as the *decidua functionalis* and is composed of a deeply situated intermediate zone (*stratum spongiosum*) and a superficial compact zone (*stratum compactum*). The *decidua basalis* is the deepest region of the endometrium and does not undergo significant monthly proliferation. Instead, it is the source of endometrial regeneration after each menses (49).

Proliferative Phase

By convention, the first day of vaginal bleeding is called day one of the menstrual cycle. After menses, the decidua basalis is composed of primordial glands and dense scant stroma in its location adjacent to the myometrium. The proliferative phase is characterized by progressive mitotic growth of the decidua functionalis in preparation for implantation of the embryo in response to rising circulating levels of estrogen (50). At the beginning of the proliferative phase, the endometrium is relatively thin (1–2 mm). The predominant change seen during this time is evolution of the initially straight, narrow, and short endometrial glands into longer, tortuous structures (51). Histologically, these proliferating glands have multiple mitotic cells, and their organization changes from a low columnar pattern in the early proliferative period to a pseudostratified pattern before ovulation. The stroma is a dense compact layer throughout this time. Vascular structures are infrequently seen.

Secretory Phase

In the typical 28-day cycle, ovulation occurs on cycle day 14. Within 48–72 hours following ovulation, the onset of progesterone secretion produces a shift in histologic appearance of the endometrium to the secretory phase, so named for the clear presence of eosinophilic protein-rich secretory products in the glandular lumen. In contrast to the proliferative phase, the secretory phase of the menstrual cycle is characterized by the cellular effects of progesterone in addition to estrogen. In general, progesterone's effects are antagonistic to those of estrogen and there is a progressive decrease in the endometrial cell's estrogen receptor concentration. As a result, in the latter half of the cycle, there is an antagonism of estrogen-induced DNA synthesis and cellular mitosis (50).

During the secretory phase, the endometrial glands form characteristic periodic acid-Schiff (PAS) positive-staining, glycogen-containing vacuoles. These vacuoles initially appear subnuclearly (by cycle day 16) and then progress toward the glandular lumen (48) (Fig. 7.10).

161

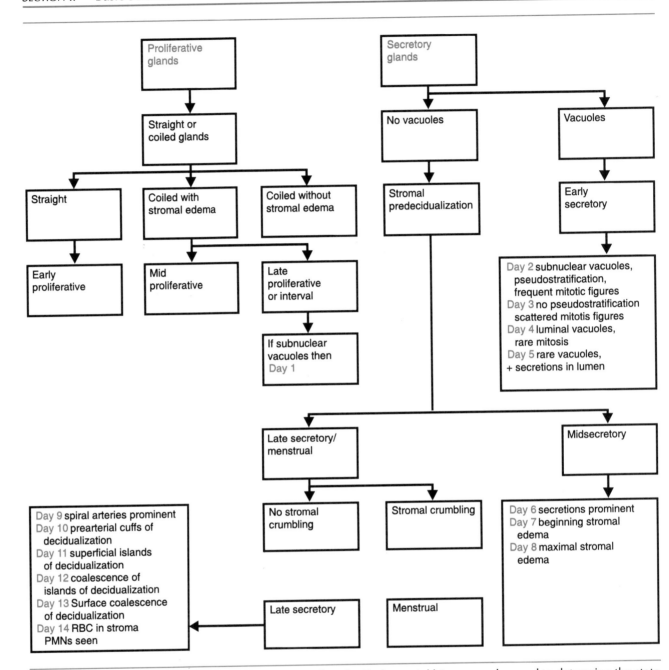

Figure 7.10   The histologic changes of the menstrual cycle. Endometrial biopsy can be used to determine the state of the endometrium corresponding to the day of the cycle.

The nuclei can be seen in the midportion of the cells by cycle day 17 and ultimately undergo apocrine secretion into the glandular lumen by cycle day 19–20. At postovulatory day 6–7, secretory activity of the glands is maximal and the endometrium is optimally prepared for implantation of the blastocyst.

The stroma of the secretory phase remains unchanged histologically until the seventh postovulatory day, when there is a progressive increase in edema. Coincident with maximal stromal edema in the late secretory phase, the spiral arteries become clearly visible and then progressively lengthen and coil during the remainder of the secretory phase. By day 24, an eosinophilic staining pattern, known as "cuffing," is visible in the perivascular stroma. Eosinophilia then progresses to form islands in the stroma followed by areas of confluence. This staining pattern of the edematous stroma is termed "pseudodecidual" because of its similarity to the pattern that occurs in pregnancy. Approximately 2 days prior to menses, there is a dramatic increase in the number of polymorphonuclear lymphocytes that migrate from the vascular system. This "leukocytic infiltration" heralds the collapse of the endometrial stroma and the onset of the menstrual flow.

Menses

In the absence of implantation, glandular secretion ceases and an irregular breakdown of the decidua functionalis occurs. The result is a shedding of this layer of the endometrium, a process termed menses. It is the destruction of the corpus luteum and its production of estrogen and progesterone that is the proximate cause of the shedding. With withdrawal of sex steroids, there is a profound spiral artery vascular spasm that ultimately leads to endometrial ischemia. Simultaneously, there is a breakdown of lysosomes and a release of proteolytic enzymes, which further promote local tissue destruction. This layer of endometrium is then shed, leaving the decidua basalis as the source of subsequent endometrial growth. Prostaglandins are produced throughout the menstrual cycle and are at their highest concentration during menses (51). Prostaglandin-$F_{2\alpha}$ ($PGF_{2\alpha}$) is a potent vasoconstrictor, causing further arteriolar vasospasm and endometrial ischemia. $PGF_{2\alpha}$ also produces myometrial contractions that decrease local uterine wall blood flow and may serve to physically expel sloughing endometrial tissue from the uterus.

Disorders of menstruation are one of the most frequent reasons women seek medical care. Although helpful in formulating a diagnostic or therapeutic plan, the specific abnormalities of menstrual flow are not directly related to unique causes.

Dating the Endometrium

The precise nature of the histologic changes that occur in secretory endometrium relative to the LH surge allows the assessment of the "normalcy" of endometrial development (Fig. 7.9). By knowing when a patient is chronologically postovulatory, it is possible to sample the endometrium with an endometrial biopsy and determine whether the state of the endometrium corresponds to the phase of the cycle (Fig. 7.10). Any large discrepancy (more than 2-day lag time) is termed a *luteal phase defect* and has been linked to both failure of implantation and early pregnancy loss (52). To perform this diagnostic test, it is first critical to determine when ovulation occurs. Once this has been established, investigators have traditionally chosen 10–12 days postovulation as the time for biopsy. However, recent data suggest that endometrial sampling at the time of implantation (6–8 days postovulation) may be more accurate (53).

Simple hematoxylin and eosin (H&E) stain evaluation is a crude, insensitive, and frequently inaccurate method of assessing endometrial receptivity. Normal implantation requires a complex set of events, many being expressed as changes within the endometrium (54). These changes include expression of specific glycoproteins and adhesion molecules, production of cytokines, and variation in tissue enzyme levels (55). As the importance of each of these factors in implantation becomes clear, it will likely be possible to subject one or more endometrial biopsies to a complex panel of stains, thereby assessing the development of individual markers. Such complex screening, already used in other tissue systems, will allow a more precise diagnosis of endometrial dysfunction than the current general diagnosis of luteal phase defect.

Ovarian Follicular Development

The number of oocytes peaks at 6–7 million by 20 weeks of gestation (56) (Fig. 7.11). Simultaneously (and peaking at the fifth month of gestation), atresia of the oogonia occurs, rapidly followed by follicular atresia. At birth, only 1–2 million oocytes remain in the ovary, and at puberty, only 300,000 of the original 6–7 million oocytes are available for ovulation (56, 57). Of these, only 400–500 will ultimately ovulate, and by the time of menopause, the ovary will be composed primarily of dense stromal tissue with only rare interspersed oocytes remaining.

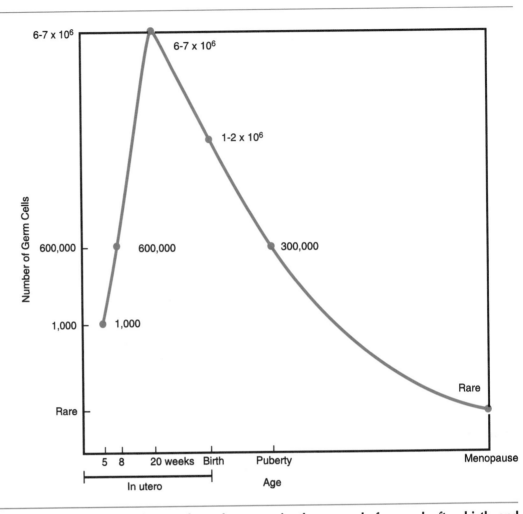

Figure 7.11   The number of oocytes in the ovary before and after birth and through menopause.

In humans, there is no further oogonial formation or mitosis postnatally. Because oocytes enter the diplotene resting stage of meiosis in the fetus and persist in this stage until ovulation, much of the deoxyribonucleic acid (DNA), proteins, and messenger ribonucleic acid (mRNA) necessary for development of the preimplantation embryo will have been synthesized by this stage. At the diplotene stage, a single layer of 8–10 granulosa cells surround the oogonia to form the primordial follicle. The oogonia that fail to become properly surrounded by granulosa cells undergo atresia (58).

Meiotic Arrest of Oocyte and Resumption

Meiosis **(the germ cell process of reduction division) is commonly divided into four phases: prophase, metaphase, anaphase, and telophase. The prophase of** *meiosis I* **is further divided into five stages: leptotene, zygotene, pachytene, diplotene, and diakinesis.** Oogonia differ from spermatogonia in that only one final daughter cell (oocyte) forms from each precursor cell with the excess genetic material discarded in three polar bodies. When the developing oogonia begin to enter meiotic prophase I, they are known as primary oocytes (59). This process begins at roughly 8 weeks of gestation. Only those oogonia that enter meiosis will survive the wave of atresia that sweeps the fetal ovary before birth. The oocytes arrested in prophase (in the late diplotene or "dictyate" stage) will remain so until the time of ovulation, when the process of meiosis resumes. The mechanism for this mitotic stasis is believed to be an oocyte maturation inhibitor (OMI) produced by granulosa cells (60). This inhibitor gains access to the oocyte via tight junctions connecting the oocyte and its surrounding cumulus of granulosa. With the midcycle LH surge, the tight junctions are disrupted and meiosis I is allowed to resume.

Follicular Development

Follicular development is a dynamic process that continues from menarche until menopause. The process is designed to allow the monthly recruitment of a cohort of follicles and, ultimately, to release a single mature dominant follicle during ovulation each month.

Primordial Follicles

The initial recruitment and growth of the primordial follicles is gonadotropin independent and affects a cohort over several months (61). However, the stimuli responsible for the recruitment of a specific cohort of follicles in each cycle is unknown. At the primordal follicle stage, shortly after initial recruitment, FSH assumes control of follicular differentiation and growth and allows a cohort of follicles to continue differentiation. This signals the shift from gonadotropin-independent to gonadotropin-dependent growth. The first changes seen are growth of the oocyte and expansion of the single layer of follicular granulosa cells into a multilayer of cuboidal cells. The decline in luteal phase progesterone and inhibin production by the now-fading corpus luteum from the previous cycle allows the increase in FSH that stimulates follicular growth (62).

Preantral Follicle

During the several days following the breakdown of the corpus luteum, growth of the cohort of follicles continues, driven by the stimulus of FSH. The enlarging oocyte then secretes a glycoprotein-rich substance, the zona pellucida, which separates it from the surrounding granulosa cells. With transformation from a primordial to a preantral follicle, there is continued mitotic proliferation of the encompassing granulosa cells. Simultaneously, theca cells in the stroma bordering the granulosa cells proliferate. Both cell types function synergistically to produce estrogens that are secreted into the systemic circulation. At this stage of development, each of the seemingly identical cohort members must either be selected for dominance or undergo atresia. It is likely that the follicle destined to ovulate has been selected prior to this point, although the mechanism for selection remains obscure.

Two-Cell Two-Gonadotropin Theory

The fundamental tenet of follicular development is the two-cell two-gonadotropin theory (63–65) (Fig. 7.12). This theory states that there is a subdivision and compartmentalization of steroid hormone synthesis activity in the developing follicle. In general, most aromatase activity (for estrogen production) is in the granulosa cells (66). Aromatase activity is enhanced by FSH stimulation of specific receptors on these cells (67, 68). However, granulosa cells lack several enzymes that occur earlier in the steroidogenic pathway and require androgens as a substrate for aromatization. Androgens, in turn, are synthesized primarily in response to stimulation by LH, and the theca cells possess most of the LH receptors at this stage (67, 68). Therefore, a synergistic relationship must exist: LH stimulates the theca cells to produce androgens (primarily androstenedione), which, in turn, are transferred to the granulosa cells for FSH-stimulated aromatization into estrogens. These locally produced estrogens create a microenvironment within the follicle that is favorable for continued growth and nutrition (69). Both FSH and local estrogens serve to further stimulate estrogen production, FSH receptor synthesis and expression, and granulosa cell proliferation and differentiation.

Androgens have two different regulatory roles in follicular development. At low concentrations (i.e., in the early preantral follicle), they serve to stimulate aromatase activity via specific receptors in granulosa cells. At higher levels of androgens, there is intense 5α-

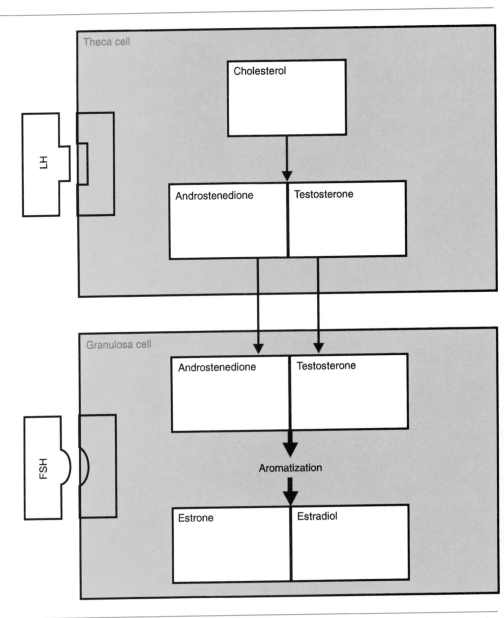

Figure 7.12   The two-cell two-gonadotropin theory of follicular development in which there is compartmentalization of steroid hormone synthesis in the developing follicle.

reductase activity that converts the androgens to forms that cannot be aromatized (63, 70). This androgenic microenvironment inhibits the expression of FSH receptors on the granulosa cells, thereby inhibiting aromatase activity and setting the follicle on the path to atresia (71). Meanwhile, as the peripheral estrogen level rises, it negatively feeds back on the pituitary and hypothalamus to decrease circulating FSH levels (72). Increased ovarian production of inhibin further decreases FSH production at this point.

The falling FSH level that occurs with the progression of the follicular phase represents a threat to continued follicular growth. The resulting adverse environment can be withstood only by follicles with a selective advantage for binding the diminishing FSH molecules; that is, those with the greatest number of FSH receptors. The dominant follicle, therefore, can be perceived as the one with a richly estrogenic microenvironment and the most FSH receptors (73). As it grows and develops, the follicle continues to produce estrogen, which results in further lowering the circulating FSH and creating a more adverse environment for competing follicles. This process continues until all members of the initial cohort have suffered atresia, with the exception of the single dominant follicle. The stage is then set for ovulation.

Preovulatory Follicle

Preovulatory follicles are characterized by a fluid-filled antrum that is composed of plasma with granulosa-cell secretions. The granulosa cells at this point have further differentiated into a heterogenous population. The oocyte remains connected to the follicle by a stalk of specialized granulosa known as the *cumulus oophorus.*

Rising estrogen levels have a negative feedback effect on FSH secretion. Conversely, LH has a biphasic regulation by circulating estrogens. At lower concentrations, estrogens are inhibitory to LH secretion. At higher levels, however, estrogen enhances LH release. This stimulation requires a sustained high level of estrogen (>200 pg/ml) for more than 48 hours (74). Once the rising estrogen level produces positive feedback, a substantial surge in LH secretion occurs. Concomitant to these events, the local estrogen/FSH interactions in the dominant follicle induce LH receptors on the granulosa cells. Thus, exposure to high levels of LH results in a specific response by the dominant follicle—the end result is luteinization of the granulosa cells, progesterone production, and triggering of ovulation. In general, ovulation will occur in the single mature, or Graafian, follicle 10–12 hours after the LH peak or 32–35 hours after the initial rise in midcycle LH (75–77).

Activin and Inhibin   It has been determined that the gonadotropins are not the only ovarian regulators of follicular development. Two related granulosa-cell-derived peptides have been identified that play opposing roles in pituitary feedback (78). The first of these, inhibin, is secreted in a pattern similar to estradiol and acts to inhibit FSH secretion. It is secreted in the greatest amounts after ovulation. As with estrogen, FSH stimulates the release of inhibin, which in turn negatively feeds back on FSH release (79, 80). The second peptide, activin, stimulates FSH release from the pituitary gland and potentiates its action in the ovary (81, 82). It is likely that there are numerous other intraovarian regulators similar to inhibin and activin, each of which may play a key role in promoting the normal ovulatory process (83). Some of these include ILGF-1, EGF/TGF-α, TGF-β1, β-FGF, IL-1, TNF-α, LI, OMI, and renin-angiotensin.

Ovulation

The midcycle LH surge is responsible for a dramatic increase in local concentrations of prostaglandins and proteolytic enzymes in the follicular wall (84). These substances progressively weaken the follicular wall and ultimately allow a perforation to form. Ovulation most likely represents a slow extrusion of the oocyte through this opening in the follicle rather than a rupture of the follicular structure (85). In fact, direct measurements of intrafollicular pressures have been recorded and have failed to demonstrate such an explosive event.

Luteal Phase

Structure of Corpus Luteum   After ovulation, the remaining follicular shell is transformed into the primary regulator of the luteal phase—the corpus luteum. Membranous granulosa cells remaining in the follicle begin to take up lipids and the characteristic yellow lutein pigment for which the structure is named. These cells are active secretory structures that produce progesterone, which supports the endometrium of the luteal phase. In addition, estrogen and inhibin are produced in significant quantities. Unlike the developing follicle, the basement membrane of the corpus luteum degenerates and proliferating blood vessels invade the granulosa-luteal cells in response to secretion of local factors. This angiogenic response allows large amounts of luteal hormones to enter the systemic circulation.

Hormonal Function and Regulation   The hormonal changes of the luteal phase are characterized by a series of negative feedback interactions designed to lead to regression of the corpus luteum if pregnancy does not occur. Corpus luteum steroids (estradiol and progesterone) negatively feed back centrally and cause a decrease in FSH and LH secretion. Continued secretion of both steroids will decrease the stimuli for subsequent follicular recruitment. Similarly, luteal secretion of inhibin also potentiates FSH withdrawal. In the ovary, local production of progesterone is inhibitory to the further development and recruitment of additional follicles.

Continued corpus luteum function depends on continued LH production. In the absence of this stimulation, the corpus luteum will invariably regress after 12–16 days and form the scar-like corpora albicans (86). The exact mechanism of luteolysis, however, is unclear and most likely also involves local paracrine factors. In the absence of pregnancy, the corpus luteum regresses and estrogen and progesterone levels wane. This, in turn, removes central inhibition on gonadotropin secretion and allows FSH and LH levels to again rise and recruit another cohort of follicles.

If pregnancy does occur, placental human chorionic gonadotropin (hCG) will mimic LH action and continually stimulate the corpus luteum to secrete progesterone. Thus, successful implantation results in hormonal support to allow continued maintenance of the corpus luteum and the endometrium. Evidence from patients undergoing oocyte donation cycles has demonstrated that continued luteal function is essential to continuation of the pregnancy until approximately 5 weeks of gestation, when sufficient progesterone is produced by the developing placenta (87). This switch in the source of regulatory progesterone production is referred to as the *luteal-placental shift*.

Summary of Menstrual Cycle Regulation

Following is a summary of the regulation of the menstrual cycle:

1. GnRH is produced in the arcuate nucleus of the hypothalamus and secreted in a pulsatile fashion into the portal circulation, where it travels to the anterior pituitary.

2. Ovarian follicular development moves from a period of gonadotropin independence to a phase of FSH dependence.

3. As the corpus luteum of the previous cycle fades, luteal production of progesterone and inhibin decreases, allowing FSH levels to rise.

4. In response to FSH stimulus, the follicles grow and differentiate and secrete increasing amounts of estrogen.

5. Estrogens stimulate growth and differentiation of the functional layer of the endometrium, which prepares for implantation. Estrogens work with FSH in stimulating follicular development.

6. The two-cell two-gonadotropin theory dictates that with LH stimulation the ovarian theca cells will produce androgens that are converted by the granulosa cells into estrogens under the stimulus of FSH.

7. Rising estrogen levels negatively feed back on the pituitary gland and hypothalamus and decrease the secretion of FSH.

8. The one follicle destined to ovulate each cycle is called the dominant follicle. It has relatively more FSH receptors and produces a larger concentration of estrogens than the follicles that will undergo atresia. It is able to continue to grow despite falling FSH levels.

9. Sustained high estrogen levels will cause a surge in pituitary LH secretion that triggers ovulation, progesterone production, and the shift to the secretory, or luteal, phase.

10. Luteal function is dependent on the presence of LH. Without continued LH secretion, the corpus luteum will regress after 12–16 days.

11. If pregnancy occurs, the embryo secretes hCG, which mimics the action of LH by sustaining the corpus luteum. The corpus luteum continues to secrete progesterone and supports the secretory endometrium, allowing the pregnancy to continue to develop.

References

1. **Bloom FE.** Neuroendocrine mechanisms: cells and systems. In: **Yen SCC, Jaffe RB,** eds. *Reproductive Endocrinology.* Philadelphia: WB Saunders Co., 1991: 2–24.

2. **Simerly RB, Chang C, Muramatsu M, Swanson LW.** Distribution of androgen and estrogen receptor mRNA-containing cells in the rat brain: an in situ hybridization study. *J Comp Neurol* 1990;294:76–95.

3. **Brown TJ, Hochberg RB, Naftolin F, MacLusky NJ.** Pubertal development of estrogen receptors in the rat brain. *Molecular Cellular Neurosciences.* 1994;5:475–83.

4. **Bergland RM, Page RB.** Can the pituitary secrete directly to the brain? Affirmative anatomical evidence. *Endocrinology* 1978;102:1325–38.

5. **Duello TM, Halmi NS.** Ultrastructural-immunocytochemical localization of growth hormone and prolactin in human pituitaries. *J Clin Endocrinol Metab* 1979;49:189–96.

6. **Blackwell RE, et al.** Concomitant release of FSH and LH induced by native and synthetic LRF. *Am J Physiol* 1973;244:170–5.

7. **Krey LC, Butler WR, Knobil E.** Surgical disconnection of the medial basal hypothalamus and pituitary function in the rhesus monkey. I. Gonadotropin secretion. *Endocrinology* 1975;96: 1073–87.

8. **Plant TM, Krey LC, Moossy J, McCormack JT, Hess DL, Knobil E.** The arcuate nucleus and the control of the gonadotropin and prolactin secretion in the female rhesus monkey (Macaca mulatta). *Endocrinology* 1978;102:52–62.

9. **Amoss M, Burgus R, Blackwell RE, Vale W, Fellows R, Guillemin R.** Purification, amino acid composition, and N-terminus of the hypothalamic luteinizing hormone releasing factor (LRF) of ovine origin. *Biochem Biophys Res Commun* 1971;44:205–10.

10. **Schwanzel-Fukuda M, Pfaff DW.** Origin of luteinizing hormone releasing hormone neurons. *Nature* 1989;338:161–4.

11. **Dierschke DJ, Bhattacharya AN, Atkinson LE, Knobil E.** Circhoral oscillations of plasma LH levels in the ovariectomized rhesus monkey. *Endocrinology* 1970;87:850–3.

12. **Knobil E.** Neuroendocrine control of the menstrual cycle. *Recent Prog Horm Res* 1980; 36:53–88.

13. **Belchetz PE, Plant TM, Nakai Y, Keogh EJ, Knobil E.** Hypophyseal responses to continuous and intermitent delivery of hypothalamic gonadotropin-releasing hormone. *Science* 1978;202:631–3.

14. **Nakai Y, Plant TM, Hess DL, Keogh EJ, Knobil E.** On the sites of the negative and positive feedback actions of estradiol and the control of gonadotropin secretion in the rhesus monkey. *Endocrinology* 1978;102:1008–14.

15. **Rabin D, McNeil LW.** Pituitary and gonadal desensitization after continuous luteinizing hormone-releasing hormone infusion in normal females. *J Clin Endocrinol Metab* 1980,51:873–6.

16. **Hoff JD, Lasley BL, Yen SSC.** Functional relationship between priming and releasing actions of luteinizing hormone-releasing hormone. *J Clin Endocrinol Metab* 1979;49:8–11.

17. **Soules MR, Steiner RA, Cohen NL, Bremner WJ, Clifton DK.** Nocturnal slowing of pulsatile luteinizing hormone secretion in women during the follicular phase of the menstrual cycle. *J Clin Endocrinol Metab* 1985;61:43–9.

18. **Filicori M, Santoro N, Marriam GR, Crowley WF Jr.** Characterization of the physiological pattern of episodic gonadotropin secretion throughout the human menstrual cycle. *J Clin Endocrinol Metab* 1986;62:1136–44.

19. **Karten MJ, Rivier JE.** Gonadotropin-releasing hormone analog design. Structure function studies towards the development of agonists and antagonists: rationale and perspective. *Endocr Rev* 1986;7:44.

20. **Conn PM, Crowley WF Jr.** Gonadotropin-releasing hormone and its analogs. *Annu Rev Med* 1994;45:391–405.

21. **Loy RA.** The pharmacology and potential applications of GnRH antagonists. *Curr Opin Obstet Gynecol* 1994;6:262–8.

22. **Hughes J, Smith TW, Kosterlitz LH, Fothergill LA, Morgan BA, Morris HR.** Identification of two related pentapeptides from the brain with potent opiate agonist activity. *Nature* 1975;258:577–80.

23. **Howlett TA, Rees LH.** Endogenous opioid peptide and hypothalamo-pituitary function. *Annu Rev Physiol* 1986;48:527–36.

24. **Facchinetti F, Petraglia F, Genazzani AR.** Localization and expression of the three opioid systems. *Semin Reprod Endocrinol* 1987;5:103.

25. **Goldstein A.** Endorphins: physiology and clinical implications. *Ann N Y Acad Sci* 1978;311:49–58.

26. **Grossman A.** Opioid peptides and reproductive function. *Semin Reprod Endocrinol* 1987; 5:115–24.

27. **Reid Rl, Hoff JD, Yen SSC, Li CH.** Effects of exogenous β-endorphin on pituitary hormone secretion and its disappearance rate in normal human subjects. *J Clin Endocrinol Metab* 1981;52:1179–84.

28. **Gindoff PR, Ferin M.** Brain opioid peptides and menstrual cyclicity. *Semin Reprod Endocrinol* 1987;5:125–33.

29. **Halbreich U, Endicott J.** Possible involvement of endorphin withdrawal or imbalance in specific premenstrual syndromes and postpartum depression. *Med Hypotheses* 1981;7:1045–58.

30. **Fiddes JC, Talmadge K.** Structure, expression and evolution of the genes for human glycoprotein hormones. *Recent Prog Horm Res* 1984;40:43–78.

31. **Vaitukaitis JL, Ross JT, Bourstein GD, Rayford PL.** Gonadotropins and their subunits: basic and clinical studies. *Recent Prog Horm Res* 1976;32:289–331.

32. **Lalloz MRA, Detta A, Clayton RN.** GnRH desensitization preferentially inhibits expression of the LH beta-subunit gene in vivo. *Endocrinology* 1988;122:1689–94.

33. **Brun del Re R, del Pozo E, de Grandi P, Friesen H, Hinselmann M, Wyss H.** Prolactin inhibition and suppression of puerperal lactation by a Br-ergocriptine (CB 154): a comparison with estrogen. *Obstet Gynecol* 1973;41:884–90.

34. **Suh HK, Frantz AG.** Size heterogeneity of human prolactin in plasma and pituitary extracts. *J Clin Endocrinol Metab* 1974:39:928–35.

35. **MacLeod RM.** Influence of norepinepherine and catecholamine depletion agents synthesis in release of prolactin growth hormone. *Endocrinology* 1969;85:916–23.

36. **Vale W, Blackwell RE, Grant G, Guillemin R.** TRF and thyroid hormones on prolactin secretion by rat pituitary cell in vitro. *Endocrinology* 1973;93:26–33.

37. **Matsushita N, Kato Y, Shimatsu A, Katakami H, Yanaihara N, Imura H.** Effects of VIP, TRH, GABA and dopamine on prolactin release from superfused rat anterior pituitary cells. *Life Sci* 1983;32:1263–9.

38. **Dufy-Barbe L, Rodriguez F, Arsaut J, Verrier D, Vincent JD.** Angiotensin-II stimulates prolactin release in the rhesus monkey. *Neuroendocrinology* 1982;35:242–7.

39. **Burrow GN.** The thyroid gland and reproduction. In: **Yen SCC, Jaffe RB,** eds. *Reproductive Endocrinology.* Philadelphia: WB Saunders Co., 1991: 555–75.

40. **Katz E, Ricciarelli E, Adashi EY.** The potential relevance of growth hormone to female reproductive physiology and pathophysiology. *Fertil Steril* 1993;59:8–34.

41. **Yen SCC.** The hypothalamic control of pituitary hormone secretion. In: **Yen SCC, Jaffe RB,** eds. *Reproductive Endocrinology.* Philadelphia: WB Saunders Co., 1991: 65–104.

42. **Insel TR.** Oxyocin and the neuroendocrine basis of affiliation. In: **Schulkin J,** ed. *Hormonally Induced Changes in Mind and Brain.* New York: Academic Press, 1993: 225–51.

43. **McNeilly AS, Roinson CAF, Houston MJ, Howie PW.** Release of oxytocin and PRL in response to suckling. *BMJ* 1983;286:257–9.

44. **Dunn FL, Brennan TJ, Nelson AE, Roberton GL.** The role of blood osmolality and volume in regulating vasopressin secretion in the rat. *J Clin Invest* 1973;52:3212–9.

45. **Vollman RF.** The menstrual cycle. In: **Friedman E,** ed. *Major Problems in Obstetrics and Gynecology.* Philadelphia: WB Saunders Co., 1977: 1–193.

46. **Treloar AE, Boynton RE, Borghild GB, Brown BW.** Variation of the human menstrual cycle through reproductive life. *Int J Fertil* 1967;12:77–126.

47. **Collett ME, Wertenberger, GE, Fiske VM.** The effects of age upon the pattern of the menstrual cycle. *Fertil Steril* 1954;5:437–48.

48. **Noyes RW, Hertig AW, Rock J.** Dating the endometrial biopsy. *Fertil Steril* 1950;1:3–25.

49. **Flowers CE Jr, Wilbron WH.** Cellular mechanisms for endometrial conservation during menstrual bleeding. *Semin Reprod Endocrinol* 1984;2:307–41.

50. **Ferenczy A, Bertrand G, Gelfand MM.** Proliferation kinetics of human endometrium during the normal menstrual cycle. *Am J Obstet Gynecol* 1979;133:859.

51. **Schwarz BE.** The production and biologic effects of uterine prostaglandins. *Semin Reprod Endocrinol* 1983;1:189.

52. **Olive DL.** The prevalence and epidemiology of luteal-phase deficiency in normal and infertile women. *Clin Obstet Gynecol* 1991;34:157–66.

53. **Castelbaum AJ, Wheeler J, Coutifaris CB, Mastroianni L Jr, Lessey BA.** Timing of the endometrial biopsy may be critical for the accurate diagnosis of luteal phase deficiency. *Fertil Steril* 1994;61:443–7.

54. **Ilesanmi AO, Hawkins DA, Lessey BA.** Immunohistochemical markers of uterine receptivity in the human endometrium. *Microsc Res Tech* 1993;25:208–22.

55. **Tabibzadeh S.** Human endometrium: an active site of cytokine production and action. *Endocr Rev* 1991;12:272–90.

56. **Peters H, Byskov AG, Grinsted J.** Follicular growth in fetal and prepubertal ovaries in humans and other primates. *J Clin Endocrinol Metab* 1978;7:469–85.

57. **Himelstein-Braw R, Byskov AG, Peters H, Faber M.** Follicular atresia in the infant human ovary. *J Reprod Fertil* 1976;46:55–9.

58. **Wassarman PM, Albertini DF.** The mammalian ovum. In: **Knobil E, Neill JD,** eds. *The Physiology of Reproduction.* New York: Raven Press, 1994:240–4.

59. **Gondos B, Bhiraleus P, Hobel CJ.** Ultrastructural observations on germ cells in human fetal ovaries. *Am J Obstet Gynecol* 1971;110:644–52.

60. **Tsafriri A, Dekel N, Bar-Ami S.** A role of oocyte maturation inhibitor in follicular regulation of oocyte maturation. *J Reprod Fertil* 1982;64:541–51.

61. **Halpin DMG, Jones A, Fink G, Charlton HM.** Post-natal ovarian follicle development in hypogonadal (HPG) and normal mice and associated changes in the hypothalamic-pituitary axis. *J Reprod Fertil* 1986;77:287–96.

62. **Vermesh M, Kletzky OA.** Longitudinal evaluation of the luteal phase and its transition into the follicular phase. *J Clin Endocrinol Metab* 1987;65:653–8.

63. **Erickson GF, Magoffin DA, Dyer CA, Hofeditz C.** Ovarian androgen producing cells: a review of structure/function relationships. *Endocr Rev* 1985;6:371–99.

64. **Erickson GF.** An analysis of follicle development and ovum maturation. *Semin Reprod Endocrinol* 1986;46:55–9.

65. **Halpin DMG, Jones A, Fink G, Charlton HM.** Post-natal ovarian follicle development in hypogonadal (HPG) and normal mice and associated changes in the hypothalamic-pituitary axis. *J Reprod Fertil* 1986;77:287–96.

66. **Ryan KJ, Petro Z.** Steroid biosynthesis of human ovarian granulosa and thecal cells. *J Clin Endocrinol Metab* 1966;26:46–52.

67. **Kobayashi M, Nakano R, Ooshima A.** Immunohistochemical localization of pituitary gonadotropin and gonadal steroids confirms the two cells two gonadotropins hypothesis of steroidogenesis in the human ovary. *J Endocrinol* 1990;126:483–8.

68. **Yamoto M, Shima K, Nakano R.** Gonadotropin receptors in human ovarian follicles and corpora lutea throughout the menstrual cycle. *Horm Res* 1992;37(Suppl 1):5–11.

69. **Hseuh AJ, Adashi EY, Jones PB, Welsh TH Jr.** Hormonal regulation of the differentiation of cultured ovarian granulosa cells. *Endocr Rev* 1984;5:76–127.

70. **McNatty KP, Makris A, Reinhold BN, DeGrazia C, Osathanondh R, Ryan KG.** Metabolism of androstenedione by human ovarian tissues in vitro with particular reference to reductase and aromatase activity. *Steroids* 1979;34:429–43.

71. **Hillier SG, Van Den Boogard AMJ, Reichert LE, Van Hall EB.** Intraovarian sex steroid acute hormone interaction and the regulation of follicular maturation: aromatization of androgens by human granulosa cells in vitro. *J Clin Endocrinol Metab* 1980;50:640–7.

72. **Chappel SC, Resko JA, Norman RL, Spies HG.** Studies on rhesus monkeys on the site where estrogen inhibits gonadotropins: delivery of 17 β-estradiol to the hypothalamus and pituitary gland. *J Clin Endocrinol Metab* 1981;52:1–8.

73. **Chabab A, Hedon B, Arnal F, Diafouka F, Bressot N, Flandre O, et al.** Follicular steroids in relation to oocyte development in human ovarian stimulation protocols. *Hum Reprod* 1986; 1:449.

74. **Young SR, Jaffe RB.** Strength-duration characteristics of estrogen effects on gonadotropin response to gonadotropin-releasing hormone in women: II. Effects of varying concentrations of estradiol. *J Clin Endocrinol Metab* 1976;42:432–42.

75. **Pauerstein CJ, Eddy CA, Croxatto HD, Hess R, Siler-Khodr TM, Croxatto HB.** Temporal relationship of estrogen, progesterone, luteinizing hormone levels to ovulation in women and infra-human primates. *Am J Obstet Gynecol* 1978;130:876–86.

76. **World Health Organization Task Force Investigators.** Temporal relationship between ovulation and defined changes in the concentration of plasma estradiol-17β luteinizing hormone, follicle stimulating hormone and progesterone. *Am J Obstet Gynecol* 1980;138:383.

77. **Hoff JD, Quigley NE, Yen SSC.** Hormonal dynamics in mid-cycle: a re-evaluation. *J Clin Endocrinol Metab* 1983;57:792–6.

78. **Demura R, Suzuki T, Tajima S, Mitsuhashi S, Odagiri E, Demura H, et al.** Human plasma free activin and inhibin levels during the menstrual cycle. *J Clin Endocrinol Metab* 1993;76:1080–2.

79. **McLachlan RI, Robertson DM, Healy DL, Burger HG, De Kretser DM.** Circulating immunoreactive inhibin levels during the normal human menstrual cycle. *J Clin Endocrinol Metab* 1987;65:954–61.

80. **Buckler HM, Healy DL, Burger HG.** Purified FSH stimulates inhibin production from the human ovary. *J Endocrinol* 1989;122:279–85.

81. **Ling N, Ying S, Ueno N, Shimasaki S, Esch F, Hotta M, et al.** Pituitary FSH is released by hetrodimer of the beta-subunits from the two forms of inhibin. *Nature* 1986;321:779–82.

82. **Braden TD, Conn PM.** Activin-A stimulates the synthesis of gonadotropin-releasing hormone receptors. *Endocrinology* 1992;130:2101–5.

83. **Adashi EY.** Putative intraovarian regulators. *Semin Reprod Endocrinol* 1988;7:1–100.

84. **Yoshimura Y, Santulli R, Atlas SJ, Fujii S, Wallach EE.** The effects of proteolytic enzymes on in vitro ovulation in the rabbit. *Am J Obstet Gynecol* 1987;157:468–75.

85. **Yoshimura Y, Wallach EE.** Studies on the mechanism(s) of mammalian ovulation. *Fertil Steril* 1987;47:22–34.

86. **Lenton EA, Landgren B, Sexton L.** Normal variation in the length of the luteal phase of the menstrual cycle: identification of the short luteal phase. *Br J Obstet Gynaecol* 1994;91:685.

87. **Scott R, Navot D, Hung-Ching L, Rosenwaks Z.** A human in vivo model for the luteal placental shift. *Fertil Steril* 1991;56:481–4.

PREVENTIVE AND PRIMARY CARE

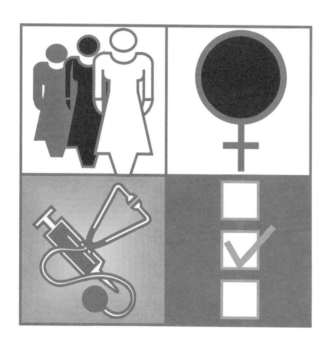

8 Preventive Health Care and Screening

Paula A. Hillard

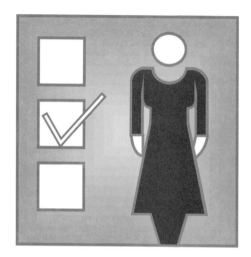

While traditionally gynecologists focus on the treatment of illnesses and abnormal conditions that can be managed in the office or in the operating room, many provide primary and preventive care that is oriented toward health maintenance and prevention or early detection of disease. The value of preventive services is apparent in trends such as the reduced mortality of cervical cancer, in part resulting from the increased use of Papanicolaou (Pap) tests. Neonatal screening for phenylketonuria (PKU) and hypothyroidism are examples of effective mechanisms for prevention of mental retardation. Women often regard their gynecologist as their primary care provider; indeed, many women of reproductive age have had no other physician. In this role, some gynecologists are extending their practices to include screening for certain medical conditions, such as hypertension, diabetes mellitus, and thyroid disease, as well as management of those conditions in the absence of complications.

Some traditional aspects of gynecologic practice, such as family planning, can be considered preventive health care. Although hormone replacement therapy can be prescribed to relieve the relatively time-limited symptoms of menopause, it also offers long-term benefits in the prevention of osteoporosis and cardiovascular disease. As primary care physicians, gynecologists provide ongoing care for women through all stages of their lives—from reproductive age to postmenopause. Preventive medical services encompass screening and counseling for a broad range of health behaviors and risks, including family planning, sexual practices, sexually transmitted diseases (STDs), smoking, alcohol and other drug use, diet, and exercise.

The Gynecologist as Primary Care Provider

Primary-preventive health care in obstetrics and gynecology has been defined as including the following elements (1):

1. The entry point to the health care system

2. Direct involvement in the patient's health care

3. Continuity in relationship between the physician and patient

4. Care managed with an awareness of the relationship of disease to the family structure

5. Dedication to long-term prevention of serious illness and for its early detection

6. General health care (i.e., concerned with diseases other than those of the reproductive tract)

7. Application of skill and judgment regarding consultation and referral, when required, for assurance of complete care by multiple health care providers

8. Available on a 24-hour basis.

In addition, the American College of Obstetricians and Gynecologists (ACOG) has defined educational objectives that outline what practicing physicians who chose to provide primary preventive care should be able to do (2):

1. Establish a physician-patient relationship that creates a health-promoting alliance, including helping patients to control their own health choices, to recognize the benefits of avoiding high-risk behavior, and to acquire the necessary attitudes and skills to change behaviors that place their health at risk

2. Be familiar with the leading causes of death and morbidity within different age groups in order to incorporate a holistic approach to assessing patients' risks

3. Apply the knowledge and skills needed to identify underlying problems; counsel patients; and educate patients, adapting to their individual needs, communication skills, age, race, sex, and socioeconomic status

4. Encourage patient follow-up

5. Incorporate a team approach to patient care, using the expertise of nurses, health educators, other allied health professionals, and relevant social services.

The leading causes of death and morbidity within different age groups are listed in Tables 8.1 and 8.2 (3).

In 1991, the president of the American College of Obstetricians and Gynecologists (ACOG) appointed a task force on primary and preventive health care. This task force reviewed previous ACOG documents and reports as well as four documents from other organizations: the Guide to Clinical Preventive Services, a report of the U.S. Preventive Services Task Force (4); the age charts for periodic health examination from the American Academy of Family Physicians (4); the American College of Physicians Preventive Care Guidelines: 1991 (5); and Healthy People 2000: National Health Promotion and Disease Prevention Objectives (3). In recognition of the wide range of practice patterns of obstetricians and gynecologists, the ACOG task force described three categories of services provided by obstetricians and gynecologists (6):

1. *Obstetric and Gynecologic Services*—include the medical and surgical care related to the female reproductive system that traditionally has been provided by obstetrician and gynecologists.

2. *Primary-Preventive Care*—describes a broader range of services, including health screening and preventive medicine.

Table 8.1   Leading Causes of Death By Age Group

Ages 13–18 Years

Motor vehicle accidents
Homicide
Suicide
Leukemia

Ages 19–39 Years

Motor vehicle accidents
Cardiovascular disease
Homicide
Coronary artery disease
Acquired immunodeficiency syndrome (AIDS)
Breast cancer
Cerebrovascular disease
Uterine cancer

Ages 40–64 Years

Cardiovascular disease
Coronary artery disease
Breast cancer
Lung cancer
Cerebrovascular disease
Colorectal cancer
Obstructive pulmonary disease
Ovarian cancer

Ages 65 Years and Older

Cardiovascular disease
Coronary artery disease
Cerebrovascular disease
Pneumonia/influenza
Obstructive lung disease
Colorectal cancer
Breast cancer
Lung cancer
Accidents

Modified with permission from **ACOG.** *The Obstetrician–Gynecologist and Primary-Preventive Health Care.* Washington, DC: American College of Obstetricians and Gynecologists, 1993:1–22.

3. *Extended Primary Care*—includes the management of diseases and conditions beyond those that pertain to the reproductive system.

The ACOG task force concluded that the practice of extended primary care should be based on each physician's education and experience (6). Books specific to the provision of primary health care by obstetrician gynecologists are now available (7).

In 1992 in the U.S., there were more than 7 million ambulatory care visits to all physicians; 455 million of these visits were made by women. Nine percent of the visits (69 million) were made to gynecologists (8). Eighty-three percent of these visits were made by individuals between the ages of 15 and 44 years (9). The most frequently cited reason for an office visit to a gynecologist by women older than 15 years of age was routine prenatal examination. The second most frequently cited reason was "general medical examination." For women in this age group, gynecologists provided more general medical examinations than general/family practitioners and internists combined. For women of reproductive age (15–44 years), gynecologists provided nearly four times as many general medical examinations than did general/family practitioners, and almost 12 times as many examinations as internists (10).

In a survey of physicians who were asked to categorize themselves as a primary care physician, a specialist, or a consultant, nearly one-half of obstetricians/gynecologists (48%) con-

Table 8.2 Leading Causes of Morbidity By Age Group

Ages 13–18 Years

Nose, throat, and upper respiratory conditions
Viral, bacterial, and parasitic infections
Sexual abuse
Injuries (musculoskeletal and soft tissue)
Acute ear infections
Digestive system conditions
Acute urinary conditions

Ages 19–39 Years

Nose, throat, and upper respiratory conditions
Injuries (musculoskeletal and soft tissue, including back and upper and lower extremities)
Viral, bacterial, and parasitic infections
Acute urinary conditions

Ages 40–64 Years

Nose, throat, and upper respiratory conditions
Osteoporosis/arthritis
Hypertension
Orthopedic deformities and impairments (including back and upper and lower extremities)
Heart disease
Hearing and vision impairments

Ages 65 Years and Older

Nose, throat, and upper respiratory conditions
Osteoporosis/arthritis
Hypertension
Urinary incontinence
Heart disease
Injuries (musculoskeletal and soft tissue)
Hearing and vision impairments

Modified with permission from **ACOG.** *The Obstetrician–Gynecologist and Primary-Preventive Health Care.* Washington, DC: American College of Obstetricians and Gynecologists, 1993:1–22.

sidered themselves to be primary care providers (10). Gynecologists younger than 35 years of age, those in the South Atlantic census region, and those who were paid by hospitals and medical centers were more likely to consider themselves as primary care providers.

Obstetricians and gynecologists are less likely than other primary care physicians to refer their patients. Data compiled by the National Center for Health Statistics (NCHS) from 1989–90 indicate that gynecologists had a referral rate of 4%, general internists 7.3%, and family and general practitioners 7.3% (11).

In 1993, ACOG commissioned a Gallop poll to assess how women viewed the care provided by their obstetricians/gynecologists (12). When compared with other physicians, obstetricians/gynecologists were more likely to perform a Pap test, pelvic examination, and breast examination than were other physicians. Obstetricians/gynecologists were as likely as other physicians to have checked blood pressure and referred patients for mammography. When compared with other physicians, they were slightly less likely to have checked cholesterol levels. Obstetricians/gynecologists are somewhat more likely than other physicians to have discussed family planning, preconception issues, and STDs, including human immunodeficiency virus. Other physicians were more likely to discuss medication use than were obstetricians/gynecologists. Other physicians were as likely as obstetricians/gynecologists to have discussed diet and exercise, smoking, alcohol use, hormone replacement therapy, osteoporosis, emotional problems, illegal drug use, and physical abuse (12). More than one-half of all women who reported seeing an obstetrician/gynecologist considered him or her to be their primary physician. As expected, the percentage was highest among

178

women aged 18–29 years (69%), and lowest among women older than 40 years of age (45%) (12).

Approaches to Preventive Care

Currently, there is a shift in health care from a focus on disease to a focus on prevention. Efforts are under way to promote effective screening measures that can have a beneficial effect on public and individual health. Following is a brief description of programs developed by the ACOG, the U.S. Preventive Services Task Force, and the American Medical Association to provide guidelines for preventive care.

Guidelines for Primary-Preventive Care

In the approach outlined by ACOG, the physician and patient first reach an understanding that a primary care relationship has been established. Patients should be aware of the services available and whether the obstetrician/gynecologist is serving as a specialist or a primary care physician. For patients with whom a primary care relationship has been established, the initial evaluation involves a complete history, physical examination, routine and indicated laboratory studies, evaluation and counseling, appropriate immunizations, and relevant interventions. Risk factors should be identified and arrangements should be made for continuing care or referral, as needed. Subsequent care should follow a specific schedule, yearly or as appropriate based on the patient's needs and age. The ACOG recommendations for periodic evaluation, screening, and counseling by age groups are shown in Tables 8.3–8.6. These tables also include recommendations for patients who have high-risk factors that require targeted screening of treatment (4). High-risk factors are listed in Table 8.7. Recommendations for immunizations are included in Table 8.8.

Guide to Clinical Preventive Services

The U.S. Preventive Services Task Force, commissioned in 1984, was a 20-member nongovernment panel of experts in primary care medicine, epidemiology, and public health, and its report was published in 1989 (4). A similar panel had been convened in 1976 in Canada—the Canadian Task Force on the Periodic Health Examination—it issued its report in 1979 (13). The charge of both panels was to develop recommendations on the appropriate use of preventive interventions based on a systematic review of evidence of clinical effectiveness.

The task force used several criteria for selecting conditions to evaluate, including the burden of suffering posed by a given condition, its prevalence (proportion of the population affected), and its incidence (number of new cases per year) (4). The task force reviewed only those preventive services that would be provided for asymptomatic individuals. Primary preventive measures are those that involve intervention before the disease develops, for example, quitting smoking, increasing physical activity, good nutrition, quitting alcohol and other drug use, seat belt use, and immunizations. Secondary preventive measures are those used to identify and treat asymptomatic persons who have risk factors or preclinical disease but in whom the disease itself has not become clinically apparent. Examples of secondary preventive measures are well known in gynecology: screening mammography and Pap tests.

The Preventive Services Task Force analyzed the effectiveness of various screening measures and tests. For screening tests, they assessed the accuracy of the test, including its sensitivity, specificity, and positive and negative predictive values. The task force also reviewed the methodologic quality of the studies. Because the design of a study influences the interpretation of the data and the weight given to its results, the U.S. Preventive Services Task Force established a hierarchy of the types of studies available to assess the effectiveness of various interventions. This hierarchy is listed in Table 8.9. The strength of the task force's recommendations regarding the value of a screening or preventive inter-

Table 8.3   Periodic Evaluation Ages 13–18

Screening	Evaluation and Counseling
History	**Sexuality**
Reason for visit	Development
Health status: medical, surgical, family	High-risk behaviors
Dietary/nutritional assessments	Contraceptive options 　Genetic counseling 　Prevention of unwanted pregnancy
Physical activity	Sexually transmitted diseases 　Partner selection 　Barrier protection
Tobacco, alcohol, other drugs	
Abuse/neglect	**Fitness**
Sexual practices	Hygiene (including dental)
	Dietary/nutritional assessment
Physical	Exercise: discussion of program
Height	
Weight	**Psychosocial evaluation**
Blood pressure	Interpersonal/family relationships
Secondary sexual characteristics 　(Tanner staging)	Sexual identity
Pelvic examination (yearly when 　sexually active or by age 18)	Personal goal development
Skin*	Behavioral/learning disorders
	Abuse/neglect
Laboratory tests	**Cardiovascular risk factors**
Pap test (yearly when sexually active 　or by age 18)	Family history
High-risk groups	Hypertension
Hemoglobin*	Hyperlipidemia
Bacteriuria testing*	Obesity/diabetes mellitus
Sexually transmitted disease testing*	
Human immunodeficiency virus 　testing*	**Health-risk behaviors**
Rubella titer*	Injury prevention
Tuberculosis skin test*	Safety belts and helmets
Lipid profile*	Recreational hazards
	Firearms
	Hearing
	Skin exposure to ultraviolet rays
	Suicide: depressive symptoms
	Tobacco, alcohol, other drugs

*In the presence of high-risk factors.
Modified with permission from **ACOG.** *The Obstetrician–Gynecologist and Primary-Preventive Health Care.* Washington, DC: American College of Obstetricians and Gynecologists, 1993:1–22.

Table 8.4   Periodic Evaluation Ages 19–39

Screening	Evaluation and Counseling
History	**Sexuality**
Reason for visit	High-risk behaviors
Health status: medical, surgical, family	Contraceptive options
Dietary/nutritional assessments	Genetic counseling
Physical activity	Prevention of unwanted pregnancy
Tobacco, alcohol, other drugs	Sexually transmitted diseases
Abuse/neglect	Partner selection
Sexual practices	Barrier protection
	Sexual functioning
Physical	
Height	**Fitness**
Weight	Hygiene (including dental)
Blood pressure	Dietary/nutritional assessment
Neck; adenopathy, thyroid	Exercise: discussion of program
Breasts	
Abdomen	**Psychosocial evaluation**
Pelvic examination	Interpersonal/family relationships
Skin*	Domestic violence
	Job satisfaction
	Lifestyle/stress
	Sleep disorders
Laboratory tests	
Pap test (physician and patient discretion after three consecutive normal tests)	
Cholesterol (Every 5 years)	**Cardiovascular risk factors**
High-risk groups	Family history
Hemoglobin*	Hypertension
Bacteriuria testing*	Hyperlipidemia
Mammography*	Obesity/diabetes mellitus
Fasting glucose test*	Lifestyle
Sexually transmitted disease testing*	
Human immunodeficiency virus testing*	**Health/risk behaviors**
Genetic testing/counseling*	Injury prevention
Rubella titer*	—Safety belts and helmets
Tuberculosis skin test*	—Occupational hazards
Lipid profile*	—Recreational hazards
Thyroid-stimulating hormone*	—Firearms
	—Hearing
	Breast self-examination

Table 8.4—*continued*

Evaluation and Counseling
Skin exposure to ultraviolet rays
Suicide: depressive symptoms
Tobacco, alcohol, other drugs

*In the presence of high-risk factors.
Modified with permission from **ACOG.** *The Obstetrician–Gynecologist and Primary-Preventive Health Care.* Washington, DC: American College of Obstetricians and Gynecologists, 1993:1–22.

vention is based on the quality of the evidence available. In some circumstances, there is good evidence to recommend for or against an intervention, whereas in others, there is only fair or poor evidence regarding the effectiveness of an intervention. The strength of the task force's recommendations were graded according to a system used by the Canadian Task Force on the Periodic Health Examination (13) (Table 8.10).

The U.S. Preventive Services Task Force drew a number of conclusions based on review of the data (4):

1. The data suggest that among the most effective interventions available to clinicians for reducing the incidence and severity of the leading causes of disease and disability in the U.S. are those that address the personal health practices of patients.

2. There is a need for greater selectivity in ordering tests and providing preventive services; the proper selection of screening tests requires careful consideration of the age, sex, and other individual risk factors of the patient in order to minimize the risk of adverse effects and unnecessary expenditures caused by screening.

3. Conventional clinical activities (e.g., diagnostic testing) may be of less value to patients than activities once considered outside the traditional role of clinician (e.g., counseling and patient education). This finding suggests a new paradigm in defining the responsibilities of the primary care provider, shifting from the treatment of illness to a concern with keeping asymptomatic individuals healthy through a focus on personal health behaviors.

4. The shifting responsibility of clinicians also implies a changing role for patients. The increasing evidence of the importance of personal health behaviors and primary prevention means that patients must assume greater responsibility for their own health. Although the clinician is often the key figure in the treatment of acute illnesses and injuries, the patient is the principal agent in primary prevention.

5. Preventive services need not be delivered exclusively during visits devoted entirely to prevention. Although preventive checkups often provide more time for counseling and other preventive services and healthy individuals may be more receptive to such interventions than those who are sick, a visit for treatment of an illness is an equally important time to practice prevention.

6. The gaps in evidence identified by the task force underscore the size of the research agenda in preventive medicine. For most topics examined in the report, the task force found inadequate evidence to evaluate effectiveness or to determine the optimal frequency of a preventive service.

7. The process used by the U.S. and Canadian task forces to evaluate effectiveness may be as important a contribution to medical policy as the recommendations themselves.

Table 8.5   Periodic Evaluations Ages 40–64

Screening	Evaluation and Counseling
History	**Sexuality**
Reason for visit	High-risk behaviors
Health status: medical, surgical, family	Contraceptive options
Dietary/nutritional assessment	Genetic counseling
Physical activity	Prevention of unwanted pregnancy
Tobacco, alcohol, other drugs	Sexually transmitted disease
Abuse/neglect	Partner selection
Sexual practices	Barrier protection
	Sexual functioning
Physical	
Height	**Fitness**
Weight	Hygiene (including dental)
Blood pressure	Dietary/nutritional assessment
Oral cavity	Exercise: discussion of program
Neck: adenopathy, thyroid	
Breasts, axillae	**Psychosocial evaluation**
Abdomen	Family relationships
Pelvic and rectovaginal examination	Domestic violence
Skin*	Job/work satisfaction
	Retirement planning
	Lifestyle/stress
	Sleep disorders
Laboratory tests	
Pap test (physician and patient discretion after three consecutive normal tests)	**Cardiovascular risk factors**
Mammography (Every 1–2 years until age 50, yearly beginning at 50)	Family history
Cholesterol (every 5 years)	Hypertension
Fecal occult blood test	Hyperlipidemia
Sigmoidoscopy (every 3–5 years after age 50)	Obesity/diabetes mellitus
High-risk groups	Life style
Hemoglobin*	
Bacteriuria testing*	**Health/risk behaviors**
Mammography	Hormone replacement therapy
Fasting glucose test*	Injury prevention
Sexually transmitted disease testing*	Safety belts and helmets
Human immunodeficiency virus testing*	Occupational hazards
Tuberculosis skin test*	Recreational hazards
	Sports involvement

Table 8.5—continued

Screening	Evaluation and Counseling
Lipid profile*	Firearms
Thyroid-stimulating hormone*	Hearing
Colonoscopy	Breast self-examination
	Skin exposure to ultraviolet rays
	Suicide: depressive symptoms
	Tobacco, alcohol, other drugs

*In the presence of high-risk factors.
Modified with permission from **ACOG.** *The Obstetrician–Gynecologist and Primary-Preventive Health Care.* Washington, DC: American College of Obstetricians and Gynecologists, 1993:1–22.

Guidelines for Adolescent Preventive Services

Around the same time that clinicians were evaluating the primary health care needs of adults, clinicians who practice adolescent medicine (with backgrounds in pediatrics, internal medicine, family medicine, gynecology, nursing, psychology, nutrition, and other professions) recognized that the guidelines for adult and pediatric health services did not always fit the needs and health risks of adolescence. Neither the ACOG Guidelines for Primary-Preventive Care (6) nor the U.S. Preventive Services Task Force recommendations (4) are sufficiently comprehensive or focused on this age group, although both documents include many important aspects of adolescent health care. The American Medical Association, with the assistance of a national scientific advisory board, developed the Guidelines for Adolescent Preventive Services (GAPS) in response to this perceived need for recommendations for delivering comprehensive adolescent preventive services (14, 15).

Obstetricians/gynecologists typically see adolescents in crisis: to provide care for unintended pregnancies or STDs, including pelvic inflammatory disease. The need for preventing these crises is evident. The ACOG guidelines recognize the role that obstetricians/gynecologists potentially could play in providing preventive services for adolescents. They suggest a schedule of visits that is "yearly or as appropriate" (6). The GAPS report goes beyond this recommendation and extends the framework of services provided. The impetus for developing GAPS was the belief that a fundamental change in the delivery of adolescent health services was necessary. Gynecologists could easily provide most, if not all, of the recommended services; annual preventive visits to a gynecologist might well lead to the prevention of gynecologic health problems. There are numerous opportunities for primary preventive care of adolescents in a gynecologist's office.

The GAPS report includes 24 recommendations (Table 8.11). These recommendations address the delivery of health care, focus on the use of health guidance to promote the health and well-being of adolescents and their families, promote the use of screening to identify conditions that occur relatively frequently in adolescents and cause significant suffering either during adolescence or later in life, and provide guidelines for immunizations for the primary prevention of specific infectious diseases (15).

The GAPS recommendations stem from the conclusion that the current health threats to adolescents are predominantly behavioral rather than biomedical, that more of today's adolescents are involved in health behaviors with the potential for serious consequences, that today's adolescents are involved in health-risk behaviors at younger ages than previous generations, that many adolescents engage in multiple health risk behaviors, and that most adolescents engage in at least some type of behavior that threatens their health and well-being (15). Gynecologists are in a good position to detect high-risk behaviors and to determine whether multiple risk-taking behaviors exist; for example, the early initiation of sexual activity and unsafe sexual practices are associated with

Table 8.6   Periodic Evaluations Ages 65 Years and Older

Screening	*Evaluation and Counseling*
History	**Sexuality**
Reason for visit	Sexual functioning
Health status: medical, surgical, family	Sexual behaviors
Dietary/nutritional assessment	Sexually transmitted diseases
Physical activity	
Tobacco, alcohol, other drugs, polypharmacy	**Fitness**
Abuse/neglect	Hygiene (general and dental)
Sexual practices	Dietary/nutritional assessment
	Exercise: discussion of program
Physical	
Height	**Psychosocial evaluation**
Weight	Neglect/abuse
Blood pressure	Life style/stress
Oral cavity	Depression/sleep disorders
Neck: adenopathy, thyroid	Family relationships
Breasts, axillae	Job/work/retirement satisfaction
Abdomen	
Pelvic and rectovaginal examination	**Cardiovascular risk factors**
Skin*	Hypertension
	Hypercholesterolemia
	Obesity/diabetes mellitus
Laboratory Tests	Sedentary lifestyle
Pap test (physician and patient discretion after three consecutive normal tests)	
Urinalysis/dipstick	**Health/risk behaviors**
Mammography	Hormone replacement therapy
Cholesterol (every 3–5 years)	Injury prevention
Fecal occult blood test	Safety belts and helmets
Sigmoidoscopy (every 3–5 years)	Occupational hazards
Thyroid-stimulating hormone test (every 3–5 years)	Recreational hazards
High-risk groups	Hearing
Hemoglobin*	Firearms
Fasting glucose test*	Visual acuity/glaucoma
Sexually transmitted disease testing*	Hearing
Human immunodeficiency virus testing*	Breast self-examination
Tuberculosis skin test*	Skin exposure to ultraviolet rays
Lipid profile*	Suicide: depressive symptoms
Colonoscopy*	Tobacco, alcohol, other drugs

*In the presence of high-risk factors.
Modified with permission from **ACOG**. *The Obstetrician–Gynecologist and Primary-Preventive Health Care*. Washington, DC: American College of Obstetricians and Gynecologists, 1993:1–22.

Table 8.7 High-Risk Factors

Bacteriuria Testing

Persons with diabetes mellitus

Colonoscopy

Personal history of:
  Inflammatory bowel disease
  Colonic polyps
Family history of:
  Familiar polyposis
  Colorectal cancer
  Cancer family syndrome

Fasting Glucose Test

Every 3–5 years for persons with family history of diabetes mellitus (one first- or two
  second-degree relatives)
Marked obesity
History of gestational diabetes mellitus

Fluoride Supplement

Persons living in areas with inadequate water fluoridation < 0.7 parts/million)

Genetic Testing/Counseling

Women of reproductive age who are exposed to teratogens
Women of reproductive age who contemplate pregnancy at 35 years of age or older
Patient, partner, or family member with history of genetic disorder or birth defect
Persons of African-American, Eastern European, Jewish, Mediterranean, or Southeast
  Asian ancestry

Hemoglobin

Caribbean, Latin American, Asian, Mediterranean, or African descent
Menorrhagia

Hepatitis B Vaccine

Intravenous drug users
Current recipients of blood products
Persons in health-related jobs with exposure to blood or blood products
Household and sexual contacts of hepatitis B virus carriers
Prostitutes
Persons with history of multiple sexual partners in the last 6 months

HIV testing

Person seeking treatment for sexually transmitted disease
Past or present intravenous drug use
History of prostitution
Past or present sexual partner HIV +, bisexual, intravenous user
Persons from area of high prevalence HIV infection
History transfusion 1978–1985

Influenza Vaccine

Residents of chronic care facilities
Persons with chronic cardiopulmonary disorders
Persons with metabolic diseases including:
  Diabetes mellitus
  Hemoglobinopathies
  Immunosuppression
  Renal dysfunction

Lipid Profile

Persons with elevated cholesterol level
History of parent or sibling with cholesterol ≥ 240 mg/dl
History of sibling parent, or grandparent with documented premature (younger than 55
years of age) coronary artery disease
Persons with diabetes mellitus
Smoker

Table 8.7—*continued*

Mammography

Women aged 35 years and older with a family history of premenopausally diagnosed breast cancer in a first-degree relative

Pneumococcal Vaccine

Chronic cardiac/pulmonary disease
Sickle cell disease
Nephrotic syndrome
Hodgkin's disease
Asplenia
Diabetes mellitus
Alcoholism
Cirrhosis
Multiple myeloma
Renal disease
Immunosuppression

Rubella Titer/Vaccine

Women of childbearing age lacking evidence of immunity
Immunization (MMR) for all women unable to show proof of immunity

Skin

Recreational or occupation exposure to sunlight
History/family history skin cancer
Precursor lesions (dysplastic nevi, some congenital nevi)

Sexually Transmitted Disease (STD)

Multiple partners/partner with multiple partners
Sexual contacts of persons with culture proven STDs
History repeated episodes STDs
Persons attending STD clinics

Tuberculin (TB) Skin Test

Patients with HIV
Close contacts (household or enclosed environments) of known or suspected persons with TB
Persons with medical risk factors known to increase the risk of disease if infection occurred
Foreign-born persons from countries with high TB prevalence
Medically underserved, low-income populations
Alcoholics and intravenous drug users
Residents of long-term care facilities, jails, mental institutions, nursing homes and facilities, other long-term residential facilities
Health-professional working in high-risk health care facilities

Thyroid-Stimulating Hormone

Individuals with strong family history thyroid disease
Patients with autoimmune disease

Modified with permission from **ACOG.** *The Obstetrician–Gynecologist and Primary-Preventive Health Care.* Washington, DC: American College of Obstetricians and Gynecologists, 1993:1–22.

substance use (16). Adolescents who are sexually active are much more likely to have used alcohol (6.3 times greater risk), four times more likely to have used drugs other than marijuana, and nearly 10 times more likely to have been a passenger in a motor vehicle with a driver who was using drugs than were adolescents who were not sexually active (17). Thus, by being aware of comorbidities, gynecologists can screen for these behaviors and potentially intervene before there are serious harmful health consequences.

Table 8.8   Immunizations

Ages 13–18 Years

Periodic
  Tetanus-diphtheria booster (once between ages 14 and 16)
High-Risk Groups
  Measles, mumps, rubella (MMR) (HR7)
  Hepatitis B vaccine (HR 10)
  Fluoride supplement (HR 11)

Ages 19–39 Years

Periodic
  Tetanus-diphtheria booster (every 10 years)
High-Risk Groups
  Measles, mumps, rubella (MMR) (HR7)
  Hepatitis B vaccine (HR 10)
  Influenza vaccine (HR 15)
  Pneumococcal vaccine (HR 16)

Age 40–64 Years

Periodic
  Tetanus-diphtheria booster (every 10 years)
  Influenza vaccine (annually beginning at age 55)
High-Risk Groups
  Mumps, measles, rubella (MMR) (HR 7)
  Hepatitis B vaccine (HR 10)
  Influence vaccine (HR 15)
  Pneumococcal vaccine (HR 16)

Ages 65 Years and Older

Periodic
  Tetanus-diphtheria booster (every 10 years)
  Influenza vaccine (annually)
  Pneumococcal vaccine (once)
High-Risk Groups
  Hepatitis B vaccine (HR 10)

Modified with permission from **ACOG.** *The Obstetrician–Gynecologist and Primary-Preventive Health Care.* Washington, DC: American College of Obstetricians and Gynecologists, 1993:1–22.

Table 8.9   Quality of Evidence—U.S. Preventive Services Task Force

---

I: Evidence obtained from at least one properly designed randomized, controlled trial.

II-1: Evidence obtained from well-designed controlled trials without randomization.

II-2: Evidence obtained from well-designed cohort or case-control analytic studies, preferably from more than one center or research group.

II-3: Evidence obtained from multiple time series with or without the intervention. Dramatic results in uncontrolled experiments (such as the results of the introduction of penicillin treatment in the 1940s) could also be regarded as this type of evidence.

III: Opinions of respected authorities, based on clinical experience, descriptive studies, or reports of expert committees.

From **Canadian Task Force on the Periodic Health Examination.** The periodic health examination. *Can Med Assoc J* 1979;121:1193–254.

Table 8.10   U.S. Preventive Services Task Force—Strength Of Recommendations

A.	There is good evidence to support the recommendation that the condition be specifically considered in a periodic health examination.
B.	There is fair evidence to support the recommendation that the condition be specifically considered in a periodic health examination.
C.	There is poor evidence regarding the inclusion of the condition in a periodic health examination, but recommendations may be made on other grounds.
D.	There is fair evidence to support the recommendation that the condition be excluded from consideration in a periodic health examination.
E.	There is good evidence to support the recommendation that the condition be excluded from consideration in a periodic health examination.

Modified with permission from **ACOG.** *The Obstetrician–Gynecologist and Primary-Preventive Health Care.* Washington, DC: American College of Obstetricians and Gynecologists, 1993:1–22.

Counseling for Health Maintenance

During periodic assessments, yearly or as appropriate, patients should be counseled about preventive care depending on their age and risk factors. Obesity, smoking, and alcohol abuse are preventable problems that can have a major long-term impact on health. Thus, patients should be counseled about smoking cessation and moderation in alcohol use and directed to appropriate community resources as necessary. Positive health behaviors, such as eating a healthy diet and engaging in regular exercise, should be reinforced. Adjustments may be necessary based on the presence of risk factors and the woman's current lifestyle and condition. Efforts should focus on weight control, cardiovascular fitness, and reduction of risk factors associated with cardiovascular disease and diabetes (18–21).

Nutrition

Patients should be given general nutritional information and referred to other professionals if they have special needs. **Assessment of the patient's body mass index (weight [in kilograms] divided by height [in meters] squared [kilograms per square meter]) will give valuable information about the patient's nutritional status. Patients who are 20% above or below the normal range (normal = 22) require evaluation and counseling and should be assessed for systemic disease or an eating disorder.**

Central obesity—measured as waist:hip ratio—is a risk factor for coronary heart disease and some forms of cancer. When the waist:hip ratio exceeds 0.76, there is a greater relative risk of death from cancer or cardiovascular disease in women aged 55–69 years.

The Food Guide Pyramid developed by the U.S. Department of Agriculture helps women choose food from five groups to provide needed nutrients (Fig. 8.1) (22). The pyramid stresses eating a variety of foods to get adequate energy, protein, vitamins, minerals, and fiber. It also stresses a diet that is high in vegetables, fruits, and grain products.

Fiber content of the diet is being studied for its potential role in the prevention of several disorders, particularly colon cancer. Currently, it is recommended that the average diet contain 20–30 g of fiber per day. Foods high in dietary fiber include whole-grain breads and cereals, green and yellow vegetables, citrus fruits, and some legumes.

Adequate calcium intake is important in the prevention of osteoporosis. A postmenopausal woman should receive 1500 mg/day. There is no evidence that moderate caffeine intake causes osteoporosis when calcium intake is inadequate. Because it is difficult to ingest 1500 mg of calcium daily in an average diet, the use of supplements may be required.

Table 8.11   Guidelines For Adolescent Preventive Services (GAPS)

1. From ages 11 to 21 years, all adolescents should have an annual routine health visit.

2. Preventive services should be age and developmentally appropriate, and they should be sensitive to individual and sociocultural differences.

3. Physicians should establish office policies regarding confidential care for adolescents and how parents will be involved in that care. These policies should be made clear to adolescent and the parents.

4. Parents or other adult caregivers of adolescents should receive health guidance at least once during early adolescence, once during middle adolescence, and preferably, once during late adolescence.

5. All adolescents should receive health guidance annually to promote a better understanding of their physical growth, psychosocial and psychosexual development, and the importance of becoming actively involved in decisions regarding their health care.

6. All adolescents should receive health guidance annually to promote the reduction of injuries.

7. All adolescents should receive health guidance annually about dietary habits, including the benefits of a healthy diet, ways to achieve a healthy diet, and safe weight management.

8. All adolescents should receive health guidance annually about the benefits of exercise and should be encouraged to engage in safe exercise on a regular basis.

9. All adolescents should receive health guidance annually regarding responsible sexual behaviors, including abstinence. Latex condoms to prevent sexually transmitted diseases (STDs) (including HIV infection) and appropriate methods of birth control should be made available with instructions on how to use them effectively.

10. All adolescents should receive health guidance annually to promote avoidance of the use of tobacco, alcohol, abusable substances, and anabolic steroids.

11. All adolescents should be screened annually for hypertension according to the protocol developed by the National Heart, Lung, and Blood Institute Second Task Force on Blood Pressure Control in Children (18).

12. Selected adolescents should be screened to determine their risk of developing hyperlipidemia and adult coronary heart disease following the protocol by the Expert Panel on Blood Cholesterol Levels in Children and Adolescents (19).

13. All adolescents should be screened annually for eating disorders and obesity by determining weight and stature and asking about body image and dieting patterns.

14. All adolescents should be asked annually about their use of tobacco products, including cigarettes and smokeless tobacco.

15. All adolescents should be asked annually about their use of alcohol and other abusable substances and about their use of over-the-counter or prescription drugs for nonmedical purposes, including anabolic steroids.

16. All adolescents should be asked annually about involvement in sexual behaviors that may result in unintended pregnancies and STDs, including HIV infection.

17. Sexually active adolescents should be screened for STDs.

18. Adolescents at risk for HIV infection should be offered confidential HIV screening with the enzyme-linked immunosorbent assay and confirmatory testing.

19. Female adolescents who are sexually active or any female 18 years of age or older should be screened annually for cervical cancer by use of a Pap test.

20. All adolescents should be asked annually about behaviors or emotions that indicate recurrent or severe depression or risk of suicide.

21. All adolescents should be asked annually about a history of emotional, physical, and sexual abuse.

22. All adolescents should be asked annually about learning or school problems.

Table 8.11—*continued*

23. Adolescents should receive a tuberculin skin test if they have been exposed to active tuberculosis, have lived in a homeless shelter, have been incarcerated, have lived in or come from an area with a high prevalence of tuberculosis, or currently work in a health care setting.

24. All adolescents should receive prophylactic immunizations according to the guidelines established by the federally convened Advisory Committee on Immunization Practices: a bivalent tetanus-diphtheria vaccine 10 years after their previous diphtheria vaccination (usually 5–6 years old). All adolescents should receive a second trivalent measles–mumps–rubella vaccination, unless there is documentation of two vaccinations earlier during childhood. A measles–mumps–rubella vaccination should not be given to adolescents who are pregnant—susceptible adolescents who engage in high-risk behaviors should be vaccinated against hepatitis B virus. This includes adolescents who have had more than one sexual partner during the previous 6 months, have exchanged sex for drugs or money, are males who have engaged in sex with other males, or have used intravenous drugs. Widespread use of the hepatitis B vaccine is encouraged because risk factors are often not easily identifiable among adolescents.

From **Elster AB, Kuznets NJ.** *AMA Guidelines for Adolescent Preventive Services (GAPS): Recommendations and Rationale.* Baltimore: Williams & Wilkins, 1994:1–191.

Figure 8.1   The Food Guide Pyramid. A Guide to Daily Food Choices. This is a guide to help men and nonpregnant women choose foods that will give them the nutrients they need. Because a pregnant woman needs extra calories, she should get at least the number of servings shown in parentheses after the standard servings.

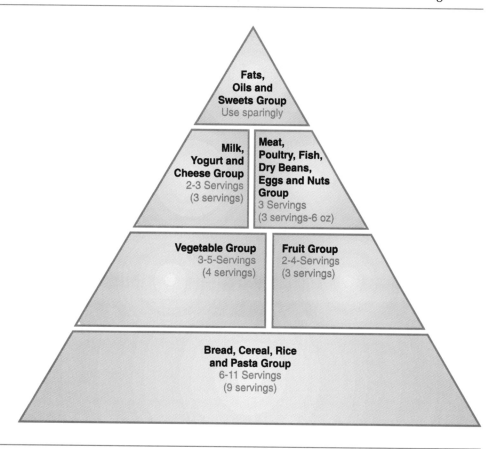

The Centers for Disease Control and Prevention has recommended that women of reproductive age who are capable of becoming pregnant take supplemental folic acid (0.4 mg daily) to help prevent neural tube defects (23). Women who are contemplating pregnancy should be counseled about the risk of neural tube defects and the role of folic acid in their prevention.

Following are some general nutritional guidelines for all women issued by the Committee on Diet and Health of the National Research Council (24):

1. Total fat intake should be 30% of calories or less. Saturated fatty acid intake should be less than 10% of calories, and the intake of cholesterol should be <300 mg daily

2. Every day, five or more servings of a combination of vegetables and fruits, especially green and yellow vegetables and citrus fruit, should be eaten. The daily intake of starches and other complex carbohydrates should be increased by eating six or more servings of a combination of breads, cereals, and legumes

3. Protein should be maintained at moderate levels (<1.6 g/kg of body weight)

4. Total daily intake of salt should be limited to 6 g or less

5. Vitamin-mineral supplement intake should not exceed the recommended dietary intake per day.

Alcohol

Alcoholic beverages should be limited to <1 oz of absolute alcohol per day (equivalent to two cans of beer, two glasses of wine, or two average cocktails).

A simple device called the T-ACE questionnaire can be used to elicit information about alcohol use and identify problem drinkers (Table 8.12). Women should be questioned in a nonjudgmental fashion about their alcohol use and directed to counseling services as required.

Exercise

Exercise can help control or prevent hypertension, diabetes mellitus, and cardiovascular disease. Moderate exercise along with calcium supplementation and hormone replacement therapy can help retard bone loss in postmenopausal women (21).

Table 8.12   T-ACE Questionnaire

Do you have a drinking problem?

Experts in treating alcohol abuse use the T-ACE questions below to help them find out whether a person has a drinking problem. These questions can also apply to other drugs.

T	How many drinks does it take to make you feel high (**TOLERANCE**)?
A	Have people **ANNOYED** you by criticizing your drinking?
C	Have you ever felt you ought to **CUT DOWN** on your drinking?
E	Have you ever had a drink first thing in the morning to steady your nerves or get rid of a hangover (**EYE OPENER**)?

If your answer to the tolerance questions is *more than two drinks,* give yourself a score of 2. If you answer *yes* to any of the other questions, give yourself a score of 1 each. *If your total score is 2 or more, you may have a drinking problem.*

Modified from **Sokol RJ, Martier SS, Ager JW.** The T-ACE questions: practical prenatal detection of risk-drinking. *Am J Obstet Gynecol* 1989;160:865.

Before beginning an exercise program, patients should be examined to ensure that exercise will not pose a risk to their health. Women should be counseled about safety guidelines for exercise. Factors that should be considered in establishing an exercise program include medical limitations and selection of activities that promote health and enhance compliance. A variety of physical activities (e.g., gardening, raking leaves, walking to work, taking the stairs) can be incorporated easily into an individual's daily routine. Emphasis should be placed on regular physical activity (e.g., 30 min/day) rather than episodic vigorous exercise, especially in sedentary individuals (21). High-impact exercise is not necessary to achieve benefits, and it may be harmful. Regular low-impact or moderate aerobic exercise has been associated with improved long-term compliance and adequate health maintenance benefits.

Cardiovascular fitness can be evaluated by measurement of heart rate during exercise. As conditioning improves, the heart rate stabilizes at a fixed level. The heart rate at which conditioning will develop is called the target heart rate (21). **The formula for calculating the target heart rate is 220 minus the patient's age times 0.75.** For example, a 50-year-old woman would target her heart rate at 119 ($220 - 50 = 170 \times 0.75 = 119$).

Smoking Cessation

Smoking is a major cause of preventable illness, and every opportunity should be taken to encourage patients who smoke to quit. The effectiveness of smoking cessation programs varies, however, and numerous approaches have been used. The American Cancer Society suggests the following five-step approach:

1. Begin by obtaining a patient history of smoking habits and assessing the patient's motivation to stop smoking.

2. Give clear advice to stop smoking, emphasizing the benefits of cessation.

3. Set a specific goal (e.g., a realistic date to stop smoking).

4. Suggest cessation strategies.

5. Arrange a visit or phone call to monitor process.

Patient education about the benefits of smoking cessation, clear advice to quit smoking, and physician support improve smoking cessation rates, although 95% of smokers who successfully quit do so on their own. Self-help materials are available from the National Cancer Institute as well as community-based support groups and local chapters of the American Cancer Society and the American Lung Association. To aid in cessation, nicotine replacement therapy may be offered in the form of chewing gum or a transdermal patch. This should be prescribed only in conjunction with, not as a replacement for, ongoing visits for counseling and support.

References

1. **ACOG.** *Obstetrician–Gynecologists: Specialists in Reproductive Health Care and Primary Physicians for Women.* ACOG Statement of Policy. Washington, DC: American College of Obstetricians and Gynecologists, 1986.

2. **ACOG.** *PROLOG.* Units 1–5. Washington, DC: American College of Obstetricians and Gynecologists, 1991.

3. **U.S. Department of Health and Human Services.** *Healthy People 2000: National Health Promotion and Disease Prevention Objectives.* Washington, DC: U.S. Government Printing Office, 1991.

4. **U.S. Preventive Services Task Force.** *Guide to Clinical Preventive Services: An Assessment of the Effectiveness of 169 Interventions.* Baltimore: Williams & Wilkins, 1989:1–419.

5. **Hayward RS, Steinberg EP, Ford DE, Roizen MF, Roach KW.** Preventive care guidelines: 1991. *Ann Intern Med* 1991;114:758–83.

6. **ACOG.** *The Obstetrician-Gynecologist and Primary-Preventive Health Care.* Washington, DC: American College of Obstetricians and Gynecologists, 1993:1–22.

7. **Seltzer VL, Pearse WH.** *Women's Primary Health Care: Office Practice and Procedures.* New York: McGraw-Hill, Inc., 1995:1–825.

8. **Schappert SM.** *National Ambulatory Medical Care Survey: 1992 Summary.* Hyattsville, MD: National Center for Health Statistics, 1994.

9. **Schappert SM.** National ambulatory medical care survey: 1991 summary. *Vital Health Stat* 1994;13:116.

10. **Leader S, Perales PJ.** Provision of primary-preventive health care services by obstetrician-gynecologists. *Obstet Gynecol* 1995;85:391–5.

11. **ACOG.** *Obstetrics and Gynecology: Primary Care—A Guide to Communicating the Lawmakers, the Public, and Patients.* Washington, DC: American College of Obstetricians and Gynecologists, 1993:1–20.

12. **The Gallop Organization.** *A Gallop Study of Women's Attitudes Toward the Use of OB/GYN for Primary Care.* Washington, DC: ACOG, 1993:1–52.

13. **Canadian Task Force on the Periodic Health Examination.** The periodic health examination. *Can Med Assoc J* 1979;121:1193–254.

14. **American Medical Association.** Guidelines for adolescent preventive services (GAPS). Chicago: American Medical Association, 1992.

15. **Elster AB, Kuznets NJ.** *AMA Guidelines for Adolescent Preventive Services (GAPS): Recommendations and Rationale.* Baltimore: Williams & Wilkins, 1994:1–191.

16. **Zabin LS, Hardy JB, Smith EA, Hirsch MB.** Substance use and its relation to sexual activity among inner-city adolescents. *J Adolesc Health* 1986;7:320–31.

17. **Orr DP, Beiter M, Ingersoll G.** Premature sexual activity as an indicator of psychosocial risk. *Pediatrics* 1991;87:141–7.

18. **National Heart, Lung, and Blood Institute.** Report of the Second Task Force on blood pressure control in children—1987. *Pediatrics* 1987;79:1–25.

19. **National Cholesterol Education Program.** Report of the Expert Panel on Blood Cholesterol Levels in children and Adolescents. *Pediatrics* 1992;89:S525–84.

20. **American College of Obstetricians and Gynecologists.** *Guidelines for Women's Health Care.* Washington, DC: ACOG, 1995.

21. **American College of Obstetricians and Gynecologists.** *Women and Exercise.* ACOG Technical Bulletin 173. Washington, DC: ACOG, 1992.

22. **U.S. Department of Agriculture.** *The Food Guide Pyramid.* Home and Garden Bulletin No. 252. Washington, DC: U.S. Department of Agriculture, Human Nutrition Information Service, 1992.

23. **Centers for Disease Control.** Recommendations for the use of folic acid to reduce the number of cases of spina bifida and other neural tube defects. *MMWR* 1992;41(RR-14):1–7.

24. **National Research Council.** *Subcommittee on the Tenth Edition of the RDAs, Food and Nutrition Board, Commission on Life Sciences. Recommended Dietary Allowances.* 10th ed. Washington, DC: National Academy Press, 1989.

9

Primary Medical Care

Thomas E. Nolan

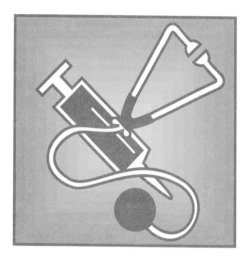

As health care providers for women, gynecologists have become responsible for care that extends beyond diseases of the reproductive organs and includes much of the general medical care of their patients. Broadening the spectrum of care requires adjustment in practice and places emphasis on the caring nature rather than the surgical procedural aspects of the specialty. Early diagnosis and treatment of medical illnesses can have a major impact on a woman's health. Although timely referral is important for complex and advanced diseases, many conditions may be treated initially by the gynecologist.

Respiratory problems are the most common reasons patients seek care from a physician, so gynecologists should be aware of their pathophysiology. **Cardiovascular disease has a significant impact on overall morbidity and is the main cause of death in women. Cardiovascular illness is associated with cigarette smoking, hypertension, hypercholesterolemia, and diabetes mellitus.** These conditions are responsive to screening, behavior modification, and control to lower risk factors. A major cause of morbidity for women is thyroid disease and, because of the interaction of hormones and the overall effect on the endocrine system, thyroid disease can be of special significance in women. The gynecologist should provide screening and the first level of therapy for these conditions.

Respiratory Infections

Infections of the respiratory system can range from the common cold to life-threatening illness. Those with risk factors should be counseled about preventive measures. Vaccines against flu and pneumonia should be offered as indicated.

Sinusitis

A problem frequently encountered in women is self-diagnosed "sinus problems" (1). Many medical problems—headaches, dental pain, postnasal drainage, halitosis, and dyspepsia—may be related to sinus conditions. The sinuses are not an isolated organ, and diseases of the sinuses are often related to conditions that affect other portions of the respiratory system (i.e., the nose, bronchial tree, and lung) (2). The entire respiratory system may be infected by one particular virus or pathogen (the sinobronchial or sinopulmonary syndrome);

195

however, the most prominent symptoms are usually produced in one anatomical area. Therefore, during the evaluation of complaints attributed to sinusitis, the presence of other infections should be investigated.

Multiple infectious and chemical agents, as well as reactions to nervous, physical, emotional, or hormonal stimuli, may cause an inflammatory response in the respiratory system (3). Systemic diseases such as connective tissue syndromes and malnutrition may contribute to chronic sinusitis. Environmental factors in the workplace and geographic conditions (e.g., cold and damp weather) may aggravate or accelerate the development of sinusitis. Contributing factors for the development of sinus disease include atmospheric pollutants, allergy, tobacco smoke, skeletal deformities, dental conditions, barotrauma from scuba diving or airline travel, and neoplasms.

Most infections begin with a viral agent in the nose or nasopharynx that causes inflammation that blocks the draining ostia. The location of symptoms varies by anatomic site: maxillary sinus over the cheeks, ethmoid sinus across the nose, frontal sinus in the supraorbital area, and sphenoid sinus to the vertex of the head. Viral agents impede the sweeping motion of cilia in the sinus and, in combination with edema from inflammation, lead to superinfection with bacteria.

Common bacteria that infect the sinuses include: *Streptococcus pyogenes, Streptococcus pneumoniae, Haemophilus influenzae, Staphylococcus aureus,* and α-*Streptococci species.* Infection with gram-negative organisms is usually limited to compromised hosts in intensive care units. Chronic sinusitis develops from either inadequate drainage or compromised local defense mechanisms. The flora in chronic disease are usually polymicrobial, consisting of aerobic and anaerobic organisms.

Sinus ailments frequently occur in middle-aged individuals. Acute infection is usually located in the maxillary and frontal sinuses. Classically, infection in the maxillary sinus is caused by obstruction of the ostia found in the medial wall of the nose. Fever, malaise, a vague headache, and pain in the maxillary teeth are early symptoms. Complaints include "fullness" in the face or pressure behind the eyes. Pressure and percussion over the malar areas result in complaints of pain. Purulent exudate in the middle meatus of the nose or in the nasopharynx are commonly observed. Initial episodes of sinusitis do not require imaging studies. When persistent infections occur, studies and referral are indicated. Therapy is usually empiric because, unless culture material is obtained by direct needle drainage, cultures are contaminated by oropharyngeal flora.

Broad antibiotic coverage is necessary to treat infection by common aerobes and anaerobes but should be limited to patients with acute pain and purulent discharge. *Ampicillin/clavulanic acid* combinations (*Augmentin*), *amoxicillin, erythromycin* with *sulfonamide,* and *cefaclor* are reasonable choices for initial therapy. Decongestant drops containing *phenylephrine* and antihistamines are useful in shrinking the obstructive ostia, but treatment should be limited to the first few days of therapy. Measures that relieve symptoms include facial hot packs and analgesics. Improvement should be apparent by 48 hours, but 10 days may be necessary for complete resolution. When improvement does not occur rapidly, other classes of antibiotics should be used because of presumed resistance. In patients who do not respond to treatment, referral to an otolaryngologist for sinus irrigation may be necessary.

Chronic sinusitis may result from repeated infections with inadequate drainage. The interval between infections becomes shorter until there are no remissions. Symptoms are recurrent pain in the malar area or chronic postnasal drip. In the preantibiotic era, chronic sinusitis was the result of repeated acute sinusitis with incomplete resolution, whereas currently allergy is more common. Surface-ciliated epithelia are injured, which results in impaired mucus removal. A vicious cycle occurs beginning with incomplete resolution of infection, followed by reinfection, and ending with the emergence of opportunistic organisms.

Allergies have become important in the etiology of chronic sinusitis. Swelling and edema of the mucosa and hypersecretion of mucus lead to ductal obstruction and infection. Chronic sinusitis is associated with chronic cough and laryngitis, with intermittent acute infections. Treatment is directed at the underlying etiology, either allergy control or aggressive management of infections. Resistant cases will require computed tomography (CT) and endoscopic surgery with polyp removal. Nasoantral window formation is radical surgery that is necessary occasionally in difficult cases.

Untreated sinus infections may have severe consequences such as orbital cellulitis leading to orbital abscess, subperiosteal abscess formation of the facial bones, cavernous sinus thrombosis, and acute meningitis. Brain and dural abscesses are rare and usually occur as a result of direct spread from a sinus. The most accurate diagnostic tool at present is CT scanning. Aggressive surgical approaches with broad-spectrum antibiotics are necessary for adequate drainage.

Otitis Media

Otitis media remains primarily a disease of children but may affect adults. Serous otitis media is usually secondary to a concurrent viral infection of the upper respiratory tract. The diagnosis rests on the visualization of fluid behind the tympanic membrane. Treatment includes antihistamines, decongestants, and glucocorticoids, but few data exist to support the use of these medications. Acute otitis media is usually a bacterial infection (most commonly *Streptococcus pneumoniae* and *Hemophilus influenza*). Initial symptoms are pain, fever, and leukocytosis; acute purulent otorrhea and hearing loss also may occur (4). Physical examination of the ear will reveal a red, bulging, or perforated membrane. Treatment is broad-spectrum antibiotics such as *amoxicillin/clavulanic acid, cefuroxime-axetil,* and *trimethoprim-sulfamethoxazole.* The role of antihistamines in the treatment of otitis media is unclear.

Bronchitis

Acute bronchitis is an inflammatory condition of the tracheobronchial tree. It is most commonly viral, usually occurring in winter. Common cold viruses (rhinovirus and coronavirus), adenovirus, influenza virus, and *Mycoplasma pneumoniae* (a nonviral pathogen) are the most common pathogens. Bacterial infections are less common and may occur as secondary pathogens. Cough, hoarseness, and fever are the usual presenting symptoms. In the initial 3–4 days, the symptoms of rhinitis and sore throat are prominent; however, coughing may last as long as 3 weeks. The prolonged nature of these infections often results in use of antibiotics to "clear up the infection." Sputum production is common and may be prolonged in cigarette smokers. Bacterial infections are most serious in cigarette smokers because of underlying damage to the lining of the upper respiratory tree and changes in the host flora.

Physical examination demonstrates a variety of upper airway sounds, usually coarse rhonchi. Rales are usually not present on auscultation, and signs of consolidation and alveolar involvement are absent. During auscultation of the chest, signs of pneumonia such as fine rales, decreased breath sounds, and egophony ("E to A changes") should be sought. In patients in whom the results of the physical examination are equivocal and who appear to have an infection, chest radiographs should be obtained to determine the presence of parenchymal disease. Paradoxically, as the initial acute syndrome subsides, sputum production may become more purulent. Sputum cultures are of limited value because of the polymicrobial nature of infections. In cases without complications, treatment is aimed at providing symptomatic relief; the use of antibiotics is reserved for situations in which chest x-ray findings are consistent with pneumonia. Cough is usually the most aggravating symptom and may be treated with antitussive preparations containing either *dextromethorphan* or *codeine.* The efficacy of expectorants has not been proven.

Chronic bronchitis is defined as a productive cough from excessive secretions for at least 3 months in a year for 2 consecutive years. It is estimated that between 10 and

197

25% of the adult population is affected by chronic bronchitis. Previously, the disease occurred less often in women than men; because cigarette smoking has increased among women, so has the incidence of bronchitis in women. Chronic bronchitis is usually classified as a form of chronic obstructive lung disease (COPD). Other contributing factors include chronic infections and environmental pathogens found in dust. The cardinal manifestation of disease is an incessant cough, usually in the morning with expectoration of sputum. Because many of these patients have frequent exacerbations and may require hospitalization, and because of the complexity of medical management required, they should be referred to an internist.

Pneumonia

Etiology

Pneumonia is defined as inflammation of the distal lung, which includes terminal airways, alveolar spaces, and the interstitium. Pneumonia may have multiple causes, including viral and bacterial infections or aspiration. *Aspiration pneumonia* is usually the result of depressed awareness commonly associated with use of drugs and alcohol or anesthesia. *Viral pneumonias* are caused by multiple infectious agents, including influenza A or B, parainfluenza virus, or respiratory syncytial virus. Most viral infections are spread by aerosolization associated with coughing, sneezing, and even conversation. Incubation is short, usually only 1–3 days before the acute onset of fever, chills, headache, fatigue, and myalgia. Symptom intensity is directly related to the intensity of the host febrile reaction. Pneumonia develops in only 1% of patients who have a viral infection, but mortality rates may reach 30% in immunocompromised individuals and the elderly. An additional risk is the development of *secondary bacterial pneumonias* after the initial viral insult. These infections are more common in elderly individuals, which explains the high fatality rate associated with pneumonia in this age group (5). *Staphylococcal* pneumonias, more commonly arising from a previous viral infection, are extremely lethal regardless of patient age. The best treatment for viral pneumonia is prevention by immunization. Flu immunization should be offered to patients over 55 years of age, as well as those who have diabetes mellitus, connective tissue syndromes, and cardiac, pulmonary, or renal disease. In epidemics, *amantadine* has been used for nonvaccinated individuals. Treatment remains supportive with antipyretics and fluids.

Bacterial pneumonia is classified as either *community-acquired* or *nosocomial,* which determines the prognosis and antibiotic therapy in many cases. Risk factors that contribute to mortality include chronic cardiopulmonary diseases, alcoholism, diabetes mellitus, renal failure, malignancy, and malnutrition. Prognostic features associated with poor outcome include greater than two-lobe involvement, respiratory rate greater than 30 breaths/minute on presentation, severe hypoxemia (<60 mm Hg on room air), hypoalbuminemia, and septicemia (6). Pneumonia is a common cause of adult respiratory distress syndrome (ARDS), which has a mortality rate between 50 and 70% (7).

Signs and Symptoms

Signs and symptoms of pneumonia vary and depend on the infecting organism and the patient's immune status (8). In typical pneumonia, symptoms include high fever, rigors, productive cough, chills, and pleuritic chest pain. Chest x-rays often show infiltration. Two-thirds of all bacterial pneumonias are caused by *Streptococcus pneumoniae* (formally referred to as *"pneumococcal pneumonia"*), *Haemophilus influenza,* and *Kelbsiella pneumoniae,* as well as gram-negative organisms and other anaerobic bacteria. *Streptococcal pneumoniae* classically presents with a sudden onset of fever and chills, rusty sputum with gram-positive cocci (so-called "coffee bean" cocci). Bacteremia may be present in up to 25% cases, and on some occasions the diagnosis is actually made on the basis of blood culture results.

Atypical pneumonia is more insidious in onset, with moderate fever without the characteristic rigors and chills. Additional symptoms include a nonproductive cough, headache, myalgias, and mild leukocytosis. Chest x-ray reveals a bronchopneumonia with a diffuse interstitial pattern, and characteristically, the patient is not nearly as ill as the x-ray suggests. Common causes of atypical pneumonia include *Mycoplasma pneumoniae,* viruses, *Legionella pneumophila, Chlamydia pneumoniae* (also called the *TWAR* agent), and other rare agents. *Legionella pneumoniae* usual presents with systemic symptoms, including severe headaches and diarrhea.

Diagnosis

A strong index of suspicion of pneumonia is required for diagnosis, especially in elderly patients and immunocompromised individuals who have altered response mechanisms. In elderly individuals, subtle clues include changes in mentation, confusion, and exacerbation of other illnesses. The febrile response may be entirely absent. Even in high-risk groups, an increased respiratory rate of more than 25 breaths per minute remains the most reliable sign. Mortality in these high-risk groups of patients is strongly correlated with the ability of the host to mount normal defenses to the symptoms of fever, chills, and tachycardia.

Laboratory Studies

Laboratory studies helpful in identifying community-acquired pneumonia are sputum gram-stain, sputum culture, and blood culture. An "adequate sputum specimen" (defined as >25 neutrophils with <10 epithelial cells per low-powered field on microscopic examination) may be difficult to obtain. Respiratory therapists are an excellent resource in obtaining an induced sputum specimen. The isolation of *Legionella pneumoniae* requires specialized laboratory techniques, including direct fluorescent antibody staining of organisms in the sputum or indirect serological tests using enzyme-linked immunosorbent assay (ELISA) technology. *Mycoplasma pneumoniae* should be suspected when the cold agglutinins test positive, the appropriate clinical symptoms are present, and diffuse bronchopneumonia is observed by on chest x-ray.

Therapy

Therapy of pneumonia should be directed at the responsible or most likely pathogen. *Procaine penicillin G,* 600,000 units intramuscularly every 12 hours, is the treatment of choice for *Streptococcal pneumoniae.* Alternate therapy is 2.4–4.8 million units of *penicillin G* daily given intravenously every 4 hours. Most patients respond within 48 hours of initiation of therapy and, once clinical resolution is achieved, oral *penicillin V-K* 500 mg four times daily may be substituted to complete 10 days of therapy. Individuals who are allergic to *penicillin* should receive intravenous *erythromycin* 500 mg every 6 hours until improvement, at which time oral preparations at the same dosage can be substituted. *Penicillin*-resistant strains of *S. pneumoniae* have emerged in the past decade and are associated with either nosocomial infections or patients treated with beta-lactam antibiotics.

Mycoplasma pneumoniae, the most common cause of atypical pneumonia, should be treated with *erythromycin* 500 mg four times daily. Hospitalization is rarely necessary, depending on the severity of the patient's condition and the need for intravenous antibiotics. High-dose *erythromycin,* 2–4 grams intravenously daily is recommended for treatment of *Legionella pneumoniae.* Once the patient becomes afebrile and her condition remains stable for 2 days, oral *erythromycin* 500 mg four times daily is substituted for a total of 3 weeks of therapy. In severe, life-threatening infections, *rifampin* 600 mg every 12 hours is added to high-dose *erythromycin* therapy.

In many cases of pneumonia, the exact causative organism cannot be determined and empiric therapy should be initiated. *Erythromycin* is active against the three most likely community-acquired organisms: *Streptococcus, Mycoplasma,* and *Legionella. Erythromycin* should only be used as a single agent in immunocompetent and young patients. In elderly or immunocompromised patients, second- or third-generation cephalosporin should be added to expand coverage of gram-negative organisms. Hospitalization is necessary in patients who are very ill, elderly, or immunocompromised. Oxygen therapy and hydration should be initiated, in addition to antibiotic therapy. Chest physiotherapy should be reserved for patients who have copious sputum or who have an ineffective cough.

Pneumococcal vaccines should be given to patients at high risk for pneumonia: elderly individuals (defined as older than 55 years of age), cigarette smokers, or patients with chronic pulmonary disease. The vaccine is active against 23 different strains of pneumococcus, which covers 85% of organisms usually cultured. If possible, the vaccine should be given prophylactically, but it may be given with antibiotic therapy in established infections. Repeat vaccination is suggested every 6 years because of a lack of antibody formation in the elderly. These patients should be vaccinated for influenza in the Fall prior to flu season.

Cardiovascular Disease

The risk factors for coronary artery disease are presented in Table 9.1. Central to treating cardiovascular disease is the control of contributing diseases and risk factors (Table 9.2). Aerobic exercise protects against cardiovascular disease (9). Additional aspects of prevention of myocardial disease, renal disease, and stroke include control of hypertension, identification and control of diabetes and obesity, and control of dietary fats, especially cholesterol, in susceptible individuals (Fig. 9.1).

Hypertension

The relationship between hypertension and cardiovascular events such as stroke, coronary artery disease, congestive heart disease, and renal disease is well known. More than 50 million people in the U.S. have hypertension. It is found in 15% of the population between the ages of 18 and 74 years; the incidence increases with age and varies with race. After 50 years of age, women have a higher incidence of hypertension than males; however, this may be a confounding variable related to the overall mortality of men at an earlier age (10). Sixty-five percent of those in the age group of 65–74 years can be classified as hypertensive (11). The contribution of hypertension to overall cardiovascular morbidity and mortality in women has been believed to be less important than in males, but this may reflect

Table 9.1   Risk Factors for Coronary Heart Disease

Positive Risk Factors
Male: Age older than 45 years
Female: Age older than 55 years
No estrogen replacement therapy (ERT)
Premature menopause without ERT
Cigarette smoking
Hypertension (blood pressure of > 140/90 or on treatment)
Diabetes
HDL cholesterol < 35 mg/dl
Family history of myocardial infarction or sudden death before 55 years of age in a first-degree male relative, or before 65 years of age in a first-degree female relative
Negative Risk Factor
HDL cholesterol > 600 mg/dl (also allows subtraction of one risk factor)

Modified from **National Institutes of Health.** *Second Report of the Expert Panel on Detection, Evaluation, and Treatment of High Blood Cholesterol in Adults.* Publication 93-3095. Bethesda, MD: National Institutes of Health, 1993:1–11.

Table 9.2   Life-style Adjustment for Cardiovascular Risk Reduction and Hypertensive Therapy

Weight reduction if overweight
Limit alcohol use to less than 1 ounce of absolute alcohol per day (2 beers, 8 ounces of wine, 2 ounces of 100-proof whiskey)
Regular aerobic exercise (30 minutes fast walking 3 times/week)
Decrease salt intake to less than 6 g/day
Stop cigarette smoking
Reduce dietary saturated fat and cholesterol
Maintain adequate intake of calcium, potassium, and magnesium
If diabetic, control glucose

the relative absence of research in women. Recognition and treatment of hypertension may decrease the development of renal and cardiac disease.

Epidemiology

The incidence of hypertension is twice as high in African-Americans than in whites. Geographic variations are present: the southeastern U.S. has a higher prevalence of hypertension and stroke, regardless of race (12). One multi-institutional study confirmed not only that there is an increased incidence in African-Americans but also that lower levels of education increase the incidence of hypertension (13). Preventive measures can be most effective in those at highest risk, such as in African-American women and individuals from the lowest socioeconomic levels (13). The influence of genetic predisposition is poorly understood. Studies of women have been limited to those that determine side effects of medication and the impact of certain medications on long-term lipid status (10).

Diagnosis

Classically, hypertension is defined as blood pressures higher than 140/90 when measured on two separate occasions. However, therapy may be indicated only for individuals at high risk. Individuals at low risk, such as white women with no other risk factors, may

Figure 9.1   Disease and risk factors contributing to cardiovascular disease.

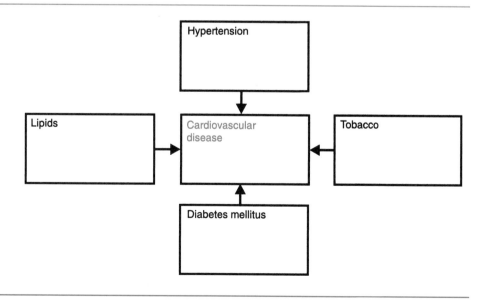

benefit from lifestyle modification only (13). What constitutes a significant systolic or diastolic pressure that requires therapy? Elevation of systolic blood pressure in middle-aged and elderly patients was once considered innocuous; however, recent studies suggest that control of systolic blood pressure is more important than control of diastolic blood pressure (14). Life insurance risk tables indicate that when blood pressure is controlled to lower than 140/90, normal survival occurs over a 10- to 20-year follow-up, regardless of gender. Published recommendations are based on sustained blood pressures higher than 140/90.

Most individuals (>95%) with hypertension have primary or essential hypertension (cause unknown), whereas less than 5% have secondary hypertension resulting from another disorder. Key factors should be determined in the history and physical. The presence of prior elevated readings, previous use of antihypertensive agents, a family history of cardiovascular death prior to age 55, and excessive alcohol and sodium use constitute important historical information. Lifestyle modification is becoming appreciated in the therapy of hypertension; thus, a detailed history of diet and physical activity should be obtained (15). Baseline laboratory evaluations to rule out reversible causes of hypertension (secondary hypertension) are listed in Table 9.3. Diagnosis and management are based on the classification of blood pressure readings (Table 9.4).

1. Patients with high normal readings (systolic 130–139 mm Hg, diastolic 85–89 mm Hg) are at high risk for developing hypertension and should be monitored yearly; consideration should be given to nonpharmacologic interventions (16). A scheme for follow-up is found in Figure 9.2.

Table 9.3 Minimal Laboratory Determinations in the Evaluation of Uncomplicated Hypertension

Dipstick urinalysis (microscopic examination indicated if any values are abnormal)

Hemoglobin or hematocrit

Creatinine, potassium, fasting glucose concentration

Total cholesterol, high-density lipoprotein cholesterol, and fasting triglycerides

Electrocardiogram

*If any of the above are abnormal, consultation or referral to an internist is indicated.

Table 9.4 Classification of Blood Pressure for Adults Aged 18 Years and Older*†

Category	Systolic (mm Hg)	Diastolic (mm Hg)
Normal	< 130	< 85
High normal	130–139	85–89
Hypertension:*†		
Stage 1 (mild)	140–159	90–99
Stage 2 (moderate)	160–179	100–109
Stage 3 (severe)	180–209	110–119
Stage 4 (very severe)	≥ 210	≥ 120

*All measurements are in patients who are otherwise asymptomatic and on medications. If measurements fall in two different categories, then the highest category should be used for classification purposes. Additionally, if other diseases are present, such as diabetes, then it should be noted in parenthesis.
†Requires the performance of two additional measures after initial reading.
Modified from **The Fifth Report of the Joint National Committee on the Detection, Evaluation, and Treatment of High Blood Pressure.** *Arch Intern Med* 1993;153:154–83.

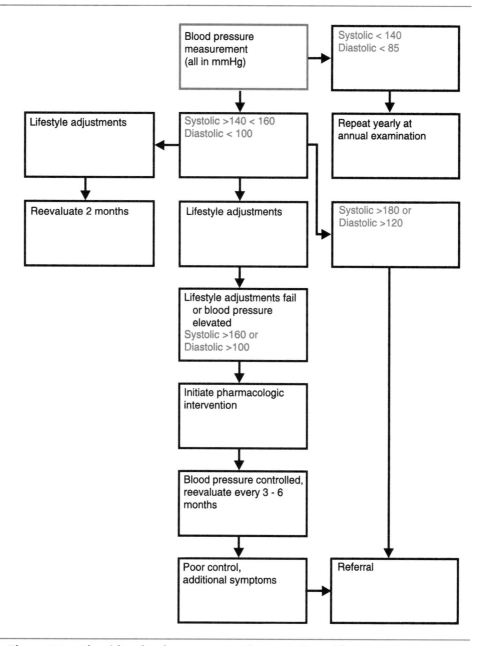

Figure 9.2   Algorithm for the treatment of uncomplicated hypertension.

2. A single elevated diastolic blood pressure reading of less than 100 torr (mm Hg) should be rechecked within 2 months before initiating therapy. Elevated readings will spontaneously resolve during the observation period in 33% of patients.

3. If blood pressure control is not easily achieved, systolic blood pressure is higher than 180 mm Hg, or the diastolic reading is higher than 110 mm Hg, referral to an internist is recommended. Referral is also indicated if secondary hypertension is suspected or evidence of end-organ damage (renal insufficiency or congestive heart failure) is detected.

The definition of what constitutes systolic hypertension requiring treatment has been hotly contested for years. Recently, a report noted that patients with systolic blood pressure higher than 160 mm Hg benefit from antihypertensive therapy regardless of their diastolic pressure (17). Middle-aged to elderly patients treated for systolic hypertension had a significant decrease in cerebral vascular accidents and coronary artery disease.

Measurement of Blood Pressure

An often overlooked but essential variable in evaluation of hypertension is the method used to obtain measurements and the need to standardize measurements (18). "White coat" or office hypertension may occur in up to 30% of patients. With patients who have elevated readings in the office but repeated normal readings outside of the office, it is reasonable to use ambulatory or home monitoring devices. In most patients, office readings are to diagnose and monitor hypertension and eliminate problems of reliability with commercial devices and patient interpretation skills.

Blood pressure measurement protocols should be standardized. The patient should be allowed to rest for 5 minutes in a seated position and the right arm should be used for measurements (for unknown reasons, the right arm has higher readings). The cuff should be applied 20 mm above the bend of the elbow and the arm should be positioned parallel to the floor. The cuff should be inflated to 30 mm Hg above the disappearance of the brachial pulse (or 220 mm Hg). The cuff should be deflated slowly, at a rate no higher than 2 mm Hg per second.

The cuff size is important, and most cuffs are marked with "normal limits" for the relative size they can accommodate. The most common clinical problem encountered is the use of a small cuff on an obese patient, resulting in "cuff hypertension." Phase IV Korotkoff sounds are described as the point at which pulsations are muffled, and phase V is characterized as complete disappearance of pulse. Most experts advocate the use of phase V Korotkoff sounds, but phase IV sounds may be used in special circumstances, with the reason documented.

The use of automated devices may help eliminate discrepancies in measurements. Regardless of the method or device used, two measurements should be obtained with less than 10 mm Hg disparity to be judged adequate. When repeated measures are performed, there should be a 2-minute rest period between readings. Blood pressure has a diurnal pattern, so determinations preferably should be performed at the same time of day. Ambulatory monitoring is not cost effective in all patients but should be used to evaluate resistance to therapy, to determine the presence of "white coat" hypertension, and to assess whether syncopal episodes are related to hypotension or episodic hypertension (19).

Cholesterol

In predicting cardiovascular morbidity, the trio of tobacco abuse, lipid disorders, and hypertension are the most significant risk factors. Cholesterol measurements are important in the assessment of the hypertensive patient (20). Both high-density lipoprotein (HPL) and low-density lipoprotein (LDL), as well as triglycerides, play a role in cardiovascular disease and should be monitored in patients with risk factors. Hypercholesterolemia, especially when combined with hypertension and a strong family history of cardiovascular events at an early age, should be managed with dietary intervention and possible pharmacologic manipulations (21). Certain medications, such as beta-blocking agents and diuretics, have a negative impact on serum cholesterol and should be avoided in individuals with lipid disorders (22). If the patient has low HDL cholesterol, antihypertensive therapy should be chosen accordingly, and more aggressive blood pressure control is indicated. Laboratory tests should be repeated as indicated by initial studies to assess cholesterol levels and on an annual basis to monitor side effects of certain medications.

Therapy

Nonpharmacologic interventions or lifestyle modifications should be attempted prior to initiation of medication unless diastolic blood pressure exceeds 110 mm Hg. An im-

204

portant element in lifestyle modifications is to modify factors contributing to cardiovascular disease. Only after these therapies fail should pharmacologic intervention be considered.

1. Weight loss in obese patients, especially in individuals with truncal and abdominal obesity, is critical to prevent the development of atherosclerosis (23). A loss of just 10 pounds has been reported to lower blood pressure (26).

2. Inquiries into dietary practices, specifically the use of certain foods that are high in sodium (such as canned goods, snack food, pork products, and soy sauce), are necessary to help the patient eliminate sources of excess salt from the diet. British researchers estimate that mortality in the U.K. would decrease by 70,000 deaths per year if individuals would decrease salt intake to 3 grams per day (25).

3. Cholesterol and fat intake should be limited in the diet.

4. Alcohol intake should be limited to no more than 2 drinks per day.

5. Exercise contributes to overall cardiovascular health. Aerobic exercise alone may prevent hypertension in 20–50% of normotensive individuals (25).

The goal of therapy is to lower blood pressure into the "normal range:" a systolic reading less than 140 mm Hg and a diastolic reading less than 85 mm Hg. If lifestyle modifications are not sufficient to control blood pressure, pharmacologic intervention should be implemented. An increasing number of antihypertensive groups and agents has become available during the past decade. Currently, only diuretics and beta blockers have been proven to reduce mortality and morbidity, although this may be related to the short duration of follow-up on the efficacy of newer agents (27).

Classes of Drugs

Diuretics **The most commonly used medication for initial blood pressure reduction is the thiazide diuretic.** The mechanism of action is to reduce plasma and extracellular fluid volume. This lowering of volume is believed to decrease peripheral resistance. Cardiac output initially decreases and then normalizes. The important long-term effect is a slight decrease in extracellular fluid volume. The maximum therapeutic dose of thiazide should be 25 mg, rather than the commonly used 50 mg. The benefit of higher doses is eliminated by the corresponding increase in side effects. Potassium-sparing diuretics (*spironolactone, triamterene,* or *amiloride*) are available in fixed-dosage combinations and should be prescribed to prevent the development of hypokalemia. Because of compliance problems, potassium supplementation is less effective than using potassium-sparing agents. Thiazide diuretics are best used in patients whose creatinine levels are less than 2.5 g/l. Loop diuretics (e.g., *furosemide*) work better than thiazide diuretics at lower glomerular filtration rates and higher serum creatinine levels. Control of hypertension in patients with renal insufficiency is difficult and is probably best handled by an internist or nephrologist. Thiazides and loop diuretics should not be used concurrently because profound diuresis may lead to renal impairment. Concurrent use of nonsteroidal anti-inflammatory drugs (NSAIDs) limit the effectiveness of thiazide diuretics. Side effects that further limit the use of thiazide diuretics include hyperuricemia (which may precipitate acute gout attacks), glucose intolerance, and hyperlipidemia (28).

Adrenergic Inhibitors Beta blockers have been used extensively for years to treat hypertension. They act by decreasing cardiac output and plasma renin activity, with some increase in total peripheral resistance. As a class, they are an excellent choice for first-line therapy, especially for migraine suffers, because they have a beneficial effect on vascular headache. The original formulation, *propranolol,* was highly lipid soluble and had a relative lack of beta specificity, which contributed to bothersome side effects such as depression, sleep disturbances (nightmares in the elderly), and constipation in higher doses. Newer β_1 selective formulations, such as *atenolol,* are water soluble and have fewer side effects. At higher doses, however, β_2 effects emerge. Despite speculation that β_1-selective agents may be safe in patients who have asthma, many experts believe that they should not be used for these patients. An additional advantage of water-soluble agents is a longer half-life. Reduced frequency of dosing improves compliance. Metabolic changes, similar to those of thiazide diuretics, have reduced the popularity of these drugs. These side effects include an increase in triglyceride levels, a decrease in HDL cholesterol, and blunting of adrenergic release in response to hypoglycemia. These metabolic problems far outweigh the benefits of these drugs for patients with diabetes (29). The effectiveness of beta-blocking agents also may decrease with the use of NSAIDS. Additional contraindications are COPD, congestive heart failure, sick sinus syndrome, or any bradyarrhythmia. Beta blockers have been used for the treatment of angina. However, if these drugs are acutely withdrawn, a rebound phenomenon of ischemia may occur and may lead to acute myocardial infarction. Beta blockers continue to be useful, despite these potential problems, especially to counteract reflex tachycardia common with smooth-muscle relaxing drugs.

Alpha$_1$-adrenergic drugs became popular for males because of minimal effects on potency and their interaction with lipids. Interestingly, they may contribute to stress urinary incontinence in women due to altered urethral tone (30). As single agents, they decrease total cholesterol and LDL cholesterol while increasing HDL cholesterol. Their mechanism of action is the promotion of vascular relaxation by blocking postganglionic norepinephrine vasoconstriction in the peripheral vascular smooth muscle. *Prazosin* and *doxazosin* are currently the most popular preparations in this class. A serious side effect of these drugs, called the "first-dose effect," is most commonly described in elderly individuals. In susceptible individuals, severe orthostasis may occur when therapy is initiated and subsides after several days. When combined with diuretics, hypotension may be exacerbated. Other side effects that may limit usefulness in some patients include tachycardia, weakness, dizziness, and mild fluid retention. Therapy should begin with small doses at bedtime followed by incremental increases.

Angiotensin-Converting Enzyme Inhibitors   Angiotensin-converting enzyme (ACE) inhibitors have rapidly become a first-line drug in the treatment of hypertension. The introduction of new formulations that allow for once- or twice-daily dosing with a good therapeutic response has increased the popularity of these drugs. There are relatively few side effects; chronic cough is the most worrisome and is a common reason for discontinuation of therapy. Other side effects are occasional first-dose hypotension and blood dyscrasias. Occasionally, patients will suffer from rashes, loss of taste, fatigue, or headaches. Other agents should be considered for women who are having intercourse and not using contraception (pregnancy is a strict contraindication). ACE inhibitors can be used in combination with other agents, including diuretics, calcium channel antagonists, and beta blockers. In contrast to beta blockers, these medications can be used in patients who have asthma, chronic obstructive airway disease, depression, diabetes, or peripheral vascular disease. For unknown reasons, they are less effective in African-Americans, unless a diuretic is used concomitantly. Use with diuretics increases the effectiveness of both drugs, but hypovolemia may result. If renal failure is present, hyperkalemia may result from potassium supplementation and altered renal tubular metabolism. Any NSAID, including **aspirin,** may decrease the antihypertensive effectiveness.

Calcium Channel Blockers   Calcium channel blockers have been a major therapeutic breakthrough for patients with coronary artery disease and have been found to be effective in patients with hypertension and peripheral vascular disease. The mechanism of action is to block calcium movement across smooth muscle, thus promoting vessel wall relaxation. Calcium channel blockers are especially useful in treating concurrent hypertension and coronary artery disease. Additionally, these drugs have been shown to be particularly effective in elderly and African-American patients. Side effects include headache, dizziness, constipation, and peripheral edema. The development of long-acting calcium channel blockers has made these preparations more useful in the treatment of hypertension. These drugs have a relative contraindication for use in patients with heart failure or conduction disturbances.

Direct Vasodilators *Hydralazine* is a potent vasodilator that has been used for years in obstetrics for treatment of severe hypertension associated with preeclampsia and eclampsia. The mechanism of action is direct relaxation of vascular smooth muscle, primarily arterial. Major side effects include headaches, tachycardia, and fluid (sodium) retention, which may result in paradoxical hypertension. Several combinations have been used to counter the side effects and enhance antihypertensive effects. Diuretics may be added to reverse fluid retention caused by sodium retention. Used in combination with beta blockers, tachycardia and headaches may be controlled without compromising the objective of lowering blood pressure. Drug-induced lupus has been widely stated as a potential side effect, but it is rare in normal therapeutic doses of 25–50 mg three times per day. *Minoxidil* is another extremely potent drug in this class, but it is of limited use in women because of its side effects (beard growth).

Central Acting Agents Central acting agents (*methyldopa* and *clonidine*) have long been used in gynecology. The mechanism of action is to inhibit the sympathetic nerves in the central nervous system, resulting in peripheral vascular relaxation. The side effects of this group of drugs (taste disorders, dry mouth) has markedly limited their popularity. The need for frequent dosing (except for the transdermal form of *clonidine*) is also a problem. Sudden withdrawal of *clonidine* may be associated with precipitation of a hypertensive crisis and induction of angina. The *clonidine* withdrawal syndrome is more likely to occur with the concomitant use of beta blockers. The side effects of this class of drugs contribute to patients' poor adherence to the treatment regimen. With the introduction of new classes of drugs with improved efficacy and reduced side effects, medications in this class are expected to decline in use.

Monitoring Therapy

Lifestyle modification should be initiated for patients with mild or moderate (stages 1 or 2) hypertension with close observation over a 3- to 6-month period. Blood pressure readings should be monitored frequently by an industrial nurse, the patient, or medical office staff at 1- to 2-week intervals. If the patient has other diseases (cardiovascular or renal), therapy should be initiated earlier and should be directed to the target organ. If lifestyle modifications alone are successful, close monitoring is necessary at 3- to 6-month intervals. When lifestyle modification is unsuccessful, medication should be administered to decrease target organ disease.

When beginning therapy, it is preferable to use a common agent that can be used to treat hypertension as well as concurrent medical conditions. Gender has not been found to be important in the choice of an antihypertensive agent. Certain conditions or patient characteristics may help guide therapeutic choices. In the presence of migraine headaches, beta blockers or calcium channel agonists may be the best choice. African-Americans may respond better to a combination of diuretics and calcium channel blockers.

Once antihypertensive medications are initiated, their effects should be monitored frequently. Selected agents and dosages for therapy are listed in Table 9.5, which is not meant to be all inclusive but rather to provide example to guide therapy. Patients capable of home blood pressure monitoring should be encouraged to measure blood pressure at the same time of day on a twice-weekly basis (31). They should maintain a log for physician review of effectiveness of therapy. A return appointment should be scheduled in 2–4 weeks to monitor effectiveness and side effects. When possible, single agents (monotherapy) should be used to improve compliance. Monotherapy should be adequate to control mild-to-moderate hypertension in 50–60% of patients. If initial doses are ineffective, a higher

Table 9.5   Selected Medications and Dosage for Control of Essential Hypertension

Medication (Class)	Normal Daily Dosage (mg/day) and Interval	Dispensing Unit (mg)
Angiotensin-converting enzyme (ACE) inhibitors		
Enalapril	5–40 (qd, bid)	2.5, 5, 10, 20
Calcium channel blockers		
Nifedipine sustained release	30–90 (qd)	30, 60, 90
Diltiazem sustained release	120–240 (bid)	60, 90, 120
Alpha blockers		
Terazosin	1–20 (qd)	1, 2, 5, 10
Mixed alpha and beta blockers		
Labetalol	200–800 (bid)	100, 200, 300
Diuretics		
Hydrochlorothiazide	12.5–50 (qd)	25, 50
Triamterene (potassium-sparing)	50–100 (bid)	50, 100
Beta blockers		
Propranolol (lipid soluble)	60–160 (qd)	60, 80, 120, 160
Atenolol (water soluble)	50–100 (qd)	50, 100
Smooth muscle relaxant		
Hydralazine	25–75 (tid, qid)	10, 25, 50, 100

Table 9.6   Schemes for Control of Essential Hypertension

Angiotensin-converting enzyme (ACE) inhibitor
Beta blockers, diuretics, central agents
Calcium channel blockers
Diuretics, beta blockers, central agents
Alpha blockers
Diuretics, beta blockers

Primary Medications are in bold, *Secondary drugs to add in combination with primary are in italics.*
Monotherapy and long-acting agents are recommended for sustained release and compliance. Fixed combinations have an advantage of compliance but are discouraged due to the inability to selectively modify doses.
Reproduced with permission from **Nolan T.** Evaluation and treatment of uncomplicated hypertension. *Clin Obstet Gynecol,* 1995;38:156–65.

dose should be used prior to changing agents. If resistance to therapy continues, a different class of medication may be used or a second drug should be added (Table 9.6).

If intolerable side effects develop, a different class of medications should be initiated and monitored. In the past, step therapy was used, starting with thiazides, followed by the addition of beta-blocking agents, and finally followed by vasodilator drugs. The newer drugs (ACE inhibitors, postadrenergic ganglionic blockers, and calcium channel blockers) are more potent than older preparations, have longer half-lives, and may be used as single agents. Referral should be considered for patients whose blood pressure is difficult to control with monotherapy. Causes of resistance to therapy include diseases missed during the initial evaluation, unrecognized early end-stage disease and poor compliance. Patients with evidence of target organ disease should be considered for transfer or referral to the appropriate specialist for more intensive diagnostic workup and therapy.

Cholesterol

"Cholesterol is the most highly decorated small molecule in biology" (32). The dietary influence of cholesterol on atherosclerosis and its relationship to hypertension and cardiovascular events (myocardial infarction and stroke) have been widely debated in both the scientific and lay communities (33). The controversy centers on how much of a role dietary cholesterol plays in the risk and prevention of cardiovascular disease (34). Many people assume that any cholesterol or fat in the diet has negative health consequences; the necessary role that cholesterol plays in normal metabolic function is not appreciated. Cholesterol metabolism is complex and, in some cases, our understanding is extrapolated from animal models. The role of cholesterol testing (who, when, and at what age) is hotly debated among health care professionals, and cholesterol testing is fraught with multiple variables that affect results.

Cholesterol metabolism is not determined exclusively by LDL and HDL cholesterol. Cholesterol is usually found in an esterized form with various proteins and glycerides that characterize the stages of metabolism. The following components are important lipid particles in cholesterol metabolism.

Chylomicrons   Chylomicrons are large lipoprotein particles that consist of dietary triglycerides and cholesterol. Chylomicrons are secreted in the intestinal lumen, absorbed into lymphatic fluid, and then passed into general circulation. In adipose tissue and skeletal muscle, they adhere to binding sites on the capillary wall and are metabolized for energy production.

Lipoprotein Particle   A lipoprotein particle has three major components. The core consists of nonpolar lipids (triglycerides and cholesterol esters), which are present in varying amounts depending on the stage of the metabolic pathway in which they are found. Surrounding the nonpolar core is a surface coat of phospholipids, apoproteins, and structural proteins.

Apoprotein   Attached to each lipoprotein particle is an apoprotein, which is a specific recognition protein exposed at the surface of a lipoprotein particle. Apoproteins have specific receptors and demarcate the stage of cholesterol metabolism. Certain apoproteins are associated with specific types of cholesterol. For example, apoprotein A-I and apoprotein A-II are associated with HDL cholesterol, the so-called "scavenger cholesterol." Apoprotein CII has additional activity as a cofactor for lipoprotein lipase.

Lipoprotein Classes

Lipoprotein particles are separated into five classes based on physical characteristics. Lipoprotein classes are determined by the separation of lipids in an electrophoretic field; however, *in vivo* they exist in a continuum. The various cholesterol metabolites are separated by density. As lipoprotein particles are metabolized and lipids are removed for energy production, they become more dense. Additionally, attached apoproteins are modified as cholesterol moves from the so-called "exogenous pathway" (dietary) to the "endogenous pathway" (postabsorption and metabolization by the liver). Subdivisions of the lipoprotein classes are described in the following section and summarized in Figure 9.3.

Prehepatic Metabolites

Chylomicrons and Remnants   Chylomicrons are composed of major lipids and apoproteins of the A, B-48, C, and E classes. Their density is 1.006 g/ml. These are large particles made up of dietary cholesterols that are absorbed with triglycerides.

209

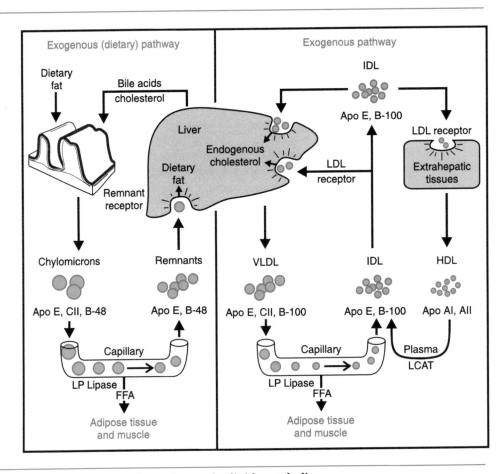

Figure 9.3   Metabolic pathways for lipid metabolism.

Posthepatic Metabolites

Very-Low-Density Lipoprotein   Very-low-density lipoproteins (VLDL) are transient remnants found after initial liver metabolism. They comprise only 10–15% of cholesterol particles and consist of endogenously synthesized triglycerides with a density of 1.006 g/ml. The diameter is considerably smaller than that of the chylomicrons, ranging from 300 to 800 nm.

Intermediate-Density Lipoprotein   Intermediate-density lipoproteins (IDL) consist of cholesterol esters, which are posthepatic remnants but are derived from dietary sources. Associated apoproteins are B-100, CIII, and E. Apoprotein B-48 is lost after the initial hepatic metabolism and B-100 is substituted. Apoprotein E, which is a liver-recognition apoprotein, is found only in VLDL and IDL. IDL metabolites are transient lipoproteins and are measured only in certain pathologic conditions. The density is 1.019 g/ml with a diameter of 250 nm—a very significant decrease from VLDL (800 nm).

LDL and HDL Cholesterol   The major lipid in the LDL cholesterol group is the cholesterol ester, which is associated with B-100 apoprotein. Approximately 60–70% of total cholesterol consists of LDL cholesterol. Elevated levels of LDL cholesterol have been associated with increased risk of myocardial infarction in women over 65 years of age. There is a structural class called LDL(a') that is associated with myocardial infarction (35). Several families with structurally abnormal B-100 apoprotein have been described. Individuals with this abnormal protein are at high risk for myocardial infarction, as a result of lipid buildup and premature atherosclerosis (35). The density of these particles ranges from 1.019 to 1.063 g/ml, and they have a diameter of 180–280 nm.

High-density cholesterol is composed of cholesterol esters with apoproteins A-I and A-II. These particles make up 20–30% of total cholesterol and are the most dense, with a weight of 1.063 to 1.120 g/ml. The diameter of this group of proteins is 50–120 nm.

Metabolism

Cholesterol metabolism is divided into two pathways. The first pathway is the *exogenous pathway,* through which dietary sources of cholesterol are metabolized. The second pathway is called the *endogenous pathway* or the *lipid transport pathway.* Individual variations exist in the ability to metabolize cholesterol: those who are normal, those who hyporespond, and those who hyperrespond (36). An individual who hyporesponds may be given cholesterol-loaded diets with no effect on serum cholesterol measurements, whereas one who hyperresponds has a high serum cholesterol regardless of dietary intake. Explanations for these differences are well described in animal models, but not in humans.

Once a meal is eaten, cholesterol is transported as dietary fat. The average American diet includes approximately 100 grams of triglyceride and approximately one gram of cholesterol daily. Dietary fats are saponified in the intestinal lumen by pancreatic lipases and synthesized into chylomicrons, which are first absorbed by active transport into intestinal lymph and then absorbed into the general circulation. Capillaries in the adipose tissue and skeletal muscle are able to incorporate triglycerides and fats by the action of lipoprotein lipase. As schematically depicted in Figure 9.3, metabolic utilization may occur during either phase of metabolism, e.g., dietary or endogenous. During absorption and synthesis of chylomicrons, apoproteins are incorporated. Apoprotein CII is important as a cofactor to activate lipoprotein lipase, which enzymatically liberates fatty acids (for energy) and monoglycerides. These fatty acids may enter endothelial, adipose, or muscle cells, where they are either oxidized into active metabolic products or re-esterified to triglycerides.

Triglycerides are found in the core lipoprotein particles and are removed through the capillary endothelium and the chylomicron. Predominant apoproteins are B-48 or B-100 and E apoproteins. When chylomicron synthesis occurs in the intestine, the primary B apoprotein is B-48; upon leaving adipose cells, muscle cells, or the liver, the second B apoprotein (B-100) is substituted. Abnormal forms of B-100 are associated with premature cardiovascular disease and are currently used as genetic markers in research laboratories (37).

Another apoprotein added during cellular metabolism is apoprotein E. Apoprotein E is important in liver recognition of chylomicron remnants. Theories suggest that hypo- and hyperresponse to dietary cholesterol may be secondary to the liver's ability to recognize and metabolize apoprotein E (38). In the animal model, populations with large numbers of liver receptors for apoprotein E easily metabolize cholesterol and are labeled hyporesponders. Individuals with a reduced number of apoprotein E receptors are unable to metabolize cholesterol as readily and thus hyperrespond. Despite dietary cholesterol modification, these individuals continue to have high serum cholesterol levels.

After metabolic degradation of dietary chylomicrons, apoprotein substitution occurs and liver metabolism of cholesterol esters begins. Lipid transport now continues in the *endogenous pathway.* Carbohydrates are synthesized to fatty acids and esterified with glycerol to form triglycerides. These newly formed triglycerides are not of dietary origin and are placed in the core of VLDL. The VLDL particles are relatively large and carry five to 10 times more triglyceride than cholesterol esters with apoprotein B-100. Hypertriglyceridemia is an independent risk factor for cardiovascular disease (39). The relationship between hypertriglyceridemia and cardiovascular disease is well known but poorly defined.

The VLDL particles are transported to tissue capillaries, where they are broken down to usable fuels, monoglycerides, and fatty acids. Apoproteins C and E are still present within this lipoprotein particle. After metabolic enzymatic degradation in the peripheral tissues, the IDL particles remain. The IDL particles are either catabolized in the liver by binding to LDL receptors or are modified in the peripheral tissues. As noted previously, they are associated with apoprotein E (liver recognition) receptors. During the transformation from IDL to LDL cholesterol, all apoproteins are removed, except apoprotein B-100. The LDL cholesterol, or the so-called "high risk" cholesterol, is found in high circulating levels.

Despite the negative implications of an elevated LDL cholesterol level, LDL cholesterol is a very important cellular metabolite as precursor for adrenocortical cells, lymphocytes and renal cells. LDL receptors on cell surfaces allow for LDL cholesterol entry into cells. In target cells, these lipid particles are hydrolyzed to form cholesterol for use in membrane synthesis and as precursors for steroid hormones (such as estrogen and progesterone). Once the cell has incorporated the necessary cholesterol, the cell surface receptor reforms, limiting further absorption. The liver uses LDL cholesterol for the synthesis of bile acids and free cholesterol, which is secreted into the bile. In a normal human, 70–80% of LDL is removed from the plasma each day and secreted in the bile via the LDL receptor pathway.

The final metabolic pathway is the transformation of HDL cholesterol in extrahepatic tissue. HDL cholesterol carries the plasma enzyme lecithin cholesterol acyltransferase (LCAT). LCAT allows HDL cholesterol to resynthesize lipids to VLDL cholesterol and recycle the lipid cascade. The fate of newly synthesized VLDL cholesterol is the same as absorbed VLDL, and it eventually becomes LDL cholesterol. HDL cholesterol acts as a "scavenger" and therefore reverses the deposit of cholesterol into tissues. There is good evidence that HDL cholesterol is responsible for the reversal of atherosclerotic changes in vessels, hence the term "good cholesterol" (40, 41).

Hyperlipoproteinemia

When cholesterol is measured, various fractions are reported. Plasma cholesterol, or *total cholesterol,* consists of cholesterol and unesterified cholesterol fractions. If triglycerides are analyzed in conjunction with cholesterol, conclusions can be drawn regarding which metabolic pathway may be abnormal. An elevation of both total cholesterol and triglycerides signifies a problem with chylomicrons and VLDL synthesis. If the triglyceride:cholesterol ratio is greater than 5:1, the predominant fractions are chylomicrons and VLDL. When the triglyceride:cholesterol ratio is less than 5:1, the problem exists in the VLDL and LDL fractions. Hyperlipoproteinemias are defined by establishing a "normal population" and then setting various limits at the 10th and 90th percentiles. Recent standards for women set the 80th percentile for cholesterol at 240 mg/dl and the 50th percentile at 200 mg/dl (Table 9.7). Researchers continue to argue that the population being studied may have different cutoff limits depending on the amount of fat versus vegetable and fiber consumption within the diet (41).

Table 9.7   Initial Classification Based on Total Cholesterol and HDL Cholesterol Levels*

Cholesterol Level	*Initial Classification*
Total Cholesterol	
< 200 mg/dl (5.2 mmol/l)	Desirable blood cholesterol
200–239 mg/dl (5.2–6.2 mmol/l)	Borderline high blood cholesterol
≥ 240 mg/dl (6.2 mmol/l)	High blood cholesterol
HDL Cholesterol	
< 35 mg/dl (0.9 mmol/l)	Low HDL Cholesterol

*HDL, high-density lipoprotein.
Reproduced with permission **Expert Panel on Detection, Evaluation and Treatment of High Blood Cholesterol in Adults.** Summary of the NCEP Adult Treatment Plan II Report. *JAMA* 1993;269:3017.

Plasma elevations of chylomicrons, LDL, VLDL, and various remnants of these entities are classified by the elevated fraction. This adds to the confusion of an already difficult topic. The study of disease states rests on this classification of hyperlipoproteinemias.

Laboratory Testing

In the past decade, cholesterol testing has become something of a fad. The consensus of most researchers is that office laboratory analysis of total cholesterol is virtually worthless as an accurate measure of cholesterol. The measurement techniques and standardization of equipment are difficult to maintain. In well-controlled studies, it has been shown that there is a wide variation in readings (42). Therefore, despite their popularity, these office analyzers are totally inadequate for either screening or monitoring treatment of patients with hypercholesterolemia. There are multiple causes of variation in cholesterol measurements (43), which include diet, obesity, smoking, ethanol intake, exercise, hypothyroidism, diabetes, acute or recent myocardial infarction, recent weight changes, and fasting state. In addition, the method of blood collection can influence the measurement, including patient positioning during blood draw, use and duration of venous occlusion, blood collection tube anticoagulants, and storage and shipping.

If a single individual has total cholesterol measured four times daily, the variation is 2.5%. If an individual is retested within 1 month, on a twice-weekly basis, the coefficient of variation increases to 4.8%. Monthly measurements over 1 year may result in a variation as high as 6.1%. Therefore, at least two and preferably four specimens should be collected 1 month apart in the same dietary state for a lipid value to be considered accurate.

Women under 50 years of age have lower lipid values than men. The rise after 50 years of age may be modified by the use of exogenous oral estrogens. The genetic basis for variability is believed to be mediated by apolipoprotein receptors.

Some researchers believe that the effect of diet and obesity may be related to hypo- and hyperresponder status. However, weight reduction in an obese individual generally affects the triglyceride level, which may decrease as much as 40%. Total cholesterol and LDL cholesterol decrease less than 10% with diet; however, HDL cholesterol increases approximately 10%. Weight gain negates any benefit from prior weight loss. Therefore, consistency of lipid measurements depends on the stability of the patient's weight.

Alcohol and cigarette smoking are well-known modifiers of cholesterol. Moderate alcohol intake (defined as approximately 2 ounces of absolute alcohol per day) is noted to increase HDL cholesterol and decrease LDL cholesterol; however, there is a complimentary increase in triglycerides. Higher intake negates this effect. The increase in HDL cholesterol is in the HDL^3 fraction, which is important to the scavenger mechanism of removing LDL cholesterol. Smoking ($>$15–20 cigarettes/day) has the opposite effect: increasing LDL cholesterol and triglyceride levels and decreasing HDL cholesterol. HDL^3 decreases with cigarette smoking. Caffeine has a mixed effect on lipoprotein measurements but should be avoided in the 12 hours prior to blood collection.

Moderate levels of exercise are as important in overall cardiovascular health as control of hypertension and cessation of cigarette smoking. Strenuous exercise lowers the concentrations of triglycerides and LDL and increases HDL in the serum. Vigorous exercise should not be performed within 12 hours of blood collection because of these acute changes. To minimize variations in cholesterol measurement, patients should be instructed as follows:

1. Avoid caffeine

2. Avoid vigorous exercise

3. Continue to smoke the usual number of cigarettes

213

4. Fast for 12 hours prior to testing

5. Avoid consuming excessive quantities of water

Because of the diurnal variation of blood triglycerides, blood samples should be collected in the morning after a 12-hour fast. The following technique can be used for the collection of blood for cholesterol measurements:

1. Request that the patient sit quietly for 15 minutes prior to testing

2. Minimize tourniquet time (to <5 minutes)

3. Collect cholesterol sample first, if multiple samples are required

4. Use blood collection tubes with ethylenediaminetetraacetic acid (EDTA) as anticoagulant

5. If samples are not to be analyzed immediately
   • store at 0°C for up to 4 days,
   • at −20°C for 6 months,
   • at −50° to −80°C indefinitely

6. Transport by mail on dry ice

One of the most important aspects of overall standardization of lipoprotein measurements is the laboratory used. Laboratory levels should be within ±5% of the Centers for Disease Control and Prevention (CDC) standards for lipoprotein measurements. In one study, approximately 80% of laboratories met this criteria (44). Therefore, to accurately assess cholesterol values, the clinician should be knowledgeable about the laboratory used. It may be of interest to speak to the clinical pathologist to see if the laboratory complies with CDC standards for cholesterol and lipoprotein measurements.

Disease States and Medication Effects   Certain disease states and medications affect cholesterol measurements. Diuretics and propranolol are noted to increase triglyceride and decrease HDL cholesterol measurements. Diuretics may also increase total cholesterol levels. Individuals with diabetes, especially those whose condition is poorly controlled, may have very high levels of triglycerides and LDL cholesterol and low levels of HDL cholesterol. This affect may explain why these individuals are prone to cardiovascular diseases. Patients whose diabetes is well controlled generally have improved lipoprotein profiles.

Pregnancy is associated with decreased total cholesterol in the first trimester and continuous increases of all fractions during the second and third trimesters (45). Low-density lipoprotein and triglyceride concentrations are those most affected by pregnancy. Because of the short duration of pregnancy, interventions are of little clinical significance. Patients with hypothyroidism are also noted to have increased levels of total cholesterol and LDL cholesterol.

Management

The first approach to therapy in obese patients is a suggested algorithm for cholesterol control (Fig. 9.4). Cholesterol fat-lowering diets are readily available in most bookstores and allow the patient to choose a diet she will be more likely to follow. The role of exercise and smoking cessation should be stressed to all patients. Those with a family history of pre-

Figure 9.4   Classification of total cholesterol, HDL cholesterol, and LDL cholesterol.

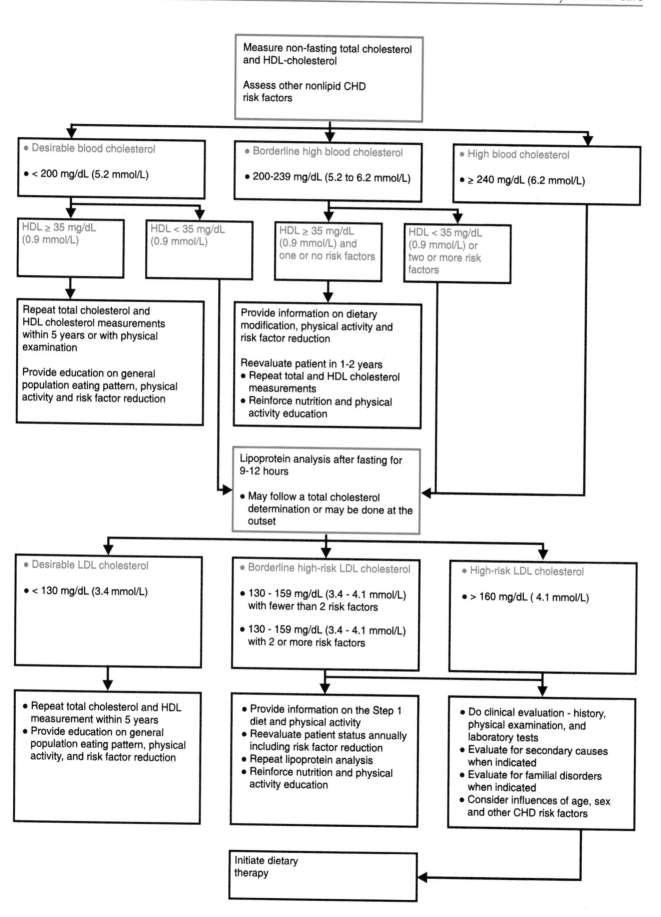

mature coronary artery problems or strokes should be tested, and conservative programs should be initiated in patients in their twenties. After 3–6 months, if the LDL cholesterol remains higher than 190 mg/dl, or higher than 160 mg/dl with risk factors, medical therapy should be initiated.

Bile acid binding resins were the mainstay of therapy for years but were associated with abdominal bloating and gas, which limited their usefulness (46). Currently, there are two drugs commonly used: *lovastatin* and *nicotinic acid* (50). The usual dose of *nicotinic acid* is 500 mg three times a day, with a maximum dose of 1.0 g four times a day. Facial flushing is a significant side effect but can be controlled with administration of 325 mg of aspirin prior to dosing. *Lovastatin,* a relatively new drug, should be initiated with a single 20-mg dose at bedtime and may be increased to 40 mg twice daily. *Lovastatin* may cause muscle necrosis if combined with *nicotinic acid, erythromycin, cyclosporin,* or fibric acid derivatives (*clofibrate* or *gemfibrozil*); therefore, creatinine kinase levels should be monitored. For patients taking either medication, serum glutamic oxaloacetic transaminase should be measured 6 and 12 weeks after initiation of therapy and semiannually once therapeutic levels are reached (47). In difficult to control cases, bile acid resins may be added to either medication.

Diabetes Mellitus

Diabetes mellitus (DM) is a chronic disorder of altered carbohydrate, protein, and fat metabolism from a deficiency in the secretion or function of insulin. The disease is defined by either fasting hyperglycemia or elevated plasma glucose levels after an oral glucose tolerance test (OGTT). Of an estimated 13 million Americans with diabetes, only 50% have been diagnosed. The prevalence of DM is higher in women and certain ethnic groups, although a background rate in the general population is 2.5% (57). Risk factors for DM are:

1. Age older than 40 years

2. Adiposity or obesity

3. A family history of diabetes.

The major complications of DM are primarily vascular and metabolic complications. They include blindness, renal disease, gangrene of an extremity, heart disease, and stroke. Diabetes is a major risk factor for cardiovascular disease (54).

Classification

After long periods of controversy regarding the classification of diabetes mellitus, a consensus group sponsored by the National Institutes of Health developed the National Diabetes Data Group classifications in 1979, presented in Table 9.8.

Type I

With insulin-dependent diabetes mellitus (IDDM) the major metabolic disturbance is the absence of insulin as a result of the destruction of beta cells in the pancreas. Insulin is necessary for glucose metabolism and cellular respiration. When insulin is absent, ketosis results. The etiology of IDDM is unknown; however, data suggest an autoimmune factor from either a viral infection or toxic components in the environment. Studies in the past decade have shown a correlation between many autoimmune diseases and the human leukocyte antigens (HLA). Insulin-sensitive tissues (muscle, liver, and fat) fail to metabolize glucose efficiently in the absence of insulin. In uncontrolled DM, additional excess counterregulatory hormones (cortisol, catecholamines, and glucagon) contribute to further metabolic dysfunction. In the absence of adequate amounts of insulin, increasing breakdown of muscle (amino acid-proteolysis), fat (fatty acid-lipolysis), and glycogen (glucose-

Table 9.8   Classification of Diabetes Mellitus

Type I:	Insulin-dependent diabetes mellitus (IDDM)
Type II:	Noninsulin-dependent diabetes mellitus (NIDDM) (Subgroups may be classified as obese or nonobese)

Other types of diabetes:

Impaired glucose tolerance (IGT)
    Subgroups—obese or nonobese

Pancreatic disease
    Secondary to destruction of islet cells

Endocrinopathies
    Cushing's, acromegaly, pheochromocytoma, hyperaldosteronism

Drug-induced

glycogenolysis) results in the presence of breakdown products. Additionally, there is an increase in glucose production from noncarbohydrate precursors because of gluconeogenesis and ketogenesis in the liver. If not promptly treated, severe metabolic decompensation (i.e., diabetic ketoacidosis or DKA) will occur and may lead to death.

Type II

Noninsulin-dependent diabetes mellitus (NIDDM) is a heterogeneous form of diabetes that commonly occurs in older age groups (>40 years), and which is more likely than IDDM to have a familial tendency. In contrast to the absence of insulin that occurs with IDDM, altered metabolism of insulin in NIDDM results in insulin resistance. This condition is characterized by impaired glucose uptake in target tissues. The compensatory increase in insulin secretion results in higher than normal circulating insulin levels (55). Obesity is present in 85% of affected patients. The cause of NIDDM is unknown, but defects in both the secretion and action of insulin are suspected.

Many patients diagnosed with NIDDM at an early age of life eventually exhaust endogenous pancreatic insulin and require injected insulin. These patients are classified as insulin-requiring diabetics as opposed to insulin-dependent diabetics (i.e., type I). When under severe stress, such as infection or surgery, they may develop diabetic ketoacidosis or a hyperglycemic hyperosmolar nonketotic state (HHNS). Risk factors for NIDDM include ethnicity (Native Americans, Hispanics, African-Americans), obesity, family history of diabetes mellitus, sedentary lifestyle, impaired glucose tolerance, upper body adiposity, and history of gestational diabetes and hyperinsulinemia. The presence of risk factors strongly influences the development of NIDDM in susceptible populations.

Diagnosis

The diagnosis of DM in nonpregnant adults rests on one of the following three methods:

1. A single fasting blood glucose level >140 mg/dl on two separate occasions.

2. A random blood glucose level >200 mg/dl in an individual with classic signs and symptoms of diabetes (polydipsia, polyuria, polyphagia, and weight loss).

3. A 2-hour OGTT (fasting sample, 30-, 60-, 90-, and 120-minute samples), after a 75-g load of glucose. A 2-hour OGTT should not be performed if the first two criteria are present.

Diagnostic criteria for HIDDM are:
- Fasting glucose <140 mg/dl
- Two-hour sample >200 mg/dl
- One additional timed sample >200 mg/dl

The 2-hour OGTT should be performed under the following conditions:

1. A 10-hour fast should precede morning testing.

2. The patient should sit throughout the procedure.

3. No smoking is permitted during the test interval.

4. Caffeinated beverages should not be consumed.

5. More than 150 g of carbohydrates should be ingested for 3 days prior to the test.

6. No drugs should be taken prior to the test.

7. The patient should not be bedridden or under stress.

Patients who should be considered for testing are:

- those with classic signs and symptoms of diabetes (i.e., polyuria, polydipsia, polyphagia, and weight loss)
- those with a family history of diabetes, especially NIDDM
- ethnic groups at high risk (Pima Indians, Native Americans, African-Americans, Hispanics)
- those who have an obstetrical history of macrosomia or shoulder dystocia
- those who have a history of recurring skin, genital, or urinary tract infections, especially monilia.

Assessment of Glycemic Control

The only acceptable method for assessment of glycemic control is determination of blood glucose by the direct enzymatic method; urine values do not correlate with blood values. In the past decade, multiple techniques using test strips and meters have been introduced. These machines work well but reflect whole blood determinations, not serum values. Upgrades of testing strips (in which blood does not need to be wiped away) and glucometers with memory have made home glucose monitoring more reliable. Urine tapes to test for ketones are a useful and quick method of assessing ketosis. If the urine is consistently positive for ketones and blood glucose values remain higher than 300 mg/dl, the patient should seek medical advice.

Treatment guidelines for physicians (Table 9.9) and patients (Table 9.10) are presented. A 10-year multicenter study, the Diabetes Control and Complication Trial, performed under the auspices of the National Institutes of Health, showed a marked reduction (40–50%) in complications of neuropathy, retinopathy, and nephropathy when patients with IDDM received intensive therapy (accomplished by a team approach) as compared with those who received standard therapy.

Treatment of NIDDM

Diet is the most important component of DM management and usually the hardest way to achieve control (54). Three major strategies are used: weight loss, low-fat diet (≤30% of calories from fat), and physical exercise. Obese patients should reduce their weight to ideal body weight. Metabolic advantages of weight reduction are improved lipid profile and glucose control secondary to increased insulin sensitivity and decreased insulin resistance. The greater the weight loss, the greater the improvement in lipid disorders. Physical exercise promotes weight loss and improves insulin sensitivity and dyslipidemia in those people who are in high-risk groups for cardiovascular and microvascular diseases (55).

Oral Hypoglycemic Agents—Sulfonylureas

Oral hypoglycemic agents are recommended for many NIDDM patients (56). First- and second-generation sulfonylureas are currently the only agents approved by the Food and

Table 9.9   Physician Guidelines in the Therapy of Diabetes Mellitus

- Establish diagnosis and classify type of diabetes mellitus (DM).

- If diagnosis of DM is already established, additional oral glucose tolerance tests should not be performed.

- Initiate diabetes education classes to learn blood glucose monitoring and diabetic medications, to learn signs, symptoms, and complications, and to learn how to manage sick days.

- Place patient on American Diabetes Association (ADA) diet with appropriate caloric, sodium, and lipid restrictions.

- Establish cardiac risk factors, kidney function (serum creatinine, 24-hour urine albumin).

- If neuropathy is present, refer to a neurologist.

- Establish extent of fundoscopic lesion (refer to ophthalmologist as needed).

- Check feet and toenails at each visit.

- Use finger stick blood glucose for daily diabetic control and urine check for ketones (but do not use first morning void).

- Follow chronic glycemic control by HgA_{1c} every 2–3 months (every 6 months in elderly) in the office.

- Initial general health evaluation should consist of history and physical examination and the following laboratory tests: Complete blood count (CBC) with differential, chemistry profile, lipid profile, urinalysis, thyroid function tests, and electrocardiogram (base line at 40 years of age or older; repeat yearly).

- Oral hypoglycemic agents (OHA) may be considered if fasting blood glucose (FBG) does not decline or increase, if the patient has had diabetes for less than 10 years, does not have severe hepatic or renal disease, and is not pregnant or allergic to sulfonylurea.

- Fasting blood sugar (FBS) (on diet) $\geq$ 250 mg/dl are not suitable candidates for oral hypoglycemic agents.

- While on oral hypoglycemic agents, check FBS and 2-hour postprandial in the office every 2 months (in conjunction with daily home glucose monitoring).

- If postprandial glucose < 200 mg/dl, omit oral hypoglycemic agents and place on diet alone and follow every 1–2 months.

- If FSG > 200 mg/dl consistently, place patient on insulin.

- If insulin is required, consider sending to an internist, especially if obese.

- If the gynecologist continues to follow patient, the amount of insulin necessary is far less than pregnant patients.

Table 9.10   Patient Guidelines for Treatment of NIDDM

Initiate an American Diabetes Association reducing diet (50% carbohydrate, 30% fat, 20% protein, high fiber) with 3 meals a day.

Maintain ideal body weight or to reduce weight by 5–15% in 3 months if obese.

Modify risk factors (smoking, exercise, fat intake)

Check fasting blood glucose (FBG) by finger stick daily for 2 months.

- If plasma blood sugar declines, no other therapy is needed.

- If FBG does not decline or increases, use of oral hypoglycemic agents may be considered.

Table 9.11   Commonly Used Oral Hypoglycemic Agents

Oral Hypoglycemic Agents	Trade Name	Daily Dose	Duration of Action (Hrs)
Tolbutamide	Orinase	750 mg—3.0 g/divided doses	6–12
Tolazamide	Tolinase	200–1000 mg/divided doses	12–24
Acetohexamide	Dymelor	250–1500 mg/single dose	12–24
Chlorpropamide	Diabinese	100–500 mg	up to 60
Glyburide	Micronase, DiaBeta	2.5–20 mg variable dose	10–24
Glipizide	Glucotrol	2.5–40 mg variable dose	3–8

Drug Administration. Currently available formulations are listed in Table 9.11. The mode of action of sulfonylureas is based on two different mechanisms: 1) enhanced insulin secretion from the pancreas, and 2) an extrapancreatic effect that is poorly understood. Endogenous insulin secretion (as measured by C-peptide) is necessary for oral hypoglycemic agents to work. Additionally, if the fasting blood glucose level on an adequate diabetic diet is higher than 250 mg/dl, there is little effect. Oral agents fail to control glucose in 3–5% of patients annually. Frequent evaluation to monitor control (every 2 months) is important. If glucose levels cannot be controlled with oral hypoglycemic agents, insulin should be administered and referral should be considered because of the increased rate of complications experienced by this group.

Thyroid Diseases

Thyroid disorders are more common in women and some families, although the exact pattern of inheritance is unknown (57). In geriatric populations, the incidence may be as high as 5% (58). Unfortunately, the laboratory diagnosis of thyroid disease can be difficult because of altered hormonal states such as pregnancy and use of exogenous hormones. Thyroid hormones act in target tissues by binding to nuclear receptors, which induces change in gene expression (59). Extrathyroidal conversation of thyroxine (T4) to triiodothyronine (T3) takes place in target tissue. T3 binds the nuclear receptor with higher affinity than T4, which makes T3 more biologically active. Pituitary thyroid-stimulating hormone (TSH) and hypothalamic thyrotropin-releasing hormone (TRH) regulate hormone production and thyroid growth by normal feedback physiology. Thyroid-stimulating immunoglobulins (TSI), once known as long-acting thyroid stimulator (LATS), bind to the TSH receptor, which results in hyperthyroid Graves' disease. Over 99% of circulating T4 and T3 are bound by plasma proteins, predominantly to thyroxine-binding globulin (TBG), and the remaining 1% of thyroid hormones are free. Free levels of thyroid hormones remain constant despite physiologic or pharmacologic alterations. Regardless of total serum protein levels, active thyroid hormone remains stable. In healthy women, transitions from puberty to menopause do not alter free thyroid hormone concentrations. Excess endogenous or exogenous sources of estrogen increase TBG plasma concentration by decreasing hepatic clearance. Androgens (especially testosterone) and corticosteroids have the opposite effect, increasing hepatic TBG clearance.

Thyroid function tests may be misleading in women receiving exogenous sources of estrogen because of altered binding characteristics. In euthyroid individuals, elevations of thyroid hormone concentrations arise from three mechanisms: 1) increased protein binding because of altered albumin and estrogen states, 2) decreased peripheral conversion of T4 to T3, or 3) rarely occurring congenital tissue resistance to thyroid hormones. The most common cause of abnormal findings is altered estrogen states (hormonal replacement therapy, pregnancy), which complicate interpretation of thyroid function studies. Most laboratories compensate by reporting a free T4 index or a "T7," which mathematically corrects for physiologic alterations. If a question arises, consultation with the clinical pathologist should be sought.

Hypothyroidism

Overt hypothyroidism occurs in 2% of women, and at least an additional 5% of women develop subclinical hypothyroidism. This is especially true in elderly individuals, in whom many of the signs and symptoms are subtle. The principal cause of hypothyroidism is autoimmune thyroiditis (Hashimoto's thyroiditis). A familial predisposition is observed in many cases, but the specific genetic or environmental trigger is unknown. The incidence of autoimmune thyroiditis increases with age, affecting up to 15% of women over 65 years of age. Many have subclinical hypothyroidism, which is defined as an elevated serum TSH concentration with a normal serum free T4 level. Thyroid replacement therapy usually reverses this condition. Autoimmune thyroiditis may be associated with other endocrine (e.g., type I diabetes, primary ovarian failure, adrenal insufficiency, and hypoparathyroidism) and nonendocrine (e.g., vitiligo and pernicious anemia) autoimmune disorders (60). Therefore, when autoimmune diseases are present, there should be a high degree of suspicion for concurrent thyroid disorders. Iatrogenic causes of hypothyroidism include surgical removal of the thyroid gland or radioactive iodine therapy for hyperthyroidism or thyroid cancer. Thirty years ago, radiation was used to treat acne and other dermatologic disorders; these patients have an increased risk of thyroid cancer and require close monitoring. Hypothyroidism rarely occurs secondary to pituitary or hypothalamic diseases from TSH or TRH deficiency but must be considered if symptoms occur after neurosurgical procedures.

Clinical Features

Manifestations of hypothyroidism include a broad range of signs and symptoms: fatigue, lethargy, cold intolerance, nightmares, dry skin, hair loss, constipation, periorbital carotene deposition (causing a yellow discoloration), carpal tunnel syndrome, and weight gain (usually less than 5–10 kg). Menstrual dysfunction is common, either as menorrhagia or amenorrhea. Infertility may arise from anovulation, but the administration of exogenous thyroid hormone is not useful for anovulatory euthyroid women. Empirical use of thyroid extract, common many years ago, should be discouraged. Common neuropsychiatric symptoms that may be early signs of hypothyroidism include depression, irritability, impaired memory, and, in the elderly, dementia. Hypothyroidism is not a cause of premenstrual syndrome (PMS), but worsening PMS may be a subtle manifestation of hypothyroidism (61). Hypothyroidism may cause precocious or delayed puberty. Hyperprolactinemia and galactorrhea are unusual manifestations of hypothyroidism. A TSH level assessment should be obtained in cases of amenorrhea, galactorrhea, and hyperprolactinemia to distinguish primary hypothyroidism from a prolactin-secreting pituitary adenoma.

Diagnosis

Hypothyroidism should always be confirmed with laboratory studies. Primary hypothyroidism is characterized by the combination of an elevated serum TSH with a low serum free T4 or free T4 index. Autoimmune thyroiditis can be confirmed by the presence of serum antithyroid peroxidase (formerly referred to as antimicrosomal) antibodies. Central hypothyroidism, although rare, is distinguished by a low or low-normal serum free T4 with either a low or inappropriate normal serum TSH concentration.

Therapy

L-thyroxine (T4) is the treatment of choice for hypothyroidism and is available as *Levothroid* **or** *Synthroid* (62). The mode of action is conversion of T4 to T3 in peripheral tissues. A parenteral formulation is available but seldom needed because of the long half-life (7 days) of oral preparations. Because binding or chelation may occur, absorption may be poor when L-thyroxine is taken in combination with aluminum hydroxide (common in antacids), cholestyramine, ferrous sulfate, or sucralfate. The usual T4 requirement is weight-related (approximately 1.6 μg/kg), but a smaller amount is needed for elderly patients. Normal daily dosage is 0.1–0.15 mg, but it should be adjusted to maintain TSH levels within the normal range.

In the early 1980s, many clinicians believed that increasing the serum T4 to mildly elevated levels would enhance conversion of T4 to T3. Subsequent data have shown that even a mild increase of T4 was associated with cortical bone loss and atrial fibrillation, particularly in older women (63). A low initial T4 dose (0.025 mg/day) should be initiated in patients with known or suspected coronary artery disease. Rapid replacement may worsen angina and, in some cases, induce myocardial infarction.

Hyperthyroidism

Hyperthyroidism affects 2% of women during their lifetime, most often during their childbearing years. The most common disorder is Graves' disease, which is associated with orbital inflammation causing the classic exophthalmus associated with the disease and a characteristic dermopathy, pretibial myxedema. The etiology of Graves' disease in genetically susceptible women is unknown. Autonomously functioning benign thyroid neoplasias are less common causes of hyperthyroidism and are associated with toxic adenomas and toxic multinodular goiter. Transient thyrotoxicosis may be the result of unregulated glandular release of thyroid hormone in postpartum (painless, silent, or lymphocytic) thyroiditis and subacute (painful) thyroiditis. Other rare causes of thyroid overactivity include: human chorionic gonadotropin-secreting choriocarcinoma, TSH-secreting pituitary adenoma, and struma ovarii. Factitious ingestion or iatrogenic overprescribing of thyroid hormones should be considered in patients with eating disorders.

Clinical Features

Symptoms of thyrotoxicosis include fatigue, diarrhea, heat intolerance, palpitations, dyspnea, nervousness, and weight loss. In young patients, there may be paradoxical weight gain from an increased appetite. Thyrotoxicosis may cause vomiting in pregnant women, which may be confused with hyperemesis gravidarum (64). Physical findings include tachycardia, tremors, proximal muscle weakness, and warm moist skin. The most dramatic physical changes are ophthalmologic and include lid retraction and lag, periorbital edema, and proptosis. These findings, however, occur in less than one-third of women. In elderly adults, symptoms are often more subtle, such as weight loss, atrial fibrillation (65), or new-onset angina pectoris. Menstrual abnormalities may include light flow or anovulatory menses and infertility. Goiter is common in most younger women with Graves' disease but may be absent in older women. Toxic nodular goiter is associated with nonhomogeneous glandular enlargement, whereas in subacute thyroiditis the gland is tender, hard, and enlarged.

Diagnosis

Most thyrotoxic patients have elevated total and free T4 and T3 concentrations (measured by radioimmunoassay). In thyrotoxicosis, serum TSH concentrations are virtually undetectable, even with very sensitive assays (sensitivity measured to 0.1 units). Sensitive serum TSH measurements may aid in the diagnosis of hyperthyroidism. Radioiodine uptake scans are useful in the differential diagnosis of established hyperthyroidism. Scans that show homogeneous uptake of radioactive iodine are suggestive of Graves' disease, whereas heterogeneous tracer uptake is suggestive of a diagnosis of toxic nodular goiter. In distinction, glandular radioisotope concentration is diminished with thyroiditis and medication-induced thyrotoxicosis.

Therapy

Antithyroid medications, either *propylthiouracil* (*PTU* 50–300 mg every 6–8 hours) or methimazole (*Tapazole*, 10–30 mg per day) are initial therapies. After metabolic control is obtained, definitive therapy is thyroid ablation with radioiodine, which results

in permanent hypothyroidism. Both antithyroid drugs block thyroid hormone biosynthesis and may have additional immunosuppressive effects on the gland. The primary difference between oral medications is that PTU partially inhibits extrathyroidal T4-to-T3 conversion and methimazole does not. However, methimazole has a longer half-life and permits single daily dosing, which may encourage compliance. Euthyroidism is typically restored in 3–10 weeks, and treatment with oral antithyroid agents is continued for 6–24 months, unless total ablation with radioiodine or surgical resection is performed. Surgery has become less popular because it is invasive and may result in inadvertent parathyroid removal, which commits the patient to lifelong calcium therapy. The relapse rate with oral antithyroid medications is 50% over a lifetime. When medical therapy is used, lifelong follow-up is important solely because of the high relapse rate. Both medications have infrequent (5%) minor side effects that include fever, rash, or arthralgias. Major toxicity (e.g., hepatitis, vasculitis, and agranulocytosis) is rare (<1%). Strep throat is a serious side effect with agranulocytosis and any patient with aerophagia should be evaluated and given antibiotics. The most common time for relapses is in the postpartum period. Therapy with 131-Iodine provides a permanent cure of hyperthyroidism in 70–80% of patients. The principal drawback to radioactive iodine therapy is the high rate of postablative hypothyroidism, which occurs in at least 50% of patients immediately after therapy, with additional cases developing at a rate of 2–3% per year. Based on the assumption that hypothyroidism will develop, patients should be given lifetime thyroid replacement. β-Adrenergic blocking agents such as *propranolol* are useful adjunctive therapy for control of sympathomimetic symptoms such as tachycardia (66). An additional benefit of beta blockers is the blocking of peripheral conversion of T4 to T3. In rare cases of thyroid storm, *PTU,* beta blockers, glucocorticoids, and high-dose iodine preparations (SSKI or intravenous sodium iodide) should be administered immediately and patients should be sent to an intensive care unit.

Thyroid Nodules and Cancer

Thyroid nodules are common and found on physical examination in up to 5% of patients. Nodules may be demonstrated on ultrasound in as many as 30% of unselected patients. Most nodules are asymptomatic and benign; however, the possibility of malignancy and hyperthyroidism must be excluded. Previous radiation in childhood, regardless of dose, is associated with a higher risk of malignancy. Virtually all nodules require histological evaluation. In the past decade, this has been accomplished by fine-needle aspiration biopsy (FNA) rather than open surgical biopsy. Thyroid function tests should be performed prior to FNA and if abnormal, the underlying disease should be treated. In many cases, the nodule will regress during therapy, eliminating the need for FNA. Nodules that persist after treatment should be biopsied. Because most nodules are "cold" on scanning, it is more cost effective to proceed with tissue sampling rather than scanning. Biopsy provides a diagnosis in 95% of cases; however, in the 5% of patients in whom a diagnosis cannot be established, surgical biopsy is necessary. Only 20% of surgical biopsies of an "indeterminate aspiration" are found to be malignant (67).

Papillary thyroid carcinoma, the most common malignancy, is found in 75% of cases. Patients younger than 50 years of age who have a primary tumor smaller than 4 cm at presentation, even with associated cervical lymph node metastasis, are usually cured. Anaplastic tumors in the elderly have a poor prognosis and progress rapidly despite therapy. Radioiodine therapy or surgical ablation are the most common methods of therapy. After therapy, the patient should be given lifetime suppression therapy and should be monitored periodically by assessing TBG levels.

References

1. **Evans FO Jr, Sydnor JB, Moore WE, Manuaring JL, Brill AH, Jackson RT, et al.** Sinusitis of maxillary antrum. *N Engl J Med* 1975;293:735–9.

2. **Slavin RG.** Sinopulmonary relationships. *Am J Otolaryngol* 1994;15:18–25.

3. **Mabry RL.** Allergic rhinosinusitis. In: **Bailey BJ,** ed. *Head and Neck Surgery—Otolaryngology.* Philadelphia: JB Lippincott, 1993:290–301.

4. **Ruben RJ, Bagger-Sjoback D, Downs MP, Gravel JS, Karakashian M, Klein JO, et al.** Recent advances in otitis media. Complications and sequela. *Ann Otol Rhinol Laryngol Suppl* 1989;139:46–55.

5. **Douglas RG Jr.** Prophylaxis and treatment of influenza. *N Engl J Med* 1990;322:443–50.

6. **Woodhead MA, MacFarlane JT, McCraken JS, Rose DH, Finch RG.** Prospective study of the aetiology and outcome of pneumonia in the community. *Lancet* 1987;1:671–4.

7. **Nolan TE, Hankins GDV.** Adult respiratory distress. In: **Pastorek JG,** ed. *Infectious Disease in Obstetrics and Gynecology.* Rockville: Aspen Publications, 1994:197–206.

8. **Farr BM, Kaiser DL, Harrison BD, Connolly CK.** Prediction of microbial aetiology at admission to hospital for pneumonia from the presenting clinical features. *Thorax* 1989;44:1031–5.

9. **Blair SN, Kohl HW III, Pafferbarger RS Jr, Clark DG, Cooper KH, Gibbons LW.** Physical fitness and all-cause mortality. *JAMA* 1989;262:2395–401.

10. **Anastos K, Charney P, Charon RA, Cohen E, Jones CY, Marte C, et al.** Hypertension in women: what is really known. *Ann Intern Med* 1991;115:287–93.

11. **The Fifth Report of the Joint National Committee on the Detection, Evaluation, and Treatment of High Blood Pressure.** *Arch Intern Med* 1993;153:154–83.

12. **Roccella EJ, Lenfant C.** Regional and racial differences among stroke victims in the United States. *Clin Cardiol* 1989;12:IV4–8.

13. **Moorman PG, Hames CG, Tyroler HA.** Socioeconomic status and morbidity and mortality in hypertensive blacks. *Cardiovasc Clin* 1991;21:179–94.

14. **Stamler J, Stamler R, Neaton JD.** Blood pressure, systolic and diastolic, and cardiovascular risks. *Arch Intern Med* 1993;153:598–615.

15. **Preuss HG.** Nutrition and diseases of women: cardiovascular disorders. *J Am Coll Nutr* 1993;12:417–25.

16. **Stamler R, Stamler J, Gosch FC, Civinelli J, Fishman J, McKeever P, et al.** Primary prevention of hypertension by nutritionally-hygienic means: final report of a randomized, controlled trial. *JAMA* 1989;262:1801–7.

17. **SHEP Cooperative research group.** Prevention of stroke by antihypertensive drug treatment in older persons with isolated systolic hypertension. *JAMA* 1991;265:3255–64.

18. **American Society of Hypertension.** Recommendations for routine blood pressure measurement by indirect cuff sphygmomanometry. *Am J Hypertens* 1992;5:207–9.

19. **The National High Blood Pressure Education Program Working Group Report on Ambulatory Blood Pressure Monitoring.** *Arch Intern Med* 1990;150:2270–80.

20. **National Education Program Working Group.** Report on management of patients with hypertension and high blood cholesterol. *Ann Intern Med* 1991;114:224–37.

21. **LaRosa JC.** Lipoproteins and coronary artery disease risk in women. *J Myocard Ischemia* 1991;5:35–42.

22. **Lardinois CK, Neuman SL.** The effects of anti-hypertensive agents on serum lipids and lipoproteins. *Arch Intern Med* 1988;148:1280–8.

23. **Selby JV, Friedman GD, Quensenberry CP Jr.** Precursors of essential hypertension: the role of body fat distribution pattern. *Am J Epidemiol* 1989;129:43–53.

24. **Schotte DE, Stunkard AJ.** The effects of weight reduction on blood pressure in 301 obese patients. *Arch Intern Med* 1990;150:1701–4.

25. **Law MR, Frost CD, Wald NJ.** By how much does dietary salt reduction lower blood pressure? Analysis of data from trials of salt reduction. *BMJ* 1991;302:819–24.

26. **Blair SN, Goodyear NN, Gibbons LW, Cooper KH.** Physical fitness and incidence of hypertension in healthy normotensive men and women. *JAMA* 1989;262:2395–401.

27. **Alderman MH.** Which antihypertensive drugs first—and why! *JAMA* 1992:2786–7.

28. **Freis ED.** Critique of the clinical importance of diuretic-induced hypokalemia and elevated cholesterol level. *Arch Intern Med* 1989;149:2640–8.

29. **Garber AJ.** Effective treatment of hypertension in patients with diabetes mellitus. *Clin Cardiol* 1992;15:715–9.

30. **Dwyer PL, Teele JS.** Prazosin: a neglected cause of genuine stress incontinence. *Obstet Gynecol* 1992;79:117–21.

31. **National high blood pressure education program working group report on ambulatory blood pressure monitoring.** *Arch Intern Med* 1990;150:2270–80.

32. **Brown MS, Goldstein JL.** A receptor-mediated pathway for cholesterol homeostasis. *Science* 1986;232:34–47.

33. **Smith GD, Pekkanen J.** Should there be a moratorium on the use of cholesterol lowering drugs? *BMJ* 1992;304:431–4.

34. **Boyd NF, Cousins M, Beaton M, Kruikov V, Lockwood G, Tritchler D.** Quantitative changes in dietary fat intake and serum cholesterol in women: results from a randomized controlled trial. *Am J Clin Nutr* 1990;52:470–6.

35. **Austin MA, Breslow JL, Hennekens CH, Buring JE, Willett WC, Krauss RM.** Low-density lipoprotein subclass patterns and risk of myocardial infarction. *JAMA* 1988;260:1917–21.

36. **Genest J Jr, McNamara JR, Ordovas JM, Jenner JL, Silberman SR, Anderson KM, et al.** Lipoprotein cholesterol, apolipoprotein A-I and B and lipoprotein (a) abnormalities in men with premature coronary artery disease. *J Am Coll Cardiol* 1992;19:792–802.

37. **Ladias JAA, Kwiterovich PO Jr, Smith HH, Miller M, Bachorik PS, Forte T, et al.** Apolipoprotein B-100 Hopkins (Arginin 4019-Tryptophan). *JAMA* 1989;262:1980–8.

38. **Katan MB, Beynen AC.** Characteristics of human hypo-and hyperresponders to dietary cholesterol. *Am J Epidemiol* 1987;125:387–99.

39. **Rauh G, Keller C, Kormann B, Spengel F, Schuster H, Wolfram G, et al.** Familial defective apolipo-protein B-100: clinical characteristics of 54 cases. *Atherosclerosis* 1992;92:233–41.

40. **Mahley RW, Weisgraber KH, Innerarity TL, Rall SC Jr.** Genetic defects in lipoprotein metabolism. *JAMA* 1991;265:78–83.

41. **Avins, AL, Haber RJ, Hulley SB.** The status of hypertrigly-ceridemia as a risk factor for coronary heart disease. *Clin Lab Med* 1989;9:153–68.

42. **Goldbourt U, Holtzman E, Neufeld HN.** Total and high density lipoprotein cholesterol in the serum and risk of mortality: evidence of a threshold effect. *BMJ* 1987;290:1239–43.

43. **Gordon DJ, Rifkind BM.** High-density lipoprotein—the clinical implications of recent studies. *N Engl J Med* 1989;321:1311–6.

44. **Ramsey LE, Yeo WW, Jackson PR.** Dietary reduction of serum cholesterol concentration: time to think again. *BMJ* 1991;303:953–7.

45. **Naughton MJ, Luepker RV, Strickland D.** The accuracy of portable cholesterol analyzers in public screening programs. *JAMA* 1990;263:1213–7.

46. **Irwig L, Glaszious P, Wilson A, Macaskill P.** Estimating an individual's true cholesterol level and response to intervention. *JAMA* 1991;266:1678–85.

47. **McManus BM, Toth AB, Engel JA, Myers GL, Maito HK, Wilson JE, et al.** Progress in lipid reporting practices and reliability of cholesterol measurement in clinical laboratories in Nebraska. *JAMA* 1989;262:83–8.

48. **van Stiphout WAHJ, Hofman A, de Bruijn AM.** Serum lipids in young women before, during, and after pregnancy. *Am J Epidemiol* 1987;126:922–8.

49. **Blum CB, Levy RI.** Current therapy for hypercholesterolemia. *JAMA* 1989;261:3582–7.

50. **Bradford RH, Shear CL, Chremos AN, Dujoune C, Downton M, Franklin FA, et al.** Expanded clinical evaluation of Lovastatin (EXCEL) study results. *Arch Intern Med* 1991;151:43–9.

51. **Centers for Disease Control and Prevention.** *Diabetes Surveillance, 1993.* Washington, DC: U.S. Dept. of Health and Human Services, Public Health Service, 1993.

52. **Jarrett RJ.** Risk factors for coronary heart disease in diabetes mellitus. *Diabetes* 1992;41 (Suppl 2):1–3.

53. **Bogardus C, Lilloja S, Howard VV, Reaven G, Mott D.** Relationships between insulin secretion, insulin action, and fasting plasma glucose concentration in non-diabetic and non-insulin-dependent diabetic subjects. *J Clin Invest* 1984;74:1238–46.

54. **Tinker LF.** Diabetes mellitus-A priority health care issue for women. *J Am Diet Assoc* 1994;94:976–85.

55. **Wood PD, Stefanick ML, Williams PT, Haskell WL.** The effects on plasma lipoproteins of a prudent weight-reducing diet, with or without exercise, in overweight men and women. *N Engl J Med* 1991;325:461–6.

56. **Tal A.** Oral hypoglycemic agents in the treatment of type II diabetes. *Am Fam Physician* 1993;43:1089–95.

57. **Tunbridge WM, Evered DC, Hall R, Appleton D, Brewis M, Clark F, et al.** The spectrum of thyroid disease in a community: the Whickham survey. *Clin Endocrinol (Oxf)* 1977; 7:481–93.

58. **Helfand M, Crapo LM.** Screening for thyroid disease. *Ann Intern Med* 1990;112:840–9.

59. **Brent GA, Moore DD, Larsen RP.** Thyroid hormone regulation of gene expression. *Annu Rev Physiol* 1991;53:17–35.

60. **Volpé R.** Autoimmunity causing thyroid dysfunction. *Endocrinol Metab Clin North Am* 1991;20:565–87.

61. **Schmidt PJ, Grover GN, Roy-Byrne PP, Rubinow DR.** Thyroid function in women with pre-menstrual syndrome. *J Clin Endocrinol Metab* 1993;76:671–4.

62. **Mandel SJ, Brent GA, Larsen PR.** Levothyroxine therapy in patients with thyroid disease. *Ann Intern Med* 1993;119:492–502.

63. **Schneider DL, Barrett-Connor EL, Morton DJ.** Thyroid hormone use and bone mineral density in elderly women. Effects of estrogen. *JAMA* 1994;271:1245–9.

64. **Mori M, Amino N, Tamaki H, Miyai K, Tanizawa O.** Morning sickness and thyroid function in normal pregnancy. *Obstet Gynecol* 1988;72:355–9.

65. **Siebers MJ, Drinka PJ, Vergauwen C.** Hyperthyroidism as a cause of atrial fibrillation in long-term care. *Arch Intern Med* 1992;152:2063–4.

66. **Zonszein J, Santangelo RP, Mackin JF, Lee TC, Coffey RJ, Canary JJ.** Propranolol therapy in thyrotoxicosis. *Am J Med* 1979;66:411–6.

67. **McHenry CR, Walfish PG, Rosen IB.** Non-diagnostic fine needle aspiration biopsy: a dilemma in management of nodular thyroid disease. *Am Surg* 1993;59:415–9.

226

10 Family Planning

Phillip G. Stubblefield

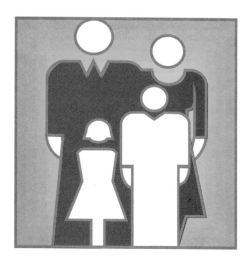

The history of contraception is a long one; however, the voluntary control of fertility is even more important in modern society (1). With each woman expected to have only one or two children, most of the reproductive years are spent trying to avoid pregnancy. Effective control of reproduction is essential to a woman's ability to accomplish individual goals beyond childbearing. From a larger perspective, the rapid growth of human populations in this century threatens survival. At its present rate, the population of the world will double in 40 years and that of many of the poorer countries of the world will double in little more than 20 years (2) (Fig. 10.1). For the individual and for the planet, reproductive health requires careful use of effective means to prevent both pregnancy and sexually transmitted diseases (STDs) (3).

From puberty until perimenopause, women are faced with concerns about childbearing or its avoidance: the only options are sexual abstinence, contraception, or pregnancy. The contraceptive choices made by American couples in 1988, when the last national fertility survey was conducted by the U.S. government from a large national probability sample, are shown in Table 10.1 (4). For couples over 35 years of age, sterilization is the number one choice. For younger couples, oral contraceptives are the most used method, and the condom ranks second. Although use of contraception is high, a significant proportion of sexually active couples do not use contraception: 13%, according to the 1988 National Fertility Survey (4), and 19%, based on a 1993 private survey (5). The percentage of women using no contraception is highest among the youngest group (i.e., adolescents).

It is estimated that 55% of births in the U.S. are unplanned (6). A major indication of unplanned pregnancy is the prevalence of induced abortion. Abortion ratios by age group indicate that the use of abortion is greatest for the youngest women and least for women in their late twenties and early thirties (Fig. 10.2). Use increases again as women become older. Young people are much more likely to experience contraceptive failure because their fertility is greater than in older women and because they are more likely to have intercourse without contraception. The effect of age on pregnancy rates with different contraceptive methods is shown in Figure 10.3.

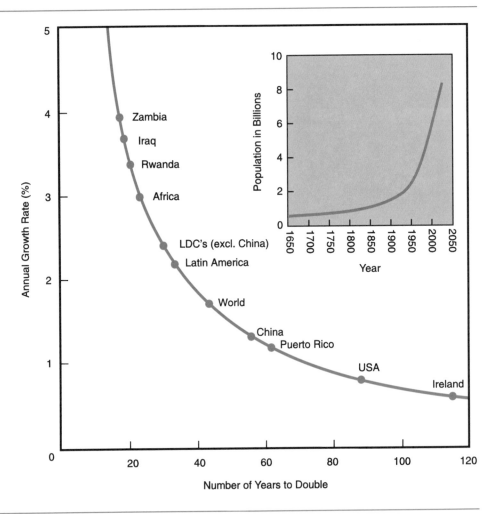

Figure 10.1   Doubling time at different rates of population growth, with representative countries, and world population growth curve. (With permission from **Hatcher RA, Trussell J, Stewart F, et al.** *Contraceptive Technology.* 16th ed. New York: Irvington Publishers, 1994:622.)

Efficacy of Contraception

Factors affecting whether pregnancy will occur include the fertility of both partners, the timing of intercourse in relation to the time of ovulation, the method of contraception used, the intrinsic effectiveness of the contraceptive method, and the correct use of the method. It is impossible to assess the effectiveness of a contraceptive method in isolation from the other factors. The best way to assess effectiveness is long-term evaluation of a group of sexually active women using a particular method for a period of time to observe how frequently pregnancy occurs. **A pregnancy rate per 100 women per year is then calculated by the *Pearl formula* (dividing the number of pregnancies by the total number of months contributed by all couples, and then multiplying the quotient by 1200).** With most methods, pregnancy rates decrease with time as the more fertile or less careful couples become pregnant and drop out. More accurate information is provided by the *life-table method,* which calculates the probability of pregnancy in successive months, which are then added over a given time interval. Problems relate to which pregnancies are counted: those occurring among all couples or those who the investigators deem to have used the method correctly. Because of this complexity, rates of pregnancy with different methods are best calculated by reporting two different rates derived from multiple studies (i.e., the lowest rate) and the usual rate as shown in Table 10.2.

Table 10.1   Current Contraceptive Status and Method: United States, 1982 and 1988

	1988	*1982*
All women	54,009,000	57,900,000
	Percent Distribution	
Total	100.0	100.0
Sterile	29.7	27.2
Surgically sterile	28.3	25.7
Contraceptively sterile	23.6	19.0
Female	16.6	12.9
Male	7.0	6.1
Noncontraceptively sterile	4.7	6.6
Female	4.7	6.3
Male	0.0	0.3
Nonsurgically sterile	1.4	1.5
Pregnant or postpartum	4.8	5.0
Seeking pregnancy	3.8	4.2
Nonuser	25.0	26.9
Never had intercourse	11.5	13.6
No intercourse in last 3 months	6.2	5.9
Intercourse in last 3 months	6.5	7.4
Nonsurgical contraception	36.7	36.7
Pill	18.5	15.6
Intrauterine device	1.2	4.0
Diaphragm	3.5	4.5
Condom	8.8	6.7
Foam	0.6	1.3
Periodic abstinence	1.4	2.2
Withdrawal	1.3	1.1
Douche	0.1	0.1
Other methods	1.2	1.3

From **Mosher WD, Pratt WF.** *Contraceptive Use in the United States, 1973–1988.* Advance Data from Vital and Health Statistics of the National Center for Health Statistics. All races combined. Washington, DC: National Center for Health, 1990:182.

Safety

Some contraceptive methods have associated health risks; areas of concern are listed in Table 10.3. All of the methods are safer than the alternative (pregnancy with birth), with the possible exception of oral contraceptive use by cigarette smokers over 35 years of age (7). Most methods provide noncontraceptive health benefits in addition to contraception. Oral contraceptives reduce the risk of ovarian and endometrial cancer and ectopic pregnancy. Barrier methods and spermicides provide some protection against STDs, cervical cancer, and tubal infertility.

Cost

Some methods, such as intrauterine devices and subdermal implants, require an expensive initial investment but provide prolonged protection for a low annual cost. The results of a

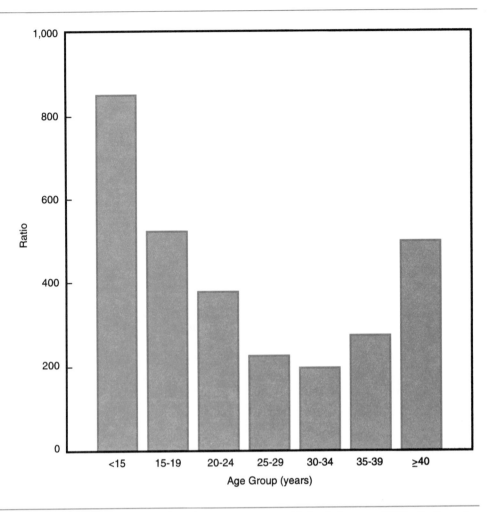

Figure 10.2   Abortion ratios, by age groups—United States, 1989. Ratio = induced abortions/1000 live births. (With permission from **Koonin LM, Smith JC, Ramick M, Lawson HW.** Abortion surveillance, 1989. *MMWR* 1992;41:1–33.)

complex cost analysis based on the cost of the method plus the cost of pregnancy if the method fails are shown in Table 10.4. Sterilization and the long-acting methods are least expensive over the long term (8).

Nonhormonal Contraceptive Methods

Coitus Interruptus

Coitus interruptus is withdrawal of the penis from the vagina before ejaculation. This method, along with induced abortion and late marriage, is believed to account for most of the decline in fertility of preindustrial Europe (9). Coitus interruptus remains a very important means of fertility control in the third world. This method has obvious advantages: immediate availability and no cost. Theoretically, the risk of STDs should be reduced, although it has not been studied. The Oxford Study reported a failure rate of 6.7 per 100 women years for this method (10). The penis must be completely withdrawn both from the vagina and from the external genitalia, as pregnancy has occurred from ejaculation on the female external genitalia without penetration.

Lactation Amenorrhea

Ovulation is suppressed during lactation. The suckling of the infant elevates prolactin levels and reduces gonadotropin-releasing hormone (GnRH) from the hypothalamus, reducing

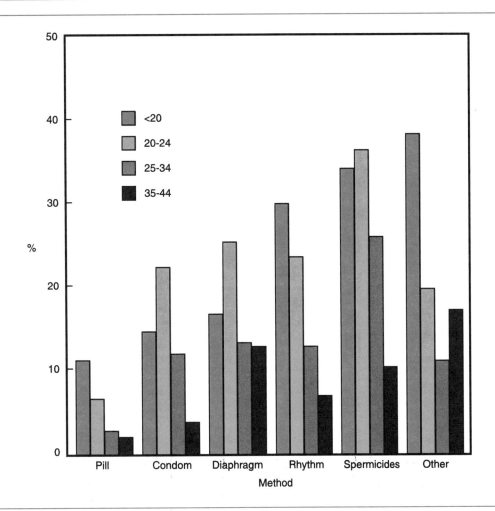

Figure 10.3   Percentage of women experiencing contraceptive failure during the first 12 months of use, by age and method, standardized by race and marital status. (With permission from **Jones EF, Forrest JD.** Contraception failure in the United States. Revised estimates from the 1982 National Survey of Family Growth. *Fam Plann Perspect* 1989;21:103–109.)

luteinizing hormone (LH) release so that follicular maturation is inhibited (11). The duration of this suppression is variable and is influenced by the frequency and duration of nursing, length of time since birth, and probably by the mother's nutritional status. Even with continued nursing, ovulation eventually returns but is unlikely before 6 months, especially if the woman is ammenorheic, is fully breast feeding, and no supplemental foods are given to the infant (12). If pregnancy is to be delayed, another method of contraception should be used from 6 months after birth, when menstruation resumes, or as soon as supplemental feeding is given. The risk of breast cancer may be reduced in women who have lactated, but whether this apparent benefit exists independent of early first pregnancy is not clear.

Combination oral contraceptives are generally not advised during lactation because they reduce the amount of milk produced by some women. Hormonal methods without estrogen can be used. These include progestin-only oral contraceptives, *Norplant,* and *Depo-Provera,* none of which decreases milk production. Barrier methods, spermicides, and intrauterine devices are also good options for nursing mothers (13).

Periodic Abstinence or "Natural Family Planning"

With periodic abstinence methods, couples attempt to avoid intercourse during the fertile period around the time of ovulation. A variety of methods are taught: the calendar method, the mucus method (Billings or ovulation method), and the symptothermal method, which is

231

Table 10.2   Percentage of Women Experiencing a Contraceptive Failure During the First Year of Use and the Percentage Continuing Use at the End of the First Year

Method	Women Experiencing Accidental Pregnancy within the First Year of Use (%)		Women Continuing Use at 1 Year (%)
	Typical Use	Perfect Use	
Chance	85	85	
Spermicides	21	6	43
Periodic abstinence			67
Calendar		9	
Ovulation method		3	
Symptothermal		2	
Postovulation		1	
Withdrawal	19	4	
Cap			
Parous women	36	26	45
Nulliparous women	18	9	58
Diaphragm	18	6	58
Condom			
Female (Reality)	21	5	56
Male	12	3	63
Pill	3		72
Progestin Only		0.5	
Combined		0.1	
Intrauterine device			
Progesterone T	2.0	1.5	81
Copper T380A	0.8	0.6	78
Levonorgestrel T20	0.1	0.1	81
DepoProvera	0.3	0.3	70
Norplant*	0.3	0.3	85
Female Sterilization	0.4	0.4	100
Male Sterilization	0.15	0.10	100

*Cumulative 5-year pregnancy rate for pliable tubing, divided by 5.
Reproduced with permission from **Hatcher RA, Trussell J, Stewart F, et al.** *Contraceptive Technology.* 16th ed. New York: Irvington Publishers Inc., 1994:113.

a combination of the first two methods. The *calendar method* is the least effective. With the *mucus method,* the woman attempts to predict the fertile period by feeling the cervical mucus with her fingers. Under estrogen influence, the mucus increases in quantity and becomes progressively more slippery and elastic until a peak day is reached. Thereafter, the mucus becomes scant and dry under the influence of progesterone until onset of the next menses. Intercourse may be allowed during the "dry days" immediately after menses until mucus is detected. Thereafter, the couple must abstain until the fourth day after the "peak" day.

In the *symptothermal method,* the first day of abstinence is predicted either from the calendar, by subtracting 21 from the length of the shortest menstrual cycle in the preceding 6

Table 10.3   Overview of Contraceptive Methods

Method	Advantages	Disadvantages	Risks	Noncontraceptive Benefits
Coitus interruptus	Available, free	Depends on male control	Pregnancy	?Decreased STD risk
Lactation	Available, free	Unreliable duration of effect	Pregnancy	?Decreased breast cancer
Periodic abstinence	Available, free	Complex methodology; motivation is essential	Pregnancy	None
Condoms	Available, no prescription needed	Motivation is essential; must be used each time; depends on male	Pregnancy	Proven to decrease STDs and cervical cancer
Spermicides	Available, no prescription needed	Must be used each time	Pregnancy	Some decrease in STDs
Diaphragm/ cap	Nonhormonal	Must be used each time; fitting required	Pregnancy, cystitis	Proven to decrease STDs and cervical cancer
IUD T380A	High efficacy for 10 years, unrelated to coitus	Initial cost; skilled inserter; pain and bleeding	Initial mild risk of PID and septic abortion	None
Progestasert	Reasonable efficacy	Initial cost; skilled inserter; replace every year	Initial mild risk of PID, ectopic pregnancy	Reduced dysmenorrhea and menstrual blood loss
Oral contraceptives	High efficacy	Motivation to take daily; cost	Thrombosis; older smokers have increased risk of MI and stroke	Many benefits (see text)
DMPA	High efficacy, convenience	Injection required; bleeding pattern	Probably none	Many (see text)
Implants	High efficacy, convenience	Surgical insertion and removal; initial cost; bleeding pattern	Functional cysts	Unknown
Postcoital hormones	Moderate efficacy	Frequent use disrupts menses; nausea	None	Unknown

STDs, sexually transmitted diseases; IUD, intrauterine device; PID, pelvic inflammatory disease; MI, myocardial infarction; *DMPA, depomedroxyprogesterone acetate.*

months, or the first day mucus is detected, whichever comes first. The end of the fertile period is predicted by use of basal body temperature. The woman takes her temperature every morning and resumes intercourse 3 days after the thermal shift, the rise in body temperature that signals that the corpus luteum is producing progesterone and that ovulation has occurred.

Efficacy   The ovulation method was evaluated by the World Health Organization in a five-country study. Women who successfully completed three monthly cycles of teaching were then enrolled in a 13-cycle efficacy study. Trussell and Grummer-Strawn calculated a 3.1%

Table 10.4   Cost per Patient per Year of Contraceptive Methods

Method	Cost ($)	Cost Multiple ($)*
Vasectomy	55	1.0
Tubal ligation	118	2.14
Intrauterine device	150	2.71
Norplant	202	3.66
Depomedroxyprogesterone acetate	396	7.19
Oral contraceptives	456	8.27
Condoms	776	14.08
Diaphragm	1147	20.81

*For every $1.00 spent on vasectomy, the amount shown would be spent on the method indicated. Reproduced with permission from **Ashraf T, Arnold SB, Maxfield M.** Cost effectiveness of levonorgestrel subdermal implants: comparison with other contraceptive methods available in the United States. *J Reprod Med* 1994:39:791–8.

probability of pregnancy in 1 year for the small proportion of couples who used the method perfectly and 86.4% probability of pregnancy for the rest (14). Because sperm may survive several days in the female genital tract, even a week's abstinence around the time of actual ovulation offers no guarantee against pregnancy. Pregnancies have occurred after a single act of coitus 7 days prior to apparent ovulation indicated by basal body temperature. Vaginal infections increase vaginal discharge, complicating the use of the method.

Accurate advance prediction of the time of ovulation would greatly facilitate both the use and efficacy of periodic abstinence. Devices that combine an electronic thermometer with small computers are being explored in an effort to improve the accuracy of basal body temperature as a predictor of the fertile phase (15). Home monitoring of estrogen provides 4 or more days warning before ovulation and allows intercourse to be resumed 1–3 days after ovulation (16). Another approach is the identification of microcrystals in saliva as an indication of approaching ovulation (17).

Risks   Conceptions resulting from intercourse remote from the time of ovulation more often lead to spontaneous abortion than conceptions from midcycle intercourse (18). However, malformations are not more common (19).

Condoms

Condoms made of animal intestine were used by the aristocracy of Europe in the 1700s, but large-scale availability of condoms began with the vulcanization of rubber in the 1840s (1). Modern condoms are usually made of latex rubber, although condoms made from animal intestine are still sold and are preferred by some who feel they afford better sensation. The condom captures and holds the seminal fluid, thus preventing its deposition in the vagina. Until recently, condoms in the U.S. were made with a relatively thick wall (0.065–0.085 mm) to prevent breakage. Japanese condoms as thin as 0.02 mm are now available in the U.S. (2). Condoms prelubricated with the spermicide *nonoxynol-9* are more effective than condoms without spermicide (20). The risk of condom breakage is about 3% (21) and is believed to be related to friction (2). Water-based lubricants may reduce the risk of breakage. Petroleum-based products such as mineral oil must be avoided because they markedly reduce the strength of condoms with only brief exposure (22).

Sexually Transmitted Disease

Latex condoms and other barrier methods reduce the risk of STDs. Gonorrhea, ureaplasma, and pelvic inflammatory disease and its sequela (tubal infertility) are reduced with consistent use of barrier methods (23, 24). A comparison of infertile women to postpartum women showed a 40% reduction in infertility with use of condoms or the diaphragm. The greatest benefit was noted with a combination of the barrier method and a spermicide (25).

Tested *in vitro, Chlamydia trachomatis,* herpes virus type 2, human immunodeficiency virus (HIV), and hepatitis B did not penetrate latex condoms but did cross through condoms made from animal intestine (26). Additional protection is provided by the addition of the spermicide *nonoxynol-9* (27). Follow-up of sexual partners of HIV-infected individuals has shown considerable protection when condoms are used (28). Consistent condom use provides more protection than inconsistent use (29). Studies of HIV-negative, high-risk women who used both condoms and spermicidal suppositories of *nonoxynol-9* demonstrated a high degree of protection from HIV seroconversion during follow-up (30). Vaginal spermicide should be used in addition to condoms when prevention of infection is of prime concern. Condoms also offer some protection from cervical neoplasia. In one study, the relative risk of severe dysplasia among users of condoms or diaphragms was 0.4 at 5–9 years of use and only 0.2 when the barriers had been used for 10 years or more, which is a 60–80% reduction (31). Another study compared women with invasive cervical cancer to controls. The relative risk of invasive cervical cancer was 0.4 when those who had used condoms or diaphragms were compared with those who had never used them (32).

Female Condom

Vaginal pouches made of polyurethane are now available as a "female condom." Efficacy trials have not matched historical trials with other barrier methods, but no randomized trial of the new method has been published. Initial U.S. trials showed a pregnancy rate of 15% in 6 months; however, reanalysis suggests that with perfect use, the pregnancy rate may be only 2.6%. This rate is comparable to perfect use of the diaphragm and cervical cap, the other female barrier methods (33). Colposcopic studies of women using the female condom demonstrate no signs of trauma, and the bacterial flora are not changed (34).

Vaginal Spermicides

Vaginal spermicides combine a spermicidal chemical, either *nonoxynol-9* or *octoxynol* with a base of cream, jelly, aerosol foam, foaming tablet, film, or suppository. Spermicides are nonionic surface-active detergents that immobilize sperm. In simulated intercourse under laboratory conditions, aerosol foams provided rapid dispersal throughout the vagina and offered the best protection. Jellies and melting suppositories provided poor distribution (35). Spermicides alone appear considerably less effective than condoms or a diaphragm with spermicide. *Nonoxynol-9* is not absorbed from the human vagina (36), and several large studies have found no greater risk for miscarriage, birth defects, or low birth weight for spermicide users than for other women (37, 38).

Nonoxynol-9 is toxic to the lactobacilli that normally colonize the vagina. Women who use spermicides regularly have increased vaginal colonization with the bacterium *Escherichia coli* and may be predisposed to *E. coli* bacteriuria after intercourse (39).

Vaginal Barriers

At the beginning of the 20th century, four types of vaginal barriers were used in Europe: vaginal diaphragm, cervical cap, vault cap, and vimule (Fig. 10.4). All of these barriers are still made and sold in England. Vaginal diaphragms and cervical caps are used in the U.S. When used consistently, vaginal barriers can be highly effective. They are safe and, as condoms, they have the noncontraceptive benefit of relative protection from STDs, tubal infertility, and cervical neoplasia.

Diaphragm

The diaphragm consists of a circular spring covered with fine latex rubber (Fig. 10.5). There are several types of diaphragm, as determined by the spring rim: coil, flat, or arcing. Coil-spring and flat-spring diaphragms become a flat oval when compressed for insertion. Arcing diaphragms form an arc or half moon when compressed; they are easiest to insert cor-

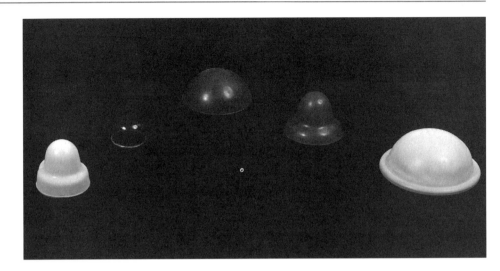

Figure 10.4   Vaginal barriers (left to right): Prentiff cavity rim cervical cap, plastic cap, vault cap, vimule, and vaginal diaphragm. (With permission from **Copeland LJ.** *Textbook of Gynecology.* Philadelphia: WB Saunders Co., 1993:159.)

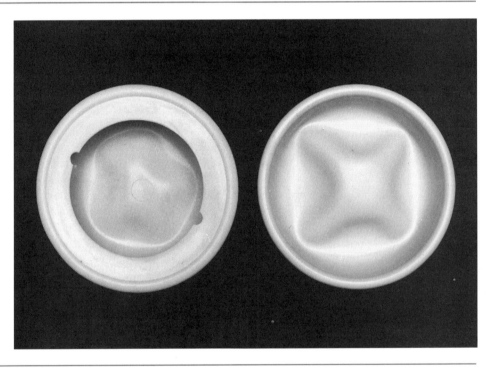

Figure 10.5   Wide seal diaphragm. (With permission from **Copeland LJ.** *Textbook of Gynecology.* Philadelphia: WB Saunders Co., 1993:162.)

rectly. The practitioner must not only fit the diaphragm for the patient, but must instruct her in its insertion and verify by examination that she can insert it correctly to cover the cervix and upper vagina. The diaphragm should be used in combination with a spermicide. One study suggests this may not be essential to the contraceptive efficacy of the diaphragm. Women who wore their diaphragms constantly, removing, washing, and reinserting the diaphragm daily without using a spermicide, had lower pregnancy rates than women who used them in the conventional fashion, with a spermicide, only when needed (40).

Fitting Diaphragms   Fitting of a diaphragm should be performed as follows:

1. To properly fit a diaphragm, a vaginal examination should be performed. With the first and second fingers in the posterior fornix, the thumb of the examining hand is placed against the first finger to mark where the first finger touches the pubic bone. The distance from the tip of the middle finger to the tip of the thumb is the diameter of the diaphragm that should first be tried.

2. A set of test diaphragms of various sizes is used, and the test diaphragm is inserted and checked by palpation. The diaphragm should open easily in the vagina and fill the fornices without pressure. The largest diaphragm that fits comfortably should be selected. A size 65, 70, or 75 diaphragm will fit most women.

3. The patient should practice insertion and should be reexamined to confirm proper position of the device. Approximately 1 teaspoon of water-soluble spermicidal jelly or cream is placed in the cavity of the dome. The diaphragm is inserted with the dome downward so that the cervix will sit in a pool of the spermicide.

4. The diaphragm can be inserted several hours prior to intercourse. If intercourse is repeated, additional spermicidal jelly should be inserted into the vagina without removing the diaphragm. The diaphragm should be left in place at least 6 hours after intercourse to allow for immobilization of sperm. It is then removed, washed with soap and water, allowed to dry, and stored away from heat. It should not be dusted with talc because genital exposure to talc may predispose ovarian cancer.

Risks   Diaphragm use, especially prolonged use during multiple acts of intercourse, appears to increase the risk of bladder infections. A smaller-sized, wide-seal diaphragm or a cervical cap can be used if recurrent cystitis is a problem, although the problem may relate not only to mechanical obstruction but to alterations in vaginal flora produced by the spermicide. An epidemiologic study comparing cases of toxic shock with controls found no increased risk from diaphragm use (41).

Cervical Cap

The cap is much smaller than the diaphragm, does not contain a spring in the rim, and covers only the cervix. Caps are used with spermicide, but the contribution of the spermicide to the efficacy is not known. Studies of the efficacy of cervical caps have revealed a range of results. The Prentiff cap has one of the best results—a pregnancy rate of eight per 100 women years with the cap left in place for as long as 5 days at a time (42). A multicenter study of 3433 women found a first-year pregnancy rate of 11.3 per 100 women. Women whose pattern of use was described as "near perfect" had a first-year pregnancy rate of 6.1 per 100, half that of the overall rate (43). The pregnancy rate increased when the cap was worn for more than 72 hours at a time. Dislodgement of the cap during intercourse or at other times was reported by 27.5% of the users after 3 months of use; dislodgement and accidental pregnancy were the main reasons that women discontinued use of the cap. By 1 year, 49% of women discontinued use or were lost to follow-up. In randomized trials, the cervical cap was as effective as the diaphragm overall, but the failure rates with "perfect use" were considerably higher for the cap than for the diaphragm (44). Parous women using the cap had more failures than nulliparous women. The Femcap, a new version of the cervical cap made of silicone rubber, is being studied. The Femcap looks like a sailor's hat. Its dome covers the cervix, while its brim fits into the vaginal fornices (45). It is made in three sizes—24-, 28-, and 32-mm diameter—and is expected to be reusable for 2–3 years. It is used with spermicide and is left in place as long as 48 hours.

Fitting Cervical Caps   The Prentiff cavity rim cervical cap is available in the U.S. in sizes 22, 25, 28, and 31 (internal diameter of the rim in mm). A cervical cap should be fitted as follows:

1. The cervical size is estimated by inspection and palpation. Nulliparous women usually require a size 22, while parous women generally are fitted with a size 25.

2. The cap is inserted by compressing it between finger and thumb and placing it through the introitus, dome outward. It is then pushed gently upward to fit over the cervix. The dome is indented with the examiner's finger to create suction against the cervix. The dome should remain compressed for several seconds, indicating a good fit, and gentle lateral pressure on the rim should not dislodge the cap. The smallest Prentiff cap (22 mm) is too large for many nulliparous women and a good fit may not be obtained.

3. Prior to use, the cap is one-third filled with spermicidal jelly or cream. It can be left in place as long as 72 hours. The patient is instructed to check for dislodgement of the cap after intercourse, and use of an additional contraceptive method such as a condom is advised until it is clear that the cap will not be dislodged.

Risks   In one large trial, negative cervical cytology progressed to dysplasia in 4% of cap wearers and in 2% of diaphragm wearers (46). Other studies have not found this effect (43) and, in contrast, Koch found cap wearers to be protected from developing dysplasia compared with controls using other methods (42). In the Femcap study, the results of cervical cytology appeared to improve during use (45). Cap use has not been associated with cystitis (42, 43).

Intrauterine Devices

Intrauterine devices (IUDs) are very important worldwide but play a minor role in contraception for the U.S. population because of a fear of infection that is no longer justified. Copper IUDs provide safe, long-term contraception with effectiveness equivalent to tubal sterilization. Hormone-releasing IUDs need to be replaced every year. Two IUDs are available in the U.S.: the Copper T380 (*Paraguard*) and the progesterone-releasing T (*Progestasert*). The Copper T380 has bands of copper on the cross arms of the T in addition to copper wire around the stem, providing a total surface area of 380 mm of copper, almost double the surface area of copper of earlier copper devices (Fig. 10.6). The copper T380 is approved by the U.S. Food and Drug Administration (FDA) for up to 10 years of continuous use.

Mechanism of Action   Intrauterine devices cause the formation of a "biological foam" within the uterine cavity that contains strands of fibrin, phagocytic cells, and proteolytic enzymes. Copper IUDs continuously release a small amount of the metal, producing an even greater inflammatory response. All IUDs stimulate the formation of prostaglandins within the uterus, consistent with both smooth muscle contraction and inflammation. Scanning electron microscopy studies of the endometrium of women wearing IUDs show alterations in the surface morphology of cells, especially of the microvilli of ciliated cells (47). There are major alterations in the composition of proteins within the uterine cavity, and new proteins and proteinase inhibitors are found in washings from the uterus (48). The altered intrauterine environment interferes with sperm passage through the uterus, preventing fertilization.

The IUD is not an abortifacient. The contraceptive effectiveness does not depend on interference with implantation, although this phenomenon also occurs and is the basis for using copper IUDs for emergency contraception. Sperm can be obtained via laparoscopy in washings from the fallopian tubes of control women at midcycle, whereas no sperm are present in the tubal washings from women wearing IUDs (49). Ova flushed from the tubes at tubal sterilization showed no evidence of fertilization in women wearing IUDs (50), and studies of serum β-human chorionic gonadotropin (hCG) do not indicate pregnancy in women wearing IUDs (51).

The progesterone-releasing IUD (*Progestasert*) contains natural progesterone in its stem inside a polymer capsule that allows sustained, slow release of the hormone. It is approved

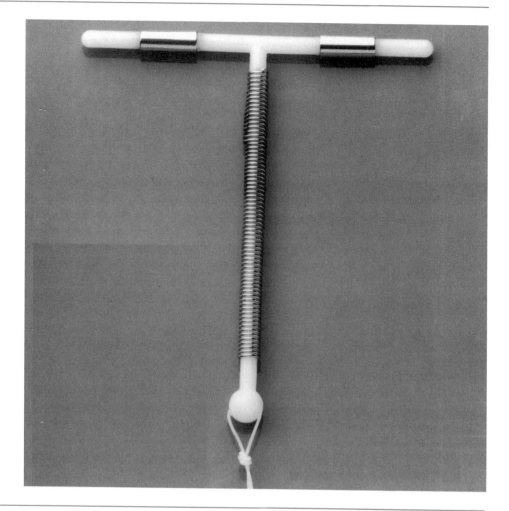

Figure 10.6   The Copper T380A (ParaGard) IUD (Courtesy, Gynopharma, Inc.).

for 1 year of use. This produces an atrophic endometrial lining. A "T" device that releases the more potent progestin, *norgestrel,* is available in Europe. It produces high local concentrations of the progestin in the uterine cavity and produces blood levels about one-half those seen with the *levonorgestrel* implant, which are sufficient to inhibit ovulation in some women (51).

Effectiveness   The Copper T380 and the *levonorgestrel* T have remarkably low pregnancy rates, less than 0.2 per 100 women years. Total pregnancies over a 7-year period were only 1.1 per 100 for the *levonorgestrel* T and 1.4 for the Copper T380 in a comparative study (52). The *Progestasert* has a higher failure rate, about three per 100 women per year.

Infection   The Women's Health study found the Dalkon Shield device (now withdrawn from the market) to increase the risk of pelvic inflammatory disease (PID) by eightfold when women hospitalized for PID were compared to control women hospitalized for other illnesses. In contrast, risk from the other IUDs was markedly less: relative risk of PID was 2.2 for the *Progestasert,* 1.9 for the Copper 7, 1.3 for the Saf-T-Coil, and 1.2 for the Lippes Loop (53). Increased risk was detectable only within 4 months of insertion of the IUD. A still larger, prospective World Health Organization Study revealed that PID increased only during the first 20 days after insertion. Thereafter, the rate of diagnosis of PID was about 1.6 cases per 1000 women per year, the same as in the general population (54).

239

Exposure to sexually transmitted pathogens is a more important determinant of PID than the wearing of an IUD. In the Women's Health Study, women who were currently married or cohabiting and who said they had only one sexual partner in the past 6 months had no increase in PID. In contrast, previously married or single women had marginal increase in risk, even though they had only one partner in the previous 6 months (55). The only pelvic infection that has been unequivocally related to IUDs is actinomycosis (56). It appears that PID with actinomycosis has been reported only in women wearing IUDs. Rates of colonization with actinomycosis increase with duration of use for plastic devices but appear to be much less for copper-releasing IUDs.

Management of PID   When PID is suspected in an IUD-wearing woman, the IUD should be immediately removed, appropriate cultures should be taken, and high-dose antibiotic therapy should be started. Pelvic abscess should be suspected and ruled out by ultrasound examination.

Ectopic Pregnancy   If pregnancy occurs in an IUD wearer, it will be ectopic in about 5% of cases. This is because the fallopian tubes are less well protected against pregnancy than the uterus. Compared with women using no contraception, however, women wearing either the Copper T380 or the *levonorgestrel* T have an 80–90% reduction in the risk of ectopic pregnancy (52), which is a greater reduction than that seen for users of barrier methods. Women using oral contraceptives have a 90% reduction of risk (57). In contrast, the Progestasert increases risk slightly, probably because the progesterone affects tubal motility and does not inhibit ovulation (58).

Fertility   Case-control studies of infertile women in the U.S. have revealed that a history of IUD use is associated with a twofold increase in the risk of tubal infertility. The risk applies to methods other than the copper IUD, for which there is no increased risk (59–61). Risk was not increased among women who reported only one sexual partner (59). The Oxford Study found that women gave birth just as promptly after IUD removal as they did after discontinuing use of the diaphragm (62). Exposure to sexually transmitted pathogens confers risk for infertility. Modern IUDs are, at most, a small risk factor (61).

Clinical Management

Contraindications to IUD use include pregnancy, a history of PID, undiagnosed genital bleeding, uterine anomalies (although a woman with separate uterine cavities might wear two IUDs), and large fibroid tumors. Chronic immune suppression should be considered a contraindication. Women with such conditions are considered to be at greater risk for PID, but in addition, the effectiveness of the IUD may be compromised. A number of pregnancies have occurred in renal transplant patients soon after IUD insertion. Copper allergy or Wilson's disease are contraindications to the use of copper IUDs.

IUD Insertion

At the initial visit, the patient's history is taken and a physical exam, cervical culture for *Neisseria gonorrhea,* and a test for chlamydia are performed, along with detailed counseling regarding risks and alternatives. The patient should avoid intercourse until returning for insertion of the device at a second visit. Premedication with oral prostaglandin inhibitors such as *ibuprofen* is strongly advised, and consideration should be given to antibiotic prophylaxis with a *tetracycline.* IUDs are usually inserted during menses in order to be sure the patient is not pregnant, but they can be inserted at any time in the cycle (63). Insertion is preceded by a sensitive urine pregnancy test and a pelvic exam to determine uterine size and position.

The technique of insertion is as follows:

1. The cervix is exposed with a speculum. The vaginal vault and cervix are cleansed with a bacteriocidal solution, such as an iodine-containing prep solution.

2. The uterine cavity should be measured with a uterine sound. The depth of the cavity should measure at least 6 cm from the external os. A smaller uterus is not likely to tolerate currently available IUDs.

3. A paracervical block with 10 ml of 1% *lidocaine* mixed with *atropine* (0.5 mg) can be used to avoid vasovagal syncope and minimize discomfort. In some women, serious cardiac arrhythmia can occur with cervical stimulation and can be avoided by these measures.

4. Use of a tenaculum for insertion is mandatory to prevent perforation. The cervix is grasped with a tenaculum, and gently pulled downward to straighten the angle between the cervical canal and the uterine cavity. The IUD, previously loaded into its inserter, is then gently introduced through the cervical canal.

5. With the "T" type of devices such as the *Paragard* and the *Progestasert,* the outer sheath of the insert is withdrawn a short distance to release the arms of the T and is then gently pushed inward again to elevate the now opened T against the fundus (64).

6. The outer sheath and the inner stylet of the inserter are withdrawn, and the strings are cut to project about 2 cm from the external cervical os.

IUDs in Pregnancy   A woman who presents with an IUD in place and an amenorrhea should have a pregnancy test and exam. If an intrauterine pregnancy is diagnosed and the IUD strings are visible, the IUD should be removed as soon as possible in order to prevent later septic abortion, premature rupture of the membranes, and premature birth (65). When the strings of the IUD are not visible, an ultrasound exam should be performed to localize the IUD and determine whether expulsion has occurred. If the IUD is present, there are three options for management:

1. Therapeutic abortion

2. Ultrasound-guided intrauterine removal of the IUD

3. Continuation of the pregnancy with the device left in place

If the patient wishes to continue the pregnancy, ultrasound evaluation of the location of the IUD is advised (66). If the IUD is not in a fundal location, ultrasound-guided removal using small alligator forceps is advised. If the location is fundal, the IUD should be left in place. If pregnancy continues with an IUD in place, the patient must be warned of the symptoms of intrauterine infection and should be cautioned to seek care promptly for fever or flu-like symptoms, abdominal cramping, or bleeding. At the earliest sign of infection, high-dose intravenous antibiotic therapy should be given and the pregnancy should be evacuated promptly.

Duration of Use   Annual rates of pregnancy, expulsions, and medical removals *decrease* with each year of use (67, 68). Therefore, a woman who has had no problem by year 5, for example, is very unlikely to experience problems in the subsequent years. As noted, the *Progestasert* should be replaced at the end of 1 year, but the T380 is approved for 10 years. Actinomyces can be detected by cervical cytology. Should actinomyces-like particles be reported, removal of the IUD and treatment with oral *penicillin* are advised.

Choice of IUDs   Of the two IUDs currently available in the U.S., the *copper T380A* is preferred for most women who want intrauterine contraception. It provides protection for 10 years, has a remarkably low pregnancy rate, and decreases risk for ectopic pregnancy. The *Progestasert* must be replaced annually, theoretically exposing the patient to some risk for infection with each insertion, and increasing cost markedly. It is less effective, and increases risk for ectopic pregnancy slightly. However, it also reduces the amount of menstrual bleeding and dysmenorrhea, whereas the *copper T380A* can be expected to increase menstrual bleeding and pain.

Hormonal Contraception

Hormonal contraceptives are female sex steroids, synthetic estrogen and a synthetic progesterone (progestin), or a progestin only. They can be administered in the form of oral contraceptives, implants, and injectables.

The most widely used hormonal contraceptive is the combination oral contraceptive (OC). Combination OCs can be monophasic, with the same dose of estrogen and progestin administered each day, or multiphasic, in which varying doses of steroids are given through a 21-day cycle. Typically, they are administered for 21 days beginning on the Sunday after a menstrual period then discontinued for 7 days to allow for withdrawal bleeding that mimics the normal menstrual cycle. The 28-day version provides placebo tablets for the last 7 days of the cycle so the user simply takes one pill a day and starts a new pack as soon as the first pack is completed. Progestin-only formulations contain no estrogen. These are taken every day without interruption. Other forms of hormonal contraception include injectable progestins and estrogen-progestin combinations, subdermal implants releasing progestin, and the experimental vaginal rings that release either estrogen-progestin or progestin alone.

Silastic rings worn in the vagina release steroid hormones that are absorbed at a constant rate, allowing contraception with blood levels of steroids well below the peak levels that are seen with OCs. Rings containing *levonorgestrel* or combinations of *levonorgestrel* and estrogens are being studied (69).

Steroid Hormone Action   Sex steroids were originally defined by their biological activity. They are characterized by their affinity for specific estrogen, progesterone, or androgen receptors, as well as by their biologic effects in different systems (70). Steroids are rapidly absorbed in the gut but go directly into the liver via the portal circulation, where they are rapidly metabolized and inactivated. Therefore, large doses of steroids are required when they are administered orally. The addition of the ethinyl group to carbon 17 of the steroid molecule hinders degradation by the liver enzyme 17-hydroxysteroid dehydrogenase.

Progestins   Progestins are synthetic compounds that mimic the effect of natural progesterone but differ from it structurally (Fig. 10.7). There are two main classes, the estrane or 19-nor progestins, which are structurally similar to testosterone but lacking a carbon at position 19, and the pregnane or 17-acetoxy compounds, which are structurally similar to progesterone. Only the estrane compounds are used in oral contraceptives in the U.S., but *medroxyprogesterone acetate (Provera)*, one of the pregnane compounds, is the major injectable progestin. The progestins differ from each other in their affinities for estrogen, androgen, and progesterone receptors; their ability to inhibit ovulation; and their ability to substitute for progesterone and antagonize estrogen. Some are directly bound to the receptor (*levonorgestrel, norethindrone*), whereas others require bioactivation as, for example, desogestrel, which is converted in the body to its active metabolite, *3-keto-desogestrel*. The 17-acetoxy progestins (e.g., *medroxyprogesterone acetate*) are bound by the progesterone receptor. *Norgestrel* exists as two stereoisomers, identified as dextronorgestrel and levonorgestrel. Only levonorgestrel is biologically active. Three newer progestins (*norgestimate, desogestrel,* and *gestodene*) are viewed as more "selective" than the other 19-nor progestins, in that they have little or no androgenic effect at doses that inhibit ovulation

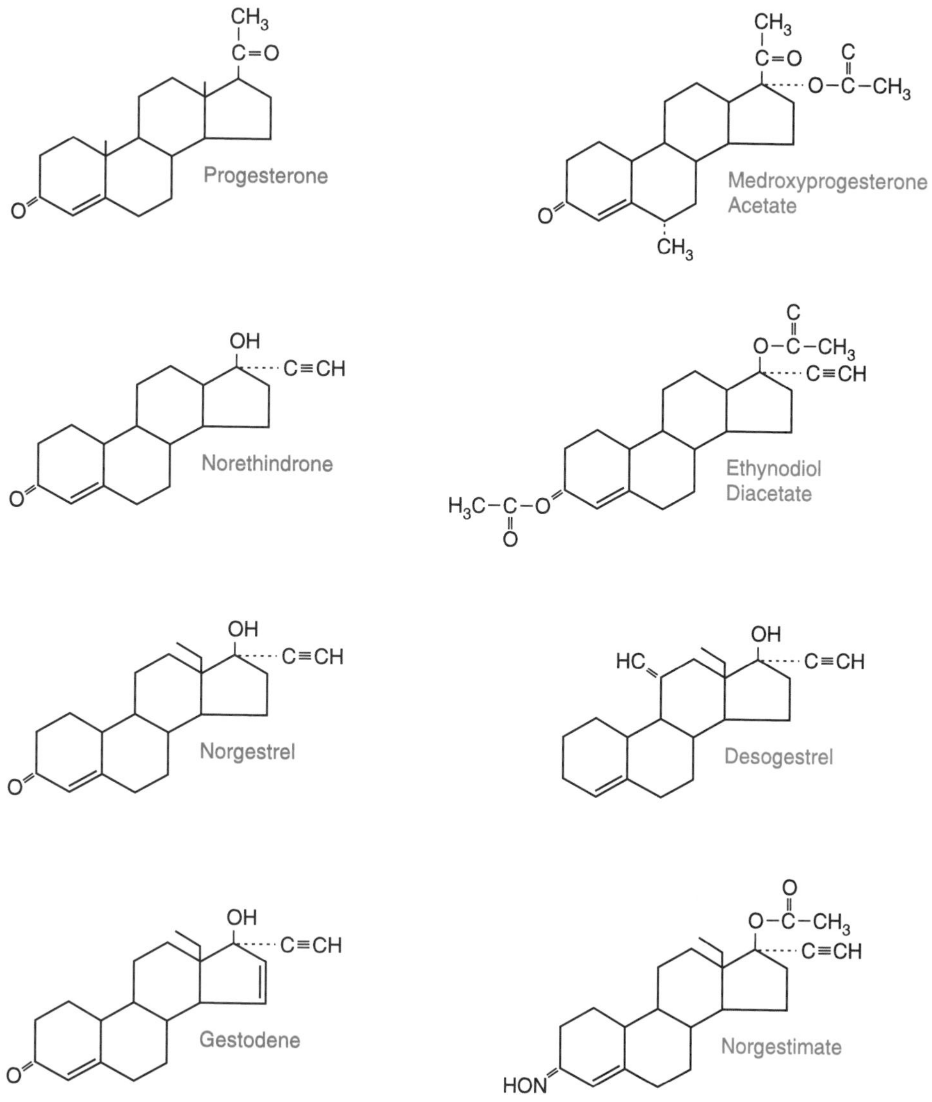

Figure 10.7   Progestins of interest for contraception. (With permission from **Copeland LJ.** *Textbook of Gynecology.* Philadelphia: WB Saunders Co., 1993.)

(71). *Norgestimate-* and *desogestrel*-containing OCs are approved by the FDA, and *gestodene* is available in Europe. *Gestodene* is a derivative of *levonorgestrel* that is more potent than the other preparations (i.e., very little of it is required for antifertility effects). Androgenic potency is considered undesirable because of the adverse effect of androgen and androgenic progestins on lipid and glucose metabolism. Androgenic progestins reduce levels of circulating high-density lipoprotein (HDL), elevate low-density lipoprotein (LDL), and adversely effect glucose tolerance in a dose-dependent fashion (72).

Estrogens

In the U.S., OCs contain either of two estrogens: *mestranol* (ME) or *ethinyl estradiol* (EE). *Mestranol* is ethinyl estradiol with an extra methyl group. It requires bioactivation in the liver, where the methyl group is cleaved, releasing the active agent, ethinyl estradiol. **Oral contraceptives with 35 μg of *ethinyl estradiol* provide the same blood levels of hormone as do OCs containing 50 μg of *mestranol*** (73).

Antifertility Effects

Combination Oral Contraceptives

Ovulation can be inhibited by oral estrogen or by oral progestin alone, but large doses are required. Pharmacologic synergism is exhibited when the two hormones are combined and ovulation is suppressed at a much lower dose of each agent. Combination OCs suppress basal FSH and LH. Oral contraceptives diminish the ability of the pituitary gland to synthesize gonadotropins when it is stimulated by the hypothalamic gonadotropin-releasing hormone (GnRH) (74). Ovarian follicles do not mature, little estradiol is produced, and there is no midcycle LH surge. Ovulation does not occur, the corpus luteum does not form, and progesterone is not produced. This blockade of ovulation is dose related. Newer low-dose OCs do not provide as dense a block and allow somewhat higher base line FSH and LH levels than higher-dose formulations (75). This makes ovulation somewhat more likely to occur if pills are missed or if the patient takes another medication that interferes with OC action.

Progestin-Only Preparations

The mode of action of progestin-only contraceptives depends very much on the dose of the compound (76). At low blood levels of progestin, ovulation will occur part of the time. With the progestin-only "minipill," which supplies 0.3 mg of *norethindrone* per day (*Micronor*), 40% of cycles are ovulatory, 25% have inadequate luteal function, 18% have follicular maturation without ovulation, and 18% have complete suppression of follicle development (76). At moderate blood levels of the progestin, normal basal levels of FSH and LH are seen and some follicle maturation may occur. Estradiol production is present and the surge of estradiol that would normally trigger pituitary release of LH occurs; there is no answering LH surge, however, and hence no ovulation. At higher blood levels of progestin, basal FSH is reduced, there is less follicular activity, less estradiol production, and no LH surge.

Hormonal Implants

With the subdermal implant that releases *levonorgestrel* (*Norplant*), there is some follicular maturation and estrogen production, but LH peak levels are low and ovulation is often inhibited. In the first year of use, ovulation is believed to occur in about 20% of cycles. The proportion of ovulatory cycles increases with time, probably as a result of the decline in hormone release. By the fourth year of use, 41% of cycles are ovulatory. The mechanisms of contraception with low-dose progestins are believed to include effects on the cervical mucus, endometrium, and tubal motility. The scant, dry cervical mucus in women using these preparations inhibits sperm migration into the upper tract. Progestins decrease nuclear estrogen receptor levels, decrease progesterone receptors, and induce activity of the enzyme 17-hydroxysteroid dehydrogenase that metabolizes natural estradiol 17β (77).

The sustained release offered by contraceptive implants allows for highly effective contraception at relatively low blood levels of the steroid. Fig. 10.8 depicts expected steroid blood levels with implants, injectables, and oral contraceptives. An additional mechanism for contraception has been discovered with the antiprogesterone *mefipristone (RU486)*. In the normal cycle, there is a small amount of progesterone production from the follicle just before ovulation. This progesterone appears essential to ovulation, because if the antiprogesterone is given prior to ovulation, it can be delayed for several days (77, 78).

Oral Contraceptives

When used consistently, combination OCs have pregnancy rates as low as 2–3 per 1000 women per year. Progestin-only OCs are less effective, with best results of 3–4 pregnancies per 100 women years. Both methods have the potential for user error; therefore, there may be a 10-fold difference between the best results and results in typical users for pregnancy prevention. Injectable progestins and implants are much less subject to user error. The difference between the best results and results in typical users is small and is comparable to pregnancy rates after tubal sterilization (Table 10.2).

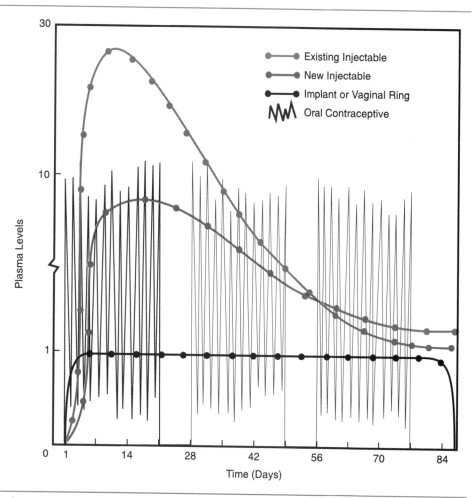

Figure 10.8   Schematic representation of the expected pharmacokinetic profiles of progestogens administered in different formulations. (Modified with permission from **Landgren BM.** Mechanism of action of gestagens. *Int J Gynecol Obstet* 1990; 32:95–110.)

Metabolic Effects and Safety

Venous Thrombosis   Older studies linked OC use to venous thrombosis and embolism, cerebral vascular accidents, and heart attack (79, 80). More recent studies have found a much lower risk (81). Critical rereading of the older literature on venous thrombosis revels that absolute risk was strongly determined by other very obvious predisposing causes of thrombosis that are now considered contraindications to OC use: previous thrombosis, preexisting vascular disease, coronary artery disease, leukemia, cancer, and serious trauma (82).

Normally, the coagulation system maintains a dynamic balance of procoagulant and anticoagulant systems in the blood. Estrogens affect both systems in a dose-related fashion. For most women, fibrinolysis (anticoagulation) is increased as much as coagulation, maintaining the dynamic balance at increased levels of production and destruction of fibrinogen (83, 84) (Fig. 10.9). Current low-dose OCs have less measurable effect on the coagulation system, and fibrinolytic factors increase at the same rate as procoagulant factors (85, 86). The lower estrogen dose (30–35 μg *ethinyl estradiol*) reduces the risk of a thromboembolic event when compared with higher-dose (50 μg estrogen) OCs (87) (Table 10.5). Smokers taking low-dose OCs demonstrate more marked activation of the coagulation system than nonsmokers—shortening of the prothrombin time, increased fibrinogen levels, and decreased antithrombin III—but also have increased fibrinolysis as measured by plasminogen activity (87). Use of OCs is not associated with a detectable hypercoagulable state for most women, but individ-

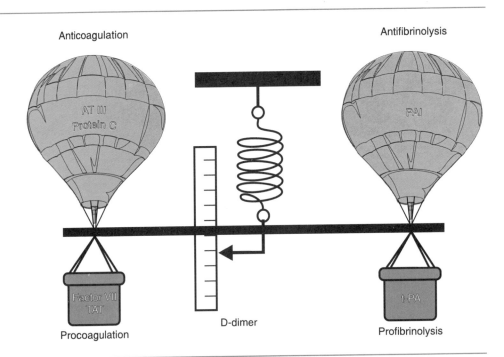

Anticoagulation

Antifibrinolysis

AT III
Protein C

PAI

D-dimer

Factor VII
TAT

t-PA

Procoagulation

Profibrinolysis

Figure 10.9   Dynamic balance of hemostasis. (With permission from **Winkler UH, Buhler K, Schlinder AE.** The dynamic balance of hemostatsis: implications for the risk of oral contraceptive use. In: **Runnebaum B, Rabe T, Kissel L,** eds. *Female Contraception and Male Fertility Regulation. Advances in Gynecological and Obstetric Research Series.* Confort, England: Parthenon Publishing Group, 1991:85–92.

Table 10.5   Oral Contraceptive Estrogen Dose and Risk of Deep Vein Thrombosis (DVT)

Estrogen (dose)	*(Rate/10,000 person years)*	*Relative Risk (all cases)*	*Relative Risk (proven diagnosis)*
<50 μg	4.2	1.0	1.0*
50 μg	7.0	1.5	2.0 (0.0–4.0)
>50 μg	10.0	1.7	3.2 (2.4–4.3)

*Base line risk used to calculate risk for higher doses.
From **Gerstman BB, Piper JM, Tomita DK, Ferguson WJ, Stadel BV, Lundin FE.** Oral contraceptive dose and the risk of deep venous thrombosis. *Am J Epidemiol* 1991;133:32–7.

ual variations may occur. Women with a family history of thrombosis have been found to have somewhat reduced levels of the anticoagulant antithrombin III, whereas levels of fibrinogen and fibronectin (a measure of endothelial damage) were significantly increased in women who were obese and hypertensive (88). Women with familial deficiency of antithrombin III, protein C, or protein S are highly likely to suffer thromboembolic episodes if given estrogen-containing OCs (88, 89). These abnormalities are rare, but a mutation of the gene for blood-clotting factor V (factor V Leiden) recently has been identified in 3–5% of the population. The abnormal factor V resists cleavage by the natural anticoagulant protein C, producing a syndrome described as "activated protein C resistance" (90). The risk of a first thromboembolic episode among women using OCs is estimated to be 2.2 per 10,000 women years for women who do not have the factor V mutation and 27.7 per 10,000 women years for women with the mutation (91). For women homozygous or heterozygous for the mutation who do not use OCs, the risk is estimated to be 4.9 per 10,000 women years. The effect of estrogen dose was not examined. Cigarette smoking did not affect risk of thrombosis.

Pregnancy is an even greater challenge for women with inherited defects of anticoagulation (92). A woman who sustains a venous event while using OCs should be evaluated

246

thoroughly after she has recovered. Assessment should include measurement of antithrombin III, protein C, and protein S levels and, when it becomes clinically feasible, identification of the factor V Leiden mutation. It should not be assumed that the oral contraceptive was the only cause of the thromboembolic episode.

Heart Disease and Stroke   Ischemic heart disease and stroke were the major causes of deaths attributed to OCs. The principal determinants of risk for myocardial infarction (MI) are advancing age and cigarette smoking (93). Past use of OCs does not increase risk of heart attack, which was clearly demonstrated by the U.S. Nurses' Study, the largest such study ever reported (94). Current users did have an age-adjusted relative risk of 2.5. Seven of the 10 current users with major coronary heart disease were smokers, severely limiting the ability of this study to determine the role of OCs. Another large U.S. study found no relationship between OC use and heart attack (81). With higher-dose preparations, women smoking 25 cigarettes or more per day had a 30-fold increased risk of heart attack (95) (Fig. 10.10). In a recent study from Finland, from 1975 until 1984 all deaths of women aged 15–39 from pulmonary embolism, heart attack, or stroke were identified, and risk while using either oral contraceptives or copper IUDs was determined (96). Neither the risk for pulmonary embolism nor the risk of death from myocardial infarction or intracranial hemorrhage was increased while taking OCs.

Angiographic studies of women who sustained cerebrovascular attacks while using OCs show that most such cases are arterial ischemic attacks rather than cerebral hemorrhage or

Figure 10.10   Risk of myocardial infarction in women younger than 50 years of age: effect of oral contraceptives and smoking. (From **Rosenberg L, Kaufman DW, Helmrich SP, et al.** Myocardial infarction and cigarette smoking in women younger than 50 years of age. *JAMA* 1985;253:2965–9.)

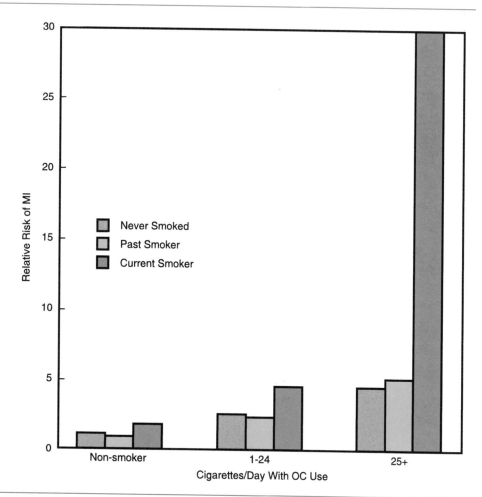

venous thrombosis (97). Most of these women exhibit one of a variety of arterial lesions (for example, stenosis, mural irregularities, and beaded arteries). Cerebral hemorrhage accounts for about 20% of strokes associated with OC use. Most of these cases are secondary to arterial or arteriovenous malformation.

Two recent studies suggest that the risk of stroke with OC use may still be present. A British case-control study of women having strokes between 1968 and 1990 revealed current users to have double the risk of stroke after adjusting for smoking and other risk factors (98). A Danish study investigated strokes occurring in women aged 15–44 years between 1985 and 1989 and included information on effects of modern low-dose OCs (99). A multivariate analysis that included smoking found women taking 50-μg estrogen OCs to have a 2.9 odds ratio for stroke, whereas women on 30- to 40-μg preparations had an odds ratio of 1.8. Progestin-only pills did not increase risk (odds ratio, 0.9). Smoking increased risk by 50%, independent of pill use. Heavy smokers were not identified as a separate group.

A rare form of cerebrovascular insufficiency, Moyamoya disease, has been reported to be linked to use of OCs (100). The risk of stroke from current low-dose OCs is very small for healthy women, but it has not been demonstrated that there is no risk. As in the case of venous thrombosis, women who sustain strokes while taking OCs should be fully evaluated for other causes, including antiphospholipid syndrome and defects in the anticoagulation system.

Blood Pressure   Oral contraceptives have a dose-related effect on blood pressure. With the older high-dose pills, as many as 5% of patients could be expected to have blood pressure elevations of higher than 140/90. The mechanism is believed to be an estrogen-induced increase in renin substrate in susceptible individuals. Current low-dose pills have minimal blood pressure effects, but surveillance of blood pressure is still advised to detect the occasional idiosyncratic response.

Glucose Metabolism   Oral estrogen alone has no adverse effect on glucose metabolism, but progestins exhibit insulin antagonism (101). Older OC formulations with higher doses of progestins produced abnormal glucose tolerance tests with elevated insulin levels in the average patient. The effect on glucose metabolism, as the effect on lipids, is related to androgenic potency of the progestin and to its dose (72).

Lipid Metabolism   Higher-dose OCs could have significant adverse effects on lipids (102). Androgens and estrogens have competing effects on hepatic lipase, a liver enzyme critical to lipid metabolism. Estrogens depress LDL and elevate HDL, which are changes that can expected to reduce risk of atherosclerosis (103). Androgens and androgenic progestins can antagonize these beneficial changes, reducing HDL and elevating LDL levels. Estrogens elevate triglyceride levels. Low-dose formulations have minimal adverse effect on lipids (104), and the newer formulations (with *desogestrel* and *norgestimate* as the progestin) produce potentially beneficial changes by elevating HDL and lowering LDL (72) (Fig 10.11). Although average values of a large group show only small lipid changes with current OCs, patients occasionally can have exaggerated effects. Women whose lipid

Figure 10.11   Percent differences in HDL and LDL cholesterol levels and in the incremental area for insulin in response to the oral glucose tolerance test (OGTT) between women taking one of seven combination oral contraceptives and those not taking oral contraceptives. The T bars indicate 1 S.D., and the double daggers ($P < 0.05$) indicate significant differences between users and nonusers in the mean values for the principal metabolic variables. EE, *ethinyl estradiol;* LG, *levonorgestrel;* NE, norethindrone; DG, desogestrel. (With permission from **Godsland IF, Crook D, Simpson R, Proudler T, Felton C, Lees B, et al.** The effects of different formulations of oral contraceptive agents on lipid and carbohydrate metabolism. *N Engl J Med* 1990;323:1375–82.)

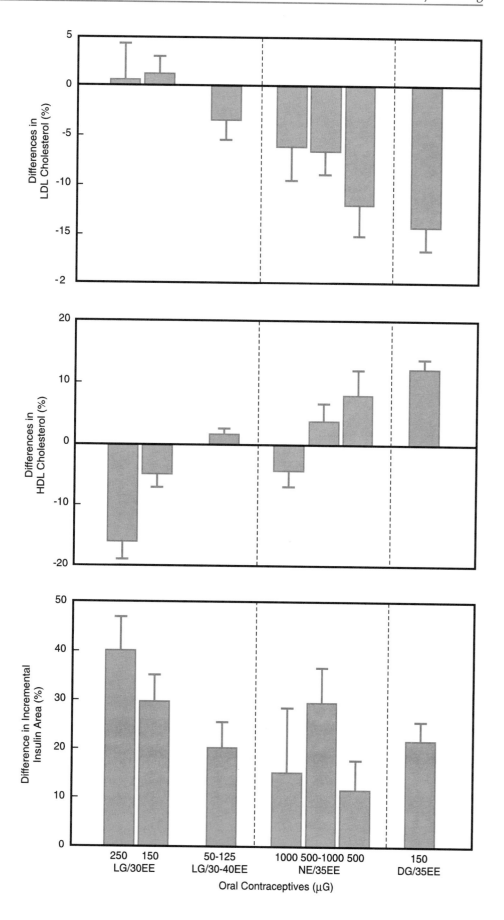

values are higher than the mean before treatment are more likely to become abnormal during treatment (104). At the doses used in current preparations, there is no evidence that any specific progestin is safer than any other in risk of vascular disease.

Other Metabolic Effects   Oral contracptives can produce changes in a broad variety of proteins synthesized by the liver. The estrogen in OCs increases circulating-thyroid-binding globulin, thereby affecting tests of thyroid function that are based on binding, increasing total thyroxine (T_4) and decreasing T_3 resin uptake. The results of actual thyroid function tests, as measured by free thyroxine and radioiodine tests, are normal (105).

OCs and Neoplasia

Endometrial Cancer and Ovarian Cancer   **Combination OCs reduce the risk for subsequent endometrial cancer and ovarian cancer (106, 107). Two years of OC use reduces the risk of subsequent endometrial cancer by 40% and 4 or more years of use reduces the risk by 60%. A 50% reduction in ovarian cancer risk was observed for women who took OCs for 3–4 years, and an 80% reduction was seen with 10 or more years of use. There was some benefit from as little as 3–11 months of use.** The benefit continues for at least 15 years since last use, and it does not diminish even at 15 years from use (107). National vital statistics data from England support these observations. Ovarian cancer mortality is declining in England and Wales for women younger than 55 years of age, and this decline has been attributed to OC use (108).

Cervical Cancer   There may be a weak association between OC use and squamous cancer of the cervix. Important risk factors are early sexual intercourse and exposure to human papillomavirus (109). Women who have used OCs typically started sexual relations at younger ages than women who have not used OCs and, in some studies, report more partners. Because barrier contraceptives reduce risk for cervical cancer, use of alternative choices for contraception can compound the difficulty in establishing an association. A comparison of IUD wearers and OC users revealed that preneoplastic lesions of the cervix progressed more rapidly among OC users (110).

Adenocarcinomas of the cervix are rare, but they are not as easily detected as other lesions by screening cervical cytology and the incidence appears to be increasing. A 1994 study found a doubling of risk of adenocarcinoma with OC use that increased with duration of use, reaching a relative risk of 4.4 if total use of OCs exceeded 12 years (111). This study adjusted for history of genital warts, number of sexual partners, and age at first intercourse. Because adenocarcinoma of the cervix is rare, absolute risk is low. If this apparent association is real, the cumulative risk of long-term OC use to 55 years of age would be about one in 1000 patients (112). Use of OCs is, at most, a minor factor in causation of cervical cancer; however, women who have used OCs should have annual Papanicolaou (Pap) tests.

Breast Cancer   The prevalence of breast cancer in the U.S. has increased, but the increase has occurred among women who are too old to have taken OCs (113). A very large study showed no overall relation between OC use and breast cancer (114). Another large study, the U.S. Nurses Health Study, reported 1,127,415 person years of observation and found no increase overall among OC users compared with nonusers (115). Some studies have revealed apparent risk to subgroups of users; for example, young women, nulligravid women, and women who used OCs before a first-term pregnancy. A British study that revealed a small but statistically stable increase in breast cancer diagnosed before 36 years of age among OC users also found that risk was lower for OCs with less than 50 μg of estrogen. Progestin-only OCs appeared to have a protective effect. Significantly, OC users who developed breast cancers had somewhat lower-stage tumors and were less likely to have positive lymph nodes than controls (116). One explanation for the apparent paradox of no overall increase but possible increased risk for small subgroups of young women is that OC use may promote growth of preexisting breast cancers, allowing early diagnosis but not increasing the lifetime risk (117). A small increase in the incidence of breast cancer prior to 44 years of age may be offset by decreased risk for women developing breast cancer at an older age, when many more cases occur. Oral contraceptive use by women with a first-degree relative who had breast cancer does not increase risk regardless of the duration of use before first-term pregnancy (118).

Liver Tumors   OCs have been implicated in the causation of benign adenomas of the liver. These hormonally responsive tumors can cause fatal hemorrhage. They usually regress when OC use is discontinued; risk is related to prolonged use (119). There is a strong correlation between OC use and hepatocellular adenoma, but fortunately, the tumors are rare; about 30 cases per 1,000,000 users per year have been predicted with older formulations (120). Presumably, newer lower-dose products are safer. A link to hepatic carcinoma has been proposed. The incidence of liver cancer has increased only slightly in England, however, and not at all in the U.S., despite many years of widespread OC use by a major proportion of women of reproductive age (120).

Health Benefits of Oral Contraceptives

OCs have important health benefits (Table 10.6). OC use produces strong and lasting reduced risk for endometrial and ovarian cancer. A 50% reduction in rates of hospitalization for pelvic infection has been reported. Chlamydial colonization of the cervix appears more likely in OC users than in nonusers but, despite this, there is a 40–50% reduction in risk for chlamydial PID (121). Combination OCs confer marked reduction in risk for ectopic pregnancy, although the progestin-only OCs appear to increase risk. Other documented benefits include a significant reduction in need for breast biopsies for benign disease, as well as reduction in surgery for ovarian cysts, dysmenorrhea, and anemia from menstrual blood loss (122). All combination OCs offer some protection from functional ovarian cysts, but this protection is less with multiphasic preparations (123). If progestin-only OCs are truly protective against breast cancer, the levonorgestrel implants also could be expected to confer this benefit.

Table 10.6   Non-contraceptive Benefits of Oral Contraception

Clearly Established Benefits

Reduced ovarian cancer

Reduced endometrial cancer

Reduced ectopic pregnancy

Reduced benign breast disease

Reduced functional ovarian cysts

Reduced uterine fibroids

Less dysmenorrhea

Less anemia

Regular menstrual cycle

Reduced pelvic inflammatory disease

Less Clearly Established Benefits

Fewer new cases of rheumatoid arthritis

Less osteopenia

Less endometriosis

Less atherosclerosis

From **Stubblefield PG.** Health benefits beyond contraception. *Int J Fertil* 1994;39(Suppl 3):132–8.

Fertility After OC Use

There may be a delay of a few months in return to ovulatory cycles after discontinuing OCs. Women with amenorrhea for more than 6 months after stopping use of OCs should undergo a full evaluation, because of the risk of prolactin-producing pituitary tumors. This risk is not related to OC use but rather to the probability that the slow-growing tumor was already present and produced menstrual irregularity, prompting the patient to take OCs (124).

Sexuality

In a study that recorded all episodes of female-initiated sexual behavior throughout the menstrual cycle, an increase at the time of ovulation was noted. This increase was abolished in women who were taking OCs (125).

Teratogenicity

A meta-analysis of 12 prospective studies, including 6102 women exposed to OCs and 85,167 unexposed women, revealed no increase in overall risk of malformation, congenital heart defects, or limb reduction defects with the use of OCs (126). Progestins have been used to prevent miscarriage. A large study compared women indicating signs of threatened abortion who were treated with progestins (primarily *medroxyprogesterone acetate*) with women who were not treated. The rate of malformation was the same among the 1146 exposed infants as among the 1608 unexposed infants (127). Conversely, estrogens taken in high doses in pregnancy can induce vaginal cancer in exposed female offspring *in utero*.

Interactions of Oral Contraceptives with Other Drugs

Some drugs reduce the effectiveness of oral contraceptives, e.g., *rifampin;* conversely, OCs can augment or reduce the effectiveness of other drugs, e.g., benzodiazepines. *Phenytoin, phenobarbital,* and *rifampin* induce synthesis of cytochrome P450 enzymes in the liver and reduce plasma levels of *ethinyl estradiol* in women taking OCs, which may cause contraceptive failure (128). *Ampicillin* and *tetracycline* have been implicated in numerous case reports of OC failure. They kill gut bacteria (primarily clostridia) that are responsible for hydrolysis of steroid glucuronides in the intestine, which allows reabsorption of the steroid via the enterohepatic circulation. However, in human studies, it has not been possible to demonstrate reduced plasma levels of *ethinyl estradiol*. Increased spotting and bleeding may indicate interference with OC effect and probably should suggest the need for additional contraception.

Certain drugs actually appear to increase plasma levels of contraceptive steroids. *Ascorbic acid (Vitamin C)* and *acetaminophen* may elevate plasma *ethinyl estradiol*.

An example of the second type of interaction (i.e., OCs affecting metabolism of other drugs) is seen with *diazepam* and related compounds. OCs reduce the metabolic clearance and increase the half-life of those benzodiazepines that are metabolized primarily by oxidation: *chlordiazepoxide, alprazolam, diazepam* and *nitrazepam*. *Caffeine* and *theophylline* are metabolized in the liver by two of the P450 isozymes, and their clearance is also reduced in OC users. *Cyclosporine* is hydroxylated by another of the P450 isozymes, and its plasma concentrations are increased by OCs. Plasma levels of some analgesic drugs are decreased in OC users. *Salicyclic* acid and *morphine* clearances are enhanced by OC use; therefore, higher doses could be needed for adequate therapeutic effect. Clearance of *ethanol* may be reduced in OC users.

Clinical Chemistry Alterations with Oral Contraceptives

Oral contraceptives have the potential to alter a number of clinical laboratory tests as a result of estrogen-induced changes in hepatic synthesis; however, a large study comparing OC users to pregnant and nonpregnant controls found minimal changes (129). Hormone users took a variety of OCs containing 50–100 μg of estrogen. Compared with nonpregnant women who were not using OCs, the OC users had an increase in thyroxine that is explained by increased circulating thyroid-binding protein, no change in creatinine, a slight reduction in mean fasting glucose values, a reduction in total bilirubin, a modest reduction in serum glutamic oxaloacetic transaminase, a decrease in alkaline phosphatase, and no change in globulin.

Choice of Oral Contraceptives

For the average patient, the first choice of preparation for contraceptive purposes is the 0.030–0.035 mg estrogen combination OCs.

1. Breakthrough bleeding and spotting are common at first, and generally improve with time. If the problem persists, one can change from a multiphasic to monophasic version at the same estrogen level.

2. If bleeding remains a problem, a temporary increase in estrogen should be tried: 20 μg of *ethinyl estradiol* daily for 7 days while continuing the OC (130).

Side effects—nausea, breast tenderness, mood changes, and weight gain—are less common with current formulations than with previous pills and usually resolve after the first few cycles.

1. If symptoms persist, the lowest dose highly effective formulations could be tried: *ethinyl estradiol* 35 μg with *norethindrone* 0.5 mg, or *ethinyl estradiol* 20 μg with *norethindrone acetate* 1.0 mg.

2. In patients who have persistent breast tenderness, the type of OC could be changed to one with more progestin activity, such as 30 μg *ethinyl estradiol* with 250 μg of *levonorgestrel*. High-progestin potency OCs produce fewer breast symptoms (131).

3. Nausea is generally related to the estrogen component, and changing to the 20 μg ethinyl estradiol preparation may be beneficial.

Injectable Hormonal Contraceptives

Depomedroxyprogesterone acetate (DMPA), a suspension of microcrystals of a synthetic progestin, is the only injectable hormonal contraceptive available in the U.S. Marketed for more than 20 years for other uses, it was finally approved for contraception in 1992. A single 150-mg intramuscular dose will suppress ovulation in most women for 14 weeks or longer (132). The regimen of 150 mg every 3 months is highly effective, producing pregnancy rates of approximately 0.3 per 100 women per year. Probably because of the high blood levels of the progestin, efficacy appears not to be reduced by administration of other drugs and is not dependent on the patient's weight. Women treated with *DMPA* experience disruption of the menstrual cycle and have initial spotting and bleeding at irregular intervals. Eventually, total amenorrhea develops in most women who take *DMPA;* with continued administration, amenorrhea develops in 50% of women by 1 year and in 80% by 3 years (Fig. 10.12). Persistent irregular bleeding can be treated by giving the next dose of *DMPA* ahead of schedule or by adding low-dose estrogen temporarily; for example, conjugated estrogens, 1.25 mg per day, can be given for 10–21 days at a time. *DMPA* persists in the body for several months in women who have used it for long-term contraception and return to fertility may be delayed; however, in a large study, 70% of former users desiring pregnancy had conceived within 12 months and 90% conceived within 24 months (133).

Safety of DMPA

Long-term users of *DMPA* have lower bone density than nonusers, probably reflecting reduced estrogen levels; however, this effect has not been associated with increased fractures (134). The effect of *DMPA* on plasma lipids has been inconsistent, but in general, *DMPA* users appear to have reduced total cholesterol and triglycerides, slight reduction in HDL cholesterol,

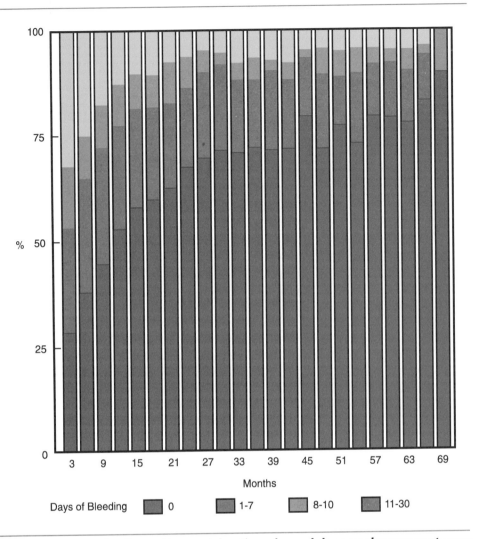

Figure 10.12   Bleeding pattern and duration of use of *depo-medroxyprogesterone acetate (DMPA):* percent of women who have bleeding, spotting, or amenorrhea while taking DMPA 150 mg every 3 months. (From **Schwallie PC, Assenzo JR.** Contraceptive use-efficacy study utilizing *medroxyprogesterone acetate* administered as an intramuscular injection once every 90 days. *Fertil Steril* 1973;24:331–9.)

and no change or slight increase in LDL cholesterol, all of which are consistent with a reduction in circulating estrogen levels. In some studies, the decrease in HDL and increase in LDL are statistically significant, although the values remain within normal ranges (135). The use of *DMPA* has not been associated with myocardial infarction. Glucose tolerance tests disclose a small elevation of glucose in *DMPA* users. There is no change in hemostatic parameters, with the exception that antithrombin III is sometimes found to be reduced with chronic therapy (135). DMPA has not been linked to thrombotic episodes in women of reproductive age. However, thrombotic episodes have occurred in elderly women with advanced cancer who were treated with a variety of agents, including *DMPA* and tamoxifen (136, 137). Such patients are at high risk for thrombosis regardless of the use of *DMPA*. Women taking *DMPA* appear to experience a weight gain of 2–3 pounds more than nonusers over several years. Its use has not been associated with teratogenesis. It is safe for use by lactating women and, as with other progestin-only hormonal methods, appears to increase milk production.

Benefits of DMPA   *DMPA* appears to have many of the noncontraceptive benefits of combination oral contraceptives. A decrease in anemia, PID, ectopic pregnancy, and endometrial cancer have been reported (138). No association between *DMPA* and cervical cancer has been demonstrated (139). Ovarian cancer has been found to be unrelated to the use of *DMPA* (140). The risk of breast cancer diagnosis during the first 4 years of use appears to be slightly increased, but there is no relation to long-term use and no overall increase in breast cancer risk; hence, any causal relationship between *DMPA* and breast cancer is unlikely (141).

Other Injectables

Other injectable contraceptives are available in other countries. Two injectables are being developed by the World Health Organization: the combination of 25 mg *medroxyproges-terone acetate* and 5 mg *estradiol cypionate* (*Cyclofem*) and the combination of 50 mg *norethindrone enanthate* plus 5 mg *estradiol valerate* (*Mesigyna*). Given once a month, both produce excellent contraceptive effects. Monthly withdrawal bleeding is like a normal menses, leading to high continuation rates (142).

Subdermal Implants

The *levonorgestrel* implant (*Norplant*) consists of six rods, each measuring 34 mm in length and 2.4 mm in outside diameter and containing 36 mg of the progestin *levonorgestrel* (143, 144). Approximately 80 µg/day is released during the first 6–12 months after insertion. The release rate then gradually declines to 30–35 µg/day. Blood levels of the steroid are about 0.35 ng/ml at 6 months and remain above 0.25 ng/ml for 5 years. Plasma levels less than 0.20 ng/ml result in higher pregnancy rates. The level of progestin present for *Norplant* users produces very effective contraception; the total number of pregnancies over 5 years is only one in 100 (144). The progestin blocks the LH surge necessary for ovulation, so that over 5 years, only about one-third of cycles are ovulatory. In response to the progestin, the cervical mucus becomes scant and thick and does not allow sperm penetration. An older, thicker-walled version of the implants was studied in the U.S. and had less contraceptive efficacy for women weighing 70 kg or more. Current devices have a pliable, less dense wall and the release rate of levonorgestrel is 15% higher than with earlier versions, so weight is less of a problem (Table 10.7). Some advise that obese women should have the implants replaced after 3 years in order to maintain a high level of pregnancy protection.

Bleeding Patterns   The implant produces endometrial atrophy. The normal menstrual cycle is disrupted, resulting in a range of possible bleeding patterns, from reasonably regular monthly bleeding, to frequent spotting and almost daily bleeding, to complete amenorrhea. The bleeding pattern changes over time and eventually tends to become more like a normal menstrual pattern. Women who have monthly bleeding are more likely to be ovulating and should be evaluated for pregnancy if they become amenorrheic. Irregular bleeding and spotting can be treated with low-dose oral estrogen, low-dose oral *levonorgestrel,* or *ibuprofen* (2). *Norplant* has no adverse effect on lactation and can be used by lactating women. Its effects are immediately reversed by removing the implants and the return to fertility is generally prompt.

Metabolic Effects   Implants do not alter glucose metabolism. There are minimal lipid changes. Total cholesterol and triglycerides are reduced and there is either no change or

Table 10.7   Pregnancy Rates with Norplant. Gross Cumulative Pregnancy Rates at 5 Years by Patient's Weight and Type of Tubing

Weight at Insertion (kg)	N	Total	Pliable Tubing	Rigid Tubing
<50	552	0.2	0	0.3
50–59	1041	3.5	2.0	4.3
60–69	585	3.5	1.5	4.5
>70	309	7.6	2.4	9.3
Total	2469	3.5	1.6	4.9

Reproduced with permission from **Darney PD.** Hormonal implants: contraception for a new century. *Am J Obstet Gynecol* 1994;170:1536–43.

minimal decrease in HDL, but the same ratio of total cholesterol to HDL is maintained. Therefore, it is very unlikely that implants promote development of atherosclerosis (144).

Adverse Events and Side Effects   Irregular bleeding and headache are the main reasons given for discontinuing use of implants. Side effects that are occasionally reported include acne, weight gain or loss, mastalgia, mood change, depression, hyperpigmentation over the implants, hirsutism, and galactorrhea. Symptomatic functional cysts occasionally occur. These usually resolve spontaneously over a few weeks without surgery. If pregnancy occurs, the probability of it being ectopic is increased compared to conceptions in other women; however, because pregnancy is so rare with implants, the total rate of ectopic pregnancies (0.28 per 1000 women years) is well below that of the U.S. population (144).

Insertion and Removal

Norplant is inserted just beneath the skin of the inner surface of the upper arm using a 10-gauge trocar as an inserter. Insertion is readily accomplished in a few minutes with local anesthesia. Removal of *Norplant* can be time consuming. The end of the rod should be manipulated into a small incision in the skin, using a scalpel to nick the fibrous sheath that forms around the rod and then pushing it out with finger pressure (143). With the Emory technique, a somewhat longer (10-mm) incision is used, and hemostat forceps are used to disrupt the fibrous capsule around the ends of all of the implants before removal with an instrument (144).

New Implants

A two-rod version of *Norplant, Norplant II,* has undergone extensive testing. It is as effective as *Norplant* and is easier to insert and remove (145). Single-rod systems containing a new progestin, *3-keto-desogestrel* (*Implanon*) are in the final phase of U.S. trials. In preliminary studies, *Implanon* appears to be even more effective than *Norplant* (146).

Postcoital Contraception

Implantation of the fertilized ovum is believed to occur on the sixth day after fertilization. This interval provides an opportunity to prevent pregnancy even after fertilization.

Estrogens

High-dose estrogen taken within 72 hours of coitus prevents pregnancy. The mechanism of action of postcoital estrogen use may involve altered tubal motility, interference with corpus luteum function mediated by prostaglandins, or alteration of the endometrium. In an analysis of more than 3000 women treated after coitus with 5 mg of *ethinyl estradiol* daily for 5 days, the pregnancy rate was 0.15% (147).

Estrogen/Progestin Combinations

The most used regimen for postcoital contraception is the combination of *ethinyl estradiol* 200 μg and *d,l norgestrel* 2 mg (two *Ovral* tablets followed by two more 12 hours later) within 72 hours of coitus (148). The average pregnancy rate with this method is 1.8% but is 1.2% if taken within 12 hours of intercourse (149). A randomized trial concluded that the *Ovral* method was just as effective as estrogen alone (147). Nausea and vomiting are common with both regimens and an antiemetic is usually prescribed.

Copper IUDs

Postcoital insertion of a copper IUD within 72 hours appears to be even more effective than sex steroids (150). Of 879 patients treated in this fashion, only one pregnancy occurred (147). No pregnancies occurred during the first month after insertion of copper IUDs as long as 7 days after coitus. Copper is toxic to the embryo.

Danazol

Danazol, a weak androgen, has also been used for emergency contraception. The pregnancy rate was 2% among 998 women (147).

256

Mifepristone

The antiprogesterone *mifepristone (RU486)* is also highly effective for postcoital contraception and appears to have no significant side effects. A three-way trial of the *Ovral* method, *danazol* (600 mg repeated after 12 hours), and *mifepristone* (600 mg as a single dose) yielded pregnancy rates of 2.62, 4.66, and 0%, respectively (151). *Mifepristone* is also highly effective in inducing menstruation when taken on day 27 of the menstrual cycle, well beyond the 72-hour window usually considered for postcoital contraception. Of 62 women treated in this fashion, only one conceived (147).

Contraception for Women with Chronic Illness

Women with chronic illness may present special problems that should be considered in the choice of a method of contraception. The illness may make pregnancy more complicated and dangerous for these women, thus making effective contraception all the more important. Some common conditions and considerations about contraception are listed in Table 10.8.

Table 10.8   Contraception for Women with Chronic Illness

Psychiatric disorders

- Oral contraceptives, implants, *DMPA,* and copper IUD are good choices.
- Use of barrier methods should be encouraged to decrease risk of STDs.

Coagulation disorders

- Hemorrhagic disorders: OCs may be indicated to prevent hemorrhagic ovarian cysts and menstrual hemorrhage.
- Thrombotic disorders: avoid estrogen-containing OCs.

Dyslipidemia

- May use low-dose OCs if lipid abnormality successfully managed by diet or drug therapy, but lipids should be monitored at 3–6 months.
- Avoid OCs if triglycerides are elevated.
- Select less androgenic OCs.
- Progestin-only OCs, *DMPA,* and IUDs are acceptable.

Hypertension

- Young women with no other risk factors with well-controlled hypertension may use low-dose OCs under close supervision.
- Older women, smokers, and those with poorly controlled hypertension should probably avoid combination OCs.
- *DMPA, Norplant,* IUDs, and progestin-only OCs are good alternatives.

Diabetes

- Young diabetic women without vascular disease can use low-dose OCs.
- Older women or women with vascualr disease probably should not use combination OCs.
- *DMPA, Norplant,* IUDs, and progestin-only OCs are good alternatives.

Headache

- Migraine without aura, without neurologic symptoms, does not rule out OCs if use is closely supervised.
- *Norplant* and *DMPA* may be used safely.

Epilepsy

- OCs do not increase the risk of seizure, but antiseizure drugs reduce efficacy of OCs and *Norplant.*
- OCs with 50 μg estrogen can be used, as can *DMPA.* IUDs, are not contraindicated.

DMPA, depomedroxyprogesterone acetate; IUD, intrauterine device; OCs, oral contraceptives.
From **Association of Reproductive Health Professionals.** *Clinical Challenges in Contraception: A Program on Women with Special Medical Conditions.* Clinical Proceedings. Washington, DC: ARHP, 1994.

Hormonal Contraception for Men

The same negative feedback of sex steroids that can block ovulation in women will also suppress spermatogenesis in men, but it will produce loss of libido and potentially extinguish sexual performance. Replacement testosterone therapy restores libido and performance without restoring spermatogenesis. The principle was first demonstrated in 1974 using oral estrogen and methyl testosterone (152). Testosterone alone will suppress pituitary release of LH and FSH to very low levels and depress or abolish spermatogenesis, whereas the testosterone in systemic circulation maintains normal sexual behavior and body habitus. Weekly doses of 200 mg achieve azoospermia in only 40–70% of white men; the rest become oligospermic (153). Pregnancy has occurred in partners of androgen-treated oligospermic men with sperm counts as low as 3 million/ml (154). Asian men may be treated more effectively than white men. One hundred mg weekly produced azoospermia in all seven Indonesian men studied (155). Combinations of *DMPA* plus androgen have been widely studied but also fail to achieve 100% sperm suppression in white men (156). Current interest is in using GnRH analogues to suppress spermatogenesis with long-acting androgens used for replacement. One of these regimens will likely prove clinically useful, but at present, costs are high and long-term safety remains to be established. Adverse lipid changes have been noted with *DMPA*-androgen combinations, raising concern about vascular disease with prolonged use. Liver cancer is a concern with long-term androgen therapy (157).

Sterilization

Surgical sterilization is the most common method of fertility control among U.S. couples (4). Laparoscopic techniques for women and vasectomy for men are safe and readily available throughout the U.S. The mean age at sterilization is 30 years. Age younger than 30 years when sterilized or divorce and remarriage are predictors of sterilization regret, which may lead to a request for reversal of sterilization (158).

Female Sterilization

Hysterectomy is no longer considered for sterilization because morbidity and mortality are too high in comparison with tubal sterilization. Four procedures are common in the U.S.:

1. Tubal sterilization at the time of laparotomy for a cesarean delivery or other abdominal operation

2. Postpartum minilaparotomy soon after vaginal delivery

3. Interval minilaparotomy

4. Laparoscopy

Vaginal tubal sterilization, which has been associated with occasional pelvic abscess, is rarely performed in the U.S.

At Cesarean Delivery   Tubal sterilization at the time of cesarean delivery adds no risk, other than a slight prolongation of operating time; however, cesarean birth has more risk that vaginal birth, and planned sterilization should not influence the decision to perform a cesarean delivery. Sterilization is no more likely to fail if done with a cesarean delivery than at other times (159).

Postpartum Minilaparotomy   In the immediate postpartum state, the uterus is enlarged and the fallopian tubes lie in the midabdomen, easily accessible through a small, 3- to 4-cm subumbilical incision.

Interval Minilaparotomy   This procedure was first described by Uchida (160). It was rediscovered and popularized in the early 1970s in response to the increased demand for sterilization procedures as a simpler alternative to laparoscopy. In the nongravid state, the uterus and tubes lie deep in the pelvis. A short transverse suprapubic incision is made, and the uterus and tubes are then elevated upward, just beneath the incision by use of a uterine-elevating probe placed into the uterine cavity through the vagina. Interval minilaparotomy is usually performed as an outpatient procedure and can be accomplished readily with local anesthesia and conscious sedation.

Surgical Techniques for Minilaparotomy or Cesarean Sterilization

The tubal lesion usually elected is the *Pomeroy* or *modified Pomeroy* technique (Fig. 10.13). In the classic Pomeroy procedure, a loop of tube is excised after ligating the base of the loop with single absorbable suture. A modification of the procedure is excision of the midportion of the tube after ligation of the segment with two separate absorbable sutures. This modified procedure has several names: partial salpingectomy, *Parkland Hospital technique,* separate sutures technique, and *modified Pomeroy.* In the *Madlener technique,* now abandoned because of too many failures, a loop of tube is crushed by cross-clamping its base, ligated with permanent suture, and then excised. *Pomeroy* and partial salpingectomy procedures have failure rates of 1–4 per 1000 cases (160). In contrast, pregnancy is almost unheard of after tubal sterilization by the *Irving* or *Uchida methods* (160, 161). In the *Irving method,* the midportion of the tube is excised, and the proximal stump of each tube is turned back and led into a small stab wound in the wall of the uterus and sutured in place, creating a blind loop. With the *Uchida method,* a saline-*epinephrine* solution (1:1000) is injected beneath the mucosa of the midportion of the tube, separating the mucosa from the underlying tube. The mucosa is incised along the antimesenteric border of the tube, and a tubal segment is excised under traction so that the ligated proximal stump will retract beneath the mucosa when released. The mucosa is then closed with sutures, burying the proximal stump and separating it from the distal stump. In Uchida's personal series of more than 20,000 cases, there were no pregnancies.

Figure 10.13   The Pomeroy technique for tubal sterilization.

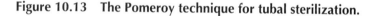

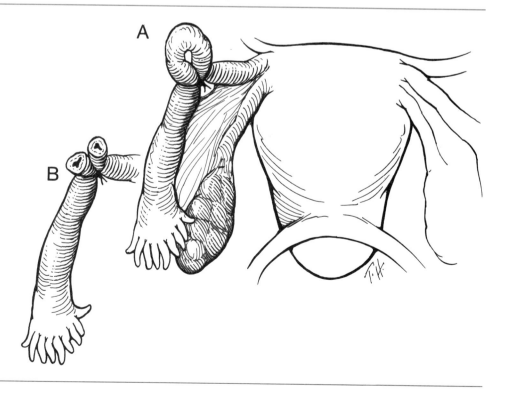

Laparoscopy

With the standard laparoscopy technique, the abdomen is inflated with a gas (carbon dioxide or nitrous oxide) via a special needle inserted at the lower margin of the umbilicus (162). A hollow sheath containing a pointed trocar is then pushed through the abdominal wall at the same location, the trocar is removed, and the laparoscope is inserted into the abdominal cavity through the sheath to visualize the pelvic organs. A second, smaller trocar is inserted in the suprapubic region to allow the insertion of special grasping forceps. Alternatively, an operating laparoscope that has a channel for the instruments can be used; thus, the procedure can be performed through a single small incision. Laparoscopic sterilization is usually performed in the hospital under general anesthesia, but can be performed under local anesthesia with conscious sedation. Overnight hospitalization for laparoscopy is rarely needed.

Open Laparoscopy   Standard laparoscopy carries with it a small but definite risk of injury to major blood vessels with insertion of the sharp trocar. With the alternative technique of open laparoscopy, neither needle nor sharp trocar is used, but instead the peritoneal cavity is opened directly through an incision at the lower edge of the umbilicus (163). A special funnel-shaped sleeve, the Hasson cannula, is then inserted and the laparoscope is introduced through it.

Techniques of Laparoscopic Sterilization   Sterilization is accomplished by any of three techniques: bipolar electrical coagulation, application of a small silastic rubber band *(Falope ring)* (164), or application of a plastic and metal clip *(Hulka clip)* across each tube (162). The *Filshie clip,* used in the U.K. and Canada, is a simple, mechanical device for occluding the tube that is not available in the U.S. In the bipolar electrocoagulation technique, the mid-isthmic portion of the tube and adjacent mesosalpinx are grasped with special bipolar forceps and radiofrequency electric current is applied to three adjacent areas, coagulating 3 cm of tube (Fig. 10.14). The tube alone is then recoagulated in the same places. The radiofrequency generator must deliver at least 25 watts into a 100-ohm resistance at the probe tips to ensure coagulation of the complete thick-

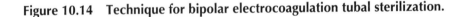

Figure 10.14   Technique for bipolar electrocoagulation tubal sterilization.

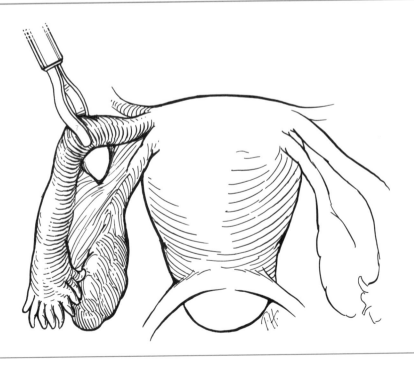

ness of the fallopian tube and not just the outer layer; otherwise, the sterilization will fail (165). To apply the *Falope ring,* the mid-isthmic portion of the tube is grasped with tongs advanced through a cylindrical probe that has the ring stretched around it. A loop of tube is pulled back into the probe and the outer cylinder is advanced, releasing the silastic ring around the base of the loop of tube, producing ischemic necrosis (Fig. 10.15). If the tube cannot be pulled easily into the applicator, the operator should stop and change to electrical coagulation rather than persist and risk lacerating the tube with the *Falope ring* applicator. The banded tube must be inspected at close range through the laparoscope to demonstrate that the full thickness of the tube has been pulled through the *Falope ring.* The *Hulka clip* is also placed across the mid-isthmis, ensuring that the applicator is at right angles to the tube and that the tube is completely contained within the clip before the clip is closed.

Figure 10.15   Placement of the Falope Ring for tubal sterilization.

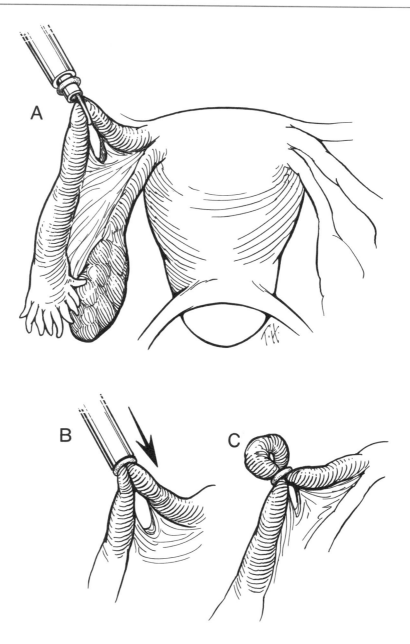

The electric and band or clip techniques each have advantages and disadvantages. Bipolar coagulation can be used with any fallopian tube. The ring and the clip cannot be applied if the tube is thickened from previous salpingitis. There is more pain during the first several hours after ring application and more analgesia will be required. Failures of the *Falope ring* or *Hulka clip* generally result from misapplication, and pregnancy, if it occurs, usually is intrauterine. Pregnancy after bipolar sterilization may occur from tuboperitoneal fistula and is ectopic in more than 50% of cases. If inadequate electrical energy is used, a thin band of fallopian tube remains that contains the intact lumen and allows intrauterine pregnancy to occur. Thermocoagulation, the use of heat probes rather than electrical current, is used extensively in Germany for laparoscopic tubal sterilization but has had little use in the U.S.

Risks of Tubal Sterilization

Tubal sterilization is remarkably safe. In 1983, the total complication rate in a large series from several institutions was 1.7 per 100 (166). Complications were increased by use of general anesthesia, previous pelvic or abdominal surgery, history of PID, obesity, and diabetes mellitus. The most common significant complication was unintended laparotomy for sterilization after intra-abdominal adhesions were found. In a more recent series, 2827 laparoscopic sterilizations were performed using local anesthesia and intravenous sedation with the silastic band. Only four cases could not be completed (a technical failure rate of 0.14%), and laparotomy was not needed (167). Rarely, salpingitis can occur as a complication of the surgery. This occurs more often with electric coagulation than nonelectric techniques. From 1977 until 1981, there were four deaths per 100,000 procedures in the U.S., less than the risk of one pregnancy; almost half of the deaths were from complications of general anesthesia, usually related to the use of mask ventilation (168). When general anesthesia is used for laparoscopy, endotracheal intubation is mandatory because the pneumoperitoneum increases the risk of aspiration. International data from the Association for Voluntary Surgical Contraception shows a similar record of safety from Third World programs: 4.7 deaths per 100,000 female sterilizations and 0.5 per 100,000 vasectomies (169).

Benefits of Sterilization

In addition to providing excellent contraception, tubal ligation is associated with reduced risk for ovarian cancer that persists for as long as 20 years after surgery and then diminishes (170).

Sterilization Failure

Many "failures" occur during the first month after laparoscopy and are the result of a pregnancy already begun when the sterilization was performed. Contraception should be continued until the day of surgery, and a sensitive pregnancy test should be performed routinely on the day of surgery. Because implantation does not occur until 6 days after conception, however, a woman could conceive just before her surgery and there would be no way to detect it. Scheduling sterilization early in the menstrual cycle obviates the problem but adds to the logistic difficulty. Another cause of failure is the finding of anatomic abnormalities, usually adhesions surrounding and obscuring one or both tubes. An experienced laparoscopic surgeon with proper instruments can usually lyse the adhesions, restore normal anatomic relations, and positively identify the tube. In some circumstances, however, successful sterilization will not be possible by laparoscopy, and the surgeon must know prior to surgery whether the patient is prepared to undergo laparotomy to accomplish sterilization, if necessary. Table 10.9 lists pregnancy rates after tubal sterilization from several sources. The range is 1–4 pregnancies per 1000 women sterilized. No difference has been demonstrated between risk of failure after tubal sterilization by open surgical techniques as compared with laparoscopy, with the exception that the *Irving* and *Uchida* techniques are considered least likely to fail.

Most studies of sterilization failure are short term. The Centers for Disease Control and Prevention is conducting a long-term study of tubal sterilization. The preliminary findings

Table 10.9 Pregnancies after Tubal Sterilization

	Pregnancies/1000	*Sterilizations*
Laparoscopy*		
Bipolar coagulation	2.1–4.0	65,971
Endocoagulation	1.1	40,425
Falope ring	0.8–4.0	498,232
Hulka clip	1.8–5.9	5503
Filshie clip	0–2	2317
Minilaparotomy†		
Modified Pomeroy	1.46	2050
Pomeroy	2	6717
Cesarean Section		
Pomeroy	3	1739
Interval laparotomy‡	6	1115

*From **Khandwala SD.** Laparoscopic sterilization: a comparison of current techniques. *J Reprod Med* 1988;33:463–7.
†From **Rimdusit P.** Separate stitches tubal sterilization, a modified Pomeroy's technique. An analysis of the procedure, complaints and failures. *J Med Assoc Thai* 1984;67:602–5.
‡From **Shephard MK.** Female contraceptive sterilization. *Obstet Gynecol Surv* 1974; 29:739–87.

indicate a 3-year failure rate of eight pregnancies per 1000 women, considerably higher than the 1–6 per 1000 shown in Table 10.9. The late failures after bipolar coagulation were usually ectopic (162).

Reversal of Tubal Sterilization

Reversal of sterilization is more successful after mechanical occlusion than after electrocoagulation, because the latter method destroys much more of the tube. With modern microsurgical techniques and an isthmus-to-isthmus anastomosis, pregnancy follows in approximately 75% of cases (171). A substantial risk for ectopic pregnancy exists after reversal.

Late Sequelae of Tubal Sterilization

Increased menstrual irregularity and pain have been blamed on previous tubal sterilization. In patients who underwent the older laparoscopy technique with unipolar electrical destruction of a major portion of the tube, these concerns may be warranted (172). Study of the problem is complicated by the facts that many women develop these symptoms even though they have not had tubal surgery, and OCs reduce pain and create an artificially normal menstrual cycle. Therefore, women who discontinued OC use concurrent with tubal sterilization will experience more dysmenorrhea, which is entirely unrelated to the sterilization. One large study found no change in menstrual function, excluding women who discontinued use of OCs and IUDs (173). In the Collaborative Review of Sterilization (CREST) of the Centers for Disease Control and Prevention (174), interviews of 2546 women were conducted before tubal sterilization and 2 years later. Fewer women reported having irregular cycles after sterilization than before sterilization. Menstrual bleeding did not increase. Women who had bipolar electrocoagulation or silastic band sterilization more often reported *decreased* menstrual pain at the 2-year interview, but women who had unipolar electrocoagulation of the tubes had *increased* pain. Bipolar cautery, the newer of the two electrosurgery techniques, is safer than unipolar electrosurgical tubal sterilization and has largely replaced it. Another long-term study compared 500 women undergoing tubal sterilization with a control group of women interviewed prior to sterilization, at 6–10 months, and then 3–4.5 years later (175). After excluding women using OCs, there were no long-term differences in menstrual cycles, intermenstrual bleeding, heavy bleeding, dysmenorrhea, or noncyclic pelvic pain. Sterilizations were performed as *modified Pomeroy,* laparoscopy with bipolar cautery, or laparoscopy with *Falope ring* application.

Male Sterilization

Vasectomy, excision of a portion of the vas deferens, is readily accomplished with local anesthesia in an office setting. It does not decrease sexual performance (176). The basic technique is to palpate the vas through the scrotum, grasp it with fingers or atraumatic forceps, make a small incision over the vas, and pull a loop of the vas into the incision. A small segment is removed, and then a needle electrode is used to coagulate the lumen of both ends. Improved techniques include the "no scalpel" vasectomy, in which the pointed end of the forceps is used to puncture the skin over the vas. This small variation reduces the chance of bleeding and avoids the need to suture the incision. Another variation is the "open-ended vasectomy," in which only the abdominal end of the severed vas is coagulated while the testicular end is left open. This is believed to prevent congestive epididymitis (2).

Reversibility   Vasectomy must be regarded as a permanent means of sterilization; however, with microsurgical techniques, vasovasostomy will result in pregnancy about half the time. The longer the interval since vasectomy, the poorer the chance of reversal.

Safety of Vasectomy   Operative complications include scrotal hematomas, wound infection, and epididymitis, but serious sequelae are very rare. There have been no reports of deaths from vasectomy in the U.S. in many years, and the death rate in a large Third World series was only 0.5 per 100,000. Studies of vasectomized monkeys showed accelerated atherosclerosis, but several large-scale human studies have found no connection between vasectomy and vascular disease (177, 178). Concerns about long-term safety have been renewed, with the report of a possible association between prostate cancer and vasectomy (179). A recent large case-control study comparing 355 cases and 2048 controls revealed no increased risk of cancer from vasectomy (180), but another large study found a weak association (relative risk 1.89) (181). An expert panel convened by the National Institutes of Health concluded that there is insufficient evidence of an association to warrant changing practice (182).

Abortion

Given the desire in developed countries to limit families to one or two children and the efficacy of contraception in general use, it is extremely likely that any normal couple will experience at least one unwanted pregnancy at some time during their reproductive years. In Third World countries, desired family size is larger, but access to effective contraception is limited. As a result, abortion is common. Worldwide, approximately 26–31 million legal abortions and an estimated 10–22 million clandestine abortions are performed every year (183). Where abortion is legal, it is generally reasonably safe; where it is illegal, complications are common, and approximately 150,000 women die every year from these complications (184). Societies cannot prevent abortion, but they can determine whether it will be illegal and dangerous or legal and safe. Many countries in which abortion is completely illegal have very high rates of clandestine abortion. Abortion rates in representative countries are given in Table 10.10 (185).

Death from illegal abortion was once common in the U.S. In the 1940s, more than 1000 women died each year of complications from abortion (186). In 1987, the last year for which complete data are available, there were 12 deaths from spontaneous abortion, six deaths from legally induced abortion, and only two deaths from illegal abortion (abortion induced by a nonprofessional) in the entire U.S. (187). The American Medical Association's Council on Scientific Affairs has reviewed the impact of legal abortion and attrib-

Table 10.10   Rates of Induced Abortion in Representative Countries 1985–1991 per 1000 Women Aged 15–44

Legal Abortion*		Illegal Abortion†	
Netherlands, 1986	5.3	Brazil, 1991	36.5
Canada, 1985	12.0	Columbia, 1989	32.7
England/Wales, 1987	14.2	Chile, 1990	45.4
U.S., 1985	28.0	Mexico, 1990	22.3
Cuba, 1988	58.0	Peru, 1990	51.9
Former USSR, 1987	181.0	Dominican Republic	43.7

*From **Henshaw SK, Morrow E.** Induced abortion: a world review. *Fam Plann Perspect* 1990;22:76–120.
†From **The Alan Guttmacher Institute.** *Aborto Clandestino: Un Realidad Latinoamericana.* New York: The Alan Guttmacher Institute, 1994;24.

utes the decline in deaths during this century to the introduction of antibiotics to treat sepsis; the widespread use of effective contraception beginning in the 1960s, which reduced the number of unwanted pregnancies; and more recently, the shift from illegal to legal abortion (188). Much of the continued decline in nonabortion-related maternal mortality of recent years can be attributed to choice of legal abortion by women at high risk for pregnancy mortality. The U.S. has a serious problem with teenage pregnancy. Without legal abortion, there would be twice as many teenage births each year.

The number of abortions reported each year in the U.S.—approximately 1,400,000 abortions according to the Centers for Disease Control and Prevention—a number that has been stable since 1980. In 1991, the national abortion ratio was 339 abortions for every 1000 live births, and the national abortion rate was 24 per 1000 women aged 15–44 years (189). Most women who obtain abortions are unmarried (79.7% in 1991), and the ratio of abortions to live births is almost 10 times higher for unmarried women than for married women. Use of abortion varies markedly with age. In 1991, 21% of women obtaining abortions were 19 years of age or younger, and 55.2% were 24 years of age or younger. In 1990, the last year for which detailed information is available, the abortion ratio for women under 15 years of age was 844 per 1000 live births, almost as many abortions as births (Fig. 10.2) (190). Abortion ratios reached their highest in the early 1980s and have declined somewhat since, especially for the youngest women (Fig. 10.16).

Duty of Health Professionals   Regardless of personal feelings about the ethics of interrupting pregnancy, health professionals have a duty to know the medical facts about abortion and to share them with their patients (191). Providers are not required to perform abortions against their ethical principles, but they have a duty to help patients assess pregnancy risks and to make appropriate referrals.

Safety of Legal Abortion: Overview of U.S. Experience

The risk of death from legal abortion is 0.4 per 100,000 induced abortions, whereas total maternal mortality is approximately 7–8 per 100,000 live births. The risk of death from legal abortion prior to 16 weeks is five- to 10-fold less than that from continuing the pregnancy on to delivery. As shown in Table 10.11, the risk of death increases with gestational age (187). For individual women with high-risk conditions (for example, cyanotic heart disease), even late abortion is a safer alternative to birth. Because of the availability of low-cost, out-of-hospital first-trimester abortion, 87% of legal abortions are performed during the first trimester, when abortion is the safest (190). The type of procedure is another determinant of risk. First-trimester abortions are virtually all performed by vacuum curettage; however, in the midtrimester, a variety of techniques can be used. Risk of death from abortion by the various techniques at different gestational ages is given in Table 10.12. The data clearly show the greater safety of instrumental evacuation of the

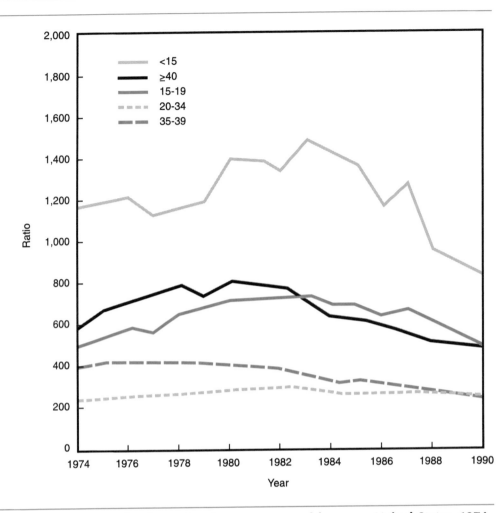

Figure 10.16   Abortion ratios, by age group and by year—United States, 1974–1989. Ratio = induced abortions/1000 live births. (With permission from **Koonin LM, Smith JC, Ramick M, Lawson HW.** Abortion surveillance, 1989. *MMWR* 1993;41:55–9.)

uterus (D & E) performed in the early midtrimester. Another determinant of risk is anesthesia. Use of general anesthesia increases the risk of perforation of the uterus, visceral injury, hemorrhage, hysterectomy, and death (192). The preferred alternative is paracervical block with local anesthetic, augmented with conscious sedation when needed.

Techniques for Abortion

Most abortions are performed by vacuum curettage. Early procedures (5–7 weeks from beginning of last normal menses) are readily performed in an office setting with these simple instruments: a 5- to 6-mm flexible plastic cannula and a modified 50-ml plastic syringe as vacuum source (193). After 7 weeks, somewhat larger rigid plastic cannulae (8–12 mm in diameter) are generally used, depending on gestational age, with an electric pump as the vacuum source. Most abortions in the U.S. are performed outside of hospitals, usually in freestanding specialty clinics, at a cost far below that of hospital services. General anesthesia is unnecessary. Adequate pain relief is provided by infiltrating the cervix with local anesthetic, augmented with intravenous sedatives and analgesics for conscious sedation (194).

Medical Means for Abortion

Mifepristone (RU486), an analogue of the progestin *norethindrone,* has strong affinity for the progesterone receptor but acts as an antagonist, blocking the effect of natural progesterone. Women with amenorrhea of less than 50 days and pregnancy confirmed by serum

Table 10.11   Death to Case Rates for Legal Abortion Mortality by Weeks of Gestation, United States, 1972–1987

Weeks of Gestation	Deaths	Abortions	Rate*	Relative Risk
≤8	33	8,673,759	0.4	1.0
9–10	39	4,847,321	0.8	2.1
11–12	33	2,360,768	1.4	3.7
13–15	28	962,185	2.9	7.7
16–20	74	794,093	9.3	24.5
≥21	21	175,395	12.0	31.5

*Legal abortion deaths per 100,000 procedures, excludes deaths from ectopic pregnancies or pregnancy with gestation length unknown.
From **Lawson HW, Frye A, Atrash HK, Smith JC, Shulman RB, Ramick M, et al.** Abortion mortality, United States, 1972–1987. *Am J Obstet Gynecol* 1994;171:1365–72.

Table 10.12   Rates for Legal Abortions by Type of Procedure and Weeks of Gestation, United States, 1974–1987*

Procedure	≤8	9–10	11–12	13–15	16–20	≥21
Vacuum curettage[†]	0.3	0.7	1.1	—	—	—
Dilation and evacuation	—	—	—	2.0	6.5	11.9
Instillation[‡]	—	—	—	3.8	7.9	10.3
Hysterectomy/ hysterotomy	18.3	30.0	41.2	28.1	103.4	274.3

*Legal induced abortion deaths per 100,000 legal induced abortions.
[†]Includes all suction and sharp curettage procedures.
[‡]Includes all instillation methods (saline, prostaglandin).
From **Lawson HW, Frye A, Atrash HK, Smith JC, Shulman HB, Ramick M, et al.** Abortion mortality, United States, 1972–1987. *Am J Obstet Gynecol* 1994;171:1365–72.

βhCG or ultrasonography receive an oral dose of 600 mg of *mifepristone* on day 1. On day 3, the patient returns for administration of a prostaglandin (195). If treatment fails or if the patient bleeds excessively, vacuum curettage is performed. In a series of almost 17,000 cases, 600 mg of *mifepristone* orally followed in 36–48 hours by either *sulprostone* or *gemeprost* produced complete abortion in 95% of cases (196). The only significant complications to date have been three myocardial infarctions, with one death. All three myocardial infarctions occurred in women over 35 years of age who were heavy smokers and occurred at the time of administration of *sulprostone*, a prostaglandin E_2 analogue. No myocardial infarctions have occurred with the prostaglandin E_1 analogue, *gemeprost*. Misoprostol, another E_1 analogue seems to have fewer side effects and a greater margin of safety than *sulprostone*. It is very effective when combined with *mifepristone* and is the prostaglandin used in U.S. trials now in progress (196).

Methotrexate and Misoprostol

The antifolate *methotrexate* provides another medical approach to pregnancy termination. Widely used to treat ectopic pregnancies without surgery (197), it can also be used with intrauterine gestations. *Methotrexate* (50 mg/M^2 intramuscularly) followed by *misoprostol* (800 mg vaginally) produced abortion in six pregnancies up to 56 days from the last menstrual period (198). *Methotrexate* alone without the *misoprostol* is also successful, although bleeding does not begin until an average of 24 days after treatment (199). These drugs are available in the U.S., where they are approved by the FDA for other indications.

Second Trimester Abortion

Most legal abortions are performed prior to 13 menstrual weeks. Abortions performed after 13 weeks include those done because of fetal defects, medical or psychiatric illness that had not manifested earlier in pregnancy, and changed social circumstances such as abandonment by the spouse. The single greatest factor determining the need for late abortion is young age. In 1990, 22.3% of abortions for women under 15 years of age were midtrimester, whereas 16% of abortions for women 15–19 years of age and only 8.0% of abortions for women 30–34 years of age were performed after 12 weeks of gestation (189).

Dilation and Evacuation

Dilation and evacuation (D & E) is the most commonly used method of abortion through 20 menstrual weeks. After that time, methods that induce labor are more common (187). Typically, the cervix is prepared by insertion of some type of hygroscopic dilator, the stem of the seaweed *laminaria japonicum* (laminaria), or a synthetic version made of polyacrilonitrile (*Dilapan*). Placed in the cervical canal as small sticks, these devices take up water from the cervix and swell, triggering dilation. When these are removed the following day, sufficient cervical dilation is accomplished to allow insertion of strong forceps and a large-bore vacuum cannula to extract the fetus and placenta (200).

Labor Induction Methods

Hypertonic Solutions   Amnioinfusion of hypertonic saline is historically important as one of the oldest labor induction methods for abortion. Saline has serious hazards: cardiovascular collapse, pulmonary and cerebral edema, and renal failure occur if the solution is injected intravenously. All patients are at risk for serious disseminated intravascular coagulopathy (201). However, attention to proper technique for amnioinfusion, with the saline instilled by gravity flow through connecting tubing from a single dose bottle under ultrasound guidance, reduces the frequency of such mishaps. Hypertonic urea is safer than saline. It is combined with low doses of prostaglandin to increase efficacy and shorten the interval from injection to abortion (202).

Prostaglandins   Prostaglandins, oxygenated metabolites of C_{20} carboxylic acid, are found naturally in most biologic tissues, where they act as modulators of cell function. They act via specific receptors of the G-protein family that are coupled to a variety of intracellular signal mechanisms, which may stimulate or inhibit adenyl cyclase, or phosphatidylinositol (203). Prostaglandins of the E and F series can cause uterine contraction at any stage of gestation. These agents can be given by intra-amniotic infusion, by intramuscular injection, or by vaginal suppository. The 15 methyl analogues of prostaglandin $F_{2\alpha}$ (*carboprost*) and prostaglandin E_2 (*dinoprostone*) are highly effective but frequently produce side effects of vomiting and diarrhea. Recently, the prostaglandin E_1 analogue *misoprostol* has been administered vaginally for midtrimester abortion. A randomized comparison of vaginal *dinoprost* suppositories (20 mg every 3 hours) and vaginally administered *misoprostol* (200 μg every 12 hours) in patients who were 12–22 weeks pregnant showed equal efficacy. The patients receiving *misoprostol* had fewer side effects of fever, uterine pain, vomiting, and diarrhea. The *misoprostol* is much less expensive and was easier to administer (204). Retained placenta is common with all prostaglandin abortions, and instrumental extraction is necessary in about half of cases. *Oxytocin* in very high doses is as effective as *dinoprostone* at 17–24 weeks of pregnancy (205). Patients initially receive an infusion of 50 units *oxytocin* in 500 ml of 5% dextrose and normal saline over 3 hours, 1 hour of no *oxytocin* followed by 100-unit/500-ml solution over 3 hours, another hour of rest, and then a 150-unit/500-ml solution over 3 hours, alternating 3 hours of *oxytocin* with 1 hour of rest. The *oxytocin* is increased by 50 units in each successive period until a final concentration of 300 units per 500 ml has been reached.

Complications   The labor induction methods share common hazards: failure of the primary procedure to produce abortion within a reasonable time, incomplete abortion, retained placenta, hemorrhage, infection, and embolic phenomena. Failed abortion can lead to serious infection and continued blood loss. Intramuscular injections of *carboprost* or vaginal suppositories of PGE$_2$ are important second-line therapies when the primary method has not produced abortion within a reasonable time period.

Induced Abortion and Subsequent Reproduction

Legal abortion, as currently practiced in the U.S., has no measurable adverse effect on later reproduction (206). Even two or more induced abortions have no detectable adverse effect (207). Abortion as practiced in the U.S. is not associated with low birth weight, prematurity, or increased perinatal loss (208). Concerns about infertility as a result of induced abortion are unfounded, except for the rare severe complication managed by hysterectomy (209). The lack of adverse effects on later pregnancy probably reflects the safety of current abortion technology in the U.S.

The Future

Contraceptive development is extremely slow in the U.S. because of the legal climate, the great cost of meeting U.S. FDA requirements, and the low priority given this area by the medical community. On the international scene, a number of new approaches to contraception are in development. The two-rod version of *Norplant* (*Norplant II*) should soon be available. *Levonorgestrel* in a biodegradable rod of caprolactone that does not require removal is currently being tested, as is the single-rod implant releasing *3-keto-desogestrel*. The once-a-month injectable combinations of estrogen and progestin are now in use outside the U.S. Silastic vaginal rings releasing either progestin or progestin-estrogen combinations have been studied for years and are now undergoing field trials in a number of countries. All of these methods for steroid delivery have the advantage of greater ease of compliance for the user. The *levonorgestrel*-releasing IUD will probably be available soon.

Perhaps one of the most promising new approaches is the use of the antiprogesterone *mefipristone* as a daily or once-a-month contraceptive in addition to its already proven efficacy as a safe abortifacient in early pregnancy.

Current methods of tubal sterilization require abdominal surgery. To meet the coming demand for vast numbers of sterilizations worldwide, easier means must be devised. Considerable effort has gone into developing transuterine methods of female sterilization that would avoid the need to open the abdominal cavity to gain access to the fallopian tubes. Hysteroscopy with tubal cannulation and electrofulgeration or the injection of silastic that forms in place into tubal plugs have been explored and now are largely abandoned (210). Another approach is the *Femcept* device to instill the biological adhesive methyl cyanoacrylate into the tubes. The device is placed blindly into the uterine cavity without hysteroscopy. A rapidly expanding intrauterine balloon pushes a measured amount of the adhesive out into the tubes. In a trial of 1279 women, one treatment accomplished bilateral closure in 71.4%, and two treatments increased this to 89.4%. The 3-year pregnancy rate was 1.7 per 100 women years (211). A simpler option is quinine pellets placed in the uterus. It has been known for years that intrauterine *quinine* can produce sclerosis of the proximal fallopian tube. This method has recently been rediscovered and is being seriously explored. A pellet containing 252 mg of *quinacrine* is inserted into the uterus during the proliferative phase of the cycle and again 1 month later. In a large trial, the 1-year pregnancy rate for 9461 women who received two doses was 2.63 per 100 women years. The rate of ectopic pregnancy was 0.89 per 1000 women years (212).

Immunological contraception/sterilization has been pursued for many years. Researchers in India coupled the beta fraction of hCG to tetanus toxoid or diphtheria toxoid as an adjuvant and produced anti-hCG antibody in monkeys and in humans (213). It is effective and has no reported side effects; however, repeated dosing is needed to keep antibody levels in the required range. The method is reversible. Whether there will be any adverse effects on pregnancy in previously vaccinated women is not known. The possibility of vaccinating men or women against specific sperm antigens and the zona pellucida is also being pursued (214).

Chinese researchers have developed a method of percutaneous occlusion of the vas that has been used in more than 100,000 men, is effective, and appears to be reversible. Polyurethane elastomer is injected into the vas, where it solidifies and forms a plug, providing an effective block to sperm. The plugs are removed using local anesthesia, and fertility returns in most cases after as long as 4 years with the plugs *in situ* (215).

References

1. **Haymes NE.** *Medical History of Contraception.* New York: Gamut Press, 1963.

2. **Hatcher RA, Trussell J, Stewart F, Stewart GK, Kowal D, Guest F, et al.** *Contraceptive Technology.* 16th ed. New York: Irvington Publishers, 1994:622.

3. **Cates W Jr.** Family planning, sexually transmitted diseases and contraceptive choice: a literature update—Part I. *Fam Plann Perspect* 1992;24:75–84.

4. **Mosher WD, Pratt WF.** *Contraceptive Use in the United States. Advance Data.* Washington, DC: National Center for Health Statistics, 1990:183.

5. *1993 Annual Birth Control Study.* Raritan, NJ: Ortho Pharmaceutical Corp., 1993.

6. **Harlap S, Kost K, Forrest JD.** *Preventing Pregnancy, Protecting Health: A New Look at Birth Control Choices in the United States.* New York: The Alan Gutmacher Institute, 1991:33.

7. **Ory HW.** Mortality associated with fertility and fertility control: 1983. *Fam Plann Perspect* 1983;15:57–63.

8. **Ashraf T, Arnold SB, Maxfield M.** Cost effectiveness of levonorgestrel subdermal implants. Comparison with other contraceptive methods available in the United States. *J Reprod Med* 1994;39:791–8.

9. **Potts M.** Coitus interruptus. In: **Corson SL, Derman RJ, Tyrer L,** eds. *Fertility Control.* Boston: Little, Brown & Co., 1985:299–306.

10. **Vessey M, Lawless M, Yeates D.** Efficacy of different contraceptive methods. *Lancet* 1982; 1:841–3.

11. **McNeilly AS.** Suckling and the control of gonadotropin secretion. In: **Knobil E, Neil JD, Ewing LI, Greenwald GS, Markert CL, Pfaff DW.,** eds. *The Physiology of Reproduction.* New York: Raven Press, 1988:2323–49.

12. **Short RV, Lewis PR, Renfree MB, Shaw G.** Contraceptive effects of extended lactational amenorrhoea: beyond the Bellagio Consensus. *Lancet* 1991:337:715–7.

13. **Saarikoski S.** Contraception during lactation. *Ann Med* 1993;25:181–4.

14. **Trussell J, Grummer-Strawn L.** Contraceptive failure of the ovulation method of periodic abstinence. *Fam Plann Perspect* 1990;22:65–75.

15. **Flynn A, Pulcrano J, Spieler, J.** An evaluation of the Bioself 110 electronic fertility indicator as a contraceptive aid. *Contraception* 1991;44:125–39.

16. **Brown JB, Holmes J, Barker G.** Use of the Home Ovarian Monitor in pregnancy avoidance. *Am J Obstet Gynecol* 1991;165:2008–11.

17. **Rotta L, Matechova E, Cerny M, Pelak Z.** Determination of the fertile period during the menstrual cycle in women by monitoring changes in crystallization of saliva with the PC2000 IMPCON minimicroscopoe. *Cesk Gynekol* 1992;57:340–52.

18. **Guerrero R, Rojas OI.** Spontaneous abortion and aging of human ova and spermatozoa. *N Engl J Med* 1975;293:

19. **Labbock MH, Queenan JT.** The use of periodic abstinence for family planning. *Clin Obstet Gynecol* 1989;32:387–402.

20. **Potts M, McDevitt J.** A use-effectiveness trial of spermicidally lubricated condoms. *Contraception* 1975;11:701–10.

21. **Grady WR, Tanfer K.** Condom breakage and slippage among men in the United States. *Fam Plann Perspect* 1994;26:107–12.

22. **Voeller B, Coulson AH, Bernstein GS, Nakamura RM.** Mineral oil lubricant causes rapid deterioration of latex condoms. *Contraception* 1989;39:95–102.

23. **Stone KM, Grimes DA, Magder LS.** Personal protection against sexually transmitted diseases. *Am J Obstet Gynecol* 1986;155:180–8.

24. **Kelaghan J, Rubin GL, Ory HW, Loyde PM.** Barrier-method contraceptives and pelvic inflammatory disease. *JAMA* 1982;248:184–7.

25. **Cramer DW, Goldman MB, Schiff I, Belisle S, Albrecht B, Stadel B, et al.** The relationship of tubal infertility to barrier method and oral contraceptive use. *JAMA* 1987;257:2246–50.

26. **Connell EB.** Barrier contraceptives. *Clin Obstet Gynecol* 1989;32:377–86.

27. **Judson FN, Ehret JM, Bodin GF, Levin MJ, Rietmeijer CA.** In vitro evaluations of condoms with and without nonoxynol 9 as physical and chemical barrier against Chlamydia trachomatis, herpes simplex virus Type 2 and human immunodeficiency virus. *Sex Transm Dis* 1989;16:251–6.

28. **Fischl MA, Dickinson GM, Scott GB, Klimus N, Fletcher MA, Parks W.** Evaluation of heterosexual partners, children, and household contacts of adults with AIDS. *JAMA* 1987;257:640–4.

29. **deVincenzi I.** A longitudinal study of human immunodeficiency virus transmission by heterosexual partners. European Study Group on Heterosexual Transmission of HIV. *N Engl J Med* 1994;331:341–6.

30. **Zekeng L, Feldblum PJ, Oliver RM, Kaptue L.** Barrier contraceptive use and HIV infection among high-risk women in Cameroon. *AIDS* 1993;7:725–31.

31. **Harris RW, Brinton LA, Cowdell RH, Skegg DC, Smith PG, Vessey MP, et al.** Characteristics of women with dysplasia or carcinoma in situ of the cervix uteri. *Br J Cancer* 1980;42:359–69.

32. **Parazzini F, Negri E, La Vecchia C, Fedele L.** Barrier methods of contraception and the risk of cervical neoplasia. *Contraception* 1989;40:519–30.

33. **Trussel J, Sturgen K, Strickler J, Dominik, R.** Comparative efficacy of the female condom and other barrier methods. *Fam Plann Perspect* 1994;26:66–72.

34. **Soper DE, Brockwell NJ, Dalton HP.** Evaluation of the effects of a female condom on the female genital tract. *Contraception* 1991;44:21–9.

35. **Johnson V, Masters WH.** Intravaginal contraceptive study. Phase II. Physiology. *West J Surg Obstet Gynecol* 1963;71:144–53.

36. **Malyk B.** *Nonoxynol-9: Evaluation of Vaginal Absorption in Humans.* Raritan, NJ: Ortho Pharmaceutical Corp., 1983.

37. **Linn S, Schoenbaum SC, Monson RR, Rosner B, Stubblefield PG, Ryan KJ.** Lack of association between contraceptive usage and congenital malformation in offspring. *Am J Obstet Gynecol* 1983;147:923–8.

38. **Harlap S, Shiono PH, Ramcharon S, Golbus M, Bachman R, Mann J, et al.** Chromosomal abnormalities in the Kaiser-Permanente birth defects study, with special reference to contraceptive use around the time of conception. *Teratology* 1985;31:381–7.

39. **Hooton TM, Hillier S, Johnson C, Roberts PL, Stamm WE.** Esherichia coli bacteriuria and contraceptive method. *JAMA* 1991;265:64–9.

40. **Ferreira AE, Araujo MJ, Regina CH, Diniz SG, Faundes A.** Effectiveness of the diaphragm, used continuously without spermicide. *Contraception* 1993;48:29–35.

41. **Davis JP, Chesney J, Wand PJ, Laventure M.** Toxic shock syndrome: epidemiologic features, recurrence, risk factors and prevention. *N Engl J Med* 1980;303:1429–35.

42. **Koch JP.** The Prentiff contraceptive cervical cap: a contemporary study of its clinical safety and effectiveness. *Contraception* 1982;25:135–9.

43. **Richwald MA, Greenland S, Gerber MM, Potik R, Kersey L, Comas MA.** Effectiveness of the cavity rim cervical cap: results of a large clinical study. *Obstet Gynecol* 1989;74:143–8.

44. **Trussell J, Strickler J, Vaughan B.** Contraceptive efficacy of the diaphragm, the sponge and the cervical cap. *Fam Plann Perspect* 1993;25:100–5.

45. **Shihata AA, Gollub E.** Acceptability of a new intravaginal barrier contraceptive device (Femcap). *Contraception* 1992;46:511–9.

46. **Centers for Disease Control.** Leads from MMWR 1984:33(4). *JAMA* 1984;251:1015.

47. **El Badrawi HH, Hafez ES, Barnhart MI, Fayad M, Shafeek A.** Ultrastructural changes in human endometrium with copper and nonmedicated IUD's in utero. *Fertil Steril* 1981;36:41–9.

48. **Umapathysivam K, Jones WR.** Effects of contraceptive agents on the biochemical and protein composition of human endometrium. *Contraception* 1980;22:425–40.

49. **Habashi M, Sahwi S, Gawish S, Osman M.** Effect of Lippes Loop on sperm recovery from human fallopian tubes. *Contraception* 1980;22:549–55.

50. **Alvarez F, Guiloff E, Brache V, et al.** New insights on the mode of action of intrauterine devices in women. *Fertil Steril* 1989;49:768–73.

51. **Segal S, Alvarez-Sanchez F, Adejeuwon CA, Brache de Mejia V, Leon P, Faundes A.** Absence of chorionic gonadotropin in sera of women who use intrauterine devices. *Fertil Steril* 1985;44:214–8.

52. **Sivin I, Stern J.** Health during prolonged use of levonorgestrel 20 micrograms/d and the copper TCu 380A intrauterine contraceptive devices: a multicenter study. *Fertil Steril* 1994;61:70–7.

53. **Burkeman RT, the Womens' Health Study.** Association between intrauterine devices and pelvic inflammatory disease. *Obstet Gynecol* 1981;57:269–76.

54. **Farley TMM, Rosenberg MJ, Rowe PJ, Chen JH, Meirik O.** Intrauterine devices and pelvic inflammatory disease: an international perspective. *Lancet* 1992;339:785–8.

55. **Lee NC, Rubin GL Borucki R.** The intrauterine device and pelvic inflammatory disease revisited. New results from the Women's Health Study. *Obstet Gynecol* 1988;72:721–6.

56. **Kriplani A, Buckshee K, Relan S, Kapila K.** Forgotten intrauterine device leading to actinomycotic pyometra, 13 years after menopause. *Eur J Obstet Gynecol Reprod Biol* 1994;53: 215–6.

57. **Ory HW. The Womens' Health Study.** Ectopic pregnancy and intrauterine contraceptive devices: new perspectives. *Obstet Gynecol* 1981;57:137–40.

58. **Snowden R.** The progestasert and ectopic pregnancy. *BMJ* 1977;1:1600–1.

59. **Cramer DW, Schiff I, Schoenbaum SC.** Tubal infertility and the intrauterine device. *N Engl J Med* 1985;312:941–7.

60. **Daling JR, Weiss N, Metch BJ.** Primary tubal infertility in relation to the use of an intrauterine device. *N Engl J Med* 1985;312:937–41.

61. **Grimes DA.** The intrauterine device, pelvic inflammatory disease, and infertility: the confusion between hypothesis and knowledge. *Fertil Steril* 1992;58:670–3.

62. **Vessey M, Doll R, Peto R, Johnson B, Wiggins P.** A long term follow up study of women using different methods of contraception—an interim report. *J Biosoc Sci* 1974;8:373–420.

63. **White MK, Ory HW, Rooks JB, Rochat RW.** Intrauterine device termination rates and the menstrual cycle day of insertion. *Obstet Gynecol* 1980;55:220–4.

64. **Burnhill MS.** Intrauterine contraception. In: **Carson SL, Derman RJ, Tyrer LB,** eds. *Fertility Control.* Boston: Little, Brown, 1985:272–88.

65. **Tatum HJ, Schmidt FH, Jain AK.** Management and outcome of pregnancies associated with copper-T intrauterine contraceptive device. *Am J Obstet Gynecol* 1976;126:869–77.

66. **Stubblefield PG, Fuller AF, Foster SG.** Ultrasound guided intrauterine removal of intrauterine contraceptive device in pregnancy. *Obstet Gynecol* 1988;72:961–4.

67. **Tietze C, Lewit S.** Evaluation of intrauterine devices: ninth progress report of the Cooperative Statistical Program. *Stud Fam Plann* 1970;1:1–40.

68. **Lippes J, Zielezny M.** The loop decade. *Mt Sinai J Med* 1975;4:353–6.

69. **Mishell DR Jr.** Vaginal contraceptive rings. *Ann Med* 1993;25:191–7.

70. **Spelsberg TC, Rories C, Rejman JJ.** Steroid action on gene expression. Possible roles of regulatory genes and nuclear acceptor sites. *Biol Reprod* 1989;40:54–69.

71. **Phillips A.** The selectivity of a new progestin. *Acta Obstet Gynecol Scand* 1990;152(Suppl): 21–4.

72. **Godsland IF, Crook D, Simpson R, Proudler T, Felton C, Lees B, et al.** The effects of different formulations of oral contraceptive agents on lipids and carbohydrate metabolism. *N Engl J Med* 1990;323:1375–81.

73. **Brody SA, Turkes A, Goldzieher JW.** Pharmacokinetics of three bioequivalent norethindrone/mestranol-50mcg and three norethindrone/ethinyl estradiol-35 µg formulations: are "low dose" pills really lower? *Contraception* 1989;40:269–84.

74. **Dericks-Tan JSE, Kock P, Taubert HD.** Synthesis and release of gonadotropins: effect of an oral contraceptive. *Obstet Gynecol* 1983;62:687–90.

75. **Gaspard UJ, Dubois M, Gillain D, Franchimont P, Duvivier J.** Ovarian function is effectively inhibited by a low dose triphasic oral contraceptive containing ethinyl estradiol and levonorgestrel. *Contraception* 1984;29:305–18.

76. **Landgren BM.** Mechanism of action of gestagens. *Int J Gynaecol Obstet* 1990;32:95–110.

77. **Luukkainen T, Heikinheimo O, Haukkamaa M, Lahteenmaki, P.** Inhibition of folliculogenesis and ovulation by the antiprogesterone RU 486. *Fertil Steril* 1988;49:961–3.

78. **Van Uem JF, Hsiu JG, Chillik CF, Danforth DR, Ulmann A, Baulieu EE, et al.** Contraceptive potential of RU486 by ovulation inhibition: I. Pituitary versus ovarian action with blockade of estrogen-induced endometrial proliferation. *Contraception* 1989,40:171–84.

79. **Stadel BV.** Oral contraceptives and cardiovascular disease. I. *N Engl J Med* 1981;305:612–8.

80. **Stadel BV.** Oral contraceptives and cardiovascular disease. II. *N Engl J Med* 1981;305:672–8.

81. **Porter JB, Hunter JR, Jick H, Stergachis A.** Oral contraceptives and nonfatal vascular disease. *Obstet Gynecol* 1985;66:1–4.

82. **Maguire MG, Tonascia J, Sartwell PE, Stolley PD, Tockman MS.** Increased risk of thrombosis due to oral contraceptives: a further report. *Am J Epidemiol* 1979;110:188–95.

83. **Ambrus JL, Mink IB, Courey NG, Niswander K, Moore RH, Ambrus CM, et al.** Progestational agents and blood coagulation. VII. Thromboembolic and other complications of oral contraceptive therapy in relationship to pretreatment levels of blood coagulation factors: summary report of a ten year study. *Am J Obstet Gynecol* 1976;125:1057–62.

84. **Winkler UH, Buhler K, Schindler AE.** The dynamic balance of hemostasis: implications for the risk of oral contraceptive use. In: **Runnebaum B, Rabe T, Kissel L,** eds. *Female Contraception and Male Fertility Regulation. Advances in Gynecological and Obstetric Research Series.* Confort, England: Parthenon Publishing Group, 1991:85–92.

85. **Notelovitz M, Kitchens CS, Coone L, McKenzie L, Carter R.** Low dose oral coantraceptive usage and coagulation. *Am J Obstet Gynecol* 1981;141:71–5.

86. **Notelovitz M, Levenson I, McKenzie L, Lane D, Kitchens CS.** The effect s of low dose oral contraceptives on coagulation and fibrinolysis in two high risk populations: young female smokers and older premenopausal women. *Am J Obstet Gynecol* 1985;152:995–1000.

87. **Gerstman BB, Piper JM, Tomita DK, Ferguson WJ, Stadel BV, Lundin FE.** Oral contraceptive dose and the risk of deep venous thromboembolic disease. *Am J Epidemiol* 1991;133:32–7.

88. **Farag AM, Bottoms SF, Mammen EF, Hosni MA, Ali AA, Moghissi KS.** Oral contraceptives and the hemostatic system. *Obstet Gynecol* 1988;71:584–8.

89. **Alving BM, Comp PC.** Recent advances in understanding clotting and evaluating patients with recurrent thrombosis. *Am J Obstet Gynecol* 1992;167:1184–9.

90. **Bertina RM, Koeleman BP, Koster T, Rosendaal FR, Dirven RJ, de Ronde H, et al.** Mutation in blood coagulation factor V associated with resistance to activated protein C. *Nature* 1994;369:64–7.

91. **Vandenbroucke JP, Koster T, Briet E, Reitsma PH, Bertina RM, Rosendaal FR.** Increased risk of venous thrombosis in oral contraceptive users who are carriers of factor V Leiden mutation. *Lancet* 1994;344:1453–57.

92. **Trauscht-Van-Horn JJ, Capeless EL, Easterling TR, Bovill EG.** Pregnancy loss and thrombosis with protein C deficiency. *Am J Obstet Gynecol* 1992;167:968–72.

93. **Mant D, Villard-Mackintosh, Vessey MP, Yeates D.** Myocardial infarction and angina pectoris in young women. *J Epidemiol Community Health* 1987;41:215–9.

94. **Stampfer MJ, Willett WC, Colditz GA, Speizer FE, Hennekens CH.** A prospective study of past use of oral contraceptive agents and risk of cardiovascular diseases. *N Engl J Med* 1988;319:1313–7.

95. **Rosenberg L, Kaufman DW, Helmrich SP, Miller DR, Stolley PD, Shapiro S.** Myocardial infarction and cigarette smoking in women younger than 50 years of age. *JAMA* 1985;253:2965–9.

96. **Hirvonen E, Heikkila-Idanpaan J.** Cardiovascular death among women under 40 years of age using low-estrogen oral contraceptives and intrauterine devices in Finland from 1975-1984. *Am J Obstet Gynecol* 1990:163:281–4.

97. **Godon-Hardy S, Meder JF, Dilouya A, Monsaingeon V, Fredy D.** Ischemic strokes and oral contraception. *Neuroradiology* 1985;27:588–92.

98. **Hannaford PC, Croft PR, Kay CR.** Oral contraception and stroke; evidence from the Royal College of General Practitioners' Oral Contraception Study. *Stroke* 1994;25:935–42.

99. **Lidegaard O.** Oral contraceptives and risk of a cerebral thromboembolic attack: results of a case-control study. *BMJ* 1993;306:956–63.

100. **Bruno A, Adams HP, Biller J, Rezai K, Cornell S, Aschenbrener CA.** Cerebral infarction due to moyamoya disease in young adults. *Stroke* 1988;19:826–31.

101. **Spellacy WN, Buhi WC, Birk SA.** The effect of estrogens on carbohydrate metabolism. Glucose, insulin, and growth hormone studies on 171 women ingesting Premarin, mestranol and ethinyl estradiol for six months. *Am J Obstet Gynecol* 1972;114:378–92.

102. **Lipson A, Stoy DB, La Rosa JC, Muesing RA, Cleary PA, Miller VT, et al.** Progestins and oral contraceptive-induced lipoprotein changes: a prospective study. *Contraception* 1986;34: 121–34.

103. **Knopp RH.** Cardiovascular effects of endogenous and exogenous sex hormones over a woman's lifetime. *Am J Obstet Gynecol* 1988;158:1630–43.

104. **Burkman RT, Zacur HA, Kimball AW, Kwiterovich P, Bell WR.** Oral contraceptives and lipids and lipoproteins: part II—relationship to plasma steroid levels and outlier status. *Contraception* 1989;40:675–89.

105. **Mishell DR Jr, Colodyn SZ, Swanson LA.** The effect of an oral contraceptive on tests of thyroid function. *Fertil Steril* 1969;20:335–9.

106. **Centers for Disease Control Cancer and Steroid Hormone Study.** Oral contraceptive use and the risk of ovarian cancer. *JAMA* 1983;249:1596–9.

107. **Centers for Disease Control Cancer and Steroid Hormone Study.** Oral contraceptive use and the risk of endometrial cancer. *JAMA* 1983;249:1600–4.

108. **Villard-Mackintosh L, Vessey MP, Jones L.** The effects of oral contraceptives and parity on ovarian cancer trends in women under 55 years of age. *Br J Obstet Gynaecol* 1989;96:783–8.

109. **Swann SH, Petitti DB.** A review of problems of bias and confounding in epidemiologic studies of cervical neoplasia and oral contraceptive use. *Am J Epidemiol* 1982;115:10–8.

110. **Vessey M, McPherson K, Lawless M, Yeates D.** Neoplasia of the cervix uteri and contraception: a possible adverse effect of the pill. *Lancet* 1983;2:930–4.

111. **Ursin G, Peters RK, Henderson BE, d'Ablaing G III, Monroe KR, Pike MC.** Oral contraceptive use and adenocarcinoma of cervix. *Lancet* 1994;344:1390–4.

112. **Chilvers C.** Oral contraceptives and cancer. *Lancet* 1994;344:1378–9.

113. **Schlesselman JJ.** Cancer of the breast and reproductive tract in relation to use of oral contraceptives. *Contraception* 1989;40:1–38.

114. **Center for Disease Control Cancer and Steroid Hormone Study.** Long term oral contraceptive use and the risk of breast cancer. *JAMA* 1983;249:1591–1604.

115. **Romieu I, Willett WC, Colditz GA, Stampfer MJ, Rosner B, Hennekens CH, et al.** Prospective study of oral contraceptive use and risk of breast cancer in women. *J Natl Cancer Inst* 1989,81:1313–21.

116. **Caygill CP, Hill MJ.** Oral contraceptives and breast cancer. *Lancet* 1989;1:1258–60.

117. **Stadel BV, Schlesselman JJ, Murray PA.** Oral contraceptives and breast cancer. *Lancet* 1989;1:1257–8.

118. **Murray PM, Stadel BV, Schlesselman JJ.** Oral contraceptive use in women with a family history of breast cancer. *Obstet Gynecol* 1989;73:977–83.

119. **Rooks JB, Ory HW, Ishak KG, Strauss LT, Greenspan JR, Hill AP, et al.** Epidemiology of hepatocellular adenoma: the role of oral contraceptive use. *JAMA* 1979;262:644–8.

120. **Forman D, Doll R, Peto R.** Trends in mortality from carcinoma of the liver and the use of oral contraceptives. *Br J Cancer* 1983;48:349–54.

121. **Wolner-Hanssen P, Eschenbach DA, Paavonen J, Kiviat N, Stevens CE, Critchlow C, et al.** Decreased risk of symptomatic chlamydial pelvic inflammatory disease associated with oral contraceptives. *JAMA* 1990;263:54–9.

122. **Vessey M, Doll R, Peto R, Johnson B, Wiggins PA.** A long term follow up study of women using different methods of contraception an interim report. *J Biosoc Sci* 1974;8:373–427.

123. **Lanes SF, Birmann B, Walker AM, Singer S.** Oral contraceptive type and functional ovarian cysts. *Am J Obstet Gynecol* 1992;166:956–61.

124. **Shy KK, McTiernan AM, Daling JR, Weiss NS.** Oral contraceptive use and the occurrence of pituitary prolactinoma. *JAMA* 1983;249:2204–7.

125. **Adams DB, Gold AR, Burt AD.** Rise in female initiated sexual activity at ovulation and its suppression by oral contraceptives. *N Engl J Med* 1978;299:1145–50.

126. **Bracken MP.** Oral contraception and congenital malformations in offspring: a review and meta-analysis of the prospective studies. *Obstet Gynecol* 1990;76:552–7.

127. **Katz Z, Lancet M, Skornik J, Chemke J, Mogilner BM, Klinberg M.** Teratogenicity of progestogens given during the first trimester of pregnancy. *Obstet Gynecol* 1985;65:775–80.

128. **Back DJ, Orme ML'E.** Pharmacokinetic drug interactions with oral contraceptives. *Clin Pharmacokinet* 1990;18:472–84.

129. **Knopp RH, Bergelin RO, Wahl PW, Walden CE, Chapman MB.** Clinical chemistry alterations in pregnancy and with oral contraceptive use. *Obstet Gynecol* 1985;66:682–90.

130. **Speroff L.** A brief for low-dose pills. *Contemp Ob/Gyn* 1981;17:27–32.

131. **Kay CR.** The happiness pill. *J R Coll Gen Pract* 1980;30:8–10.

132. **Kaunitz AM.** Long-acting injectable contraception with depot medroxyprogesterone acetate. *Am J Obstet Gynecol* 1994;170:1543–9.

133. **Pardthaisong T.** Return of fertility after use of the injectable contraceptive Depo-Provera: updated analysis. *J Biosoc Sci* 1984;16:23–34.

134. **Cundy T, Reid OR, Roberts H.** Bone density in women receiving depot medroxyprogesterone acetate for contraception. *BMJ* 1991;303:13–6.

135. **Fahmy K, Khairy M, Allam G, Gobran F, Alloush M.** Effect of depo-medroxyprogesterone acetate on coagulation factors and serum lipids in Egyptian women. *Contraception* 1991;44:431–4.

136. **Okada Y, Horikawa K.** A case of phlebothrombosis of lower extremity and pulmonary embolism due to progesterone. *Kokyu To Junkan* 1992;40:819–22.

137. **Ishizaki T, Itoh R, Yasuda J, Yamamoto T, Okada H.** Effect of high dose medroxyprogesterone acetate on coagulative and fibrinolytic factors in patients with gynecological cancers. *Gan To Kagaku Ryoho* 1992;19:837–42.

138. **Kaunitz AM, Rosenfield A.** Injectable contraception with depot medroxyprogesterone acetate: current status. *Drugs* 1993;45:857–65.

139. **La Vecchia C.** Depot-medroxyprogesterone acetate, other injectable contraceptives, and cervical cancer. *Contraception* 1994;49:223–9.

140. **World Health Organization.** Depot medroxyprogesterone acetate (DMPA) and the risk of epithelial ovarian cancer. The WHO Collaborative Study of Neoplasia and Steroid Contraceptives. *Int J Cancer* 1991;49:191–5.

141. **Chilvers C.** Breast cancer and depot-medroxyprogesterone acetate: a review. *Contraception* 1994;49:211–22.

142. **Guo-wei S.** Pharmacodynamic effects of once a month combined injectable contraceptives. *Contraception* 1994;49:361–85.

143. **Speroff L, Darney PD.** *A Clinical Guide for Contraception.* Baltimore: Williams & Wilkins, 1992:117–56.

144. **Darney PD.** Hormonal implants: contraception for a new century. *Am J Obstet Gynecol* 1994;170:1536–43.

145. **Gao J, Wang SL, Wu SC, Sun BL, Allonen H, Luukkainen T.** Comparison of the clinical performance, contraceptive efficacy and acceptability of levonorgestrel releasing IUD, and Norplant 2 implants in China. *Contraception* 1990;41:485–94.

146. **Davies GC, Li XF, Newton JR, van Beek A, Coelingh-Bennink HJT.** Release characteristics, ovarian activity and menstrual bleeding pattern with a single contraceptive implant releasing 3 keto desogestrel. *Contraception* 1993;47:251–61.

147. **Haspells AA.** Emergency contraception: a review. *Contraception* 1994;50:101–8.

148. **Yuzpe AA.** Postcoital contraception. *Clin Obstet Gynecol* 1984;11:787–97.

149. **Kane LA, Sparrow MJ.** Postcoital contraception: a family planning study. *N Z Med J* 1989;102:151–3.

150. **Lippes J, Malik T, Tautum HJ.** The postcoital copper-T. *Adv Plann Parent* 1976;11:24–9.

151. **Webb AMC, Russell J, Elstein M.** Comparison of Yuszpe regimen, Danazol and Mifepristone (RU486) in oral postcoital contraception. *BMJ* 1992;305:927–31.

152. **Briggs MH, Briggs M.** Oral contraceptives for men. *Nature* 1974;252:585–6.

153. **Wallace EM, Gow SM, Wu FC.** Comparison between testosterone enanthate-induced azoospermia and oligozoospermia in a male contraceptive study. I: Plasma luteinizing hormone, follicle stimulating hormone, testosterone, estradiol, and inhibin concentrations. *J Clin Endocrinol Metab* 1993;77:290–3.

154. **Wallace EM, Aitken RJ, Wu FC.** Residual sperm function in oligozoospermia induced by testosterone enanthate administered as a potential steroid male contraceptive. *Int J Androl* 1992;15:416–24.

155. **Arsyad KM.** Sperm function in Indonesian men treated with testosterone enanthate. *Int J Androl* 1993;16:355–61.

156. **Swerdloff RS, Wang C, Bhasin S.** Developments in the control of testicular function. *Baillieres Clin Endocrinol Metab* 1992;6:451–83.

157. **Murad F, Haynes RC.** Androgens and anabolic steroids. In: **Gilman AG, Goodman LS, Gilman A,** eds. *Goodman and Gilman's The Pharmacological Basis of Therapeutics.* 6th ed. New York: MacMillan, 1980:1448–65.

158. **Marcil-Gratton N.** Sterilization regret among women in metropolitan Montreal. *Fam Plann Perspect* 1988;20:222–7.

159. **Shepard MK.** Female contraceptive sterilization. *Obstet Gynecol Surv* 1974;29:739–87.

160. **Uchida H.** Uchida tubal sterilization. *Am J Obstet Gynecol* 1975;121:153–9.

161. **Irving FC.** A new method of insuring sterility following cesarean section. *Am J Obstet Gynecol* 1924;8:335–7.

162. **Hulka JF.** Methods of female sterilization. In: **Nichols DH,** ed. *Gynecologic and Obstetric Surgery.* St. Louis: Mosby, 1993:640–51.

163. **Hasson HM.** Open laparosocopy. In: **Zatuchni GI, Daly MJ, Sciarra JJ,** eds. *Gynecology and Obstetrics.* Vol. 6. Philadelphia: Harper & Row, 1982:1–8.

164. **Yoon IB, King TM, Parmley TH.** A two-year experience with the Falope ring sterilization procedure. *Am J Obstet Gynecol* 1977;127:109–12.

165. **Soderstrom RM, Levy BS, Engel T.** Reducing bipolar sterilization failures. *Obstet Gynecol* 1989;74:60–3.

166. **DeStefano F, Greenspan JR, Dicker RC, Peterson HB, Strauss LT, Rubin GL.** Complications of interval laparoscopic tubal sterilization. *Obstet Gynecol* 1983;61:153–8.

167. **Poindexter AN, Abdul-Malak M, Fast JE.** Laparoscopic tubal sterilization under local anesthesia. *Obstet Gynecol* 1990;75:5–8.

168. **Peterson HB, DeStefano F, Rubin GL, Greenspan JR, Lee NC, Ory HW.** Deaths attributable to tubal sterilization in the United States, 1977–1981. *Am J Obstet Gynecol* 1983;146:131–6.

169. **Khairullah Z, Huber DH, Gonzales B.** Declining mortality in international sterilization services. *Int J Gynaecol Obstet* 1992;39:41–50.

170. **Weiss NS, Lee NC, Peterson HB.** Tubal sterilization, hysterectomy, and the subsequent occurrence of epithelial ovarian cancer. *Am J Epidemiol* 1991;134:362–9.

171. **Corson SL.** Female sterilization reversal. In: **Corson SL, Derman RJ, Tyrer LB,** eds. *Fertility Control.* Boston: Little, Brown, 1985:107–18.

172. **Neil JR, Hammond GT, Noble AD, Rushton L, Letchworth AT.** Late complications of sterilization by laparoscopy and tubal ligation: a controlled study. *Lancet* 1975;2:669–71.

173. **Kwak HM, Chi IC, Gardner SD, Lau FE.** Menstrual pattern changes in laparoscopic sterilization patients whose last pregnancy was terminated by therapeutic abortion. *J Reprod Med* 1980;25:67–71.

174. **DeStefano F, Huezo C, Peterson HB, Rubin GL, Layde PM, Ory HW.** Menstrual changes after tubal sterilization. *Obstet Gynecol* 1983;62:673–81.

175. **Rulin MC, Davidson AR, Philliber SG, Graves WL, Cushman LF.** Long-term effect of tubal sterilization on menstrual indices and pelvic pain. *Obstet Gynecol* 1993;82:118–21.

176. **Liskin LS, Pile JM, Quillin WF.** Vasectomy—safe and simple. Baltimore, population information program. *Popul Rep D* 1983;11(5):62–99.

177. **Walker AM, Jick H, Hunter JR, Danford A, Watkins RN, Alhaoeff L.** Vasectomy and non-fatal myocardial infarction. *Lancet* 1981;1(8210):13–5.

178. **Goldacre MJ, Holford TR, Vessey MP.** Cardiovascular disease and vasectomy. *N Engl J Med* 1982;308:805–8.

179. **Rosenberg L, Palmer JR, Zauber AG, Warshauer ME, Stolley PD, Shapiro S.** Vasectomy and the risk of prostate cancer. *Am J Epidemiol* 1990;132;1051–5.

180. **Rosenberg L, Palmer JR, Zauber AG, Warshauer ME, Strom BL, Harlap S.** The relation of vasectomy to the risk of cancer. *Am J Epidemiol* 1994;140:431–8.

181. **Giovannucci E, Tosteson TD, Speizer FE, Ascherio A, Vessey MP, Colditz BA.** A retrospective cohort study of vasectomy and prostate cancer in U.S. men. *JAMA* 1993;269:878–82.

182. **Pollack AE.** Vasectomy and prostate cancer. *Adv Contracept* 1993;9:181–6.

183. **Henshaw SK, Morrow E.** Induced abortion. A world review. *Fam Plann Perspect* 1990;22:76–120.

184. **Mahler H.** The safe motherhood initiative: a call to action. *Lancet* 1987;1:668–70.

185. **Alan Guttmacher Institute.** *Aborto Clandestino: Una Realidad Latinoamericana.* New York: The Alan Guttmacher Institute, 1994.

186. **Cates W Jr, Rochat RW.** Illegal abortions in the United States: 1972–1974. *Fam Plann Perspect* 1976;8:86–92.

187. **Lawson HW, Frye A, Atrash HK, Smith JL, Shulman HB, Ramick M.** Abortion mortality, United States, 1972–1987. *Am J Obstet Gynecol* 1994;171:1365–72.

188. **Council on Scientific Affairs, American Medical Association.** Induced termination of pregnancy before and after Roe v Wade: trends in the mortality and morbidity of women. *JAMA* 1992;268:3231–9.

189. **Abortion surveillance: preliminary data—United States 1991.** *MMWR* 1994;43(3):42–4.

190. **Koonin LM, Smith JC, Ramick M, Lawson HW.** Abortion surveillance—United States, 1989. *MMWR* 1992;41(5):1–33.

191. **Susser M.** Induced abortion and health as a value. *Am J Public Health* 1992;82:1323–4.

192. **Atrash HK, Cheek TG, Hogue CJ.** Legal abortion mortality and general anesthesia. *Am J Obstet Gynecol* 1988;158:420–4.

193. **Karman H, Potts M.** Very early abortion using syringe as vacuum source. *Lancet* 1972;1:1051–2.

194. **Stubblefield PG.** Control of pain for women undergoing abortion. *Int J Gynaecol Obstet* 1989;3(Suppl):131–140.

195. **Ulmann A, Silvestre L, Chemama L, Rezvani Y, Renault M, Aguillaume CJ, Baulieu EE.** Medical termination of early pregnancy with mifepristpone (RU486) followed by a prostaglandin analogue: study in 16,639 women. *Acta Obstet Gynecol Scand* 1992;71:278–83.

196. **Peyron R, Aubeny E, Targosz V, Silvestre L, Renault M, Elkik F.** Early termination of pregnancy with mifeprisone (RU486) and the orally active prostaglandin misoprostol. *N Engl J Med* 1993;328:1509–13.

197. **Stovall TG, Ling FW.** Single dose methotrexate: an expanded clinical trial. *Am J Obstet Gynecol* 1993;168:1759–65.

198. **Creinin MD, Darney PD.** Methotrexaate and misoprostol for early abortion. *Contraception* 1993;48:339–48.

199. **Creinin, MD, Darney PD.** Methotrexate for abortion at ≤42 days gestation. *Contraception* 1993;48:519–25.

200. **Wapner RJ, Davis GH, Johnson A, Weinblatt VJ, Fischer RL, Jackson LG.** Selective reduction of multifetal pregnancies. *Lancet* 1990;335:90–3.

201. **Hern WM.** *Abortion Practice.* Philadelphia: JB Lippincott, 1984.

202. **Binkin NJ, Schulz KF, Grimes DA, Cates W Jr.** Urea-prostaglandin versus hypertonic saline for instillation abortion. *Am J Obstet Gynecol* 1983;146:947–52.

203. **Negishi M, Sugimoto Yl, Ichikawa A.** Prostanoid receptors and their biological actions. *Prog Lipid Res* 1993;32:417–34.

204. **Jain JK, Mishell DR.** A comparison of intravaginal misoprostol with prostaglandin E_2 for termination of second trimester pregnancy. *N Engl J Med* 1994;331:290–3.

205. **Winkler CL, Gray SE, Hauth JC, Owen J, Tucker JM.** Mid-second-trimester labor induction: Concentrated oxytocin compared with prostaglandin E_2 suppositories. *Obstet Gynecol* 1991;77:297–300.

206. **Hogue CJR, Cates W Jr, Tietze C.** The effects of induced abortion on subsequent reproduction. *Epidemiol Rev* 1982;4:66–94.

207. **Chung CS, Steinhoff PG, Smith RG, Mi MP.** The effects of induced abortion on subsequent reproductive function and pregnancy. In: *Papers of the East-West Population Institute.* Honolulu: East-West Institute, 1983;86.

208. **Linn S, Schoenbaum SC, Monson RR, Rosner R, Stubblefield PC, Ryan KJ.** The relationship between induced abortion and outcome of subsequent pregnancies. *Am J Obstet Gynecol* 1983;146:136–40.

209. **Stubblefield PG, Monson RR, Schoenbaum SC, Wolfson CE, Cookson DJ, Ryan KJ.** Fertility after induced abortion: a prospective follow-up study. *Obstet Gynecol* 1984;63:186–93.

210. **Thatcher SS.** Hysteroscopic sterilization. *Obstet Gynecol Clin North Am* 1988;15:51–9.

211. **Richart RM, Neuwirth RS, Goldsmith A, Edelman DA.** Intrauterine administration of methyl cyanoacrylate as an outpatient method of permanent female sterilization. *Am J Obstet Gynecol* 1987;156:981–7.

212. **Hieu DT, Tan TT, Tan DN, Nguyet PT, Than P, Vinh DQ.** 33,781 cases of non-surgical female sterilization with quinacrine pellets in Vietnam. *Lancet* 1993;342:213–7.

213. **Talwar GP, Singh O, Pal R, Chatterjee N, Upadhyay SN, Kaushic C, et al.** A birth control vaccine is on the horizon for family planning. *Ann Med* 1993;25:207–12.

214. **Aitken RJ, Peterson M, Koothan PT.** Contraceptive vaccines. *Br Med Bull* 1993;49:88–99.

215. **Zhao SC.** Vas deferens occlusion by percutaneous injection of polyurethane elastomer plugs: clinical experience and reversibility. *Contraception* 1990;41:453–9.

11 Sexuality and Sexual Function

David A. Baram

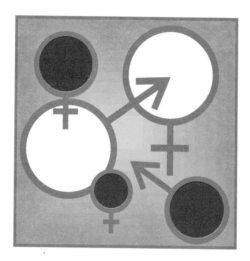

Sexuality and sexual function are a part of a woman's overall health and well-being. Aspects of a woman's sexual function should be included in the general assessment of her health, and appropriate counseling should be offered as needed.

Sexual concerns and sexual dysfunction are common in the general population. According to the results of several recent surveys, approximately 60% of the women questioned had concerns about their sexuality (1, 2). One-third of the women lacked interest in sex, 20% said that sex was not pleasurable, 15% experienced pain with intercourse, up to 50% experienced difficulty becoming aroused, 50% noted difficulty reaching orgasm, and up to 25% were unable to reach orgasm.

One of eight women in the U.S. will be forcibly raped during her lifetime (3), and nearly one-half of women in the U.S. report some type of contact sexual victimization (4). Sexual assault can have long-term effects on a woman's mental and sexual function as well as her general health and well-being.

Despite the importance of these issues to their health care, many women find it difficult to talk to their physicians about sexual concerns, and many physicians are uncomfortable discussing sexual issues with their patients (5). Surveys of primary care physicians reveal that fewer than one-half ask their new patients about sexual practices and concerns and that many physicians make incorrect assumptions about their patients' sexual activity based on age, race, or socioeconomic status (6, 7). Physicians may be concerned that patients will be offended by questions about their sexual practices or may believe that little useful information will be gained by asking patients about sexual concerns or a history of sexual assault. In addition, some physicians may have anxiety about their perceived inability to treat sexual concerns, may believe that they have too little time to obtain a sexual history, or may experience personal discomfort when discussing sexual matters with their patients (8). However, **surveys of patients reveal that they expect their physician to be able to address sex-related concerns and believe it is appropriate for questions about sexuality to be included as a routine part of the gynecologic history** (5).

279

Sexuality

Physicians will feel more comfortable talking to their patients about sex if they have an understanding of the normal sexual response and know how to approach the evaluation and treatment of common sexual dysfunctions. Asking about sexual concerns gives physicians an opportunity to educate patients and dispel sexual myths and misconceptions and gives patients permission to address sexual issues in a professional, confidential, and nonjudgmental setting (9). A few open-ended questions are all that is necessary to elicit a basic sexual history from patients. These questions should be a part of the medical history taken during a routine examination (8):

1. "Are you currently sexually active?" "With men, women, or both?"

2. "Are you or your partner having any sexual difficulties at this time?"

3. "Have you ever experienced any unwanted or harmful sexual activity?"

Further inquiries about specific sexual dysfunction or the sequelae of sexual abuse can be addressed when appropriate, and the patient can be referred for psychologic counseling or sex therapy when necessary (10).

Sexual Practices

Two recent comprehensive surveys provide an interesting and useful description of the sexual behavior of Americans (2, 11). Sexual activity among adolescents in the U.S. has increased significantly during the past 20 years. By 19 years of age, 66–75% of women and 79–86% of men will have had intercourse. Most young men and women have multiple, serial sexual partners. They use condoms infrequently and inconsistently, thus exposing themselves to sexually transmitted diseases and unintended pregnancy. A survey of American men and women between the ages of 18 and 59 years revealed that (2):

- Since 18 years of age, men had an average of six partners and women had an average of two.
- Women have sex with a partner from a few times per month (47%) to 2–3 times per week (32%) to 4 or more times a week (7%). Twelve percent of women have sex a few times per year, and 3% have never been sexually active.
- The most appealing sexual activity for both men and women is vaginal intercourse. Watching their partner undress and receiving and giving oral sex were also considered very pleasurable. Other sexual practices, such as anal sex, group sex, or sex with a stranger were far less appealing.
- Most Americans are monogamous. Seventy-five percent of married men and 85% of married women said they had never been unfaithful.
- There are fewer homosexuals than previously believed—2.7% of men and 1.3% of women had a homosexual partner in the past year. Since puberty, 7.1% of men and 3.8% of women had same-gender sexual partners.
- Twenty-two percent of women said they had been forced to do something sexual, usually by someone they loved, but only 3% of men admitted to forcing themselves on a woman. Perhaps men and women have different ideas about what constitutes sexual coercion.

The Sexual Response Cycle

The sexual response cycle in women is mediated by the complex interplay of psychologic, environmental, and physiologic (hormonal, vascular, muscular, and neurological) factors. **The initial phase of the sexual response cycle is *desire,* followed by the four successive phases originally described by Masters and Johnson (12), *arousal, plateau, orgasm,* and *resolution.*** There is wide variability in the way women respond sexually, and each phase can be affected by aging, illness, medication, alcohol, illicit drugs, and relationship factors.

For most women, the clitoris is the most sexually sensitive part of their anatomy, and stimulation of the clitoris produces the greatest sexual arousal and the most intense orgasms. Other sexually sensitive areas are the nipples, breasts, labia, and, to a lesser extent, the vagina. Although the lower third of the vagina is responsive to touch, the upper two-thirds of the vagina is sensitive primarily to pressure.

There has been speculation about the existence of a G spot (named after Ernest Graefenberg, who first described it in 1944), an area of the vagina located anteriorly midway between the symphysis pubis and the cervix that is believed to be exquisitely sensitive to deep pressure. This area, believed to be similar to the male prostate, has been described as glandular tissue capable of secreting prostatic acid phosphatase into the urethra, sometimes in such copious amounts that women seem to ejaculate during orgasm (13). However, analysis of the fluid "ejaculate" has proven that it is probably urine, not prostatic fluid. It is not uncommon for women who are normally continent to leak urine during orgasm. These women should be reassured that this is a common phenomena and does not require medical intervention.

Desire Phase

Sexual desire is the motivation and the inclination to be sexual. It is a "subjective feeling state" that may be triggered by both internal (fantasy) and external (an interested partner) sexual cues and is dependent on adequate neuroendocrine functioning (14). Desire is influenced by sexual orientation, preferences, psychologic mind-set, and environmental setting.

Arousal (Excitement) Phase

The arousal phase is mediated by the parasympathetic nervous system and is characterized by erotic feelings and the appearance of vaginal lubrication. Sexual arousal increases blood flow to the vagina, and the resulting vasocongestion and possible changes in capillary permeability create a condition that increases the capillary filtration fraction. The filtered capillary fluid transudates between the intercellular spaces of the vaginal epithelium, causing droplets of fluid to form on the walls of the vagina. In addition to feelings of sexual tension, sexually excited women experience tachycardia, rapid breathing, an elevation in blood pressure, a generalized feeling of warmth, breast engorgement, generalized muscle tension (myotonia), nipple erection, mottling of the skin, and a maculopapular erythematous rash ('sex flush') over the chest and breasts. During this phase, the clitoris and labia become swollen; the vagina lengthens, distends, and dilates; and the uterus elevates out of the pelvis (12, 13).

Plateau Phase

During the plateau phase, sexual tension and erotic feelings intensify and vasocongestion reaches maximum intensity. The skin becomes more mottled, the breasts become more engorged, and the nipples become more erect. The labia become more swollen and turn dark red and the lower third of the vagina swells and thickens to form the "orgasmic platform" (12, 13). The clitoris becomes more swollen and elevates to lie nearer the symphysis pubis. The uterus elevates fully out of the pelvis. With adequate sexual stimulation, women reach the point of orgasm.

Orgasm Phase

Orgasm is a myotonic response mediated by the sympathetic nervous system. It is experienced as a sudden release of the tension that has built up during the arousal and plateau stages. Orgasm is the most intensely pleasurable of the sexual sensations. It consists of multiple (3–15) 0.8-second reflex rhythmic contractions of the muscles surrounding the vagina, perineum, anus, and orgasmic platform. Uterine contractions are also experienced by many women during orgasm (12, 13). Thus, some women describe the sensation of an orgasm as different following hysterectomy. Many women who are orgasmic prefer to have orgasms prior to intercourse, during the time when clitoral stimulation is most intense. Unlike men, who are unresponsive to sexual stimulation after orgasm (refractory period), women are potentially multiorgasmic and capable of experiencing more than one orgasm during a single sexual cycle. Thus, they can experience orgasms both before and during intercourse if adequate clitoral stimulation is provided.

Resolution Phase

Following the sudden release of sexual tension brought about by orgasm, women experience a feeling of relaxation and well-being. The physiologic changes that took place during arousal are reversed and the body returns to a resting state. Complete uterine descent, detumescence of the clitoris and orgasmic platform, and decongestion of the vagina and labia takes about 5–10 minutes.

Factors Affecting Sexual Response

Aging

Aging and the cessation of ovarian function accompanying menopause have a significant effect on the sexual response cycle of women. **Sexual desire and the frequency of intercourse decrease as women age, although women retain interest in sex and continue to have the potential for sexual pleasure for their entire lives.** The need for closeness, love, and intimacy does not change with age. The way women function sexually as they grow older is largely dependent on partner availability and how frequently they had sex and how much they enjoyed sex when they were younger (15).

Anatomic changes that accompany aging are noted in Table 11.1. These changes predispose women to more frequent episodes of vulvovaginitis and urinary tract infections that, along with decreased vaginal lubrication, may cause dyspareunia. The effects of aging on sexual physiology are noted in Table 11.2. Women who remain coitally active after menopause have less vulvar and vaginal atrophy than abstinent women (16).

Illnesses that accompany aging may also have an impact on sexual function. Arteriosclerosis may decrease vaginal blood flow and cause decreased arousal, lubrication, and orgasmic intensity. Chronic obstructive pulmonary disease may cause lowered testosterone levels, impairing sexual desire. Pain from an arthritic hip may make it difficult for a woman to find a comfortable position for intercourse.

Table 11.1   Anatomic Changes of Aging

Reduced vaginal size

Thinning of vaginal walls

Decreased elasticity of vaginal walls

Shrinkage of the labia majora

Thinning of the labia minora

Decreased clitoral sensitivity

Decreased clitoral size

Reduced perineal muscle tone

Thinner orgasmic platform

Breast atrophy

Decreased breast engorgement during arousal

Sensory changes in the nipple and areola

From **Masters WH, Johnson VE.** *Human Sexual Response.* Boston: Little, Brown and Company, 1966.

Table 11.2   Sexual Physiology—Effects of Aging

Increased time required to become sexually aroused

Longer time needed to lubricate

Production of less vaginal lubrication

Less intense orgasms

Increased need for stimulation to become orgasmic

No change in the ability to have orgasms

Less likely to be multiorgasmic

From **Mooradian AD, Greiff V.** Sexuality in older women. *Arch Intern Med* 1990;150:1033–8.

Several psychosocial factors may influence an older woman's sexual activity. Older women may lack a sexual partner or their partner may develop erectile dysfunction. The couple may have had an unsatisfactory sexual relationship earlier in life and may not be able to successfully negotiate the changes and possible sexual dysfunctions that can come with aging. Couples may find that they can no longer function sexually as they did in the past and are unable to make the transition to a new (noncoital) way of lovemaking. Other factors include privacy issues (such as living in a nursing home), reluctance to masturbate if a partner is not available, and the negative attitudes of society toward sexuality in older women (15).

Management of sexual difficulties in older women should include local or systemic estrogen supplementation to alleviate vaginal dryness, urinary tract symptoms, and dyspareunia. The sexual expectations of the patient and her partner and an assessment of their current level of sexual functioning should also be evaluated. Myths they may have about sexuality in the elderly should be dispelled. If the couple is interested in retaining sexual function, they should be instructed in alternative forms of sexual expression and ways of alleviating discomfort. However, aging patients may have difficulty changing their sexual expectations and ways of making love. They may not easily adapt to change and may resist reevaluating long-held sexual beliefs, attitudes, behavior, and gender roles. In some cases, couples may be comfortable not having sexual intercourse as a part of their relationship.

Drugs

A variety of prescription and nonprescription medications, including alcohol and illicit drugs, can alter the normal sexual response (Table 11.3) (17–19). The patient's use of these drugs should be assessed as part of the medical history and adjustments in dosage or formulation may be suggested, if appropriate.

Illness

Both acute (e.g., myocardial infarction) and chronic illnesses (e.g., chronic renal disease or arthritis) can create depression, a distorted body image, physical discomfort, and disturbances in the hormonal, vascular, and neurologic integrity needed for sexual functioning (20). Neurologic disorders that impair sexual functioning include multiple sclerosis, alcoholic neuropathy, and spinal cord injury. Endocrine and metabolic disorders, such as diabetes mellitus, hyperprolactinemia, testosterone deficiency, estrogen deficiency states, and hypothyroidism can affect the sexual response.

Infertility evaluation and treatment can have a significant effect on a woman's body image and feelings of self-worth and self-esteem. Infertility may cause her to feel depressed, helpless, hopeless, unattractive, and sexually undesirable. The loss of sexual spontaneity, a goal-directed approach to sex, and the need for scheduled intercourse may lead to sexual dysfunction and relationship difficulties (21).

Table 11.3   Drugs That Can Interfere With Sexual Functioning

Antihypertensives
Thiazide diuretics
Antidepressants
Antipsychotics
Antihistamines
Barbiturates
Narcotics
Benzodiazepines
Hallucinogens
Amphetamines
Cocaine
Oral contraceptives

Breast cancer diagnosis and treatment can affect sexuality. However, most women cope well with the stress of treatment and do not develop major psychiatric disorders or significant sexual dysfunction. A number of studies have compared women who undergo mastectomies to women who have conservative surgery with breast conservation and have revealed little difference between the two groups in postoperative marital satisfaction, psychologic adjustment, frequency of sex, or incidence of sexual dysfunction. The frequency of breast stimulation with sexual activity does decrease after mastectomy (12). Women who undergo lumpectomy have more positive feelings about their bodies, especially their appearance when naked, than do women who have mastectomies (22). The strongest predictor of postcancer sexual satisfaction is not the extent of the surgery but rather the woman's overall psychologic health, relationship satisfaction, and precancer level of sexual functioning (23).

Common gynecologic procedures performed for either benign or malignant conditions can affect psychosexual functioning (24). An oophorectomy in a premenopausal woman can have a deleterious effect on sexual desire and feelings of sexual arousal. These effects can be reversed by estrogen replacement therapy and, when indicated, androgen replacement (25, 26). **A number of studies have demonstrated that abdominal hysterectomy does not have an adverse effect on sexual functioning if the vagina is not shortened excessively and if the ovaries are preserved.** Many women report a decrease in dyspareunia and an increase in libido and frequency of intercourse following hysterectomy for benign disease (25, 27, 28).

Women who undergo surgery for gynecologic cancer experience more sexual dysfunction (inhibited sexual desire, decreased arousal, dyspareunia, and anorgasmia) and are less sexually active than healthy women of the same age (29, 30). Dyspareunia may be related to a decrease in vaginal lubrication secondary to surgical menopause or to vaginal scarring from radiation therapy. Some patients, especially those with cervical cancer, may worry that resumption of sexual activity may provoke a recurrence of their disease (31). Among patients with gynecologic cancer, sexual activity following treatment does not seem related to the type of cancer or the stage of the disease.

Physicians should discuss sexual concerns with the patient and her partner prior to surgery, attempt to dispel myths and misconceptions, and continue to offer counseling to patients after treatment. Specific technical advice (the use of water-based lubricating jelly, noncoital sexual activity for patients with severe dyspareunia, the use of vaginal dilators, and Kegel's exercises) should also be provided (32). Women who function well prior to surgery and have a positive self-image will be better able to cope with the sexual difficulties caused by gynecologic cancer treatment than women with poor precancer sexual adjustment (30).

Sexual Dysfunction

The sexual dysfunctions include:

1. Sexual desire disorders (hypoactive or inhibited sexual desire and sexual aversion)

2. Sexual arousal disorders

3. Orgasmic disorders

4. Sexual pain disorders (vaginismus and dyspareunia)

5. Sexual disorders due to general medical conditions and substance abuse.

Each disorder can be further classified as either (32):

1. Lifelong or acquired (after a period of normal sexual functioning)

2. Generalized (i.e., not limited to a specific partner or situation)

3. Situational.

A comprehensive history is an important part of the evaluation of patients with sexual dysfunction. The following areas should be included (33, 34):

1. A specific description of the dysfunction and an analysis of current sexual functioning

2. When the dysfunction began and how it progressed over time

3. Any precipitating factors

4. The patient's theory about what caused the dysfunction

5. What effect the dysfunction has had on her relationship

6. Past treatment and outcomes

7. Expectations and goals for treatment

8. Understanding of sexual physiology and sexual behavior

9. Any myths or misinformation

Although many physicians have some anxiety about discussing sexual issues with their patients and believe that they lack the basic skills to provide sexual counseling, most sexual concerns can be treated by the general gynecologist. The **PLISSIT** model (35) is a useful sexual counseling and therapy method consisting of four levels of therapeutic intervention. Using the first three levels of this model, approximately 80–90% of sexual concerns can be addressed (34). The **PLISSIT** model is as follows:

1. *Permission* validates the patient's feelings and gives her permission to address her sexual concerns.

2. *Limited Information* provides the patient with information about sexual physiology and behavior.

3. *Specific Suggestions* involve specific reeducation regarding the patient's sexual attitudes and practices.

4. *Referral for Intensive Therapy* is reserved for those patients who do not respond to the first three levels of intervention and who may require intensive individual or couple therapy.

As an example of a specific suggestion, a woman with primary anorgasmia is first given permission to look at her genitalia and touch her clitoris. She is then given limited information about genital anatomy and the physiology of the sexual response. Specific suggestions are then offered about using fantasy and directed masturbation, encouraging her to make use of self-help books such as Heiman and LoPiccolo's *Becoming Orgasmic: A Sexual and Personal Growth Program for Women*. Patients who have been sexually abused or who have significant anxiety or depression, sexual aversion, or significant marital dysfunction should be referred to a therapist who specializes in these areas.

Desire Phase Disorders (Hypoactive or Inhibited Sexual Desire)

Hypoactive sexual desire is a deficiency or absence of sexual fantasies and desire for sexual activity causing marked distress and interpersonal difficulty. Patients with desire phase disorders have little interest in seeking sexual stimuli but often retain the ability to become sexually aroused and experience orgasm if they are approached sexually by their partner. This disorder usually develops in adulthood, often after a period of adequate sexual interest and functioning. Some individuals may experience sexual aversion, a complete avoidance of all sexual activity with a partner (32). Desire phase disorder is the most common sexual dysfunction in both women and men and is the most difficult to treat (36, 37).

Physiologic causes of hypoactive sexual desire include medications (Table 11.3), chronic medical illnesses, depression, stress, substance abuse, aging, and hormonal alterations (18, 38). Serum testosterone and prolactin levels should be evaluated in any patient presenting with the recent onset of a desire phase disorder because elevated prolactin levels (from a pituitary adenoma) or low testosterone levels (sometimes following natural or surgical menopause) could be responsible. Some postmenopausal patients who experience dyspareunia secondary to vaginal atrophy may avoid intercourse. This condition will resolve with systemic or vaginal estrogen replacement therapy.

Individual causes of inhibited sexual desire include religious orthodoxy, anhedonic or obsessive-compulsive personality (these patients may lack the capacity for play and find it difficult to display emotion), masked sexual deviation (e.g., transvestism), fear of pregnancy or sexually transmitted diseases, and object choice issues (i.e., the patient may be a homosexual trying to function sexually in a heterosexual relationship). Some individuals experience an unconscious and involuntary suppression of sexual desire and actively avoid sexual situations. They may suppress their desire by evoking negative thoughts or by allowing spontaneously emerging negative thoughts to intrude when they have a sexual opportunity (38). Sexual desire can also be inhibited by performance anxiety, low self-esteem, depression, the anticipation of an unpleasant sexual experience, fear of intimacy, or residual guilt about sex and pleasure. Women who have been sexually abused as children or sexually assaulted as adults may experience sexual avoidance or aversion. Some patients may fear loss of control over their sexual feelings and, therefore, may suppress them completely. If a patient is experiencing another form of sexual dysfunction, such as dyspareunia or anorgasmia, she may also be experiencing decreased sexual desire (38).

Relationship causes of low sexual desire include lack of sexual attraction for the partner (due to factors such as poor hygiene), poor sexual skills, inexperience of one or both partners, marital conflict, or fear of closeness due to distrust of the partner or a sense of vulnerability. Some couples experience sexual difficulties because of differences in feelings regarding how close one partner would like to be to the other. One partner may want to be very close, whereas the other desires more distance (39). Couples may be sexually incompatible, with one partner making sexual demands the other is unable or unwilling to accommodate. Couples may have difficulty with the timing or the way they initiate sexual activity, or they may have incompatible levels of sexual desire (40). Spouse abuse, financial problems, and marital power and control issues can affect sexual desire. It is difficult for anyone to feel sexual if they are depressed about the relationship, angry with their partner, or feeling unloved.

Treatment of patients with inhibited sexual desire may require both individual therapy and relationship counseling. Insight-oriented psychotherapy may allow the patient to identify the negative feelings that inhibit her erotic impulses and to gain insight into the underlying causes of her low sexual desire (38). Individual "homework" assignments include identifying erotic feelings, body awareness exercises, reading about human sexuality and sexual techniques, and fantasy training (41). In addition, the couple is instructed in how to perform structured sexual exercises known as *sensate focus exercises* (42). These behavior modification exercises are designed to reduce sexual anxiety and to provide the couple with a nondemanding, nonthreatening, and reassuring environment in which they can address performance anxiety, sexual communication issues, and lack of sexual experience and knowledge (38).

Orgasmic Dysfunction

Orgasmic dysfunction in women is characterized by persistent or recurrent delay in or absence of orgasm following a normal sexual excitement phase, resulting in distress or interpersonal difficulty. Orgasmic dysfunction is more prevalent in younger and less sexually experienced women. Primary (lifelong) anorgasmia is found in approximately 5–10% of women (37) and is more common than secondary (acquired) anorgasmia. Some women develop secondary anorgasmia due to relationship problems, depression, substance abuse, prescription medication (e.g., *fluoxitine*), chronic medical illness (e.g., diabetes), estrogen deficiency, or neurologic disorders (e.g., multiple sclerosis) (32). Many women who are orgasmic with masturbation and during noncoital sex may be distressed because they are not orgasmic during intercourse, do not have multiple orgasms or an orgasm with every sexual encounter, or do not have an orgasm at the same time as their partner. Surveys of sexual behavior demonstrate, however, that most couples do not experience orgasm simultaneously, and that many women are more likely to be orgasmic during foreplay, when they receive more direct and intense clitoral stimulation, than during intercourse (37).

The most common psychologic cause of anorgasmia is obsessive self-observation and monitoring during the arousal phase, often accompanied by anxiety and distracting, negative, and self-defeating thoughts (43, 44). A woman with orgasmic dysfunction may be so busy monitoring her own and her partner's response and so concerned about "failing" that she is unable to relax enough to allow her natural reflexes to take over and trigger an orgasm (38, 45). Masters and Johnson call this form of performance anxiety "spectatoring" (38). Inhibited orgasm may be related to a history of sexual abuse, negative feelings toward sexuality, relationship problems, low self-esteem, poor body image, or fear of losing control (44).

Numerous programs have been proposed for the treatment of orgasmic dysfunction (44). Approaches include evaluation and treatment of medical and psychiatric disorders (including substance abuse), sex education, communication and sexual skills training, marital therapy, group therapy, erotic fantasy, and counseling to reduce sexual anxiety and performance anxiety. The Masters and Johnson approach (37) uses sensate focus exercises aimed at reducing anxiety, improving sexual technique, reawakening natural sensuality, and eliminating the goal-oriented approach to sexuality. Although Masters and Johnson have claimed an 80% success rate for their program, others were not always able to replicate their results (44).

The most effective treatment for primary anorgasmia is a program of directed masturbation while employing erotic fantasy. Success rates of 80–90% have been reported using this technique (45). Several excellent self-help books are available to help women learn how to become orgasmic through masturbation. These include Heiman and LoPiccolo's *Becoming Orgasmic* and Barbach's *For Yourself.* A vibrator may be useful if the patient is unable to have an orgasm without one. Once the patient has experienced orgasm through masturbation, she may want to have orgasms while she is with her partner, either during foreplay or intercourse. Manual stimulation of the clitoris while having intercourse (the bridge technique) may help women become orgasmic with their partner.

Sexual Pain Disorders

Vaginismus

Vaginismus is the recurrent or persistent involuntary contraction of the perineal muscles surrounding the outer third of the vagina when vaginal penetration with a penis, finger, tampon, or speculum is attempted (32). Vaginismus is an involuntary reflex precipitated by real or imagined attempts at vaginal penetration. It can be *global,* in which the woman is unable to place anything inside her vagina, or *situational,* in which she is able to use a tampon and can tolerate a pelvic examination but cannot have intercourse. Many women with vaginismus have normal sexual desire, experience vaginal lubrication, and are orgasmic but are unable to have intercourse. Vaginismus can be *primary,* in which the woman has never been able to have intercourse, or *secondary,* which is often due to acquired dyspareunia. Some couples may cope with this difficulty for years before they seek help. They usually seek treatment because they desire children or decide they would like to consummate their relationship. Vaginismus is relatively rare, affecting approximately 1% of women (37).

Vaginismus can be a conditioned response to an unpleasant experience such as past sexual abuse, a painful first pelvic examination, or a painful first attempt at intercourse. It may occur secondary to religious orthodoxy or sexual orientation concerns (46, 47). Many women with vaginismus have an extreme fear of penetration and misconceptions about their anatomy and about the size of their vagina. They may believe that their vagina is too small to accommodate a tampon or penis and that great physical harm will result from placing anything inside the vagina.

Although medical conditions are rarely the cause of vaginismus, conditions such as endometriosis, chronic pelvic inflammatory disease, partially imperforate hymen, and vaginal stenosis must be ruled out by a careful pelvic examination. The pelvic examination, which should be performed, if possible, in the presence of the woman's partner, allows the physician to help educate the couple about normal female anatomy and may help dispel misconceptions about the size of the introitus and vagina. Providing the patient with a mirror to observe the examination is helpful. Because the etiology of vaginismus is usually psychophysiologic, patients with this condition should not have surgery to "enlarge" their introitus unless they have a partially imperforate hymen or other valid indication for surgery.

Treatment of vaginismus is directed toward extinguishing the conditioned involuntary vaginal spasm. This can be accomplished by the following:

1. Help the woman become more familiar with her anatomy and more comfortable with her sexuality.

2. Teach her techniques to help her relax when she anticipates vaginal penetration.

3. Instruct her in the use of Kegel's exercises in order to gain control over the muscles surrounding her introitus.

4. Instruct her how to use graduated rubber dilators (fingers can also be used as dilators).

The protocol for use of the dilators is explained to the patient while she is in the office, but the actual placement of the dilators is done by the patient when she is at home. It is important for the patient to maintain total control over the use the dilators and to use them in an environment that is comfortable and safe. The dilators should be covered with a warm, water-soluble lubricant. She should initially try to place the dilators (or her finger) in her vagina when she is alone and relaxed. If she is unable to relax enough to place to smallest dilator in her vagina, she may be able to reduce her anxiety by learning relaxation or self-hypnosis techniques. Medications, such as *propranolol* or *alprazolam,* may also help reduce anxiety. Once the patient has been able to place the smallest dilator in her vagina, she can progressively insert the larger dilators, practicing Kegel's exercises while the dilators are in place. When she is comfortable inserting the larger dilators, she can instruct her partner how to place the dilators in her vagina while she maintains control over how quickly the dilators are placed. She may then be ready to proceed to intercourse. Again, this must be under her control, with her sitting or kneeling over her partner and inserting his penis herself. Most couples (90%) who follow this protocol are successful and able to have intercourse.

Dyspareunia

Dyspareunia ("difficult mating") is genital pain that occurs before, during, or after intercourse in the absence of vaginismus. The repeated experience of pain during intercourse can cause marked distress, anxiety, and interpersonal difficulties, leading to anticipation of a negative sexual experience and eventually to sexual avoidance (32). As with other forms of sexual dysfunction, dyspareunia can be generalized or situational, lifelong or acquired. Secondary dyspareunia occurs, on the average, about 10 years after the onset of sexual activity. **Dyspareunia is one of the most common sexual dysfunctions seen by gynecologists and is estimated to affect about two-thirds of women during their lifetime** (48). Women with dyspareunia usually discuss the pain with their sexual partner, but fewer than one-half of these women consult a physician. Because dyspareunia is a psychophysiologic condition, both psychologic and physical factors must be considered in patient assessment.

A careful history should be directed toward a complete chronology of the discomfort, an assessment of the impact of the dyspareunia on the patient and her partner, and any prior attempts to treat the condition (46, 47, 49). During the physical examination, attempts should be made to identify any often subtle organic factors contributing to the discomfort. Physiologic changes that take place during sexual arousal may account for pain that is present during intercourse but absent at other times, such as during a routine pelvic examination. Examples are Bartholin gland cysts, which swell during intercourse, and adhesive bands that form between portions of the hymenal ring only during arousal (46).

Causes of pain on stimulation of the external genitalia include chronic vulvitis and clitoral irritation and hypersensitivity. Pain at the introitus caused by penile entry can be caused by a rigid hymenal ring, scar tissue in an episiotomy repair, a Müllerian abnormality, vaginitis caused by one of the many common vaginal pathogens such as candida, trichomonas, or Gardnerella, or by irritation from over-the-counter vaginal sprays, douches, or contraceptive devices. Vaginal infection is the most common cause of successfully treated dyspareunia (50). A common cause of dyspareunia is friction due to inadequate sexual arousal. This situation can be resolved by counseling the couple to spend more time with foreplay, ensuring that the woman has adequate lubrication prior to intercourse. Use of a water-soluble lubricant (e.g., *Astroglide*) also is helpful. Vaginal atrophy resulting from hypoestrogenic states (menopause and lactation) can be treated with systemic or vaginal estrogen replacement.

289

Vulvar vestibulitis syndrome is a constellation of symptoms consisting of severe pain or burning on touching the vestibule and attempting vaginal entry. The treatment of this syndrome is empiric because the etiology is unknown (48). A comprehensive multimodality approach may be necessary, as outlined in Chapter 14. Associated infections should be treated, vulvovaginal irritants should be eliminated, and surgery (vestibulectomy with vaginal advancement) should be reserved for patients with severe dyspareunia who have not responded to conservative management (48).

Causes of midvaginal pain include a congenitally shortened vagina, interstitial cystitis, and urethritis. Pain with orgasm may be associated with uterine contractions. Dyspareunia with deep vaginal penetration can be associated with inadequate vaginal lengthening and lubrication secondary to inadequate sexual arousal, chronic pelvic inflammatory disease, endometriosis, a fixed retroverted uterus, a pelvic mass, an enlarged uterus as a result of myomas or adenomyosis, inflammatory bowel disease, irritable bowel syndrome, or pelvic relaxation (49).

Psychological factors contributing to dyspareunia include:

1. *Developmental factors,* e.g., an upbringing that invested sex with guilt and shame

2. *Traumatic factors,* e.g. childhood sexual abuse or other sexual assault

3. *Relationship factors,* e.g., anger or resentment toward a sexual partner.

Lazarus (51) uses the mnemonic **BASIC ID** to describe his multimodal approach to the assessment of dyspareunia. This approach addresses the issues noted in Table 11.4.

Sexual Assault

Sexual assault of children and adult women has reached epidemic proportions in the U.S. and is the fastest growing, most frequently committed, and most underreported crime (52, 53). Sexual assault is a crime of violence, not passion, and encompasses a continuum of sexual activity that ranges from sexual coercion to contact abuse (unwanted kissing, touching, or fondling) to forcible rape. In a survey of female family practice patients, 47% reported some type of contact sexual victimization during their lifetime. Twenty-five percent reported attempted rape and 13% had been forcibly raped, many as children (4). **The terms *sexual abuse survivor* or *assault survivor* are preferable to *victim*.**

Table 11.4 Assessment of Dyspareunia	
Behavior	Faulty technique
Affect	Guilt, anger, fear and shame
Sensation	Where is the pain?
Imagery	Do intrusive thoughts or negative images disrupt sexual enjoyment?
Cognition	Are there dysfunctional beliefs or misinformation that play a role in undermining sexual participation?
Interpersonal	How do the partners communicate and relate in both sexual and nonsexual settings?
Drugs	Is the patient on any medication that would diminish vaginal lubrication?

From **Lazarus AA.** Dyspareunia: a multimodal psychotherapeutic perspective. In: **Leiblum SR, Rosen RC,** eds. *Principles and Practice of Sex Therapy.* 2nd ed. New York: The Guilford Press, 1989:89–112.

Childhood Sexual Abuse

Childhood sexual abuse has a profound and potentially lifelong effect on the survivor. Whereas most cases of childhood sexual abuse are not reported by the survivor or her family, it is estimated that as many as one-third of adult women were sexually abused as children. Younger children are more often exposed to genital fondling or noncontact abuse (exhibitionism or forced observation of masturbation), and children older than 10 years of age are more likely to be forced to have intercourse or oral sex (54). As children age, they are more likely to experience sexual abuse outside the home and more likely to be victimized by strangers. As adolescents, women survivors of childhood sexual abuse are at risk for early unplanned pregnancy, prostitution, antisocial behavior, running away from home, eating disorders, and multiple somatic symptoms. These women are more likely to engage in health risk behaviors such as smoking, substance abuse, and early sexual activity with multiple partners (55). They may be unable to trust or establish rapport with adults. Women survivors of childhood sexual abuse often develop feelings of powerlessness and helplessness and may become chronically depressed. There is a high incidence of self-destructive behavior, including suicide and deliberate self-harm such as cutting or burning themselves (56, 57). They are also at risk of becoming victimized again later in life (58).

Women who have been sexually abused as children or sexually assaulted as adults often experience sexual dysfunction and difficulty with intimate relationships and parenting (59). Compared to women who have not been sexually assaulted, they are more likely to experience depression, chronic anxiety, anger, substance abuse problems, multiple personality disorder, borderline personality disorder, fatigue, low self-esteem, feelings of guilt, and sleep disturbance (60). They often experience social isolation, phobias, and feelings of vulnerability and loss of control (3, 61). Survivors of sexual assault represent a disproportionate number of patients with chronic headaches and chronic pelvic pain (62). They may develop *posttraumatic stress disorder (PTSD),* defined as development of characteristic symptoms following a psychologically traumatic event outside of normal human experience. Symptoms of PTSD include blunting of affect, intrusive reexperiencing of the incident, avoidance of stimuli associated with the assault, and intense psychologic distress and agitation in response to reminders of the event (52, 56). Women affected by PTSD are more likely to commit suicide. The cognitive sequelae include flashbacks, nightmares, disturbances in perception, and dissociative experiences (63). These women may not be able to tolerate pelvic examinations and may avoid seeking routine gynecologic care; however, they are more likely to use the medical care system for nongynecologic concerns (64). Women with PTSD are at greater risk for being overweight and having gastrointestinal disturbances (55).

Rape

Although the legal definition of sexual assault may vary from state to state, most definitions of rape include:

1. **The use of physical force, deception, intimidation, or the threat of bodily harm**

2. **Lack of consent or inability to give consent because the survivor is very young or very old, impaired by alcohol or drug use, unconsciousness, or mentally or physically impaired**

3. **Oral, vaginal, or rectal penetration with a penis, finger, or object.**

The National Women's Study provides the best statistics available about the incidence of forcible rape in the U.S. (3). This study revealed that 13%, or one of eight adult women, are survivors of at least one completed rape during their lifetime. Of the women they surveyed, 0.7% had been raped during the past year, equaling an estimated 683,000 adult women who were raped during a 12-month period. Of the women surveyed, 39% were raped more than once. Most disturbing, however, is the finding that most of rapes occurred during childhood and adolescence; 29% of all forcible rapes occurred when the survivor was younger than 11 years of age, and 32% occurred between the ages of 11 and 17 years. Indeed, "rape in America is a tragedy of youth" (3). Twenty-two percent of rapes occurred between the ages of 18 and 24 years, 7% between the ages of 25 and 29 years, and only 6% occurred when the survivor was older than 30 years of age.

There are many myths about rape. Perhaps the most common is that women are raped by strangers. In fact, only about 20–25% of women are raped by someone they do not know. Most women are raped by a relative or acquaintance (9% by husbands or ex-husbands, 11% by fathers or stepfathers, 10% by boyfriends or ex-boyfriends, 16% by other relatives, and 29% by other nonrelatives) (3). Although acquaintance rape may seem to be less traumatic than stranger rape, survivors of acquaintance rape often take longer to recover. Another common misconception about rape is that most survivors sustain serious physical injury. Seventy percent of rape survivors report no physical injury, and only 4% sustain serious injury. Serious injury is rare, although almost one-half of the rape survivors report being fearful of serious injury or death during the assault (3). About 1% of sexual assaults result in death.

There are at least four types of rapists (65).

1. *Opportunist rapists (30%)* **exhibit no anger toward the women they assault and usually use little or no force.** These rapes are impulsive and may occur in the context of an existing relationship ("date" or acquaintance rape).

2. *Anger rapists (40%)* **usually batter the survivor and use more physical force than is necessary to overpower her.** This type of sexual assault is episodic, impulsive, and spontaneous. The rapist is angry or depressed and is often seeking retribution—for perceived wrongs or injustices he imagines have been done to him by others, especially women. He may victimize the very young or the very old.

3. *Power rapists (25%)* **do not intend to harm their victim but rather to possess or control her in order to gain sexual gratification.** However, a power rapist may use force or the threat of force to overcome his victim. These assaults are premeditated, repetitive, and may increase in aggression over time. The rapist is usually anxious and may give orders to his victim, ask her personal questions, or inquire about her response during the assault. This assault may occur over an extended period of time while the victim is held captive. These rapists are insecure about their virility and are trying to compensate for their feelings of inadequacy and low self-esteem.

4. *Sadistic rapists (5%)* **become sexually excited by inflicting pain on their victim.** These rapists may have a thought disorder and often exhibit other forms of psychopathology. This type of assault is calculated and planned. The victim is often a stranger. The rape may involve bondage, torture, or bizarre acts and may occur over an extended period of time. The survivor often suffers both genital and nongenital injuries and may be murdered or mutilated. Other rapists may act out of impulse, as when they encounter a victim during the course of another crime such as burglary. Some rapists believe they are entitled to their victim, as in acquaintance rape or father-daughter incest (52). A consistent finding among all types of rapists is a lack of empathy for the survivor.

Even when sexual assaults are reported (only 16% of rapes are ever reported to the police) few rapists are arrested and even fewer are brought to trial and convicted. Fewer than 1% of rapists ever serve a prison term (65). Many women do not report the assault to the police because they are concerned about their name being disclosed by the news media, fear retaliation from the perpetrator, are afraid they will not be believed, or do not trust the judicial process.

292

Only 17% of rape survivors seek medical attention after an assault. Many rape survivors do not inform their physicians about the assault and may never volunteer information about the assault unless they are directly asked. Therefore, when obtaining a medical history, physicians should routinely ask, "Has anyone ever forced you to have sexual relations when you did not want to?"

Effects of Rape

Following sexual assault, women have many concerns, including pregnancy, sexually transmitted diseases (including human immunodeficiency virus [HIV] infection), being blamed for the assault, having their name made public, and having their family and friends find out about the assault. The initial reactions to sexual assault may be shock, numbness, withdrawal, and possibly denial. It is difficult to predict how any assaulted individual will react. Despite their recent trauma, women presenting for medical care may appear calm and detached.

The *Rape Trauma Syndrome* is a constellation of physical and psychologic symptoms including fear, helplessness, disbelief, shock, guilt, humiliation, embarrassment, anger, and self-blame. The acute, or disorganization, phase of the syndrome lasts from days to weeks. Survivors may experience intrusive memories of the assault, blunting of affect, and hypersensitivity to environmental stimuli. They are anxious, do not feel safe, have difficulty sleeping, and experience nightmares and a variety of somatic symptoms (52, 66). They may fear that their assailant will return to rape them again.

In the weeks to months following the sexual assault, survivors often return to normal activities and routines. They may appear to have dealt successfully with the assault, but they may be repressing strong feelings of anger, fear, guilt, and embarrassment. In the months following the assault, survivors begin the process of integration and resolution. During this phase, they begin to accept the assault as part of their life experience, and somatic and emotional symptoms may decrease progressively in severity. However, the sequelae of rape are often persistent and longlasting (56). Over the long term, survivors may have difficulty with work and with family relationships. Disruption of existing relationships is not uncommon. Nearly one-half of the survivors lose their jobs or are forced to quit in the year following the rape (61).

Examination and Treatment

The responsibilities of physicians providing immediate treatment for sexual assault survivors are listed in Table 11.5. **Because of the legal ramifications, consent must be obtained from the patient prior to obtaining the history, performing the physical examination, and collecting evidence. Documentation of the handling of specimens is especially important, and the "chain of evidence" for collected material must be care-**

Table 11.5   Physician Responsibilities in Treating Sexual Assault Survivors

1. Obtaining an accurate gynecologic history, including a recording of the sexual assault.

2. Assessing, documenting, and treating physical injuries.

3. Obtaining appropriate cultures (including samples for forensic tests), treating any existing infection, and providing prophylaxis for sexually transmitted diseases.

4. Providing therapy to prevent unwanted pregnancy.

5. Providing counseling for the patient and her partner and/or family.

6. Arranging for follow-up medical care and counseling.

7. Reporting to legal authorities as required by state law.

From **American College of Obstetricians and Gynecologists.** *Sexual Assault.* Technical Bulletin. Washington, DC: ACOG, 1992:172.

fully maintained. Everyone who handles the evidence must sign for it and hand it directly to the next person in the chain. The patient should be interviewed in a quiet and supportive environment by an examiner who is objective and nonjudgmental. Support personnel and patient advocates, such as family, friends, or, if available, a counselor from a rape crisis service, should be encouraged to accompany the patient. It is important not to leave the survivor alone and to give her as much control as possible over the examination.

The history should include the following information:

1. A general medical history and a gynecologic history, including last menstrual period, prior pregnancies, past gynecologic infections, contraceptive use, and last voluntary intercourse prior to the assault.

2. It is important to ascertain whether the survivor bathed, douched, urinated, defecated, brushed her teeth, or changed her clothes after the assault.

3. A detailed description of the sexual assault should be obtained, including the date and time of the assault, number of assailants, use of weapons, threats, and restraints, and any physical injuries that may have occurred.

4. A detailed description of the type of sexual contact must be obtained, including whether vaginal, oral, or anal contact or penetration occurred, whether the assailant used a condom, and whether there were other possible sites of ejaculation, such as the hands, clothes, or hair of the survivor.

5. The emotional state of the survivor should be observed and recorded.

The survivor should undress while standing on clean examination table paper in order to catch any hair or fibers falling from her clothing. All of her clothing should be placed in individually labeled paper bags, sealed, and given to the proper authorities. Wet or damp clothing should be air dried before packaging. During the physical examination, the degree of injury to the survivor should be assessed and any injuries should be documented for use as evidence. The nature, size, and location of all injuries should be carefully documented, using photographs or drawings if possible. Nongenital injuries occur in 20–50% of all rapes (67). The most common injuries are bruises and abrasions of the head, neck, and arms (52) and genital injuries accompanied by bleeding and pain. The most common genital findings are erythema and small tears of the vulva, perineum, and introitus. There may be bleeding, mucosal tears, erythema, or a hematoma noted around the rectum if penetration has occurred. Identification of small lacerations of the genitalia or rectum may be aided by colposcopy or by staining with toluidine blue. Bite marks are not uncommon and frequently are found on the breasts or genitalia. Foreign bodies may be found in the vagina, rectum, or urethra. If oral penetration has taken place, injuries of the mouth and pharynx may occur (68).

Evidence must be properly collected for legal purposes as follows:

1. Examination of the patient with a Wood's light may help identify semen, which will fluoresce. Areas of fluorescence should be swabbed with a cotton-tipped applicator moistened with sterile water. Swabs of the vagina, mouth, and rectum may be obtained to test for the presence of sperm or semen.

2. A Papanicolaou smear may also be useful to document the presence of sperm.

3. A sample of the vaginal secretions should be obtained for examination for motile sperm, semen, or pathogens. Motile sperm in the vagina indicate ejaculation within 6 hours.

4. Vaginal secretions should also be collected to test for the presence of acid phosphatase, an enzyme found in high concentrations in seminal fluid, and for DNA fingerprinting (69).

5. The survivor's pubic hair should be combed over a sheet of paper in an attempt to obtain pubic hair from the assailant.

6. Fingernail scrapings from the survivor should be collected and evaluated for evidence of the assailant's blood, hair, or skin. DNA fingerprinting may also be used on this evidence.

7. Saliva should be collected from the survivor to document whether she is a secretor of major blood group antigens (80% of the population are secretors). If the patient is not a secretor and blood group antigens are found in vaginal washings, the antigens are probably from the semen of the assailant (69).

Laboratory tests that should be performed on all sexual assault survivors are listed in Table 11.6.

Treatment of sexual assault survivors should be directed to prevention of possible pregnancy and provision of prophylactic treatment for sexually transmitted diseases. Approximately 5% of fertile rape survivors will become pregnant (70). Options include 1) awaiting the next expected menses; 2) repeating the serum pregnancy test in 1–2 weeks; and 3) postcoital contraception. If the patient desires postcoital contraception, a preexisting pregnancy can usually be ruled out by performing a sensitive human chorionic gonadotropin assay. Pregnancy prophylaxis can be provided by the immediate administration of two tablets of a combination oral contraceptive (each containing 50 μg of ethinyl estradiol and 0.5 mg norgestrel, i.e., *Ovral* birth control pills) followed by two more tablets 12 hours later. The regimen is effective if it is administered within 72 hours after the sexual assault. Some patients experience nausea and vomiting when given postcoital contraception; these symptoms can be controlled with an antiemetic agent such as *promethazine* (12.5 mg every 4–6 hours). Postcoital contraception has a small failure rate and potential teratogenicity, which should be explained to the patient (71).

The risk of acquiring a sexually transmitted disease is difficult to assess, because the prevalence of preexisting sexually transmitted diseases is high (43%) in rape survivors (72):

1. Prophylaxis for sexually transmitted disease should be offered to all survivors and should cover infections with *neisseria gonorrhoeae, chlamydia trachomatis,* and

---

Table 11.6   Laboratory Studies In The Evaluation Of Sexually Assaulted Adults

Cultures of the cervix, mouth, and rectum for:
Neisseria gonorrhoeae
Chlamydia trachomatis
Herpes simplex
Cytomegalovirus
Serologic test for syphilis
Wet prep for trichomonas
Hepatitis B surface antigen
Antibody human immunodeficiency virus antibody
Pregnancy test

incubating syphilis. Current recommendations include *ceftriaxone* (250 mg intramuscularly) or *cefixime* (400 mg orally) followed by *doxycycline* (100 mg twice daily) or *tetracycline* (500 mg four times daily) for 7 days (73). If the patient is allergic to *cephalosporins, spectinomycin* 2 g intramuscularly may be used.

2. Hepatitis B prophylaxis should be offered if the assailant is believed to be in a high-risk group for carrying the virus and the survivor has experienced vaginal or anal trauma with bleeding. The treatment is *hepatitis immune globulin (HBIG)* 0.06 ml/kg intramuscularly immediately followed by another dose 1 month later, if the survivor is hepatitis B antibody negative. Another alternative, which provides both short- and long-term protection, is a single dose of HBIG and initiation of hepatitis B vaccination (52).

3. Tetanus prophylaxis (5 ml intramuscularly) should also be administered if indicated.

4. The patient should be instructed to return for repeat serologic tests (syphilis and hepatitis) and sexually transmitted disease cultures in 4 weeks.

5. The HIV test should be repeated in 6 and 12 months.

6. Ongoing supportive counseling for the patient should be arranged, and the patient should be referred to a sexual assault center or a therapist who specializes in the treatment of sexual assault survivors.

References

1. **Frank E, Anderson C, Rubinstein D.** Frequency of sexual dysfunction in "normal couples. *N Engl J Med* 1978;299:11–115.

2. **Michael RT, Gagnon JH, Laumann EO, Kolata G.** *Sex in America.* Boston: Little, Brown and Company, 1994.

3. **Kilpatrick DG, Edmunds CN, Seymour AK.** *Rape in America.* New York: National Victim Center, 1992.

4. **Walch AG, Broadhead WE.** Prevalence of lifetime sexual victimization among female patients. *J Fam Pract* 1992;35:511–6.

5. **Ende J, Rockwell S, Glasgow M.** The sexual history in general medical practice. *Arch Intern Med* 1984;144:558–61.

6. **Hunt AD, Litt IF, Loebner M.** Obtaining a sexual history from adolescent girls. *J Adolesc Health* 1988;9:52–4.

7. **Bowman M.** The new sexual history: inquiring about sexual practices. *Am Fam Physician* 1989;40:82–3.

8. **Bachman GA, Leiblum SR, Grill J.** Brief sexual inquiry in gynecologic practice. *Obstet Gynecol* 1989;73:425–7.

9. **Stevenson RWD, Szasz G, Maurice WL, Miles JE.** How to become comfortable talking about sex to your patients. *Can Med Assoc J* 1983;128:797–800.

10. **Reamy K.** Sexual counseling for the nontherapist. *Clin Obstet Gynecol* 1984;27:781–8.

11. **Seidman SN, Rieder RO.** A review of sexual behavior in the United States. *Am J Psychiatry* 1994;151:330–41.

12. **Masters WH, Johnson VE.** *Human Sexual Response.* Boston: Little Brown and Company, 1966.

13. **Weisberg M.** Physiology of female sexual response. *Clin Obstet Gynecol* 1984;27:697–705.

14. **Leiblum SR, Rosen RC.** *Sexual Desire Disorders.* New York: The Guilford Press, 1988.

15. **Mooradian AD, Greiff V.** Sexuality in older women. *Arch Intern Med* 1990;150:1033–8.

16. **Bachmann GA.** Sexual issues at menopause. *Ann N Y Acad Sci* 1990;592:87–94.

17. Drugs that cause sexual dysfunction: an update. *Med Lett Drugs Ther* 1992;34:73–8.

18. **Kaplan HS.** *The Evaluation of Sexual Disorders: Psychological and Medical Aspects.* New York: Brunner/Mazel, 1983.

19. **Buffum J.** Prescription drugs and sexual function. *Psychiatr Med* 1992;10:181–98.

20. **Wincze JP, Carey MP.** *Sexual Dysfunction.* New York: Guilford Press, 1991.

21. **Keye WR.** Psychosexual responses to infertility. *Clin Obstet Gynecol* 1984;27:760–6.

22. **Schover LR.** The impact of breast cancer of sexuality, body image, and intimate relationships. *CA Cancer J Clin* 1991;41:112–20.

23. **Schover LR, Jensen SB.** *Sexuality and Chronic Illness: A Comprehensive Approach.* New York: Guilford Press, 1988.

24. **Bachman GA.** Psychosexual aspects of hysterectomy. *Womens Health Issues* 1990;1:41–9.

25. **Nathorst-Boos J, von Schoultz B.** Psychological reactions and sexual life after hysterectomy with and without oophorectomy. *Gynecol Obstet Invest* 1992;34:97–101.

26. **Bellarose SB, Yitzchak MB.** Body image and sexuality in oophorectomized women. *Arch Sex Behav* 1993;5:435–59.

27. **Virtanen H, Makinen J, Tenho T, Kiilholma P, Pitkanen Y, Hirvonen T.** Effects of abdominal hysterectomy on urinary and sexual symptoms. *Br J Urol* 1993;72:868–72.

28. **Helmstrom L, Lundberg PO, Sorbom D, Backstrom T.** Sexuality after hysterectomy: a factor analysis of women's sexual lives before and after subtotal hysterectomy. *Obstet Gynecol* 1993;81:357–62.

29. **Thranov I, Klee M.** Sexuality among gynecologic cancer patients—a cross-sectional study. *Gynecol Oncol* 1994;52:14–9.

30. **Anderson BL.** Yes, there are sexual problems. Now, what can we do about them? *Gynecol Oncol* 1994;52:10–3.

31. **Cull A, Cowie VJ, Farquharson DIM, Livingstone JRB, Smart GE, Elton RA.** Early stage cervical cancer: psychosocial and sexual outcomes of treatment. *Br J Cancer* 1993;68:216–20.

32. **American Psychiatric Association.** *Diagnostic and Statistical Manual of Mental Disorders.* 4th ed. Washington, DC: American Psychiatric Association, 1994.

33. **Sanderson MO, Maddock JW.** Guidelines for assessment and treatment of sexual dysfunction. *Obstet Gynecol* 1989;73:130–5.

34. **Franger AL.** Taking a sexual history and managing common sexual problems. *J Reprod Med* 1988;33:639–43.

35. **Pion R, Annon J.** The office management of sexual problems: brief therapy approaches. *J Reprod Med* 1975;15:127–44.

36. **Hawton K, Catalan J, Fagg J.** Low sexual desire: sex therapy results and prognostic factors. *Behav Res Ther* 1991;29:217–24.

37. **Spector IP, Carey, MP.** Incidence and prevalence of the sexual dysfunctions: a critical review of the empirical literature. *Arch Sex Behav* 1990;19:389–408.

38. **Kaplan HS.** *Disorders of Sexual Desire and Other New Concepts and Techniques in Sex Therapy.* New York: Brunner/Mazel, 1979.

39. **Lazarus AA.** A multimodal perspective on problems of sexual desire. In: Leiblum SR, Rosen RC, eds. *Sexual Desire Disorders.* New York: The Guilford Press, 1988:145–67.

40. **Levine SB.** Intrapsychic and individual aspects of sexual desire. In: Leiblum SR, Rosen RC, eds. *Sexual Desire Disorders.* New York: The Guilford Press, 1988:21–44.

41. **LoPiccolo J, Friedman JM.** Broad-spectrum treatment of low sexual desire: integration of cognitive, behavioral, and systemic therapy. In: Leiblum SR, Rosen RC, eds. *Sexual Desire Disorders.* New York: The Guilford Press, 1988:107–44.

42. **Masters WH, Johnson VE.** *Human Sexual Inadequacy.* New York: Bantam Books, 1970.

43. **Wincze JP, Carey MP.** *Sexual Dysfunction: A Guide for Assessment and Treatment.* New York: The Guilford Press, 1991.

44. **McCabe MP, Delaney SM.** An evaluation of therapeutic programs for the treatment of secondary inorgasmia in women. *Arch Sexual Behavior* 1992;21:69–89.

45. **Heiman JR, Grafton-Becker V.** Orgasmic disorders in women. In: **Leiblum SR, Rosen RC,** eds. *Principles and Practice of Sex Therapy.* 2nd ed. New York: The Guilford Press, 1989:51–88.

46. **Steege J.** Dyspareunia and vaginismus. *Clin Obstet Gynecol* 1984;27:750–9.

47. **Lamont J.** Vaginismus. *Am J Obstet Gynecol* 1978;131:632–8.

48. **Marinoff SC, Turner MLC.** Vulvar vestibulitis syndrome: an overview. *Am J Obstet Gynecol* 1991;165:1228–33.

49. **Steege JF, Ling FW.** Dyspareunia. *Obstet Gynecol Clin North Am* 1993;20:779–93.

50. **Glatt AE, Zinner SH, McCormack WM.** The prevalence of dyspareunia. *Obstet Gynecol* 1990;75:433–6.

51. **Lazarus AA.** Dyspareunia: a multimodal psychotherapeutic perspective. In: **Leiblum SR, Rosen RC,** eds. *Principles and Practice of Sex Therapy.* 2nd ed. New York: The Guilford Press, 1989:89–112.

52. **Dunn SFM, Gilchrist VJ.** Sexual assault. *Prim Care* 1993;20:359–73.

53. **Sorenson SB, Stein JA, Siegel JM, Golding JM, Burnam MA.** The prevalence of adult sexual assault. *Am J Epidemiol* 1987;126:1154–64.

54. **Bachman GA, Moeller TP, Bennet J.** Childhood sexual abuse and the consequences in adult women. *Obstet Gynecol* 1988;71:631–42.

55. **Springs FE, Friedrich WN.** Health risk behaviors and medical sequelae of childhood sexual abuse. *Mayo Clin Proc* 1992;67:527–32.

56. **Council on Scientific Affairs, American Medical Association.** Violence against women: relevance for medical practitioners. *JAMA* 1992;267:3184–9.

57. **Wyatt GE, Guthrie D, Notgrass CM.** Differential effects of women's child sexual abuse and subsequent sexual revictimization. *J Consult Clin Psychol* 1992;60:167–73.

58. **Polit DF, White CM, Morton TD.** Child sexual abuse and premarital intercourse among high-risk adolescents. *J Adolesc Health* 1990;11:231–4.

59. **Mackey TF, Hacker SS, Weissfeld LA, Ambrose NC, Fisher MG, Zobel DL.** Comparative effects of sexual assault on sexual functioning of child sexual abuse survivors and others. *Issues Mental Health Nurs* 1991;12:89–112.

60. **Laws A.** Does a history of sexual abuse in childhood play a role in women's medical problems? A review. *J Womens Health* 1993;2:165–72.

61. **Ellis E, Atkeson B, Calhoun K.** An assessment of long term reaction to rape. *J Abnorm Psychol* 1981;90:263–6.

62. **Walling MK, Reiter RC, O'Hara MW, Milburn AK, Lilly G, Vincent SD.** Abuse history and chronic pain in women. 1. Prevalences of sexual abuse and physical abuse. *Obstet Gynecol* 1994;84:193–9.

63. **Hendricks-Matthews MK.** Survivors of abuse. *Prim Care* 1993;20:391–406.

64. **Felitti VJ.** Long-term medical consequences of incest, rape, and molestation. *South Med J* 1991;84:328–31.

65. **Groth AN.** *Men Who Rape: The Psychology of the Offender.* New York: Plenum Press, 1979.

66. **Burgess A, Holmstrom L.** Rape trauma syndrome. *Am J Psychol* 1974;131:981–6.

67. **Geist F.** Sexually related trauma. *Emerg Med Clin North Am* 1988;6:439–66.

68. **Dupre AR, Hampton HL, Morrison H, Meeks GR.** Sexual assault. *Obstet Gynecol Surv* 1993;48:640–7.

69. **American College of Obstetricians and Gynecologists.** *Sexual Assault.* Technical Bulletin. Washington, DC: ACOG, 1992:172.

70. **Beckmann CR, Groetzinger LL.** Treating sexual assault victims. A protocol for health professionals. *Female Patient* 1989;14:78–83.

71. **Beebe DK.** Emergency management of the adult female rape victim. *Am Fam Physician* 1991;43:2041–6.

72. **Jenny C, Hooton TM, Bowers A, Copass MK, Krieger JN, Hillier SL, et al.** Sexually transmitted diseases in victims of rape. *N Engl J Med* 1990;322:713–6.

73. **Abramowicz M.** Drugs for sexually transmitted diseases. *Med Lett Drugs Ther* 1991;33:119–22.

12

Common Psychiatric Problems

Nada L. Stotland

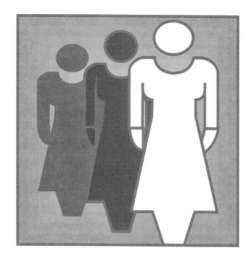

Psychiatric problems are a central or major complicating factor in many outpatient visits for medical care (1, 2). Psychiatric diagnoses are extremely common and account for considerable morbidity and mortality in the population. Unfortunately, psychiatric disorders may be un- or misdiagnosed and under- or mistreated in a nonpsychiatric setting (3–6). Clinical depression, for example, affects up to one-fourth of women at some point in their lives (7, 8), but the 80% of cases are undiagnosed and untreated (9). More than one-half of patients who commit suicide have seen a nonpsychiatric physician within 1 month preceding the act (10).

The Context of Psychiatric Conditions

Attitudes

Few gynecologists feel fully comfortable diagnosing and treating psychiatric problems. Undergraduate medical education does not prepare students for the psychosocial demands of clinical practice, and there is a huge and constantly increasing array of technical knowledge and skills that must be encompassed in gynecologic training programs. Patients who have psychiatric problems provoke various kinds of negative reactions in practitioners (Table 12.1). These reactions are inaccurate and counterproductive. Psychiatric diagnoses are now as reliable and valid as other medical diagnoses, and psychiatric treatments can be specific and effective. When embraced as a ubiquitous and worthy component of practice, psychiatric problems can offer the intellectual challenge and professional gratification that comes with alleviating suffering.

History

There is a long history of association between gynecologic and psychiatric problems. The psychiatric term "hysteria" is derived from the belief of ancient Greek physicians that unexplainable losses of motor and special sensory function in women were caused by the wanderings of unanchored uteri to distant body parts, where they interfered with normal physiology (11). The history of medicine is replete with explanations linking gynecologic and psychiatric pathology. Presumed associations have included premenstrual syndrome, postpartum depression, involutional melancholia, unexplained pelvic pain, and vaginismus. Before the recent advances in knowledge about the causes and treatments of infertil-

299

Table 12.1   Practitioners' Negative Reactions Toward Patients with Psychiatric Problems

1. Social stigma attached to psychiatric diagnoses, patients, and practitioners.

2. Belief that individuals with psychiatric disorders are weak, unmotivated, manipulative, or defective.

3. Belief that the criteria for psychiatric diagnoses are intuitive rather than empirical.

4. Belief that psychiatric treatments are ineffective and unsupported by medical evidence.

5. Fear that patients with psychiatric problems will demand and consume inordinate and limitless time from a medical practice.

6. Precipitation in others, including doctors, of feelings that are complementary to the strong and unpleasant emotions experienced by patients with psychiatric disorders.

7. Gynecologists' own uncertainty about their skills at psychiatric diagnosis, referral, and treatment.

8. Failure to view psychiatric problems as legitimate grounds for medical attention.

ity, including habitual spontaneous abortion, most cases of infertility were ascribed to unconscious emotional conflict. There are still many misconceptions about relationships between psychiatric and gynecologic processes. Some of these are real and situational, whereas others have no basis. Certain gynecologic and medical disorders can have an emotional component (i.e., cancer), and some situations unique to women may precipitate depression.

Impact of Society

Reproductive anatomy and physiology are perceived as central in women's development and psychology in a way that is not true of men. Menstruation and menopause are widely believed to cause depressive symptoms or personality changes. The major changes in women's social roles in North America over the past several decades put these beliefs into new perspectives. Beliefs that women typically exaggerate or imagine physical symptoms may lead to underdiagnosis and neglect of serious medical conditions. The specter of "bored housewives" draining the nation's coffers by spending endless hours in medically needless psychotherapy is adduced in efforts to forestall equitable coverage for legitimate psychiatric care under national health insurance plans. The gynecologist is immersed in a culture (and various subcultures) like every other human being and shares that culture's beliefs and attitudes. It is neither necessary nor possible for a clinician to be divested of cultural context, but it is possible and necessary to be aware of it, its interaction with the patient's social background, and the impact on clinical care. It is valuable for the gynecologist to reflect on his or her attitudes toward psychiatric illness and treatment, on the appropriate roles of women in society and the family, and on the relationships between femaleness and psychological functioning.

Psychiatric Assessment and Diagnosis

Diagnostic System

In the past, psychiatric diagnosis was based at least partially on speculations about a patient's unconscious psychological conflicts. In the absence of verifiable criteria, a patient might receive different diagnoses from different physicians. The current edition of the *Diagnostic and Statistical Manual (DSM IV)*, produced and published by the American Psychiatric Association, is based on empirical, valid, and reliable evidence. Use of the DSM system results in interrater reliability fully comparable to that of other diagnostic systems in medicine in general. In addition, *DSM IV* diagnoses are strongly correlated with response to treatment. Criteria in *DSM IV* are the basis for the diagnostic entities described in this chapter.

The use of *DSM IV* criteria simplifies psychiatric assessment for the nonpsychiatric clinician, because *DSM IV* offers straightforward lists of signs and symptoms requisite for each diagnosis. In addition, the American Psychiatric Association has published a special edition of *DSM IV* for the primary care provider: *DSM IV PC*. This volume is organized by presenting symptoms rather than psychiatric nosology and uses algorithms and decision trees to facilitate the diagnostic process. Accurate diagnosis is critical to successful management. When referring a patient to a specialist, it is helpful to assess signs and symptoms systematically in order to identify questions of relevance to mental health professionals.

Approach to the Patient

The fact that *DSM IV* provides diagnostic criteria in the form of lists of specific signs and symptoms does not imply that the interaction with a patient should be reduced to a series of rapid-fire questions and answers. A wealth of valuable information can be obtained from the spontaneous statements of the patient about her concerns and distress and from her response to the physician's open-ended, facilitating questions. This in no way means that the physician and the other patients awaiting care should be held hostage by the talkative patient. The patient with extensive complaints and a detailed account of each can be informed of the total time realistically available, invited to focus on her most pressing problem, and offered a continuing dialogue at another appointment.

On the physician's side, however, it is critical neither to jump to diagnostic conclusions nor to pass over them to therapeutic interventions. One study found that many primary care physicians, feeling that they had too little time or training, tended to minimize verbal interactions with patients and rely quickly and heavily on the prescription of psychotropic drugs to treat psychiatric problems (12). Because of perceived time pressures, primary care physicians may be quick to proceed to specific questions before the patient has an opportunity to explain the problem in her own words. A patient who is allowed, or encouraged, to talk for 3–5 minutes before being asked specific questions may reveal information that is useful, even vital, to her care: a thought disorder or psychosis, a predominant mood, abnormally great anxiety, personality style or disorder, and attitudes toward her diagnosis and treatment. Such information may emerge only much later, or not at all, in a question-and-answer format (13).

Techniques of Psychiatric Referral

The issue of referral to a mental health professional comes up repeatedly in the discussion of psychiatric illness in gynecologic practice. The first question that arises is when to refer. Most mild psychiatric disorders are treated by nonpsychiatric physicians (1, 14). Most antidepressants and antianxiety agents are prescribed by nonpsychiatric physicians. However, most psychiatric disorders are overlooked or misdiagnosed in primary care practice. When they are diagnosed, the treatments often are not used in the most scientific or efficacious manner (3, 4). Each gynecologist must decide whether to assume the responsibility for the treatment of psychiatric illness in general as well as for each individual patient.

There are no absolutes in the decision to refer a patient. The following issues relate to the referral decision:

1. Nature and severity of the patient's disorder

2. The gynecologist's knowledge

3. Time available in the gynecologic practice

4. Patient's preference

5. Availability and choices of mental health professionals

6. The gynecologist's degree of comfort with the patient and the disorder.

Most gynecologists will refer patients who are suicidal, homicidal, or psychotic. Patients should be referred for evaluation when the psychiatric diagnosis is not clear and when they fail to respond to a first attempt at treatment. For many patients, the gynecologist can resume the responsibility for ongoing care after an initial or periodic assessment by a psychiatrist.

Uneasiness with the referral process stems logically from stigmas and misconceptions. Clinicians fear that patients will be insulted, alienated, or alarmed by a recommendation that they seek psychiatric care. There are several straightforward and effective techniques for decreasing the discomfort of both the gynecologist and patient and for enhancing the likelihood of a clinically successful referral.

It is essential to base the reasons for the referral on the patient's own signs and symptoms; that is, the reasons should reflect some aspect of her subjectively experienced distress. For a patient suffering from clinical depression, this might be her difficulty sleeping, her loss of appetite, or her lack of energy. For a patient with an anxiety disorder, it might be her palpitations, shortness of breath, or nervousness. For a patient with mild Alzheimer's disease, it might be forgetfulness or frightening episodes in which she finds herself in a neighborhood she does not recognize.

It is advisable to emphasize the distress produced by a diagnostic dilemma rather than the physician's hypothesis that the patient's symptoms are the result of psychological conflict. This is especially true in patients with somatization disorders. For example, the physician may chose one of the following statements: "It is very stressful to be suffering so badly and to have the doctors unable to figure out what is wrong. I would like you to see one of our staff who specializes in helping people to cope with these difficult situations," or "It must be difficult to function when you have been so sickly all your life, have seen so many doctors, have had so many diagnostic tests and medical treatments, and still don't have an answer or feel well."

Two indications for referral are especially difficult for gynecologists to communicate to patients: suicidal or homicidal behavior and psychosis. Both are social taboos, even more stigmatized than other symptoms of mental illness. **Many physicians fear that discussion of suicide or homicide will precipitate an enactment of this behavior that otherwise would not have taken place. The opposite is the case** (15, 16). An open discussion of impulses to hurt oneself or others helps the patient to regain control, recognize the need for psychological help, or obtain necessary emergency intervention such as psychiatric hospitalization. Avoiding the subject intensifies her belief that she must try to cope with unbearable feelings alone, whereas pursuing the subject conveys the message that someone can tolerate and try to understand her feelings, lend her emotional strength, help her think through her situation, and keep her and others safe from danger. Specific techniques for the evaluation and referral of possibly suicidal patients are addressed in the following section on Mood Disorders.

Psychosis is the other condition that nonpsychiatrists assume will be difficult to discuss with patients. In fact, most psychotic patients have had previous experience not only with their psychotic symptoms, but also with psychiatric referral and treatment. They recognize that society at large views their signs and symptoms as unacceptable and requiring psychiatric intervention. Their symptoms may also be distressing to them. They can often discuss their "voices" or delusional beliefs quite matter-of-factly.

Conversely, patients who are acutely psychotic tend to be acutely distressed. Although they may not realize that their changes in behavior and thinking are the result of mental illness, they usually know that something is very wrong and accept referral to an expert. The clinician can tell the psychotic patient that her observable signs and symptoms are a cause of concern and advise her that a specialist will be best able to help understand and treat her problem. Patients who are either acutely or chronically paranoid tend to be most resistant to referral.

Some patients, although decreasing in number, believe that any mention of mental health intervention implies either that they are "crazy" or that the referring physician is convinced that their physical symptoms are imaginary or even deliberately manufactured. The gynecologist may wish to state explicitly that this is not the case. Again, making the real reason for the referral clear and founded in signs and symptoms known to the patient will nearly always allay anxiety over a psychiatric referral.

Under no circumstances is it acceptable to refer the patient to a psychiatrist without informing her in advance. Unless the patient is acutely psychotic and functionally incompetent or there is a psychiatric emergency, she must be asked rather than told. A referral that begins with an unexpected clinical encounter with a psychiatrist is unfair to the psychiatrist and the patient and is unlikely to end in a satisfactory collaboration.

In light of a patient's possible perception that mental health referral is an indication of the gynecologist's disdain or disinterest, and in the interest of good patient care in general, the referring gynecologist should make it clear to the patient that he or she will remain involved in her care. Two concrete ways to accomplish this are asking the patient to call after her consultation with the mental health professional and making an appointment for her to return to the gynecologist's office after that visit. In the inpatient setting, the gynecologist can indicate an intention to hear about a psychiatric consultation during rounds. The mental health professional can be presented to the patient as an integral and standing member of the health care team, one with whom the gynecologist will collaborate, rather than as a last resort for patients without *bona fide* gynecologic problems.

Selection of a Mental Health Professional

Mental disturbances are treated by social workers, psychologists, members of the clergy, and various kinds of "counselors" as well as by psychiatrists. The distinctions among mental health professionals are not generally well known or understood by the lay public. In addition, the criteria for membership in each profession vary from place to place and institution to institution. Social workers and psychologists can be educated at the Bachelor's, Master's, or doctoral level. In some states, licensure is required; generally, social workers must have a Master's degree and clinical psychologists must have a doctorate degree to qualify. "Counselors" include a wide variety of practitioners, including marriage counselors, pastoral counselors, school counselors, family counselors, and others. The training of social workers may focus on social policy, institutional work, the psychosocial aspects of medical illness, or individual psychotherapy.

Practitioners of all mental health disciplines may be trained in psychotherapy. For a patient who does not meet criteria for a serious psychiatric disorder and who is able to carry out her responsibilities, supportive psychotherapy is probably sufficient and can be provided by any trained mental health professional. Doctoral-level clinical psychologists and neuropsychologists can also perform testing that can be helpful diagnostically, especially in identifying and localizing brain pathology and in defining intelligence levels, which may be an unrecognized cause of a patient's noncompliance.

Trained social workers are often particularly knowledgeable about community resources for patients and their families and about the impact of gynecologic disease and treatment on both. Self-help or professionally led therapy groups are extremely helpful for patients whose distress is limited to the circumstances of a gynecologic condition or treatment such as infertility or a malignancy. There is substantive evidence that participation in a supportive group lengthens the survival time and improves the quality of life for some cancer patients (17, 18).

Psychiatrists are the only medically trained mental health professionals. They are particularly helpful with diagnostic dilemmas, especially when there is a question of psychological or behavioral manifestations of medical illness or pharmacologic treatment and when a medical understanding of the gynecologic condition and treatment is necessary for clinical care. Psychiatrists are the only mental health professionals who can prescribe psychoactive medications and other biological interventions as well as psychotherapies. They treat seriously ill patients and take responsibility for emergency situations.

The choice of mental health referral for a particular patient depends on many factors. Factors that help determine the type of mental health referral are as follows:

1. Clinical diagnosis

2. Clinical situation

3. Choices available in the area

4. Constraints of the patient's health care coverage/finances

5. Interest, knowledge, and experience of the available mental health professionals in the psychological aspects of gynecologic practice

6. Nature of the relationship between the referring gynecologist and the individual mental health professional.

Considering the frequency of psychiatric problems in gynecologic practice, it is worthwhile for the gynecologist to develop a relationship with one or more mental health care professionals. The availability of familiar and trusted resources enhances the likelihood that problems will be identified and addressed, whereas the clinician will be inclined to overlook or minimize problems with solutions that appear to be overly time-consuming or out of reach altogether. Similarly, it is also useful to know about local hotlines and resources for battered women and for mothers who fear they pose a danger to their children.

Specific Disorders

In every patient whose emotions or behaviors cause concern, a nonpsychiatric medical disorder or a reaction to prescribed or illicit drugs should first be considered. The diagnosis can then focus on determining whether an emotional disorder is psychiatric or situational in nature.

Mood Disorders

Definitions and Diagnostic Criteria

Mood **is the emotional coloration of a patient's experience.** *Mood disorders* are frequently confused with the ubiquitous ups and downs of everyday experience and with inevitable responses to life difficulties. Patients with mood disorders encounter frustration and rejection when others' well-meaning attempts to reason with or distract them fail to influence their moods. Mood may be pathologically elevated (*mania*) or lowered (*depression*) or may alternate between the two (*bipolar disorders*).

Mania   *Mania* is characterized by:

1. Elevated mood, sometimes with euphoria and sometimes with irritability

2. Grandiosity

3. Decreased sleep

4. Increased energy

5. Reckless behavior, as with expenditures of money

6. Speeding of speech and physical activity.

Mania can be acute or subacute (*hypomania*). Hypomanic patients may enjoy their condition and may be the envy of others, because of their self-confidence, ebullience, energy, and productivity. Acute mania is a life-threatening condition; patients literally exhaust themselves, disinterested in either food or sleep.

Depression   *Depression* is characterized by:

1. Sad mood, crying

2. Irritability

3. Hopelessness and helplessness

4. Decreased ability to concentrate

5. Decreased energy

6. Interference with sleep, early awakening

7. Decreased appetite

8. Withdrawal from social relationships

9. Inability to enjoy previously gratifying activities

10. Guilt

11. Decreased libido

12. Speeding or slowing of speech and activity

13. Thoughts of death or suicide.

The patient who has five or more of the signs and symptoms of depression for a significant part of each day for 2 weeks or more has a clinical depression. Depression may be acute or chronic (*dysthymic disorder*) and may occur once, recurrently, or cyclically. Depression is believed to have an underlying biochemical and biological etiology as well as a behavioral component. It is accompanied by abnormal regulation of norepinephrine and decreased serotonin activity, and treatment is directed toward correcting these factors. Psychological factors such as unexpressed anger, unresolved grief, and learned helplessness also can play a role in depression.

Depression may or may not be related to a discernible precipitating factor such as a negative life event. The presence of a "depressing" situation, such as a serious, disfiguring, or life-threatening gynecologic condition, does not make depression inevitable and in no way precludes a psychiatric diagnosis or treatment. In such a situation, the clinical depression can be considered a secondary complication of the gynecologic disease, and it is as fully deserving of treatment as any other painful and disabling complication. Significant medical illness may cause changes in energy, sleep, and appetite but does not make the patient feel pessimistic or guilty. Patients who meet criteria for depression respond to treatment for depression; this treatment has a major impact on quality of life, regardless of the prognosis of any coexisting medical illness.

Epidemiology

The overall lifetime prevalence of affective disorders is 8.3%; the 6-month prevalence is 5.8% (19). In adolescents and adults, depression is two to three times more common in women than in men (7,19–24). Women have a lifetime risk of 10–25% and a point prevalence of 5–9% (7). Depression is the single most common reason for psychiatric hospitalization in the U.S. (9). The natural course of an untreated major depressive episode is approximately 9 months. As many as 15% of individuals with severe depressive disorders are successful in committing suicide (7, 25, 26).

The highest incidence of depression is in the age group of 25–44 years (7). There is no evidence that employment outside the home increases vulnerability to depression, although the assumption of multiple roles, especially in the absence of adequate social support, may be stressful (27–29).

Related Illnesses Relevant to Gynecologic Practice

External pressures may bring about a major depressive disorder. Although these episodes may be situational, they may signal the beginning of a problem. A number of factors may predispose a woman to depression: early childhood loss, physical or sexual abuse (including abuse by a spouse or partner), socioeconomic deprivation, genetic predisposition, and lifestyle stress of multiple roles.

Women are more susceptible to depression during certain times of their lives. Certain life cycle events, such as infertility or reproductive loss, may be a source of stress and may contribute to depression. Relationships between a history of major depression and reproductive events, menstrual cycle mood changes, and postpartum depression are likely to be predictors of psychologic problems. The physician should be alert to these events and the accompanying risk of depression.

Adolescents and Young Adults   Adolescents and young adults often suffer a form of depression, called *atypical depression,* in which their levels of sleep and appetite are enhanced rather than decreased.

Premenstrual Syndrome   Many women, perhaps a majority, experience mood and behavioral changes during the premenstrual phase of their cycles (30–32). Many women present to their gynecologist with self-diagnosed "premenstrual syndrome." About 3–5% of all women may suffer from symptoms so marked or debilitating that they warrant a psychiatric diagnosis of *premenstrual dysphoria* (7, 31). Mood and behavioral changes related to the menstrual cycle have been the subject of much debate. They are considered inherent to the menstrual cycle and are often associated with negative feelings and behaviors. No specific hormonal levels, treatments, or markers associated with premenstrual symptoms have been identified.

Women who have premenstrual symptoms may be suffering from a specific psychiatric illness such as depression or personality disorders. Therefore, women who experience premenstrual symptoms should undergo a thorough psychologic evaluation to identify any other underlying disorders that can then be treated. They must also rate their symptoms prospectively on forms, separate from the record of their menses, for at least two consecutive cycles before the diagnosis of premenstrual dysphoria can be confirmed by a clear association with symptoms during the luteal phase of the cycle. A very small percentage of patients who describe premenstrual changes qualify for the strict diagnosis of premenstrual dysphoric disorder (7). In these cases, the premenstrual dysphoria interferes with the patient's functioning in her daily activities.

Initial treatment of premenstrual symptoms that are not disabling is directed of lifestyle changes. Nonpharmacologic treatments with few or no negative side effects and the potential for overall positive effects include the following:

- elimination of caffeine intake
- smoking cessation
- regular exercise
- regular, nutritious diet
- adequate sleep
- active stress reduction.

Patients with the psychiatric diagnosis of premenstrual dysphoric disorder have been reported to respond to selective serotonin reuptake inhibitors. Because these agents require several weeks for therapeutic effect, they must be administered on an ongoing basis. Other medications that have been studied as treatment for PMS are listed in Table 12.2.

Reproductive Events   Women who experience a perinatal loss undergo a natural grieving process, which may be misdiagnosed as depression. Many of the symptoms are similar; however, self-esteem is usually preserved with perinatal loss, whereas in depression it is not. Counseling and support should be provided and, if the mood disturbance is intense or longstanding, psychiatric consultation should be obtained.

Mild feelings of depression often occur following pregnancy but usually do not represent major clinical depression. Women at risk for significant postpartum depression are more likely to have a history of depression or adjustment problems. Postpartum blues and the increased vulnerability for postpartum depression are believed to be precipitated by the emotional and possibly the endocrinologic changes associated with this time.

Women who are infertility patients report a higher level of stress, but there is no evidence that they have a higher prevalence of major depression. Repeated failed attempts at pregnancy, particularly those associated with the use of assisted reproductive technology, are the most emotionally difficult events. Such couples may benefit from counseling and group treatment, especially after repeated interventions or termination of medical care.

Menopause and Aging   As a physiologic process, menopause is not associated with depression (33). The notion of an increase in depression at the time of menopause, so-called involutional melancholia, has been dispelled. Menopause and midlife adjustment disorders should be considered within their social, cultural, and psychologic contexts.

Women in families or social groups in which status and social roles are lost in later life are more vulnerable to depression than older women who fulfill gratifying social functions (34, 35). Depression in elderly patients can cause a "pseudodementia," characterized by decreased activity and interest and seeming forgetfulness. Unlike patients with organically based dementia, these patients complain of memory loss rather than trying to compensate and cover up for it.

Functional Assessment   The diagnosis of depression is straightforward, using the aforementioned criteria. If diagnostic criteria are fulfilled, there is a high likelihood of response to treatment for depression. Some individuals have a chronic, mild form of depression that assumes the quality of a character style. They, too, often respond to antidepressant treatment.

The severity of depression is determined by the subjective emotional pain experienced by the patient and the degree of interference with her normal functioning. Acute depression is

Table 12.2   Scientific Basis of Selected Medications Used to Treat PMS

Treatment	Scientific Basis	Advantages	Disadvantages	Notes
Alprazolam	Several double-blind, placebo-controlled, randomized crossover studies. Results were mixed. Placebo was as effective as alprazolam in some studies.	Oral medication appears to be more effective in alleviating depression and anxiety symptoms than physical symptoms.	Potential for dependence, requires tapering, drowsiness reported by many subjects; long-term effects unknown, safety during pregnancy unknown.	The studies involved highly selective groups of women. There was a high dropout rate in one of the positive studies. In one study that found alprazolam effective, 87% of the women had a history of major depression or an anxiety disorder. Different doses were used in the studies (0.75–2.25 mg); the standard effective dose is unknown.
Fluoxetine (Prozac)	Several double-blind, randomized, placebo-controlled, crossover trials. All found fluoxetine effective.	Well tolerated, single daily oral dose. Significant decrease in psychic and behavioral symptoms.	Long-term effects unknown. Safety during pregnancy unknown. Appears less effective in controlling physical symptoms.	Trials involved very small, highly select groups of women. Duration of treatment did not exceed 3 months. All trials used 20 mg orally daily.
Gonadotropin-releasing hormone agonist	Several small, double-blind, randomized, placebo-controlled, crossover trials. Most patients experienced improvement.	Rapidly reversible, many patients report being virtually symptom-free during therapy.	Produces pseudomenopause, expensive, risk for osteoporosis, hypoestrogenic symptoms. Usually given for only short periods of time.	An "add-back" regimen of estrogen-progestin in addition to gonadotropin-releasing hormone agonist has been reported. If replicated, it may have potential for an effective, long-term treatment for premenstrual syndrome.
Spironolactone	Several double-blind, randomized, placebo-controlled trials. Mixed results.	May alleviate bloating and improve symptoms related to mood. Oral medication taken once or twice a day. Nonaddictive.	Effectiveness not proven consistently across studies.	Spironolactone is the only diuretic that has shown effectiveness in treating premenstrual syndrome in controlled, randomized trials. Method of action may be antiandrogen properties.
Vitamin B_6	Ten randomized double-blind trials. About one-third of the trials reported positive results, one-third reported negative results, and one-third reported ambiguous results.		No conclusive evidence that vitamin B_6 is more effective than placebo.	Doses ranged from 50 to 500 mg. Only one study involved more than 40 subjects. The large multicenter trial (N = 204) reported similar results for placebo and vitamin B_6.

Reproduced with permission from **The American College of Obstetricians and Gynecologists.** *Committee Opinion.* Washington, DC: ACOG, 1995.

an agonizingly painful disease. Patients and their friends and families, reluctant to consider a psychiatric disorder, often attribute the signs and symptoms of depression to life circumstances or to a medical condition, either diagnosed or undiagnosed. The persistence of symptoms in the face of a pleasant life situation or the failure to respond to attempts at cheering the patient, such as changes of scene, often provoke guilt in the patient and disapproval by her significant others. The patient is more likely to complain of a low energy level and general malaise than of a depressed mood. She must be questioned specifically about diagnostic signs and symptoms.

Management

Both antidepressant medication and psychotherapy are effective in the treatment of depression. There is evidence that a combination of the two treatments results in the best outcomes (25). The most effective psychotherapies for depression are specifically targeted at the negative thought processes associated with the disease (*cognitive therapy*) (25, 36, 37). Supportive psychotherapies, which help the patient identify stresses and mobilize her existing strengths to deal with them, is a useful adjunct to medication (36).

Because of the stigma of psychiatric disorders, the confusion between ordinary transient sad moods and the clinical disorder of depression, and the tendency of patients to blame themselves for this condition, some care must be taken to explain the disease to the patient. It can be useful to show her the diagnostic criteria in a textbook. She must understand that her condition is not due to weakness but to a biochemical alteration in her brain. She must also understand that antidepressant medications are not "uppers," which artificially elevate mood, but substances that restore the normal balance of neurotransmitters in the brain. Cognitive therapy is also associated with biochemical change. It is often helpful or necessary to explain the condition to the patient's significant others as well.

There are several classes of antidepressant medication, which are outlined in Table 12.3. All of these agents have comparable therapeutic efficacy and require 2–4 weeks for therapeutic effect. Responses are individual; a patient who does not respond to one medication may respond to another, even one in the same class. The choice of antidepressant is based on side effects, dosage schedule, cost, physician familiarity, and individual therapeutic response. If the patient has relatives who suffer from depressive disorders and have responded to particular medications, there is increased likelihood that she will respond similarly. She is also more likely to respond to agents that have been effective during past episodes. The potential side effects of the most frequently used drugs are presented in Table 12.4

Tricyclic Antidepressants   *Tricyclic antidepressants* have been available for nearly 30 years. They are well studied and available inexpensively in generic form. They all have anticholinergic side effects that may be problematic in medically ill and elderly patients. They cause some degree of slowing of intracardiac conduction; this side effect can be tolerated and managed in all but a few patients, and it can be therapeutic for those with pathologically enhanced conduction. Although several times a day dosing is often prescribed, especially at the beginning of treatment, bedtime dosing, especially for patients who have difficulty sleeping, is effective and may be preferable. A significant problem with these drugs is their lethal potential, given the association between depression and suicide (38). Some of these medications, such as *nortriptyline,* have "therapeutic windows"—drug blood levels above or below which they are not effective—that must be monitored by assessing drug levels in the blood. The average dose for tricyclics is about 225 mg/day in divided doses.

Monoamine Oxidase Inhibitors   *Monoamine oxidase (MAO) inhibitors* are especially effective for atypical depression (39, 40). They require dietary restrictions and can be used only in patients who are able to understand and comply with those restrictions.

Selective Serotonin Reuptake Inhibitors   The newest class of antidepressants is the selective serotonin reuptake inhibitors (SSRIs). These medications have few if any medically severe side effects; side effects that occur include anxiety, tremor, headache, and gastrointestinal upset (41). They are administered on a once-a-day regimen, with little need for dosage adjustments in most cases. SSRIs have long half-lives, so that occasional missed doses and withdrawal do not constitute problems. It is difficult or impossible to use SSRIs

309

Table 12.3   Pharmacology of Antidepressant Medications

Drug	Therapeutic Dosage Range (mg/day)	Average (Range) of Elimination Half-Lives (hours)*	Potentially Fatal Drug Interactions
Tricyclics			
Amitriptyline (Elavil, Endep)	75–300	24 (16–46)	Antiarrhythmics, MAO inhibitors
Clomipramine (Anafranil)	75–300	24 (20–40)	Antiarrhythmics, MAO inhibitors
Desipramine (Norpramin, Pertofrane)	75–300	18 (12–50)	Antiarrhythmics, MAO inhibitors
Doxepin (Adapin, Sinequan)	75–300	17 (10–47)	Antiarrhythmics, MAO inhibitors
Imipramine (Janimine, Tofranil)	75–300	22 (12–34)	Antiarrhythmics, MAO inhibitors
Nortriptyline (Aventyl, Pamelor)	40–200	26 (18–88)	Antiarrhythmics, MAO inhibitors
Protiptyline (Vivactil)	20–60	76 (54–124)	Antiarrhythmics, MAO inhibitors
Trimipramine (Surmontil)	75–300	12 (8–30)	Antiarrhythmics, MAO inhibitors
Heterocyclics			
Amoxapine (Asendin)	100–600	10 (8–14)	MAO inhibitors
Bupropion (Wellbutrin)	225–450	14 (8–24)	MAO inhibitors (possibly)
Maprotiline (Ludiomil)	100–225	43 (27–58)	MAO inhibitors
Trazodone (Desyrel)	150–600	8 (4–14)	—
Selective serotin reuptake inhibitors			
Fluoxetine (Prozac)	10–40	168 (72–360)[†]	MAO inhibitors
Paroxetine (Paxil)	20–50	24 (3–65)	MAO inhibitors[‡]
Sertraline (Zoloft)	50–150	24 (10–30)	MAO inhibitors[‡]
Monoamine oxidase inhibitors (MAO inhibitors)[§]			
Isocarboxazid (Marplan)	30–50	Unknown	For all three MAO inhibitors: vasoconstrictors,[‖] decongestants,[‖] meperidine, and possibly other narcotics
Phenelzine (Nardil)	45–90	2 (1.5–4.0)	
Tranylcypromine (Parnate)	20–60	2 (1.5–3.0)	

*Half-lives are affected by age, sex, race, concurrent medications, and length of drug exposure.
†Includes both fluoxetine and norfluoxetine.
‡By extrapolation from fluoxetine data.
§MAO inhibition lasts longer (7 days) than drug half-life.
‖Including pseudoephedrine, phenylephrine, phenylpropanolamine, epinephrine, norepinephrine, and others.
From **Depression Guideline Panel.** *Depression in Primary Care: Detection, Diagnosis, and Treatment.* Quick Reference Guide for Clinicians, No. 5. AHCPR Publication No. 93-0552. Rockville, MD: U.S. Department of Health and Human Services, Public Health Service, Agency for Health Care Policy and Research, 1993:15.

to commit suicide (40, 41). They are, however, much more expensive than the tricyclics. Little is known about their use in the elderly; caution should be taken, and treatment should begin with low doses in older women.

Lithium Salts   *Lithium* salts are the treatment of choice for bipolar conditions and are also useful in the enhancement of other antidepressants in patients who are resistant to treatment (42, 43). They have potentially toxic effects on kidney, heart, thyroid, and liver; treatment must be preceded and punctuated by determinations of the appropriate laboratory values. Certain anticonvulsants are also efficacious in some cases of mania. Both lithium and

Table 12.4   Side-Effect Profiles of Antidepressant Medications

		Central Nervous System		Cardiovascular			
	Anticholinergic†	Drowsiness	Insomnia/ Agitation	Orthostatic Hypotension	Cardiac Arrhythmia	Gastrointestinal Distress	Weight Gain (over 6 kg)
Amitriptyline	4+	4+	0	4+	3+	0	4+
Desipramine	1+	1+	1+	2+	2+	0	1+
Doxepin	3+	4+	0	2+	2+	0	3+
Imipramine	3+	3+	1+	4+	3+	1+	3+
Nortriptyline	1+	1+	0	2+	2+	0	1+
Protriptyline	2+	1+	1+	2+	2+	0	0
Trimipramine	1+	4+	0	2+	2+	0	3+
Amoxapine	2+	2+	2+	2+	3+	0	1+
Maprotiline	2+	4+	0	0	1+	0	2+
Trazodone	0	4+	0	1+	1+	1+	1+
Bupropion	0	0	2+	0	1+	1+	0
Fluoxetine	0	0	2+	0	0	3+	0
Paroxetine	0	0	2+	0	0	3+	0
Sertraline	0	0	2+	0	0	3+	0
Monoamine oxidase inhibitors	1	1+	2+	2+	0	1+	2+

*Numerals indicate the likelihood of side effect occuring ranging from 0 for absent or rare to 4+ for relatively common.
†Dry mouth, blurred vision, urinary hesitancy, constipation.
From **Depression Guideline Panel.** *Depression in Primary Care: Detection, Diagnosis, and Treatment.* Quick Reference Guide for Clinicians, No. 5. AHCPR Publication No. 93-0553. Rockville, MD: U.S. Department of Health and Human Services, Public Health Service, Agency for Health Care Policy and Research, 1993:14.

anticonvulsants are used for complex psychiatric cases; therefore, they are more likely to be prescribed by psychiatrists than by gynecologists.

Bupropion   *Bupropion* is an antidepressant that does not fall into any of the major categories. It has fewer anticholinergic effects than tricyclics, but it is more effective in lowering the seizure threshold.

Referral

The most critical issue in referral of depressed patients is the evaluation of suicide risk. Risk factors for suicide include the following (44):

1. Recent losses

2. Family history of suicide

3. Previous suicide attempts

4. Impulsivity

5. Concurrent substance abuse

6. Current or past physical or sexual abuse

7. The availability of means to commit suicide.

Women attempt suicide more frequently than men, but men complete the act more frequently than women (45, 46). This is probably due at least in part to the fact that men tend to use more drastic or irreversible means, such as firearms, while women tend to overdose on medication.

The association between past self-destructive behavior and successful suicide is counterintuitive. It would seem that someone who had repeatedly made suicidal gestures is more interested in the responses of others than in actually committing suicide. The data do not bear out this assumption; a past suicide attempt is associated with an increased risk of completed suicide. A physician may dismiss suicidal ideation or behavior in a patient with a history of suicide gestures. This may be part of the reason why most individuals who commit suicide have consulted a nonpsychiatric physician within the preceding month (10). Another factor contributing to suicide is the reluctance of the physician to bring up or pursue the subject.

Inquiry about suicidal ideation and behavior is a proper part of every mental status examination and is mandatory for every patient with past or current depression or evidence of self-destructive behavior. The subject need not be awkward to discuss. When discussing difficulties in the patient's situation or mood, the clinician can comment that almost everyone has at some time felt so bad as to wish that he or she were dead and then ask whether the patient has had such thoughts in the present or past. Nonsuicidal patients generally react by acknowledging the thought and offering the reasons why they would not act on it: "I knew it wasn't really that bad," "I would never do that to my family," or "My religion forbids suicide." If the patient has ongoing or recent suicidal ideation, the clinician must determine whether the patient may act on her feelings and whether she has a specific plan and the means to carry it out. Such plans include arranging time to be alone and undisturbed, making wills or other financial arrangements, and setting up care for dependents.

It is important to distinguish between the wish to be dead and the intention to kill oneself. They may coexist, but they may also be entirely separate. A patient in a painful life situation—a chronic, painful, or terminal medical condition; the birth of a severely damaged child; or a grievous loss—may feel and express a wish to die, and even refuse recommended medical care, but clearly and genuinely disavow any intention of actively harming herself. Most patients who are actively suicidal also give accurate answers about their feelings, but only if they are asked.

If the patient has previously engaged in self-destructive behavior without a plan or warning, it is wise to consult a psychiatrist. If a patient is actively suicidal, she should be referred *immediately* to a psychiatrist. Other mental health professionals may be helpful but are less likely to have dealt extensively with and assumed responsibility for suicidal patients, to be able decide whether the patient should be hospitalized, and to be legally privileged to put into effect psychiatric hospitalization when indicated.

Until she is in the physical presence of a psychiatrist, a suicidal patient should be observed and protected at all times—every second—whether she is in the consulting room or the bathroom. The staff member assigned to remain with her may not leave to make a telephone call, go to the bathroom, or have a snack. If help must be summoned, by the gynecologist or an assigned staff member, a call can be made in the patient's hearing from a telephone in the consulting room, by shouting from the doorway, or by taking the patient along to wherever it is necessary to go to arrange a psychiatric consultation. Family members may offer to monitor the patient and can sometimes do so effectively and humanely, but the restrictions just mentioned are not always obvious to them and must be emphasized. It is better to risk inconvenience and possible embarrassment to both the gynecologist and the patient than to risk a fatal outcome.

Psychiatric referral can also be useful in less dramatic cases. The gynecologist may feel inexperienced in the area of depression or may be overloaded with other patients requiring psychological attention and support. Other indications for referral include failure to respond, or to respond fully, to an adequate first trial of antidepressant medication; diagnostic questions; other concurrent problems, such as relationship difficulties, domestic violence, or substance abuse; recurrent depressive episodes; and patient request.

Anxiety Disorders

Definition and Diagnostic Criteria

Anxiety is a sense of dread without objective cause for fear, accompanied by the usual physical concomitants of fear. Although some anxiety is a ubiquitous and inescapable part of human experience, anxiety and anxiety disorders are severely painful and deserving of medical attention. The anxiety disorders include *generalized anxiety, panic disorder, agoraphobia, specific phobias, obsessive-compulsive disorder,* **and** *posttraumatic stress disorder.*

Generalized Anxiety Disorder *Generalized anxiety disorder,* as the name implies, consists of anxiety pervading the patient's life. The patient suffers from restlessness, easy fatigability, difficulty concentrating, irritability, muscle tension, and sleep disturbances. Whereas depressed patients fall asleep more or less normally and then awaken earlier than intended, anxious patients have difficulty with sleep onset.

Panic Disorder *Panic disorder* is characterized by panic attacks with acute periods of intense fear and at least four of the following symptoms:

1. Palpitations

2. Diaphoresis

3. Trembling

4. Shortness of breath

5. A choking sensation

6. Chest discomfort

7. Gastrointestinal distress

8. Lightheadedness

9. Sense of unreality

10. Fear of going crazy or dying

11. Paresthesias

12. Chills or hot flushes.

The attacks recur without specific precipitating events and occasion ongoing concern and behavioral changes meant to avert the possibility of future attacks. These include avoidance of specific situations, assuring oneself of the possibility of escape from the situations, or refusing to be alone.

The symptoms of panic attacks are often confused, by both patients and care providers, with the symptoms of serious cardiac or pulmonary disease. They lead to many fruitless trips to the emergency department and costly, even invasive, medical investigations. A careful history can establish the correct diagnosis in most cases.

Agoraphobia   *Agoraphobia* involves the avoidance of situations in which the patient fears she will be trapped, such as the center of a row in the theater or driving over a bridge. She fears that the situation will trigger panic. Agoraphobia and panic disorder can exist separately or together.

Specific Phobias   *Specific phobias* are irrational fears of certain objects or situations, despite the patient's awareness that the object or situation poses no real danger. Of particular concern in gynecology are fear of needles and fear of vomiting. Social phobia causes the patient to fear and avoid situations in which the patient imagines she will be observed by others in a humiliating light. Patients may alter their lives to avoid these anxieties, thereby damaging their interpersonal relationships or ability to carry out their responsibilities, or they may manage to carry on while enduring considerable psychic pain.

Obsessive-Compulsive Disorder   *Obsessive-compulsive disorder* produces obsessions (recurrent impulses, images, or thoughts that the patient recognizes as her own but cannot control) or compulsions (intrusive, repetitive behaviors that the patient feels are essential to avoid some irrelevant negative outcome). The disorder can be mild or totally crippling. In one-half the cases, it becomes chronic. Neurobiologically, it is associated with disregulation of serotonin.

Posttraumatic Stress Disorder   *Posttraumatic stress disorder* is the result of exposure to an event that threatens the life or safety of the patient or others. At the time of the trauma, the patient experiences horror, terror, or a sense of helplessness. Afterward, the patient may lose conscious memory of all or part of the event, avoid situations reminiscent of it, and become acutely distressed when she cannot avoid them. She feels numb and detached, often without a sense of the future. She is hyperarousable and irritable and experiences difficulty sleeping and concentrating. She reexperiences the event through nightmares, "flashbacks," and intrusive thoughts.

Epidemiology

Panic disorder without agoraphobia is two times more common in women than in men; with agoraphobia, panic disorder is three times more common in women (7, 47). Onset is most common in young adults, often following a stressful event (47). The lifetime prevalence is 1.5–3.5%; the 1-year prevalence is 1–2% (7). A substantial percentage of patients experience depressive episodes as well (47, 48). Phobias are somewhat more common in women, depending on the object of the phobia (7, 20, 48). The 1-year prevalence is 9%, and the lifetime prevalence is 10–11% (7). Obsessive-compulsive disorder is equally common in men and women, and there is evidence of familial transmission (7, 48). Prevalences are 2.5% for lifetime and 1.5–2.1% for 1 year (7, 19). Posttraumatic stress disorder has a lifetime prevalence of 1–14% (7); victims of violence (including child abuse and wife battering) and war are at increased risk (7).

Functional Assessment

Given the relationship between anxiety disorders and traumatic experiences, signs and symptoms of anxiety disorder are a warning that the patient may have been abused. For effective treatment planning and prognostication, it is important to know how long the patient has suffered from the disorder, what previous attempts have been made to diagnose and treat it, and the effect it has had on the patient's psychological development, life choices, lifestyle, and relationships. In some cases, an entire family will have organized schedules and activities around the patient's symptoms. She and they may accept the necessity for this distortion and may not comment on it unless specifically asked. It is similarly essential to inquire specifically about the patient's daily activities and the circumstances under which anxiety symptoms occur. Rapidly deteriorating function signals the need for prompt intervention.

Management

Many physicians equate the management of anxiety with the use of antianxiety medication. This equation has resulted in a situation in which the overprescription of benzodiazepines, particularly for women, is a concern in the lay media and a source of ammunition for critics of current medical practice (49). Managing, even tolerating, patient anxiety is an anxiety-provoking process, because the patient's anxiety is contagious and the gynecologist fears confrontation with a limitless demand on time and energy. Prescribing medication is a familiar and comfortable, if not optimal, way to end a medical interview. Benzodiazepines are effective and relatively benign when used for a focused problem, but they are not without significant negative effects and they are not the only or best approach to treatment of all cases of anxiety (50). It is often important to defer the administration of pharmacologic anxiolytics so that the impact of the clinical interaction can be assessed without that confounding variable.

Benzodiazepines are most useful in time-limited situations, whether single or repeated. Use can quickly become chronic, with escalating dosages and diminishing therapeutic effects (50). So many women are taking benzodiazepines and take them so for granted, that their use may not be noted in medical histories. Patients admitted to the hospital may suffer unrecognized withdrawal symptoms that complicate their treatment or may continue to take medications from a personal supply without informing the medical staff. For chronic anxiety and many cases of acute anxiety, there are alternative approaches that are highly effective and largely free of side effects (51–54).

It is important to ascertain the source of anxiety or obsessiveness. Many patients and their families are anxious because of misinformation or misunderstandings about care of a medical problem. Few patients can absorb information about their gynecologic conditions and treatments at a single visit, but most hesitate to burden the physician or risk humiliation by asking that it be repeated. Patients also suffer anxiety when there is disagreement among family members or medical staff about the diagnosis or recommended treatment. Many patients dread certain specific aspects of medical or surgical care, sometimes on the basis of information or experience that is not current. Not uncommonly, a simple explanation or alteration in procedure will allay the patient's anxiety significantly. For example, a reassuring family member or friend can be allowed to remain with the patient, sedation can be administered orally or by inhalation before an intravenous line is inserted, or the patient can be allowed control over her own analgesia.

Behavioral interventions are extremely useful in managing anxiety (51–55). They include hypnosis, desensitization, and relaxation techniques. They have no deleterious side effects. Whereas the use of medications prescribed by the physician tends to foster the patient's dependence, relaxation techniques provide her with tools to cope with her own anxiety. Specialists in behavioral medicine, usually psychologists, are expert in these techniques, which also can be mastered and taught by gynecologists.

It is easy to be trapped into a cat-and-mouse game with an anxious and needy patient. Faced with an obsessional or anxious, talkative, and needy patient in the midst of bedside rounds, clinic, or office hours, the clinician can develop a pattern of attempted avoidance, sometimes alternating with overindulgence stemming from feelings of guilt. This kind of behavior, which results in sporadic, unpredictable reinforcement of the patient's anxiety symptoms and demands for attention, is most likely to lead to increased incidence of symptoms and demands. Attempting to escape by appearing distracted or harassed, or yielding

315

with despair to the destruction of the day's schedule and the care of other patients, simply heightens the patient's anxiety. It is preferable to develop a plan prospectively after considering one's own tolerance and the needs of the patient.

Gynecologists tend to underrate the power of their personal interactions with patients and their own ability to structure and limit those interactions appropriately. The patient should be informed of the time available and asked to focus on the problem about which she has most concern, with other problems to be discussed at future, scheduled visits. Instead of scheduling appointments and returning telephone calls grudgingly in response to patient demands, the gynecologist should inform the patient that her condition requires regular, brief, scheduled visits. She should be asked to call the office or clinic staff between visits, at convenient prearranged times, to advise the team of her progress.

It is also important to help the patient's significant others to support her and cope with her symptoms without organizing their lives around her. Self-help and professionally led groups focused on specific disorders lessen patients' feelings of isolation and offer education about the disorder, treatment, and coping styles for the patient and her family. It is important to choose the group carefully. Although groups focused on victimization can validate patients' experiences and pain, they can also interfere with patients' motivation and ability to continue their development and find other forms of identification and gratification.

Medication does have a place in the management of anxiety disorders. Table 12.5 provides a description of many of the compounds that are used in managing these disorders. *Clomipramine* is a specific, effective treatment for obsessive-compulsive disorder (56). Selective serotonin reuptake inhibitors are useful as well. *Buspirone,* although marketed for chronic anxiety, has not proven effective in most controlled studies (57). Benzodiazepines are effective when taken for acute anxiety or during relatively brief, time-limited (up to several days) stressful situations. The specific agent should be chosen on the basis of onset of action and half-life. The patient must be admonished to avoid concomitant use of alcohol. She should also exercise extreme care when driving or engaging in other potentially dangerous activities requiring attention, concentration, and coordination while taking benzodiazepines.

Referral

As with all other conditions, criteria for referral depend largely on the tolerance, interest, time, and expertise of the gynecologist. Patients who fail to respond to a trial of office counseling or medication, who are unable to fulfill their responsibilities, who exhaust the patience and resources of significant others, who pose a diagnostic dilemma, who consume inordinate quantities of medical resources, or who are becoming more symptomatic should be evaluated by a psychiatrist.

Somatizing Disorders

Definitions and Diagnostic Criteria

Somatizing disorders are those in which psychological conflicts are expressed in the form of physical symptoms. There is a spectrum of somatizing disorders based on the degree to which the patient is consciously aware of or responsible for the symptoms. The spectrum ranges from the malingerer to the so-called "hysteric," who is completely unaware of the link between her psyche and her physical problem.

Malingering   *Malingering* consists of the deliberate mimicking of signs and symptoms of physical or mental illness in order to achieve a tangible personal gain, such as exemption from dangerous military duties or exoneration from criminal responsibility. *Factitious disorder,* **or** *Münchhausen syndrome,* **is a related and poorly understood condition in which the patient actively causes somatic damage or feigns somatic symptoms that result in hospital admission and painful, dangerous, and invasive diagnostic and thera-**

Table 12.5   Compounds Used for Anxiety

Medication	Trade Name	Rate of Absorption*	Half-Life†	Active Long-Acting Metabolite	Comments
Benzodiazepines					
					Metabolism of benzodiazepines is inhibited by cimetidine, disulfiram, isoniazid, and oral contraceptives. Metabolism of benzodiazepines is enhanced by rifampin.
Alprazolam	Xanax	Intermediate	Intermediate	No	Preferred in elderly patients or patients with poor hepatic functions.
Chlordiazepoxide	Librium, others	Intermediate	Intermediate	Yes	
Clonazepam	Klonopin	Long	Long	No	
Clorazepate	Tranxene, others	Short	Short	Yes	
Diazepam	Valium, others	Short	Long	Yes	Half-life increased three or four times in elderly patients.
Lorazepam	Ativan, others	Intermediate	Intermediate	No	Preferred in elderly patients or patients with poor hepatic function.
Oxazepam	Serax	Long	Intermediate	No	Preferred in elderly patients or patients with poor hepatic function.
Prazepam	Centrax	Long	Short	Yes	
Atypical agent					
Buspirone	BuSpar				Not effective in panic disorder, little sedation, little risk of dependence/tolerance.

*Long ≥ 2 hours; Intermediate = 1–2 hours; Short ≤ 1 hour.
†Long > 20 hours; Intermediate = 6–20 hours; Short < 6 hours.
Adapted from **Gilman AG, Rall TW, Nies AS, Taylor P.** *The Pharmacological Basis of Therapeutics.* 8th ed. New York: McGraw-Hill, 1990.
From **Stotland NL.** Psychiatric and psychosocial issues in primary care for women. In: **Seltzer VL, Pearse WH,** ed. *Women's Primary Health Care: Office Practice and Procedures.* New York: McGraw-Hill, 1995.

peutic procedures. Significant iatrogenic conditions, such as adhesions or Cushing's syndrome, may develop. These patients are initially engaging but eventually frustrate the staff. When suspicion develops and a psychiatrist is called in for consultation, the patient generally flees, only to reappear elsewhere. As a result, there is little data about etiology, incidence, and management. Often, these patients are medically sophisticated by virtue of medical training, previous serious medical illnesses, or significant others in medical professions. Mothers may enact this disorder through their children, which is referred to as "Münchhausen by proxy."

Somatization Disorder   *Somatization disorder* begins before 30 years of age and continues for many years. The patient has a multiplicity of symptoms for which adequate medical bases cannot be established; these symptoms lead either to repeated medical visits or to impairment in the performance of life responsibilities. To qualify for the diagnosis, the patient must at some time have experienced pain related to four different anatomical sites or physiologic functions, two gastrointestinal symptoms, one sexual or reproductive symptom, and one pseudoneurologic symptom or deficit other than pain. The patient's perception is that she is "sickly." She responds accurately to questions about her past symptoms and treatments but may not volunteer information about them unless she is asked.

Conversion Disorder   *Conversion disorder,* formerly termed "hysteria," results in a loss of voluntary motor or sensory function that cannot be explained by medical illness, that is not deliberately produced by the patient, and that appears to be related to psychological stress or conflict. The prognosis is directly related to the length of time from onset to diagnosis.

Other Somatizing Disorders   In *pain disorder,* the symptom consists of pain. *Body dysmorphic disorder* consists of preoccupation with a trivial or imagined defect in bodily appearance, which is seldom assuaged by attempts at medical or surgical correction. *Hypochondriasis* is not a matter of particular numbers or types of symptoms but of a patient's nonpsychotic conviction or fear that she suffers from a serious disease. This conviction causes her to amplify normal bodily sensations and is not responsive to medical reassurance.

Epidemiology

Somatization is believed to be the most common and most difficult psychological symptom in office practice. It has been estimated that 60–80% of the general population experiences one or more somatic symptoms in a given week (58). Somatization disorder occurs almost exclusively in women; menstrual complaints may be an early sign (7, 19, 58). Lifetime prevalence in women is 0.2–2.0% (7, 59). Conversion disorder is two to 10 times more frequent in women than in men (there is no gender difference in children) (7, 60–63), and it is more common in rural and disadvantaged populations with little medical sophistication (7). Conversion disorder may develop into somatization disorder. Reported rates of somatization disorder is 11–300 per 100,000 (7, 60, 64). Pain disorder is extremely common in both genders (7). Hypochondriasis is equally distributed between men and women; prevalence in general medical practice is estimated to be 4–9% (7). There are few statistics about body dysmorphic disorder, but it seems equally distributed between men and women, with an average age of first occurrence at about 30 years (7, 58).

Functional Assessment

Most somatizing disorders are chronic. The point is not so much the fact that the patient has somatic symptoms, but rather how she copes with them. The clinician needs to know how many other health care providers the patient has previously consulted for her current or past symptoms, what diagnostic and therapeutic maneuvers were performed, and what outcomes resulted. How handicapped has she been by her complaints and for how long? What does she believe is wrong with her, and what treatment and prognosis does she expect?

Management

Management of somatizing disorders is focused on the avoidance of unnecessary medical interventions, iatrogenic medical or psychological complications, and disability. Patients with these disorders cause the primary practitioner much anxiety, not only because of their demands but also because it is never possible to rule out completely a significant medical illness. Clinical experience is full of examples of patients with multiple sclerosis and other diseases who endure months or years labeled as "neurotic" before the correct diagnosis is made. Patients with years of psychologically based gastrointestinal symptoms can get appendicitis. Each instance requires clinical judgment.

As with anxious patients, it is important not to structure the doctor-patient relationship so that the patient receives attention inconsistently and only in response to escalating demands. It is best to schedule frequent, brief, regular visits during which the clinician allots a small amount of time to listen to and sympathize with the patient's somatic complaints and spends the bulk of the time reinforcing the patient's successful efforts to function despite her chronic symptoms. Family counseling should also focus on the family's role in facilitating function rather than invalidism.

It is often tempting to attempt to unmask patently psychologically based symptoms by tricking the patient: shouting "fire!" in the vicinity of a "paralyzed" patient, searching the patient's hospital room or belongings for paraphernalia used to cause symptoms, documenting the patient's behavior when she believes she is not observed. Some of these maneuvers are unethical, and others are useful diagnostically but not therapeutically. Humiliating a frustrating patient may be momentarily gratifying, may force her to relinquish a symptom, or may even provoke her to seek care elsewhere, but it does not solve her problem or prevent further drain on medical resources.

Patients with conversion, somatizing, and hypochondriacal disorders often derive benefit from prescriptive behavioral regimens aimed at saving face and restoring function. It was once believed that a patient relieved of one symptom would soon substitute another, but data do not bear out this assumption. The behavioral regimen should consist of health-promoting activities relevant to the target symptoms, planned in a step-wise progression, and recommended with reasonable conviction and authority. For example, the patient with difficulty swallowing can be prescribed a regimen progressing from clear liquids through purees to soft foods and finally a regular diet. The patient with difficulties in the extremities can undertake an exercise regimen. The patient's preoccupation with her symptoms can be channeled into focused documentation of her progress in a log that she brings to her medical appointments; she can be advised not to dwell on her symptoms apart from this important notation.

It is critical to remember that patients with somatic complaints due to clinical depression, posttraumatic stress disorder, anxiety disorders, and domestic violence frequently seek care from gynecologists. In the case of physical abuse, the gynecologist is often virtually the only contact the patient is allowed to have with the world outside the battering situation. These possibilities must be considered and eliminated before care is directed to the management of symptoms.

There is considerable cross-cultural variation in the extent to which feelings and conflicts are somatized. In Asian cultures, for example, direct complaints about feelings, behaviors, and interpersonal relationships are almost unheard of; these complaints are expressed and treated somatically. On the other hand, some very sophisticated and psychologically informed patients may interpret serious somatic signs as symptoms of unconscious conflict.

Referral

Patients with somatizing disorders may resist psychiatric referral more adamantly than any other single class of patients. Focused as they are on physical symptoms, these patients may regard suggestions of mental health consultation as an indication that their complaints are not taken seriously and as a sign of contempt and rejection by the gynecologist. It is particularly useful with these patients to emphasize the inseparable links between mind and body in all human beings; we all speak of "butterflies in the stomach," situations that "give us a headache," and responding to unwelcome or shocking news by "having a heart attack."

It is also useful to frame the referral in terms of an offer of support for the patient's distress rather than a statement that her troubles are "all in her head." It is enormously helpful to have a mental health professional as a more or less constant member of the clinical team, both to facilitate working alliances and to lessen any negative feelings about referral. Some medical institutions have dedicated "medical psychiatry" services for both inpatients and outpatients; these services offer expertise in the psychological complications of disease and in somatization. Because "somatic" and "psychological" symptoms often coexist and interact, the gynecologist should work in collaboration with the mental health professional.

Personality Disorders

Definitions and Diagnostic Criteria

Personality disorders are pervasive, lifelong, maladaptive patterns of perception and behavior. Patients do not experience themselves as symptomatic, but as put upon by circumstances and other people. They view their own behaviors, which can wreak havoc in the health care setting as well as in patients' lives, as normal, expectable, inevitable reactions to these perceptions. In fact, their behaviors generally provoke in others responses that confirm their expectations. For example, a patient who is convinced that people always abandon her clings desperately to others, driving them eventually to run away.

Personality disorders are organized into clusters. Patients often manifest characteristics of several diagnoses within and without the cluster:

1. **Cluster A—Personality Disorders**
   - Paranoid
   - Schizoid
   - Schizotypal

2. **Cluster B—Personality Disorders**
   - Narcissistic
   - Histrionic
   - Borderline
   - Antisocial

3. **Cluster C—Personality Disorders**
   - Avoidant
   - Dependent
   - Obsessive-compulsive

Individuals who fit in cluster A are isolated, suspicious, detached, and odd. Narcissistic patients are grandiose, arrogant, envious, and entitled. Histrionic individuals are flamboyant and provocative. Antisocial behavior disregards laws and rules of common decency toward others. Borderline patients have difficulty controlling impulses and maintaining stable affects and consistent, realistic perceptions of and relationships with others. They fluctuate between overvaluation and castigation of the same person or direct these feelings alternately between one person and another. When this happens on a gynecology service, it can precipitate major tensions among the staff. These patients also engage in self-destructive behaviors.

Epidemiology

Overall, lifetime prevalence of personality disorders is 2.5% (19). Cluster A disorders are more common in males (7). Within cluster B, 75% of cases are female; the prevalence is 2% in the general population (7). Personality disorders such as narcissistic personality are more common in the clinical population than in the general population (7). Among cluster C disorders, dependent personality is one of the most frequently diagnosed disorders (7); obsessive-compulsive personality is twice as common in males as in females (7). There is a strong association between personality disorders and a history of abuse in childhood (65–68). A current abusive situation should also be considered.

Functional Assessment

The functional results of personality disorders range widely. At one end of the spectrum, the disorder is merely a somewhat exaggerated benign personality style. At the other end, the individual suffers terrible emotional pain and is unable to function in work roles or relationships, spending significant periods of time in psychiatric hospitals or penal institutions. The patient will not present with the signs and symptoms listed in the diagnostic criteria but instead will have complaints about her treatment by others, their responses to her, and the unfairness and difficulties of life in general. Personality disorders do not directly bring patients to gynecologists' offices, but they greatly complicate things once patients arrive there. In the assessment of function, the patient need not be confronted with the origins of her complaints, but rather questions can be asked in her own language: how long has she experienced these troubles, and how much do they hamper her ability to learn, work, and form and maintain relationships?

Management

Significant change is effected rarely in individuals with personality disorders, and often it occurs only after years of expert psychotherapy. The challenge in the gynecology setting is to minimize contention and drain on medical staff while maximizing the likelihood of effective diagnosis and treatment of the patient's gynecologic and primary care conditions. The most helpful single step is identification of the personality disorder. This step enables the gynecologist to recognize when the patient's behaviors result from her personality disorder, to avoid becoming entangled in fruitless interactions with the patient, and to set limits that are neither withholding nor overindulgent.

There is increasing evidence that psychotropic medications are useful for some patients with personality disorders; however, treatment should be given in consultation with a psychiatrist. For example, the treatment of depressive or anxious symptoms in borderline patients is fraught with danger of overdose because of the patients' impulsive and self-destructive tendencies and unstable, often rageful relationships.

Low doses of major tranquilizers are sometimes helpful. Because personality disorders are by definition chronic, minor tranquilizers pose significant risk of habituation. They can be prescribed for temporary stresses, but the gynecologist should take care to prescribe only enough for the intended period of use and indicate "no refill." At the same time, some patients' anxiety, demands, and power struggles are eased when they are given control over their own use of medication. Such an approach requires sufficient familiarity with the patient to ensure safety.

Referral

Personality disorders, by definition, do not directly cause symptoms, so those symptoms cannot generally be used to explain the need for referral to the patient. She attributes her suffering to the misdeeds of others or the cruelty of the world in general, but she does suffer. The stressful effects of this suffering often constitute the most effective basis for referral to a mental health professional. With personality disorders, as with any other conditions, it is not wise to avoid the truth if the patient asks about her diagnosis. If the correct diagnosis is entered on the chart or billing forms, as it should be, many people, including the patient, will have access to it. It is helpful to go over the DSM IV criteria with the patient; this approach puts the diagnosis into a neutral, scientific, and therapeutic context.

Adjustment Disorders

Definitions and Diagnostic Criteria

Adjustment disorders are temporary, self-limited responses to life stressors that are part of the normative range of human experience (in contrast to those that precipitate posttraumatic stress disorder). The patient has symptoms of anxiety or depression that are sufficient to lead her to seek medical care but that do not meet criteria of quantity or quality to establish another psychiatric diagnosis. This diagnosis requires an identifiable stressor, onset within 3 months after the stress begins, and spontaneous resolution within 6 months after the stressor ends. Adjustment disorders must be distinguished from the normal grieving process, which tends to be underestimated in U.S. society and medicine.

Epidemiology

Adjustment disorders affect males and females equally (7) and account for 5–20% of patients in outpatient mental health treatment (7, 69). Very little has been published about these illnesses and prevalences are unknown, although one study did find a 2.3% prevalence among a sample of patients receiving care in a walk-in health clinic (70).

Functional Assessment

The important issue with adjustment disorders is the differentiation between the disorder, an even milder reaction not worthy of a diagnostic label, and a more serious psychiatric disorder. The clinician will want to know the nature of the stressor, whether the patient is able to eat, sleep, and carry out her responsibilities, what coping skills she has used in the past and is able to use currently, and whether she is becoming better or worse each day.

Management

Patients with adjustment disorders can be treated by primary care physicians. The most effective intervention is brief office counseling. Often, the medical setting is the only place the patient can vent her feelings and think through her situation. Although the gynecologist can offer suggestions, it is important that the patient brings her own coping skills to bear and makes autonomous decisions about how to proceed.

Referral

Psychiatric referral is seldom necessary. If the gynecologist prefers not to undertake brief office counseling, the patient can be seen by a nurse clinician, social worker, or psychologist, preferably a member of the office or hospital staff who is familiar with the gynecologist and the practice. The referring gynecologist should follow the patient's progress and facilitate transfer of the mental health portion of care to a psychiatrist if symptoms do not resolve.

Eating Disorders

Definitions and Diagnostic Criteria

Preoccupation, even obsession, with thinness is a major problem for women in North America. Only a small minority of women profess to be satisfied with their weights and body shapes; nearly all admit to current or recent attempts to limit food intake. Physicians share social prejudices and can easily exacerbate patients' concerns.

Anorexia Nervosa   *Anorexia nervosa* is associated with severe restrictions on food intake, often accompanied by excessive physical exercise and the use of diuretics or laxatives. Clinical features include menstrual irregularities; intense, irrational fear of becoming fat; preoccupation with body weight as an indicator of self-worth; and inability to acknowledge the realities and dangers of the condition.

Bulimia   Patients with *bulimia* are overcome by eating binges, which they attempt to counteract by inducing vomiting or using laxatives. They may be of normal or excessive weight. They have a high incidence of associated depression and low self-esteem.

Epidemiology

More than 90% of cases of anorexia and bulimia occur in females (7); the prevalence is 0.5–1.0% in late adolescence and 1–3% in early adulthood (7, 71). There is some evidence of familial transmission (7, 72). No statistics are available for overeating, which is frequently overlooked; obesity is an increasingly prevalent clinical problem (73, 74). Some cases of anorexia are diagnosed when patients seek care from gynecologists for infertility or amenorrhea.

Functional Assessment

One vital index of functional impairment is the patient's nutritional, hormonal, and general health status, as well as specific medical complications of an eating disorder. Untreated anorexia poses significant risk of death, often from cardiac complications of electrolyte ab-

322

normalities. The repeated induction of vomiting can cause erosion of tooth enamel by gastric juices. The other index is the patient's psychiatric status: her insight into her problem, her mood, her self-esteem, her relationships, her general level of function. Eating disorders, like several other psychiatric illnesses, may be associated with a history of childhood abuse and with current domestic violence (75). Inquiry should be made about these factors.

Management

Patients with anorexia or bulimia should be treated by mental health professionals, preferably individuals with specific expertise in this area. Anorexia, in particular, is a life-threatening and not easily treated disease. A specific contract for weight gain must be made with the patient; if she fails to comply, hospitalization may be required. Patients sometimes resort to elaborate subterfuges to conceal their failure to eat and gain weight. Some patients with bulimia respond to antidepressant medication. Eating disorders should be treated by a mental health professional before instituting gynecologic interventions such as ovulation induction. Attention to the risks of osteopenia or osteoporosis is essential in amenorrheic patients with anorexia nervosa and warrants a collaborative effort between the psychiatrist and gynecologist.

Psychotic Disorders

Definitions and Diagnostic Criteria

Psychotic disorders are characterized by major distortions of thinking and behavior. They include *schizophrenia, schizophreniform disorders, schizoaffective disorders, delusional disorders,* and *brief psychotic disorders*. General medical and toxic conditions should always be considered first. Distinctions between the disorders are based on symptoms, time course, severity, and associated affective symptoms. **The hallmark of psychosis is the presence of delusions or hallucinations.** Hallucinations are sensory perceptions in the absence of external sensory stimuli. Delusions are bizarre beliefs about the nature or motivation of external events. Because there is no universal definition of "bizarre," the diagnostician working with a patient from an unfamiliar culture must determine whether a given belief is normal in that culture. Delusions and hallucinations are the so-called "positive symptoms" of schizophrenia. The "negative symptoms" include apathy and loss of connections to others and to activities. These symptoms are often more disabling than the so-called positive ones.

Epidemiology

Schizophrenia occurs in approximately 1% of the population worldwide (7, 76). Onset is in the late teens to midthirties; women succumb later and have more prominent mood symptoms and a better prognosis than men (7, 77–79). The risk is 10 times greater for first-degree biological relatives (7) and for individuals of low socioeconomic status (7, 76, 78). It is unclear whether indigent status is a precipitating stress or a result of psychotic illness.

Functional Assessment

There is wide variability in the functional impact of psychotic disorders. Clinicians must be careful not to assume that patients are incompetent to make decisions or to maintain independent lives, especially if they comply with treatment. A relentlessly downhill course is not inevitable; some psychotic disorders remit, and a significant percentage of patients recover. Therefore, mental status should be carefully examined for each patient, regardless of whether the patient has had a previously diagnosed psychiatric condition. It is equally important to include in every medical history an inquiry about past psychiatric diagnoses and treatments. Gynecologists who avoid this part of the history because of stigma or concern about complex clinical problems may find themselves confronted later with life-threatening psychiatric emergencies.

In the rapid-fire interview context imposed by some medical settings, it is entirely possible to overlook florid psychosis. Patients who believe that conspiracies or Martians are responsible for their gynecologic symptoms can seem reasonable when answering "yes or no" questions. Open-ended questions focused on the patient's conception of the history of present illness and the reasons for it, the expected treatment, and the patient's real-life functioning (i.e., living situation, money management, self-care, employment) are more fruitful and relevant.

When psychotic women have responsibility for the care of children or other dependents, their ability to do so should probably be assessed in consultation with an expert. This is also true for other severely impaired patients. This is not to imply that they are invariably incompetent to carry out these duties. The assessment should be performed with sensitivity to avoid damaging patients' already compromised self-esteem and threatening what is often a major source of emotional gratification and a sense of worthiness and identity.

Sensationalized media accounts of some violent crimes exacerbate public misconceptions about psychotic illness. In fact, individuals with psychoses are not much more likely than members of the general population to commit crimes (they are more likely to be victims of crimes) or to engage in violent behavior. The best predictor of risk is previous history. Special caution must be taken with paranoid patients who believe, without good evidence, that others are determined to harm them. Because of their painful suspicions, paranoid patients may not easily confide these beliefs or other critical historical data.

Management

Psychotic illnesses are nearly always managed by psychiatrists. However, a primary care practitioner can readily assume responsibility, in consultation with a psychiatrist, for a stable patient who complies with treatment. It is important to concentrate on the patient's strengths and to avoid humiliating her by the thoughtless use of stigmatizing epithets among staff or by behaviors that betray an unwarranted expectation of dangerousness or incompetence. The most effective approach is a multidisciplinary one, integrating social services, family support, rehabilitative efforts, and general medical, psychopharmacologic, and psychotherapeutic care (78, 80).

Referral

Chronically psychotic patients are accustomed to the fact that psychiatrists are consulted when they seek medical care. Acutely psychotic patients are often very frightened and sometimes very agitated. In either case, the patient should be told that her symptoms necessitate consultation with an expert who will very likely to able to mitigate them. With a paranoid patient, the clinician should focus on her distress and avoid debates about the nature of her suspicions. It is important to be clear, matter-of-fact, open, and confident. If the patient becomes increasingly agitated or threatening during the course of a medical interaction, the physician should not reply in kind but should firmly summon enough help to subdue the patient if necessary, inform the patient that steps must be taken to ensure her safety and that of others, and obtain emergency psychiatric consultation.

Summary

Psychiatric disorders are real, diagnosable, and treatable. The effective identification and management of psychiatric conditions can save the gynecologist considerable grief, the health care system useless expenditure, and the patients significant suffering, morbidity, disability, and mortality. It can be intellectually challenging and professionally gratifying. The foundations for successful interventions are an open mind, an interest in the patient's replies to open-ended questions, inquiries about past psychiatric symptoms and treatments, knowledge of the straightforward criteria for making accurate psychiatric diagnoses, and a working relationship with one or more mental health experts.

References

1. **Schurman RA, Kramer PD, Mitchell JB.** The hidden mental health network: treatment of mental illness by nonpsychiatrist physicians. *Arch Gen Psych* 1985;42:89–94.

2. **Dubovsky SL.** *Psychotherapeutics in Primary Care.* New York: Grune & Stratton, 1981.

3. **Smith I, Adkins S, Walton J.** *Pharmaceuticals: Therapeutic Review.* New York: Shearson, Lehman, Hutton International Research, 1988.

4. **Pierce C.** Failure to spot mental illness in primary care is a global problem. *Clin Psych News* 1993;21(8):5.

5. **Margolis RL.** Nonpsychiatric house staff frequently misdiagnose psychiatric disorders in general hospital inpatients. *Psychosomatics* 1994;35(5):485–91.

6. **Perez-Stable EJ, Miranda J, Munoz RF, Ying DW.** Depression in medical outpatients: underrecognition and misdiagnosis. *Arch Intern Med* 1990;150:1083–8.

7. **American Psychiatric Association.** *Diagnostic and Statistical Manual of Mental Disorders.* 4th ed. Washington, DC: American Psychiatric Press, 1994.

8. **Depression Guideline Panel.** *Depression in Primary Care: Vol. 1, Detection and Diagnosis.* Clinical Practice Guideline No. 5. AHCPR Publication No. 93-0550. Rockville, MD: US Department of Health and Human Services, Public Health Service, Agency for Health Care Policy and Research, 1993.

9. **Cassem NH.** Depression. In: **Cassem NH,** ed. *Massachusetts General Hospital Handbook of General Hospital Psychiatry.* St. Louis: Mosby Year Book, 1991:237–68.

10. **Murphy GE.** The physician's responsibility for suicide. II: Errors of omission. *Ann Intern Med* 1975;82:305–9.

11. **Veith I.** *Hysteria: The history of a Disease.* Chicago: The University of Chicago Press, 1965.

12. **Orleans CT, George LK, Houpt JL, Brodie HKH.** How primary care physicians treat psychiatric disorders: a national survey of family practitioners. *Am J Psych* 1985;142(1):52–7.

13. **Beckman HB, Frankel RM.** The effect of physician behavior on the collection of data. *Ann Intern Med* 1984;101:692–6.

14. **McGrath E, Keita GP, Strickland BR, Russo NF.** *Women and Depression: Risk Factors and Treatment Issues.* Final report of the American Psychological Association's National Task Force on Women and Depression. Washington, DC: American Psychological Association, 1990.

15. **Dubovsky SL, Weissberg MP.** *Clinical Psychiatry in Primary Care.* 3rd ed. Baltimore: Williams & Wilkins, 1986.

16. **Scheiber SC.** The psychiatric interview, psychiatric history, and mental status examination. In: **Hales RE, Yudofsky SC, Talbott JA,** eds. *Textbook of Psychiatry.* 2nd ed. Washington, DC: The American Psychiatric Press, 1994:187–219.

17. **Spiegel D, Bloom JR, Kraemer HL, Gottheil E.** Effect of psychosocial treatment on survival of patients with metastatic breast cancer. *Lancet* 1989;2:888–91.

18. **Fawzy FI, Cousins NI, Fawzy NW, Kemeny ME, Elashoff R, Morton D.** A structured psychiatric intervention for cancer patients. I: Changes over time in methods of coping and affective disturbance. *Arch Gen Psych* 1990;47:720–5.

19. **Regier DA, Boyd JK, Burke JD Jr, Rae DS, Myers JK, Kramer M, et al.** One-month prevalence of mental disorders in the United States—based on five Epidemiologic Catchment Area sites. *Arch Gen Psych* 1988;45:977–85.

20. **Robins LN, Helzer JE, Weissman MN, Orvaschel H, Graenberg E, Burke JD Jr, et al.** Lifetime prevalence of specific psychiatric disorders in three sites. *Arch Gen Psych* 1984;41:949–58.

21. **Boyd JH, Weissman MM.** Epidemiology of affective disorders: a reexamination and future directions. *Arch Gen Psych* 1981;38:1039–46.

22. **Goldman N, Ravid R.** Community surveys: sex differences in mental illness. In: **Guttentag M, Salasin S, Belle D,** eds. *The Mental Health of Women.* New York: Academic Press, 1980.

23. **Nolen-Hoeksema S.** *Sex differences in depression.* Stanford, CA: Stanford University Press, 1990.

24. **Weissman MM, Leaf PJ, Holzer CE, Myers JK, Tischler GL.** The epidemiology of depression: an update on sex differences in rates. *J Affect Dis* 1984;7:179–88.

25. **Jefferson JW, Greist JH.** Mood disorders. In: **Hales RE, Yudofsky SC, Talbott JA,** eds. *Textbook of Psychiatry.* 2nd ed. Washington, DC: American Psychiatric Press, 1994:465–94.

26. **Sainsbury P.** Depression, suicide, and suicide prevention. In: **Baltimore RA,** ed. *Suicide.* Baltimore: Williams & Wilkins, 1990:17–38.

27. **Perlin LI.** Sex roles and depression. In: **Datan N, Ginsberg L,** eds. *Life-Span Developmental Psychology: Normative Life Crises.* New York: Academic Press, 1975:191–207.

28. **Radloff LS.** Sex differences in depression: the effects of occupation and marital status. *Sex Roles* 1975;1:249–65.

29. **Roberts RE, O'Keefe SJ.** Sex differences in depression reexamined. *J Health Soc Behav* 1981;22:394–9.

30. **Hamilton JA, Parry BL, Blumenthal SL.** The menstrual cycle in context: I. Affective syndromes associated with reproductive hormonal changes. *J Clin Psych* 1988;49:474–80.

31. **Jensvold MF.** Psychiatric aspects of the menstrual cycle. In: **Stewart DE, Stotland NL,** eds. *Psychological Aspects of Women's Health Care.* Washington, DC: American Psychiatric Press, 1993:165–92.

32. **Tavris C.** *The mismeasure of women: why women are not the better sex, the inferior sex, or the opposite sex.* New York: Simon & Schuster, 1992.

33. **McKinlay JB, McKinlay SM, Brambilla DJ.** Health status and utilization behavior associated with menopause. *Am J Epidemiol* 1987;125:110–21.

34. **Hamilton JA.** Psychobiology in context: reproductive-related events in men's and women's lives (review of motherhood and mental illness). *Contemp Psych* 1984;3:12–6.

35. **Nadelson C, Notman MT, Ellis EA.** Psychosomatic aspects of obstetrics and gynecology [special issue]. *Psychosomatics* 1983:24(10).

36. **Andrews G, Harvey R.** Does psychotherapy benefit neurotic patients? A reanalysis of the Smith, Glass, and Miller data. *Arch Gen Psych* 1981;38:1203–8.

37. **Wright JK, Beck AT.** Cognitive therapy. In: **Hales RE, Yudofsky SC, Talbott JA,** eds. *Textbook of Psychiatry.* 2nd ed. Washington, DC: American Psychiatric Press, 1994:1083–114.

38. **Noll KM, Davis JM, De Leon-Jones F.** Medication and somatic therapies in the treatment of depression. In: **Beckman EE, Leber WR,** eds. *Handbook of Depression: Treatment, Assessment, and Research.* Homewood, IL: Dorsey Press, 1985.

39. **Liebowitz MR, Quitkin FM, Stewart JW, McGrath PJ, Harrison W, Rabkin J, et al.** Phenelzine v imipramine in atypical depression: a preliminary report. *Arch Gen Psych* 1984;41:669–77.

40. **Schatzberg AF, Cole JO.** Antidepressants. In: *Manual of Clinical Pharmacology.* Washington, DC: American Psychiatric Press, 1986:3–65.

41. **Stark P, Hardison D.** A review of multicenter controlled studies of fluoxetine vs. imipramine and placebo in outpatients with major depressive disorder. *J Clin Psych* 1985;46:53–8.

42. **Goodwin FK, Jamison KR.** Medical treatment of acute bipolar depression. In: **Goodwin FK, Jamison KR,** eds. *Manic-Depressive Illness.* New York: Oxford University Press, 1990:630–64.

43. **Goodwin FK, Jamison KR.** Medical treatment of manic episodes. In: **Goodwin FK, Jamison KR,** eds. *Manic-Depressive Illness.* New York: Oxford University Press, 1990:603–29.

44. **Hirschfeld RMA, Goodwin FK.** Mood disorders. In: **Talbott JA, Hales RE, Yudofsky SC,** eds. *Textbook of Psychiatry.* Washington, DC: American Psychiatric Press, 1988:403–41.

45. **Klerman GL.** Clinical epidemiology of suicide. *J Clin Psychiatry* 1987;48:12(Suppl):33–8.

46. **Buda M, Tsuang MT.** The epidemiology of suicide: implications for clinical practice. In: **Blumenthal SJ, Kupfer DJ,** eds. *Suicide Over the Life Cycle: Risk Factors, Assessment, and Treatment of Suicidal Patients.* Washington, DC: American Psychiatric Press, 1990:17–38.

47. **Rosenbaum JF, Pollack MH.** Anxiety. In: **Cassem NH,** ed. *Massachusetts General Hospital Handbook of General Hospital Psychiatry.* St. Louis: Mosby Year Book, 1991:159–90.

48. **Hollander E, Simeon D, Gorman JM.** Anxiety disorders. In: **Hales RE, Yudofsky SC, Talbott JA,** eds. *Textbook of Psychiatry.* 2nd ed. Washington, DC: American Psychiatric Press, 1994:495–564.

49. **Baldessrini RJ.** Drugs and the treatment of psychiatric disorders. In: **Gilman AG, Rall TW, Nies AS, Taylor P,** eds. *Goodman and Gilman's The Pharmacological Basis of Therapeutics.* 8th ed. New York: Pergamon Press, 1990:383–435.

50. **Roy-Byrne PP, Cowley DS.** *Benzodiazepines in Clinical Practice: Risks and Benefits.* Washington, DC: American Psychiatric Press, 1991.

51. **Barlow DH, Craske MG, Cerny JA, Klosko JS.** Behavioral treatment of panic disorder. *Behav Ther* 1989;20:261–82.

52. **Foa EB, Steketee G, Grayson JB, Turner RM, Latimer PR.** Deliberate exposure and blocking of obsessive-compulsive rituals: immediate and long-term effects. *Behav Ther* 1984;15:450–72.

53. **Cooper NA, Clum GA.** Imaginal flooding as a supplementary treatment for PTSD in combat veterans: a controlled study. *Behav Ther* 1989;20:381–91.

54. **Butler G.** Issues in the application of cognitive and behavioral strategies to the treatment of social phobia. *Clin Psychol Rev* 1989;9:91–106.

55. **Craske MG, Brown TA, Barlow DH.** Behavioral treatment of panic disorder: a two-year followup. *Behav Ther* 1991;22:289–304.

56. **Jenike MA, Baer L, Summergrad P, Weilburg JB, Holland A, Seymour R.** Obsessive-compulsive disorder: a double-blind, placebo-controlled trial of clomipramine in 27 patients. *Am J Psychol* 1989;146:1328–30.

57. **Jenike MA, Baer L.** An open trial of buspirone in obsessive-compulsive disorder. *Am J Psychol* 1988;145:1285–6.

58. **Cassem NH, Barsky AJ.** Functional symptoms and somatoform disorders. In: **Cassem NH,** ed. *Massachusetts General Hospital Handbook of General Hospital Psychiatry.* St. Louis: Mosby Year Book, 1991:131–57.

59. **Cloninger CR, Reich T, Guze SB.** The multifactorial model of disease transmission. III: Familial relationship between sociopathy and hysteria (Briquet's syndrome). *Br J Psych* 1975;127:23–32.

60. **Ford CV, Folks DG.** Conversion disorders: an overview. *Psychosomatics* 1985;26:371–7, 380–3.

61. **Ljundberg L.** Hysteria: clinical, prognostic, and genetic study. *Acta Psych Scand Suppl* 1957;32:1–162.

62. **Stefansson JH, Messina JA, Meyerowitz S.** Hysterical neurosis, conversion type: clinical and epidemiological considerations. *Acta Psychol Scand* 1976;59:119–38.

63. **Raskin M, Talbott JA, Meyerson AT.** Diagnosis of conversion reactions: predictive value of psychiatric criteria. *JAMA* 1966;197:530–4.

64. **Toone, BK.** Disorders of hysterical conversion. In: **Bass C,** ed. *Physical Symptoms and Psychological Illness.* London: Blackwell Scientific, 1990:207–34.

65. **Beck JC, van der Kolk B.** Reports of childhood incest and current behavior of chronically hospitalized psychotic women. *Am J Psychol* 1987;144:1474–6.

66. **Koss MP.** The women's mental health research agenda: violence against women. *Am Psychol* 1990;45:257–63.

67. **Bryer JB, Nelson BA, Miller JB, Krol PA.** Childhood sexual and physical abuse as factors in adult psychiatric illness. *Am J Psychol* 1987;114:1426–30.

68. **van der Kolk BA, Herman JL, Perry C.** *Traumatic Antecedents of Borderline Personality Disorder.* Presented at the Fourth Annual Meeting of the Society for Traumatic Stress Studies, Baltimore, 1987.

69. **Andreasen NC, Wasek P.** Adjustment disorders in adolescents and adults. *Arch Gen Psych* 1980;37:1166–70.

70. **Fabrega H Jr, Mezzich JE, Mezzich AC.** Adjustment disorder as a marginal or transitional illness category in DSM-III. *Arch Gen Psychol* 1987;44:567–72.

71. **Stewart DE, Robinson GE.** Eating disorders and reproduction. In: **Stewart DE, Stotland NL,** eds. *Psychological Aspects of Women's Health Care.* Washington, DC: American Psychiatric Press, 1993:411–24.

72. **Strober M, Morell W, Burroughs J, Salkin B, Jacobs C.** A controlled family study of anorexia nervosa. *J Psych Res* 1985;19:329–46.

73. **Bray GA.** Definitions, measurements, and classification of the syndromes of obesity. *Int J Obes* 1978;2:99–112.

74. **VanItallie TB.** Health implications of overweight and obesity in the United States. *Ann Intern Med* 1985;103:983–8.

75. **Root MP, Fallon P.** The incidence of victimization experiences in a bulimic sample. *J Interpersonal Violence* 1986;3:161–73.

76. **Goff DC, Manschreck TC, Groves JE.** Psychotic patients. In: **Cassem NH,** ed. *Massachusetts General Hospital Handbook of General Hospital Psychiatry.* St. Louis: Mosby Year Book, 1991:217–36.

77. **Von Korff M, Nestadt G, Romanoski A, Anthony J, Eaton W, Merchant A, et al.** Prevalence of treated and untreated DSM-III schizophrenia: results of a two-stage community survey. *J Nerv Ment Dis* 1985;173:577–81.

78. **Black DW, Andreasen NC.** Schizophrenia, schizophreniform disorder, and delusional (paranoid) disorder. In: Hales RE, Yudofsky SC, Talbott JA, eds. *Textbook of Psychiatry.* 2nd ed. Washington, DC: American Psychiatric Press, 1994:411–63.

79. **Beiser M, Iacono WG.** Update on the epidemiology of schizophrenia. *Can J Psych* 1990;35:657–68.

80. **Michels R, Marzuk PM.** Progress in psychiatry (first of two parts). *N Engl J Med* 1993;329(8):552–60.

81. **Stotland NL.** Psychiatric and psychosocial issues in primary care for women. In: **Seltzer VL, Pearse WH,** ed. *Women's Primary Health Care: Office Practice and Procedures.* New York: McGraw-Hill, 1995.

GENERAL GYNECOLOGY

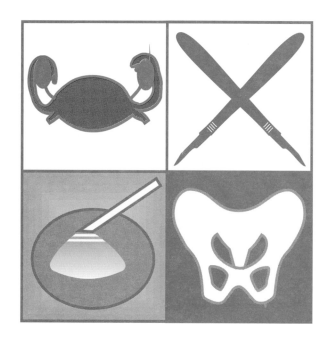

13 Benign Diseases of the Female Reproductive Tract: Symptoms and Signs

Paula A. Hillard

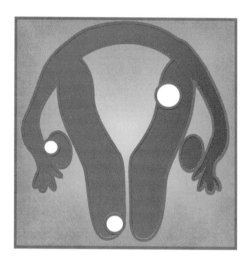

Benign conditions of the female genital tract include lesions of the uterine corpus and cervix, ovaries and fallopian tubes, and the vagina and vulva. Classification of the benign lesions of the vulva, vagina, and cervix are listed in Table 13.1. Leiomyoma, polyps, and hyperplasia are the most common benign conditions of the uterus. Benign tumors of the ovaries are listed in Table 13.2.

A symptom is subjective evidence of disease or of a patient's condition as perceived by the patient; a sign is objective evidence of the existence of disease as perceived by the patient. Common gynecologic problems include abnormal bleeding, a pelvic mass, and vulvovaginal symptoms. The causes of vaginal bleeding and a pelvic mass vary by age group (Table 13.3). For each age group, the most common causes of these problems are described, along with techniques of diagnosis and principles of management. Malignant diseases are presented in Chapters 30 through 37.

Abnormal Bleeding

Prepubertal Age Group

To appropriately evaluate a young girl with vaginal bleeding, the events of puberty must be understood (1, 2). The hormonal changes that eventuate in the cyclic functioning of the hypothalamic-pituitary-ovarian axis are described in Chapter 7. An understanding of the normal sequence and timing of these events is critical to an appropriate assessment of a girl at the onset of bleeding (see Chapter 23).

Differential Diagnosis of Prepubertal Bleeding

Slight vaginal bleeding can occur within the first few days of life because of withdrawal from the high level of maternal estrogens. After the neonatal period, a number of causes of bleeding should be considered in this age group (Table 13.4). The onset of menses before

331

Table 13.1   Classification of Benign Conditions of the Vulva, Vagina, and Cervix

Vulva

Skin conditions
Pigmented lesions
Tumors and cysts
Ulcers
Dystrophies

Vagina

Embryonic origin
    Mesonephric, paramesonephric, and urogenital sinus cysts
    Adenosis (related to diethylstilbestrol)
    Vaginal septa/duplications
Disorders of pelvic support
    Cystocele
    Rectocele
    Urethrocele
Other
    Condyloma
    Urethral diverticuli
    Fibroepithelial polyp
    Vaginal endometriosis

Cervix

Infectious
    Condyloma
    Herpes simplex virus ulceration
    Chlamydial cervicitis
    Other cervicitis
Other
    Endocervical polyps
    Nabothian cysts
    Columnar epithelium eversion

Table 13.2   Benign Ovarian Tumors

Functional

Follicular
Corpus luteum
Theca lutein

Inflammatory

Tubo-ovarian abscess or complex

Neoplastic

Germ cell
    Benign cystic teratoma
    Other and mixed
Epithelial
    Serous cystadenoma
    Mucinous cystadenoma
    Fibroma
    Cystadenofibroma
    Brenner tumor
    Mixed tumor

Other

Endometrioma

Table 13.3   Causes of Bleeding and Pelvic Mass By Approximate Frequency and Age Group

Bleeding

Prepubertal	Adolescent	Reproductive	Perimenopausal	Postmenopausal
Vulvovaginal and external lesions Foreign body Precocious puberty Tumor	Anovulation Pregnancy Exogenous hormone use Coagulopathy	Pregnancy Anovulation Exogenous hormone use Fibroids Cervical and endometrial polyps Thyroid dysfunction	Anovulation Fibroids Cervical and endometrial polyps Thyroid dysfunction	Endometrial lesions, including cancer Exogenous hormone use Atrophic vaginitis Other tumor—vulvar, vaginal, cervical

Pelvic Mass

Infancy	Prepubertal	Adolescent	Reproductive	Perimeno-pausal	Postmeno-pausal
Functional ovarian cyst Germ cell	Germ cell tumor	Functional cyst Pregnancy Dermoid/other germ cell tumors Obstructing vaginal/uterine anomalies Epithelial ovarian tumors	Functional cyst Pregnancy Uterine fibroids Ovarian epithelial tumors	Fibroids Ovarian epithelial tumors Functional cysts	Ovarian tumor (malignant or benign) Bowel, malignant tumor or inflammatory Metastases

Table 13.4   Causes of Vaginal Bleeding in Prepubertal Girls

Vulvar and external

Vulvitis with excoriation
Trauma (e.g., straddle injury)
Lichen sclerosus
Condylomas
Molluscum contagiosum
Urethral prolapse

Vaginal

Vaginitis
Vaginal foreign body
Trauma (abuse, penetration)
Vaginal tumor

Uterine

Precocious puberty

Ovarian tumor

Exogenous estrogens

Topical
Enteral

breast budding is unusual (1). Vaginal bleeding in the absence of secondary sexual characteristics should be evaluated carefully (2).

The causes of bleeding in this age group range from the medically mundane to malignancies that may be life-threatening. The source of the bleeding is sometimes difficult to identify, and parents who observe blood in a child's diapers or panties may be unsure of the source. Pediatricians will usually look for urinary causes of bleeding, and gastrointestinal factors should also be considered (3, 4).

Vulvar Lesions   Vulvar irritation can lead to pruritus with excoriation, maceration of the vulvar skin, or fissures that can bleed. Other visible external causes of bleeding in this age group include urethral prolapse, condylomata, or molluscum contagiosum (2–5). Urethral prolapse can present acutely with a tender mass that may be friable or bleed slightly. It may be confused with a vaginal mass. The classical presentation is a mass symmetrically surrounding the urethra. This condition can be managed medically with the application of topical estrogens. The presence of condyloma may prompt questioning about abuse, although it has been suggested that condyloma that appears during the first 2 years of life may have been acquired perinatally from a mother with human papillomavirus infection (5). Excoriation and hemorrhage into the skin can cause bleeding.

Foreign Body   A foreign body in the vagina is a common cause of vaginal discharge, which may appear purulent or bloody. Young children explore all orifices and may place all varieties of small objects inside their vaginas (Fig. 13.1). An object, such as a small plastic object, can sometimes be palpated on rectal examination. The most common foreign bodies are small pieces of toilet paper that find their way into the vagina (6). One recent study suggests that the presence of vaginal foreign bodies may be a marker for sexual abuse; although this remains to be confirmed, the possibility of abuse must be kept in mind for any child with vulvovaginal symptoms (7).

Precocious Puberty   Precocious puberty (see Chapter 23) occasionally can present with vaginal bleeding in the absence of other secondary sexual characteristics, although the

Figure 13.1   Foreign body (plastic toy) in the vagina of an 8-year-old girl.

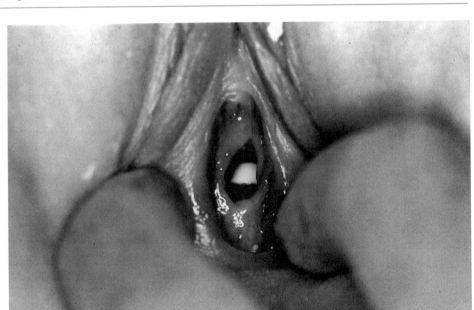

more common occurrence is the onset of breast budding or pubic hair growth before vaginal bleeding.

Trauma   Trauma can be a cause of genital bleeding. **A careful history should be obtained from one or both parents or caretakers and the child herself, because trauma caused by sexual abuse is often not recognized.** Physical findings that are inconsistent with the description of the alleged accident should prompt consideration of abuse and appropriate consultation or referral to an experienced social worker or sexual abuse team. **There is a mandatory legal obligation to report suspected child physical abuse in all states;** most states specifically require reporting child sexual abuse as well, but even in those that do not, the laws are broad enough to encompass sexual abuse implicitly (8). Even the suspicion of sexual abuse requires notification. In general, straddle injuries affect the anterior vulvar area, whereas penetrating injuries with lesions of the fourchette or lesions that extend through the hymenal ring are less likely to occur as a result of accidental trauma (Fig. 13.2) (9). Pediatric genital findings in cases of suspected sexual abuse have been classified as follows.

1. Normal

2. Nonspecific (consistent with either abuse or other causes)

3. Specific findings (strongly suggesting abuse)

4. Definitive findings (the presence of sperm within the vagina)

Figure 13.2   Straddle injury—vulva hematoma in a 13-year-old girl.

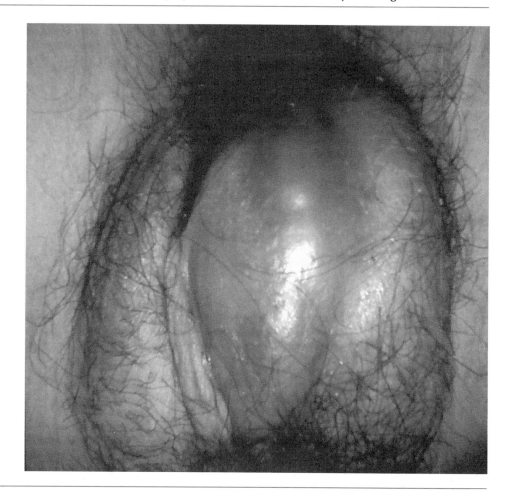

Most cases of child sexual abuse do not come to light with an acute injury and instead are associated with normal or nonspecific genital findings (9, 10). Forms of abuse such as fondling or digital penetration may not result in lasting visible genital lesions (11).

Other Causes   Other serious but rare causes of true vaginal bleeding include vaginal tumors. The most common tumor in the prepubertal age group is a rhabdomyosarcoma ("sarcoma botryoides"), which presents with bleeding and a grape-like clustered mass (Chapter 32). Other forms of vaginal tumor are also rare but should be ruled out if no other obvious source of bleeding is found externally.

Hormonally active ovarian tumors can lead to endometrial proliferation and bleeding. Exogenously administered estrogens can result in bleeding. This can be caused by the overuse of topical estrogens prescribed as therapy for vulvovaginitis or labial adhesions or can result from accidental ingestion of prescription estrogens.

Diagnosis

A careful examination is indicated when a child presents with genital complaints (12). The technique of examining the prepubertal child is described in Chapter 1. **If no obvious cause of bleeding is visible externally or within the distal vagina, an examination under anesthesia with an endoscope may be needed to completely visualize the vagina and cervix** (13).

Imaging Studies   If an ovarian or vaginal mass is suspected, a pelvic ultrasound examination can provide useful information. The appearance of the ovaries (normal prepubertal size, follicular development, cystic or solid) can be noted, as well as the size and configuration of the uterus. **The prepubertal uterus has a distinctive appearance, with equal proportions of cervix and fundus and a size of approximately 2–3.5 cm in length and 0.5–1 cm in width** (Fig. 13.3). The fundus enlarges with estrogen stimulation. An ultrasound examination should be the first imaging study performed; more sophisticated imaging techniques such as magnetic resonance imaging (MRI) or computed tomography (CT) scanning are rarely indicated.

Management

The management of bleeding in the prepubertal age group is directed to the cause of bleeding. If bloody discharge believed to be due to nonspecific vulvovaginitis persists despite therapy, further evaluation to rule out the presence of a foreign body may be necessary. Skin lesions (chronic irritation) and lichen sclerosus may be difficult or frustrating to manage but can be treated with a short course of topical mild steroids. Vaginal and ovarian tumors should be managed in consultation with a gynecologic oncologist.

Adolescence

Normal Menses

To assess vaginal bleeding during adolescence, it is necessary to have an understanding of the range of normal menstrual cycles (see Chapter 7). **During the first 2 years after menarche, most cycles are anovulatory.** Despite this, they are somewhat regular, within a range of approximately 21–40 days (14–16). In more than one-quarter of girls, a pattern of +10 days and a cycle length of 20–40 days are established within the first three cycles; in one-half of girls, the pattern is established by the seventh cycle; and in two-thirds of girls, such a pattern is established within 2 years of menarche (16).

The mean duration of menses is 4.7 days; 89% of cycles last ≤7 days. The average blood loss per cycle is 35 ml (17), and the major component of menstrual discharge is endometrial tissue. Recurrent bleeding in excess of 80 ml/cycle results in anemia.

Quantitative information about the volume of menstrual blood loss is of little clinical use, however. The common clinical practice of asking how many pads or tampons are soaked

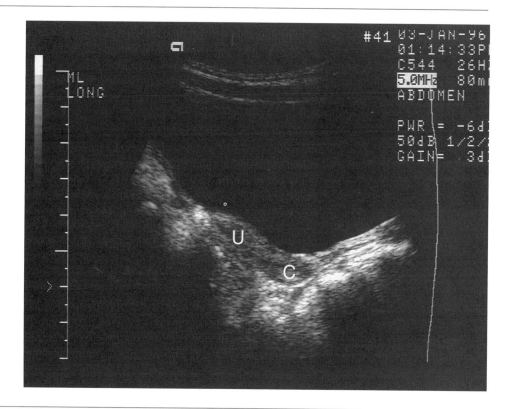

Figure 13.3   Pelvic ultrasound (transabdominal) of a premenarchal 10-year-old girl. U = uterine corpus; C = cervix. Note that the body of the uterus is about the same size as the cervix.

on a heavy day or per cycle can give a rough approximation of blood loss (3–5 pads per day is typical). Individual variations in fastidiousness, lack of familiarity with the volume of blood loss other than one's own, and errors in estimation or recollection result in inaccuracies in estimations of menstrual volume. One study found that one-third of individuals who estimated their cycles to be moderate or light had bleeding in excess of 80 ml/cycle, whereas nearly one-half of those who described the bleeding as heavy had flow less than 80 ml/cycle (18). In addition, the amount of menstrual blood contained in each tampon or pad may vary both within brands as well as from one brand to another.

The transition from anovulatory to ovulatory cycles takes place during the first several years after menarche. It results from the so-called "maturation of the hypothalamic-pituitary-ovarian axis," characterized by positive feedback mechanisms in which a rising estrogen level triggers a surge of luteinizing hormone and ovulation. **Most adolescents have ovulatory cycles by the end of their second year of menstruation, although most cycles (even anovulatory ones) remain within a rather narrow range of 21–42 days.**

Cycles that are longer than 42 days, cycles that are shorter than 21 days, and bleeding that lasts more than 7 days should be considered out of the ordinary, particularly after the first 2 years from the onset of menarche. The variability in cycle length is greater during adolescence than adulthood; thus, greater irregularity is acceptable if significant anemia or hemorrhage is not present. However, consideration should be given to an evaluation of possible causes of abnormal menses (particularly underlying causes of anovulation such as androgen excess syndromes) for girls whose cycles are consistently outside normal ranges.

Differential Diagnosis   *Anovulation*   **Anovulatory bleeding can be too frequent, prolonged, or heavy, particularly after a long interval of amenorrhea.** The physiology of this phenomenon relates to a failure of the feedback mechanism in which rising estrogen levels result in a decline in follicle-stimulating hormone (FSH) with subsequent decline of estrogen levels. Thus, estrogen secretion continues, resulting in endometrial proliferation with subsequent unstable growth and incomplete shedding. The clinical result is irregular, prolonged, and heavy bleeding. Conditions that are associated with anovulation are listed in Table 13.5 and more fully discussed in Chapters 24, 25, and 27.

Studies of adolescent menses show differences in rates of ovulation, based on number of months or years postmenarche. **The younger the age at menarche, the sooner regular ovulation is established.** In one study, the time from menarche until 50% of the cycles were ovulatory was 1 year for girls whose menarche occurred when they were younger than 12 years of age, 3 years for girls whose menarche occurred between 12 and 12.9 years of age, and 4.5 years for girls whose menarche occurred at 13 years of age or older (19).

Pregnancy-Related Bleeding   **The possibility of pregnancy must be considered when an adolescent presents with abnormal bleeding.** Bleeding in pregnancy can be associated with a spontaneous abortion, ectopic pregnancy, or other pregnancy-related complications such as a molar pregnancy. In the U.S., 50% of 17-year-old females have had sexual intercourse (20). Issues of confidentiality for adolescent health care are addressed in Chapter 1.

Exogenous Hormones   Abnormal bleeding that is experienced while an individual is taking exogenous hormones often has a very different cause from bleeding that occurs without hormonal manipulation. **Oral contraceptive use is associated with breakthrough bleeding, which occurs in as many as 30% of individuals during the first cycle of combination pill use. In addition, irregular bleeding can result from missed pills** (21). Strict compliance with correct and consistent pill-taking is difficult for many individuals who take oral contraceptives; one study reported that only 40% of women took a pill every day (22). Other studies suggest that adolescents have an even more difficult time taking oral contraceptives, missing an average of three pills per month (23). With this many missed pills, it is not surprising that some individuals experience irregular bleeding. The solution is to emphasize consistent pill-taking; if the individual is unable to comply with daily pill use, perhaps an alternative contraceptive method may be preferable.

Other methods of contraception can also produce irregular bleeding. Irregular bleeding occurs frequently in users of *depo medroxyprogesterone acetate (DMPA),* although at the end of 1 year, more than 50% of users will be amenorrheic (24). The implantable subdermal *levonorgestrel* implant (*Norplant*) is also associated with relatively high rates of irregular and unpredictable bleeding (25). Although the mechanism of bleeding associated

Table 13.5   Conditions Associated with Anovulation and Abnormal Bleeding

Eating disorders
  Anorexia nervosa
  Bulimia nervosa

Excessive physical exercise
Chronic illness
Alcohol and other drug abuse
Stress

Thyroid disease
  Hypothyroidism
  Hyperthyroidism

Diabetes mellitus
Androgen excess syndromes

with these hormonal methods is not well established, many believe that bleeding occurs from an atrophic endometrium, suggesting options for therapy. However, it should not be assumed that any bleeding occurring while an individual is using a hormonal method of contraception is caused by that method. Other local causes of bleeding, such as from a cervicitis or endometritis, can also occur during hormonal therapy.

Hematologic Abnormalities   In the adolescent age group, the possibility of a hematologic cause of abnormal bleeding must be considered. One study reviewed all patient visits of adolescents to an emergency room with the complaint of excessive or abnormal bleeding (Fig. 13.4) (26). The most common coagulation abnormality diagnosed was idiopathic thrombocytopenic purpura, followed by von Willebrand's disease.

Infections   Irregular or postcoital bleeding can be associated with chlamydial cervicitis. **Adolescents have the highest rates of chlamydial infections of any age group, and screening for chlamydia should be performed routinely among sexually active teens** (27).

Patients who present with menorrhagia have been found to have a higher incidence of sexually transmissible organisms (28). **Adolescents have the highest rates of pelvic inflammatory disease (PID) of any age group when only sexually experienced individuals are considered** (29) (see Chapter 15).

Figure 13.4   Etiology of menorrhagia in adolescents. (Adapted from **Claessens AE, Cowell CA.** Acute adolescent menorrhagia. *Am J Obstet Gynecol* 1981;139: 277–80.)

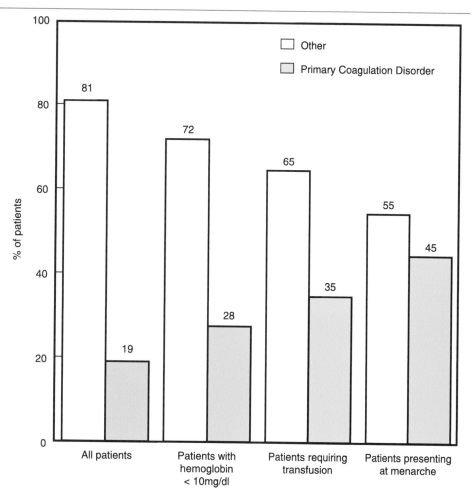

Other Endocrine or Systemic Problems   Abnormal bleeding can be associated with thyroid dysfunction. Signs and symptoms of thyroid disease can be somewhat subtle in teens (Chapter 25). Hepatic dysfunction can lead to abnormalities in clotting factor production and should be suspected and ruled out.

Polycystic ovarian syndrome can occur during adolescence, and manifestations of excess androgen effect (hirsutism, acne) should prompt evaluation (30). **Androgen disorders occur in about 5–10% of women, making them the most common endocrinopathy in women** (Chapter 25). Classical polycystic ovarian syndrome, functional ovarian hyperandrogenism, or partial, late-onset congenital adrenal hyperplasia all can occur in adolescence (31). **These disorders are often overlooked, unrecognized, or untreated.** Women with even mild disorders are candidates for intervention. These disorders may be a harbinger of diabetes, endometrial cancer, and cerebrovascular disease. Apparently normal adolescent changes in skin, hair, and menstrual cyclicity can be indicators of androgen abnormality. If the androgen abnormality is ignored, it is likely to persist beyond adolescence, and additional weight gain with significant psychosocial costs is likely (32). Androgenic changes are partially reversible if detected early and managed appropriately. Behavioral changes (diet and exercise) also are desirable.

Anatomic Causes   Obstructive or partially obstructive genital anomalies can present during adolescence. Müllerian abnormalities such as obstructing longitudinal vaginal septa or uterus didelphis can cause hematocolpos or hematometra. If these obstructing anomalies have or develop a small outlet, the presentation may be of persistent dark-brownish discharge (old blood) rather than or in addition to a pelvic mass. Many varieties of uterine and vaginal anomalies can be seen. Figure 13.5 illustrates situations in which abnormal bleeding can occur as a result of obstructing septa.

Diagnosis

Any adolescent with abnormal bleeding should undergo sensitive pregnancy testing, regardless of her statements about whether she has had intercourse. The medical consequences of failing to diagnose a pregnancy are too severe to risk missing the diagnosis. Complications of pregnancy should then be managed accordingly.

Figure 13.5   The types of obstructive or partially obstructive genital anomalies that can occur during adolescence.

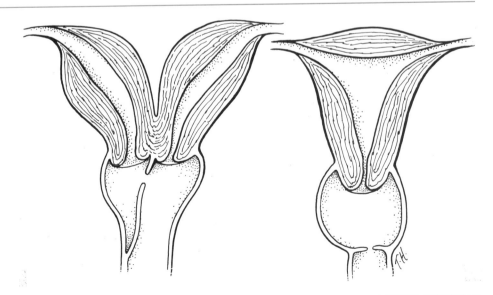

Laboratory Testing   In addition to a pregnancy test, laboratory testing should include a complete blood count with platelets, coagulation studies, and bleeding time. During the examination, cultures for gonorrhea and tests for chlamydia infection are appropriate if the patient has been sexually active. Thyroid studies may also be appropriate as indicated.

Imaging Studies   If the pregnancy test is positive, pelvic imaging using ultrasound may be necessary to confirm a viable intrauterine pregnancy and rule out a spontaneous abortion or ectopic pregnancy. If a pelvic mass is suspected on examination, or if the examination is inadequate (more likely to be the case in an adolescent than an older woman) and additional information is required, pelvic ultrasound may be helpful. **Although transvaginal ultrasound examination can be more helpful than transabdominal ultrasound in ascertaining details of pelvic anatomy, the use of the vaginal probe may not be possible in a young girl or one who has not used tampons or had intercourse.** Direct communication between the clinician and the radiologist can be helpful in identifying candidates for transvaginal ultrasound examination.

Other imaging studies are not indicated as initial testing but may be helpful in selected instances. If a pelvic ultrasound examination does not lead to clarification of the anatomy when vaginal septa, uterine septa, uterine duplication, or vaginal agenesis are suspected, MRI can be helpful in delineating anatomic abnormalities. It has been suggested that this imaging technique can often replace laparoscopy in the evaluation of uterine and vaginal developmental anomalies (33). CT scanning may be helpful in detecting nongenital intraabdominal abnormalities.

Management

The goal of management is to base therapy on the appropriate diagnosis. Thus, management of bleeding abnormalities related to pregnancy, thyroid dysfunction, hepatic abnormalities, hematologic abnormalities, or androgen excess syndromes should be directed to treating the underlying condition. Oral contraceptives, particularly the progestin formulation agents that may be less androgenic, can be extremely helpful in managing androgen excess syndromes. In the absence of a specific diagnosis, the assumption is that of anovulation or dysfunction bleeding.

Anovulation: Mild Bleeding

Adolescents who have mildly abnormal bleeding, as defined by adequate hemoglobin levels, are best treated with frequent reassurance, close follow-up, and supplemental iron. If the patient has been bleeding heavily or for a prolonged interval, however, an apparent decrease in the bleeding does not necessarily mean that therapy is not required. This type of bleeding characterizes anovulatory bleeding and is likely to continue in the absence of therapy.

A patient who is mildly anemic will benefit from hormonal therapy. If the patient is not bleeding heavily at the time of evaluation, a combination low-dose oral contraceptive can be prescribed to be used in the manner in which it is used for contraception (21 days of hormonally active pills, followed by 7 days of placebo, during which time withdrawal bleeding is expected). If the patient is not sexually active, she should be reevaluated after three to six cycles to determine whether this regimen should be continued. Parents may sometimes object to the use of oral contraceptives if their daughter is not sexually active (or if they believe her not to be or even if they would like her not to be). These objections are frequently based on misconceptions about the potential risks of the pill and can be overcome by careful explanation of the pill's role as medical therapy. Similarly, if the medication is discontinued when the young woman is not sexually active and she subsequently becomes sexually active and requires contraception, it may be difficult to explain the reinstitution of oral contraceptives to the parents. Consideration can certainly be given to continuing the pill, and parents should be reassured that this is not medically dangerous.

Sometimes, providing parents with accurate information about the safety of oral contraceptives, emphasizing that currently available oral contraceptive preparations contain lower doses of estrogens and progestins than those used in the 1960s and 1970s and emphasizing the hormonal rather than contraceptive function, may not be persuasive. In such cases, **cyclic progestins are an alternative. *Medroxyprogesterone acetate*, 5–10 mg/day for 10–13 days every 1–2 months, prevents excessive endometrial buildup and irregular shedding caused by unopposed estrogen stimulation.** This therapy also should be reevaluated regularly and accompanied by oral administration of iron. Eventual maturation of the hypothalamic-pituitary-ovarian axis usually will eventually establish regular menses.

Acute Bleeding: Moderate

Patients who are bleeding acutely but who are stable and do not require hospital admission will require doses of hormones that are much higher than those in oral contraceptives. An effective regimen is the use of combination monophasic oral contraceptives (every 6 hours for 4–7 days). After that time, the dose should be tapered or stopped to allow withdrawal flow. With this therapy, the patient and her parents should be given specific written and verbal instructions warning them about the potential side effects of high-dose hormonal therapy—nausea, breast tenderness, and breakthrough bleeding. The patient should be instructed to call with any concerns rather than discontinue the pills, and she must understand that stopping the prescribed regimen may result in a recurrence of heavy bleeding.

Both the patient and her mother should be warned to expect heavy withdrawal flow for the first period. It will be controlled by the institution of combination low-dose oral contraceptive therapy given once daily and continued for three to six cycles to allow regular withdrawal flow. If the patient is not sexually active, the pill may be discontinued and the menstrual cycles may be reassessed.

Acute Bleeding: Emergency Management

The decision to hospitalize the patient depends on the rate of current bleeding and the severity of any existing anemia. The actual acute blood loss may not adequately be reflected in the initial blood count but will be revealed with serial hemoglobin assessments. The cause of acute menorrhagia may be a primary coagulation disorder (26), **so measurements of coagulation and hemostasis, including bleeding time, should be performed for any adolescent patients with acute menorrhagia.** Von Willebrand's disease, platelet disorders, or hematologic malignancies can all present with menorrhagia. Depending on the patient's level of hemodynamic stability or compromise, a blood sample can be analyzed for type and screen. The decision to transfuse must be considered carefully, and the benefits and risks should be discussed with the adolescent and her parents. Generally, there is no need for transfusion unless the patient is hemodynamically unstable.

In patients who, by exclusion, have been diagnosed as having dysfunctional bleeding, hormonal therapy usually makes it possible to avoid surgical intervention (dilation and curettage (D&C), operative hysteroscopy, or laparoscopy). A patient who has been hospitalized for severe bleeding requires aggressive management as follows.

1. **After stabilization, when appropriate laboratory assessment and an examination have established a working diagnosis of anovulation, hormonal management will usually control bleeding.**

2. ***Conjugated estrogens*, either 25–40 mg given intravenously every 6 hours or 2.5 mg given orally every 6 hours, will usually be effective.**

3. **If estrogens are not effective, the patient should be reevaluated, and the diagnosis should be reassessed.** The failure of hormonal management suggests

that a local cause of bleeding is more likely. In this event, consideration should be given to a pelvic ultrasound examination to determine any unusual causes of bleeding (such as uterine leiomyomas or endometrial hyperplasia) and to assess the presence of intrauterine clots that may impair uterine contractility and prolong the bleeding episode.

4. **If intrauterine clots are detected, evacuation of the clots (suction curettage or D&C) is indicated.** Although a D&C will provide effective immediate control of the bleeding (34), it is unusual to reach this step in management for in adolescents.

More drastic forms of treatment than a D&C (such as ablation of the endometrium by laser or rollerball devices) are considered inappropriate for adolescents because of concerns about future fertility.

If intravenous or oral administration of estrogen controls the bleeding, oral progestin therapy should be instituted and continued for several days to stabilize the endometrium. This therapy can be accomplished by using a combination oral contraceptive, usually one with 50 μg of estrogen, or by using the tapering regimen previously described. The medication can be tapered and ultimately stopped to allow withdrawal bleeding. Low-dose combination oral contraception can be continued for three to six cycles.

In general, the prognosis for regular ovulatory cycles and subsequent normal fertility in young women who experience an episode of abnormal bleeding is good, particularly for patients who develop abnormal bleeding as a result of anovulation within the first years after menarche. A few girls, including those in whom there is an underlying medical cause such as polycystic ovary syndrome or coagulopathy, will continue to have abnormal bleeding into middle and late adolescence and adulthood and will require continued evaluation and management. Ovulation induction may be necessary to achieve fertility.

Long-Term Hormonal Suppression

For patients with underlying medical conditions, such as coagulopathies or a malignancy requiring chemotherapy, long-term therapeutic amenorrhea with menstrual suppression using the following regimens may be necessary.

1. Progestins, such as oral *norethindrone, norethindrone acetate,* or *medroxyprogesterone acetate,* on a continuous daily basis

2. Continuous (noncyclic) combination regimens of oral estrogen and progestins (birth control pills) that do not include a withdrawal bleeding-placebo week

3. Depot formulations of progestins (*DMPA*), with or without concurrent estrogens

4. Gonadotropin-releasing hormone (GnRH) analogs

The choice of regimen depends on any contraindications (such as active liver disease precluding the use of estrogens, or thrombocytopenia precluding intramuscular injections) and the clinician's experience. Although the goal of these long-term suppressive therapies is amenorrhea, all of these regimens may be accompanied by breakthrough bleeding. They require regular follow-up visits and continued patient encouragement. Occasional episodes of spotting and mild breakthrough bleeding that do not result in a lowered hemoglobin level may be managed expectantly. When breakthrough bleeding affects the hemoglobin level, it should be evaluated with respect to the underlying disease. For example, in a patient with underlying platelet dysfunction, breakthrough bleeding may reflect a lowered platelet count. Bleeding in a patient with hepatic disease may reflect worsening hepatic function. Supplemental estrogen can be helpful in the management of excessive breakthrough bleeding that has no specific cause other than the hormonal therapy.

Reproductive Age Group

Normal Menses   Beyond the first 1–2 years after menarche, menstrual cycles generally conform to a cycle length of 21–40 days, with a duration of less than 7 days of menstrual flow. As a woman approaches menopause, cycle length becomes more irregular as more cycles become anovulatory. Although the most frequent cause of irregular bleeding is hormonal, other causes occur more often than during the adolescent years. Pregnancy-related bleeding (spontaneous abortion, ectopic pregnancy) should always be considered, and a pregnancy test should always be obtained as part of the evaluation of abnormal bleeding. Although a variety of terms has been used to describe abnormal menses (Table 13.6), a complete description of the menstrual pattern may be more important than the use of the correct term.

Differential Diagnosis   *Dysfunctional Uterine Bleeding*   **The term dysfunctional uterine bleeding has been used to describe abnormal bleeding for which no specific cause has been found. It most often implies a mechanism of anovulation, although not all bleeding that is outside the normal range (either in cycle length or duration) is anovulatory. The term is a diagnosis of exclusion, which is probably more confusing than enlightening**.

Most anovulatory bleeding is a result of what has been termed "estrogen breakthrough." In the absence of ovulation and the production of progesterone, the endometrium responds to estrogen stimulation with proliferation. This endometrial growth without periodic shedding results in eventual breakdown of the fragile endometrial tissue. Healing within the endometrium is irregular and dysynchronous. Relatively low levels of estrogen stimulation will result in irregular and prolonged bleeding, whereas higher sustained levels result in episodes of amenorrhea followed by acute, heavy bleeding.

Pregnancy-Related Bleeding   Spontaneous abortion can present with excessive or prolonged bleeding. In the U.S., more than 50% of pregnancies are unintended (29), and 10% of women are at risk for unintended pregnancy but use no method of contraception. About one-half of unintended pregnancies are a result of nonuse of contraception; however, the other one-half are contraceptive failures (35). Unintended pregnancies are most likely to occur among adolescents and women over 40 years of age (Chapter 10). A woman may be unaware that she has conceived and may seek care because of abnormal bleeding. If an ectopic pregnancy is ruled out, the management of spontaneous abortion may include either observation, if the bleeding is not excessive, or curettage or D&C, depending on the clinician's judgment and the patient's preference (36).

Exogenous Hormones   Irregular bleeding that occurs while a woman is using contraceptive hormones should be considered differently than bleeding that occurs in the absence of exogenous hormone use. Breakthrough bleeding during the first 1–3 months of oral contraceptive use occurs in up to 30–40% of users and should almost always be managed expectantly with

Table 13.6 Abnormal Menses—Terminology

Term	Interval	Duration	Amount
Menorrhagia	Regular	Prolonged	Excessive
Metrorrhagia	Irregular	± Prolonged	Normal
Menometrorrhagia	Irregular	Prolonged	Excessive
Hypermenorrhea	Regular	Normal	Excessive
Hypomenorrhea	Regular	Normal or less	Less
Oligomenorrhea	Infrequent and/or irregular	Variable	Scanty

reassurance because the frequency of breakthrough bleeding decreases with each subsequent month of use. Irregular bleeding can also result from inconsistent pill taking (37–39).

Not all bleeding that occurs while an individual is taking oral contraceptives is a consequence of hormonal factors. In one study, women who experienced irregular bleeding while taking oral contraceptives were found to have a higher frequency of chlamydia infection (40).

Irregular bleeding is almost invariably present during the first year of use of both the subdermal implant *levonorgestrel* (*Norplant*) and *DMPA* (24, 25). Because irregular bleeding is so often present with these two methods of contraception, contraceptive counseling prior to the use of the method is imperative. Women who do not believe that they can cope with irregular, unpredictable bleeding may not be good candidates for these methods. As with oral contraceptives, the possibility of nonhormonal causes of bleeding (e.g., chlamydial cervicitis) should be considered (41). When an individual is using one of these methods, reassurance and counseling should be provided. The exact mechanism of irregular bleeding associated with progestin-only methods is not well established but may related to incomplete suppression of follicular activity with periodic elevations of estradiol (42). The additional oral use of estrogen has been reported to improve bleeding with both *DMPA* and the subdermal *levonorgestrel* (24, 42, 43). Combination oral contraceptives have also been used in patients with the subdermal *levonorgestrel* implants (43). For a patient who is considering removal of the implants because of irregular bleeding and who may choose an oral contraceptive as an alternative, the use of combination pills can allow both the clinician and the patient to assess the patient's tolerance of and compliance with oral contraceptive therapy. The use of nonsteroidal anti-inflammatory drugs has been shown to result in decreased bleeding (43).

Endocrine Causes   Both hypothyroidism and hyperthyroidism can be associated with abnormal bleeding. With hypothyroidism, menstrual abnormalities including menorrhagia are common (Chapter 25). The most common cause of thyroid hyperfunctioning in premenopausal women is Graves' disease, which occurs 4–5 times more often in women than men. Hyperthyroidism can result in oligomenorrhea or amenorrhea, and it can also lead to elevated levels of plasma estrogen.

Diabetes mellitus can be associated with anovulation, obesity, insulin resistance, and androgen excess. Androgen disorders are very common among women of reproductive age and should be evaluated and managed. Because androgen disorders are associated with significant cardiovascular disease, the condition should be diagnosed promptly. This condition becomes more immediately of concern in older women of reproductive age. Management of bleeding disorders associated with androgen excess consists of an appropriate diagnostic evaluation followed by the use of oral contraceptives (in the absence of significant contraindications), coupled with dietary and exercise modification.

Anatomic Causes   Anatomic causes of abnormal bleeding in women of reproductive age occur more frequently than in women in other age groups. **Uterine leiomyomas occur in as many as one-half of all women older than 35 years of age, although they are asymptomatic in many or even most women. The mechanism of abnormal bleeding related to leiomyomas is not well established.** Several theories have been postulated (44).

1. Ulceration over a submucous tumor

2. Anovulation

3. Increased endometrial surface area

4. Interference of leiomyomas with normal uterine contractility

5. Compression of venous plexi of the adjacent myometrium and endometrium

Diagnosis is based on the characteristic findings of an irregularly enlarged uterus. The size and location of the usually multiple leiomyomas can be confirmed and documented with pelvic ultrasound (Fig. 13.6). If the examination is adequate and symptoms are absent, ultrasound is not always necessary unless an ovarian mass cannot be excluded.

Endometrial polyps are a cause of intermenstrual bleeding, irregular bleeding, and menorrhagia. The diagnosis is based on either visualization with hysteroscopy or on the microscopic assessment of an office biopsy or curettage specimen. Cervical lesions can result in abnormal bleeding, either intermenstrual or postcoital. Endocervical polyps can cause bleeding. Infectious cervical lesions, such as condyloma, herpes simplex virus ulcerations, chlamydial cervicitis, or cervicitis caused by other organisms, can cause bleeding. Other benign cervical lesions, such as wide eversion of endocervical columnar epithelium or Nabothian cysts, may be noted on examination but are rarely symptomatic.

Coagulopathies and Other Hematologic Causes   The presence of excessively heavy menses should prompt an evaluation of hematologic status. A complete blood count will be helpful in detecting anemia, significant problems such as leukemia, or disorders associated with thrombocytopenia. Abnormal liver function, which can be seen with alcoholism or other chronic liver diseases, results in inadequate production of clotting factors and can lead to excessive menstrual bleeding. Coagulation abnormalities such as von Willebrand's disease can have a variable clinical picture and may escape diagnosis until the reproductive years. Oral contraceptives, which increase the level of factor VIII, can be helpful and newer therapies, including *desmopressin acetate,* may be necessary, particularly before surgical procedures.

Infectious Causes   Women with a cervicitis, particularly chlamydial cervicitis, can present with irregular bleeding and postcoital spotting (see Chapter 15). Therefore, cervical testing for chlamydia should be considered, especially for sexually active adolescents, women in their twenties, and women who are not in a monogamous relationship. Endometritis can cause excessive menstrual flow. Thus, a woman who presents with menor-

Figure 13.6   Transvaginal pelvic ultrasound demonstrating multiple uterine leiomyomas.

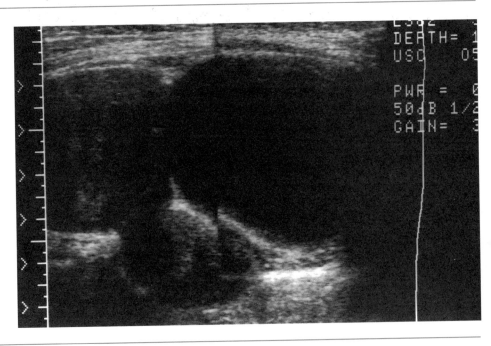

rhagia and increased menstrual pain and a history of light-to-moderate previous menstrual flow may have an upper genital tract infection or PID (endometritis/salpingitis/oophoritis). Occasionally, chronic endometritis will be diagnosed when an endometrial biopsy is obtained for evaluation of abnormal bleeding in a patient without specific risk factors for PID.

Neoplasia   Abnormal bleeding is the most frequent symptom of women with invasive cervical cancer. An obvious cervical lesion should be biopsied, because the results of a Papanicolaou (Pap) test may be falsely negative with invasive lesions as a result of tumor necrosis. Unopposed estrogen has been associated with a variety of abnormalities of the endometrium, from cystic hyperplasia to adenomatous hyperplasia, hyperplasia with cytologic atypia, and invasive carcinoma. **Endometrial hyperplasia, hyperplasia with atypia, and invasive endometrial cancer can be diagnosed by endometrial sampling or D&C. Such sampling is mandatory in the evaluation of abnormal bleeding in women older than 35–40 years of age, obese women, and those with a history of anovulation.** Although vaginal neoplasia is uncommon, a careful examination of the vagina is mandatory in evaluating abnormal bleeding. This includes attention to all surfaces of the vagina, including anterior and posterior areas that may be obscured by the vaginal speculum on examination.

Diagnosis

For all women, the evaluation of excessive and abnormal menses includes a thorough medical and gynecologic history, the exclusion of pregnancy, and a careful gynecologic examination. For women of normal weight between the ages of approximately 20 and 35 years who do not have clear risk factors for sexually transmitted diseases (STDs), who have no signs of androgen excess, who are not using exogenous hormones, and who have no other findings on examination, management may be based on a clinical diagnosis.

Laboratory Studies   In any patients with excessive bleeding, an objective measurement of hematologic status should be performed with a complete blood count to detect anemia or thrombocytopenia. A sensitive pregnancy test must be performed to rule out pregnancy-related problems. In addition, because of the possibility of a primary coagulation problem, screening coagulation studies such as a protime and partial thromboplastin time should be considered; an assessment of bleeding time may help diagnose von Willebrand's disease, although if this diagnosis is strongly suspected, further testing may be necessary, including measurement of von Willebrand factor activity and antigen levels, factor VIII activity, and a multimer analysis of a von Willebrand factor subtype (45).

Imaging Studies   Women with abnormal bleeding who have a history consistent with chronic anovulation, who are obese, or who are older than 35–40 years of age require further evaluation. A pelvic ultrasound may be helpful in delineating anatomic abnormalities if the examination results are suboptimal or if an ovarian mass is suspected. A pelvic ultrasound examination is the best technique for evaluating the uterine contour, endometrial thickness, and ovarian structure. Ultrasound is particularly valuable in determining whether a pelvic mass is cystic or solid. The use of a vaginal probe transducer allows better assessment of endometrial and ovarian disorders, particularly in women who are obese. A new technique of sonohysterography involves the infusion of saline into the uterine cavity during transvaginal ultrasonography. This technique has been reported to be especially helpful in visualizing intrauterine problems such as polyps (46). Transvaginal ultrasonography alone has also been reported to have value in differentiating benign polyps from malignant lesions (47). Other techniques, such as CT scanning and MRI, are not as helpful in the initial evaluation and should be reserved for specific indications such as exploring the possibility of other intra-abdominal disorders or adenopathy.

Endometrial Sampling   **Endometrial sampling should be performed to evaluate abnormal bleeding in women who are at risk for endometrial polyps, hyperplasia, or carcinoma. The technique of D&C, which in the past was used extensively for the**

evaluation of abnormal bleeding, has been replaced largely by the office endometrial biopsy. The classic study in which a D&C was performed before hysterectomy with the conclusion that less than one-half of the endometrium was sampled in more than one-half of the patients has led to the questioning of D&C as the "gold standard" for endometrial diagnosis (48, 49).

It has been argued that there is no longer a place for a "blind" D&C, because hysteroscopy can direct a biopsy to a specific area of the uterus (50). In most cases, however, office endometrial biopsy can be performed instead of a D&C. **Indications for a D&C or hysteroscopy include the following:**

1. Cervical stenosis precluding adequate endometrial biopsy

2. Patient intolerance of endometrial biopsy

3. Anatomic factors (e.g., massive obesity) precluding adequate endometrial biopsy

4. Patient has abnormal bleeding and is having another surgical procedure performed under general anesthesia

A number of devices are designed for endometrial sampling (Fig. 13.7), including an inexpensive disposable flexible plastic sheath with an internal plunger that allows tissue aspiration, disposable plastic cannulae of varying diameters that attach to a manually locking syringe that allows the establishment of a vacuum, and cannulae (both rigid metal and plastic) with tissue traps that attach to an electric vacuum pump. Several studies comparing the adequacy of sampling using these devices with D&C have shown a comparable ability to detect abnormalities. It should be noted that these devices are designed to obtain a tissue sample rather than a cytologic washing. Devices designed to obtain endometrial sample for assessment of cytology are also available; they have been shown to detect invasive cancer as well as D&C but to have a lower sensitivity for detecting premalignant lesions.

Management

Nonsurgical The management of abnormal bleeding during the reproductive years depends on the cause of the problem. Most bleeding problems can be managed nonsurgically.

Figure 13.7   Devices used for sampling endometrium. From top to bottom: Serrated Novak, Novak, Kevorkian, Explora (Mylex), and Pipelle (Unimar). (Reproduced from **Berek JS, Hacker NF.** *Practical Gynecologic Oncology.* 2nd ed. Baltimore: Williams & Wilkins, 1994:286.)

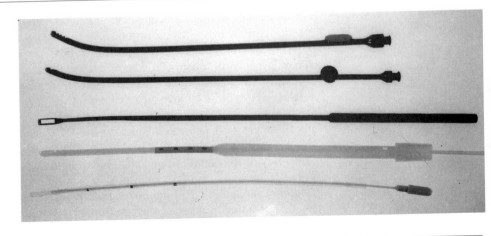

Treatment with nonsteroidal anti-inflammatory drugs (NSAIDs) such as *ibuprofen* and *mefenamic acid* has been shown to decrease menstrual flow by 30–50% (51, 52).

Hormonal management of abnormal bleeding can frequently control excessive or irregular bleeding. Oral contraceptives have long been known to result in decreased menstrual flow and thus a lower risk of iron-deficiency anemia (53). Although this effect was first demonstrated with oral contraceptive formulations that contained higher doses of both estrogens and progestins than the agents used today, low-dose combined oral contraceptives have been shown to have a similar effect (54). Low-dose oral contraceptives may be used during the perimenopausal years in healthy nonsmoking women who have no major cardiovascular risk factors. The benefits of menstrual regulation in such women often override the potential risks.

For patients in whom estrogen use is contraindicated, progestins, both oral and parenteral, can be used to control excessive bleeding. Cyclic oral *medroxyprogesterone acetate,* administered in a dose of 10 mg/day for 10 days per month, will induce withdrawal bleeding and prevent the development of endometrial hyperplasia with anovulation and resultant amenorrhea. The benefits to the patient include a regular flow and the prevention of long intervals of amenorrhea, which may end in unpredictable, profuse bleeding. This therapy reduces the risk of hyperplasia resulting from persistent, unopposed estrogen stimulation of the endometrium. Depot formulations of *medroxyprogesterone acetate* have also been used to establish amenorrhea in women at risk of excessive bleeding.

In Europe, the intrauterine device containing *norgestrel* has been used therapeutically to deliver progestin locally to the endometrium in women with abnormal bleeding who have been diagnosed with dysfunctional uterine bleeding (55, 56). In the U.S., the *norgestrel*-containing device is not available; a device containing progesterone is available and approved for contraception for 1 year's use. It has been shown to decrease menstrual flow and dysmenorrhea (57, 58). Some clinicians are using this device therapeutically for women with abnormal bleeding.

Surgical Therapy **The surgical management of abnormal bleeding should be reserved for situations in which medical therapy has been unsuccessful or is contraindicated. The D&C, although sometimes appropriate as a diagnostic technique, is questionable as a therapeutic modality.** One study reported a measured reduction in menstrual blood loss for the first menstrual period only (59). Other studies have suggested a longer-lasting benefit (34).

The surgical options range from hysteroscopy with resection of submucous leiomyomas to laparoscopic techniques of myomectomy to endometrial ablation (Chapter 21) to hysterectomy (Chapter 22). The assessment of the relative advances, risks, benefits, complications, and indications of these procedures is a subject of ongoing clinical research (60). The proposed advantages of techniques other than hysterectomy include a shorter recovery time and less early morbidity. However, symptoms can recur or persist.

Much has been written about the psychologic sequelae of hysterectomy, and some of the aforementioned surgical techniques have been developed in an effort to provide less drastic management options. Most well-controlled recent studies have suggested that, in the absence of preexisting psychopathology, indicated but elective surgical procedures for hysterectomy have few if any significant psychologic sequelae (including depression) (61, 62) (Chapter 12).

Postmenopausal Women

Differential Diagnosis The causes of postmenopausal bleeding and the percentage of patients who present with different conditions are presented in Table 13.7.

Table 13.7   Etiology of Postmenopausal Bleeding

Factor	Approximate Percentage
Exogenous estrogens	30
Atrophic endometritis/vaginitis	30
Endometrial cancer	15
Endometrial or cervical polyps	10
Endometrial hyperplasia	5
Miscellaneous (e.g., cervical cancer, uterine sarcoma, urethral caruncle, trauma)	10

Reproduced with permission from **Hacker NF, Moore JG.** *Essentials of Obstetrics and Gynecology.* Philadelphia: WB Saunders, 1986:467.

Benign Women who are taking hormone replacement therapy during menopause may be using a variety of hormonal regimens that can result in bleeding (see Chapter 28). In the classic sequential method of administration, estrogens are given for the first 25 days of each month. A progestin, often 5–10 mg/day of *medroxyprogesterone acetate,* is added to the last 10–13 days of this regimen in an effort to reduce the risk of endometrial hyperplasia and neoplasia. Most women who take these hormones in this way will experience withdrawal bleeding, which is perceived by the patient as a menstrual period. Although the incidence of withdrawal bleeding does decline somewhat with age and duration of therapy, more than 50% of women continue to experience bleeding after 65 years of age.

Because some women become symptomatic during the days when they are not taking estrogens, as in the previously described classic regimen, many clinicians have modified this regimen to include continuous (every day) estrogen therapy. In addition, studies have assessed endometrial response to varying durations of progestin regimens; treatment with progestins for 10 days per month reduced the incidence of endometrial hyperplasia to 2%, and treatment for 13 days reduced the incidence to 0% in one study (63). It has been suggested that endometrial sampling is indicated for any bleeding that occurs beyond the expected time of withdrawal following the progestin therapy. Bleeding before or on day 10 has been described as being associated with endometrial proliferation and should prompt biopsy (64). A significant change in withdrawal bleeding (e.g., absence of withdrawal bleeding for several months followed by resumption of bleeding or a marked increase in the amount of bleeding) should prompt endometrial sampling.

Patient compliance has been a significant issue with hormone replacement therapy (65). Missed doses of medication and failure to take the medication in the prescribed fashion can lead to irregular bleeding or spotting that is benign in origin.

The primary problems that women report with hormone replacement therapy include vaginal bleeding and weight gain (66). The use of a continuous low-dose combined regimen of therapy has the advantage that, for many women, bleeding will ultimately cease after a period of several months during which irregular and unpredictable bleeding may occur (67, 68). Some women are unable to tolerate these initial months of irregular bleeding. The risk of endometrial hyperplasia or neoplasia with this regimen appears to be low.

Other benign causes of bleeding include atrophic vaginitis and cervical polyps, which may present as postcoital bleeding or spotting. Women who experience bleeding after menopause may attempt to minimize the extent of the problem; they may describe only "spotting" or "pink or brownish discharge." However, any indication of bleeding or spotting should be evaluated. In the absence of hormone therapy, any bleeding after menopause (classically defined as absence of menses for 1 year) should prompt evaluation with endometrial sampling. At least one-fourth of postmenopausal women with bleeding have a neoplastic lesion.

Endometrial polyps and other abnormalities can be seen in women who are taking *tamoxifen*. These polyps can be benign, although they must be distinguished from endometrial malignancies, which may also occur with this drug.

Neoplasia   Endometrial, cervical, and ovarian malignancies must be ruled out in cases of postmenopausal bleeding. A Pap test is essential when postmenopausal bleeding is noted, although the Pap test is an insensitive diagnostic test for detecting endometrial cancer. **Only about 50% of women with endometrial cancer will have a positive Pap test result** (69). About 5–10% of women with normal endometrial cells on Pap test will have endometrial hyperplasia or carcinoma (70), whereas about one-fourth of those with atypical endometrial cells indicated on Pap test results will have carcinoma (71). The Pap test results are negative in some cases of invasive cervical carcinoma because of tumor necrosis (72).

Cervical malignancy is diagnosed by cervical biopsy of grossly visible lesions and colposcopically directed biopsy for women with abnormal Pap test results (Chapter 16). Functional ovarian tumors may produce estrogen and lead to endometrial hyperplasia or carcinoma, which may present with bleeding.

Diagnosis

Pelvic examination to detect local lesions and Pap test to assess cytology are essential first steps in finding the cause of postmenopausal bleeding. Endometrial sampling, through office biopsy, hysteroscopy, or D&C, is usually considered essential. Pelvic ultrasound examination and, in particular, vaginal ultrasonography can suggest the cause of bleeding. Initial office biopsy is more cost-effective than D&C, surgery, or observation alone (73). The cost-effectiveness of other screening strategies, including transvaginal ultrasound, has not been well studied. It has been suggested that **an endometrial thickness of less than 6 mm (4–5 mm in some reports) on transvaginal ultrasound is unlikely to indicate endometrial cancer** (74–76).

Management

The management of atrophic vaginitis includes topical or systemic use of estrogens after other causes of abnormal bleeding have been excluded. Cervical polyps can easily be removed in the office.

Endometrial Hyperplasia   The terminology that has been used to describe endometrial hyperplasia is confusing, and the clinician must consult with the pathologist to ensure an understanding of the diagnosis. **The following lesions are considered to be benign:** *anovulatory, proliferative, cystic glandular hyperplasia, simple cystic hyperplasia* (Fig. 13.8), *simple hyperplasia, and adenomatous hyperplasia without atypia.* **These terms reflect and describe an exaggerated proliferative response of the endometrium. In most cases, benign endometrial hyperplasia is resolved with D&C or progestin therapy.** Repeat surveillance with endometrial biopsy may be warranted.

The presence of atypia with abnormal proliferation, including features of "back-to-back" crowding of the glands, with epithelial activity demonstrated by papillary projections into the glands, is associated with an increased risk of progression to endometrial carcinoma (Fig. 13.9). These architectural abnormalities may be associated with individual cellular atypia (enlarged, irregular nuclei, chromatin clumping, and prominent nucleoli). The presence of mitotic activity also can be variable (77).

The management of endometrial hyperplasia rests on an understanding of the natural history of the lesion involved. In one study, only 2% of 122 patients with hyperplasia without cytologic atypia progressed to carcinoma, whereas 23% of those with atypical hyperplasia sub-

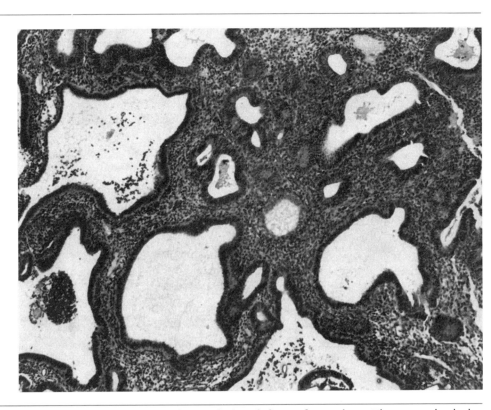

Figure 13.8   Simple cystic hyperplasia of the endometrium. The normal tabular pattern is replaced by cystically dilated proliferative endometrial glands. (Reproduced from **Berek JS, Hacker NF.** *Practical Gynecologic Oncology.* 2nd ed. Baltimore: Williams & Wilkins, 1994:126.)

sequently developed carcinoma (78). Architectural complexity and crowding appears to place patients at greater risk for progression than does the presence of cytologic atypia alone.

These data suggest that **most women with endometrial hyperplasia will respond to progestin therapy and are not at increased risk of developing cancer.** Patients who do not respond are at a significantly increased risk of progressing to invasive cancer and should be advised to have a hysterectomy. Patients who are unlikely to respond can be identified on the basis of cytologic atypia. A suggested scheme of management is outlined in Figure 13.10. This treatment is discussed in more detail in Chapter 31.

Pelvic Mass

The probable causes of a pelvic mass found on physical examination or through radiologic studies are vastly different in a prepubertal child than they are during adolescence or during the postmenopausal years (Table 13.3). A pelvic mass may be gynecologic in origin or it may arise from the urinary tract or bowel. The gynecologic causes of a pelvic mass may be uterine, adnexal, or more specifically ovarian.

Prepubertal Age Group

Differential Diagnosis   Fewer than 5% of ovarian malignancies occur in children and adolescents. Ovarian tumors account for approximately 1% of all tumors in these age groups. Germ cell tumors make up one half two-thirds of ovarian neoplasms in individuals younger than 20 years of age. A review of studies conducted from 1940 until 1975 concluded that 35% of all ovarian

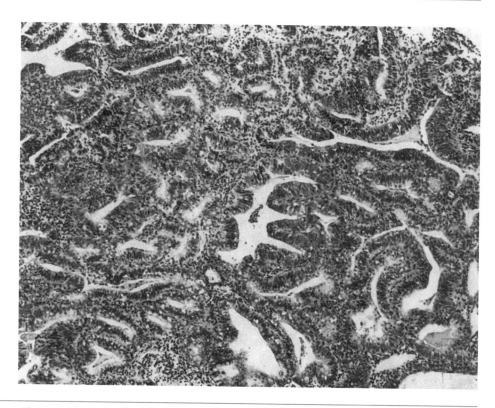

Figure 13.9 Aypical hyperplasia (complex hyperplasia with severe nuclear atypia). The proliferative endometrial glands reveal considerable crowding and papillary infoldings. The endometrial stroma, although markedly diminished, can still be recognized between the glands. (Reproduced from **Berek JS, Hacker NF.** *Practical Gynecologic Oncology.* 2nd ed. Baltimore: Williams & Wilkins, 1994:127.)

neoplasms occurring during childhood and adolescence were malignant (79). **In girls younger than 9 years of age, approximately 80% of the ovarian neoplasms were found to be malignant** (80, 81). Germ cell tumors account for approximately 60% of ovarian neoplasms in children and adolescents, compared with 20% of these tumors in adults (79). Epithelial neoplasms are rare in the prepubertal age group.

Because neoplastic tumors are rare, data are usually reported from referral centers. However, some reports include only neoplastic masses, whereas others include nonneoplastic masses. One community survey of ovarian masses revealed that the frequency of malignancy was much lower than previously reported; of all ovarian masses confirmed surgically in childhood and adolescence, only 6% of masses were malignant neoplasms, and only 10% of neoplasms were malignant (82). In one series, nonneoplastic masses in young women and girls younger than 20 years of age constituted two-thirds of the total (83). Even in girls younger than 10 years of age, 60% were of the masses were nonneoplastic, and two-thirds of the neoplastic masses were benign. Functional, follicular cysts can occur in fetuses, newborns, and prepubertal children. They may be associated with sexual precocity.

Abdominal or pelvic pain is one of the most frequent presenting symptoms. In a prepubertal child, a pelvic mass very quickly becomes abdominal in location as it enlarges, because of the small size of the pelvic cavity. The diagnosis of ovarian masses in the prepubertal age group is difficult because of the rarity of the diagnosis (and therefore a low index of suspicion), as well as the fact that many symptoms are nonspecific and acute symptoms are more likely to be attributed to more common entities such as appendicitis. Abdominal palpation and bimanual rectoabdominal examination are important in any child who has nonspecific abdominal or pelvic complaints. An ovarian mass that is abdominal in location can be con-

353

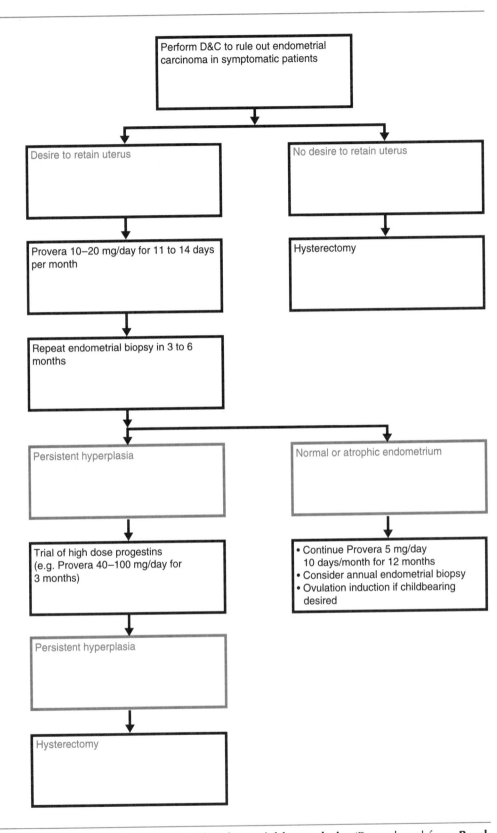

Figure 13.10   Management of endometrial hyperplasia. (Reproduced from **Berek JS, Hacker NF.** *Practical Gynecologic Oncology.* 2nd ed. Baltimore: Williams & Wilkins, 1994:299.)

fused with other abdominal masses occurring in children, such as Wilms' tumor or neuroblastoma. Acute pain is often associated with torsion. The ovarian ligament becomes elongated as a result of the abdominal location of these tumors, thus predisposing to torsion.

Diagnosis and Management

In recent years, ultrasonography has become an excellent tool for predicting the presence of a simple ovarian cyst. Figure 13.11 outlines a plan of management for pelvic masses in the prepubertal age group. **Unilocular cysts are virtually always benign and will regress in 3–6 months;** thus, they do not require surgical management with

Figure 13.11   Management of pelvic masses in premenarchal and adolescent girls.

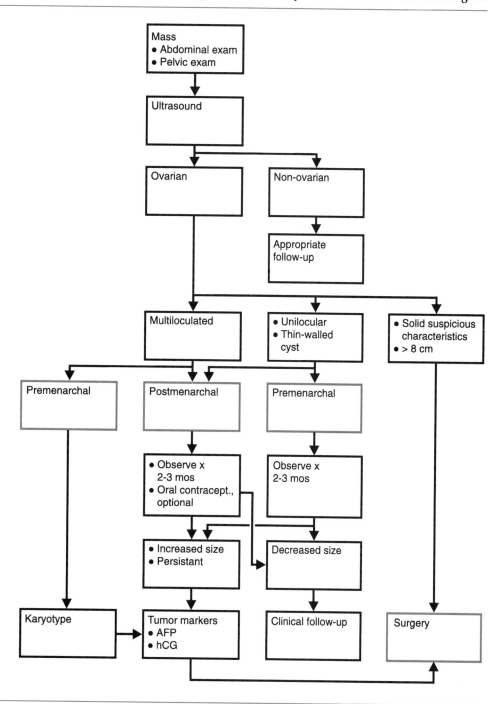

oophorectomy or oophorocystectomy. Close observation is recommended, although there is a risk of ovarian torsion that must be discussed with the child's parents. Recurrence rates after cyst aspiration (either ultrasonographically guided or with laparoscopy) may be as high as 50%. Attention must be paid to long-term effects on endocrine functioning as well as future fertility; preservation of ovarian tissue is a priority for patients with benign tumors.

Additional imaging studies, such as CT scanning, MRI, or Doppler flow studies, may suggest the diagnosis. Because the risk of a germ cell tumor is high, the finding of a solid component mandates surgical assessment.

Adolescent Age Group

Differential Diagnosis

Ovarian Masses

Many series report ovarian tumors occurring in both children and adolescents. Some reports divide their findings by age group, although this is less helpful than a division by pubertal development. The clinician's response to a pelvic or abdominal mass varies in relation to the patient's pubertal status, because the likelihood of functional masses increases after menarche. **The risk of malignant neoplasms is lower among adolescents than among younger children. Epithelial neoplasms occur with increasing frequency with age. Germ cell tumors are the most common tumors of the first decade of life but occur less frequently during adolescence** (Chapter 33). **Mature cystic teratoma is the most frequent neoplastic tumor of children and adolescents, accounting for more than one-half of ovarian neoplasms in women younger than 20 years of age** (79).

It is well established that neoplasia can arise in dysgenetic gonads. Malignant tumors have been found in about 25% of dysgenetic gonads of patients with a Y chromosome (84). Gonadectomy is recommended for patients with XY gonadal dysgenesis or its mosaic variations (85).

Functional ovarian cysts occur frequently in adolescence. They may be an incidental finding on examination or may present with pain caused by torsion, leakage, or rupture. Endometriosis is less common during adolescence than in adulthood, although it can occur during adolescence. In series of adolescents referred with chronic pain, 50–65% have been found to have endometriosis (86, 87). Although endometriosis can occur in young women with obstructive genital anomalies (presumably as a result of retrograde menstruation), one review of pelvic pain and dysmenorrhea found that most adolescents with endometriosis did not have associated obstructive anomalies (88). Endometriosis occurring in young women may have an atypical appearance, with nonpigmented or vesicular lesions, peritoneal windows, and puckering.

Uterine Masses

Other causes of pelvic masses, such as uterine abnormalities, are rare in adolescence. Uterine leiomyomas are not commonly seen in this age group. Obstructive uterovaginal anomalies present during adolescence, at the time of menarche or shortly thereafter. The diagnosis is frequently neither suspected nor delayed, particularly when the patient is seen by a general surgeon (89). A wide range of anomalies can be seen, from imperforate hymen to transverse vaginal septa, to vaginal agenesis with a normal uterus and functional endometrium, vaginal duplications with obstructing longitudinal septa, and obstructed uterine horns. Patients may present with cyclic pain, amenorrhea, vaginal discharge, or an abdominal, pelvic, or vaginal mass (Fig. 13.5). A hematocolpos, hematometra, or both will frequently be present, and the resulting mass can be quite large.

356

Inflammatory Masses

Adolescents have the highest rates of PID of any age group, if one considers only individuals at risk for STDs (i.e., those who have had sexual intercourse) (29). Thus, an adolescent presenting with pelvic pain may be found to have an inflammatory mass. The diagnosis of pelvic inflammatory disease is primarily a clinical diagnosis based on the presence of lower abdominal, pelvic, and adnexal tenderness; cervical motion tenderness; a mucopurulent discharge; and the signs of elevated temperature, white blood cell count, or sedimentation rate (Chapter 15). PID is clearly associated with the risks of acquiring sexually transmissible infections, and methods of contraception may decrease the risk (spermicides, oral contraceptives, male latex condoms) or increase the risk (the intrauterine device). Inflammatory masses may consist of a tubo-ovarian complex (a mass consisting of matted bowel, tube, and ovary), tubo-ovarian abscess (a mass consisting primarily of an abscess cavity within an anatomically defined structure such as the ovary), pyosalpinx, or, chronically, hydrosalpinx.

Pregnancy

In adolescents, pregnancy should always be considered as a cause of a pelvic mass. In the U.S., more than 50% of adolescent young women have experienced sexual intercourse by 17 years of age (20). More than 85% of pregnancies among adolescents are unintended (35). Adolescents may be more likely than adults to deny the possibility of pregnancy because of wishful thinking, anxiety about discovery by parents or peers, or unfamiliarity with menstrual cycles and information about fertility. Ectopic pregnancies may present with pelvic pain and an adnexal mass. With the availability of quantitative measurements of β-human chorionic gonadotropin (hCG), more ectopic pregnancies are being discovered before rupture, allowing conservative management with laparoscopic surgery or medical therapy with *methotrexate* (Chapter 17). The risk of ectopic pregnancy varies by method of contraception: users of no contraception have the highest risk, whereas oral contraceptive users have the lowest risk (90). As in older patients, paraovarian cysts and nongynecologic masses may be discovered in adolescents.

Diagnosis

A history and pelvic examination are critical in the diagnosis of a pelvic mass. Considerations in adolescents include the anxiety associated with a first pelvic examination, as well as issues of confidentiality related to questions of sexual activity. Techniques for history taking and the performance of the first examination are discussed in Chapter 1.

Laboratory studies should always include a pregnancy test (regardless of stated sexual activity), and a complete blood count may be helpful in diagnosing inflammatory masses. Tumor markers, including α-fetoprotein and hCG, may be elaborated by germ cell tumors and can be useful in preoperative diagnosis as well as follow-up (Chapter 33).

As in all age groups, the primary diagnostic technique for evaluating pelvic masses in adolescents is ultrasonography. Although transvaginal ultrasound examinations may provide more detail than transabdominal scans, a transvaginal examination may not be well tolerated by adolescents (91). For cases in which the ultrasound examination is inconclusive, CT or MRI may be helpful. An accurate preoperative assessment of anatomy is critical, particularly in cases of uterovaginal malformations. MRI can be useful for evaluating this group of rare anomalies (92, 93). Some sort of imaging technique should be used in evaluating patients who present with abdominal pain, because an unexpected ovarian mass may be difficult to manage through an incision intended for an appendectomy.

Management

The management of masses in adolescents depends on the suspected diagnosis as well as the presenting complaint. Figure 13.11 outlines a plan of management for pelvic masses in adolescents. **Asymptomatic unilocular cystic masses are best managed conservatively, because the likelihood of malignancy is low. If surgical management is required based on symptoms or uncertainty of diagnosis, attention should be paid to minimizing the risks of subsequent infertility resulting from pelvic adhesions. In addition, every effort should be made to conserve ovarian tissue. In the presence of a malignant unilateral ovarian mass, management may include unilateral oophorectomy rather than more radical surgery, even if the ovarian tumor has metastasized** (Chapter 33). Analysis of frozen sections may not be reliable. In general, conservative surgery is appropriate; further surgery can be performed if necessary after an adequate histologic evaluation of the ovarian tumor (79).

The surgical management of inflammatory masses is rarely necessary in adolescents, except to treat rupture of tubo-ovarian abscess or failure of medical management with broad-spectrum antibiotics (Chapter 15). Conservative, unilateral adnexectomy can usually be performed in these situations, rather than a "pelvic clean-out," maintaining reproductive potential (94). Percutaneous drainage and laparoscopic management of tubo-ovarian abscesses are becoming more popular, although as with the laparoscopic management of ovarian masses, the surgeon's skill and experience are critical and prospective studies are lacking.

Reproductive Age Group

Conditions diagnosed as a pelvic mass in women of reproductive age are presented in Table 13.8.

Differential Diagnosis

It is difficult to determine the frequency of diagnoses of pelvic mass in women of reproductive age because many pelvic masses are not ultimately treated with surgery. Nonovarian or

---

Table 13.8   Conditions Diagnosed as a "Pelvic Mass" in Women of Reproductive Age

Full urinary bladder

Urachal cyst

Sharply anteflexed or retroflexed uterus

Pregnancy (with or without concomitant leiomyomas)
  Intrauterine
  Tubal
  Abdominal

Ovarian or adnexal masses
  Functional cysts
  Inflammatory masses
    Tubo-ovarian complex
    Diverticular abscess
    Appendiceal abscess
  Matted bowel and omentum
  Peritoneal cyst
  Stool in sigmoid
  Neoplastic tumors
    Benign
    Malignant

Paraovarian or paratubal cysts

Intraligamentous myomas

Less common conditions that must be excluded:
  Pelvic kidney
  Carcinoma of the colon, rectum, appendix
  Carcinoma of the fallopian tube
  Retroperitoneal tumors (anterior sacral meningocele)
  Uterine sarcoma or other malignant tumors

---

nongynecologic conditions may be confused with an ovarian or uterine mass (Table 13.8). There are series in which the frequency of masses found at laparotomy is reviewed, although the varying indications for surgery, indications for referral, type of practice (gynecologic oncology vs. general gynecology), and patient populations (a higher percentage of African-Americans with uterine leiomyomas, for example) will affect the percentages. Benign masses, such as functional ovarian cysts, will often (appropriately) not require surgery.

Age is an important determinant of the likelihood of malignancy. In one series of women who underwent laparotomy for pelvic mass, malignancy was seen in only 10% of those younger than 30 years of age, and most of these tumors had low malignant potential (95). The most common tumors found during laparotomy for pelvic mass are dermoids (seen in one-third of women younger than 30 years of age) and endometriomas (approximately one-fourth of women 31–49 years of age) (95).

Uterine Masses

Uterine Leiomyomas   Uterine leiomyomas, also known as myomas or fibroids, are by far the most common benign uterine tumors. Other benign uterine growths, such as uterine vascular tumors, are rare. Uterine leiomyomas are usually diagnosed on physical examination. They may be subserosal, intramucosal, or submucosal in location within the uterus or located in the cervix, in the broad ligament, or on a pedicle (Fig. 13.12). They are estimated to be present in at least 20% of all women of reproductive age and may be discovered incidentally during routine annual examination. Leiomyomas are more common in African-American than in white women. Asymptomatic fibroids may be present in 40–50% of women older than 40 years of age. They may occur singly but often are multiple. They may cause a range of symp-

Figure 13.12   Uterine leiomyomas in various anatomic locations. (Reproduced with permission from **Hacker NF, Moore JG.** *Essentials of Obstetrics and Gynecology.* 2nd ed. Philadelphia: WB Saunders, 1992:348.)

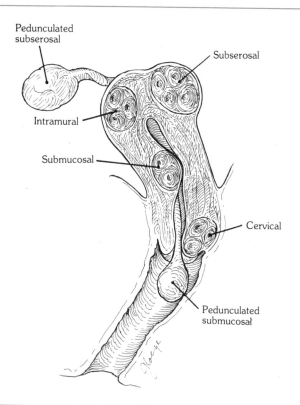

toms, from abnormal bleeding to pelvic pressure, which may lead to the diagnosis. Fewer than one-half of uterine leiomyomas are estimated to produce symptoms, however (44).

The cause of uterine leiomyomas is unknown. Several studies have suggested that each leiomyoma arises from a single neoplastic cell within the smooth muscle of the myometrium (96). There appears to be an increased familial incidence. Hormonal responsiveness and binding has been demonstrated *in vitro*. Fibroids have the potential to enlarge during pregnancy as well as to regress after menopause.

Grossly, fibroids are discrete nodular tumors that vary in size and number (Fig. 13.13). They may be microscopic or huge (a uterine weight of 74 lb has been reported). They may cause symmetric uterine enlargement or they may distort the uterine contour significantly. The consistency of an individual leiomyoma varies from hard and stony (as with a calcified leiomyoma) to soft (as with cystic degeneration), although the usual consistency is described as firm or rubbery. Although they do not have a true capsule, the margins of the tumor are blunt, noninfiltrating, and pushing and are usually separated from the myometrium by a pseudocapsule of connective tissue, which allows easy enucleation at the time of surgery. There is usually one major blood vessel supplying each tumor. The cut surface is characteristically whorled.

Degenerative changes are reported in approximately two-thirds of all specimens (97). Leiomyomas, with an increased number of mitotic figures, may occur in various forms: 1) during pregnancy or in women taking progestational agents; 2) with necrosis; and 3) as a *"smooth muscle tumor of uncertain malignant potential"* (**defined as having 5–9 mitoses/10 high-power fields (hpf) that do not demonstrate nuclear atypia or giant cells, or with a lower mitotic count (2–4 mitoses/10 hpf) that does demonstrate atypical nuclear features or giant cells**). Studies suggest that malignant degeneration of a preexisting leiomyoma is extremely uncommon, occurring in less than 0.5% (98).

Leiomyosarcoma is a rare malignant neoplasm composed of cells that have smooth muscle differentiation (Chapter 31). The typical patient with leiomyosarcoma is in her mid-

Figure 13.13   Multiple uterine leiomyomas.

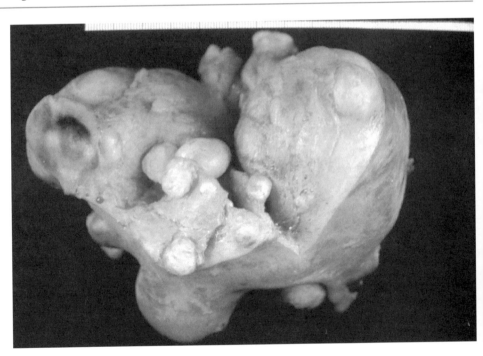

fifties and presents with abnormal bleeding. In most cases, diagnoses are made (postoperatively) after microscopic examination of a uterus removed because of suspected leiomyomas. **Sarcomas that have a malignant behavior have ≥10 mitoses/hpf.**

Uterine fibroids are frequently diagnosed on the basis of clinical findings of an enlarged, irregular uterus on pelvic examination. However, any pelvic tumor potentially can be confused with an enlarged uterus.

The most common presenting symptom associated with fibroids, and the one that most frequently leads to surgical intervention, is menorrhagia, which is reportedly present in one-third of women undergoing myomectomy (99). Chronic pelvic pain may also be present. Pain may be characterized as dysmenorrhea, dyspareunia, or pelvic pressure (Chapter 14). Acute pain may result from torsion of a pedunculated leiomyoma or infarction and degeneration. The following urinary symptoms may be present:

1. Frequency, which may result from extrinsic pressure on the bladder.

2. Partial ureteral obstruction may be caused by pressure from large tumors at the pelvic brim. Reports suggest some degree of ureteral obstruction in 30–70% of tumors above the pelvic brim. Ureteral compression is 3–4 times more common on the right, because the left ureter is protected by the sigmoid colon.

3. Rarely, complete urethral obstruction, resulting from elevation of the base of the bladder by the cervical or lower uterine leiomyoma with impingement on the region of the internal sphincter, may occur (100).

Leiomyomas are an infrequent primary cause of infertility and have been reported as a sole cause in less than 3% of infertile patients (44). One review of myomectomies performed for all indications noted a prior history of infertility in 27% of women (44). Pregnancy loss or complications can occur in women with leiomyomas, although most patients have uncomplicated pregnancies and deliveries. One study calculated a 10% rate of pregnancy complications in women with fibroids (101). **Although growth of leiomyomas may occur with pregnancy, one study noted no demonstrable change in size (based on serial ultrasound examination) in 90% of the patients** (102).

The following symptoms may infrequently be associated with leiomyomas:

1. Rectosigmoid compression, with constipation or intestinal obstruction

2. Prolapse of a pedunculated submucous tumor through the cervix, with associated symptoms of severe cramping and subsequent ulceration and infection (uterine inversion has also been reported)

3. Venous stasis of the lower extremities and possible thrombophlebitis secondary to pelvic compression

4. Polycythemia

5. Ascites

Ovarian Masses

During the reproductive years, the most common ovarian masses are benign. About two-thirds of ovarian tumors are encountered during the reproductive years (103). Most ovarian tumors (80–85%) are benign, and two-thirds of these occur in women between 20 and 44 years of age. **The chance that a primary ovarian tumor is malignant in a patient**

younger than 45 years of age is less than 1 in 15. Most tumors produce few or only mild, nonspecific symptoms. The most common symptoms include abdominal distension, abdominal pain or discomfort, lower abdominal pressure sensation, and urinary or gastrointestinal symptoms. If the tumor is hormonally active, symptoms of hormonal imbalance, such as vaginal bleeding related to estrogen production, may be present. Acute pain may occur with adnexal torsion, cyst rupture, or bleeding into a cyst. Pelvic findings in patients with benign and malignant tumors differ. Masses that are unilateral, cystic, mobile, and smooth are most likely to be benign, whereas those that are bilateral, solid, fixed, irregular, and associated with ascites, cul-de-sac nodules, and a rapid rate of growth are more likely to be malignant.

In terms of assessing ovarian masses, the distribution of primary ovarian neoplasms by decade of life can be helpful (104). Ovarian masses in women of reproductive age are probably benign, but the possibility of malignancy must be considered (Fig. 13.14).

Nonneoplastic Ovarian Masses **Follicular cysts, corpus luteum cysts, and theca lutein cysts comprise the category of functional ovarian cysts. All are benign and usually do not cause symptoms or require surgical management.** The annual rate of hospitalization for functional ovarian cysts has been estimated to be as high as 500 per 100,000 women-years in the U.S., although little is known about the epidemiology of the condition (105). **The most common functional cyst is the follicular cyst, which is rarely larger than 8 cm.** These cysts are usually found incidental to pelvic examination, although they may rupture, causing pain and peritoneal signs (Fig. 13.15). They usually resolve in 4–8 weeks.

Corpus luteum cysts are less common than follicular cysts. A corpus luteum is called a cyst when its diameter is greater than 3 cm. Before sensitive pregnancy tests were available, Halban syndrome was described, which simulated an ectopic pregnancy but consisted of a persistent corpus luteum cyst, delayed menses, the presence of an adnexal mass, and pain. Corpus luteum cysts may rupture, leading to a hemoperitoneum and requiring surgical management (Fig. 13.16). Patients taking anticoagulant therapy are at particular risk for rupture. Rupture of these cysts occurs more often on the right side and may occur during intercourse. Most ruptures occur on cycle days 20–26 (106). Culdocentesis usually reveals fluid with a hematocrit level less than 12% when a ruptured cyst is the cause of intraperitoneal bleeding (106).

Theca lutein cysts are the least common of functional ovarian cysts. They are usually bilateral and occur with pregnancy, including molar pregnancies. Up to one-fourth of molar pregnancies and 10% of choriocarcinomas may be associated with these cysts (107). They may be associated with multiple gestations, diabetes, Rh sensitization, *clomiphene citrate* and human menopausal gonadotropin/human chorionic gonadotropin ovulation induction, and the use of GnRH analogs. Theca lutein cysts may be quite large (up to 30 cm), are multicystic, and regress spontaneously.

Combination monophasic oral contraceptive therapy has been reported to markedly reduce the risk of functional ovarian cysts (108–111). Although some authors have questioned whether current low-dose oral contraceptives reduce the risk of functional ovarian cysts to the same extent as the previously available higher-dose preparations (112), other authors have found that the risk is still decreased but the protective effect may be somewhat attenuated (113, 114).

In 1987, a case report suggested that women who were taking triphasic oral contraceptives were more likely to develop functional ovarian cysts (115). This conclusion was based on seven women, with no defined denominator of users. Grimes and Hughes calculated rates of hospitalization for functional cysts from 1979 until 1986 (105). The rates remained essentially stable, whereas the number of users of multiphasic oral contraceptives grew from 0 to 3 million during this period, leading to the conclusion that, if such an association ex-

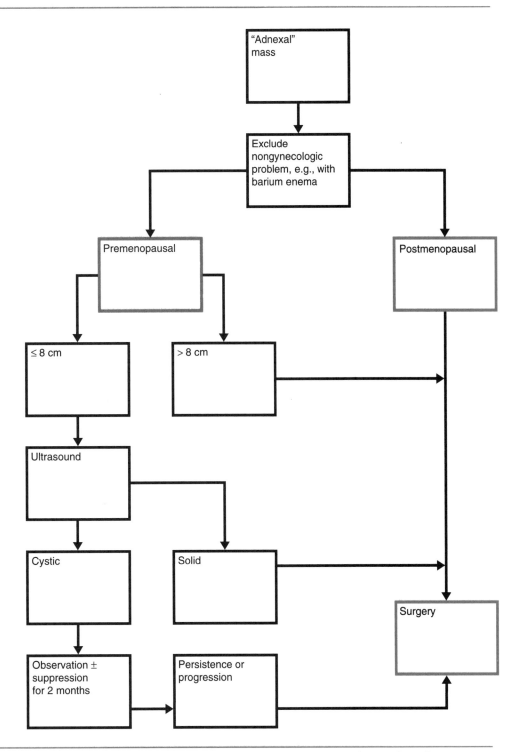

Figure 13.14   Preoperative evaluation of the patient with an adnexal mass. (Reproduced from **Berek JS, Hacker NF.** *Practical Gynecology Oncology.* 2nd ed. Baltimore: Williams & Wilkins, 1994:322.)

isted, the net public health impact was small. In addition, a population-based, case-control study did not support the speculation that use of triphasic oral contraceptives appreciably increased the risk of functional ovarian cysts (112). Other studies have also not demonstrated an increased risk (114). Smokers have a twofold increased risk of developing functional ovarian cysts, which suggests a line of investigation on the effect of smoking on ovarian function as a well as a potential cause of functional ovarian cysts (116).

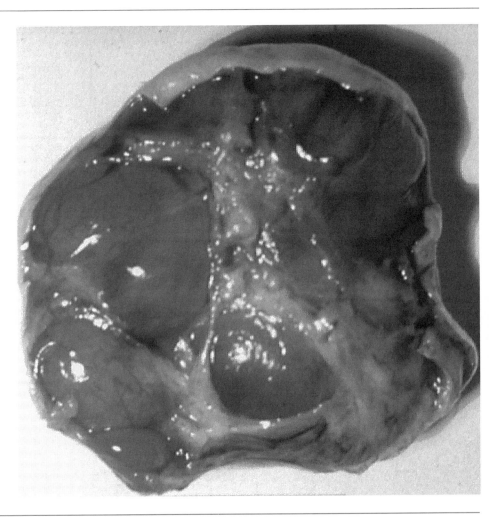

Figure 13.15   Follicular cysts of the ovary.

Figure 13.16   Corpus luteum cyst of the ovary. The left ovary is normal and the right ovary has a ruptured hemorrhagic corpus luteum cyst.

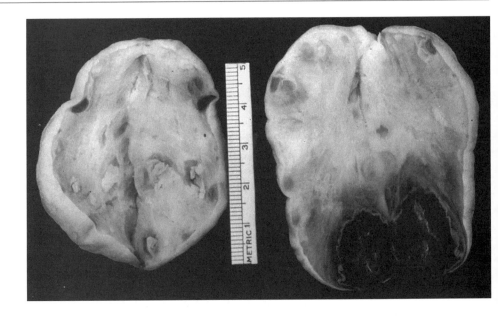

Other Benign Masses   Women with endometriosis may develop ovarian endometriomas ("chocolate" cysts), which can enlarge to 6–8 cm in size. A mass that does not resolve with observation may be an endometrioma (Chapter 26).

Although enlarged, polycystic ovaries were originally considered the *sine qua non* of polycystic ovarian syndrome (PCOS), polycystic ovaries probably represent a final common phenotype of a wide variety of causes; they have been described as a sign, not a diagnosis (117). The prevalence of PCOS among the general population depends on the diagnostic criteria used. In one study, 257 volunteers were examined with ultrasound; 22% were found to have polycystic ovaries (118). Thus, the finding of bilateral generously sized ovaries on examination or polycystic ovaries on ultrasound examination should prompt evaluation for the full-blown syndrome, which includes hyperandrogenism and chronic anovulation as well as polycystic ovaries. However, surgical intervention should not be recommended on the basis of this finding alone.

Neoplastic Masses   **More than 80% of benign cystic teratomas (dermoid cysts) occur during the reproductive years. The median age of occurrence is 30 years** (119). One-third of women younger than 30 years of age who underwent laparotomy for pelvic mass were found in one series to have a dermoid cyst (95). Histologically, benign cystic teratomas have an admixture of elements (Fig. 13.17). In one study of ovarian masses that were surgically excised, dermoid cysts represented 62% of all ovarian neoplasms in women younger than 40 years of age (104). Malignant transformation occurs in less than 2% of dermoid cysts in women of all ages; more than three-fourths of cases of malignant transformation occur in women older than 40 years of age (103). **The risk of torsion with dermoid cysts is approximately 15%, and it occurs more frequently than with ovarian tumors in general, perhaps because the high fat content of most dermoid cysts, allowing them to "float" within the abdominal and pelvic cavity** (Fig. 13.18). As a result of this fat content, on pelvic examination, a dermoid cyst frequently is described as anterior in location. They are bilateral in approximately 10% of cases, although many have advanced the argument against bivalving a normal-appearing contralateral ovary because of the risk of adhesions, which may result in fertility. **An ovarian cystectomy is almost al-**

Figure 13.17   Histologic appearance of a mature cystic teratoma of the ovary.

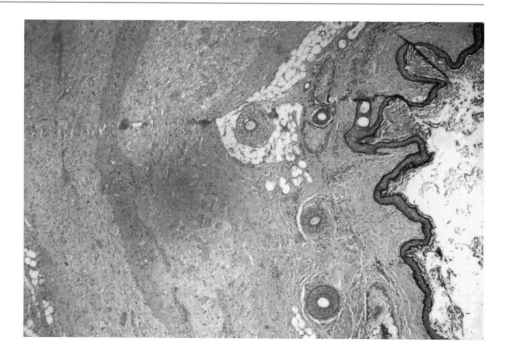

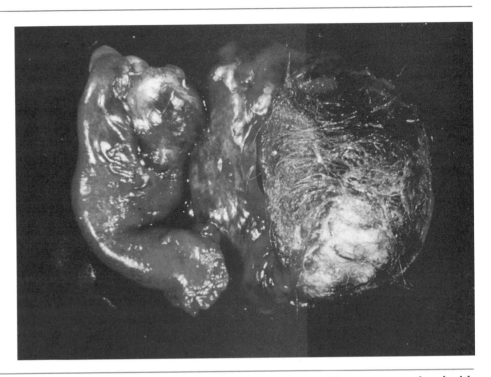

Figure 13.18   Mature cystic teratoma (dermoid cyst) of the ovary associated with adnexal torsion.

ways possible, even if it appears that only a small amount of ovarian tissue remains. Preserving a small amount of ovarian cortex in a young patient with a benign lesion is preferable to the loss of the entire ovary.

The risk of epithelial tumors increases with age. Although some texts report that serous cystadenomas are the more common benign neoplasm, a recent study indicated that benign cystic teratomas occurred most frequently, representing 66% of benign tumors in women younger than 50 years of age; serous tumors accounted for only 20% (104). **Serous tumors are generally benign; 5–10% have borderline malignant potential and 20–25% are malignant.** Serous cystadenomas are often multilocular, sometimes with papillary components (Fig. 13.19). The surface epithelial cells secrete serous fluid, resulting in a watery cyst content. Psammoma bodies, which are areas of fine calcific granulation, may be scattered within the tumor and are visible on x-ray. A frozen section is necessary to distinguish between benign (Fig. 13.20), borderline, and malignant serous tumors, because gross examination alone cannot make this distinction. Mucinous ovarian tumors may grow to large dimensions (Fig. 13.21). Benign mucinous tumors typically have a lobulated, smooth surface, are multilocular, and may be bilateral in up to 10% of cases. Mucoid material is present within the cystic loculations (Fig. 13.22). **Five to 10% of mucinous ovarian tumors are malignant.** They may be difficult to distinguish histologically from metastatic gastrointestinal malignancies. Other benign ovarian tumors include fibromas (Fig. 13.23) (a focus of stromal cells), Brenner tumors (Fig. 13.24) (which appear grossly similar to fibromas and which are frequently found incidentally), and mixed forms of tumors such as the cystadenofibroma.

Other Adnexal Masses

Masses that include the fallopian tube are related primarily to inflammatory causes in this age group. A tubo-ovarian abscess can be present in association with PID (Chapter 15). In addition, a complex inflammatory mass consisting of bowel, tube, and ovary may be present without a large abscess cavity.

366

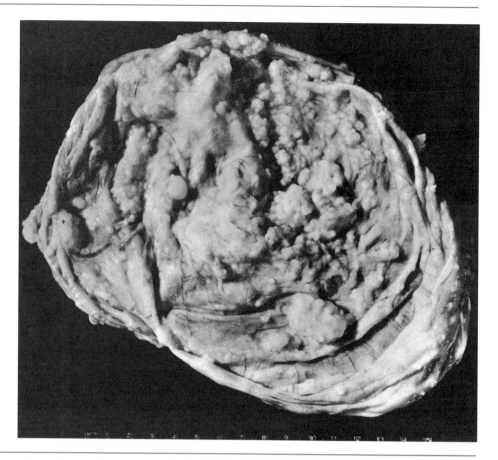

Figure 13.19   Gross appearance of a multilocular serous cystadenoma of the ovary. (Reproduced with permission from **Scully RE.** *Tumors of the Ovary and Maldeveloped Gonads.* Washington DC: Armed Forces Institute of Pathology, 1979:58.

Ectopic pregnancies can occur in the reproductive age group and must be excluded when a patient presents with pain, a positive pregnancy test, and an adnexal mass (Chapter 17).

Paraovarian cysts may be noted either on examination or on imaging studies. In many instances, a normal ipsilateral ovary can be visualized using ultrasonography (120). The frequency of malignancy in paraovarian tumors is quite low, although one review reported malignancy in 2% of patients (121).

Diagnosis

A complete pelvic examination, including rectovaginal examination and Pap test, should be performed. Estimations of the size of a mass should be presented in centimeters rather than in comparison to common objects or fruit (e.g., orange, grapefruit, tennis ball, golf ball). After pregnancy has been excluded, one simple office technique that can help determine whether a mass is uterine or adnexal includes sounding and measuring the depth of the uterine cavity.

Other Studies **Endometrial sampling with an endometrial biopsy or D&C is mandatory when both a pelvic mass and abnormal bleeding are present.** An endometrial lesion—carcinoma or hyperplasia—may coexist with a benign mass such as a leiomyoma. In a woman with leiomyomas, abnormal bleeding cannot be assumed to be caused solely by the fibroids. Clinicians differ in recommendations about the need for endometrial biopsy when the diagnosis is leiomyomas with regular menses.

Studies of the urinary tract may be necessary if urinary symptoms are prominent, including cystometric measurements if incontinence or pressure is a prominent symptom. Cys-

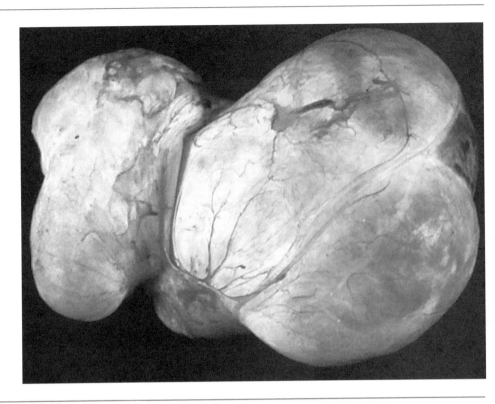

Figure 13.20   Benign serous papillary cystadenoma of the ovary.

Figure 13.21   Large benign mucinous cystadenoma of the ovary.

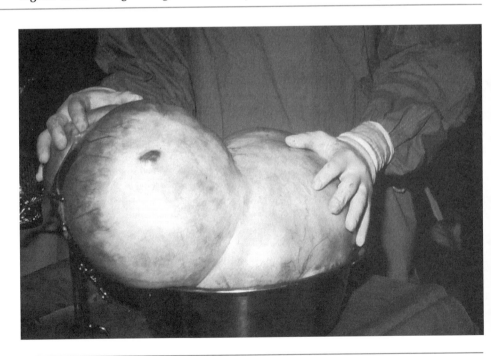

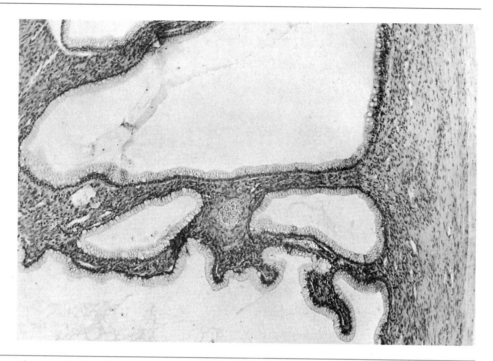

Figure 13.22   Histologic appearance of mucinous cystadenoma of the ovary. **Scully RE:** *Tumors of the Ovary and Maldeveloped Gonads.* Washington DC: Armed Forces Institute of Pathology, 1979:83.

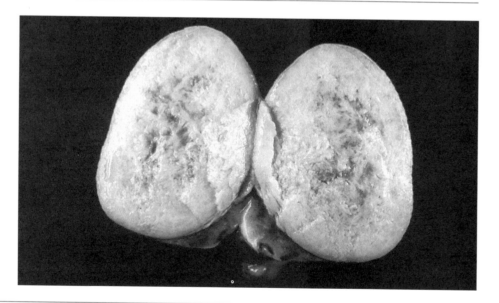

Figure 13.23   Ovarian fibroma that was removed from a patient with ascites and a right pleural effusion (*Meigs' syndrome*).

toscopy may sometimes be necessary or appropriate to rule out intrinsic bladder lesions. An ultrasound or intravenous pyelogram may be appropriate to demonstrate ureteral deviation, compression, or dilation in the presence of moderately large and laterally located fibroids or other pelvic mass. Such findings may provide an indication for surgical intervention for otherwise asymptomatic leiomyomas.

Laboratory Studies   Laboratory studies that are indicated for women of reproductive age with a pelvic mass include pregnancy test, Pap test, complete blood count, erythrocyte sed-

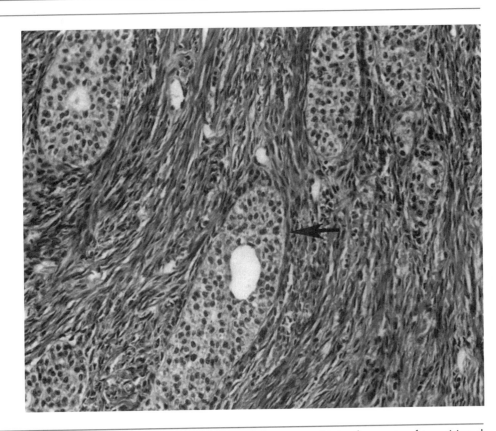

Figure 13.24   Benign Brenner tumor of the ovary. Note the nests of transitional metaplasia (arrow) found within the fibrotic stroma. (Reproduced from **Berek JS, Hacker NF.** *Practical Gynecologic Oncology.* 2nd ed. Baltimore: Williams & Wilkins, 1994:145.)

imentation rate, and testing of stool for occult blood. The value of tumor markers, such as CA125 in a premenopausal woman with a pelvic mass, has been widely debated. **A number of benign conditions, including uterine leiomyomas, PID, pregnancy, and endometriosis can cause elevated CA125, and thus may lead to unnecessary surgical intervention.**

Imaging Studies   Other studies may be necessary or appropriate. The most commonly indicated study is pelvic ultrasonography, which will help document the origin of the mass to determine whether it is uterine, adnexal, bowel, or gastrointestinal. The ultrasound examination also provides information about the size of the mass and its consistency, which can help determine management: unilocular cyst, mixed echogenicity (Fig. 13.25); multiloculated cyst, solid (Fig. 13.26).

Transvaginal and transabdominal ultrasonography have been compared in the diagnosis of pelvic masses. Transvaginal scanning has the advantage of additional information about the internal architecture or anatomy of the mass (122). Heterogeneous pelvic masses, described as tubo-ovarian abscesses on transabdominal ultrasound, can be separated on transvaginal scans into pyosalpinx, hydrosalpinx, tubo-ovarian complex, and tubo-ovarian abscess (91) (Fig. 13.27).

The diagnostic accuracy of transvaginal ultrasonography in diagnosing endometrioma can be quite high (Fig. 13.28) (123). Endometriomas can have a variety of ultrasonographic appearances, from purely cystic to varying degrees of complexity with septation or debris to a solid appearance. A scoring system that can help predict benign versus malignant adnexal masses is presented in Table 13.9.

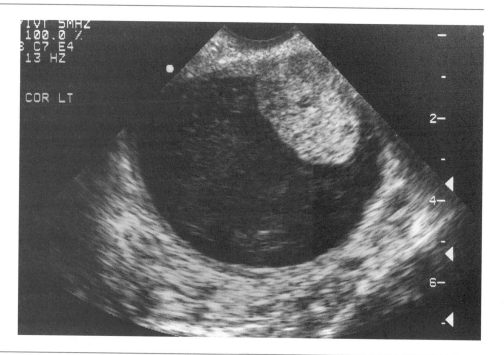

Figure 13.25   Transvaginal ultrasonogram of a unilocular ovarian cyst. This is characteristic of a benign process or corpus luteum cyst.

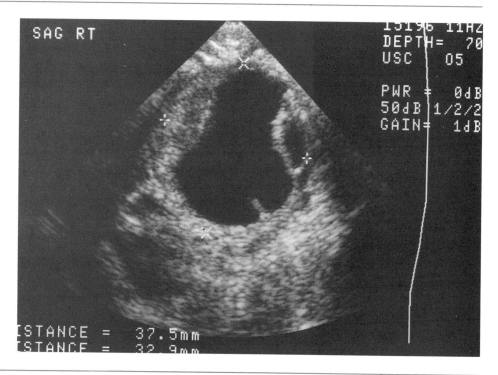

Figure 13.26   Transvaginal ultrasonogram of a complex, predominantly solid mass.

CT is seldom indicated as a primary diagnostic procedure, although it may be helpful in planning treatment when a malignancy is strongly suspected or when a nongynecologic disorder may be present. An abdominal flat plate x-ray is not a primary diagnostic procedure, although taken for other indications it may reveal calcifications that can assist in the discovery or diagnosis of a mass. Pelvic calcifications (teeth) consistent with a benign cystic teratoma (Fig. 13.29), a calcified uterine fibroid, or scattered calcifications

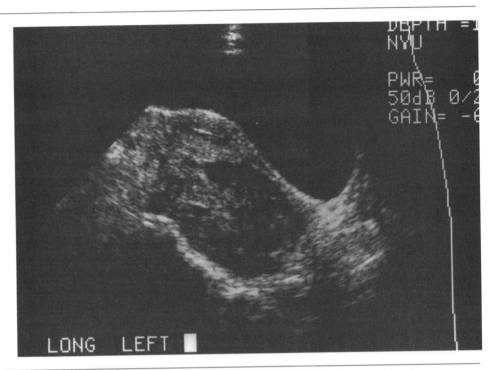

Figure 13.27   Transvaginal ultrasonogram of bilateral tubo-ovarian abscesses.

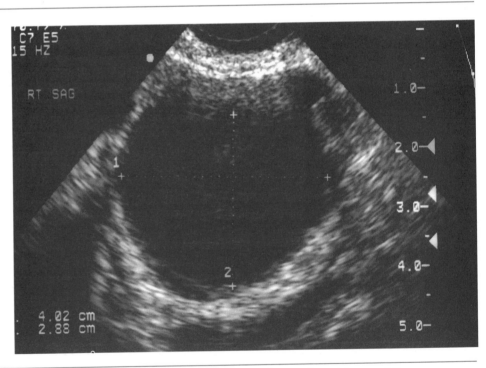

Figure 13.28   Transvaginal ultrasonogram of an endometrioma of the ovary.

consistent with psammoma bodies of a papillary serous cystadenoma can be seen on abdominal x-ray.

Hysteroscopy provides direct evidence of intrauterine pathology or submucous leiomyomas that distort the uterine cavity (see Chapter 21). Hysterosalpingography will demonstrate indirectly the contour of the endometrial cavity and any distortion or obstruction of the uterotubal junction secondary to leiomyomas, an extrinsic mass, or peritubal adhe-

Table 13.9   Ultrasound Scoring System for Adnexal Masses*

Clear cyst and smooth borders	1
Clear cyst with slightly irregular border; cyst with smooth walls but low-level echoes (i.e., endometrioma)	2
Cyst with low-level echoes with slightly irregular border but no nodularity (i.e., endometrioma); clear cyst in postmenopausal patient	3
Equivocal, nonspecific ultrasound appearance: solid ovarian enlargement or small cyst with irregular borders and internal echoes (hemorrhagic cyst or benign ovarian tumor)	4–6
Multiseptated or irregular cystic mass consistent in appearance with ovarian tumor (7 = less nodularity; 8–9 = more nodularity)	7–9
Pelvic mass as above, with ascites	10

1 = benign; 10 = malignant.
Modified from **Finkler NJ, Benacerraf B, Lavin PT, Wojciechowski C, Knapp RC.** Comparison of CA 125, clinical impression, and ultrasound in the preoperative evaluation of ovarian masses. Reprinted with permission from The American College of Obstetricians and Gynecologists (*Obstet Gynecol 1988;72:659*).

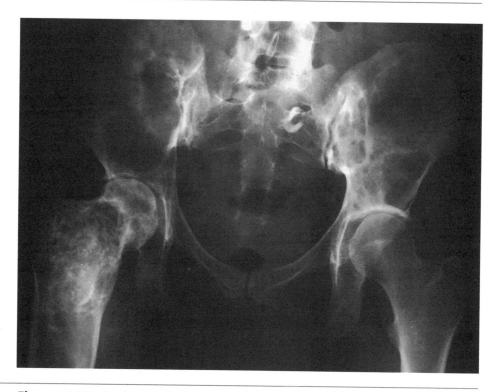

Figure 13.29   Benign cystic teratoma (dermoid cyst) of the ovary with teeth seen on abdominal x-ray.

sions. Newer studies combine the techniques of hysterosalpingography, in which fluid is instilled into the uterine cavity, with transvaginal ultrasound.

MRI may be most useful in the diagnosis of uterine anomalies (33), although its value uncommonly justifies the increased cost of the procedure over ultrasound for the diagnosis of other pelvic masses.

Management

The management of a pelvic mass is based on an accurate diagnosis. An explanation of this diagnosis should be conveyed to the patient, along with a discussion of the likely course of the disease (e.g., growth of uterine leiomyomas, regression of fibroids at menopause, regression of a follicular cyst, the uncertain malignant potential of an ovarian mass). All options for management should be presented and discussed, although it is appropriate for the physician to state a recommended approach with an explanation of the reasons for the recommendation. Management should be based on the primary symptoms and may include observation with close follow-up, temporizing surgical therapies, medical management, or definitive surgical procedures.

Management of Leiomyomas

Nonsurgical **Judicious patient observation and follow-up are indicated primarily for uterine leiomyomas; intervention is reserved for specific indications and symptoms.** Periodic repeat examinations are indicated to ensure that the tumors are not growing rapidly. Uterine size should be recorded on the patient's chart, and the location of the palpable leiomyomas should be described and diagrammed.

The use of GnRH agonists results in a 40–60% decrease in uterine volume and can be of value in some clinical situations. Hypoestrogenism results from treatment and has been associated with reversible bone loss and symptoms such as hot flashes. Thus, treatment has been limited to short-term use, although low-dose hormonal replacement may be effective in minimizing the hypoestrogenic effects. Regrowth of leiomyomas is experienced within a few months in about one-half of women treated. Some indications for the use of GnRH agonists in women with leiomyomas are as follows:

1. Preservation of fertility in women with large leiomyomas before attempting conception, or preoperative treatment before myomectomy

2. Treatment of anemia to allow recovery of normal hemoglobin levels before surgical management, minimizing the need for transfusion or allowing autologous blood donation

3. Treatment of women approaching menopause in an effort to avoid surgery

4. Preoperative treatment of large leiomyomas to make vaginal hysterectomy, hysteroscopic resection or ablation, or laparoscopic destruction more feasible

5. Treatment of women with medical contraindications to surgery

6. Treatment of women with personal or medical indications for delaying surgery

Hormonal therapy with progestational agents may result in a decrease in uterine size and amenorrhea; anemia is allowed to resolve by initiating iron therapy several weeks before definitive surgery. Success with this therapy has been limited.

Surgical Determining potential indications for surgical treatment requires careful judgment and assessment of the degree of associated symptoms. **Asymptomatic leiomyomas do not usually require surgery. Some indications for surgery include the following:**

1. Abnormal uterine bleeding with resultant anemia, unresponsive to hormonal management

2. Chronic pain with severe dysmenorrhea, dyspareunia, or lower abdominal pressure and/or pain

3. Acute pain, as in torsion of a pedunculated leiomyoma, or prolapsing submucosal fibroid

4. Urinary symptoms or signs such as hydronephrosis after complete evaluation

5. Rapid enlargement of the uterus during the premenopausal years, or any increase in uterine size in a postmenopausal woman, because of inability to exclude a uterine sarcoma

6. Infertility, with leiomyomas as the only abnormal finding

7. Enlarged uterine size with compression symptoms or discomfort

Hysterectomy is definitive surgical management of symptomatic uterine leiomyomas (Chapter 22). Abdominal myomectomy is an alternative to hysterectomy for patients who desire childbearing, who are young, or who prefer that the uterus be retained. Vaginal myomectomy is indicated in the case of a prolapsed pedunculated submucous fibroid. Hysteroscopic resection of small submucous leiomyomas is a technique that may offer benefits for a selected group of patients (Chapter 21).

Ovarian Masses

The rapid development of ultrasound technology and its frequent, if not routine, application during gynecologic examinations has led to the more frequent detection of ovarian cysts. The treatment for ovarian masses that are suspected to be functional tumors is expectant. A classic study popularized the use of oral contraceptives as suppressive therapy, although the results of this study have been misinterpreted (124). In this study, 286 patients (aged 16–48 years) with adnexal masses were treated with combination oral contraceptives. Eighty-one women had a persistent mass after this therapy; surgery was performed on these women, none of whom was found to have a physiologic cyst. This study has been interpreted to indicate that suspected functional cysts should be treated with oral contraceptives, although there are no data to indicate a more rapid resolution with oral contraceptives than with time alone. If a woman needs contraception and wishes to use oral contraceptives for birth control, it is perfectly acceptable to prescribe them in this setting. However, **a randomized prospective study showed no acceleration of the resolution of functional ovarian cysts (which were associated with the use of *clomiphene citrate* or human menopausal gonadotropins) with oral contraceptives compared with observation alone** (125). **Another study revealed that oral contraceptives are effective in leading to resolution of functional ovarian cysts, although they are no more effective than time alone** (126). However, oral contraceptives are effective in reducing the risk of subsequent ovarian cysts.

Symptomatic cysts should be evaluated promptly, although mildly symptomatic masses suspected to be functional can be managed with analgesics rather than surgery. Surgical intervention is warranted in the face of significant pain or the suspicion of malignancy. On ultrasonography, large cysts and those that have multiloculations, septa, papillae, and increased blood flow are all suspected signs of neoplasia. If a malignant cyst is suspected, at any age, explorative laparotomy should be performed promptly.

Ultrasonographic or CT scanning aspiration procedures should not be used in women in whom there is a suspicion of malignancy. Laparoscopic surgery should be reserved for diagnostic or therapeutic purposes for patients at very low risk for malignancy. One survey of gynecologic oncologists' experiences with patients who had originally undergone laparoscopic management of malignant or borderline tumors suggested that so-called "benign" characteristics do not preclude malignancy and that laparoscopic management can be associated with partial or incomplete excision and delays in definitive surgery (127). The management of ovarian dermoid cysts and other benign masses with operative laparoscopy has been described, although the surgeon's experience and skill are important in the prevention of spill of the cyst contents. The clear advantage of this technique is the shorter hospital stay, shorter recovery time, and less postoperative pain. Few controlled trials have been performed to compare the laparoscopic approach to laparotomy (128) (Chapter 21).

Postmenopausal Age Group

Differential Diagnosis

Ovarian Masses

During the postmenopausal years, the ovaries become smaller (129).

1. Before menopause, the dimensions are approximately $3.5 \times 2 \times 1.5$ cm.

2. In early menopause, the ovaries are approximately $2 \times 1.5 \times 0.5$ cm.

3. In late menopause, they are even smaller: $1.5 \times 0.75 \times 0.5$ cm.

Barber has described the postmenopausal palpable ovary (PMPO) syndrome, suggesting that any ovary that is palpable on examination beyond the menopause is abnormal and deserves evaluation (129); however, this has not been shown to be a reliable predictor of malignancy (Chapter 33). Clearly, body habitus makes a difference in the ease of examination, but a postmenopausal ovary that, on palpation, is comparable in size to a premenopausal ovary is abnormally large. The incidence of ovarian cancer increases with age and is predominantly a disease of postmenopausal women; the average patient age is 61 years (Chapter 33).

Considering the ease of pelvic ultrasound evaluation, a new problem has arisen in postmenopausal women: the discovery of a small ovarian cyst. This is particularly troublesome in a woman who is entirely asymptomatic and whose ultrasound examination was performed for indications unrelated to the pelvis. It has been suggested that **when the cyst is asymptomatic, small (<5 cm in diameter), unilocular, and thin-walled, the risk of malignancy is extremely low and these masses can be followed conservatively, without surgery** (131). Surgery may be indicated in some women with an adverse pedigree with a strong family history of ovarian, breast, endometrial, or colon cancer, or if the mass appears to be enlarging (see Chapter 33). The addition of color flow Doppler examination may be helpful in distinguishing benign from malignant masses (132). **The risk of malignancy for women older than 50 years of age or for postmenopausal women (approximately the same groups) at the time of laparotomy for a pelvic mass is approximately 50%** (95, 104).

Uterine and Other Masses

In women who have been under regular gynecologic care, the discovery of a new pelvic mass after menopause is worrisome, because the likelihood of malignant neoplasm is high if it is an ovarian tumor. However, many postmenopausal women have not had regular gynecologic care, and the discovery of a mass may reflect the persistence of uterine fibroids that had not previously been discovered. Some women may not remember having been told of a pelvic mass. Thus, a review of old medical records may be helpful in determining the preexistence of a benign pelvic mass.

Other benign masses can occur in this age group, including paraovarian cysts and unusual tumors such as benign retroperitoneal cysts of müllerian type (133).

Diagnosis

A personal and family medical history is helpful in detecting individuals at increased risk for the development of ovarian cancer. Several hereditary family cancer syndromes involve ovarian neoplasms (see Chapter 33). However, patients with hereditary forms of epithelial ovarian cancer account for only a small percentage of all cases; 95% of cases of ovarian cancer are sporadic and without identifiable heritable risk (134).

In one multicenter prospective study, the individual accuracy of pelvic examination, ultrasound, and serum CA125 in discriminating between benign and malignant pelvic masses was approximately the same (approximately 75%) (135). When the results of all three examinations were negative, no malignancy was found.

Management

The use of improved imaging techniques may allow the nonoperative management of ovarian masses that are probably benign (Table 13.9). When surgery is believed to be indicated, based on characteristics of the mass, a family or personal medical history, or the patient's desire for definitive diagnosis, selection of the appropriate surgical procedure is critical for effective therapy. The standard of care continues to be laparotomy, with appropriate staging procedures performed as necessary (Chapter 33). Ovarian cystectomy or oophorectomy may be indicated (136). Many surgeons are using a less invasive laparoscopic technique, although the assessment of this procedure and its efficacy await further confirmation and study (137).

Vulvar Conditions

Vulvar and vaginal symptoms are a common presenting complaint to gynecologists. The presence of vulvar symptoms may bring a patient to the clinician; however, this anatomic site is not one that is easily inspected by the patient. Thus, vulvar lesions may be noted on examination and may not have been noticed by the patient.

Neonatal

In the neonatal age group, various developmental and congenital abnormalities may be noted. Whereas an extensive discussion of these abnormalities is beyond the scope of this text, obstetricians will recognize that they must be prepared to deal with the parents and family when an infant is born with ambiguous genitalia. The etiology of these problems, as well as intersex disorders that may be discovered in an older child, can be complex. Chromosomal abnormalities, enzyme deficiencies (including 17- or 21-hydroxylase deficiency as causes of congenital adrenal hyperplasia), or prenatal masculinization of a female fetus resulting from maternal androgen-secreting ovarian tumors or, rarely, drug exposures can all result in genital abnormalities that are noted at birth (138). These abnormalities are addressed in Chapter 23.

The situation of ambiguous genitalia represents a social and potential medical emergency that is best handled by a team of specialists, which may include urologists, neonatologists, endocrinologists, and pediatric gynecologists. The first questions parents ask after a baby is born include "is it a boy or a girl?" In the case of ambiguous genitalia, the parents should be informed that the baby's genitals are not fully developed and, therefore, a simple examination of the external genitalia cannot determine the actual sex. The parents should be told that data will be collected but that it may take several days to determine the baby's intended sex. In some situations, it may be best to state simply that the baby has some serious medical complications.

Other genital abnormalities may be noted at birth, although few obstetricians or pediatricians carefully examine the external genitalia of female neonates. It has been argued that careful inspection of the external genitalia of all female infants should be performed, with gentle probing of the introitus and anus to determine the patency of the hymen or a possible imperforate anus. If patency is in doubt, a rectal thermometer may be used to gently test the patency (138). It has been suggested that the obstetrician-gynecologist should perform this examination on all female infants in the delivery room (139). Various types of hymenal configurations in the newborn have been described, ranging from imperforate to microperforate, to cribriform, to hymenal bands, and hymens with central anterior, posterior, or eccentric orifices (140). An examination in the neonatal period would prevent the discovery of an imperforate hymen or vaginal septum only after a young woman experiences periodic pelvic and abdominal pain with the development of a large hematometra or hematocolpos.

Congenital vulvar tumors may include "strawberry" hemangiomas, which are relatively superficial vascular lesions and large cavernous hemangiomas. Treatment is controversial; many lesions will spontaneously regress. Some clinicians have advocated cryotherapy, argon laser therapy, or sclerosing solutions (141).

Childhood

It may be difficult for a young child to describe vulvar sensations. Parents may notice the child crying during urination, scratching herself repeatedly, or complaining of vague symptoms. Often, the child's pediatrician will have evaluated the child for urinary tract infection. Evaluation for pinworms is also warranted, as pinworms can cause severe itching in the vulvar as well as perianal area. Vulvovaginitis is the most common gynecologic problem of childhood. Prepubertally, the vulva, vestibule, and vagina are anatomically and histologically vulnerable to infection. The physical proximity of the vagina and vestibule to the anus can result in overgrowth of bacteria that can cause primary vulvitis and secondary vaginitis (see Chapter 15).

The clinician should be familiar with normal prepubertal genital anatomy and hymenal configuration (142, 143). The unestrogenized vulvar vestibule is mildly erythematous and can be confused with infection. In addition, smegma around and beneath the prepuce may resemble patches of candida vulvitis. The prepubertal vulvar area is quite susceptible to chemical irritants.

Chronic skin conditions such as lichen sclerosus, seborrheic dermatitis, and atopic vulvitis may occur in children (144). Lichen sclerosus, the cause of which is not well established, has a characteristic "cigarette paper" appearance in a keyhole distribution (around the vulva and anus) (Fig. 13.30). Lichen sclerosus in the pediatric patient should be treated with reassurance that the condition will regress as the child progresses through adrenarche and menarche. Medications include *progesterone* in oil (400 mg in 4 oz. of Aquaphor) applied twice daily; *betamethasone valerate* (0.1% ointment, *Valisone*) or high-potency topical corticosteroids, *Temovate* (0.05%) cream, applied once or twice daily for 2–3 weeks, until symptoms regress, then tapered to twice per week or less often to minimize use.

Labial agglutination may occur as a result of chronic vulvar inflammation from any cause (Fig. 13.31). The treatment of labial agglutination consists of a brief course (2–4 weeks) of externally applied estrogen cream. The area of agglutination (adhesion) will become thin as a result, and separation can often be performed in the office with the use of a topical anesthetic (e.g., *lidocaine* jelly) (Fig. 13.32). Urethral prolapse may present with acute pain or bleeding, or the presence of a mass may be noted (144).

Vulvovaginal complaints of any sort in a young child should prompt the consideration of possible sexual abuse. Sexually transmitted infections may occur in prepubertal children (145). Sensitive but direct questioning of the parent or caretaker and the child should be a part of the evaluation.

Adolescence

Adolescents with gonadal dysgenesis or androgen insensitivity may present with abnormal pubertal development and primary amenorrhea (Chapter 23). Various developmental abnormalities, including vaginal agenesis, imperforate hymen, transverse and longitudinal

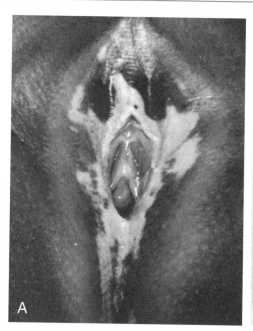
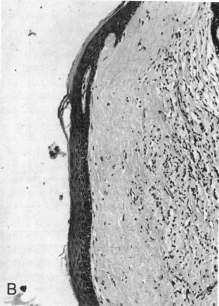

Figure 13.30   A: Lichen sclerosus in a 7-year-old girl. (Reproduced from **Novak ER, Woodruff JB,** eds. *Novak's Gynecologic and Obstetric Pathology.* 7th ed. Philadelphia: WB Saunders, 1974:21.) **B. Histologic appearance of lichen sclerosus.**

vaginal septa, vaginal and uterine duplications, hymenal bands, and septa, most commonly present in early adolescence with amenorrhea (for the obstructing abnormalities) or with concerns such as inability to use tampons (for hymenal and vaginal bands and septa). These developmental abnormalities must be evaluated carefully to determine both external and internal anatomy.

A tight hymenal ring may be discovered because of concerns about the inability to use tampons or initiate intercourse. Manual dilation can be successful, as can small relaxing incisions at 6 o'clock and 8 o'clock in the hymenal ring. This can sometimes be done in the office under local anesthesia but may require conduction or general anesthesia in the operating room. The condition of "hypertrophy of the labia minora" has been described, along with surgical procedures to correct this developmental abnormality (146). This condition is more appropriately considered a variant of normal, with reassurance as the primary therapy. Genital ulcerations may be noted in girls with leukemia or other cancers requiring chemotherapy (147). The possibility of sexual abuse, incest, or involuntary intercourse should be considered for young adolescents with vulvovaginal complaints, STDs, or pregnancy (148).

Reproductive Women

In postmenarchal individuals, vulvar symptoms are most often related to a primary vaginitis and a secondary vulvitis. The presence of vaginal discharge can lead to vulvar irritative symptoms, or candidal vulvitis may be present. The causes of vaginitis and cervicitis are addressed in Chapter 15. As noted, young children may have a difficult time describing vulvar symptoms; adult women describe vulvar symptoms using a variety of terms (itching, pain, discharge, discomfort, burning, external dysuria, soreness, pain with intercourse or sexual activity). Burning with urination from noninfection causes may be difficult to distinguish from a urinary tract infection, although some women can distinguish pain when the urine hits the vulvar area (an external dysuria) from burning pain (often suprapubic in location) during urination. A urine culture may be necessary to help make the distinction.

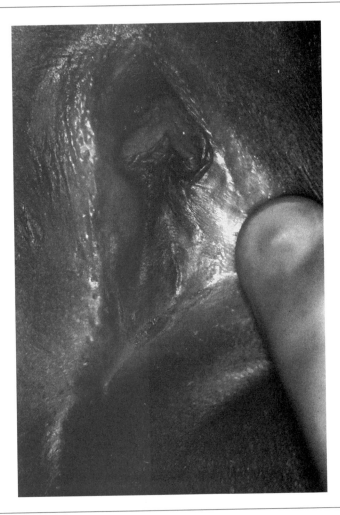

Figure 13.31   Posterior labial agglutination in a 9-year-old girl.

Itching is a very common vulvar symptom. A variety of vulvar conditions and lesions can present with pruritus (149, 150).

A number of skin conditions that occur on other areas of the body may occur on the vulvar area. Table 13.10 contains a list of these conditions classified as either infectious or noninfectious causes. Whereas the diagnosis of some of these conditions is apparent from inspection alone (e.g., a skin tag) (Fig. 13.33), any lesions that appear atypical or in which the diagnosis is not clear should be biopsied.

Pigmented vulvar lesions include benign nevi, lentigines, melanosis, seborrheic keratosis, and some vulvar intraepithelial neoplasias (VIN), especially multifocal VIN 3. Suspicious pigmented vulvar lesions, in particular, should warrant biopsy to rule out VIN or malignant melanoma (151). Approximately 10% of white women have a pigmented vulvar lesion; some of these lesions may be malignant (Chapter 34) or have the potential for progression (VIN) (Chapter 16). The behavior of some nevocellular lesions (representing about 2% of nevi) is not well established (152). Multiple hyperpigmented lesions of typical lentigo simplex and melanosis are common, and any areas with irregular borders should be biopsied (Fig. 13.34).

Vulvar Biopsy   **A vulvar biopsy is essential in distinguishing benign from premalignant or malignant vulvar lesions, especially because many lesions may have a somewhat similar ap-**

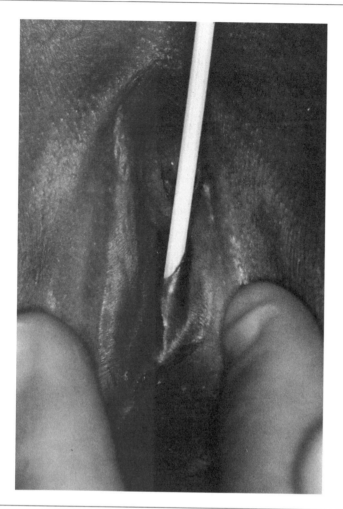

Figure 13.32 Cotton-tipped applicator placed inside the labial agglutination shown in Figure 13.31.

pearance. Vulvar biopsies should be performed liberally to ensure that these lesions are diagnosed and treated appropriately. A prospective study of vulvar lesions biopsied in a gynecologic clinic found lesions occurring in the following order of frequency: epidermal inclusion cyst (Fig. 13.35), lentigo, Bartholin duct obstruction, carcinoma *in situ,* melanocytic nevi, acrochordon, mucous cyst, hemangiomas, postinflammatory hyperpigmentation, seborrheic keratoses, varicosities, hidradenomas, verruca, basal cell carcinoma, and unusual tumors such as neurofibromas, ectopic tissue, syringomas, and abscesses (153). Clearly, the frequency with which a lesion would be reported on biopsy is related to the frequency with which all lesions of a given pathology are biopsied. Thus, the above listing probably underrepresents such common lesions as condylomas.

The biopsy is easily performed in the office using a local anesthetic. Typically, 1% *lidocaine* is infiltrated beneath the lesion using a small (25–27 gauge) needle. Disposable punch biopsy instruments come in a variety of sizes from 2 to 6 mm in diameter. They have the advantage of being sharp and thus facilitate obtaining a good specimen. Sterilizable instruments are also available and may be a more ecologically sound choice if they can be maintained and sharpened periodically. These skin biopsy instruments, along with fine forceps, scissors, and a scalpel, should be available in all outpatient gynecologic settings. For the smaller biopsies, it is usually unnecessary to place a suture. Topical silver nitrate can be used for hemostasis. Multiple biopsies may be appropriate to obtain representative areas of a lesion, if the lesion has a variable appearance or is multifocal. Although the vul-

Table 13.10   Subacute and Chronic Recurrent Conditions of the Vulva

Noninfectious	Infectious
Acanthosis nigricans	Cellulitis
Atopic dermatitis	Folliculitis
Behcet's disease	Furuncle/carbuncle
Contact dermatitis	Insect bites (e.g., chiggers, fleas)
Crohn's disease	Necrotizing fasciitis
Diabetic vulvitis*	Pubic lice
Hidradenitis suppurativa*	Scabies
Hyperplastic dystrophy	Tinea
Lichen sclerosus	
Mixed dystrophy	
Paget's disease	
Pseudo folliculitis	
Razor bumps	
Psoriasis	
Seborrheic dermatitis	
Vulvar intraepithelial neoplasia	

*Etiology unknown, often secondarily infected.

var biopsy procedure involves minimal discomfort, the biopsy sites will be painful for several days after the procedure. The prescription of a topical anesthetic such as 2% *lidocaine* jelly, to be applied periodically and before urinating, is appreciated by patients who require this procedure. Infection of the site can occur, and patients should be cautioned to report excessive erythema or purulent drainage.

Other Vulvar Conditions   *Pseudofolliculitis* similar to what has been described as pseudofolliculitis barbae (razor bumps) may occur in women who shave pubic hair to conform to a bikini (154). It consists of an inflammatory reaction surrounding an ingrown hair and occurs most commonly among individuals with curly hair, particularly African-Americans.

Fox-Fordyce disease is characterized by a chronic, pruritus eruption of small papules/cysts formed by keratin-plugged apocrine glands. It is commonly present over the lower abdomen, mons pubis, labia majora, and inner portions of the thighs. *Hidradenitis suppurativa* is a chronic condition involving the apocrine glands with the formation of multiple deep nodules, scars, pits, and sinuses that occur in the axilla, vulva, and perineum (Fig. 13.36). Hyperpigmentation and secondary infection are often seen. Hidradenitis suppurativa can be extremely painful and debilitating. It is often treated with antibiotics (with coverage of both aerobic and anaerobic bacteria). Estrogens or antiandrogen therapy has been attempted; surgical therapy with wide local excision may be necessary.

Acanthosis nigricans involves widespread velvety pigmentation in skin folds, particularly the axillae, neck, thighs, submammary area, and vulva and surrounding skin. It is of particular interest to gynecologists because of its association with androgen disorders and, as such, is associated with obesity, chronic anovulation, acne, glucose intolerance, and cardiovascular disease (155).

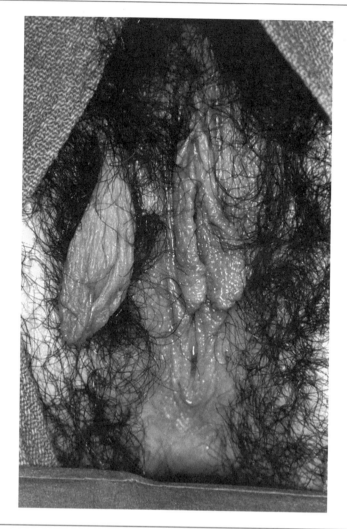

Figure 13.33   Large benign skin tag from left labium majus.

Intraepithelial Neoplasia   A classification of intraepithelial lesions of the vulva is presented in Table 16.13.

Extramammary Paget's disease of the vulva is an intraepithelial neoplasia containing vacuolated Paget's cells (Chapter 16). Clinically, it may have an appearance varying from moist, oozing ulcerations to an eczematoid lesion with scaling and crusting, to a grayish lesion (150). A biopsy to confirm the diagnosis is mandatory.

Vulvar intraepithelial neoplasia is associated with human papillomavirus infection and is increasing in frequency, particularly among young women (Chapter 16) (156). Diagnosis requires biopsy of any suspicious vulvar lesions, particularly those that are pigmented or discolored. The increasing frequency of this entity makes a careful vulvar inspection mandatory during annual gynecologic examinations.

Vulvar Tumors, Cysts, and Masses   *Condyloma acuminata* are very common vulvar lesions and are usually easily recognized and treated with topical therapies such as tri- and bichloroacetic acid. Other sexually transmitted organisms, such as the virus responsible for *molluscum contagiosum* and the lesions of *syphilis* and *condyloma lata,* may occasionally be mistaken for vulvar condyloma

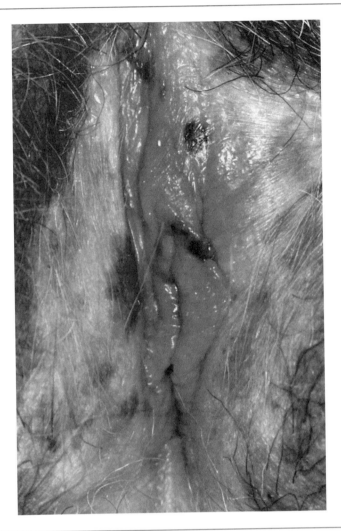

Figure 13.34   Lentigo simplex and melanosis of vulva. Note multiple hyperpigmented lesions. (Reproduced from **Wilkinson EJ, Stone IK.** Atlas of Vulvar Disease. Baltimore: Williams & Wilkins, 1995:41.)

acuminata caused by the human papillomavirus (see Chapter 15). A summary of benign vulvar tumors is listed in Table 13.11. There is argument regarding whether sebaceous cysts exist on the vulva or whether these lesions are histopathologically epidermal or epidermal inclusion cysts (138). These cysts may result from the burial of fragments of skin after the trauma of childbirth or episiotomy.

Recently, it has been argued that the commonly cited concept of milk lines extending into the vulva and accounting for lesions of mammary-like anogenital glands (e.g., fibroadenoma, lactating glands) is not supported by observations in human embryos; such studies show that primordia of the mammary glands do not extend beyond the axillary-pectoral area (157). Eccrine or apocrine glands have been suggested as the probable source of these unusual lesions.

Bartholin duct cysts are a common vulvar lesion. They result from occlusion of the duct with accumulation of mucous and are frequently asymptomatic. Infection of the gland may result in the accumulation of purulent material, with the formation of a rapidly enlarging, painful, inflammatory mass (a Bartholin abscess). An inflatable bulb-tipped catheter has been described by Word and is quite easy to use (158). The small catheter is inserted

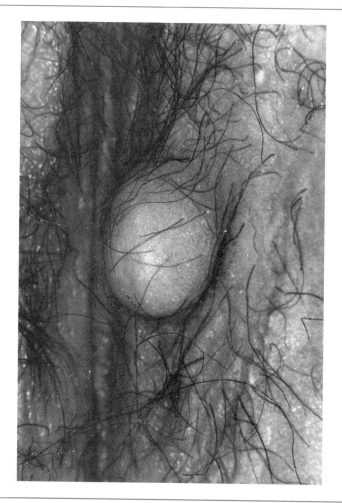

Figure 13.35   Inclusion cysts on right labium majus. (Reproduced from **Wilkinson EJ, Stone IK.** Atlas of Vulvar Disease. Baltimore: Williams & Wilkins, 1995:17.)

through a small stab wound into the abscess after infiltration of the skin with local anesthesia; the balloon of the catheter is inflated with 2–3 cc of saline and the catheter remains in place for 4–6 weeks, allowing epithelialization of a tract and the creation of a permanent gland opening.

Skene duct cysts are cystic dilations of the Skene glands typically located adjacent to the urethral meatus within the vulvar vestible (Fig. 13.37). Although most are small and often asymptomatic, they may enlarge and cause urinary obstruction, requiring excision.

The symptom of painful intercourse (dyspareunia) may be caused by many different vulvovaginal conditions, including common vaginal infections and vaginismus (Chapter 15). A careful sexual history is essential, as is a careful examination of the vulvar area and vagina. *Vulvodynia* is the term used to describe unexplained vulvar pain, sexual dysfunction, and the resultant psychological disability (159). The term *vulvar vestibulitis* has been used to describe a situation in which there is pain during intercourse, primarily during entry (160, 161). The condition is characterized by tender areas surrounding the vulvar vestibule and hymenal ring (see Chapter 14). A number of recent studies have failed to demonstrate a consistent relationship with any genital infectious organism, including chlamydia, gonorrhea, Trichomonas, mycoplasma, Ureaplasma, Gardnerella, Candida, or human papillomavirus (162–164).

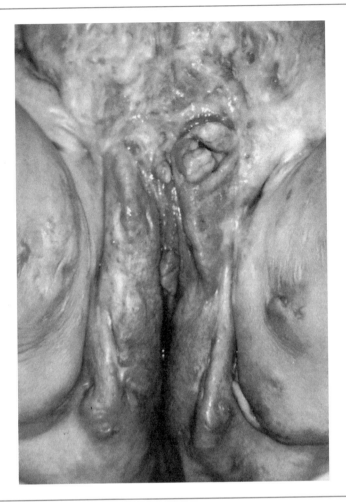

Figure 13.36   Hidradenitis suppurativa involving both labia majora and crease folds. (Reproduced from **Wilkinson EJ, Stone IK.** Atlas of Vulvar Disease. Baltimore: Williams & Wilkins, 1995:150.)

Other conditions that have been described as contributing to vulvar pain and dyspareunia include subclinical human papillomavirus infection (165). In cases of vulvar symptoms that have been studied carefully using PCR (polymerase chain reaction) technology, human papillomavirus has not been found to be causative of either the symptoms or the visible lesion of vestibular papillomatosis (165, 166). Vestibular papillomatosis may be a nonspecific response to discharge or inflammation.

Vulvar Ulcers

A number of sexually transmissible infections can cause vulvar ulcers, including herpes simplex virus, syphilis, lymphogranuloma venereum, and granuloma inguinale (Chapter 15). *Crohn's disease* can include vulvar involvement with abscesses, fistulae, sinus tracts, fenestrations, and other scarring. Although medical treatment with systemic steroids and other systemic agents is the mainstay of therapy, surgical therapy of both intestinal and vulvar disease may be required.

Behcet's disease is characterized by genital and oral ulcerations with ocular inflammation. The cause and the most effective therapy are not well established.

Lichen planus also causes oral and genital ulcerations. Typically, there is desquamative vaginitis with erosion of the vestibule. Treatment is based on the use of both topical and

Table 13.11   Types of Vulvar Tumors

1. Cystic lesions	3. Anatomic
Bartholin duct cyst	Hernia
Cyst in the canal of Nuck (hydrocele)	Urethral diverticulum
Epithelial inclusion cyst	Varicosities
Skene duct cyst	
	4. Infections
2. Solid Tumors	Abscess—Bartholin, Skene, periclitoral, other
Acrocordon (skin tag)	Condyloma lata
Angiokeratoma	Molluscum contagiosum
Bartholin gland adenoma	Pyogenic granuloma
Cherry angioma	
Fibroma	5. Ectopic
Hemangioma	Endometriosis
Hidradinoma	Ectopic breast tissue
Lipoma	
Granular cell myoblastoma	
Neurofibroma	
Papillomatosis	

systemic steroids. Plasma cell mucositis appears as erosions in the vulvar area, particularly the vestibule. Biopsy is essential in making the diagnosis.

Postmenopausal Women

Several vulvar conditions occur most commonly in postmenopausal women. Symptoms are primarily itching and vulvar soreness, in addition to dyspareunia.

Vulvar Dystrophies

In the past, numerous terms have been used to describe disorders of vulvar epithelial growth that produce a number of nonspecific gross changes. These terms have included leukoplakia, lichen sclerosus et atrophicus, atrophic and hyperplastic vulvitis, and kraurosis vulvae. The malignant potential of the vulvar dystrophies is less than 5%; at particular risk is the patient with cellular atypia on initial biopsy. The International Society for the Study of Vulvar Diseases (ISSVD) has recommended a classification of vulvar dystrophies, which is presented in Table 16.13.

Squamous Hyperplasia   Squamous hyperplasia is seem most often in postmenopausal women but may occur during the reproductive years. Pruritus is the most common symptom. The lesion appears thickened and hyperkeratotic, and there may be excoriation. Squamous hyperplasia tends to be discrete but may be symmetrical and multiple. Biopsies are necessary to make the diagnosis and to evaluate the presence of atypia and exclude malignancy.

The treatment is local application of a *fluorinated corticosteroid* ointment three times a day for 6 weeks. Typically, the lesion totally regresses. If a new lesion recurs, repeat biopsy should be performed and an additional 6 weeks of treatment with topical steroids should be given.

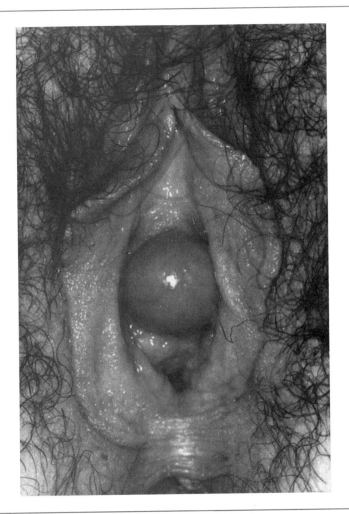

Figure 13.37   Skene duct cyst. (Reproduced from **Wilkinson EJ, Stone IK.** Atlas of Vulvar Disease. Baltimore: Williams & Wilkins, 1995:21.)

Lichen Sclerosus **Lichen sclerosus is the most common white lesion of the vulva (Fig. 13.38). Lichen sclerosus can occur at any age, although it is most common among postmenopausal women** (167). The symptoms are pruritus, dyspareunia, and burning. Lichen sclerosus characteristically presents with decreased subcutaneous fat such that the vulva is atrophic, with small or absent labia minora, thin labia majora, and sometimes phimosis of the prepuce. The surface is pale with a shiny, crinkled pattern, often with fissures and excoriation. The lesion tends to be symmetrical and often extends to the perineal and perianal areas. The diagnosis is confirmed by biopsy. Invasive cancer is only rarely associated with lichen sclerosus.

The treatment is with 2% *testosterone* cream in a petrolatum base applied twice daily for 3 weeks and then once daily for 3 weeks. A maintenance treatment of once daily or once every other day is continued, depending on the response and the persistence of the symptoms. The patient must be informed that *testosterone* can produce masculinizing side effects. Treatment must be continued indefinitely, because the *testosterone* allows the patient to live with the disease instead of curing the disease. Alternatively, 0.05% *clobetasol*, a potent steroid, can also be used, and approximately 80% of patients have a satisfactory response (168). Superficial vulvectomy can be used in severe cases or in those who are refractory to medication. Recurrences are common after surgical treatment.

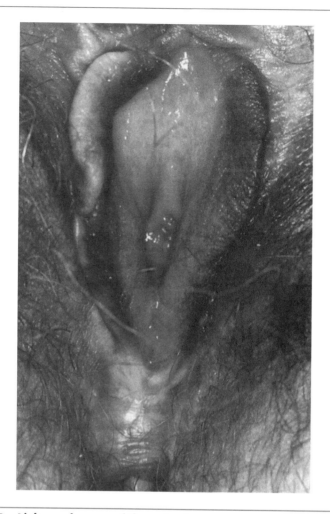

Figure 13.38   Lichen sclerosus of the vulva in a postmenopausal patient. (Reproduced from **Wilkinson EJ, Stone IK.** Atlas of Vulvar Disease. Baltimore: Williams & Wilkins, 1995:36.)

Mixed Dystrophy   Mixed dystrophy consists of varying proportions of hypoplastic and hyperplastic tissues, and accounts for about 20% of vulvar dystrophies. Atypia occurs more frequently in mixed dystrophy than in pure hyperplastic dystrophies. The symptoms are burning, pruritus, and dyspareunia. The lesion appears as keratinized, white epithelium associated with patches of pale, thin, shiny, wrinkled epithelium. The diagnosis must be made by biopsy, and multiple biopsies are necessary to exclude areas of focal atypia.

The treatment is *fluorinated corticosteroid* ointment three times daily for 6–8 weeks followed by 2% *testosterone* ointment three times daily for 6–8 weeks. Thereafter, *testosterone* ointment should be used indefinitely, usually every other day. Areas of severe atypia may be best treated by local excision.

Urethral Lesions   Vulvar lesions that may be seen in other age groups, but that occur more commonly among older women, include urethral caruncles and prolapse of the urethral mucosa. Both conditions can be treated with topical or systemic estrogen cream. Various vulvar skin lesions, including seborrheic keratoses and "cherry" hemangiomas (senile hemangiomas), occur more commonly on aging skin.

Vaginal Conditions

Vaginal discharge is one of the most common vaginal symptoms. Conditions ranging from vaginal candidiasis to chlamydia cervicitis to bacterial vaginosis to cervical carcinoma may cause vaginal discharge. Infectious vaginal conditions are addressed more completely in Chapter 15. Vaginal lesions may occasionally be palpable to a woman. More commonly, vaginal lesions are discovered on examination. They may contribute to symptoms (such as bleeding or discharge) or they may be entirely asymptomatic. Vaginitis, cervicitis, and vaginal or cervical lesions (including malignancies) can be causes of vaginal discharge. Other noninfectious causes of discharge are as follows:

1. Retained foreign body—tampon, pessary

2. Ulcerations—tampon-induced, lichen planus

3. Malignancy—cervical, vaginal

4. Postmenopausal atrophic vaginitis, postradiation vulvovaginitis

Pediatric

Sexual abuse should always be considered in prepubertal children with vaginal discharge. A vaginal culture for gonorrhea and chlamydia should be performed. Vulvovaginitis is usually caused by multiple organisms that are present in the perineal area, although a single organism such as streptococcus or Shigella may be causative. Treatment should be initiated with a focus on hygienic and cleansing measures. A short-term (<4 weeks) course of topical estrogens and broad-spectrum antibiotics may be necessary. Culture should also be performed if simple hygienic measures are ineffective in resolving symptoms. The problem can be recurrent.

Vaginal Irrigation   A technique for obtaining vaginal cultures and for performing vaginal irrigation has been described by Pokorny (13). A "catheter within a catheter" can be fashioned using the tubing from an intravenous "butterfly" setup within a sterile urethral catheter. Nonbacteriostatic saline (1 cc) can be injected, aspirated, and sent for culture. Cultures taken in this manner are almost always better tolerated than cultures obtained using a cotton-tipped applicator. A larger quantity of saline can then be used to irrigate the vagina while the catheter is still within the vagina. Small foreign bodies can often be flushed from the vagina in this manner.

Adolescence and Older

Vaginal tampons have been associated with both microscopic and macroscopic ulcerations. Healing of the macroscopic ulcerations occurs within several weeks without specific therapy if tampon use is suspended. A follow-up examination to demonstrate healing is appropriate, with biopsy of any persistent ulcerations to rule out other lesions.

Toxic shock syndrome has been associated with tampon use and vaginal *Staphylococcus aureus*-produced exotoxins. Toxic shock syndrome consists of fever, hypotension, a diffuse erythroderma with desquamation of the palms and soles, plus involvement of at least three major organ systems (169). Vaginal involvement includes mucous membrane inflammation.

Some vaginal lesions are asymptomatic and are noted incidentally on examination. *Fibroepithelial polyps* consist of polypoid folds of connective tissue, capillaries, and stroma covered by vaginal epithelium. Although they can be excised easily in the office, their vascularity can be troublesome, and excision is not necessary unless the diagnosis is in question. *Cysts of embryonic origin* can arise from mesonephric, paramesonephric, and urogenital sinus epithelium. *Gartner's duct cysts* are of mesonephric origin and are usually present on the lateral vaginal wall. They rarely cause symptoms and, therefore, do not require treatment. Other embryonic cysts can arise anterior to the vagina and beneath the bladder. Cysts that arise from the urogenital sinus epithelium are located in the area of the vulvar vestibule. *Vaginal adenosis,* the presence of epithelial-lined glands within the vagina, has been associated with *in utero* exposure to diethylstilbestrol. No therapy is necessary, other than close observation and periodic palpation to detect nodules that may need to be biopsied to rule out vaginal clear cell adenocarcinoma (Chapter 32).

Women will sometimes describe a bulging lesion of the vagina and vulvar area, variably associated with symptoms of pressure or discomfort. The most common cause of such a lesion is one of the disorders of vaginal support: cystocele, rectocele, or urethrocele. Management of these conditions is discussed in Chapter 20. Other genital lesions, such as urethral diverticuli or occasionally embryonic cysts, may present with similar symptoms.

References

1. **Marshall WA, Tanner JM.** Variations in pattern of pubertal changes in girls. *Arch Dis Child* 1969;44:291.

2. **Harlan WR, Harlan EA, Grillo GP.** Secondary sex characteristics of girls 12 to 17 years of age: the U.S. Health Examination Survey. *J Pediatr* 1980;96:1074–8.

3. **Hammerschlag MR, Alpert S, Rosner I, Thurston P, Semine D, McComb D, et al.** Microbiology of the vagina in children: normal and potentially pathogenic organisms. *Pediatrics* 1978;62:57–62.

4. **Hammerschlag MR, Alpert S, Onderdonk AB, Thurston P, Drude E, McCormack WM, et al.** Anaerobic microflora of the vagina in children. *Am J Obstet Gynecol* 1978;131:853–6.

5. **Davis AJ, Emans SJ.** Human papillomavirus infection in the pediatric and adolescent patient. *J Pediatr* 1989;115:1–9.

6. **Herman-Giddens ME.** Vaginal foreign bodies and child sexual abuse. *Arch Pediatr Adolesc Med* 1994;138:195–200.

7. **Pokorny SF.** Long-term intravaginal presence of foreign bodies in children. A preliminary study. *J Reprod Med* 1994;39:931–5.

8. **American Medical Association.** *Diagnostic and Treatment Guidelines on Child Sexual Abuse.* Chicago: American Medical Association, 1992.

9. **Emans SJ, Woods ER, Flagg NT.** Genital findings in sexually abused, symptomatic, and asymptomatic girls. *Pediatrics* 1987;79:778–85.

10. **Muram D.** Child sexual abuse—genital findings in prepubertal girls. I. The unaided medical examination. *Am J Obstet Gynecol* 1989;160:328–33.

11. **deJong AR, Rose M.** Frequency and significance of physical evidence in legally proven cases of child sexual abuse. *Pediatrics* 1989;84:1022–6.

12. **Emans SJ, Goldstein P.** The gynecologic examination of the prepubertal child with vulvovaginitis: use of the knee-chest position. *Pediatrics* 1980;65:758–60.

13. **Pokorny SF, Stormer LVN.** Atraumatic removal of secretions from the prepubertal vagina. *Am J Obstet Gynecol* 1987;156:581–2.

14. **Treloar AE, Boynton RE, Behn BG, Brown BW.** Variation of the human menstrual cycle through reproductive life. *Int J Fertil* 1970;12:77–126.

15. **Flug D, Largo RH, Prader A.** Menstrual patterns in adolescent Swiss girls: a longitudinal study. *Ann Hum Biol* 1984;495–508.

16. **World Health Organization Task Force on Adolescent Reproductive Health.** World Health Organization multicenter study on menstrual and ovulatory patterns in adolescent girls: a multicenter cross-sectional study of menarche. *J Adolesc Health* 1986;7:229–35.

17. **Fraser IS, McCarron G, Markham R, Resta T.** Blood and total fluid content of menstrual discharge. *Obstet Gynecol* 1985;61:194–8.

18. **Fraser IS, McCarron G, Markham R.** A preliminary study of factors influencing perception of menstrual blood loss volume. *Am J Obstet Gynecol* 1984;139:788–93.

19. **Apter D, Vihko R.** Early menarche, a risk factor for breast cancer, indicates early onset of ovulatory cycles. *J Clin Endocrinol Metab* 1983;57:82–6.

20. **Center for Disease Control.** Premarital sexual experience among adolescent women—United States, 1970-1988. *MMWR* 1991;39:929–32.

21. **Hillard PJA.** The patient's reaction to side effects of oral contraceptives. *Am J Obstet Gynecol* 1989;161:1312–5.

22. **Oakley D, Sereinka S, Bogue E-L.** Oral contraceptive pill use after an initial visit to the family planning clinic. *Fam Plann Perspect* 1991;23:150–4.

23. **Ballassone ML.** Risk of contraceptive discontinuation among adolescents. *J Adolesc Health* 1989;10:527–33.

24. **Kaunitz AM.** Injectable contraception. *Clin Obstet Gynecol* 1989;32:356–67.

25. **Shoupe D, Mishell DR.** Norplant: subdermal implant system for long-term contraception. *Am J Obstet Gynecol* 1989;160:1286–92.

26. **Claessens AE, Cowell CA.** Acute adolescent menorrhagia. *Am J Obstet Gynecol* 1981;139:277–80.

27. **Center for Disease Control and Prevention.** 1993 Sexually transmitted diseases treatment guidelines. *MMWR* 1993;42:1–102.

28. **Wolner-Hanssen P, Kiviat NB, Holmes KK.** Atypical pelvic inflammatory disease: subacute, chronic, or subclinical upper genital tract infection in women. In: **Holmes KK, Mardh P-A, Sparling PF, Wiesner PJ, Cates W Jr, Lemon SM, et al.,** eds. *Sexually Transmitted Diseases.* 2nd ed. New York: McGraw-Hill, 1984:615–9.

29. **Harlap S, Kost K, Forrest JD.** *Preventing Pregnancy Protecting Health: A New Look at Birth Control Choices in the United States.* New York: The Alan Guttmacher Institute, 1991.

30. **National Institute for Child Health and Development.** Androgens and women's health. *Clinician* 1994;12:1–30.

31. **Ibanez L, Potau N, Zampolli M, Prat N, Gussinye M, Saenger P, et al.** Source localization of androgen excess in adolescent girls. *J Clin Endocrinol Metab* 1994;79:1778–84.

32. **Gulekli B, Turhan NO, Senoz S, Kukner S, Oral H, Gokmen O.** Endocrinological, ultrasonographic and clinical findings in adolescent and adult polycystic ovary patients: a comparative study. *Gynecol Endocrinol* 1993;7:273–7.

33. **Olson MC, Posniak HV, Tempany CM, Dudiak CM.** MR imaging of the female pelvic region. *Radiographics* 1992;12:445–65.

34. **Nickelsen C.** Diagnostic and curative value of uterine curettage. *Acta Obstet Gynecol Scand* 1986;65:693–7.

35. **The Alan Guttmacher Institute.** *Sex and America's Teenagers.* New York: The Alan Guttmacher Institute, 1994.

36. **Nielsen S, Hahlin M.** Expectant management of first-trimester spontaneous abortion. *Lancet* 1995;345:84–6.

37. **Rosenberg MJ, Long SC.** Oral contraceptives and cycle control: a critical review of the literature. *Adv Contracept* 1992;8:35–45.

38. **Stubblefield PG.** Menstrual impact of contraception. *Am J Obstet Gynecol* 1994;170:1513–22.

39. **Rosenberg MJ Waugh MS, Long S.** Unintended pregnancies and use, misuse, and discontinuation of oral contraceptives. *J Reprod Med* 1995;40:355–60.

40. **Krettek JE, Arkin SI, Chaisilwattana P, Monif GR.** Chlamydia trachomatous in patients who used oral contraceptives and had intermenstrual spotting. *Obstet Gynecol* 1993;81:728–31.

41. **Hillard PJA.** Breakthrough bleeding associated with subdermal implants and depot medroxyprogesterone acetate. *The Contraception Report* 1994;5:13–6.

42. **Archer DF.** Management of bleeding in women using subdermal implants. *Contemp Obstet Gynecol* 1995;40:11–25.

43. **Diaz S, Croxatto HB, Pavez M, Behadj H, Stern J, Sivin I.** Clinical assessment of treatments for prolonged bleeding in users of Norplant implants. *Contraception* 1990;42:97–109.

44. **Buttram VC, Reiter RC.** Uterine leiomyomata: etiology, symptomatology, and management. *Fertil Steril* 1981;36:433–45.

45. **Rick ME.** Diagnosis and management of von Willebrand's syndrome. *Med Clin North Am* 1994;78:609–23.

46. **Parsons AK, Lense JJ.** Sonohysterography for endometrial abnormalities: preliminary results. *J Clin Ultrasound* 1993;21:87–95.

47. **Kupfer MC, Schiller VL, Hansen GC, Tessler FN.** Transvaginal sonographic evaluation of endometrial polyps. *J Ultrasound Med* 1994;13:535–9.

48. **Stock RJ, Kanbour A.** Prehysterectomy curettage. *Obstet Gynecol* 1975;45:537–41.

49. **Grimes DA.** Diagnostic dilation and curettage: a reappraisal. *Am J Obstet Gynecol* 1982;142: 1–6.

50. **American College of Obstetricians and Gynecologists.** *Hysteroscopy.* ACOG Technical Bulletin. Washington, DC: ACOG, 1994.

51. **Anderson ABM, Haynes PJ, Guillebaud J, Turnball AC.** Reduction of menstrual blood loss by prostaglandin synthetase inhibitors. *Lancet* 1976;1:774–6.

52. **Hall P, Maclachlan N, Thorn N, Nudd MW, Taylor CG, Garrioch DB.** Control of menorrhagia by the cyclo-oxygenase inhibitors naproxen sodium and mefenamic acid. *Br J Obstet Gynaecol* 1987;94:554–8.

53. **Royal College of General Practitioners.** *Oral Contraceptives and Health.* London: Pitman Medical, 1970.

54. **Larsson G, Milsom I, Lindstedt G, Rybo G.** The influence of a low-dose combined oral contraceptive on menstrual blood loss and iron status. *Contraception* 1992;46:327–34.

55. **Parmer J.** Long-term suppression of hypermenorrhea by progesterone intrauterine contraceptive devices. *Am J Obstet Gynecol* 1984;139:578–9.

56. **Chi IC, Farr G.** The non-contraceptive effects of the levonorgestrel-releasing intrauterine device. *Adv Contracept* 1994;10:271–85.

57. **Diagnostic and Therapeutic Technology Assessment (DATTA).** Intrauterine devices. *JAMA* 1989;261:2127–30.

58. **Mishell DR.** Weighing the IUD option. *Dialogues in Contraception* 1990;2:6–8.

59. **Haynes PJ, Hodgson H, Anderson AB, Turnbull AC.** Measurement of menstrual blood loss in patients complaining of menorrhagia. *Br J Obstet Gynaecol* 1977;84:763–8.

60. **Pinion SB, Parkin DE, Abramovich DR, Naji A, Alexander DA, Russelll IT, et al.** Randomised trial of hysterectomy, endometrial laser ablation, and transcervical endometrial resection for dysfunctional uterine bleeding. *BMJ* 1994;309:979–83.

61. **Bachmann GA.** Psychosexual aspects of hysterectomy. *Womens Health Issues* 1990;1:41–9.

62. **Gitlin MJ, Pasnau RO.** Psychiatric syndromes linked to reproductive function in women: a review of current knowledge. *Am J Psychiatry* 1989;136:1313–22.

63. **Studd JWW, Thom MH.** Oestrogens and endometrial cancer. In: **Studd JWW,** ed. *Progress in Obstetrics and Gynecology.* 9th ed., Vol. 1. Edinburgh: Churchill Livingstone, 1981:182–98.

64. **Padwick ML, Davies JP, Whitehead MI.** A simple method for determining the optimal dosage of progestogen in postmenopausal women receiving estrogens. *N Engl J Med* 1986; 350:930–4.

65. **Ravnikar VA.** Compliance with hormone replacement therapy: are women receiving the full impact of hormone replacement therapy preventive health benefits? *Womens Health Issues* 1992;2:75–80.

66. **Ryan PJ, Harrison R, Blake GM, Fogelman I.** Compliance with hormone replacement therapy (HRT) after screening for postmenopausal osteoporosis. *Br J Obstet Gynaecol* 1992;99: 325–8.

67. **Magos AL, Brincat M, Studd JW, Wardle P, Schlesinger P, O'Dowd T.** Amenorrhea and endometrial atrophy with continuous oral estrogen and progestogen therapy in postmenopausal women. *Obstet Gynecol* 1985;65:496–9.

68. **Prough SG, Aksel S, Wiebe RH, Shepherd J.** Continuous estrogen/progestin therapy in menopause. *Am J Obstet Gynecol* 1987;157:1449–53.

69. **Gusberg SB, Milano C.** Detection of endometrial carcinoma and its precursors. *Cancer* 1981;47:1173–5.

70. **Ng ABP, Reagan JW, Hawliczek S, Went BW.** Significance of endometrial cells in the detection of endometrial carcinoma and its precursors. *Acta Cytol* 1974;18:356–61.

71. **Zucker PK, Kasdon EJ, Feldstein ML.** The validity of Pap smear parameters as predictors of endometrial pathology in menopausal women. *Cancer* 1985;56:2256–63.

72. **van der Graaf Y, Vooijs GP, Gaillar HL, Go DM.** Screening errors in cervical cytology smears. *Acta Cytol* 1987;31:434–8.

73. **Feldman S, Berkowitz RS, Tosteson AN.** Cost-effectiveness of strategies to evaluate postmenopausal bleeding. *Obstet Gynecol* 1993;81:968–75.

74. **Bakos O, Smith P, Heimer G.** Transvaginal ultrasonography for identifying endometrial pathology in postmenopausal women. *Maturitas* 1994;20:181–9.

75. **Karlsson B, Granberg S, Hellberg P, Wikland M.** Comparative study of transvaginal sonography and hysteroscopy for the detection of pathologic endometrial lesions in women with postmenopausal bleeding. *J Ultrasound Med* 1994;13:757–62.

76. **Van den Bosch T, Vandendael A, Van Schoubroeck D, Wranz PA, Lombard CJ.** Combining vaginal ultrasonography and office endometrial sampling in the diagnosis of endometrial disease in postmenopausal women. *Obstet Gynecol* 1995;85:349–52.

77. **Kurman RJ, Norris HJ.** Endometrial hyperplasia and metaplasia. In: **Kurman RJ,** ed. *Blaustein's Pathology of the Female Genital Tract.* 3rd ed. New York: Springer-Verlag, 1987: 322–37.

78. **Kurman RJ, Kaminski PF, Norris HJ.** The behavior of endometrial hyperplasia. A long-term study of "untreated" hyperplasia in 170 patients. *Cancer* 1985;56:403–12.

79. **Breen JL, Maxson WS.** Ovarian tumors in children and adolescents. *Clin Obstet Gynecol* 1977;20:607–23.

80. **Lampkin BC, Wong KY, Kalinyak KA, Carter D, Heckel J, Zaboy KA, et al.** Solid malignancies in children and adolescents. *Surg Clin North Am* 1985;65:1351–86.

81. **Norris HJ, Jensen RD.** Relative frequency of ovarian neoplasms in children and adolescents. *Cancer* 1972;30:713–9.

82. **Diamond MP, Baxter JW, Peerman GC Jr, Burnett LS.** Occurrence of ovarian malignancy in childhood and adolescence: a community-wide evaluation. *Obstet Gynecol* 1988;71:858–60.

83. **Van Winter JT, Simmons PS, Podratz KC.** Surgically treated adnexal masses in infancy, childhood, and adolescence. *Am J Obstet Gynecol* 1994;170:1780–9.

84. **Schellhas HF.** Malignant potential of the dysgenetic gonad—Part I. *Obstet Gynecol* 1974; 44:298–309.

85. **Troche V, Hernandez E.** Neoplasia arising in dysgenetic gonads. *Obstet Gynecol Surv* 1986;41:74–8.

86. **Goldstein D, deCholnoky C, Emans SJ, Leventhal JM.** Laparoscopy in the diagnosis and management of pain in adolescents. *J Reprod Med* 1980;24:251–6.

87. **Chatman DL, Ward AB.** Endometriosis in adolescents. *J Reprod Med* 1982;27:156–60.

88. **Hurd SJ, Adamson GD.** Pelvic pain: endometriosis as a differential diagnosis in adolescents. *Adolesc Pediatr Gynecol* 1992;5:3–7.

89. **Tolete-Velcek FT, Hansbrough F, Kugaczewski J, Coren CV, Klotz DH, Price AF, et al.** Uterovaginal malformations: a trap for the unsuspecting surgeon. *J Pediatr Surg* 1989;24: 736–40.

90. **Franks AL, Beral V, Cates W, Hogue CJR.** Contraception and ectopic pregnancy risk. *Am J Obstet Gynecol* 1990;163:1120–3.

91. **Bulas DI, Ahlstrom PA, Sivit CJ, Blask AR, O'Donnell RM.** Pelvic inflammatory disease in the adolescent: comparison of transabdominal and transvaginal sonographic evaluation. *Radiology* 1992;183:435–9.

92. **Mitchell DG, Outwater EK.** Benign gynecologic disease: applications of magnetic resonance imaging. *Top Magn Reson Imaging* 1995;7:26–43.

93. **Schwartz LB, Seifer DB.** Diagnostic imaging of adnexal masses. A review. *J Reprod Med* 1992;37:63–71.

94. **Wiesenfeld HC, Sweet RL.** Progress in the management of tuboovarian abscesses. *Clin Obstet Gynecol* 1993;36:433–44.

394

95. **Hernandez E, Miyazawa K.** The pelvic mass. Patients' ages and pathologic findings. *J Reprod Med* 1988;33:361–40.

96. **Townsend DE, Sparkes RS, Baluda MC, McClelland G.** Unicellular histogenesis of uterine leiomyomas as determined by electrophoresis of glucose-6-phosphate dehydrogenase. *Am J Obstet Gynecol* 1970;107:1168–73.

97. **Persaud V, Arjoon PD.** Uterine leiomyoma: incidence of degenerative change and a correlation of associated symptoms. *Obstet Gynecol* 1969;35:432–6.

98. **Leibsohn S, d'Ablaing G, Mishell DR Jr, Schlaerth JB.** Leiomyosarcoma in a series of hysterectomies performed for presumed uterine leiomyomas. *Am J Obstet Gynecol* 1990;162:968–74.

99. **Brown JM, Malkasian GD, Symmonds RE.** Abdominal myomectomy. *Am J Obstet Gynecol* 1967;99:126–9.

100. **Lifschitz S, Buchsbaum HJ.** Urinary tract involvement by benign and malignant gynecologic disease. In: **Buchsbaum HJ, Schmidt JD,** eds. *Gynecologic and Obstetric Urology.* Philadelphia: WB Saunders, 1978.

101. **Katz Vl, Dotters DJ, Droegemueller W.** Complications of uterine leiomyomas in pregnancy. *Obstet Gynecol* 1989;73:593–6.

102. **Winer-Muram HT, Muram D, Gillieson MS.** Uterine myomas in pregnancy. *J Can Assoc Radiol* 1984;35:168–70.

103. **Scully RE.** *Atlas of Tumor Pathology: Tumors of the Ovary and Maldeveloped Gonads.* Washington, DC: Armed Forces Institute of Pathology, 1979:30.

104. **Koonings PP, Campbell K, Mishell DR Jr, Grimes DA.** Relative frequency of primary ovarian neoplasms: a 10 year review. *Obstet Gynecol* 1989;74:921–6.

105. **Grimes DA, Hughes JM.** Use of multiphasic oral contraceptives and hospitalization of women with functional ovarian cysts in the United States. *Obstet Gynecol* 1989;73:1037–9.

106. **Hallatt JG, Steele CH, Snyder M.** Ruptured corpus luteum with hemoperitoneum: a study of 173 surgical cases. *Am J Obstet Gynecol* 1983;139:6.

107. **Girouard DP, Barclay D, Collins CT.** Hyperreactio luteinalis. Review of the literature and report of 2 cases. *Obstet Gynecol* 1964;23:513–25.

108. **Ramcharan S, Pellegrin FA, Ray R, Hsu JP.** The Walnut Creek Contraceptive Drug Study. A prospecitve study of the side effects of oral contraceptives. Vol. 3, an interim report: a comparison of disease occurrence leading to hospitalization or death in users and nonusers of oral contraceptives. *J Reprod Med* 1980;25(Suppl 6):345–72.

109. **Royal College of General Practitioners.** *Oral Contraceptives and Health.* Kent, England: Pitman Medical Publishing, 1974.

110. **Vessey M, Metcalfe A, Wells C, McPherson K, Westhoff C, Yeates D.** Ovarian neoplasms, functional ovarian cysts, and oral contraceptives. *BMJ* 1987;294:1518–20.

111. **Ory H.** Functional ovarian cysts and oral contraceptives. *JAMA* 1974;228:68–9.

112. **Holt VL, Daling JR, McKnight B, Moore D, Stergachis A, Weiss NS.** Functional ovarian cysts in relation to the use of monophasic and triphasic oral contraceptives. *Obstet Gynecol* 1992;79:529–33.

113. **Lanes SF, Birmann B, Walker AM, Singer S.** Oral contraceptive type and functional ovarian cysts. *Am J Obstet Gynecol* 1992;166:956–61.

114. **Grimes DA, Godwin AJ, Rubin A, Smith JA, Lacarra M.** Ovulation and follicular development associated with three low-dose oral contraceptives: a randomized controlled trial. *Obstet Gynecol* 1994;83:29–34.

115. **Caillouette JC, Koehler AL.** Phasic contraceptive pills and functional ovarian cysts. *Am J Obstet Gynecol* 1987;156:1538–42.

116. **Holt VL, Daling JR, McKnight B, Moore DE, Stergachis A, Weiss NS.** Cigarette smoking and functional ovarian cysts. *Am J Epidemiol* 1994;139:781–6.

117. **Givens JR.** Polycystic ovaries: a sign, not a diagnosis. *Semin Reprod Endocrinol* 1984;2:271–80.

118. **Polson DW, Adams J, Wadsworth J, Franks S.** Polycystic ovaries—a common finding in normal women. *Lancet* 1988;1:870–2.

119. **Horowitz IR, de al Cuesta RS.** Benign and malignant tumors of the ovary. In: **Carpenter SE, Rock JA,** eds. *Pediatric and Adolescent Gynecology.* New York: Raven Press, 1992:397–416.

120. **Kim JS, Woo SK, Suh SJ, Morettin LB.** Sonographic diagnosis of paraovarian cysts: value of detecting a separate ipsilateral ovary. *Am J Roentgenol* 1995;164:1441–4.

121. **Stein AL, Koonings PP, Schlaerth JB, Grimes DA, d'Ablaing G.** Relative frequency of malignant paraovarian tumors: should paraovarian tumors be aspirated? *Obstet Gynecol* 1990;75:1029–31.

122. **Leibman AJ, Kruse B, McSweeney MB.** Transvaginal sonography: comparison with transabdominal sonography in the diagnosis of pelvic masses. *Am J Roentgenol* 1988;151:89–92.

123. **Fried AM, Rhodes, RA, Morehouse IR.** Endometrioma: analysis and sonographic classification of 51 documented cases. *South Med J* 1993;86:297–301.

124. **Spanos WJ.** Preoperative hormonal therapy of cystic adnexal masses. *Am J Obstet Gynecol* 1973;116:551–6.

125. **Steinkampf MP, Hammond KR, Blackwell RE.** Hormonal treatment of functional ovarian cysts: a randomized, prospective study. *Fertil Steril* 1990;54:775–7.

126. **Turan C, Zorlu CG, Ugur M, Ozcan T, Kaleli B, Gokmen O.** Expectant management of functional ovarian cysts: an alternative to hormonal therapy. *Int J Gynaecol Obstet* 1994;47:257–60.

127. **Maiman M, Seltzer V, Boyce J.** Laparoscopic excision of ovarian neoplasms subsequently found to be malignant. *Obstet Gynecol* 1991;77:563–5.

128. **Pittaway DE, Takacs P, Bauguess P.** Laparoscopic adnexectomy: a comparison with laparotomy. *Am J Obstet Gynecol* 1994;171:385–91.

129. **Barber HRK, Graber EA.** The PMPO syndrome. *Obstet Gynecol Surv* 1973;28:357.

130. **Barber HRK, Graber EA.** The PMPO syndrome (postmenopausal palpable ovary syndrome). *Obstet Gynecol* 1971;38:921–30.

131. **Kroon E, Andolf E.** Diagnosis and follow-up of simple ovarian cysts detected by ultrasound in postmenopausal women. *Obstet Gynecol* 1995;85:211–4.

132. **Bonilla-Musoles F, Ballester MJ, Simon C, Serra V, Raga F.** Is avoidance of surgery possible in patients with perimenopausal ovarian tumors using transvaginal ultrasound and duplex color Doppler sonography? *J Ultrasound Med* 1993;12:33–9.

133. **de Peralta MN, Delahoussaye PM, Tornos CS, Silva EG.** Benign retroperitoneal cysts of müllerian type: a clinicopathologic study of three cases and review of the literature. *Int J Gynecol Pathol* 1994;13:273–8.

134. **Teneriella MG, Park RC.** Early detection of ovarian cancer. *CA Cancer J Clin* 1995;45: 71–87.

135. **Schutter EM, Kenemans P, Sohn C, Kristen P, Crombach G, Westermann R, et al.** Diagnostic value of pelvic examination, ultrasound, and serum CA125 in postmenopausal women with a pelvic mass. An international multicenter study. *Cancer* 1994;74:1398–406.

136. **Curtin JP.** Management of the adnexal mass. *Gynecol Oncol* 1994;55:S42–6.

137. **Parker WH, Berek JS.** Laparoscopic management of adnexal masses. *Obstet Gynecol Clin North Am* 1994;21;79–92.

138. **Valdes CT, Malinak LR, Franklin RR.** In: **Kaufman RH, Friedrich EG, Gardner HL,** eds. *Benign Diseases of the Vulva and Vagina.* Chicago: Year Book Medical Publishers, Inc., 1989:26–54.

139. **Muram D, Buxton BH.** The importance of the gynecologic examination in the newborn. *J Tenn Med Assoc* 1983;76:239.

140. **Mor N, Merlob P, Reisner SH.** Types of hymen in the newborn infant. *Eur J Obstet Gynecol Reprod Biol* 1986;22:225–8.

141. **Kaufman RH, Friedrich EG, Gardner HL.** Solid tumors. In: **Kaufman RH, Friedrich EG, Gardner HL,** eds. *Benign Diseases of the Vulva and Vagina.* Chicago: Year Book Medical Publishers, Inc., 1989:194–236.

142. **Pokorny SF.** Configuration of the prepubertal hymen. *Am J Obstet Gynecol* 1987;157:950–6.

143. **Pokorny SF.** The genital examination of the infant through adolescence. *Curr Opin Obstet Gynecol* 1993;5:753–7.

144. **Pokorny SF.** Prepubertal vulvovaginopathies. *Obstet Gynecol Clin North Am* 1992;19:39–58.

145. **Pokorny SF.** Child abuse and infections. *Obstet Gynecol Clin North Am* 1989;16:401–15.

146. **Radman HM.** Hypertrophy of the labia minora. *Obstet Gynecol* 1976;48:78–80.

147. **Muram D, Gold SS.** Vulvar ulcerations in girls with myelocytic leukemia. *South Med J* 1993;86:293–4.

148. **The Alan Guttmacher Institute.** *Sex and America's Teenagers.* New York: The Alan Guttmacher Institute, 1994:1–88.

149. **Sobel JD.** Controversial aspects in the management of vulvovaginal candidiasis. *J Am Acad Dermatol* 1994;31:S10–3.

150. **Valdes CT, Malinak LR, Franklin RR.** Developmental anomalies of the vulva and vagina. In: **Kaufman RH, Friedrich EG, Gardner HL.** *Benign Diseases of the Vulva and Vagina.* Chicago: Year Book Medical Publishers, 1989:26–54.

151. **Rock B.** Pigmented lesions of the vulva. *Dermatol Clin* 1992;10:361–70.

152. **Rock B, Hood AF, Rock JA.** Prospective study of vulvar nevi. *J Am Acad Dermatol* 1990;22:104–6.

153. **Hood AF, Lumadue J.** Benign vulvar tumors. *Dermatol Clin* 1992;10:371–85.

154. **Halder RM.** Pseudofolliculitis barbae and related disorders. *Dermatol Clin* 1988;6:407–12.

155. **National Institute for Child Health and Development.** Androgens and women's health. *Clinician* 1994;12:1–30.

156. **Kaufman RH.** Intraepithelial neoplasia of the vulva. *Gynecol Oncol* 1995;56:8–21.

157. **van der Putte SC.** Mammary-like glands of the vulva and their disorders. *Int J Gynecol Pathol* 1994;13:150–60.

158. **Word B.** A new instrument for office treatment of cysts and abscess of Bartholin's gland. *JAMA* 1964;190:777.

159. **Paavonen J.** Vulvodynia—a complex syndrome of vulvar pain. *Acta Obstet Gynecol Scand* 1995;74:243–7.

160. **Friedrich EG.** Vulvar vestibulitis syndrome. *J Reprod Med* 1987;32:110–4.

161. **Bazin S, Bouchard C, Brisson J, Morin C, Meisels A, Fortier M.** Vulvar vestibulitis syndrome: an exploratory case-control study. *Obstet Gynecol* 1994;83:47–50.

162. **Bergeron C, Moyal-Barracco M, Pelisse M, Lewin P.** Vulvar vestibulitis. Lack of evidence for a human papillomavirus etiology. *J Reprod Med* 1994;39:936–8.

163. **Prayson RA, Stoler MH, Hart WR.** Vulvar vestibulitis. A histopathologic study of 36 cases, including human papillomavirus in situ hybridization analysis. *Am J Surg Pathol* 1995;19:154–60.

164. **Dennerstein GJ, Scurry JP, Garland SM, Brenan JA, Fortune DW, Sfameni SF, et al.** Human papillomavirus vulvitis: a new disease or an unfortunate mistake? *Br J Obstet Gynaecol* 1994;101:992–8.

165. **Pao CC, Hor JJ, Fu YL.** Genital human papillomavirus infections in young women with vulvar and vestibular papillomatosis. *Eur J Clin Microbiol Infect Dis* 1994;13:433–6.

166. **Elchalal U, Gilead L, Vardy DA, Ben-shachar I, Anteby SO, Schenker JG.** Treatment of vulvar lichen sclerosus in the elderly: an update. *Obstet Gynecol Surv* 1998;50:155–62.

167. **Carli P, Bracco G, Taddei G, Sonni L, De Marco A, Maestrini G, et al.** Vulvar lichen sclerosus. Immunohistologic evaluation before and after therapy. *J Reprod Med* 1994;39:110–4.

168. **Bracco GL, Carli P, Sonni L, Maestrini G, De Marco A, Taddei GL, et al.** Clinical and histologic effects of topical treatments of vulval lichen sclerosus: a critical evaluation. *J Reprod Med* 1993;38:37–40.

169. **Wager GP.** Toxic shock syndrome: a review. *Am J Obstet Gynecol* 1983;146:93–102.

397

14 Pelvic Pain and Dysmenorrhea

Andrea J. Rapkin

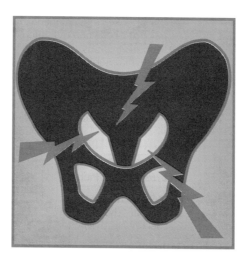

Acute cyclic, and chronic pelvic pain encompass a large proportion of gynecologic complaints and are among the most challenging problems confronting the practitioner. By definition, *acute pain* **is intense and characterized by sudden onset, sharp rise, and short course.** *Cyclic pain* **refers to pain that is associated with the menstrual cycle.** Dysmenorrhea or painful menstruation is the most common form of cyclic pain and is classified as primary or secondary on the basis of associated anatomic pathology (1). *Chronic pelvic pain* **is pain of more than 6 months' duration** (2).

Whereas acute pain often occurs in conjunction with profound autonomic reflex responses such as nausea, emesis, diaphoresis, and apprehension, obvious autonomic reflex responses are not present in chronic pelvic pain. In addition, acute pelvic pain is often associated with signs of inflammation or infection, such as fever and leukocytosis, that are absent in chronic pain states. The pathophysiology of acute pelvic pain involves mediators of inflammation present in high concentration as the result of infection, ischemia, or chemical irritation (3, 4). In contrast, the cause of chronic pelvic pain is often obscure. Additionally, chronic pain is characterized by physiological, affective, and behavioral responses that differ from those associated with acute pain (5). **Chronic pelvic pain is best managed in a multidisciplinary approach that can address its complex and interactive components.**

Acute Pain

The differential diagnosis of acute pelvic pain is outlined in Table 14.1. The character of the pain is helpful in establishing a differential diagnosis. **Rapid onset of pain is most consistent with perforation of a hollow viscus or ischemia. Colic or severe cramping pain is often associated with muscular contraction or obstruction of a hollow viscus, such as intestine or uterus. Pain perceived over the entire abdomen suggests a generalized reaction to an irritating fluid within the peritoneal cavity.**

The viscera are relatively insensitive to pain. The first perception of visceral pain is a vague, deep, poorly localized sensation with corresponding autonomic reflex responses.

399

Table 14.1   Differential Diagnosis of Acute Pelvic Pain

Gynecologic Disease or Dysfunction

Acute Pain

1. Complication of pregnancy
   a. Ruptured ectopic pregnancy
   b. Abortion, threatened or incomplete
   c. Degeneration of a leiomyoma
2. Acute infections
   a. Endometritis
   b. Pelvic inflammatory disease (acute PID)
   c. Tubo-ovarian abscess
3. Adnexal disorders
   a. Hemorrhagic functional ovarian cyst
   b. Torsion of adnexa
   c. Twisted para ovarian cyst
   d. Rupture of functional or neoplastic ovarian cyst

Recurrent Pelvic Pain

1. Mittelschmerz (midcycle pain)
2. Primary dysmenorrhea
3. Secondary dysmenorrhea

Gastrointestinal

1. Gastroenteritis
2. Appendicitis
3. Bowel obstruction
4. Diverticulitis
5. Inflammatory bowel disease
6. Irritable bowel syndrome

Genitourinary

1. Cystitis
2. Pylonephritis
3. Ureteral lithiasis

Musculoskeletal

1. Abdominal wall hematoma
2. Hernia

Other

1. Acute poryphyria
2. Pelvic thrombophlebitis
3. Aneurysm
4. Abdominal angina

Once the pain becomes localized, however, it is called referred pain. Referred pain is well localized and superficial and its pattern is related to the nerve distribution or dermatome of the spinal cord segment innervating the involved viscus. The location of the referred pain provides insight into the location of the primary disease process. The innervation of the pelvic organs is outlined in Table 14.2 (3).

History **Early diagnosis of acute pelvic pain is critical because delay can increase morbidity and mortality.** An accurate history is key to a correct diagnosis (Fig. 14.1). The date and character of the past two menstrual periods and the presence of abnormal bleeding or discharge should be ascertained. Menstrual, sexual, and contraceptive components of the history, as well as previous sexually transmitted diseases and gynecologic conditions, are important. Inquiries should be made about the medical and surgical history. A pain history should be obtained and include how and when the pain started, the presence of gastrointestinal symptoms (e.g., anorexia, nausea, vomiting, constipation, obstipation,

Table 14.2   Nerves Carrying Painful Impulses From The Pelvic Organs

Organ	Spinal Segments	Nerves
Perineum, vulva, lower vagina	S2–S4	Pudendal, inguinal, genitofemoral, posterofemoral cutaneous
Upper vagina, cervix, lower uterine segment, posterior urethra, bladder trigone, uterosacral and cardinal ligaments, rectosigmoid, lower ureters	S2–S4	Sacral afferents traveling through the pelvic plexus
Uterine fundus, proximal fallopian tubes, broad ligaments, upper bladder, cecum appendix, terminal large bowel	T11–T12, L1	Thoracolumbar splanchnic nerves through uterine and hypogastric plexes
Outer two-thirds of fallopian tubes, upper ureter	T9–T10	Thoracolumbar splanchnic nerves through mesenteric plexus
Ovaries	T9–T10	Thoracolumbar splanchnic nerves traveling with ovarian vessels via renal and aortic plexus and celiac and mesenteric ganglia

flatus pattern) or urinary tract symptoms (e.g., urgency, frequency, hematuria, or dysuria), and signs of infection (e.g., fevers, chills).

Pathology

Abnormal Pregnancy   An ectopic pregnancy is defined as implantation of the fetus in a site other than the uterine cavity (see Chapter 19). Ninety-five percent of ectopic pregnancies develop in the fallopian tube. With the advent of sensitive pregnancy tests, misdiagnosis of ectopic pregnancy is less common. However, a substantial number of maternal deaths are still attributable to ectopic gestation.

Symptoms   Ectopic pregnancy produces pain with acute dilation of the tube. If tubal rupture occurs, localized abdominal pain tends to be relieved temporarily and is replaced by generalized pelvic and abdominal pain as the hemoperitoneum develops. Typically, there has been amenorrhea for 6–8 weeks and irregular bleeding or spotting related to fluctuating levels of human chorionic gonadotropin (hCG) and low progesterone concentrations. A mass in the cul-de-sac may produce an urge to defecate. Referred pain to the right shoulder often develops if the collection of intra-abdominal blood transverses the right colic gutter and irritates the diaphragm (cervical 3–5 innervation). Dizziness or syncope can ensue if blood loss is significant.

Signs   Pulse and blood pressure taken in erect and supine positions (orthostatic vital signs) are especially helpful in documenting an early or small hemoperitoneum. In young women, there may be elevation of pulse or decrease in blood pressure only when their position is altered from supine to erect. Abdominal examination usually is notable for tenderness and guarding in one or both lower quadrants. With the development of hemoperitoneum, generalized abdominal distention and rebound tenderness are prominent and bowel sounds are often decreased. Pelvic examination usually reveals mild tenderness on motion of the cervix. Adnexal tenderness is often more pronounced on the side in which the ectopic pregnancy is located. A mass consisting of a hematosalpinx or hematoma isolated by adhesions is sometimes present; however, a palpable mass is more often the corpus luteum of pregnancy. Low-grade fever and leukocytosis are uncommon but can be present if the ectopic

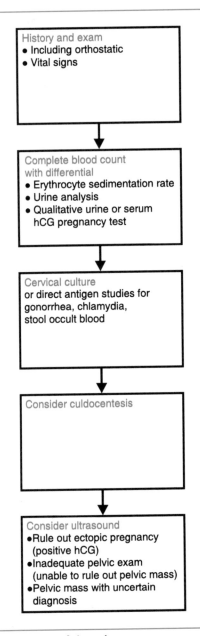

Figure 14.1   Diagnosis of acute pelvic pain.

pregnancy has ruptured the tube. The hematocrit often reveals progressive anemia, indicating internal bleeding, although low hematocrit is a late sign of blood loss in young women because of vasoconstriction and subsequent hemoconcentration. The assessment of hematocrit, therefore, must be combined with evaluation of orthostatic vital signs.

Diagnosis   The diagnosis of ectopic pregnancy is discussed in Chapter 17. In any woman of reproductive age, a serum or urine pregnancy test with a sensitivity >20 IU/ml of hCG should be performed and, if positive, the possibility of ectopic pregnancy must be excluded before the patient can be discharged or treated for another diagnosis. Acute pelvic pain during pregnancy can also result from other types of pathology. After ultrasonography has confirmed an intrauterine pregnancy, adnexal torsion, leakage or rupture of an ovarian cyst, degeneration of leiomyoma, or gastrointestinal or urinary tract pathology should be considered. Coexistent intrauterine and ectopic pregnancy is rare (1/30,000).

Leaking or Ruptured Ovarian Cyst

Functional cysts (e.g., follicle, corpus luteum) are the most common ovarian cysts and rupture more readily than benign or malignant neoplasms. The pain associated with rupture of the ovarian follicle at the time of ovulation is called *mittelschmerz.* The small amount of blood leaking into the peritoneal cavity and high concentration of prostaglandins in follicular fluid could cause this midcycle pelvic pain. However, the pain is mild or moderate and self-limited and, with an intact coagulation system, hemoperitoneum is unlikely. A hemorrhagic corpus luteum cyst can develop in the luteal phase of the menstrual cycle. Rupture of this cyst can produce either a small amount of intraperitoneal bleeding or frank hemorrhage resulting in significant blood loss and hemoperitoneum.

Nonmalignant neoplasms, most commonly cystic teratoma (dermoid) or cystadenomas, as well as inflammatory ovarian masses such as endometriomas can also leak or rupture. A history of a dermoid cyst or endometrioma that has not yet undergone surgical extirpation is not uncommon. Surgical exploration is indicated if rupture of the cyst leads to hemoperitoneum (corpus luteum) or chemical peritonitis (endometrioma, benign cyst teratoma) that could impair future fertility.

Symptoms   An ovarian cyst that is not undergoing torsion, rapidly expanding, becoming infected, or leaking does not cause acute pain. A ruptured corpus luteum cyst is the most common cyst to rupture and to produce hemoperitoneum. Symptoms of a ruptured corpus luteum cyst are similar to those of a ruptured ectopic pregnancy. The onset of pain is usually sudden and is associated with increasing generalized abdominal pain and, occasionally, dizziness or syncope if hemoperitoneum develops. A ruptured endometrioma or benign cystic teratoma (dermoid cyst) will produce similar symptoms; however, dizziness and signs of hypovolemia are not present because blood loss is minimal.

Signs   Hypovolemia will be present only if there is hemoperitoneum. The most important sign is the presence of significant abdominal tenderness, often associated with rebound tenderness due to peritoneal irritation. The abdomen can be moderately distended and there are decreased bowel sounds. On pelvic examination, a mass is often present if the cyst is leaking and not completely ruptured. Fever and leukocytosis are rare. The hematocrit is decreased only if active bleeding is present.

Diagnosis   The diagnosis is based on a pregnancy test, a complete blood count, and ultrasonography or culdocentesis. If orthostasis is not present and the peripheral hematocrit is relatively normal, a hematocrit of $\leq 16\%$ of the fluid obtained from the cul-de-sac is usually consistent with leakage of a small amount of blood into the peritoneal fluid and not hemoperitoneum.

Management   Orthostasis, anemia, or a hematocrit of the fluid obtained by culdocentesis $>16\%$ suggests hemoperitoneum, which usually requires surgical treatment using laparoscopy or laparotomy. Culdocentesis is very helpful in determining the cause of peritonitis: fresh blood suggests a corpus luteum; chocolate "old" blood suggests an endometrioma; oily sebaceous fluid suggests a benign teratoma; purulent fluid suggests pelvic inflammatory disease (PID) or tubo-ovarian abscess. Patients who are not orthostatic or anemic and who have a small amount of blood in the cul-de-sac fluid (hematocrit <16) can often be observed in the hospital without surgical intervention or even discharged from the emergency room after observation.

Torsion of Adnexa

Torsion (twisting) of the vascular pedicle of an ovary, fallopian tube, paratubal cyst, or rarely just a fallopian tube results in ischemia and rapid onset of acute pelvic pain. **A benign cystic teratoma is the most common neoplasm to undergo torsion.** Because adhesions are usually involved with ovarian carcinoma and inflammatory masses, these conditions are rarely affected by torsion. Torsion is also unusual in a normal tube and ovary, although it can occur with a polycystic ovary.

Symptoms   The pain of torsion can be severe and constant or it can be intermittent if the torsion is partial and intermittently untwists. The onset of the torsion and the symptoms of abdominal pain frequently coincide with lifting, exercise, or intercourse. Autonomic reflex responses are usually present (e.g., nausea, emesis, apprehension).

Signs   On examination, the abdomen is very tender and localized rebound tenderness can be noted in the lower quadrants. The most important sign is the presence of a large pelvic mass. Mild temperature elevation and leukocytosis may accompany the infarction. Torsion should be suspected in any woman with acute pain and a unilateral adnexal mass.

Diagnosis   Torsion occludes the lymphatic and venous drainage of the involved adnexa; therefore, the mass will rapidly increase in size, and it will not be difficult to palpate during physical examination or to visualize with ultrasonography. Ultrasonography will confirm the presence of a mass, but it is not necessary if the pelvic examination reveals a large tender adnexal mass (at least 8–10 cm in diameter).

Management   **Adnexal torsion must be treated surgically. If the tissue has not infarcted, the adnexa may be untwisted and a cystectomy may be performed. If necrosis has occurred, an oophorectomy is mandatory.** Treatment may be accomplished using laparoscopy or laparotomy, depending on the size of the mass.

Acute Salpingo-oophoritis

The presentation and management of acute salpingo-oophoritis and PID are discussed in Chapter 15. PID is a polymicrobial infection heralded by the acquisition of a sexually transmitted pathogen such as *Neisseria gonorrhea* or *Chlamydia trachomatous* and resulting in the ascending spread of aerobic and anaerobic vaginal bacteria. Endometrial biopsy such as that performed during hysterosalpingography, termination of pregnancy, or parturition also can cause endometritis/salpingo-oophoritis.

Symptoms   Gonococcal PID is manifest by the acute onset of pelvic pain that increases with movement, fever, purulent vaginal discharge, and sometimes nausea and vomiting. The pain is often associated with a menstrual period, when the upper genital tract is readily accessible to pathogens. Chlamydial salpingo-oophoritis is associated with more insidious symptoms that can be confused with the symptoms of irritable bowel.

Signs   Direct and rebound abdominal tenderness with palpation are usually notable on examination. The most important sign of acute salpingo-oophoritis is cervical motion and bilateral adnexal tenderness. Evaluation of the pelvis may be difficult because of acute pain but should be done because the absence of a discrete mass or masses will differentiate acute salpingo-oophoritis from tubo-ovarian abscess or torsion. Leukocytosis is often present, and an elevated erythrocyte sedimentation rate is a nonspecific although more sensitive sign of inflammation.

Diagnosis   Lower abdominal tenderness with or without rebound, cervical motion tenderness, and adnexal tenderness must be present to establish the diagnosis of PID (6–8). If one or more of the following objective signs are present, the diagnostic accuracy is increased: fever, leukocytosis, inflammatory mass, culdocentesis revealing white blood cells or bacteria on Gram stain, Gram-negative intracellular diplococci on Gram stain of the cervix, or positive chlamydia antigen test of the cervix. Appendicitis often is mistaken for PID.

Management   Salpingo-oophoritis may be treated on an outpatient basis with broad-spectrum and oral antibiotics (7, 9, 10). Criteria for hospitalization include suspected or undiagnosed tubo-ovarian abscess, pregnancy, presence of an intrauterine device, uncertain diagnosis, nausea and vomiting precluding oral medication, upper peritoneal signs, and failure to respond to oral antibiotics within 48 hours. Hospital treatment should also be considered for episodes of PID in a young woman who desires future childbearing. Outpatient antibiotic regimens are often successful for uncomplicated PID; however, the patient *must* be reassessed within 48 hours and, if her condition has not significantly improved, admitted to the hospital for intravenous antibiotic therapy. The details of treatment of acute PID are outlined in Chapter 15.

Tubo-Ovarian Abscess

Tubo-ovarian abscesses, sequela of acute salpingitis, are usually bilateral, although unilateral abscess formation can occur. The symptoms and signs are similar to those of acute salpingitis, although pain and fever have often been present for more than 1 week. A ruptured tubo-ovarian abscess is a life-threatening surgical emergency because Gram-negative endotoxic shock can develop rapidly.

Diagnosis   Tubo-ovarian abscesses can be palpated on bimanual examination as very firm, exquisitely tender bilateral fixed masses. The abscesses can "point" in the cul-de-sac. The clinical diagnosis can be substantiated by ultrasonography. The differential diagnosis of a unilateral mass includes not only tubo-ovarian abscess, but adnexal torsion, endometrioma, leaking ovarian cyst, or periappendiceal abscess. If examination and ultrasonography are not definitive, laparoscopy or laparotomy should be performed.

Management   Unruptured tubo-ovarian abscesses may be treated medically with intravenous antibiotics and close monitoring to detect leakage or impending rupture. **A ruptured tubo-ovarian abscess rapidly leads to diffuse peritonitis evidenced by tachycardia, rebound tenderness in all four quadrants of the abdomen, and if progressive, hypertension and oliguria. Exploratory laparotomy with resection of infected tissue is mandatory.**

Uterine Leiomyomas

Although acute pelvic pain is rare, leiomyomas may produce discomfort when they encroach on adjacent structures such as the bladder, rectum, or supporting ligaments of the uterus. Acute pelvic pain can develop if the myoma undergoes degeneration or torsion. Degeneration of myomas occurs secondary to a loss of blood supply, usually caused by rapid growth associated with pregnancy. The diagnosis of degenerating uterine leiomyoma in a nonpregnant woman is often erroneous, because this condition is frequently confused with subacute salpingo-oophoritis. A pedunculated subserosal leiomyoma can undergo torsion and ischemic necrosis and is associated with pain similar to that of adnexal torsion. If a submucous leiomyoma becomes pedunculated, the uterus will contract forcefully as if to expel a foreign body, and the resulting pain is similar to that of labor. The cramping pain is usually associated with hemorrhage.

Signs   Abdominal examination reveals an irregular solid mass or masses arising from the uterus. In the case of degeneration, the inflammation can cause abdominal tenderness on palpation and mild localized rebound tenderness. Elevation of temperature and leukocytosis can also occur. Ultrasonography is useful in distinguishing adnexal masses from those of uterine origin.

Management   Degeneration of a leiomyoma is treated with observation and pain medication. A pedunculated, twisted subserosal leiomyoma can easily be excised laparoscopically; however, surgery is not mandatory. A submucous leiomyoma associated with pain and hemorrhage should be excised transcervically with hysteroscopic guidance, if needed.

Endometriosis

A thorough discussion of endometriosis is presented in Chapter 26. Endometriosis is characterized by the presence and proliferation of endometrial tissue in sites outside the endometrial cavity. Women with endometriosis often experience dysmenorrhea (painful menses), dyspareunia (painful intercourse), and dyschezia (pain with bowel movements). Often, there is a history of luteal phase bleeding or infertility. Acute pain attributable to endometriosis is usually premenstrual and menstrual. If nonmenstrual acute generalized pain occurs, a ruptured endometrioma (chocolate endometriotic cyst within the ovary) should be considered. In this situation, hemoperitoneum is absent, although the fluid from the chocolate cyst can cause chemical peritonitis.

Signs   The abdomen is often tender in the lower quadrants. Significant distension or rebound tenderness is usually not present. Pelvic examination often reveals a fixed, retroverted uterus with tender nodules in the uterosacral region or thickening of the cul-de-sac. An adnexal mass, if present, is usually fixed to the broad ligament and cul-de-sac.

Diagnosis   Culdocentesis can identify the contents of a ruptured endometrioma. If the diagnosis is unclear, ultrasonography is helpful, and laparoscopy provides a definitive diagnosis. In patients who have an established diagnosis of endometriosis or who have recently been treated surgically, ovarian hormonal suppression (pseudomenopause) can be tried as treatment and as a means of confirming the correlation between the current pain and the underlying diagnosis of endometriosis.

Management   A ruptured endometrioma is an indication for laparoscopy or laparotomy with ovarian cystectomy or oophorectomy. If a small endometrioma (<3 cm) is suspected and there are no signs of rupture, medical management may proceed (see Chapter 26). Diagnostic laparoscopy may be performed if endometriosis or an unruptured endometrioma is suspected but unconfirmed.

Gastrointestinal Tract

Appendicitis is the most common intestinal source of acute pelvic pain in women. The symptoms and signs of appendicitis can be similar to those of PID. Typically, the first symptom of appendicitis is diffuse abdominal pain, especially epigastric pain, along with anorexia and nausea. Within a matter of hours, the pain generally shifts to the right lower quadrant. Fever, chills, emesis, and obstipation may ensue. This classic symptom pattern is often lacking, however. Atypical abdominal pain can occur when the appendix is retrocecal or entirely within the true pelvis. In this setting, tenesmus and diffuse suprapubic pain may result. The patient with appendicitis is more likely to have pronounced and persistent gastrointestinal symptoms than the patient with salpingo-oophoritis.

Signs   Local tenderness is usually detected on palpation of the right lower quadrant at *McBurney's point*. Signs of appendicitis include severe generalized muscle guarding, abdominal rigidity, rebound tenderness, a right-sided mass or tenderness on rectal examination, positive psoas sign (pain with forced hip flexion or passive extension of hip positive), and obturator signs (pain with passive internal rotation of flexed thigh). A low-grade temperature is usually present, although the temperature may be normal. Cervical motion or bilateral adnexal tenderness is usually absent on pelvic examination, but unilateral adnexal tenderness on the right side may be present.

Diagnosis   The total leukocyte count is often normal in acute appendicitis, but the differential diagnosis usually reveals a left shift. The pelvic organs may appear normal with ultrasonography, whereas the appendix may appear abnormal. Gastrograffin or barium enema with normal filling of the appendix rules out appendicitis. Diagnostic laparoscopy can be useful to rule out other sources of pelvic pathology, but occasionally it is difficult to visualize the appendix sufficiently to rule out early appendiceal inflammation.

Management   Laparotomy, with false-positive rate of 20%, is preferable to continued observation and the possibility of rupture and peritonitis. Not only is a ruptured appendix life-threatening, it also may have profound sequelae for the fertility of a woman of reproductive age.

Acute Diverticulitis

Acute diverticulitis is a condition in which there is inflammation of a diverticulum or out-pouching of the wall of the colon, usually involving the sigmoid colon. Diverticulitis typically affects postmenopausal women, but rarely it can occur in the thirties and forties.

Symptoms   The severe left lower quadrant pain of diverticulitis can follow a long history of symptoms of irritable bowel (bloating, constipation, and diarrhea), although diverticulosis is usually asymptomatic. Diverticulitis is less likely to lead to perforation and peritonitis than appendicitis. Fever, chills, and constipation usually are present; however, anorexia and vomiting are uncommon.

Signs   Abdominal examination reveals distention with left lower quadrant tenderness on direct palpation and localized rebound tenderness. Abdominal and pelvic examination may reveal an immobile, doughy inflammatory mass in the left lower quadrant. Bowel sounds are hypoactive, and they are absent if peritonitis is present. Leukocytosis is frequently observed.

Diagnosis and Management   A computed tomography (CT) scan is a useful adjunct to the history and physical examination. A barium enema is contraindicated. Initially, diverticulitis is managed medically with broad-spectrum intravenous antibiotics. A diverticular abscess often requires surgical intervention, however.

Intestinal Obstruction

The most common causes of intestinal obstruction in women are postsurgical adhesions, hernia formation, inflammatory bowel disease, and carcinoma of the bowel or ovary. Intestinal obstruction is heralded by colicky abdominal pain followed by abdominal distension, vomiting, constipation, and obstipation. Higher and more acute obstruction results in early vomiting, whereas colonic obstruction has a greater degree of abdominal distension and obstipation. Vomiting first consists of gastric contents followed by bile and then material with feculent odor, depending on the level of obstruction.

Signs   Marked abdominal distension is present. At the onset of mechanical obstruction, bowel sounds are high pitched and maximal during an episode of colicky pain. As the obstruction progresses, bowel sounds decrease and, when absent, suggest ischemic bowel. An elevated white blood cell count and fever are often present in the late stages.

Diagnosis and Management   Abdominal x-rays exhibiting a characteristic gas pattern will help rule out ileus and determine whether obstruction is partial or complete. Complete obstruction requires surgical management, whereas partial obstruction can often be treated with intravenous fluids and nasogastric suction. The cause of the obstruction should be determined.

Urinary Tract

Ureteral colic due to ureteral lithiasis is caused by a sudden increase in intraluminal pressure and associated inflammation. Urinary tract infections producing acute pain include cystitis or pyelonephritis.

Symptoms   The pain of lithiasis is typically severe and crampy and can radiate from the costovertebral angle to the groin. Hematuria is often present. Cystitis is associated with dull suprapubic pain, urinary frequency, urgency, dysuria, and occasionally hematuria. Urethritis secondary to chlamydia or gonorrhea may have similar symptoms and must be ruled out. Pyelonephritis is associated with flank and costovertebral angle pain, although lateral lower abdominal pain occasionally is present.

Signs   In patients with lithiasis or pyelonephritis, there is pain with firm pressure over the costovertebral angle. Peritoneal signs are absent. Suprapubic tenderness may accompany cystitis.

407

Diagnosis Diagnosis of a stone is made by urinalysis that shows red blood cells and ultrasonography of intravenous pyelography (IVP) that outlines the stone. In a patient with a urinary tract infection, urinalysis reveals bacteria and leukocytes, and the culture shows significant bacterial growth.

Management Expectant medical and surgical management are both options for renal lithiasis. Nonpregnant women with pyelonephritis and all women with cystitis can be treated on an outpatient basis.

Diagnostic Tests

All female patients of reproductive age with acute pelvic pain should undergo the following tests:

1. Complete blood count with hematocrit, hemoglobin, white cell count and differential

2. Erythrocyte sedimentation rate (nonspecific but often the only abnormal laboratory finding in a women with subacute PID)

3. Urinalysis

4. Sensitive qualitative urine or serum pregnancy test

Other studies that may be helpful include the following:

1. *Culdocentesis* with hematocrit if bloody fluid is obtained and Gram stain and culture if the fluid is purulent. A mass in the cul-de-sac precludes culdocentesis.

2. *Pelvic ultrasonography* is useful to rule out ectopic gestation or to assess the adnexae if the results of the examination are inconclusive or difficult to obtain because of obesity or guarding.

3. *Abdominal x-ray* or *upper or lower gastrograffin studies* are helpful to rule out gastrointestinal pathology when such symptoms predominate.

4. *CT scan* is useful for evaluation of retroperitoneal masses or abscesses related to the gastrointestinal tract.

Diagnostic laparoscopy is reserved for establishing the diagnosis in patients with acute abdomen of uncertain etiology, for elucidating the nature of an ambiguous adnexal mass, or for delineating whether a pregnancy is intrauterine or extrauterine (if the ultrasonography results are negative or equivocal). If salpingo-oophoritis is suspected, laparoscopy can improve the accuracy of the diagnosis. Visualization may be hampered if diagnostic laparoscopy is performed in the presence of a large pelvic mass (>12 cm), and laparoscopy is relatively contraindicated in patients with peritonitis, severe ileus, or bowel obstruction. In these settings, laparotomy is preferable.

Cyclic Pain: Primary and Secondary Dysmenorrhea

Dysmenorrhea is a common gynecologic disorder that affects approximately 50% of menstruating women (11). Primary dysmenorrhea is menstrual pain without pelvic pathology, whereas secondary dysmenorrhea is painful menses with underlying pathology. Primary dysmenorrhea usually appears within 1–2 years of menarche, when ovulatory cycles are established. The disorder affects younger women but may persist into the forties. Secondary dysmenorrhea usually develops years after menarche and can occur with anovulatory cycles. The differential diagnosis of secondary dysmenorrhea is outlined in Table 14.3 (2).

Table 14.3 Peripheral Causes of Chronic Pelvic Pain

Gynecologic

Noncyclic

1. Adhesions
2. Endometriosis
3. Salpingo-oophoritis
   a. Acute
   b. Subacute
4. Ovarian remnant syndrome
5. Pelvic congestion syndrome (varicosities)
6. Ovarian neoplasms
7. Pelvic relaxation

Cyclic

1. Primary dysmenorrhea
2. Secondary dysmenorrhea
   a. Imperforate hymen
   b. Transverse vaginal septum
   c. Cervical stenosis
   d. Uterine anomalies (congenital malformation, bicornuate uterus, blind uterine horn)
   e. Intrauterine synechiae (Asherman's syndrome)
   f. Endometrial polyps
   g. Uterine leiomyoma
   h. Adenomyosis
   i. Pelvic congestion syndrome (varicosities)
   j. Endometriosis
3. Atypical cyclic
   a. Endometriosis
   b. Adenomyosis
   c. Ovarian remnant syndrome
   d. Chronic functional cyst formation

Gastrointestinal

1. Irritable bowel syndrome
2. Ulcerative colitis
3. Granulomatous colitis (Crohn's disease)
4. Carcinoma
5. Infectious diarrhea
6. Recurrent partial small bowel obstruction
7. Diverticulitis
8. Hernia
9. Abdominal angina
10. Recurrent appendiceal colic

Genitourinary

1. Recurrent or relapsing cystourethritis
2. Urethral syndrome
3. Interstitial cystitis
4. Ureteral diverticuli or polyps
5. Carcinoma of the bladder
6. Ureteral obstruction
7. Pelvic kidney

Neurologic

1. Nerve entrapment syndrome
2. Neuroma

Table 14.3—*continued*

Musculoskeletal

Low back pain syndrome

1. Congenital anomalies
2. Scoliosis and kyphosis
3. Spondylolysis
4. Spondylolisthesis
5. Spinal injuries
6. Inflammation
7. Tumors
8. Osteoporosis
9. Degenerative changes
10. Coccydynia

Myofascial Syndrome

Systemic

1. Acute intermittent porphyria
2. Abdominal migraine
3. Systemic lupus erythematosis
4. Lymphoma
5. Neurofibromatosis

Primary Dysmenorrhea

The cause of primary dysmenorrhea is increased endometrial prostaglandin production (12–15). These compounds are increased in secretory as opposed to proliferative endometrium. The decline of progesterone levels in the late luteal phase triggers lytic enzymatic action, resulting in a release of phospholipids with the generation of arachidonic acid and activation of the cyclooxygenase pathway. The biosynthesis and metabolism of prostaglandins and thromboxane derived from arachidonic acid are depicted in Figure 14.2 (14). Women with primary dysmenorrhea have higher uterine tone, and high amplitude contractions result in decreased uterine blood flow (16). Vasopressin concentrations are also higher in women with dysmenorrhea (17).

Symptoms   **The pain of primary dysmenorrhea usually begins a few hours prior to or just after the onset of a menstrual period and may last as long as 48–72 hours.** The pain is labor-like with suprapubic cramping and may be accompanied by lumbosacral back ache, pain radiating down the anterior thigh, nausea, vomiting, diarrhea, and rarely syncopal episodes. The pain of dysmenorrhea is colicky in nature and, unlike abdominal pain due to chemical or infectious peritonitis, is improved with abdominal massage, counter pressure, or movement of the body.

Signs   On examination, the vital signs are normal. The suprapubic region may be tender to palpation. Bowel sounds are normal, and there is no upper abdominal tenderness and no abdominal rebound tenderness. Bimanual examination at the time of the dysmenorrheic episode often reveals uterine tenderness; however, severe pain with movement of the cervix or palpation of the adnexal structures is absent. The pelvic organs are normal in primary dysmenorrhea.

Diagnosis   To diagnose primary dysmenorrhea, it is necessary to rule out underlying pelvic pathology and confirm the cyclic nature of the pain. Pelvic examination should be performed to assess the size, shape, and mobility of the uterus; size and tenderness of adnexal structures; and nodularity or fibrosis of uterosacral ligaments or rectovaginal septum. Cervical studies for gonorrhea and chlamydia and, if relevant, a complete blood count with erythrocyte sedimentation rate are helpful to rule out subacute salpingo-oophoritis. If no abnormalities are found, primary dysmenorrhea tentatively can be diagnosed.

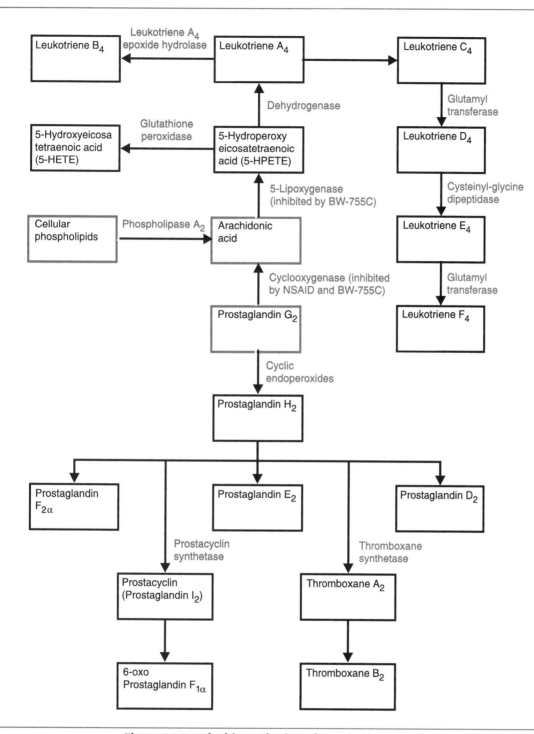

Figure 14.2   The biosynthesis and metabolism of prostaglandins and thromboxane derived from arachidonic acid. (Reproduced with permission from **Chaudhuri G.** Physiologic aspects of prostaglandins and leukotrienes. *Semin Reprod Endocrinol* 1985;3:219–30.)

Treatment   Prostaglandin synthase inhibitors are effective for the treatment of primary dysmenorrhea in approximately 80% of cases (18, 19). The inhibitors should be taken just prior to or at the onset of pain and continuously every 6–8 hours to prevent re-formation of prostaglandin by-products. The medication should be taken for the first few days of menses. A 4- to 6-month course of therapy with changes in dosages and types of inhibitors should be attempted before confirming treatment failure. The medication may be contraindicated in patients with gastrointestinal ulcers or bronchospastic hypersensitivity to *aspirin*. Side effects are usually mild and include nausea, dyspepsia, diarrhea, and occasionally fatigue.

For the patient with primary dysmenorrhea who has no contraindications to oral contraceptive agents or who desires contraception, the birth control pill is the agent of choice. Oral contraceptives decrease endometrial proliferation and create an endocrine milieu similar to the early proliferative phase when prostaglandins are lowest. **More than 90% of women with primary dysmenorrhea will have relief with birth control pills** (20). If the patient does not respond to this regimen, *hydrocodone* or *codeine* may be added for 2–3 days per month. Prior to administration of a narcotic medication, however, psychological factors and other organic pathology should be ruled out with diagnostic laparoscopy. Pain management, in particular, and acupuncture or transcutaneous electrical nerve stimulation also may be useful (21–23). Surgical approaches for primary dysmenorrhea (e.g., laparoscopic uterine nerve ablation or presacral neurectomy) should be used rarely.

Secondary Dysmenorrhea

Secondary dysmenorrhea usually occurs years after the onset of menarche. However, by definition, secondary dysmenorrhea does not reflect age of onset but is cyclic menstrual pain in association with underlying pelvic pathology. **The pain of secondary dysmenorrhea often begins 1–2 weeks prior to menses and persists until a few days after the cessation of bleeding.** The mechanisms underlying secondary dysmenorrhea are diverse and not fully elucidated, although most involve either excess prostaglandin production or hypertonic uterine contractions secondary to cervical obstruction, intrauterine mass, or a foreign body. Nonsteroidal anti-inflammatory agents and oral contraceptives are less likely to provide pain relief in secondary dysmenorrhea than in primary dysmenorrhea.

The most common cause of secondary dysmenorrhea is endometriosis, followed by adenomyosis and an intrauterine device. The differential diagnosis of secondary dysmenorrhea, which is outlined in Table 14.3, includes primary dysmenorrhea and noncyclic pelvic pain. Whereas the diagnosis of primary dysmenorrhea is based on history and presence of a normal pelvic examination, the diagnosis of secondary dysmenorrhea may require review of a pain diary and ultrasound or laparoscopy. The management of secondary dysmenorrhea is the treatment of the specific underlying disorder.

Adenomyosis

Dysmenorrhea accompanied by adenomyosis (ingrowth of the endometrium into the uterine musculature) often begins up to 1 week prior to menses and may not resolve until after the cessation of menses. Associated dyspareunia, dyschezia, and metrorrhagia increase the probability of the diagnosis of adenomyosis. Whereas endometriosis is characterized by ectopic endometrium within the peritoneal cavity, adenomyosis is defined as the presence of endometrial glands within the myometrium, at least one high power field from the basis of the endometrium. Adenomyosis, endometriosis, and uterine leiomyomas frequently coexist. Although occasionally noted in women in the younger reproductive years, the average age of symptomatic women is usually 40 years or older.

Symptoms   Adenomyosis is often asymptomatic. Symptoms typically associated with adenomyosis include excessively heavy or prolonged menstrual bleeding and dysmenorrhea, often beginning up to 1 week prior to the onset of a menstrual flow.

Signs   The uterus is diffusely enlarged, although usually <14 cm, and is often soft and tender, particularly at the time of menses. Mobility of the uterus is not restricted and there is no associated adnexal pathology.

Diagnosis   Adenomyosis is a clinical diagnosis and imaging studies, although helpful, are not definitive. Because of cost and negligible improvement in diagnostic accuracy, these studies are not routinely recommended. In women with diffuse uterine enlargement and negative pregnancy tests, secondary dysmenorrhea may be attributed to adenomyosis; however, suspected adenomyosis can be confirmed pathologically only at the time of hysterectomy. In one study, the clinical diagnosis was confirmed in only 48% of cases (24).

Management   The management of adenomyosis depends on the patient's age and desire for future fertility. Relief of secondary dysmenorrhea caused by adenomyosis can be assured after hysterectomy, but less invasive approaches can be tried initially. Nonsteroidal anti-inflammatory agents, oral contraceptives, and menstrual suppression with progestins or continuous oral contraceptive pills have been found to be useful.

Chronic Pelvic Pain

The differential diagnosis of chronic pelvic pain is outlined in Table 14.3. Patients with chronic pelvic pain are frequently anxious and depressed. Their marital, social, and occupational lives usually have been disrupted. These patients often have had poor treatment outcomes after traditionally effective gynecologic and medical therapy and may have had multiple unsuccessful surgeries for pain. Approximately 12% of hysterectomies are performed for pelvic pain and 30% of patients who seek treatment at pain clinics already have had a hysterectomy (25, 26). **Approximately 60–80% of patients undergoing laparoscopy for chronic pelvic pain have no intraperitoneal pathology, nor do they have tissue distortion that correlates with the pain (2). Additionally, the relationship between the pain response and certain types of prevalent intraperitoneal pathology, such as endometriosis, adhesions, or venous congestion can be inconsistent (2). Frequently overlooked but common causes of chronic pelvic pain are nongynecologic causes such as irritable bowel syndrome, interstitial cystitis, abdominal wall or pelvic floor myofascial syndrome, or nerve entrapment.**

"Plasticity" of the nervous system or alterations in signal processing may be involved in maintaining painful states (2, 4, 27). Various neurohumoral modulators such as prostaglandins, vasoactive intestinal peptide, substance P, and endorphins can modulate peripheral neurotransmission and affect neurotransmission at the level of the spinal cord (28). The spinal cord is more than a simple conduit between the periphery and the brain — it is an important site of "gating" mechanisms such as excitation, inhibition, convergence, and summation of neural stimuli (29). The pain sensation is also modified within the brain by neurotransmitters, such as norepinephrine, serotonin, and gamma-aminobutyric acid (GABA), as well as by endogenous endorphin and nonendorphin analgesic systems. Different regions of the brain are important in altering the sensory and affective components of the pain response. These components of pain are affected by early experience, conditioning, fear, arousal, depression, and anxiety (27, 30).

Evaluation

An approach to the patient with chronic pelvic pain is outlined in Figure 14.3. On the first visit, a thorough pain history should be elicited, including the nature of the complaint; location of the pain, radiation patterns, severity, aggravating, and alleviating factors; the effect of the menstrual cycle, stress, work, exercise, intercourse, and orgasm; the context in which pain arose; and the social and occupational toll of pain. A symptomatic history specific to all of the types of pathology listed in Table 14.3 should be obtained:

1. Genital (abnormal vaginal bleeding, discharge, dysmenorrhea, dyspareunia, infertility)

2. Enterocelic (constipation, diarrhea, flatulence, hematochezia, and relationship of pain to bowel movements)

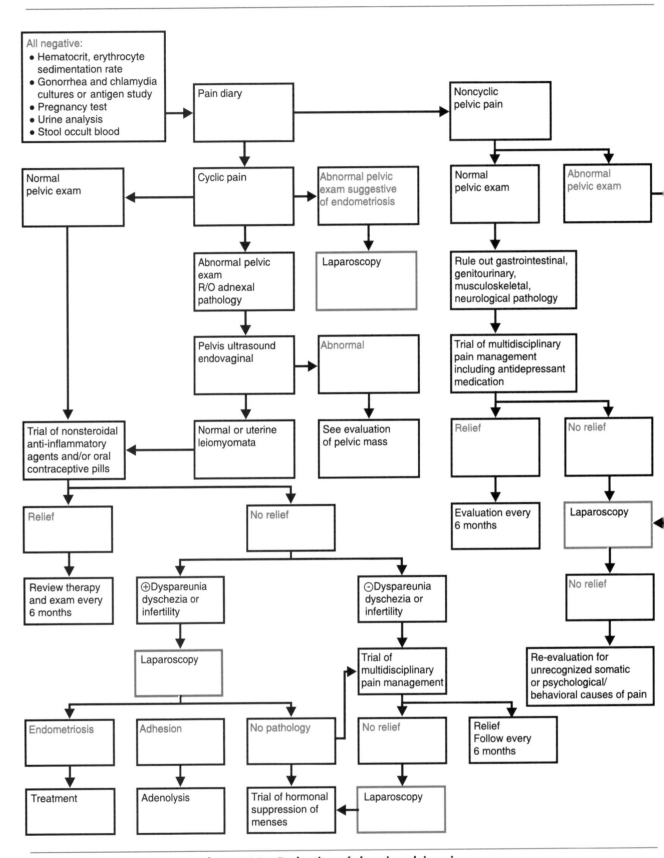

Figure 14.3   Evaluation of chronic pelvic pain.

3. Musculoskeletal (trauma, exacerbation with exercise or postural changes)

4. Urologic (urgency, frequency, nocturia, dysuria, incontinence, hematuria)

The history should include gynecologic, medical, surgical factors; medication intake; prior evaluations for the pain; and prior operative and pathology reports (2).

Symptoms of an acute process (fever, anorexia, nausea, emesis, significant diarrhea, obstipation, abdominal distension, undiagnosed uterine bleeding, pregnancy, or recent abortion) should alert the physician to the possibility of an acute condition requiring immediate medical or surgical intervention, especially if accompanied by the following factors: elevated temperature, orthostasis, peritoneal signs, pelvic or abdominal mass, abnormal complete blood count, positive genital or urinary tract cultures, or a positive pregnancy test.

Physical Examination   A complete physical examination should be performed, with particular attention to the examination of the abdomen, the lumbosacral area, the external genitalia, the vagina, the uterus, the tubes, and the ovaries (bimanual and rectovaginal examination). **The examination should include evaluation of the abdomen with muscles tensed (head raised off the table or with straight leg raising) to differentiate abdominal wall and visceral sources of pain. Abdominal wall pain is augmented and visceral pain is diminished with the above maneuvers** (31, 32). The patient should be examined while standing for hernias, both abdominal (inguinal and femoral) and pelvic (cystocele and enterocele). An attempt should be made to locate by palpation the tissues that reproduce the patient's pain. If abdominal wall sources of pain are noted, it is useful to block these areas with local anesthetics before performing the pelvic exam (31, 32).

The Psychological Component

The pain history includes a current and past psychological history that encompasses the following elements: psychosocial factors; history of past (or current) physical, sexual, or emotional abuse; history of psychiatric hospitalization; suicide attempts; and chemical dependency (2). The attitude of the patient and her family toward the pain, resultant behavior of the patient and her family, and current upheavals in the patient's life should be discussed. The part of the history that addresses sensitive issues must be reobtained after a rapport has been established with the patient.

It is vital to appreciate the various influences that can distort pain perception and expression. A distinction can be drawn between factors leading to a painful condition and those maintaining it. Regardless of the original cause of the pain, when pain has persisted for any length of time, it is likely that other facts are maintaining or at least contributing to it. The full physical evaluation should be accompanied by a review of psychosocial factors. Pain is commonly accompanied by anxiety and depression, and these conditions must be carefully assessed and treated (2). In a typical gynecologic setting, referral to a psychologist can evoke resistance, because the inference is drawn that the referring physician is ascribing the pain to psychological causes. The patient must understand the reason for this referral and must be reassured that it is a routine and necessary part of the evaluation.

Gynecologic Causes

Endometriosis and adhesions are the most common gynecologic conditions detected by laparoscopy performed for the evaluation of chronic pelvic pain.

Endometriosis

Endometriosis is detected in 15–40% of patients who undergo laparoscopy for the assessment of chronic pelvic pain (33). Endometriosis produces a low-grade inflammatory reaction (34). The cause of the pain is not well established, however. There is no correlation between the location of disease and symptoms of pain (35, 36). **There also appears to be no relationship between the incidence or severity of pain and the stage of the endometriotic lesions. Regardless of the stage of disease, as many as 30–50% of patients** have no pain, and 40–60% of patients exhibit no tenderness on examination (36). Deeply infiltrating lesions of the rectovaginal septum are strongly associated with pain (37, 38), however, which is probably neuropathic in origin. Prostaglandin (PGE and $F_{2\alpha}$) production from small petechial implants that are present in mild, low-stage disease was found to be much greater than from the powder burn or black implants, which are more common in patients with higher-stage endometriosis (39). Therefore, prostaglandin production may account for severe pain in some patients who have mild disease.

Clinically, it is possible to determine whether there is a relationship between pain and endometriosis based on the hormonal sensitivity of the disease. After induction of a hypo-estrogenic state, patients who have pelvic pain and dysmenorrhea related to endometriosis should experience relief. The pain relief usually occurs within 2 months of treatment but often returns to the pretreatment level by 18 months posttreatment (40). Intermenstrual pain is not as consistently associated with endometriosis as it is with dysmenorrhea, and it is somewhat less responsive to hormonal manipulation. A discussion of endometriosis and treatment is in Chapter 26.

Adhesions

Adhesions detected by laparoscopy are often in the same general region of the abdomen as the pelvic pain complaint (41). However, neither the specific location (i.e., adnexal structures, parietal, visceral peritoneum, or bowel) nor the density of the adhesions correlates with the presence of pain symptoms (42). Uncontrolled prospective studies of adhesiolysis have not consistently demonstrated a significant reduction in pain (43). In one study of lysis of adhesions, a subgroup of women with anxiety, depression, multiple somatic symptoms, and social and occupational disruption responded poorly to adhesiolysis. The group without these symptoms had significant improvement in pain (43). One prospective study, however, noted a significant improvement in pain, as measured by two of three methods of assessment, only if the adhesions were dense and involved the bowel (44).

Symptoms   Noncyclic abdominal pain, which may increase with intercourse or activity, is a common pain complaint in women with adhesions. There is no pattern symptom that is specific to adhesions, however. Dense adhesions involving bowel can result in a partial or complete bowel obstruction.

Signs   The abdominal wall must be carefully elevated for myofascial or neurologic causes. Most women with adhesions have undergone a previous surgical procedure with possible injury to the abdominal wall structures, which may be the cause of pain. Decreased mobility of pelvic organs or adnexal enlargement often is noted in patients with adhesions.

Diagnosis and Management   Diagnostic laparoscopy is recommended if somatic factors have been eliminated and the results of the psychological evaluation are negative. Endometriosis or subacute salpingo-oophoritis associated with adhesions should be explored.

The role of adhesions in pelvic pain is uncertain. Adhesiolysis is recommended only after a thorough multidisciplinary evaluation has been performed and an integrated treatment approach has been established to address stress, mood, and associated behavioral responses. Repeated surgical procedures to lyse adhesions are not recommended.

Pelvic Congestion

In 1954, Taylor suggested that emotional stress could lead to autonomic nervous system dysfunction manifest as smooth muscle spasm and congestion of the veins draining the ovaries and uterus (45). In women with chronic pelvic pain, transuterine venography often reveals delayed disappearance of contrast medium from the uterine and ovarian veins (46). Because pregnant and postpartum women have asymptomatic pelvic congestion, the role of congested veins as a cause of pelvic pain is uncertain. The specific neurotransmitters involved in mediating this theoretic syndrome are unknown.

Symptoms and Signs   Typical symptoms of the pelvic congestion include lower abdominal and back pain, secondary dysmenorrhea, dyspareunia, abnormal uterine bleeding, chronic fatigue, and irritable bowel symptoms. Pain usually begins with ovulation and lasts until the end of menses.

The uterus is often bulky and the ovaries are enlarged with multiple functional cysts. The uterus, parametria, and uterosacral ligaments are tender.

Diagnosis and Management   Transuterine venography is the standard method for diagnosis. Pelvic ultrasonography with Doppler flow studies or laparoscopy may show varicosities. Because these tests are expensive and have potential morbidity, they should be performed only when patients are symptomatic.

Treatment of presumptive pelvic congestion ranges from hormonal suppression and cognitive behavioral pain management to hysterectomy. Low-estrogen, progestin-dominant continuous oral contraceptives, high-dose progestins, or gonadotropin-releasing hormones often provide pain relief. Hormonal suppression is the initial mode of treatment for women with suspected pelvic congestion. *Medroxyprogesterone acetate,* 30 mg daily, has been found to be useful (47). Treatment should comprise a multidisciplinary approach that incorporates psychotherapy and behavioral pain management. For women who have completed childbearing, hysterectomy with possible oophorectomy is a reasonable option.

Salpingo-oophoritis

Patients with salpingo-oophoritis usually exhibit symptoms and signs of acute infection. Acute salpingitis is discussed in the Acute Pain section of this chapter and in Chapter 16. Atypical or partially treated infection may not be associated with fever or peritoneal signs. Menstrual irregularity, dysmenorrhea, noncyclic pelvic pain, and dyspareunia are symptoms of subclinical disease (7). Subacute or atypical salpingo-oophoritis is often a sequela of chlamydia or mycoplasma infection. Alternatively, a patient with multiple partners may develop frequent recurrent infections (48). Patients with initial gonococcal PID are more likely to develop recurrent infections (49). The mechanism for this increased susceptibility to future infections has not been delineated, although it has been suggested that the fallopian tube and cervix may lose some of their natural resistance to microorganisms.

Diagnosis   Abdominal motion, cervical motion, and bilateral adnexal tenderness are typical of pelvic infection. A complete blood count and erythrocyte sedimentation rate (ESR), as well as cervical culture for gonorrhea and chlamydia, should be performed. Laparoscopy with peritoneal fluid cultures can usually confirm the diagnosis. Patients with either an abnormal ESR or clinical examination should be treated empirically for salpingo-oophoritis before laparoscopy.

Ovarian Remnant Syndrome

Chronic pelvic pain may be caused by the ovarian remnant syndrome in patients who have had a hysterectomy and bilateral salpingo-oophorectomy for severe endometriosis or PID. Ovarian remnant syndrome results from residual ovarian cortical tissue that is left *in situ* after a difficult dissection in an attempt to perform an oophorectomy. Often, the patient has had multiple pelvic operations with the uterus and adnexa removed sequentially.

Symptoms and Signs   The patient usually complains of lateral pelvic pain, often occurring in conjunction with ovulation or the luteal phase. Symptoms tend to arise 2–5 years after initial oophorectomy. A tender mass in the lateral region of the pelvis is pathognomonic.

Diagnosis   Ultrasonography usually confirms the presence of a mass with the sonographic characteristics of ovarian tissue. In a patient who has had bilateral salpingo-oophorectomy and is not taking hormonal replacement therapy, estradiol and follicle-stimulating hormone

(FSH) assays reveal a characteristic premenopausal picture, although occasionally the remaining ovarian tissue may not be active enough to suppress FSH levels (50, 51).

Management   Initial medical treatment with either *danazol,* high-dose progestins, or oral contraceptives has produced mixed results. Patients may experience relief of pain with gonadotropin-releasing hormone agonists, although these medications are impractical for long-term therapy. Laparoscopic examination is usually nonproductive because an ovarian mass may be missed or adhesions may prevent accurate diagnosis. Laparotomy is necessary for treatment. The corrective surgery tends to be arduous and may be complicated by inadvertent cystotomy, enterotomy, postoperative small bowel obstructions, and hematoma formation. Surgical pathology usually reveals the presence of ovarian tissue sometimes accompanied by endometriosis, corpus luteal or follicular cysts, and fibrous adhesions (50, 51).

Other Gynecologic Pathology: Leiomyomas, Ovarian Tumors, Pelvic Relaxation

Patients with obvious gynecologic pathology such as benign or malignant ovarian cysts, uterine leiomyomas of sufficient size to encroach on supporting ligaments or other somatic structures, or significant pelvic relaxation should be evaluated and treated in a manner appropriate to the underlying condition (see Chapters 13 and 19). Pain associated with these conditions is generally not severe, and appropriate surgical management is therapeutic.

Gastroenterologic Causes of Chronic Pelvic Pain

The uterus, cervix, and adnexa share the same visceral innervation with the lower ileum, sigmoid colon, and rectum. Pain signals travel via sympathetic nerves to spinal cord segments T10–L1 (52). Therefore, it is often difficult to determine whether lower abdominal pain is of gynecologic or enterocelic origin. Skillful medical history and examination are necessary to distinguish gynecologic from gastrointestinal causes of pain.

Irritable Bowel Syndrome   **Irritable bowel syndrome (IBS) is one of the more common causes of lower abdominal pain and may account for up to 60% of referrals to the gynecologist for chronic pelvic pain** (52). The exact cause of irritable bowel syndrome is unknown; however, patients with IBS have pain with smaller volume of distension of the bowel than those without IBS (53). Patients with IBS also have an abnormal pain referral pattern with colonic distension. Visceral hypersensitivity or hyperalgesia has been postulated as the cause of pain, although the reasons are not known (54).

Symptoms and Signs   The predominant symptom of IBS is abdominal pain. Other symptoms include abdominal distention, excessive flatulence, alternating diarrhea and constipation, increased pain prior to a bowel movement, decreased pain after a bowel movement, and pain exacerbated by events that increase gastrointestinal motility such has high-fat diet, stress, anxiety, depression, and menses. The pain is usually intermittent, occasionally constant, and cramp-like and more likely to occur in the left lower quadrant.

A palpable tender sigmoid colon or discomfort during insertion of the finger into the rectum, as well as hard feces in the rectum, are signs suggestive of IBS (52).

Diagnosis   The diagnosis of IBS is usually based on history and physical examination. Although the findings may be suggestive, especially in young women, they are not specific. In one study, 91% of patients with IBS had two or more symptoms of IBS (abdominal distension, relief of pain with bowel movement, more frequent and looser bowel movements with the onset of pain), whereas 30% of patients with organic disease had two or more of these symptoms (55). A complete blood count, stool sampling for white blood cells and occult blood, sigmoidoscopy, colonoscopy, or barium enema are usually required, particularly in older individuals or in young women who have not responded to initial treatment. The results of these studies are normal with IBS.

Management   Medical therapy for IBS is generally unsatisfactory, and response rates to placebos are high (56). A multidisciplinary program consisting of medical and psychological approaches is recommended. The treatment comprises reassurance, education, stress reduction, bulk-forming agents, and low-dose tricyclic antidepressants. The multidisciplinary management approach addresses the cognitive, affective, and behavioral components of the pain. Therapy may decrease the intensity of nociceptor stimulation as well as change the interpretation of the pain.

Inflammatory bowel disease such as Crohn's disease or ulcerative colitis, infectious enterocolitis, intestinal neoplasms, appendicitis, and hernia must be ruled out with appropriate history and physical examination, complete blood count, stool cultures, and where appropriate, visualization of colonic mucosa.

Urologic Causes

Chronic pelvic pain of urologic origin may be related to recurrent cystourethritis, urethral syndrome, sensory urgency of uncertain etiology, and interstitial cystitis. An appropriate diagnostic workup can rule out infiltrating bladder tumors, ureteral obstruction, renal lithiasis, and endometriosis.

Urethral Syndrome

Urethral syndrome is a symptom complex including dysuria, frequency and urgency of urination, suprapubic discomfort, and often dyspareunia in the absence of any abnormality of the urethra or bladder. The cause of urethral syndrome is uncertain and has been attributed to subclinical infection, urethral obstruction, and psychogenic and allergic factors (57).

Symptoms   Urinary urgency, frequency, and suprapubic pressure are often observed. Other less frequent symptoms include bladder or vaginal pain, urinary incontinence, postvoid fullness, dyspareunia, and suprapubic pain.

Signs   Physical and neurologic examination should be performed. The anal reflex should document that sacral 2, 3, and 4 spinal cord segments have not been interrupted (57). Anatomic abnormalities, including pelvic relaxation, urethral caruncle, and hypoestrogenism, should be evaluated. Vaginitis should be excluded. The urethra should be palpated carefully for purulent discharge.

Diagnosis   A clean catch or catheterized urine specimen should be obtained to rule out urinary tract infection. Urethral and cervical cultures for chlamydia should be obtained, if indicated, and testing for vaginitis should be performed as indicated. If results of urine and urethral cultures, the evaluation for vulvovaginitis, and tests for allergic phenomena that can cause contact dermatitis of the urethra are negative, the diagnosis is presumed. Ureoplasma, chlamydia, candida, trichomonas, gonorrhea, and herpes should be excluded. Cystoscopic evaluation should be performed to rule out urethral diverticuli, interstitial cystitis, and cancer.

Management   Various forms of therapy have been suggested for urethral syndrome. Patients in whom infections have been ruled out but who have sterile pyuria have been shown to respond to a 2- to 3-week course of *doxycycline* or *erythromycin* (57). Long-term, low-dose antimicrobial prophylaxis is often used in women who have symptoms of urgency or frequency and who have had a history of recurrent urinary tract infections. Some of these women may continue to have symptoms when their urine is not infected and then becomes infected later (57). All postmenopausal women should undergo a trial of local estrogen therapy for approximately 2 months. If there is no improvement after antibiotic or estrogen therapy, urethral dilation can be considered. Positive results have been achieved with biofeedback techniques (57).

Interstitial Cystitis

Interstitial cystitis is more frequent in women than men. Most patients are between 40 and 60 years of age. The cause of interstitial cystitis is unknown, although an autoimmune basis is generally accepted (57).

Symptoms and Signs   Symptoms include severe and disabling urinary frequency and urgency, nocturia, dysuria, and occasional hematuria. Suprapubic, pelvic, urethral, vaginal, or perineal pain is common and can be partially relieved by emptying the bladder.

Pelvic examination usually reveals anterior vaginal wall and suprapubic tenderness. Urinalysis may show microhematuria without pyuria, although results may be normal.

Diagnosis   The diagnosis is made on the basis of symptoms and characteristic cystoscopic findings (57, 58). Cystoscopy performed while the patient is awake may show only bladder hypersensitivity; under anesthesia, however, with sufficient distension of the bladder, submucosal hemorrhages and cracking of the mucosa may be noted (52). Although the histologic features of the biopsy specimen are nonspecific, there is usually submucosal edema, vasodilatation, and infiltration by macrophages, plasma cells, and eosinophils.

Management   Management is empiric because the cause is uncertain. Various pharmaceutical approaches have been used, including anticholinergic, antispasmodic, and anti-inflammatory agents. Hydrostatic bladder distension may produce temporary relief by creating detrusor ischemia and enervation of the bladder wall. Biofeedback and behavioral therapy also have been used with some success (57).

Neurologic and Musculoskeletal Causes

Nerve Entrapment

Abdominal cutaneous nerve injury or entrapment may occur spontaneously or within weeks to years after transverse suprapubic skin or laparoscopy incisions (31, 59). The ilioinguinal or ileohypogastric nerves may become trapped between the transverse and internal oblique muscles, especially when the muscles contract. Alternatively, the nerve may be ligated or traumatized during the surgery. Symptoms of nerve entrapment include burning, aching pain in the dermatomal distribution of the involved nerve (60, 61). Hip flexion and exercise exacerbate pain. The pain is usually perceived as coming from inside the abdomen, not from the skin.

Signs   On examination, the pain usually can be localized with the finger tip. The maximal point of tenderness in an iliohypogastric or ilioinguinal injury is usually at the rectus margin, medial and inferior to the anterior iliac spine. A tentative diagnosis is confirmed by diagnostic nerve block with 0.25% *bupivacaine*. Patients usually report immediate relief of symptoms after injection and at least 50% of patients experience relief that lasts longer than a few hours (61).

Management   Many patients may require no further intervention if diagnostic nerve block is effective, although some patients require up to five biweekly injections. If injection is successful in producing only limited pain relief and there are no contributory visceral or psychological factors, cryoneurolysis or surgical removal of the involved nerve is recommended.

Myofascial Pain

Myofascial syndrome has been documented in approximately 15% of patients with chronic pelvic pain (62). Trigger points, initiated by pathogenic autonomic reflex of visceral or muscular origin, can be observed upon examination of these patients (63, 64). The referred pain of the trigger point occurs in a dermatomal distribution, and it is felt to be due to nerves from the muscle or deeper structures sharing a common second-order neuron in the spinal cord. Painful trigger points can be abolished with the injection of local anesthetic into the painful points (63). Trigger points are often present in women with chronic pelvic pain, irrespective of the presence or type of underlying pathology. In one study, 89% of women with chronic pelvic pain had abdominal, vaginal, or lumbosacral trigger points (63). In the absence of pathology, various factors, including psychological, hormonal, and biomechanical factors, are believed to predispose the chronicity of the myofascial syndrome (64–66).

Symptoms   Abdominal wall pain is often exacerbated by the premenstrual period or stimuli to the dermatome of a trigger point (e.g., full bladder or bowel or any stimulation to organs that share the dermatome of the involved nerve) (32).

Signs   Finger tip pressure on the trigger points evokes local and referred pain. Tensing of the rectus muscles by either straight leg lifting or raising the head off the table increases the pain. A specific jump sign can be elicited by palpation with a fingertip or a cotton-tipped swab. An electric sensation confirms correct needle placement (32, 63).

Management   Injection of the trigger point with 3 ml of 0.25% *bupivacaine* will provide relief that usually outlasts the duration of anesthetic action. After four to five biweekly injections, the procedure should be abandoned if long-lasting relief is not obtained (63). Along with the injection of trigger points, multidisciplinary pain management should be undertaken, especially if anxiety, depression, a history of physical or sexual abuse, sexual dysfunction, or social or occupational disruption are present (2).

Low Back Pain Syndrome

Women who complain of lower back pain without pelvic pain rarely have gynecologic pathology, although low back pain may accompany gynecologic pathology. Back pain may be caused by gynecologic, vascular, neurologic, psychogenic, and spondylogenic (related to the axial skeleton and its structure) pathology (2, 66, 67).

Symptoms   Women with low back pain syndrome often have pain originating after trauma or physical exertion. The pain is often experienced in the morning or upon arising or with fatigue. Nongynecologic low back pain can intensify with the menstrual cycle.

Signs   Examination includes inspection, examination with movement, and palpation. Various anatomic structures in the spine should be considered as sources of pain. Muscles, vertebral joints, and disks (including the lumbosacral junction, the paravertebral sacrospinal muscles, and the sacroiliac joints) must be examined carefully because they are common sources of spondylogenic pain (2, 67).

Diagnosis   Diagnostic imaging studies can be helpful. These tests should be performed with maximal flexion while the patient is standing, lying, and sitting. An elevated ESR suggests pain of inflammatory or neoplastic origin.

Management   Orthopedic or rheumatologic consultation is necessary prior to the initiation of management for back pain unless the back pain is suggestive of referred gynecologic pain.

Psychological Factors

From a psychological perspective, various factors may promote the chronicity of pain, including the meaning attached to the pain, anxiety, the ability to redirect attention, personality, mood state, experience, and reinforcement contingencies that may amplify or attenuate pain (2). The *Minnesota Multiphasic Personality Inventory (MMPI)* studies of women with chronic pelvic pain reveal a high prevalence of a convergence "V" profile (elevated scores on the hypochondriasis, hysteria, and depression scales). In studies comparing women who have pain and no pathology with those who have endometriosis-related pain or with controls, MMPI profiles were unable to distinguish those with obvious organic findings; however, both pain groups differed from controls (2).

There is a close relationship between depression and pain (68). Both give rise to similar behavior, such as behavioral and social withdrawal and decreased activity. Both depression and pain may be mediated by the same neurotransmitters such as norepinephrine, serotonin, and endorphins (2). Antidepressants appear to improve both pain and depression.

Childhood physical and sexual abuse has been noted to be more prevalent in women with chronic pelvic pain than those with other types of pain and control groups (52% vs. 12%) (69). Individual differences in personality and habitual coping strategies also may influence response to pain and pain recurrence.

Management of Chronic Pelvic Pain

In patients without apparent pathology or pathology that has an equivocal role in pain production, multidisciplinary therapy is usually preferable. This approach incorporates the skills of the gynecologist, psychologist, and (ideally) anesthesiologist. A low dose of a tricyclic antidepressant is combined with behavioral therapy directed toward reducing the reliance on pain medication, increasing activity, and reducing the toll the pain takes on the women's overall lifestyle (2). Women with depression should be treated with an appropriate therapeutic dose of antidepressant medication (70).

The approach to women with chronic pain must be therapeutic, supportive, and sympathetic. Regular follow-up appointments should be offered because requesting that the patient return only if pain persists can reinforce pain behavior. Specific skills are taught using cognitive behavioral approaches. Women should be offered ways to reduce uncertainty and to enhance the opportunities for control of pain. Various strategies, including relaxation techniques, stress management, sexual and marital counseling, hypnosis, and other psychotherapeutic approaches, have been found to be useful. Psychotherapy is indicated when women show pronounced depression or when there are sexual difficulties or indications of past trauma. Acupuncture may be beneficial (71). Diagnostic uterosacral, hypogastric, or epidural nerve blocks can be used (72).

Outcome of Multidisciplinary Approach

Various studies of multidisciplinary pain management have been performed. Retrospective, uncontrolled studies show relief of pain in 85% of the subjects (71, 73). One prospective randomized study had a similar response rate that was significantly better than that of traditional therapy (74).

Surgical Therapy

Laparoscopy **Women with disabling cyclic pain that does not respond to nonsteroidal anti-inflammatory agents or oral contraceptives should undergo laparoscopic evaluation. Diagnostic laparoscopy is a standard procedure in the evaluation of patients with chronic noncyclic pelvic pain; however, laparoscopy should not be performed until other nongynecologic somatic or visceral causes of pain have been excluded.** At the time of diagnostic laparoscopy, endometriotic lesions should be biopsied and, if infection is suspected, cultures should be performed. All visible endometriosis should be surgically excised or electrocoagulated. Patients with dysmenorrhea may benefit from transection of the uterosacral ligaments. The uterosacral ligaments carry the principal afferent nerve supply from the uterus to the hypogastric nerve. The original procedure was performed by colpotomy with a success rate of 70% (75). In one study, laparoscopic nerve ablation relieved dysmenorrhea in 85% of patients (76).

Lysis of Adhesions The role of pelvic adhesions in the genesis of pain is unclear (2). Adhesiolysis, even via laparoscopy, is frequently complicated by adhesion reformation (77).

Other etiologies must be treated first. Psychological consultation and management should precede or accompany the lysis of adhesions.

Presacral Neurectomy   Presacral neurectomy (PSN) or sympathectomy for dysmenorrhea was first described by 1937 (78). The discovery of highly successful medical therapies has supplanted surgery; however, primary or secondary dysmenorrhea unrelieved by traditional therapy and nonresponsive to multidisciplinary pain management is an indication for presacral neurectomy. The response rate to PSN for secondary dysmenorrhea is 50–75% (2, 77). The neurectomy will only relieve pain deriving from the cervix, uterus, and proximal fallopian tubes (via T11–L2). The nerve supply to the adnexal structures (via T9–T10) bypasses the hypogastric nerve. Therefore, lateralizing visceral pain is unlikely to be relieved by presacral neurectomy. Intraoperative complications such as hemorrhage or ureteral injury can occur in a small percentage of cases. Because the sacral nerve supply is unaffected by division of the presacral nerve, normal micturition, defecation, and parturition will be preserved. A local anesthetic hypogastric block under fluoroscopic guidance can help predict the response to this operation.

Hysterectomy   **Hysterectomy has often been performed to treat pelvic pain; however, 30% of patients seeking treatment at pain clinics have already undergone hysterectomy without pain relief** (25). Hysterectomy is particularly useful for women who have completed childbearing and who have secondary dysmenorrhea or chronic pain due to endometriosis or to uterine pathology such as adenomyosis or to pelvic congestion. Before recommending hysterectomy for pain or unilateral adnexectomy for unilateral pain, it is useful to apply the **PREPARE** mnemonic (see Chapter 3) (79). The ***Procedure*** that is being done, the ***Reason*** or indication, ***Expectation*** or desired outcome of the procedure, the ***Probability*** that the outcome will be achieved, ***Alternatives*** and nonsurgical options, and ***Risks*** as well as ***Expense*** should be discussed.

In one study, hysterectomy to treat women with central pelvic pain (including dysmenorrhea, dyspareunia, and uterine tenderness) provided pain relief in 77% of patients (80). The treatment response did not vary with specific symptoms, physical examination findings, surgical procedure, or documentation of uterine pathology. Because the study was uncontrolled and retrospective, it remains unclear which patients would have improved without surgical management.

Vulvar Pain

Vulvar pain, or *vulvodynia,* is described as chronic vulvar discomfort characterized by burning, stinging, and irritation. Vulvodynia has been associated with multiple factors, and no single treatment program is effective for all patients. Although the etiology of vulvar pain differs from that of pelvic pain, the process of obtaining the pain history and use of the pain diary is similar. Exposure to contact allergens, toxic medications (such as topical *5-fluorouracil [5-FU]*), other dermatological infections or conditions (e.g., monilia, herpes, human papillomavirus (HPV), lichen sclerosis, or psoriasis), and presence of systemic dermatologic signs (e.g., oral lesions, rash on any other part of the body, or axillary cysts) should be ascertained. Sexual history should be obtained. Questions regarding arousal, dyspareunia (including timing and location), lubrication, orgasm, and whether the problem is primary or secondary should be included. The presence of past or present physical or sexual trauma should be elicited. Any surgical trauma to the area, including hymenotomy, vaginal births, episiotomy, or vaginal surgery, should be ascertained. Miscellaneous causes of vulvar pain include dysesthesias associated with spinal disc problems, pudendal or genitofemoral neuralgia, previous episodes of herpes zoster, or referred pain from urethra, vagina, or interstitial cystitis; therefore, historical questions pertaining to these entities should be asked.

Examination   The physical examination should include meticulous investigation for the presence of erythema and lesions (ulcers and/or fissures; raised, white, or pigmented). The area of tenderness should be outlined with a cotton-tipped swab. The presence of peri-urethral or Bartholin gland tenderness should be ascertained. Pelvic floor levator ani muscle tone should be determined, and wet mount of vaginal secretions (saline and potassium hydroxide), vaginal pH, and amine "whiff" tests should be performed.

After thorough history and physical examination, it should be possible to rule out vaginosis or vaginitis (e.g., monilia, trichomonas, bacterial vaginosis, HPV, herpes) and to treat accordingly.

If erythema or hypertrophic changes or lesions are present, colposcopy should be performed and hypertrophic areas, ulcers, or lesions should be identified and biopsied to rule out lichen sclerosis or hypertrophic dystrophy, neoplasm, or other infectious processes.

Colposcopy   Colposcopic findings in women with vulvar pain syndromes usually fall into one of two categories:

1. Diffuse acetowhitening of cutaneous or mucosal surfaces

2. Painful vestibular erythema without acetowhitening

The clinical picture after acetic acid application that is most consistent with evidence of HPV infection includes patchy papillations of vestibular structures, fine florid papillomatosis of the vestibule, and on occasion, smooth epithelial surfaces with acetowhite changes with 5% acetic acid. Among women with only diffuse irritative acetowhitening or biopsy revealing HPV, intramuscular or intralesional interferon, topical *5-FU,* CO_2 laser or 30% trichloracetic acid applications controlled up to 75% of moderate to severe symptomatology (81). The side effects of interferon consisted of flu-like symptoms. In another study, 50% of patients treated with *interferon* reported relief (82).

If exam or colposcopy reveals erythema and inflammatory changes, allergens should be strongly suspected. The patient should be instructed to avoid potential allergens and initiate treatment using topical 1% *hydrocortisone* twice per day until symptoms resolve or for 1 month. If symptoms persist, a biopsy is recommended.

Vulvar Vestibulitis Syndrome

Vulvar vestibulitis syndrome is defined as "severe pain on vestibular or vaginal entry, tenderness to pressure localized within the vulvar vestibule, and physical findings confined to vestibular erythema of varying degrees." Burning, stinging, and rawness are also often present (83). The etiology of vulvar vestibulitis syndrome remains unknown. It is often associated with preceding vaginal candida infections and may be a hypersensitivity reaction or possibly an irritant or allergic reaction. In Friedrich's study, 15% of women noted onset of symptoms within 6 weeks of gynecologic surgery or childbirth; 63% reported symptoms of prior severe and repeated vulvovaginal candidiasis, and 12% had a history of sexual abuse. HPV has been demonstrated by DNA hybridization techniques in many cases. However, histological investigation has not been useful in clarifying the pathogenesis. Nonspecific chronic inflammatory infiltrate within the vestibular glands is the most frequent histologic finding (84).

Treatment   For patients with mild signs or symptoms of recent onset (within 3 months), conservative therapy consisting of warm sitz baths, lubrication with intercourse, 1% *hydrocortisone* cream, and oral *calcium carbonate* (1000 mg daily) can be helpful. If symptoms are longstanding or severe, tricyclic antidepressant such as *amitriptyline* in doses of 25–50 mg at bedtime, combined with directed psychological and behavioral pain management, should be offered. Pelvic floor muscle relaxation may also be helpful. If this approach has failed, perineorrhaphy or surgical excision of minor vestibular glands can be performed. This "Woodruff procedure" has not been subjected to controlled studies but is generally successful in relieving pain in 50% of women treated; 40% of women treated experience moderate improvement in pain, and the remaining 10% have no relief or occasionally are more symptomatic (85). Prior to surgical excision, women should undergo psychological evaluation and if abnormalities are detected on projected psychological testing, such as a *Minnesota Multiphasic Personality Inventory, Chronic Illness Problem Inventory,* or *Marital Dyadic Inventory,* psychological pain management should ensue. Previous studies have suggested that factors predictive of an improved surgical outcome include willingness to undergo psychological evaluation, as well as increased parity. Medical regimens were successful in only 8% of women with painful vestibular erythema (8).

References

1. **Dawood MY.** Dysmenorrhea. *Clin Obstet Gynecol* 1990;3(2):168–78.

2. **Rapkin AJ, Reading AE.** *Curr Probl Obstet Gynecol Fertil* 1991;14(4):99–137.

3. **Bonica JJ.** General considerations of pain in the pelvis and perineum. In: **Bonica JJ, Loeser JD, Chapman CR, Fordyce WE,** ed. *The Management of Pain II.* Philadelphia: Lea & Febiger, 1990;1283–312.

4. **Rapkin AJ.** Gynecologic pain in the clinic: is there a link with the basic research? In: **Gebhart GF,** ed. *Visceral Pain. Progress in Pain Research and Management.* Vol. 5. Seattle: IASP Press, 1995.

5. **Bonica JJ.** Neurophysiologic and pathologic aspects of acute and chronic pain. *Arch Surg* 1977;112:750–61.

6. **Kahn JG, Walker CK, Washington AE, Landers DV, Sweet RL.** Diagnosing pelvic inflammatory disease. *JAMA* 1991;266(18):2594–604.

7. **Centers for Disease Control and Prevention.** 1993 sexually transmitted diseases treatment guidelines. *MMWR* 1993;42(RR-14):1–13.

8. **Sellors J, Mahony J, Goldsmith C, Rath D, Mander R, Hunter B, et al.** The accuracy of clinical findings and laparoscopy in pelvic inflammatory disease. *Am J Obstet Gynecol* 1991; 164:113–20.

9. **Centers for Disease Control and Prevention.** Recommendations for the prevention and control of chlamydia trachomatis infections. *MMWR* 1993;42(RR-12):1–36.

10. **Holmes KK, Mårdh PA, Sparling PF, Wiesner PJ, Cates W Jr, Lemon SM, et al.** *Sexually Transmitted Diseases,* 2nd ed. New York NY: McGraw-Hill, 1990.

11. **The American College of Obstetricians and Gynecologists.** *Dysmenorrhea.* ACOG Technical Bulletin. Washington, DC: ACOG, 1983;63.

12. **Wiqvist NE, Lindblom B, Wilhelmsson L.** The patho-physiology of primary dysmenorrhea. *Res Clin Forums* 1979;1:47–54.

13. **Lundstrom V, Green K.** Endogenous levels of prostaglandin in $F_2\alpha$ and its main metabolites in plasma and endometrium of normal and dysmenorrheic women. *Am J Obstet Gynecol* 1978; 130:640–6.

14. **Chaudhuri G.** Physiologic aspects of prostaglandins and leukotrienes. *Semin Reprod Endocrinol* 1985;3(3):219–30.

15. **Rapkin AJ, Berkley KJ, Rasgon NL.** Dysmenorrhea. In: **Yaksh TL,** ed. *Anesthesia: Biologic Foundation.* New York: Raven Press, 1995.

16. **Akerlund M, Stromberg P, Forsling ML.** Primary dysmenorrhea and vasopressin. *Br J Obstet Gynaecol* 1979;86:484–7.

17. **Akerlund M, Stromberg P, Forsling ML.** Primary dysmenorrhea and vasopressin. *Br J Obstet Gynaecol* 1979;86:484–7.

18. **The Medical Letter: Drugs for Dysmenorrhea.** *Med Lett Drugs Ther* 1979;21:81–4.

19. **Filler WW, Hall WC.** Dysmenorrhea and its therapy. *Am J Obstet Gynecol* 1970;106:104–9.

20. **Chan WY, Dawood MY.** Prostaglandin levels in menstrual fluid of non-dysmenorrheic and dysmenorrheic subjects with and without oral contraceptive or ibuprofen therapy. *Adv Prostaglandin Thromboxane Res* 1980;8:1443–7.

21. **Helms JM.** Acupuncture for the management of primary dysmenorrhea. *Obstet Gynecol* 1987; 69:51–6.

22. **Lundberg T, Bondesson L, Lundstrom V.** Relief of primary dysmenorrhea by transcutaneous electrical nerve stimulation. *Acta Obstet Gynecol Scand* 1985;64:491.

23. **Mannheimer JS, Whalen EC.** The efficacy of transcutaneous electrical nerve stimulation in dysmenorrhea. *Clin J Pain* 1985;1:75.

24. **Lee NC, Dikcer RC, Rubin GL, Ory HW.** Confirmation of the preoperative diagnoses for hysterectomy. *Am J Obstet Gynecol* 1984;150:283–7.

25. **Reiter RC.** A profile of women with chronic pelvic pain. *Clin Obstet Gynecol* 1990;33:130–6.

26. **Chamberlain A, La Ferla J.** The gynecologists approach to chronic pelvic pain. In: **Burrows G, Elton D, Stanley G.,** eds. *Handbook of Chronic Pain Management.* Vol. 33. Amsterdam: Elsevier, 1987:371–82.

27. **Wall PD.** The John J. Bonica distinguished lecture. Stability and instability of central pain mechanisms. In: **Dubner R, Gebhart G, Bond M,** eds. *Proceedings of the 5th World Congress on Pain.* Amsterdam: Elsevier Science Publishers BV, 1988:13–24.

28. **Janig W, Morrison JFB.** Functional properties of spinal visceral afferents supplying abdominal and pelvic organs, with special emphasis on visceral nociception. In: **Cervero F, Morrison JFB,** eds. *Visceral Sensation. Progress in Brain Research.* New York: Elsevier Science Publications, 1986:87–114.

29. **Cervergo F, Tattersall JEH.** Somatic and visceral sensory integration in the thoracic spinal cord. In: **Cervero F, Morrison JFB,** eds. *Visceral Sensation. Progress in Brain Research.* New York: Elsevier Science Publications, 1986:189–205.

30. **Bonica JJ.** The management of pain. Biochemistry and modulation of nociception and pain. In: **Bonica JJ,** eds. *The Management of Pain II.* Philadelphia: Lea & Febiger, 1990:95–121.

31. **Greenbaum DS, Greenbaum RB, Joseph JG, Natale JE.** Chronic abdominal wall pain diagnostic validity and costs. *Dig Dis Sci* 1994;39(9):1935–41.

32. **Slocumb JC.** Chronic somatic myofascial, and neurogenic abdominal pelvic pain. *Clin Obstet Gynecol* 1990;33:145–53.

33. **Vercellini P, Fedele L, Molteni P, Arcaini L, Bianchi S, Candiani GB.** Laparoscopy in the diagnosis of gynecologic chronic pelvic pain. *Int J Gynaecol Obstet* 1990;32:261–67.

34. **Hill JA, Anderson DJ.** Lymphocyte activity in the presence of peritoneal fluid from fertile women and infertile women with and without endometriosis. *Am J Obstet Gynecol* 1989;161:861–4.

35. **Fedele L, Parazzini F, Bianchi S, Arcaini L, Candiani GB.** Stage and localization of pelvic endometriosis and pain. *Fertil Steril* 1990;53:155–8.

36. **Fukaya T, Hoshiai H, Yajima A.** Is pelvic endometriosis always associated with chronic pain? A retrospective study of 618 cases diagnosed by laparoscopy. *Am J Obstet Gynecol* 1993;169:719–22.

37. **Cornillie FJ, Oosterlynck D, Lauweryns JM.** Deeply infiltrating pelvic endometriosis: histology and clinical significance. *Fertil Steril* 1990;53:978–83.

38. **Koninckx RP, Meuleman C, Demeyere S, Lesaffre E, Cornilie FJ.** Suggestive evidence that pelvic endometriosis is a progressive disease, whereas deeply infiltrating endometriosis is associated with pelvic pain. *Fertil Steril* 1991;55:759–65.

39. **Vernon MW, Beard JS, Graves K, Wilson E.** Classification of endometriotic implants by morphologic appearance and capacity to synthesize prostaglandin F. *Fertil Steril* 1984;46:801–6.

40. **Fedele L, Bianchi S, Baglione S, Arcaini L, Candiani GB.** Stage and localization of pelvic endometriosis and pain. *Fertil Steril* 1989;73:1000–4.

41. **Stout AL, Steege JF, Dodson WC, Hughes CL.** Relationship of laparoscopic findings to self-report of pelvic pain. *Am J Obstet Gynecol* 1991;73–9.

42. **Rapkin AJ.** Adhesions and pelvic pain: a retrospective study. *Obstet Gynecol* 1986;68:13–5.

43. **Steege JF, Scott AL.** Resolution of chronic pelvic pain after laparoscopic lysis of adhesions. *Am J Obstet Gynecol* 1991;165:278–83.

44. **Peters AAW, Trimbos-Kemper GCM, Admiral C, Trimbos JB.** A randomized clinical trial on the benefit of adhesiolysis in patients with intraperitoneal adhesions and chronic pelvic pain. *Br J Obstet Gynaecol* 1992;99:59–62.

45. **Taylor HC Jr.** Pelvic pain based on a vascular and autonomic nervous system disorder. *Am J Obstet Gynecol* 1954;67:1177–96.

46. **Beard RW, Highman JH, Pearce S, Reginald PW.** Diagnosis of pelvic varicosities in women with chronic pelvic pain. *Lancet* 1984;2:946–9.

47. **Farquhar CM, Rogers V, Franks S, Pearce S, Wadsworth J, Beard RW.** A randomized controlled trial of medroxyprogesterone acetate and psychotherapy for the treatment of pelvic congestion. *Br J Obstet Gynaecol* 1989;96:1153–62.

48. **Eschenbach DA, Holmes KK.** Acute pelvic inflammatory disease: current concepts of pathogenesis, etiology, and management. *Clin Obstet Gynecol* 1975;197(18):35–6.

49. **Sweet RL, Gibbs RS.** Pelvic inflammatory disease. In: **Sweet R, Gibbs RS,** eds. *Infectious Disease of the Female Genital Tract (Part 1)*. Baltimore: Williams & Wilkins, 1985;53–77.

50. **Steege JF.** Ovarian remnant syndrome. *Obstet Gynecol* 1987;70:64–7.

51. **Price FV, Edwards R, Buchsbaum HJ.** Ovarian remnant syndrome: difficulties in diagnosis and management. *Obstet Gynecol Surv* 1990;45:151–6.

52. **Rapkin AJ, Mayer EA.** Gastroenterologic causes of chronic pelvic pain. *Obstet Gynecol Clin North Am* 1993;20(4):663–82.

53. **Hightower NC, Roberts JW.** Acute and chronic lower abdominal pain of enterologic origin in chronic pelvic pain. In: **Ranaer MR,** ed. *Chronic Pelvic Pain in Women*. New York: Springer-Verlag, 1981:110–37.

54. **Mayer EA, Gebhart GF.** Functional bowel disorders and the visceral hyperalgesia hypothesis. In: **Mayer ER, Raybould HE,** eds. *Pain Research and Clinical Management*. Vol. 9. Amsterdam: Elsevier, 1993:3–28.

55. **Whitehead WE, Schustger MM.** *Gastrointestinal Disorders*. San Diego: Academic Press, 1985.

56. **Klein KB.** Controlled treatment trials in the irritable bowel syndrome: a critique. *Gastroenterology* 1988;95:232.

57. **Karram MM.** Frequency, urgency, and painful bladder syndromes. In: **Walters MD, Karram MM,** eds. *Clinical Urogynecology*. St. Louis: Mosby, 1993:285–98.

58. **Messing EM, Stamey TA.** Interstitial cystitis: early diagnosis, pathology and treatment. *Urology* 1978;12:381.

59. **Sippo WC, Burghardt A, Gomez AC.** Nerve entrapment after Pfannenstiel incision. *Am J Obstet Gynecol* 1987;157:420–1.

60. **Bonica JJ.** Pelvic and perineal pain caused by other disorders. In: **Bonica JJ,** eds. *The Management of Pain II*. Philadelphia: Lea & Febiger, 1990;69:1383–94.

61. **Bonica JJ.** Applied anatomy relevant to pain. In: **Bonica JJ,** eds. *The Management of Pain II*. Philadelphia: Lea & Febiger, 1990:133–58.

62. **Reiter RC.** Occult somatic pathology in women with chronic pelvic pian. *Clin Obstet Gynecol* 1990;33:154–60.

63. **Slocumb JC.** Neurological factors in chronic pelvic pain: trigger points and the abdominal pelvic pain syndrome. *Am J Obstet Gynecol* 1984;149:536–43.

64. **Travell J.** Myofascial trigger points: clinical view. *Adv Pain Res Ther* 1976;1:919–26.

65. **Ling FW, Slocumb JC.** Use of trigger point injections in chronic pelvic pain. *Obstet Gynecol Clin North Am* 1993;20:809–15.

66. **Baker PK.** Musculoskeletal origins of chronic pelvic pain. *Obstet Gynecol Clin North Am* 1993;20:719–42.

67. **Renaer M, Vertommen H, Nijs P, Wagemans L, Van Hemerijck T.** Psychosocial aspects of chronic pelvic pain in women. *Am J Obstet Gynecol* 1979;134:75–80.

68. **Wood DP, Weisner MG, Reiter RC.** Psychogenic chronic pelvic pain. *Clin Obstet Gynecol* 1990;33:179–95.

69. **Rapkin AJ, Kames LD, Darke LL, Stampler FM, Naliboff BD.** History of physical and sexual abuse in women with chronic pelvic pain. *Obstet Gynecol* 1990;76:92–6.

70. **Walker EA, Sullivan MD, Stenchever MA.** Use of antidepressants in the management of women with chronic pelvic pain. *Obstet Gynecol Clin North Am* 1993;20(4):743–51.

71. **Rapkin AJ, Kames LD.** The pain management approach to chronic pelvic pain. *J Reprod Med* 1987;32:323–7.

72. **McDonald JS.** Management of chronic pelvic pain. *Obstet Gynecol Clin North Am* 1993;20(4): 817–38.

73. **Milburn A, Reiter RC, Rhomberg AT.** Multidisciplinary approach of chronic pelvic pain. *Obstet Gynecol Clin North Am* 1993;20(4):643–61.

74. **Peters AA, van Dorst E, Jellis B, van Zuuren E, Hermans J, Trimbos JB.** A randomized clinical trial to compare two different approaches in women with chronic pelvic pain. *Obstet Gynecol* 1991;77:740–4.

75. **Doyle IB.** Paracervical uterine denervation by transection of the cervical plexus for the relief of dysmenorrhea. *Am J Obstet Gynecol* 1955;70:1–16.

76. **Lichten EM, Bombard J.** Surgical treatment of primary dysmenorrhea with laparoscopic uterine nerve ablation. *J Reprod Med* 1987;32:37–41.

77. **Parsons LH, Stovall TG.** Surgical management of chronic pelvic pain. *Obstet Gynecol Clin North Am* 1993;20(4):765–78.

78. **Cotte G.** Resection of the presacral nerves in the treatment of obstinate dysmenorrhea. *Am J Obstet Gynecol* 1937;33:1034–40.

79. **Reiter RC, Lench JB, Gambone JC.** Clinical commentary: consumer advocacy, elective surgery, and the "golden era of machine." *Obstet Gynecol* 1989;74:815–7.

80. **Stovall TG, Ling FW, Crawford DA.** Hysterectomy for chronic pelvic pain of presumed uterine etiology. *Obstet Gynecol* 1990;75:676–9.

81. **Reid R, Greenberg MD, Daoud Y, Husain M, Selvaggi S, Wilkinson E.** Colposcopic findings in women with vulvar pain syndromes: a preliminary report. *J Reprod Med* 1988; 33:523–32.

82. **Mann MS, Kaufman RH, Brown D, Adam E.** Vulvar vestibulitis: significant clinical variables and treatment outcome. *Obstet Gynecol* 1992;79:122–5.

83. **Friedrich EG.** Vulvar vestibulitis syndrome. *J Reprod Med* 1987;32:110–4.

84. **Furlonge CB, Thin RN, Evans BE, McKee PH.** Vulvar vestibulitis syndrome: a clinico-pathological study. *Br J Obstet Gynaecol* 1991;98:703–6.

85. **Woodruff JD, Parmley TH.** Infection of the minor vestibular gland. *Obstet Gynecol* 1983;62: 609–12.

15

Genitourinary Infections and Sexually Transmitted Diseases

David E. Soper

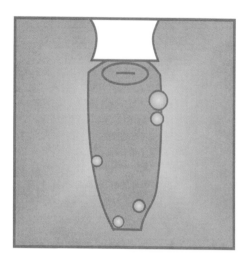

Genitourinary tract infections are among the most frequent disorders for which patients seek care from gynecologists. By understanding the pathophysiology of these diseases and having an effective approach to their diagnosis, physicians can institute appropriate antimicrobial therapy to treat these conditions and reduce long-term sequelae.

The Normal Vagina

Normal vaginal secretions are composed of vulvar secretions from sebaceous, sweat, Bartholin, and Skene glands; transudate from the vaginal wall; exfoliated vaginal and cervical cells; cervical mucous; endometrial and oviductal fluids; and microorganisms and their metabolic products. The type and amount of exfoliated cells, cervical mucous, and upper genital tract fluids are determined by biochemical processes that are influenced by hormone levels (1). Vaginal secretions may increase in the middle of the menstrual cycle because of an increase in the amount of cervical mucus. These cyclic variations do not occur when oral contraceptives are used and ovulation does not occur.

The vaginal desquamative tissue is made up of vaginal epithelial cells that are responsive to varying amounts of estrogen and progesterone. Superficial cells, the predominant cell type in women of reproductive age, predominate when estrogen stimulation is present. Intermediate cells predominate during the luteal phase because of progestogenic stimulation. Parabasal cells predominate in the absence of either hormone, a condition that may be found in postmenopausal women who are not receiving hormonal replacement therapy.

The normal vaginal flora is predominantly aerobic, with an average of six different species of bacteria, the most common of which is hydrogen peroxide producing lactobacilli. The microbiology of the vagina is determined by factors that affect the ability of bacteria to survive (2). These factors include vaginal pH and the availability of glucose for bacterial metabolism. **The pH of the normal vagina is lower than 4.5, which is maintained by the production of lactic acid.** Estrogen-stimulated vaginal epithelial cells are rich in glycogen. Vaginal epithelial cells break down glycogen to monosaccharides, which can then be converted by lactobacilli to lactic acid.

Normal vaginal secretions are floccular in consistency, white in color, and usually located in the dependent portion of the vagina (posterior fornix). Vaginal secretions can be analyzed by a wet-mount preparation. A sample of vaginal secretions is suspended in 0.4 ml of normal saline in a glass tube, transferred to a slide, covered with a slip, and assessed by microscopy. Some clinicians prefer to prepare slides by suspending secretions in saline placed directly on the slide. Secretions should not be placed on the slide without saline, because this method causes drying of the vaginal secretions and does not result in a well-suspended preparation. Microscopy of normal vaginal secretions reveals many superficial epithelial cells, few white blood cells (<1 per epithelial cell), and few, if any, clue cells. **Clue cells are superficial vaginal epithelial cells with adherent bacteria, usually *G. vaginalis,* which obliterates the crisp cell border and usually can be visualized microscopically.** Potassium hydroxide 10% (KOH) may be added to the slide, or a separate preparation can be made, to examine the secretions for evidence of fungal elements. The results are negative in women with normal vaginal microbiology. Gram stain will reveal that normal superficial epithelial cells appear normal and a predominance of gram-positive rods (lactobacilli).

Vaginal Infections

Bacterial Vaginosis

Bacterial vaginosis (BV) has previously been referred to as nonspecific vaginitis or *Gardnerella* vaginitis. It is an alteration of normal vaginal bacterial flora that results in the loss of hydrogen-peroxide-producing lactobacilli and an overgrowth of predominantly anaerobic bacteria (3, 4). The most common form of vaginitis in the U.S. is BV (5). Anaerobic bacteria can be found in less than 1% of the flora of normal women. In women with BV, however, the concentration of anaerobes, as well as *Gardnerella vaginalis* and *Mycoplasma hominis,* is 100 to 1000 times higher than in normal women. Lactobacilli are usually absent.

It is not known what triggers the disturbance of normal vaginal flora. It has been postulated that repeated alkalinization of the vagina, which occurs with frequent sexual intercourse or use of douches, plays a role. After normal hydrogen-peroxide-producing lactobacilli disappear, it is difficult to reestablish normal vaginal flora, and recurrence of BV is common.

Numerous studies have shown an association of BV with significant adverse sequelae. Women with BV have an increased risk of pelvic inflammatory disease (PID) (6), postabortal PID (7), postoperative cuff infections after hysterectomy (8), and abnormal cervical cytology (9). Pregnant women with BV are at risk for premature rupture of the membranes (10), preterm labor and delivery (10), chorioamnionitis, and postcesarean endometritis (11). It is not known whether screening for, and treatment of, BV will decrease the risk of these adverse sequelae.

Diagnosis

Bacterial vaginosis is diagnosed on the basis of the following findings (12):

1. A fishy vaginal odor, which is particularly noticeable following coitus, and vaginal discharge are present.

2. Vaginal secretions are gray and thinly coat the vaginal walls.

3. The pH of these secretions is higher than 4.5 (usually 4.7 to 5.7).

4. Microscopy of the vaginal secretions reveals an increased number of clue cells, and leukocytes are conspicuously absent. In advanced cases of BV, more than 20% of the epithelial cells are clue cells.

5. The addition of KOH to the vaginal secretions (the whiff test) releases a fishy, amine-like odor.

Treatment

Ideally, treatment of BV should inhibit anaerobes but not vaginal lactobacilli. The following treatments are effective (13):

1. *Metronidazole,* an antibiotic with excellent activity against anaerobes but poor activity against lactobacilli, is the drug of choice for the treatment of BV. A dose of 500 mg administered orally twice a day for 7 days should be used. Patients should be advised to avoid using alcohol during treatment with *metronidazole* and for 24 hours thereafter.

2. An alternative regimen uses a single, 2-g oral dose of *metronidazole.*

The overall cure rates are 95% for the 7-day regimen and 84% for the 2-g single-dose regimen (13). Following are other alternative regimens:

1. *Metronidazole* gel, 0.75%, one applicator full (5 g) intravaginally twice daily for 5 days

2. *Clindamycin* cream, 2%, one applicator full (5 g) intravaginally at bedtime for 7 days

3. *Clindamycin,* 300 mg, orally twice daily for 7 days

Many clinicians prefer intravaginal treatment because of a lack of systemic side effects such as mild-to-moderate gastrointestinal upset and unpleasant taste. Treatment of the male sexual partner has not been shown to improve therapeutic response and therefore is not recommended.

Trichomonas Vaginitis

Trichomonas vaginitis is caused by the sexually transmitted, flagellated parasite, *Trichomonas vaginalis.* The transmission rate is high; 70% of males contract the disease after a single exposure to an infected female, which suggests that the rate of male-to-female transmission is even higher. The parasite is an anaerobe that has the ability to generate hydrogen to combine with oxygen to create an anaerobic environment. It exists only in trophozoite form. Trichomonas vaginitis often accompanies bacterial vaginosis, which can be diagnosed in up to 60% of patients with *Trichomonas vaginitis.*

Diagnosis

Local immune factors and inoculum size influence the appearance of symptoms. Symptoms and signs may be much milder in patients with a smaller inoculum of trichomonads, and *Trichomonas vaginitis* is often asymptomatic (14, 15).

1. *Trichomonas vaginitis* is associated with a profuse, purulent, malodorous vaginal discharge that may be accompanied by vulvar pruritus.

2. Vaginal secretions may exude from the vagina.

3. In patients with high concentrations of organisms, a patchy vaginal erythema and colpitis macularis ("strawberry" cervix) may be observed.

431

4. The pH of the vaginal secretions is usually higher than 5.0.

5. Microscopy of the secretions reveals motile trichomonads and increased numbers of leukocytes.

6. Clue cells may be present because of the common association with BV.

7. The whiff test may also be positive.

Morbidity associated with *Trichomonas vaginitis* is related to its association with BV. Patients with *Trichomonas vaginitis* are at increased risk of postoperative cuff cellulitis following hysterectomy (8). Pregnant women with *Trichomonas vaginitis* are at increased risk for premature rupture of the membranes and preterm delivery.

Because of the sexually transmitted nature of *Trichomonas vaginitis,* women with this infection should be tested for other sexually transmitted diseases (STDs), particularly *Neisseria gonorrhoeae* and *Chlamydia trachomatis.* Serologic testing for syphilis and human immunodeficiency virus (HIV) infection should also be considered.

Treatment

The treatment of *Trichomonas vaginitis* can be summarized as follows:

1. *Metronidazole* is the drug of choice for treatment of vaginal trichomoniasis. Both a single-dose (2 g orally) and a multidose regimen (500 mg twice daily for 7 days) are highly effective and have cure rates of approximately 95%.

2. The sexual partner should also be treated.

3. *Metronidazole* gel, although highly effective for the treatment of BV, should not be used for the treatment of vaginal trichomoniasis.

4. Women who do not respond to initial therapy should be treated again with *metronidazole* 500 mg, twice daily for 7 days. If repeated treatment is not effective, the patient should be treated with a single 2-g dose of *metronidazole* once daily for 3–5 days.

5. Patients who do not respond to repeated treatment with *metronidazole* and for whom the possibility of reinfection has been excluded should be referred for expert consultation. In these uncommon refractory cases, an important part of management is to obtain cultures of the parasite to determine its susceptibility to *metronidazole.*

Vulvovaginal Candidiasis

It is estimated that as many as 75% of women experience at least one episode of vulvovaginal candidiasis (VVC) during their lifetimes (16). Almost 45% of women will experience two or more episodes per year (17). Fortunately, few will be plagued with a chronic, recurrent infection. *Candida albicans* is responsible for 85–90% of vaginal yeast infections. Other species of *Candida,* such as *C. glabrata* and *C. tropicalis,* can cause vulvovaginal symptoms and tend to be resistant to therapy. Candida are dimorphic fungi existing as blastospores, which are responsible for transmission and asymptomatic colonization, and as mycelia, which result from blastospore germination and enhance colonization and facilitate tissue invasion. The extensive areas of pruritus and inflammation often associated with minimal invasion of the lower genital tract epithelial cells suggest that an extracellular toxin or enzyme may play a role in the pathogenesis of this disease. A hypersensitivity phenomenon also may be responsible for the irritative symptoms associated with vulvovaginal candidiasis, especially for patients with chronic, recurrent disease. Patients with symptomatic disease usually have an increased concentration of these microorganisms ($>10^4$/ml) compared with asymptomatic patients ($<10^3$/ml) (18).

Factors that predispose women to the development of symptomatic VVC include antibiotic use (19, 20), pregnancy (21), and diabetes (22). Through a mechanism referred to as "colonization resistance," lactobacilli prevent the overgrowth of the opportunistic fungi. Antibiotic use disturbs the normal vaginal flora, decreasing the concentration of lactobacilli and other normal flora, and thus allowing an overgrowth of fungi. Pregnancy and diabetes are both associated with a qualitative decrease in cell-mediated immunity, leading to a higher incidence of candidiasis.

Diagnosis

The symptoms of VVC consist of vulvar pruritus associated with a vaginal discharge that typically resembles cottage cheese.

1. The discharge can vary from watery to homogeneously thick. Vaginal soreness, dyspareunia, vulvar burning, and irritation may be present. External dysuria ("splash" dysuria) may occur when micturition leads to exposure of the inflamed vulvar and vestibular epithelium to urine. Examination reveals erythema and edema of the labia and vulvar skin. There may be discrete pustulopapular peripheral lesions. The vagina may be erythematous with an adherent, whitish discharge. The cervix appears normal.

2. The pH of the vagina in patients with VVC is usually normal (<4.5).

3. Fungal elements, either budding yeast forms or mycelia, will appear within as many as 80% of cases. The results of saline preparation of the vaginal secretions usually are normal, although there may be a slight increase in the number of inflammatory cells in severe cases.

4. The whiff test is negative.

5. A presumptive diagnosis can be made in the absence of microscopy-proven fungal elements if the pH and the results of the saline preparation are normal. A fungal culture is recommended to confirm the diagnosis.

Treatment

1. Topically applied azole drugs are the most commonly available treatment for VVC and are more effective than *nystatin* (Table 15.1) (13). Treatment with azoles results in relief of symptoms and negative cultures among 80–90% of patients who have completed therapy. Symptoms usually take 2–3 days to resolve. There is a trend to shorten the duration of therapy to 1–3 days. Although the shorter period of therapy implies a shortened duration of treatment, because the short-course formulations have higher concentrations of the antifungal agent, they cause an inhibitory concentration in the vagina that persists for several days.

2. An oral antifungal agent, *fluconazole*, used in a single 150-mg dose, has been approved for the treatment of VVC. It appears to have equal efficacy when compared with topical azoles in the treatment of mild-to-moderate VVC (23). Patients should be advised that their symptoms will not disappear for 2–3 days so they will not expect additional treatment.

3. Adjunctive treatment with a weak topical steroid, such as 1% *hydrocortisone* cream, may be helpful in relieving some of the external irritative symptoms.

Table 15.1   Vulvovaginal Candidiasis—Topical Treatment Regimens

---

Butoconazole

2% cream 5 g intravaginally for 3 days[†]

Clotrimazole

1% cream 5 g intravaginally for 7–14 days[†]
100 mg vaginal tablet for 7 days[†]
100 mg vaginal tablet, two tablets for 3 days
500 mg vaginal tablet, single dose

Miconazole

2% cream 5 g intravaginally for 7 days[*†]
200 mg vaginal suppository for 3 days[*]
100 mg vaginal suppository for 7 days[*†]

Ticonazole

6.5% ointment 5 g intravaginally, single dose[*]

Terconazole

0.4% cream 5 g intravaginally for 7 days
0.8% cream 5 g intravaginally for 3 days
80 mg suppository for 3 days[*]

---

[*]Oil-based, may weaken latex condoms.
[†]Available over-the-counter
Morbidity and Mortality Weekly Report. Centers for Disease Control and Prevention. *MMWR* 1993;42: 72–3.

Chronic Vulvovaginal Candidiasis

A small number of women will develop chronic, recurrent vulvovaginal candidiasis. These women experience persistent irritative symptoms of the vestibule and vulva. Burning replaces itching as the prominent symptom in patients with chronic VVC. The diagnosis should be confirmed by direct microscopy of the vaginal secretions and by fungal culture. **Many women with chronic vaginitis presume that they have a chronic yeast infection when this is not the case. Many of these patients have chronic dermatitis or atrophic dermatitis.**

The treatment of patients with chronic VVC consists of inducing a remission of chronic symptoms with daily *ketoconazole* (400 mg/day) or *fluconazole* (200 mg/day) until symptoms resolve. Patients should then be maintained on prophylactic doses of these agents (*ketoconazole* = 100 mg/day; *fluconazole* = 150 mg weekly) for 6 months (24).

Inflammatory Vaginitis

Desquamative inflammatory vaginitis is a clinical syndrome characterized by diffuse exudative vaginitis, epithelial cell exfoliation, and a profuse purulent vaginal discharge (25). The cause of inflammatory vaginitis is unknown, but gram stain findings reveal a relative absence of normal long gram-positive bacilli (lactobacilli) and their replacement with gram-positive cocci, usually streptococci. Women with this disorder have a purulent vaginal discharge, vulvovaginal burning or irritation, and dyspareunia. A less frequent complaint is vulvar pruritus. Vaginal erythema is present, and there may be an associated vulvar erythema, vulvovaginal ecchymotic spots, and colpitis macularis. The pH of the vaginal secretions is uniformly higher than 4.5 in these patients.

Initial therapy is the use of 2% *clindamycin* cream, one applicator full (5 g) intravaginally once daily for 7 days. Relapse occurs in approximately 30% of patients, who should be retreated with intravaginal 2% *clindamycin* cream for 2 weeks. When relapse occurs in postmenopausal patients, supplementary hormonal replacement therapy should be considered.

Atrophic Vaginitis

Estrogen plays an important role in the maintenance of normal vaginal ecology. Women undergoing menopause, either occurring naturally or secondary to surgical removal of the ovaries, may develop inflammatory vaginitis, which may be accompanied by an increased, purulent vaginal discharge. In addition, they may note dyspareunia and postcoital bleeding resulting from atrophy of the vaginal and vulvar epithelium. Examination reveals atrophy of the external genitalia, along with a loss of the vaginal rugae. The vaginal mucosa may be somewhat friable in areas. Microscopy of the vaginal secretions shows a predominance of parabasal epithelial cells and an increased number of leukocytes.

This disorder is treated with topical estrogen vaginal cream. Use of 1 g of *conjugated estrogen* cream intravaginally each day for 1–2 weeks generally provides relief. Systemic estrogen replacement therapy should be considered to prevent recurrence of this disorder.

Cervicitis

The cervix is made up of two different types of epithelial cells: squamous epithelium and glandular epithelium. The cause of cervical inflammation depends on the epithelium affected. The ectocervical epithelium can become inflamed by the same microorganisms that are responsible for vaginitis. In fact, the ectocervical squamous epithelium is an extension of and is continuous with the vaginal epithelium. *Trichomonas, Candida,* and *Herpes simplex* virus can cause inflammation of the ectocervix. Conversely, *Neisseria gonorrhoeae* and *Chlamydia trachomatis* infect only the glandular epithelium and are responsible for mucopurulent endocervicitis (MPC) (26).

Diagnosis

The diagnosis of MPC is based on the finding of a purulent endocervical discharge, generally yellow or green in color and referred to as "mucopus" (27).

1. After removal of ectocervical secretions with a large swab, a small cotton swab is placed into the endocervical canal and the cervical mucus is extracted. The cotton swab is inspected against a white or black background to detect the green or yellow color of the mucopus. In addition, edema, erythema, and friability of the zone of ectopy (glandular epithelium) are present. Although edema and erythema of the endocervix can be difficult to distinguish, friability or easily induced bleeding can be assessed by touching the ectropion with a cotton swab or spatulum.

2. Placement of the mucopus on a slide that can be gram-stained will reveal the presence of an increased number of neutrophils (>30 high-power fields). The presence of intracellular gram-negative diplococci, leading to the presumptive diagnosis of gonococcal endocervicitis, also may be detected. If the gram-stain results are negative for gonococci, the presumptive diagnosis is chlamydial MPC.

3. Tests for both gonorrhea (culture on Thayer-Martin media) and chlamydia, such as cell culture, enzyme-linked immunosorbent assay (ELISA) (chlamydiazyme), or direct fluorescent antibody (MicroTrak), should be performed. The microbial etiology of endocervicitis is unknown in approximately 50% of cases in which gonococci or chlamydia are not detected.

Treatment of MPC consists of an antibiotic regimen recommended for the treatment of uncomplicated lower genital tract infection with both chlamydia and gonorrhea (13) (Table 15.2). It is imperative that all sexual partners be treated with a similar antibiotic regimen.

Pelvic Inflammatory Disease

PID is caused by microorganisms colonizing the endocervix ascending to the endometrium and fallopian tubes. PID is a clinical diagnosis implying that the patient has upper genital tract infection and inflammation. The inflammation may be present at any point along a

---

Table 15.2   Treatment Regimens for Gonococcal and Chlamydial Infections

Neisseria gonorrhoeae **endocervicitis**

> *Ceftriaxone* 125 mg intramuscularly (single dose), or
> *Ofloxacin* 400 mg orally (single dose), or
> *Cefixime* 400 mg orally (single dose), or
> *Ciprofloxacin* 500 mg orally (single dose)

Chlamydia trachomatis **endocervicitis**

> *Doxycycline* 100 mg orally b.i.d. for 7 days, or
> *Azithromycin* 1 gram orally (single dose), or
> *Ofloxacin* 300 mg orally b.i.d. for 7 days, or
> *Erythromycin* base 500 mg orally 4 times a day for 7 days, or
> *Erythromycin ethylsuccinate* 800 mg orally 4 times a day for 7 days

Morbidity and Mortality Weekly Report. Centers for Disease Control and Prevention. *MMWR* 1993;42: 51–57.

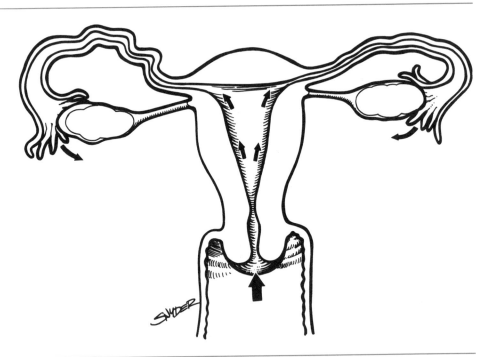

Figure 15.1   Microorganisms originating in the endocervix ascend into the endometrium, fallopian tubes, and peritoneum, causing pelvic inflammatory disease (endometritis, salpingitis, peritonitis). (Reproduced with permission from **Soper DE.** Upper genital tract infections. In: **Copeland LJ,** ed. *Textbook of Gynecology.* Philadelphia: WB Saunders, 1993:521.)

Most cases of PID are caused by sexually transmitted microorganisms, *Neisseria gonorrhoeae,* and *Chlamydia trachomatis* (28–30). Less frequently, respiratory pathogens such as *Haemophilus influenzae,* Group A streptococci, and pneumococci can colonize the lower genital tract and cause PID. Endogenous microorganisms found in the vagina, particularly the BV microorganisms, also are often isolated from the upper genital tract of women with PID. The BV microorganisms include anaerobic bacteria such as *Prevotella* and peptostreptococci as well as *Gardnerella vaginalis.* BV often occurs in women with PID, and the resultant complex alteration of vaginal flora may facilitate the ascending spread of pathogenic bacteria by enzymatically altering the cervical mucus barrier (31).

Diagnosis

Traditionally, the diagnosis of PID has been based on a triad of symptoms and signs including pelvic pain, cervical motion, and adnexal tenderness and the presence of fever. It is now recognized that there is wide variation in many symptoms and signs among women with this condition, which makes the diagnosis of acute PID difficult. Many women with PID exhibit subtle or mild symptoms that are not readily recognized as PID. Consequently, delay in diagnosis and therapy probably contributes to the inflammatory sequelae in the upper reproductive tract (32).

The goal for the diagnosis of PID is to establish diagnostic guidelines that are sufficiently sensitive to avoid missing mild cases but sufficiently specific to avoid giving antibiotic therapy to women who are not infected. Genitourinary tract symptoms may indicate PID; therefore, the diagnosis of PID should be considered in women with any genitourinary symptoms including, but not limited to, lower abdominal pain, excessive vaginal discharge, menorrhagia, metrorrhagia, fever, chills, and urinary symptoms (33). **Some women may develop PID without having any symptoms.**

Pelvic organ tenderness, either uterine tenderness alone or uterine tenderness with adnexal tenderness, is present in patients with PID. Cervical motion tenderness suggests the presence of peritoneal inflammation that causes pain when the peritoneum is stretched by moving the cervix and causing traction of the adnexa on the pelvic peritoneum. Direct or rebound abdominal tenderness may be present.

Evaluation of lower genital tract secretions, both vaginal and endocervical, is a crucial part of the workup of a patient with PID (34). In women with PID, an increased number of polymorphonuclear leukocytes may be detected in a wet mount of the vaginal secretions or in the mucopurulent discharge.

More elaborate tests may be used in women with severe symptoms because an incorrect diagnosis may cause unnecessary morbidity (35) (Table 15.3). These tests include endometrial biopsy to confirm the presence of endometritis, sonography or other radiologic tests to characterize a tubo-ovarian abscess, and laparoscopy to visually confirm salpingitis.

Treatment

Therapy regimens for PID must provide empiric, broad-spectrum coverage of likely pathogens (13, 36) including *Neisseria gonorrhoeae, Chlamydia trachomatis,* gram-negative facultative bacteria, anaerobes, and streptococci. Recommended regimens for the

---

Table 15.3   Clinical Criteria for the Diagnosis of Pelvic Inflammatory Disease (PID)

Symptoms

　None necessary

Signs

　Pelvic organ tenderness
　Leukorrhea and/or mucopurulent endocervicitis

Additional criteria to increase the specificity of the diagnosis

　Endometrial biopsy showing endometritis
　Elevated C-reactive protein or erythrocyte sedimentation rate
　Temperature higher than 38°C
　Leukocytosis
　Positive test for gonorrhea or chlamydia

Elaborate criteria

　Sonography documenting tubo-ovarian abscess
　Laparoscopy visually confirming salpingitis

treatment of PID are listed in Table 15.4. Hospitalization is recommended, especially when the diagnosis is uncertain, pelvic abscess is suspected, clinical disease is severe, or compliance with an outpatient regimen is in question. Hospitalized patients can be considered for discharge when their fever has totally lysed (<99.5°C for more than 24 hours), the white blood cell count has become normal, rebound tenderness is absent, and repeat examination shows marked amelioration of pelvic organ tenderness (37).

Sexual partners of women with PID should be evaluated and treated for urethral infection with chlamydia or gonorrhea (Table 15.2). Urethral tests from male sexual partners of women with nongonococcal, nonchlamydial PID usually will not reveal the presence of one of these STDs (38, 39).

Tubo-Ovarian Abscess

Tubo-ovarian abscess (TOA) is an end-stage process of acute PID. TOA is diagnosed when a patient with PID has a pelvic mass that is palpable during bimanual examination. The condition usually reflects an agglutination of pelvic organs (tube, ovary, bowel) forming a palpable complex. Occasionally, an ovarian abscess can result from the entrance of microorganisms through an ovulatory site. **Treatment of TOA involves the use of an antibiotic regimen administered in a hospital** (Table 15.4). **Approximately 75% of women with TOA will respond to antimicrobial therapy alone. Failure of medical therapy suggests the need for surgical exploration and drainage of the abscess (40).**

Other Major Infections

Genital Ulcer Disease

In the U.S., most patients with genital ulcers have genital herpes simplex virus (HSV) or syphilis (41–43). Chancroid is the next most common cause of sexually transmitted geni-

---

Table 15.4   CDC Guidelines for Treatment of PID

Outpatient treatment

Regimen A:

Cefoxitin 2 g intramuscularly, plus *probenecid,* 1 g orally concurrently, or *ceftriaxone,* 250 mg intramuscularly, or equivalent cephalosporin
    <PLUS>
Doxycycline 100 mg orally 2 times daily for 14 days

Regimen B:

Ofloxacin 400 mg orally 2 times daily for 14 days
    <PLUS>
Clindamycin 450 mg orally 4 times daily, or *metronidazole* 500 mg orally 2 times daily for 14 days

Inpatient treatment

Regimen A:

Cefoxitin 2 g intravenously every 6 hours, or
Cefotetan 2 g intravenously every 12 hours,
    <PLUS>
Doxycycline 100 mg intravenously or orally every 12 hours

Regimen B:

Clindamycin 900 mg intravenously every 8 hours
    <PLUS>
Gentamicin loading dose intravenously or intramuscularly (2 mg/kg of body weight) followed by a maintenance dose (1.5 mg/kg) every 8 hours

Morbidity and Mortality Weekly Report. Centers for Disease Control and Prevention. *MMWR* 1993;42: 78–80.

tal ulcers, followed by the rare occurrence of lymphogranuloma venereum (LGV) and granuloma inguinale (donovanosis). These diseases are associated with an increased risk for HIV infection. Other infrequent and noninfectious causes of genital ulcers include abrasions, fixed drug eruptions, carcinoma, and Behçet's disease.

Diagnosis

A diagnosis based on history and physical examination is often inaccurate. Therefore, evaluation of all women with genital ulcers should include a serologic test for syphilis (43). Because of the consequences of inappropriate therapy, such as tertiary disease and congenital syphilis in pregnant women, diagnostic efforts are directed at excluding syphilis. An optimal workup of the patient with a genital ulcer includes the performance of a dark-field examination or direct immunofluorescence test for *Treponema pallidum*, culture or antigen test for HSV, and culture for *Haemophilus ducreyi*. Dark-field or fluorescent microscopes and selective media to culture for *H. ducreyi* are often not available in most offices and clinics. Even after complete testing, the diagnosis remains unconfirmed in one-fourth of patients with genital ulcers. For this reason, most clinicians base their initial diagnosis and treatment recommendations on their clinical impression of the appearance of the genital ulcer (Fig. 15.2) and knowledge of the most likely cause in their patient population (42).

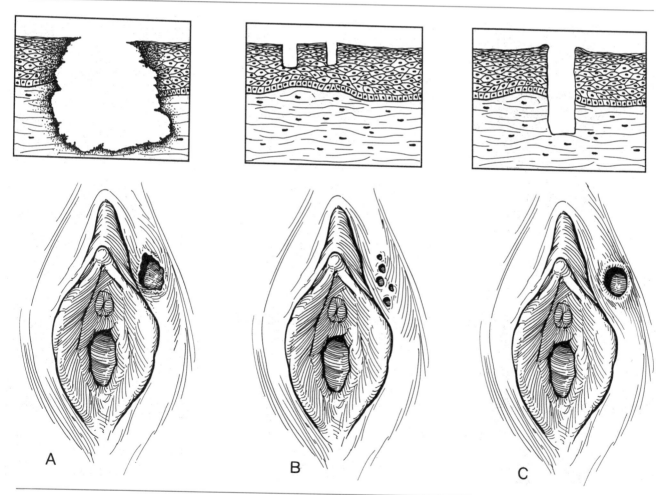

Figure 15.2   Showing the appearance of the ulcers of chancroid (A), herpes (B), and syphilis (C). The ulcer of chancroid has irregular margins and is deep with undermined edges. The syphilis ulcer has a smooth, indurated border and a smooth base. The genital herpes ulcer is superficial and inflamed. (Modified from **Schmid GP, Shcalla WO, DeWitt WE.** Chancroid. In: **Morse SA, Moreland AA, Thompson SE,** eds. *Atlas of Sexually Transmitted Diseases.* Philadelphia: JB Lippincott, 1990.)

Several clinical presentations are highly suggestive of specific diagnoses:

1. **A nonpainful and minimally tender ulcer, not accompanied by inguinal lymphadenopathy, is likely to be syphilis, especially if the ulcer is indurated.** A nontreponemal rapid plasma reagin (RPR) test, or venereal disease research laboratory (VDRL) test, and a confirmatory treponemal test—fluorescent treponemal antibody absorption (FTA ABS) or microhemagglutinin-*Treponema Pallidum* (MHA TP) should be used to presumptively diagnose syphilis. The results of nontreponemal tests usually correlate with disease activity and should be reported quantitatively.

2. **Grouped vesicles mixed with small ulcers, particularly with a history of such lesions, are almost pathognomonic of genital herpes.** Nevertheless, laboratory confirmation of the diagnosis is recommended because the diagnosis of genital herpes is traumatic for many women, alters their self image, and affects their perceived ability to enter new sexual relationships and bear children. Culture is the most sensitive and specific test; sensitivity approaches 100% in the vesicle stage and 89% in the pustular stage and drops to as low as 33% in patients with ulcers. Nonculture tests are about 80% as sensitive as culture.

3. **One to three extremely painful ulcers, accompanied by tender inguinal lymphadenopathy, are unlikely to be anything except chancroid.** This is especially true if the adenopathy is fluctuant.

4. **An inguinal bubo accompanied by one or several ulcers is most likely chancroid.** If there is no ulcer, the most likely diagnosis is LGV.

Treatment

Chancroid Recommended regimens for the treatment of chancroid include *azithromycin,* 1 g orally in a single dose; *ceftriaxone,* 250 mg intramuscularly in a single dose; or *erythromycin* base, 500 mg orally four times daily for 7 days. Patients should be reexamined 3–7 days after initiation of therapy to ensure the gradual resolution of the genital ulcer, which can be expected to heal within 2 weeks unless it is unusually large.

Herpes A first episode of genital herpes should be treated with *acyclovir,* 200 mg orally 5 times daily, for 7–10 days or until clinical resolution is attained. Although *acyclovir* provides partial control of the symptoms and signs of clinical herpes, it neither eradicates latent virus nor affects subsequent risk, frequency, or severity of recurrences after the drug is discontinued. Daily suppressive therapy (400 mg orally twice daily) reduces the frequency of HSV recurrences by at least 75% among patients with six or more recurrences of HSV per year. Suppressive treatment with oral *acyclovir* does not totally eliminate symptomatic or asymptomatic viral shedding or the potential for transmission.

Syphilis **Parenteral *penicillin G* is the preferred drug for treatment of all stages of syphilis.** *Benzathine penicillin G,* 2.4 million units intramuscularly in a single dose, is the recommended treatment for adults with primary, secondary, or early latent syphilis. The *Jarisch-Herxheimer reaction* is an acute febrile reaction—accompanied by headache, myalgia, and other symptoms—that may occur within the first 24 hours after any therapy for syphilis; patients should be advised of this possible adverse reaction.

***Latent syphilis* is defined as those periods after infection with *Treponema pallidum* when patients are seroreactive but show no other evidence of disease.** Patients with latent syphilis of longer than 1 year's duration or of unknown duration should be treated with *benzathine penicillin G,* 7.2 million units total, administered as three doses of 2.4 million units intramuscularly each, at 1-week intervals. All patients with latent syphilis should be evaluated clinically for evidence of tertiary disease (e.g., aortitis, neurosyphilis, gumma, and iritis). Quantitative nontreponemal serologic tests should be repeated at 6 months and again at 12 months. An initially high titer (>1:32) should decline at least fourfold (two dilutions) within 12–24 months.

Genital Warts

Condylomata acuminata are a manifestation of human papillomavirus (HPV) infection (44). The nononcogenic HPV types 6 and 11 are usually responsible for genital warts. The warts tend to occur in areas most directly affected by coitus, namely the posterior fourchette and lateral areas on the vulva. Less frequently, warts can be found throughout the vulva, in the vagina, and on the cervix. Minor trauma associated with coitus can cause breaks in the vulvar skin, allowing direct contact between the viral particles from an infected male and the basal layer of the epidermis of his susceptible sexual partner. Infection may be latent or may cause viral particles to replicate and produce a wart. Exophytic genital warts are highly contagious; more than 75% of sexual partners develop this manifestation of HPV infection when exposed.

The goal of treatment is removal of the warts; it is not possible to eradicate the viral infection. Treatment is most successful in patients with small warts that have been present for less than 1 year. It has not been determined whether treatment of exophytic genital warts reduces transmission of HPV. Selection of a specific treatment regimen depends on the anatomic site, size, and number of warts, as well as expense, efficacy, convenience, and potential adverse effects (Table 15.5). Recurrences more often result from reactivation of subclinical infection than reinfection by a sex partner; therefore, examination of sex partners is not absolutely necessary. However, many of these sex partners may have exophytic warts and may benefit from therapy and counseling concerning transmission of warts.

Human Immunodeficiency Virus

It is estimated that at least 20–25% of persons with HIV are women. Although intravenous drug use remains the most common risk behavior for women with AIDS (50%), heterosexual transmission is increasing, now constituting 36% of AIDS cases in women (45). Infection with HIV produces a spectrum of disease that progresses from an asymptomatic state to full-blown acquired immune deficiency syndrome (AIDS). The pace of disease progression is variable. The median time between infection with HIV and the development of AIDS is 10 years, with a range from a few months to more than 12 years. In a study of adults infected with HIV, symptoms developed in 70%–85% of infected adults, and AIDS developed in 55%–60% within 12 years after infection. Women with HIV-induced altered immune function are at increased risk for infections such as tuberculosis (TB), bacterial pneumonia, and *Pneumocystis carinii* pneumonia (PCP). Because of its impact on the immune system, HIV affects the diagnosis, evaluation, treatment, and follow-up of many other diseases and may decrease the efficacy of antimicrobial therapy for some STDs.

Diagnosis

Infection is most often diagnosed by HIV 1 antibody tests. Antibody testing begins with a sensitive screening test such as ELISA or a rapid assay. If confirmed by Western blot or

Table 15.5   Treatment Options for External Genital and Perianal Warts

Modality (%)	Efficacy (%)	Recurrence risk
Cryotherapy	63–88	21–39
Podophyllin 10–25%	32–79	27–65
Podofilox 0.5%*	45–88	33–60
Triochloroacetic acid 80–90%	81	36
Electrodesiccation or cautery	94	22
Laser†	43–93	29–95
Interferon	44–61	0–67

*May be self-applied by patients at home.
†Expensive, reserve for patients who have not responded to other regimens.

other supplemental testing, a positive antibody test result means a person is infected with HIV and is capable of transmitting the virus to others. Human immunodeficiency virus antibody is detectable in more than 95% of patients within 6 months of infection. Women diagnosed with any STD, particularly genital ulcer disease, should be offered HIV testing (42). Women at risk for STD, such as those with multiple sexual partners or whose partners have multiple sexual partners, should be offered HIV testing.

The initial evaluation of an HIV-positive woman includes screening for diseases associated with HIV such as TB and STDs, administration of recommended vaccinations (hepatitis B, pneumococcal, and influenza), and behavioral and psychosocial counseling. Intraepithelial neoplasia is strongly associated with HPV infection and has been found to occur in high frequency in women coinfected with HPV and HIV. The CD4− T-lymphocyte count is the best laboratory indicator of clinical progression, and comprehensive management strategies for HIV infection are typically stratified by CD4− count. Patients with CD4− counts from 200 to 500 CD4− cells/ul are more likely to develop HIV-related symptoms and to require medical intervention. Patients with CD4− counts <200 cells/ul are at increased risk for developing complicated HIV disease.

Treatment

Treatment of HIV infection and prophylaxis against opportunistic infections continue to evolve rapidly. Currently, the initiation of antiretroviral therapy (*zidovudine* (ZDV)) has been recommended for symptomatic women with CD4− counts less than 500 cells/ul and for asymptomatic patients with counts less than 300 cells/ul. It appears that ZDV delays progression to advanced disease. In addition, patients with less than 200 CD4− T cells/ul or with constitutional symptoms should receive PCP prophylaxis (*trimethoprim/sulfamethoxazole* or aerosol *pentamidine*).

Urinary Tract Infection

Acute Cystitis

Women with acute cystitis generally have an abrupt onset of multiple, severe urinary tract symptoms including dysuria, frequency, and urgency associated with suprapubic or low back pain. Suprapubic tenderness may be noted on physical examination. Urinalysis reveals pyuria and sometimes hematuria. Several factors increase the risk for cystitis, including sexual intercourse, the use of a diaphragm and a spermicide, delayed postcoital micturition, and a history of a recent urinary tract infection (47–49).

Esherichia coli is the most common pathogen isolated from the urine of young women with acute cystitis, and it is present in 80% of cases (50). *Staphylococcus saprophyticus* is present in an additional 5–15% of patients with cystitis. The pathophysiology of cystitis in women involves the colonization of the vagina and urethra with coliform bacteria from the rectum. For this reason, the effects of an antimicrobial agent on the vaginal flora play a role in the eradication of bacteriuria.

Treatment

High concentrations of *trimethoprim* and the fluoroquinolones in vaginal secretions result in eradicating *E. coli* but minimally altering normal anaerobic and microaerophilic vaginal flora. *Trimethoprim/sulfamethoxazole* (160–800 mg every 12 hours) or *trimethoprim* alone (100 mg every 12 hours) are the optimal choices for an empirical 3 day therapy for uncomplicated cystitis. The fluoroquinolones (i.e., *ofloxacin*, 200 mg every 12 hours) are also highly effective and are well tolerated in 3-day regimens, but these preparations are more expensive than *trimethoprim/sulfamethoxazole* and should generally be reserved for recurrent infections, treatment failures, infections in patients with allergies to other drugs, and infections caused by strains resistant to other antimicrobial agents (51).

In patients with typical symptoms, an abbreviated laboratory workup followed by empirical therapy is suggested. The diagnosis can be presumed if pyuria is detected by microscopy or leukocyte esterase testing. Urine culture is not necessary, and a short course of antimicrobial therapy should be given. No follow-up visit or culture is necessary unless symptoms persist or recur.

Recurrent Cystitis

About 20% of premenopausal women with an initial episode of cystitis will have recurrent infections. More than 90% of these recurrences are caused by exogenous reinfection. Recurrent cystitis should be documented by culture to rule out a resistant microorganism. Patients may be treated by one of three strategies: continuous prophylaxis, postcoital prophylaxis, or therapy initiated by the patient when symptoms are first noted.

Postmenopausal women may also have frequent reinfections. Hormonal replacement therapy or topically applied estrogen cream along with antimicrobial prophylaxis are helpful in treating these patients.

Urethritis

Women with dysuria caused by urethritis have a more gradual onset of mild symptoms, which may be associated with abnormal vaginal discharge or bleeding related to concurrent cervicitis. Patients may also have a new sex partner or experience lower abdominal pain. Physical examination may reveal the presence of mucopurulent cervicitis or vulvovaginal herpetic lesions. *Chlamydia trachomatis, Neisseria gonorrhoeae,* or genital herpes may cause acute urethritis. Pyuria is present on urinalysis, but hematuria is rarely seen. Treatment regimens for chlamydia and gonococcal infections are presented in Table 15.2.

Occasionally, vaginitis caused by *Candida albicans* or trichomonas is associated with dysuria. On careful questioning, patients generally describe external dysuria sometimes associated with vaginal discharge and pruritus and dyspareunia. They usually do not experience urgency or frequency. Pyuria and hematuria are absent.

Acute Pyelonephritis

The clinical spectrum of acute, uncomplicated pyelonephritis in young women ranges from gram-negative septicemia to a cystitis-like illness with mild flank pain. *Escherichia coli* accounts for more than 80% of these cases. Microscopy of unspun urine reveals pyuria and gram-negative bacteria. A urine culture should be obtained in all women with suspected pyelonephritis; blood cultures should be performed in those who are hospitalized, because results are positive in 15–20% of cases. In the absence of nausea and vomiting and severe illness, outpatient oral therapy can be given safely. Patients who have nausea and vomiting, moderate to severe illness, and who are pregnant should be hospitalized. Outpatient treatment regimens include *trimethoprim/sulfamethoxazole* (160–800 mg every 12 hours) or a quinolone (i.e., *ofloxacin,* 200–300 mg every 12 hours) for 10–14 days. Inpatient treatment regimens include the use of parenteral *ceftriaxone* (1–2 g daily), *ampicillin* (1 g every 6 hours) and *gentamicin* (especially if enterococcus species are suspected) or *aztreonam* (1 g every 8–12 hours). Symptoms should resolve after 48–72 hours. If fever and flank pain persist after 72 hours of therapy, sonography or computed tomography should be considered to rule out a perinephric or intrarenal abscess or ureteral obstruction. A follow-up culture should be obtained 2 weeks after the completion of therapy.

References

1. **Huggins GR, Preti G.** Vaginal odors and secretions. *Clin Obstet Gynecol* 1981;24:355–77.

2. **Larsen B.** Microbiology of the female genital tract. In: **Pastorek J,** ed. *Obstetric and Gynecologic Infectious Disease.* New York: Raven Press, 1994:11–26.

3. **Eschenbach DA, Davick PR, Williams BL, Klebanoff SJ, Young-Smith K, Critchlow CM, et al.** Prevalence of hydrogen peroxide-producing *Lactobacillus* species in normal women and women with vaginal vaginosis. *J Clin Microbiol* 1989;27:251–6.

4. **Spiegel CA, Amsel R, Eschenbach DA, Schoenknecht F, Holmes KK.** Anaerobic bacteria in nonspecific vaginitis. *N Engl J Med* 1980;303:601–7.

5. **Kent HL.** Epidemiology of vaginitis. *Am J Obstet Gynecol* 1991;165:1168–76.

6. **Eschenbach DA, Hillier S, Critchlow C, Stevens C, De Rouen T, Holmes KK.** Diagnosis and clinical manifestations of bacterial vaginosis. *Am J Obstet Gynecol* 1988;158:819–28.

7. **Larsson P, Platz-Christensen JJ, Thejls H, Forsum U, Pahlson C.** Incidence of pelvic inflammatory disease after first trimester legal abortion in women with bacterial vaginosis after treatment with metronidazole: a double-blind randomized study. *Am J Obstet Gynecol* 1992; 166:100–3.

8. **Soper DE, Bump RC, Hurt WG.** Bacterial vaginosis and trichomoniasis vaginitis are risk factors for cuff cellulitis after abdominal hysterectomy. *Am J Obstet Gynecol* 1990;163:1016–23.

9. **Platz-Christensen JJ, Sundstrom E, Larsson PG.** Bacterial vaginosis and cervical intraepithelial neoplasia. *Acta Obstet Gynecol Scand* 1994;73:586–8.

10. **Martius J, Eschenbach DA.** The role of bacterial vaginosis as a cause of amniotic fluid infection, chorioamnionitis and prematurity—a review. *Arch Gynecol Obstet* 1900;247:1–13.

11. **Watts DH, Krohn MA, Hillier SL, Eschenbach DA.** Bacterial vaginosis as a risk factor for postcesarean endometritis. *Obstet Gynecol* 1990;75:52–8.

12. **Amsel R, Totten PA, Spiegel CA, Chen KC, Eschenbach D, Holmes KK.** Nonspecific vaginitis: diagnostic criteria and microbial and epidemiologic associations. *Am J Med* 1983;74:14–22.

13. **Centers for Disease Control.** *The Sexually Transmitted Diseases Treatment Guidelines.* Washington, DC: Centers for Disease Control, 1993:1–102.

14. **Wolner-Hanssen P, Krieger JN, Stevens CE, Kivlat NB, Koutsky L, Critchlow C, et al.** Clinical manifestations of vaginal trichomoniasis. *JAMA* 1989;261:571–6.

15. **Krieger JN, Tam MR, Stevens CE, Nielsen IO, Hale J, Kiviat NB, et al.** Diagnosis of trichomoniasis. Comparison of conventional wet-mount examination with cytologic studies, cultures, and monoclonal antibody staining of direct specimens. *JAMA* 1988;259:1223–7.

16. **Hurley R, De Louvois J.** *Candida* vaginitis. *Postgrad Med J* 1979;55:645–7.

17. **Hurley R.** Recurrent *Candida* infection. *Clin Obstet Gynecol* 1981;8:208–13.

18. **Sobel JD.** Vulvovaginal candidiasis. In: **Pastorek J,** ed. *Obstetric and Gynecologic Infectious Disease.* New York: Raven Press, 1994:523–36.

19. **Caruso LJ.** Vaginal moniliasis after tetracycline therapy. *Am J Obstet Gynecol* 1964;90:374.

20. **Oriel JD, Waterworth PM.** Effect of minocycline and tetracycline on the vaginal yeast flora. *J Clin Pathol* 1975;28:403.

21. **Morton RS, Rashid S.** Candidal vaginitis: natural history, predisposing factors and prevention. *Proc R Soc Med* 1977;70(Suppl 4):3–12.

22. **Odds FC.** *Candida and Candidiasis.* Baltimore: University Park Press, 1979:104–10.

23. **Brammer KW.** Treatment of vaginal candidiasis with a single oral dose of fluconazole. *Eur J Clin Microbiol Infect Dis* 1988;7:364–7.

24. **Sobel JD.** Management of recurrent vulvovaginal candidiasis with intermittent ketoconazole prophylaxis. *Obstet Gynecol* 1985;65:435–60.

25. **Sobel JD.** Desquamative inflammatory vaginitis: a new subgroup of purulent vaginitis responsive to topical 2% clindamycin therapy. *Am J Obstet Gynecol* 1994;171:1215–20.

26. **Kiviat NB, Paavonen JA, Wolner-Hanssen P, Critchlow CW, Stamm WE, Douglas J, et al.** Histopathology of endocervical infection caused by *Chlamydia trachomatis,* herpes simplex virus, *Trichomonas vaginalis,* and *Neisseria gonorrhoeae. Hum Pathol* 1990;21:831–7.

27. **Brunham RC, Paavonen J, Stevens CE, Kiviat N, Kuo CC, Critchlow CW, et al.** Mucopurulent cervicitis—the ignored counterpart in women of urethritis in men. *N Engl J Med* 1984; 311:1–6.

28. **Soper DE, Brockwell NJ, Dalton HP.** Microbial etiology of urban emergency department acute salpingitis: treatment with ofloxacin. *Am J Obstet Gynecol* 1992;167:653–60.

29. **Sweet RL, Draper DL, Schachter J, James J, Hadley WK, Brooks GF.** Microbiology and pathogenesis of acute salpingitis as determined by laparoscopy: what is the appropriate site to sample? *Am J Obstet Gynecol* 1980;138:985–9.

30. **Wasserheit JN, Bell TA, Kiviat NB, Wolner-Hanssen P, Zabriskie V, Kirby BD, et al.** Microbial causes of proven pelvic inflammatory disease and efficacy of clindamycin and tobramycin. *Ann Intern Med* 1986;104:187–93.

31. **Soper DE, Brockwell NJ, Dalton HP, Johnson D.** Observations concerning the microbial etiology of acute salpingitis. *Am J Obstet Gynecol* 1994;170:1008–17.

32. **Hillis SD, Joesoef R, Marchbanks PA, Wasserheit JN, Cates W Jr, Westrom L.** Delayed care of pelvic inflammatory disease as a risk factor for impaired fertility. *Am J Obstet Gynecol* 1993;168:1503–9.

33. **Wolner-Hanssen P, Kiviat NB, Holmes KK.** Atypical pelvic inflammatory disease: subacute, chronic, or subclinical upper genital tract infection in women. In: **Holmes KK, March P-A, Sparking PF,** eds. *Sexually Transmitted Diseases.* 2nd ed. New York: McGraw-Hill, 1990: 614–20.

34. **Westrom L.** Diagnosis and treatment of salpingitis. *J Reprod Med* 1983;28:703–8.

35. **Soper DE.** Diagnosis and laparoscopic grading of acute salpingitis. *Am J Obstet Gynecol* 1991; 164:1370–6.

36. **Peterson HB, Walker CK, Kahn JG, Washington AE, Eschenbach DA, Faro S.** Pelvic inflammatory disease. Key treatment issues and options. *JAMA* 1991;266:2605–11.

37. **Soper DE.** Pelvic inflammatory disease. *Infect Dis Clin North Am* 1994;8:821–40.

38. **Gilstrap LC 3d, Herbert WN, Cunningham FG, Hauth JC, Van Patten HG.** Gonorrhea screening in the male consorts of women with pelvic infection. *JAMA* 1977;238:965–6.

39. **Potterat JJ, Phillips L, Rothenberg RB, Darrow WW.** Gonococcal pelvic inflammatory disease: case-finding observations. *Am J Obstet Gynecol* 1980;138:1101–4.

40. **Reed SD, Landers DV, Sweet RL.** Antibiotic treatment of tuboovarian abscesses: comparison of broad-spectrum B-lactam agents versus clindamycin-containing regimens. *Am J Obstet Gynecol* 1991;164:1556–62.

41. **Corey L, Adams HG, Brown ZA, Holmes KK.** Genital herpes simplex virus infection: clinical manifestations, course, and complications. *Ann Intern Med* 1983;98:958–72.

42. **Schmid GP.** Approach to the patient with genital ulcer disease. *Med Clin North Am* 1990;74: 1559–72.

43. **Hutchinson CM, Hook EW.** Syphilis in adults. *Med Clin North Am* 1990;74:1389–1416.

44. **McCance DJ.** Human papillomavirus. *Infect Dis Clin North Am* 1994;8:751–67.

45. **Dinsmoor MJ.** HIV infection and pregnancy. *Clin Perinatol* 1994;21:85–94.

46. **Sande MA, Carpenter CCJ, Cobbs CG, Holmes KK, Sanford JP.** Antiretroviral therapy for adult HIV-infected patients. Recommendations from a state-of-the-art conference. National Institute of Allergy and Infectious Disease State-of-the-Art Panel on Anti-Retroviral Therapy for Adult HIV-Infected Patients. *JAMA* 1993;270:2583–9.

47. **Remis RS, Gurwith MJ, Gurwith D, Hargrett-Beam NT, Layde PM.** Risk factors for urinary tract infection. *Am J Epidemiol* 1987;126:685–94.

48. **Fihn SD, Latham RH, Roberts P, Running K, Stamm WE.** Association between diaphragm use and urinary tract infection. *JAMA* 1985;254:240–5.

49. **Strom BL, Collins M, West SL, Kreisberg J, Weller S.** Sexual activity, contraceptive use, and other risk factors for symptomatic and asymptomatic bacteriuria: a case-control study. *Ann Intern Med* 1987;107:816–23.

50. **Stamm WE, Counts GW, Running KR, Fihn S, Turck M, Holmes KK.** Diagnosis of coliform infection in acutely dysuric women. *N Engl J Med* 1982;307:463–8.

51. **Stamm WE, Hooton TM.** Management of urinary tract infections in adults. *N Engl J Med* 1993;329:1328–34.

16   Intraepithelial Disease of the Cervix, Vagina, and Vulva

Kenneth D. Hatch
Neville F. Hacker

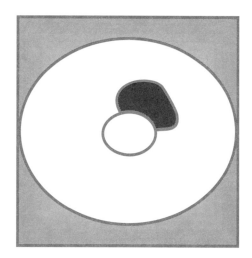

Intraepithelial disease frequently occurs and often coexists in the cervix, vagina, and vulva. The causes and epidemiologic bases are common in all three locations, and treatment typically is ablative and conservative. Early diagnosis and management are essential for the prevention of disease progression to invasive cancer.

Cervical Intraepithelial Neoplasia

The concept of *preinvasive disease* of the cervix was introduced in 1947, when it was recognized that epithelial changes could be identified that had the appearance of invasive cancer but were confined to the epithelium (1). Subsequent studies showed that if these lesions are not treated, they could progress into cervical cancer (2). Improvements in cytologic assessment led to the identification of early precursor lesions called *dysplasia,* which signaled possible development of future cancer. For a number of years, *carcinoma in situ (CIS)* was treated very aggressively (most often with hysterectomy), whereas dysplasias were believed to be less significant and were not treated or were treated by colposcopic biopsy and cryosurgery. The concept of *cervical intraepithelial neoplasia* (CIN) was introduced in 1968, when Richart indicated that all dysplasias have the potential for progression (3). It is now recognized that most early CIN lesions will regress spontaneously if untreated (4); nevertheless, CIN refers to a lesion that may progress to invasive carcinoma. This term is equivalent to the term "dysplasia." Dysplasia means "abnormal maturation;" consequently, proliferating metaplasia without mitotic activity should not be called dysplasia. Squamous metaplasia should not be diagnosed as dysplasia (or CIN) because it does not progress to invasive cancer.

The criteria for the diagnosis of intraepithelial neoplasia may vary according to the pathologist, but the significant features are cellular immaturity, cellular disorganization, nuclear abnormalities, and increased mitotic activity. The extent of the mitotic activity, immature cellular proliferation, and nuclear atypicality identifies the degree of neoplasia. If the mi-

447

toses and immature cells are present only in the lower one-third of the epithelium, the lesion usually is designated as CIN 1. Involvement of the middle and upper thirds is diagnosed as CIN 2 and CIN 3, respectively (Fig. 16.1).

Cervical Anatomy

The cervix is composed of *columnar epithelium*, which lines the endocervical canal, and *squamous epithelium*, which covers the exocervix (5). The point at which they meet is called the *squamocolumnar junction (SCJ)* (Figs. 16.2 and 16.3).

The SCJ rarely remains restricted to the external os. Instead, it is a dynamic point that changes in response to puberty, pregnancy, menopause, and hormonal stimulation (Fig. 16.4). In neonates, the SCJ is located on the exocervix. At the time of menarche, the production of estrogen causes the vaginal epithelium to fill with glycogen. Lactobacilli act on the glycogen to the pH, stimulating the subcolumnar reserve cells to undergo *metaplasia* (5).

The metaplasia advances from the original SCJ inward, toward the external os, and over the columnar villi. This process establishes an area called the *transformation zone*. The transformation zone extends from the original SCJ to the physiologically active SCJ. As the metaplastic epithelium in the transformation zone matures, it begins to produce glycogen and eventually resembles the original squamous epithelium colposcopically and histologically.

In most cases, CIN is believed to originate as a single focus in the transformation zone at the advancing SCJ. The anterior lip of the cervix is twice as likely to develop CIN as the posterior lip, and CIN rarely originates in the lateral angles. Once CIN occurs, it can progress horizontally to involve the entire transformation zone but usually does not replace the original squamous epithelium. This progression usually results in CIN with a sharp external border. Proximally, CIN involves the cervical clefts, and this area tends to have the most severe CIN lesions. The extent of involvement of these cervical glands has significant therapeutic implications because the entire gland must be destroyed to ensure elimination of the CIN (5).

The only way to determine where the original SCJ was located is to look for Nabothian cysts or cervical cleft openings, which indicate the presence of columnar epithelium. Once the metaplastic epithelium matures and forms glycogen, it is called the "healed transfor-

Figure 16.1   Diagram of the different grades of CIN.

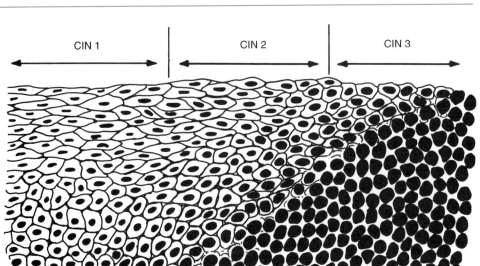

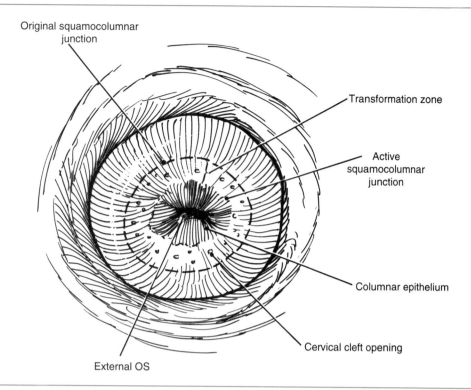

Figure 16.2   The cervix and the transformation zone.

Figure 16.3   Cross-section of the cervix and the endocervix.

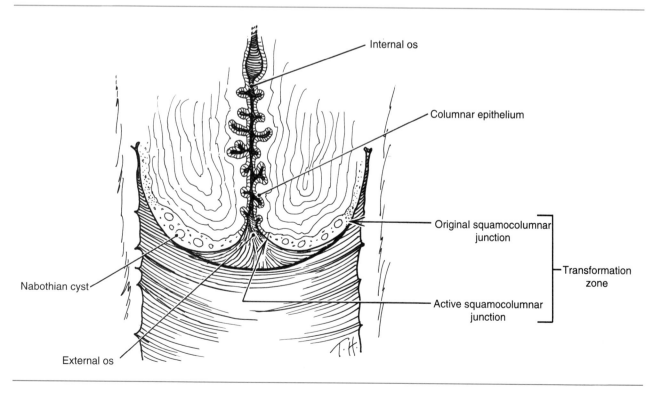

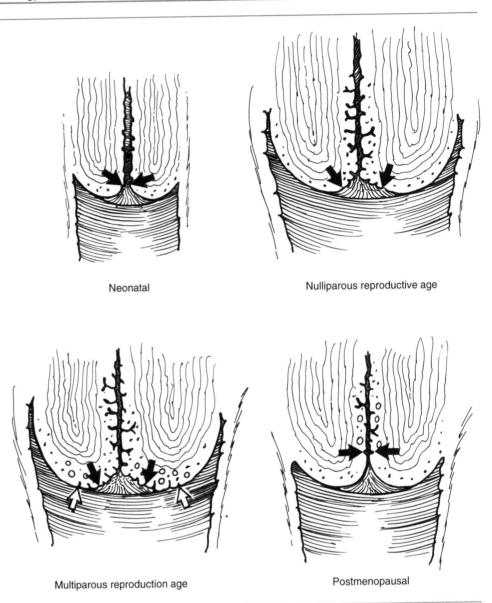

Neonatal

Nulliparous reproductive age

Multiparous reproduction age

Postmenopausal

Figure 16.4   Different locations of the transformation zone and the squamo-columnar junction during a woman's lifetime. The arrows mark the active transformation zone.

mation zone" and is relatively resistant to oncogenic stimuli. However, the entire SCJ with early metaplastic cells is more susceptible to oncogenic factors, which may cause these cells to transform into cervical intraepithelial neoplasia (CIN). Therefore, **CIN is most likely to begin either during menarche or following pregnancy, when metaplasia is most active. Conversely, a woman who has reached menopause without developing CIN has little metaplasia and is at a lower risk.** It has been established that oncogenic factors are introduced through sexual intercourse. Several agents, including sperm, seminal fluid histones, trichomonas, chlamydia, herpes simplex virus, and human papillomavirus (HPV), have been studied, and it is now known that HPV plays an important role in the development of CIN.

Normal Transformation Zone

The original squamous epithelium of the vagina and exocervix is described as having four layers (5):

1. The *basal layer* is a single row of immature cells with large nuclei and a small amount of cytoplasm.

2. The *parabasal layer* includes 2–4 rows of immature cells that have normal mitotic figures and provide the replacement cells for the overlying epithelium.

3. The *intermediate layer* includes 4–6 rows of cells with larger amounts of cytoplasm in a polyhedral shape separated by an intercellular space. Intercellular bridges, where differentiation of glycogen production occurs, can be identified with light microscopy.

4. The *superficial layer* includes 5–8 rows of flattened cells with small uniform nuclei and a cytoplasm filled with glycogen. The nucleus becomes pyknotic and the cells detach from the surface (exfoliation). These cells form the basis for Papanicolaou (Pap) testing.

Columnar Epithelium   Columnar epithelium has a single layer of columnar cells with mucus at the top and a round nucleus at the base. The glandular epithelium is composed of numerous ridges, clefts, and infoldings and, when covered by squamous metaplasia, leads to the appearance of gland openings. Technically, the endocervix is not a gland, but the term "gland openings" is often used.

Metaplastic Epithelium   Metaplastic epithelium, found at the SCJ, begins in the subcolumnar reserve cell (Fig. 16.4). Under stimulation of lower vaginal acidity, the reserve cells proliferate, lifting the columnar epithelium. The immature metaplastic cells have large nuclei and a small amount of cytoplasm without glycogen. As the cells mature normally, they produce glycogen, eventually forming the four layers of epithelium. The metaplastic process begins at the tips of the columnar villi, which are exposed first to the acid vaginal environment. As the metaplasia replaces the columnar epithelium, the central capillary of the villus regresses and the epithelium flattens out, leaving the epithelium with its typical network vasculature. As metaplasia proceeds into the cervical clefts, it replaces columnar epithelium and similarly flattens the epithelium. The deeper clefts, however, may not be completely replaced by the metaplastic epithelium, leaving mucus-secreting columnar epithelium trapped under the squamous epithelium. Some of these glands open onto the surface; others are completely encased, with mucus collecting in Nabothian cysts. Gland openings and Nabothian cysts mark the original SCJ and the outer edge of the original transformation zone (5).

Human Papillomavirus

The cytologic changes of HPV were first recognized by Koss (6) in 1956 and given the term *koilocytosis,* but their significance was not recognized until 20 years later, when Meisels and colleagues (7) reported these changes in mild dysplasia (Fig. 16.5). Molecular biologic studies have demonstrated high levels of HPV DNA and capsid antigen, indicating productive viral infection in these koilocytic cells (8). The HPV genome has been demonstrated in all grades of cervical neoplasia (9). As the CIN lesions become more severe (Fig. 16.6), the koilocytes disappear, the HPV copy numbers decrease, and the capsid antigen disappears, indicating that the virus is not capable of reproducing in less differentiated cells (10). Instead, it appears that portions of the HPV DNA become integrated into the host cell. Integration of the transcriptionally active DNA into the host cell appears to be necessary for malignant growth (11). Malignant transformation appears to require the expression of E6 and E7 oncoproteins produced by HPV (12). Because HPV will not grow in cell culture, there is no direct evidence of the carcinogenesis of HPV. However, a cell culture system has been described for growing keratinocytes that allows for stratification and will produce differentiated specific keratinase (13). When normal cells are transfected with the plasmid-containing HPV 16, the transfected cells produced cystologic abnormalities identical to those seen in intraepithelial neoplasia. The E6 and E7 oncoproteins are identifiable in the transfected cell lines, which is the strongest laboratory evidence of a cause-and-effect relationship (14).

451

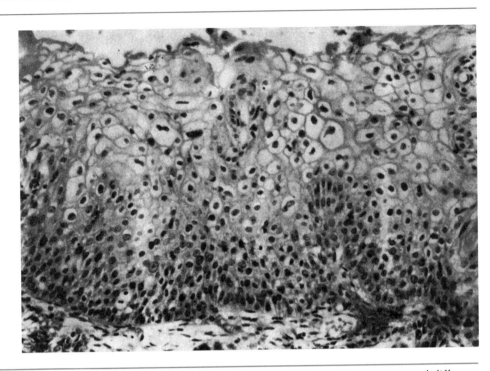

Figure 16.5   CIN 1 with koilocytosis. The normal maturation process and differentiation from the basal and parabasal layers to the intermediate and superficial layers are maintained. In the upper layers, koilocytes are characterized by perinuclear halos, well-defined cell borders, and nuclear hyperchromasia, irregularity, and enlargement. (From **Fu YS, Woodruff JD.** Pathology. In: **Berek JS, Hacker NF,** eds. *Practical Gynecologic Oncology.* 2nd ed. Baltimore: Williams & Wilkins, 1994:118.)

Figure 16.6   CIN 3 with the entire thickness of the epithelium replaced by abnormal cells that have large hyperchromatic, irregular nuclei. The normal maturation is lost. Mitotic figures are seen in the superficial layers (left upper corner). (From **Fu YS, Woodruff JD.** Pathology. In: **Berek JS, Hacker NF,** eds. *Practical Gynecologic Oncology.* 2nd ed. Baltimore: Williams & Wilkins, 1994:119.)

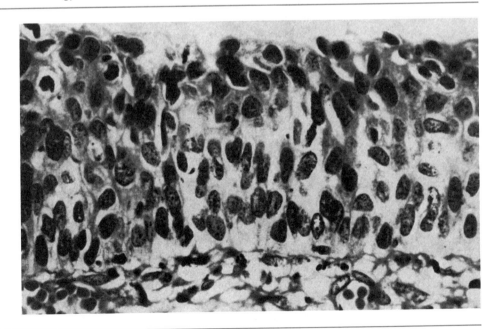

Cervical cancer cell lines that contain active copies of HPV 16 or 18 (SiHa, HeLa, C 4-11, Ca Ski) demonstrate the presence of HPV 16 E6 and E7 oncoproteins (15).

Recent case-control data have firmly established that HPV DNA can be detected in most women with cervical neoplasia (16, 17). There is a 10-fold or greater risk of cervical neoplasia associated with the detection of HPV DNA. The relative risk of neoplasia associated with HPV is as high as 40 with a lower 95% confidence limit of 15 (16). **The percentage of intraepithelial neoplasia apparently attributed to HPV infection approaches** 90% (17).

Although the number of known genital HPV types now exceeds 20, only certain types count for approximately 90% of high-grade intraepithelial lesions and cancer (HPV types 16, 18, 31, 33, 35, 39, 45, 51, 52, 56, 58) (17). **Type 16 is the most common HPV type in invasive cancer and in CIN 2 and CIN 3 and is found in 47% of women in both categories** (18). It is also the most common HPV type in women with normal cytology. Unfortunately, HPV 16 is not very specific, because it can be found in 16% of women with low-grade lesions and up to 14% of women with normal cytology. **HPV 18 is found in 23% of women with invasive cancers, 5% of women with CIN 2 and CIN 3, 5% of women with HPV and CIN 1, and fewer than 2% of patients with negative findings** (17). **Therefore, HPV 18 is more specific than HPV 16 for invasive tumors.**

Usually, HPV infections do not persist. Most women have no apparent clinical evidence of disease, and the infection is eventually suppressed or eliminated (16). Other women exhibit low-grade cervical lesions that may regress spontaneously. A minority of women exposed to HPV develop persistent infection that may progress to CIN (16, 19). Factors that may have a role in this progression include smoking, contraceptive use, infection with other sexually transmitted diseases, or nutrition (16, 18). Any factor that influences the integration of HPV DNA into the human genome may cause progression to invasive disease (20).

Pap Test Classification

In 1989, a National Cancer Institute (NCI) workshop held in Bethesda, Maryland resulted in the development of the Bethesda System for cytologic reporting (21). A standardized method of reporting cytology findings was needed to facilitate peer review and quality assurance. In the Bethesda System, potentially premalignant squamous lesions fall into three categories: *atypical squamous cells of undetermined significance (ASCUS), low-grade squamous intraepithelial lesions (LSIL),* and *high-grade squamous intraepithelial lesions (HSIL).* Low-grade squamous intraepithelial lesions include CIN 1 (mild dysplasia) and the changes of HPV, termed *koilocytotic atypia.* High-grade squamous intraepithelial lesions include CIN 2 and CIN 3 (moderate dysplasia, severe dysplasia, and carcinoma *in situ*). A comparison of the various terms as they relate is shown in Table 16.1.

Cellular changes associated with HPV (i.e., koilocytosis and CIN 1) are incorporated within the category of LSIL because the natural history, distribution of various HPV types, and cytologic features of both of these lesions are the same (20). **Long-term follow-up studies have shown that lesions properly classified as "koilocytosis" progress to high-grade intraepithelial neoplasia in 14% of cases** (22) **and that lesions classified as mild dysplasia progress to severe dysplasia/CIS in 16% of cases** (4). It was initially thought that lesions classified as koilocytosis would contain only low-risk HPV types, such as 6 and 11, whereas high-risk HPV types, such as 16 and 18, would be limited to true neoplasms, including CIN 1, thus justifying the distinction. Histopathologic and molecular virologic correlation, however, has demonstrated a similar heterogeneous distribution of low- and high-risk HPV types in both koilocytosis and CIN 1 (23). Studies evaluating the dysplasia/CIS/CIN terminology have demonstrated a lack of interobserver and intraobserver reproducibility (24). The greatest lack of reproducibility is between koilocytosis and CIN 1 (25). Thus, on the basis of clinical behavior, molecular biologic findings and morphologic features, HPV changes and CIN 1 appear to be the same disease. The rationale for combining CIN 2 and CIN 3 into the category of HSIL is similar. The biologic studies reveal the similar mix of high-risk HPV types in the two lesions, and the separation of the

453

Table 16.1   Comparison of Cytology Classification Systems

Bethesda System	Dysplasia/CIN System	Papanicolaou System
Within normal limits	Normal	I
Infection (organism should be specified)	Inflammatory atypia (organism)	II
Reactive and reparative changes		
Squamous cell abnormalities Atypical squamous cells of undetermined significance	Squamous atypia	IIR
Low-grade squamous intraepithelial lesion (LSIL)	HPV atypia	
High-grade squamous intraepithelial lesion (HSIL)	Mild dysplasia CIN 1 Moderate dysplasia CIN 2	III
	Severe dysplasia Carcinoma in situ CIN 3	IV
Squamous cell carcinoma	Squamous cell carcinoma	V

CIN, cervical intraepithelial neoplasia.
From **Berek JS, Hacker NF**, eds. *Practical Gynecologic Oncology*. 2nd ed. Baltimore: Williams & Wilkins, 1994: 205.

lesions has been shown to be irreproducible (24, 25). In addition, the management of CIN 2 and CIN 3 is similar, so separation serves no useful clinical purpose.

ASCUS

Abnormal cells that do not fulfill the criteria for low- or high-grade squamous intraepithelial lesions are described as ASCUS. This category includes many of the minor abnormalities that in the past have been termed "atypical." The undetermined significance reflects not only a lack of uniform diagnostic criteria for these cells but also the uncertain relation of these cells to subsequent cervical cancer, HPV infection, or other conditions. As a result, this diagnosis, frequently used in cytology reports, has led to some confusion about treatment and follow-up. The ASCUS category does not include the condylomatous or koilocytotic atypia, formerly included in class II of the Papanicolaou classification and now categorized as LSIL.

The ASCUS category is restricted to those test results disclosing abnormal cells that are truly of unknown significance. The ASCUS category does not include benign, reactive, and reparative changes that should be coded as normal in the Bethesda system. Because of the lack of diagnostic criteria and the fear of medicolegal action, the diagnosis has become quite common, ranging from 3 to 25% in some centers (26). It is anticipated that when standardized diagnostic criteria are used, the rate of ASCUS results should be 3–5% (26).

Diagnosis

The Pap Test

Patients should be advised not to douche for 48 hours before undergoing a Pap test, not to use vaginal creams for 1 week before the test, and to abstain from coitus for 24 hours in advance.

Technique   The Pap test should include samples from both the endocervix and the exocervix. The most widely used device for sampling the endocervical canal is a saline-moistened, cotton-tipped swab.

1. Do not use a lubricant on the vaginal speculum.

2. Place the endocervical brush or cotton-tipped swab inside the endocervix, and roll it firmly against the canal (27).

3. Remove the endocervical brush or cotton-tipped swab and place the sample on a glass slide.

4. Place the spatula against the cervix with the longer protrusion in the cervical canal.

5. Rotate the spatula clockwise 360° firmly against the cervix. If the spatula does not scrape the entire transformation zone, rotate the spatula again further out on the cervix. Rotate it enough times to cover the entire transformation zone.

6. Immediately place the sample from the spatula onto the glass slide by rotating the spatula against the slide in a clockwise manner.

7. Immediately fix the slide with a spray fixative held 9–12 inches from the slide or by placing the slide in a 95% ethanol fixative.

The smear should be thick enough that it is not transparent. If it is too thin, the result will be a drying artifact and too few cells to screen adequately. However, if the smear is too thick, the Papanicolaou stain will not penetrate.

A vaginal pool sample is not recommended for screening for cervical cancer. It has been used to collect shed endometrial cells to screen for endometrial cancer and to provide a maturation index. The technique is not helpful for either use, however, and should be abandoned.

For cytology screening, two slides may be used instead of one. If the endocervix pipette is used, two slides are preferable. With two slides, the endocervix sample can be applied immediately instead of waiting for the cervical scrape. This process reduces air-drying artifact. There are four major factors that cause sample error: improper collection, poor transfer from collecting device to slide, air drying, and contamination with lubricant.

Colposcopy

Preparation of the Patient

A woman with abnormal Pap test results may be frightened because she assumes she has cancer (5). A discussion with the patient to allay her anxiety will make the examination easier for both the patient and the physician. This discussion should emphasize the following:

1. There is a low probability of finding an invasive cancer.

2. It is likely that only "dysplasia" will be found.

3. CIN is abnormal cells but not cancer.

4. CIN can be treated by simple methods without hospitalization or major surgery.

The procedures of colposcopy and biopsy should be described to the patient. She should expect some mild cramping comparable to menstrual cramps during the performance of the endocervical curettage (ECC) and cervical biopsies. If the cramping is severe, the patient may be advised to take nonsteroidal anti-inflammatory drugs (NSAIDs) to relieve pain. Anesthesia is not necessary.

Procedure

The colposcopy procedure is performed in the following manner:

1. *Position the patient.* The patient is placed in the lithotomy position with drapes covering her legs.

2. *Bring the colposcope into position.* Use the colposcope's bright light to inspect the vulva and perianal area for signs of inflammation, ulceration, or HPV infection, first using the naked eye and then the low power of the colposcope.

3. *Insert the speculum.* While looking through the colposcope at low power, the vagina can be inspected for discharge, inflammation, ulceration, or HPV lesions.

4. *Expose the cervix.* Gently examine the cervix so the surface epithelium is not abraded.

5. *Repeat the Pap test, if necessary.* Use both an endocervical swab and a spatula to obtain the sample. This technique provides a cytologic smear that correlates with the histology. If the pathologist who will perform the histologic examination already has been provided with a smear, the repeat smear may not be necessary.

6. *Cleanse the cervix with cotton swabs.* Saline may be used to help clear excess cellular debris.

7. *Examine the cervix with the colposcope.* Begin at low power to look at color tone and topography. Note any gross lesion, excess friability, or ulceration. Identify the original squamous epithelium and the columnar villi. If white epithelium is present at this point, it is termed "leukoplakia." Progress to higher power to examine the vascular pattern.

8. *Apply acetic acid.* Apply 3–5% acetic acid with a cotton swab to the cervix and upper vagina and allow it to remain for at least 30 seconds. Continue to inspect the cervix through the colposcope at low power during this phase. The longer the acetic acid is exposed to the cervix, the more visible the lesion will be.

9. *Examine the columnar villi.* The columnar villi will swell, making them more prominent initially, and then they may fade and become harder to identify after repeated application of acetic acid. The junction of the columnar epithelium and squamous metaplastic epithelium is the *SCJ.* When the SCJ is seen in its entirety, the examination is satisfactory.

10. *Look for acetowhite epithelium.* The CIN lesions will become more apparent the longer they are exposed to acetic acid, as the acid penetrates deeper and coagulates more protein.

11. *Look for punctation and mosaic.*

12. *Look for the external border of acetowhite lesions.*

13. *Look for the internal border of the acetowhite lesions.* This border will be limited by the previously identified SCJ.

14. *Reexamine the cervix with the green filter.* This filter will accentuate the margins of acetowhite epithelium and aid in identifying abnormal vessels.

15. *Ask these questions:*
    - Is there any suggestion of invasion?
    - Is the entire lesion and the entire transformation zone visible? If so, the examination is satisfactory. If not, it is unsatisfactory.
    - Where is the most significant area to biopsy?

16. *Perform the ECC under direct colposcopic vision.* Place the curette inside the SCJ and systematically scrape the endocervix (approximately 2 cm in length).

Cervical mucus, clotted blood, and fragments of endocervical epithelium will accumulate at the exocervix. This coagulum should be recovered with forceps and submitted for evaluation.

17. *Perform colposcopically directed biopsy of the most severe area.* After the ECC has been performed, the cervix is cleaned again with acetic acid and the biopsy is performed under direct vision. The number of biopsies may vary with the size of the lesion.

18. *Apply Monsel's solution or silver nitrate for hemostasis.* Apply pressure with a cotton swab as the Monsel's solution or silver nitrate is applied with a separate cotton-tipped applicator directly onto the biopsy site.

19. *Colpophotography may be performed.* This procedure should be performed prior to the ECC and biopsy and may be used to document the findings.

20. *Document the colposcopic findings.* The location of the SCJ and the colposcopic lesions should be noted on a diagram of the cervix. The biopsy sites are identified by an "X."

Acetowhite Epithelium

Epithelium that turns white after application of acetic acid (3–5%) is called acetowhite epithelium (Fig. 16.7) (28). **The application of acetic acid coagulates the proteins of the nucleus and cytoplasm and makes the proteins opaque and white** (5).

The acetic acid does not affect mature, glycogen-producing epithelium, because the acid does not penetrate below the outer one-third of the epithelium. The cells in this region have very small nuclei and a large amount of glycogen (not protein). These areas appear pink dur-

Figure 16.7   Diagram of punctation. The central capillaries of the columnar villi are preserved and produce the punctate vessels on the surface.

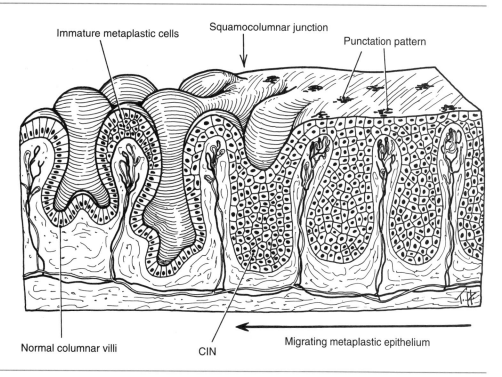

Immature metaplastic cells

Squamocolumnar junction

Punctation pattern

Normal columnar villi

CIN

Migrating metaplastic epithelium

ing colposcopy. Dysplastic cells are those most affected. They contain large nuclei with abnormally large amounts of chromatin (protein). The columnar villi become "plumper" after acetic acid is applied; these cells are then easier to see. They appear slightly white, particularly if the beginning signs of metaplasia are present. The immature metaplastic cells have larger nuclei and also show some effects of the acetic acid. Because the metaplastic epithelium is very thin, it is not as white or opaque as CIN but instead appears gray and filmy (5).

Leukoplakia   Translated literally, leukoplakia is white plaque (5). In colposcopic terminology, this plaque is white epithelium visible before application of acetic acid. Leukoplakia is caused by a layer of keratin on the surface of the epithelium. Immature squamous epithelial cells have the potential to develop into keratin-producing cells or glycogen-producing cells. In the vagina and on the cervix, the normal differentiation is toward glycogen. Keratin production is abnormal in the cervicovaginal mucosa. Several things can cause leukoplakia, including HPV; keratinizing CIN; keratinizing carcinoma; chronic trauma from diaphragm, pessary, or tampon use; and radiotherapy.

Leukoplakia should not be confused with the white plaque of a monilial infection, which can be completely wiped off with a cotton-tipped applicator. Currently, the most common reason for leukoplakia is HPV infection. Because it is not possible to see through the thick keratin layer to the underlying vasculature during colposcopy, such areas should be biopsied to rule out keratinizing carcinoma.

Punctation   **Punctation refers to dilated capillaries terminating on the surface, which appear from the ends as a collection of dots** (Fig. 16.7). When these vessels occur in a well-demarcated area of acetowhite epithelium, they indicate an abnormal epithelium—most often CIN (5). The punctate vessels are formed as the metaplastic epithelium migrates over the columnar villi. Normally, the capillary regresses; however, when CIN occurs, the capillary persists and appears more prominent.

Mosaic   **Terminal capillaries surrounding roughly circular or polygonal-shaped blocks of acetowhite epithelium crowded together are called mosaic because their appearance is similar to mosaic tile** (Fig. 16.8). These vessels form a "basket" around the blocks of abnormal epithelium. They may arise from a coalescence of many terminal punctate vessels or from the vessels that surround the cervical gland openings (5).

Atypical Vascular Pattern   **Atypical vascular patterns are characteristic of invasive cervical cancer** and include looped vessels, branching vessels, and reticular vessels. These patterns are discussed in Chapter 32.

Endocervical Curettage   The entire coagulant from the endocervical curettage, placed on a piece of filter paper or brown paper towel, is immersed in 10% buffered formalin or Bouin's solution. Absorbent paper towels should be avoided because they disintegrate when they become wet. The cheapest paper towels provide the best surface.

Cervical Biopsy   The cervical biopsy sample is placed on a dry paper towel. The biopsy should be oriented on its side with the surface at right angles to the surface of the paper. It should be allowed to dry for a minute to ensure attachment to the piece of paper and then placed in the fixative with the specimen down. The specimen and paper will float, and the specimen will stay attached to the undersurface of the paper with its proper orientation. This allows the pathologist to orient the biopsy in the paraffin block and avoid tangential sectioning.

Correlation of Findings

Ideally, both the pathologist and colposcopist should review the colposcopic findings and the results of cytologic assessment, cervical biopsy, and ECC before deciding therapy (28–31).

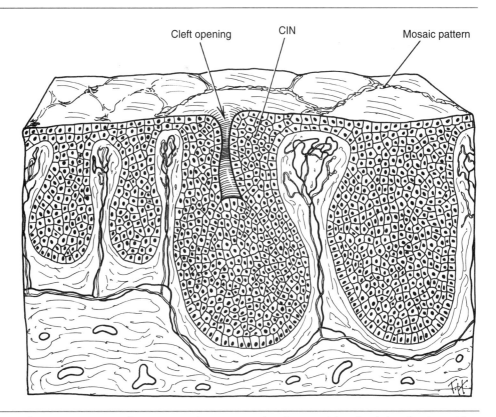

Figure 16.8   Mosaic pattern. This pattern develops as islands of dysplastic epithelium proliferate and push the ends of the superficial blood vessels away, creating a pattern that looks like mosaic tiles.

This is particularly true when operators are first learning the technique of colposcopy. The cytology results should not be sent to one laboratory and the histology results to another. The colposcopist should not treat the report but rather treat the disease. When the cytology and biopsy results correlate, the colposcopist can be reasonably certain that the worst lesion has been identified. If the cytology indicates a more significant lesion than the histology, the patient should undergo further evaluation and additional biopsies as necessary.

Human Papillomavirus Typing

Screening for HPV has been suggested as a means of secondary assessment of abnormal cytology (32). As a screening tool, HPV typing cannot be recommended, and further studies are warranted. As a secondary triage technique for assessing ASCUS and LSIL Pap test results, however, it may be reasonable to use because CIN or invasive cancer will be found in more than 80% of patients with high-risk types. Further studies are warranted before HPV typing can be recommended to determine which patients should undergo colposcopy for assessment of Pap test results that are interpreted as ASCUS or LSIL.

Cervicography

Cervicography has been investigated as a secondary means of assessment of patients with atypical Pap test results (33–35). Cervicography was used to identify lesions, and results were then compared with colposcopy examination and biopsy. More than 90% of the colposcopically diagnosed lesions were correctly identified with cervicography. There was no instance of missed invasive cancer.

August reported 586 patients with persistent atypia who underwent repeat Pap testing, cervicography, and colposcopic examination (33). Of the 43 patients with LSIL, both cervicography and colposcopy were equally effective in identifying these lesions (33 of 43, 77%). For the 40 women with HSIL, cervicography results were suspicious in 38 and colposcopy results were positive in 39. A comparison of the sensitivity, specificity, positive predictive value, and negative predictive value of cervicography versus colposcopic impression versus repeat cytology is shown in Table 16.2.

Jones et al. evaluated 236 patients with atypical Pap test results by histology, cervicography, and colposcopy (34) (Table 16.2). The repeat Pap test was successful in detecting only 17% of the 58 patients who had squamous intraepithelial lesions. A repeat Pap test is not recommended as an intermediate step assessing patients with atypical Pap results. Although the sensitivity of colposcopy and cervicography are similar, the specificity of cervicography is much greater than that for colposcopy (34).

Campion et al. prospectively evaluated 6,035 patients with cervicography, repeat cytology, and colposcopic biopsy (35). Cervicography identified 94.8% of LSIL, 96.3% of HSIL, and all six invasive cancers, whereas repeat cytology missed three of the six invasive cancers, 25.9% of HSIL, and 28.4% of the LSIL.

These three major studies reveal the importance of visualizing the cervix by either colposcopy or cervicography. Simply repeating the cytologic assessment will result in missing 26–83% of squamous intraepithelial lesions (34–36) and, most alarmingly, 50% of invasive cancers. The effectiveness of cervicography triage is approximately the same as colposcopy triage. A number of factors will lead to the choice of one modality or the other. These factors might include the cost to the patient, the training of the physician, the availability of equipment, and the expectation of the patient.

Because 70–85% of patients with atypical Pap test results will have benign histology, it is not indicated to simply excise the transformation zone of all patients with atypical smears (Table 16.3). This approach would lead to overtreatment of most women, many of whom are young with active metaplasia in the transformation zone, which can be overdiagnosed on cytologic assessment and misinterpreted on colposcopy. If colposcopy is used as a means of evaluating atypical Pap test results, one must be cautious not to overinterpret the metaplastic areas. There is also a risk that pathologists will overinterpret the colposcopically directed biopsies and the patient will be diagnosed as having low-grade lesion when metaplasia is the only finding.

Table 16.2   Comparison of Papanicolaou Smear, Colposcopy, and Cervicography for Atypical Papanicolaou Smear

Author (Ref. No.)	Sensitivity			Specificity		
	Cytology	Colposcopy	Cervicography	Cytology	Colposcopy	Cervicography
August (33)	26%	84%	82%	97%	62%	62%
Jones (34)	17%	100%	90%	98%	28%	60%

Table 16.3   Histologic Diagnosis of Patients with Atypical Cytology

Author (Ref. No.)	Number of Patients	Benign No. (%)	CIN 1 No. (%)	CIN 2 No. (%)	CIN 3 No. (%)	Cancer No. (%)
August (33)	1214	1028 (84.7)	100 (8.2)	54 (4.4)	30 (2.5)	2 (0.2)
Jones (34)	236	178 (75.4)	48 (20.4)	7 (2.9)	3 (1.3)	—
Noumoff (39)	375	267 (71.2)	70 (18.7)	20 (5.3)	18 (4.8)	—
Total	1825	1473 (80.7)	218 (11.9)	81 (4.5)	51 (2.8)	2 (0.1)

Evaluation of the Abnormal Pap Smear

An algorithm for the management of abnormal Pap test results is presented in Figure 16.9.

ASCUS

Current management of ASCUS is controversial. Cytologic assessment is an excellent screening tool but is not an effective triage procedure because results will be negative in approximately 40% of patients in whom CIN lesions have been diagnosed colposcopically (36). Colposcopy is a time-consuming and expensive form of triage and may result in

Figure 16.9   An algorithm for the evaluation, treatment, and follow-up of an abnormal Pap test.

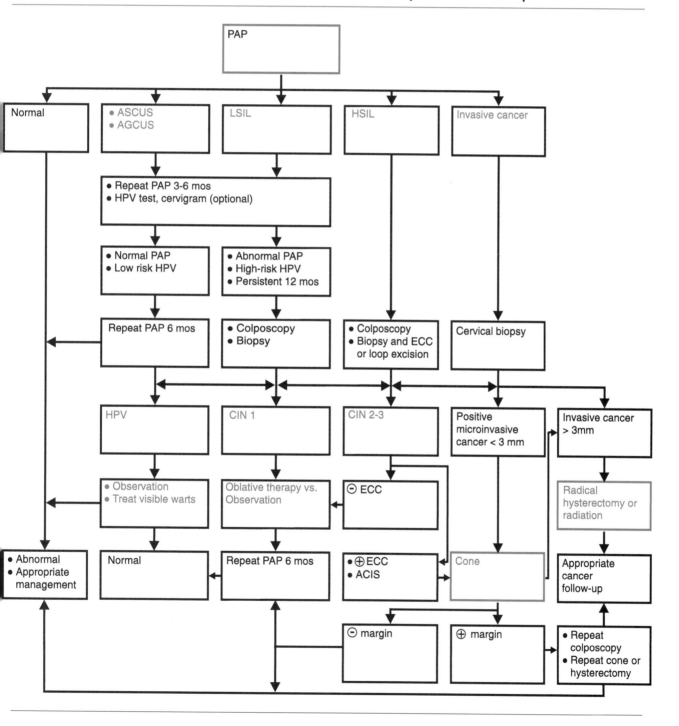

overtreatment of patients. Nevertheless, many patients with ASCUS Pap test results undergo colposcopically directed biopsy.

1. The Pap test could be repeated at intervals of 3–6 months. If the results of two consecutive tests are negative, a return to yearly Pap testing is indicated.

2. If either of the test results indicates a repeat ASCUS or more severe classification, the patient is a candidate for colposcopy or cervicography or HPV testing.

3. Alternatively, the patient who has had one ASCUS Pap test result could undergo cervicography or HPV testing. If either of these test results is positive, colposcopy should be performed immediately and, if the results are negative, yearly screenings should be resumed.

The HPV data obtained from women with ASCUS Pap test results are nearly identical to those of LSIL, indicating that ASCUS may be the earliest evidence of an HPV infection (37). No prospective studies indicating the natural history of women who have ASCUS cytology are currently available. Because of its similarity to LSIL, these data must be extrapolated. Analysis of screening programs in British Columbia indicate that in women younger than 34 years of age, 84% of lesions regress spontaneously (38). Lesions regress in 40% of women older than 34 years of age. Nasiell et al. reported 62% regression after an average follow-up period of 39 months, with 22% of lesions persisting and 16% progressing (4). Both Campion and Kataja found that HPV type 16 was associated with a greater risk of progression to HSIL (21, 38). Despite the fact that most low-grade lesions will regress spontaneously, some physicians are unwilling to expectantly manage these lesions for fear of litigation. When a woman has a colposcopically identifiable abnormal transformation zone and CIN documented by biopsy, destruction of that abnormal transformation zone is reasonable. Some patients may choose not to have the lesion treated and prefer instead to be monitored by cytologic and colposcopic examination every 4–6 months. If a lesion persists more than 2 years, treatment should be recommended because of the diminished likelihood of spontaneous regression.

LSIL

Most cytology specimens demonstrating LSIL represent processes that will revert spontaneously to normal without therapy (39). However, a few women in this category will have a lesion that will progress.

1. At a minimum, patients with cytology indicating LSIL should undergo repeat cervical cytology assessment at approximately 4–6 months and colposcopy should be performed if an abnormality persists.

2. Because of the false-negative rate of Pap testing, it is generally preferable to perform colposcopy after the initial LSIL result to determine whether a lesion is present.

3. Following histologic confirmation, if the entire lesion and the limits of the transformation zone area are seen, the lesion can be ablated or the patient can be monitored without treatment.

Management depends to a large degree on the desire and compliance of the patient. Because approximately 15% of these lesions progress (4), ablation is a reasonable treatment. Conversely, because approximately 60% of these lesions regress spontaneously (4, 40), follow-up is an appropriate form of management for a compliant patient when indicated. An LSIL result can be followed closely with repeat samples obtained with a cytobrush and an endocervical curettage without the need for a cone biopsy or other treatment. If follow-up and no treatment are selected and the lesion persists for 1 year, treatment is indicated (40). Visible HPV or CIN 1 lesions (Fig. 16.10) should be ablated. Some of these HPV-associated changes found adjacent to focal CIN 2 lesions are shown in Figure 16.11.

HSIL

Any woman with a cytology specimen suggesting the presence of high-HSIL (moderate or severe dysplasia, CIN 2 or 3, or CIS) should undergo colposcopy and directed biopsy (Figs. 16.12 and 16.13). Following colposcopically directed biopsy and determination of the distribution of the lesion, ablative therapy aimed at destruction or removal of the entire transformation zone usually should be performed. Outpatient management can be undertaken only if the entire lesion and limits of the transformation zone are seen and results of endocervical curettage are negative. **Any lesion suggestive of invasive cancer should be biopsied.** Conization may be appropriate.

Treatment of CIN

Before treatment is instituted, the histologic diagnosis must be accurate and the extent of the lesion must be determined. A variety of ablative techniques have been used to treat CIN, including surgical excision, cryosurgery, laser vaporization, and, more recently, loop electrosurgical excision. Most of these techniques can be performed in an outpatient setting, which is one of the main objectives in the management of this disease. Because all therapeutic modalities carry an inherent recurrence rate of up to 10%, cytologic follow-up at approximately 3-month intervals for 1 year is necessary. Ablative therapy is appropriate when the following conditions exist:

1. No evidence of microinvasive or invasive cancer on cytology, colposcopy, endocervical curettage, or biopsy.

Figure 16.10   CIN 1, mild dysplasia associated with human papillomavirus infection of the cervix. There is a shiny, snow-white color and a micropapillary surface contour. (From **Berek JS, Hacker NF,** eds. *Practical Gynecologic Oncology.* 2nd ed. Baltimore: Williams & Wilkins, 1994:207.)

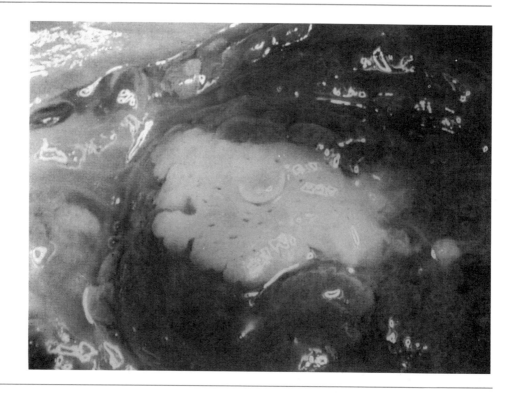

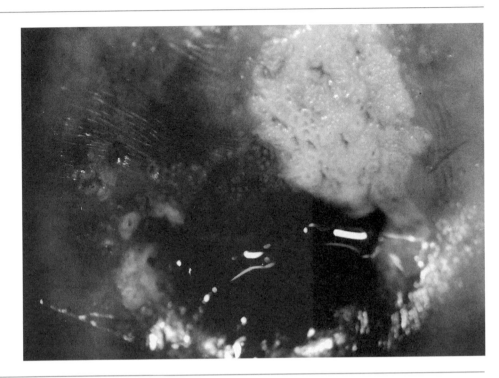

Figure 16.11   HPV/CIN 1 presents as a white lesion with surface spicules. Adjacent to the warty lesion is an area of mosaicism at the squamocolumnar junction, which is CIN 2.

2. The lesion is located on the ectocervix and can be seen entirely.

3. There is no involvement of the endocervix as determined by colposcopy and endocervical curettage.

Cryotherapy

Cryotherapy destroys the surface epithelium of the cervix by crystallizing the intracellular water, resulting in the eventual destruction of the cell. The temperature needed for effective destruction must be in the range of -20 to$-30°C$. Nitrous oxide ($-89°C$) and CO_2 ($-65°C$) produce temperatures below this range and, therefore, are the most commonly used gases for this procedure.

The technique believed to be most effective is a freeze-thaw-freeze method in which an ice ball is achieved 5 mm beyond the edge of the probe. The time required for this process is related to the pressure of the gas; the higher the pressure, the faster the ice ball is achieved.

Cryotherapy has been shown to be an effective method of treatment for CIN with very acceptable failure rates under certain conditions (41–45). It is a relatively safe procedure with few complications. Cervical stenosis is rare but can occur. Post-treatment bleeding is uncommon and is usually related to infection.

Cure rates are related to the grade of the lesion; CIN 3 has a greater chance of failure (Table 16.4). Townsend has shown that cures are also related to the size of the lesion; those "covering most of the ectocervix" have failure rates as high as 42%, compared with a 7% failure rate for lesions less than 1 cm in diameter (45). A presence of positive endocervical curettage findings also can significantly reduce the cure rate. Endocervical gland involvement is important because the failure rate in women with gland involvement was 27% compared with 9% in those who did not have such involvement (46).

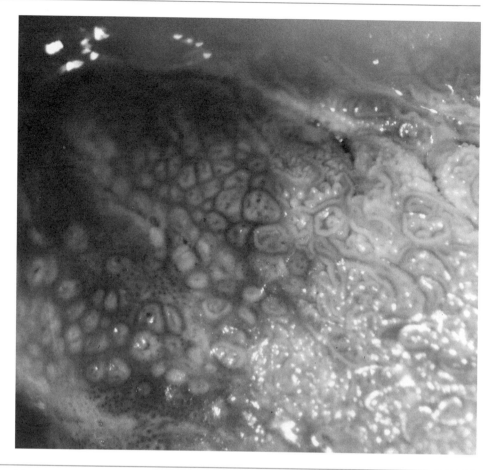

Figure 16.12   HPV/VIN 2–3. Cribriform pattern of HPV at periphery with mosaicism and punctation near the squamocolumnar junction.

Figure 16.13   CIN 3, showing a white lesion with associated punctation and coarse mosaicism.

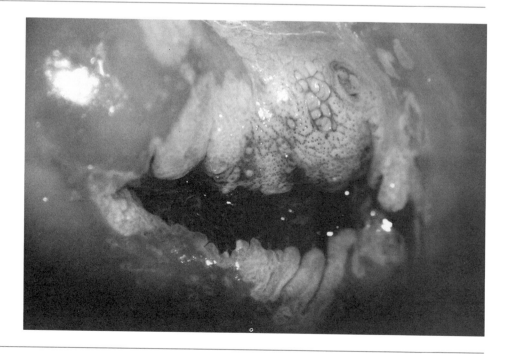

Table 16.4   Results of Cryotherapy for Cervical Intraepithelial Neoplasia (CIN) Compared to Grade of CIN

Author (Ref. No.)	CIN 1		CIN 2		CIN 3	
	No.	% Failure	No.	% Failure	No.	% Failure
Ostergard (42)	13/205	6.3%	7/93	7.5%	9/46	19.6%
Creasman (43)	15/276	5.4%	17/235	7.2%	46/259	17.8%
Andersen (41)	—	—	9/123	7.3%	17/74	23.0%
Benedet (44)	7/143	4.9%	19/448	4.2%	65/1003	6.5%
Total	35/624	5.6%	50/899	5.6%	137/1382	9.9%

Cryotherapy should therefore be considered acceptable therapy when the following criteria are met:

1. Cervical intraepithelial neoplasia, grade 1–2

2. Small lesion

3. Ectocervical location only

4. Negative endocervical curettage

5. No endocervical gland involvement on biopsy

Laser

Laser vaporization therapy may be chosen for patients in whom invasive cancer has been ruled out, the entire lesion can be seen, and endocervical curettage results are negative (48–56). Laser vaporization is particularly applicable in the following situations:

1. Large lesions that the cryoprobe cannot adequately cover

2. Irregular cervix with a "fish mouth" appearance and deep clefts

3. Extension of disease to the vagina or satellite lesions on the vagina

4. Lesions with extensive glandular involvement in which the treatment must reach beyond the deepest gland cleft

The major advantage of laser vaporization therapy is the ability to control exactly the depth and width of destruction by direct vision through the colposcope. Several studies have demonstrated that CIN can be found at an average of 1.2 mm and up to a depth of 5.2 mm inside the cervical crypts, regardless of whether the lesion is located in the exocervix or endocervix (46). Wright and Riopelle have shown that destruction or resection of the tissue to a depth of 3.8 mm will ablate all the involved glands in 99.7% of cases (47). Nevertheless, the tissue should be ablated to a depth of 7 mm, which is the location of the deepest endocervical gland. Both CIN 2 and CIN 3 with glandular involvement will have deeper crypt involvement than CIN 1 lesions without endocervical gland involvement (47).

The other major advantage of laser therapy is the rapid post-treatment healing phase. This process takes approximately 3–4 weeks, after which time a new epithelium has formed completely and, in most cases, will have a mature glycogen containing epithelium. The healed cervix has a normal appearance with a small visible transformation zone at the cervical os.

Tissue Interaction   When the laser beam contacts tissue, its energy is absorbed by the water in the cells, causing it to boil instantly. The cells explode into a puff of vapor (therefore, the term "laser vaporization"). The protein and mineral content is incinerated by the heat and leaves a charred appearance at the base of the exposed area. The depth of laser destruction is a function of the power of the beam (watts), the area of the beam (mm^2), and the length of time the laser remains in the tissue. The beam must be moved uniformly across the tissue surface to prevent deep destruction. The laser beam vaporizes a central area and leaves a narrow zone of heat necrosis surrounding the laser crater. The goal of laser vaporization is to minimize this area of tissue necrosis. This goal is accomplished by using high wattage (20 watts) with medium beam size (1.5 mm) and moving the beam uniformly but quickly over the surface. The zone of thermal necrosis will be ≤0.1 mm when the laser is used in this manner. Some lasers have a function called "super pulse," in which the laser beam is electronically switched off and on thousands of times per second, thereby allowing the tissue to cool between pulses to create less thermal necrosis.

Laser Technique   Before using the laser, the physician must be familiar with the physics of the procedure and thoroughly understand the safety precautions. If one has not had laser training, a laser course and hands-on training or a preceptorship is recommended.

To reduce vascularity and ensure that the patient is not pregnant, laser therapy should be performed during the first week following the menstrual period. Laser vaporization may be performed on an outpatient basis with local infiltration block, paracervical block, or no anesthesia. Patients uniformly agree that laser vaporization is less painful than colposcopic biopsy.

The patient should be placed in a comfortable position and should be examined colposcopically once again to ensure that she is a candidate for vaporization therapy. A solution of 1% *xylocaine* is injected either into the cervical stroma or as a paracervical block. The cervix and upper vagina is stained with Lugol's solution to ensure that all nonstaining areas will be included in the vaporization. The laser is activated to 20 watts of power with a 1.5-mm beam size. The focal length should be the same as the focal length of the colposcope (300 mm is recommended). The entire lesion should be outlined with the laser beam, allowing a 2- to 3-mm margin around the nonstaining area. Starting on the posterior lip of the cervix, tissue should be vaporized to a depth of the cervical glands. This level is identified by the appearance of the typical yellow collagen matrix and the absence of mucus bubbling onto the surface from the endocervical glands. A saline-dampened cotton-tipped applicator is used to wipe away the char frequently and to observe the yellow collagen matrix. It can also be used to apply pressure to small bleeding points while the laser beam coagulates the vessel. The laser crater is extended toward the SCJ until the entire lesion has been vaporized to the satisfactory depth.

Postlaser Instructions   A small amount of clear vaginal discharge may be present in 3–5 days. Approximately 5% of patients report spotting that abates within 2 weeks (48). If the spotting is as heavy as the menstrual period, the patient should be examined and Monsel's solution should be applied for hemostasis. The patient should refrain from tampon use, intercourse, and douching for 1 month; at 3 months after the procedure, a follow-up examination should be performed by Pap testing, colposcopy, or cervicography. The second follow-up examination should be performed at 6 months. If these evaluations are negative, routine Pap testing at 6- to 12-month intervals is recommended.

Laser Excision   When it is necessary to obtain tissue for diagnosis, the laser can be used to cut an excisional cone. For this procedure, *xylocaine* with *epinephrine* (*Pitressin*) is injected directly into the cervical stroma. The laser beam is adjusted to a watt size of 0.2–0.5 mm in diameter. The watt is set at 20–30 watts, and the peripheral margins of the cone are outlined. The incision is deepened circumferentially by passing the laser beam progressively across the tissue. Utilizing fine hooks, traction and countertraction are created at different points around the cone margin while the laser cuts deeply into the underlying stroma to a depth satisfactory to remove all of the abnormal tissue. To decrease the amount of thermal injury to the cone, the "super pulse" laser is ideal. When the appropriate depth has been obtained, the endocervical margin is incised, either with the laser, scissors, or a scalpel. An endocervical curettage may be performed to ensure that the margin is adequate. Additional hemostatic medication rarely is required. The postoperative follow-up is similar to that for vaporization. If the cone defect is significantly deep or large, there may be a higher incidence of bleeding or discharge (49).

Combination Laser Vaporization and Excision   Occasionally, the configuration of the cervix and the cervical lesion indicates that a vaporization technique be used on the exocervix and the excisional cone technique be used on the endocervix. This combination would be applicable to patients who have positive endocervical curettage findings with a very wide exocervical abnormality that is of a minor grade. Performing an excisional cone on the entire cervix would result in a large loss of cervical volume, whereas vaporizing the surface would reduce the loss of cervical stroma. The endocervical canal is the area that must be biopsied, and the excisional cone biopsy can be limited to that area.

Results of Laser Therapy   Laser therapy has extremely varied results (48–56). In general, the earlier reports showed a lower success rate; the improvement in success rate is attributed to the realization that the entire transformation zone needed to be treated, not just the individual identified lesions (Table 16.5). The therapeutic efficacy of laser conization versus knife conization is shown in Table 16.6, and a comparison of intraoperative and postoperative bleeding with the two procedures is listed in Table 16.7.

The CO_2 laser is an excellent tool for the treatment of CIN. In properly selected patients, the success rate with laser vaporization will be higher than 95% (Table 16.6). For patients

Table 16.5   Success Rate for Laser Vaporization

Author (Ref. No.)	CIN 1		CIN 2		CIN 3	
	No.	NED (%)	No.	NED (%)	No.	NED (%)
Burke (49)	49	41 (83.6)	42	36 (85.7)	40	31 (77.5)
Wright (50)	110	108 (98.2)	140	133 (95)	190	179 (94.2)
Rylander (51)	22	21 (95.5)	49	48 (97.9)	133	116 (87.2)
Jordan (52)	142	140 (98.6)	153	145 (94.7)	416	390 (93.8)
Baggish (53)	741	675 (91.1)	1048	978 (93.3)	1281	1228 (96)
Benedet (54)	312	301 (96.5)	472	428 (90.7)	773	702 (90.8)
Total	1376	1286 (93.5)	1904	1768 (92.9)	2833	2646 (93.4)

Table 16.6   Therapeutic Efficiency of Cervical Conization: Comparison Between Laser and Knife Techniques

Percentage of patients who are "cured" by conization			
Author (Ref. No.)	Laser	Author (Ref. No.)	Knife
Larsson (55)	95.6%	Larsson (55)	94.0%
Bostofte (48)	93.2%	Bostofte (48)	90.2%
Wright (50)	96.2%	Bjerre* (57)	94.8%
Baggish (56)	97.5%	Kolstad* (58)	97.6%

*Patients had negative cone margins.

Table 16.7   Perioperative and Postoperative Bleeding from Cervical Conization: Comparison Between Laser and Knife Techniques

Percentage of patients undergoing conization who develop significant vaginal bleeding			
Author (Ref. No.)	**Laser**	**Author (Ref. No.)**	**Knife**
Larsson (55)	2.3%	**Larsson** (55)	14.8%
Bostofte (48)	5.0%	**Bostofte** (48)	17.0%
Wright (50)	12.2%	**Jones** (59)	10.0%
Baggish (56)	2.5%	**Luesley** (60)	13.0%

who need diagnostic conization, the cone can be obtained by laser excision performed on an outpatient basis with less blood loss and fewer complications than with a cold knife conization (48–60).

Loop Electrosurgical Excision

Loop electrosurgical excision is a valuable tool for the diagnosis and treatment of CIN. It has the advantage of being able to perform simultaneously a diagnostic and therapeutic operation during one outpatient visit (61–71).

The tissue effect of electricity depends on the concentration of electrons (size of the wire), the power (watts), and the water content of the tissue. If low power or a large-diameter wire is used, the effect will be electrocautery and the thermal damage to tissue will be extensive. If the power is high, (35–55 watts) and the wire loop is small (0.5 mm), the effect will be electrosurgical and the tissue will have little thermal damage. The actual cutting is a result of a steam envelope developing at the interface between the wire loop and the water-laden tissue. This envelope is then pushed through the tissue, and the combination of electron flow and acoustical events separates the tissue. Following the excision, a 5-mm diameter ball electrode is used and the power is set at 50 watts. The ball is placed near the surface so a spark occurs between the ball and the tissue. This process is called electrofulguration, and it results in some thermal damage that leads to hemostasis. If too much fulguration occurs, the patient will develop an eschar with more discharge and the risk of infection and late bleeding will be higher.

Loop excision should not be used prior to identification of an intraepithelial lesion that requires treatment. The risk of the "see and treat" philosophy is that in women with only metaplasia, the entire transformation zone will be removed along with varying amounts of the cervical canal, thus potentially compromising fertility (69–71). This is particularly true of young women, who may have large, immature transformation zones with extensive acetowhite areas.

The technique for loop excision is as follows:

1. A nonconductive nylon-coated speculum with suction capability should be used. Nonconductive nylon-coated vaginal retractors are also helpful.

2. The cervix is evaluated colposcopically to delineate the lesion and determine endocervical involvement.

3. Local anesthesia (1–2% *xylocaine* with *epinephrine*) is injected at the 3, 6, 9, and 12 o'clock positions or directly into the stroma at the line of excision.

4. The grounding pad is attached to the patient's thigh.

5. The power source—electrosurgical generator—is set at 35–55 watts using a blend of cutting and coagulation.

6. Suction is attached to the speculum.

7. The selected loop is based on the size of the transformation zone, preferably to excise tissue in one piece.

8. The base is coagulated with a ball electrode (5 mm) at 50–60 watts. Application of Monsel's solution is optional.

Complications following loop electrosurgical excision are fairly minimal and compare favorably with those following laser ablation and conization. Intraoperative hemorrhage, postoperative hemorrhage, and cervical stenosis can occur but at acceptably low rates, as noted in Table 16.8. The SCJ is visible in more than 90% of patients following this procedure.

One advantage of loop excision over ablative procedures is the ability to diagnose unsuspected invasive disease (Table 16.9). The loop has several advantages over the laser:

1. Treatment time is shorter.

2. It is easier to learn.

Table 16.8   Complications of Electrosurgical Excision

Complications	Number of Patients	Operative Hemorrhage	Postoperative Hemorrhage	Cervical Stenosis
Prendeville (61)	111	2	2	—
Whiteley (62)	80	0	3	—
Mor-Yosef (63)	50	1	3	—
Bigrigg (64)	1000	0	6	—
Gunasekera (65)	98	0	0	—
Howe (66)	100	0	1	—
Minucci (67)	130	0	1	2
Wright (68)	432	0	8	2
Luesley (69)	616	0	24	7
Total	2617	3 (0.001%)	48 (1.8%)	11/6178 (1.0%)

Table 16.9   Unsuspected Invasion in Electrosurgical Excision Specimens

Author (Ref. No.)	Patients	Microinvasive	Invasive
Prendeville (61)	102	1	—
Bigrigg (64)	1000	5	—
Gunasekera (65)	98	—	1
Howe (66)	100	1	—
Chappatte (70)	100	3	—
Wright (68)	141	1	—
Luesley (69)	616	4	6 (adenocarcinoma *in situ*)
Total	2157	15 (0.7%)	1 (0.04%)

3. There is no hazard to the eyesight.

4. Equipment breakdowns occur less often.

5. The cone sample is better than with laser.

6. There is less handling of the tissues.

7. Discomfort is reduced.

One study of these two modes of therapy compared pain and operative time in a randomized fashion (65). Electrosurgical excision showed an advantage over laser therapy (Table 16.10).

The most important issue in selecting therapy is whether the loop is an effective means of eradicating CIN. A combined literature series indicated a recurrent rate of approximately 4% (Table 16.11). This rate compares favorably with the recurrence rate for other types of procedures used in the treatment of CIN.

Following are possible contraindications to the loop procedure:

1. Patient anxiety

2. Contraindication to local anesthesia or vasoconstrictor

3. Extremely large lesions

Table 16.10   Grade of Discomfort of Large Loop Excision versus Laser Conization

Side Effect	Loop Excision (n=98)	Laser (n=101)
Not unpleasant	80 (92%)	32 (32%)
Moderately unpleasant	16 (16%)	50 (50%)
Very unpleasant	2 (2%)	19 (18%)
Operative time	20–50 sec (mean 16 sec)	4–15 min (mean 6.5 min)

From **Gunasekera PC, Phipps JH, Lewis BV**. Large loop excision of the transformation zone (LLETZ) compared to carbon dioxide laser in the treatment of CIN: a superior mode of treatment. *Br J Obstet Gynecol* 1990;97:995–8.

Table 16.11   Results of Loop Electrosurgical Excision

Author (Ref. No.)	Number of Patients Treated	Number of Patients Recurred
Prendeville (61)	102	2
Whiteley (62)	80	4
Bigrigg (64)	1000	41
Gunasekera (65)	98	7
Luesley (69)	616	27
Murdoch (71)	600	16
Total	2496	97 (3.9%)

4. Vaginal extension

5. Obvious clinical carcinoma

Conization

Conization of the cervix plays an important role in the management of CIN. Before the availability of colposcopy, conization was the standard method of evaluating an abnormal Pap test result. Conization is both a diagnostic and therapeutic procedure and has the advantage over ablative therapies of providing tissue for further evaluation to rule out invasive cancer (55–60).

Conization is indicated for diagnosis in women with HSIL on the Pap test under the following conditions:

1. Limits of the lesion cannot be visualized with colposcopy.

2. The SCJ is not seen at colposcopy.

3. Endocervical curettage histologic findings are positive for CIN 2 or CIN 3.

4. There is a lack of correlation between cytology, biopsy, and colposcopy results.

5. Microinvasion is suspected based on biopsy, colposcopy, or cytology results.

6. The colposcopist is unable to rule out invasive cancer.

Lesions with positive margins are more likely to recur following conization (55–57) (Table 16.12). Dempoulos (72) has shown that endocervical gland involvement also is predictive of recurrence (23.6% with gland involvement compared with 11.3% without gland involvement).

Hysterectomy

Hysterectomy for treatment of CIN is currently considered too radical. Coppleson (73) reported 38 cases of invasive cancer occurring after hysterectomy among 8998 women (0.4%). The incidence of significant bleeding, infection, and other complications, including death, are higher with hysterectomy than with other means of treating CIN. There are some situations in which hysterectomy remains a valid and appropriate method of treatment for CIN:

1. Microinvasion

2. Cervical intraepithelial neoplasia at limits of conization specimen

3. Poor compliance with follow-up

Table 16.12   Recurrence of Cervical Intraepithelial Neoplasia (CIN) after Cone Biopsy

Author (Ref. No.)	Patients	Negative Margins	Positive Margins
Larsson (55)	683	56	246
Bjerre (57)	1226	64	429
Kolstad (58)	1121	27	291
Total	3030	147 (4.9%)	966 (31.9%)

4. Other gynecologic problems requiring hysterectomy, such as fibroids, prolapse, endometriosis, and pelvic inflammatory disease

5. Cancerphobia

Glandular Cell Abnormalities

Atypical Glandular Cells of Undetermined Significance

The Bethesda system includes a category for glandular cell abnormalities (21). These cells may be classified as 1) adenocarcinoma or 2) *atypical glandular cells of undetermined significance (AGCUS).* Atypical endocervical cells are important because of their risk of significant disease. In a series of 63 patients from whom subsequent cervical biopsy or hysterectomy specimens were evaluated, 17 women had CIN 2 or CIN 3, five women had adenocarcinoma *in situ,* and two women had invasive adenocarcinoma (74). An additional eight patients had CIN 1, and two women had endometrial hyperplasia. Overall, 32 patients (50.8%) had significant cervical lesions. This is a much higher positivity rate than that for ASCUS Pap test results.

Adenocarcinoma *In Situ*

In adenocarcinoma *in situ* (AIS), the endocervical glandular cells are replaced by tall columnar cells with nuclear stratification, hyperchromasia, irregularity, and increased mitotic activity (75–78). Cellular proliferation results in crowded, cribriform glands. However, the normal branching pattern of the endocervical glands is maintained. Most neoplastic cells resemble those of the endocervical mucinous epithelium. Endometrioid and intestinal cell types occur less often. About 50% of women with cervical AIS also have squamous CIN. Thus, some of the AIS lesions represent incidental findings in specimens removed for treatment of squamous neoplasia. Because AIS is located near or above the transformation zone, conventional cervical specimens may not be effective to sample AIS. Obtaining specimens by cytobrush may improve detection of AIS. If the focus of AIS is small, cervical biopsy and endocervical curettage may have negative findings. In such cases, a more comprehensive survey of the cervix in the form of conization is necessary. This type of specimen also allows exclusion of coexisting invasive adenocarcinoma. **The term "microinvasion" should not be used to describe adenocarcinomas.** Once the gland has been invaded, there is no definable technique for identifying the true "depth of invasion," because the invasion may have originated from the mucosal surface or the periphery of the underlying glands. The "breakthrough" of the basement membrane cannot truly be described; therefore, the tumor is either adenocarcinoma *in situ* or invasive adenocarcinoma.

With the recent apparent increase in invasive adenocarcinoma of the endocervix, more attention has been directed toward adenocarcinoma *in situ.* There is evidence that adenocarcinoma *in situ* may progress to invasive cancer (75). Boone reported a series of 52 cases of adenocarcinoma of the uterine cervix in which the results of 18 endocervical biopsies were interpreted as negative 3–7 years prior to the presentation with cancer. In five of these cases, adenocarcinoma *in situ* was found.

Bertrand studied the anatomic distribution of AIS in 23 women (76). All 23 patients had AIS involving both the surface and the glandular endocervical epithelium, often with the deepest glandular cleft also involved. The entire endocervical canal was at risk; nearly one-half of the patients had lesions between 1.5 and 3.0 cm from the external os. Fifteen patients had unifocal disease, three had multifocal disease, and five patients had AIS of undermined type. Eleven of the 23 patients had squamous intraepithelial lesions as well as AIS. Muntz reported 40 patients with AIS who had cervical conization (77). Twenty-three of 40 (58%) had coexisting squamous intraepithelial lesions and two patients had invasive squamous cell carcinoma. Of the 22 patients who underwent hysterectomy, the margins on the cone specimen were positive in 10 patients, and 70% had residual AIS, including two with foci of invasive adenocarcinoma. One of the 12 patients with negative margins had focal residual adenocarcinoma in the hysterectomy specimen. Eighteen women had conization only with negative margins and had no relapse of disease after a medium interval of 3 years. Thus, positive margins on the conization specimen are significant findings in these patients.

Poyner published the results of a more alarming study of 28 patients with AIS (78). Of the eight patients with positive margins who underwent repeat conization or hysterectomy, three had residual AIS and one patient had invasive adenocarcinoma. Four of 10 patients with negative margins who underwent hysterectomy or repeat conization had residual AIS. One patient in whom the cone margin could not be evaluated was found to have invasive adenocarcinoma. Of the 15 patients treated conservatively with repeat conization of the cervix and close follow-up, seven (47%) had a recurrent glandular lesion detected after the conization, including invasive adenocarcinomas in two women. More disturbing is the finding that a glandular lesion was not suspected in 48% of the patients, based on Pap test and endocervical curettage results obtained prior to conization of the cervix.

Adenocarcinoma *in situ* must be considered a serious cancer precursor of adenocarcinoma. The entire endocervical canal is at risk, and detection of the lesion with cytology or endocervical curettage may not be reliable. Any patient with a positive cone margin should undergo repeat conization. If fertility is not desired, a hysterectomy should be performed because of the risk of recurrence, even in the presence of negative margins.

Vaginal Intraepithelial Neoplasia

Vaginal intraepithelial neoplasia (VAIN) often accompanies CIN and is believed to have a similar cause (79). VAIN lesions may be extensions onto the vagina from the CIN or they may be satellite lesions occurring mainly in the upper vagina. Because the vagina does not have a transformation zone with immature epithelial cells to be infected by HPV, the mechanism of entry of HPV is by way of skin abrasions from coitus or tampon use. As these abrasions heal with metaplastic squamous cells, the HPV may begin its growth in a manner similar to that in the cervical transformation zone (Fig. 16.14).

Signs

Vaginal intraepithelial neoplasia lesions are asymptomatic. Because they often accompany active HPV infection, the patient may complain of vulvar warts or an odoriforous vaginal discharge from vaginal warts.

Screening

Women with an intact cervix should undergo routine cytologic screening. Because VAIN is nearly always accompanied by CIN, the Pap test result is likely to be positive when VAIN is present. The vagina should be carefully inspected by colposcopic examination at the time of colposcopy for any CIN lesion. Particular attention should be paid to the upper vagina. Women who have persistent positive Pap test results after treatment of CIN should be examined carefully for VAIN. For women in whom the cervix has been removed for cervical neoplasia, Pap testing should be performed at regular intervals initially, depending on the diagnosis and severity of lesion, and yearly thereafter.

Diagnosis

Colposcopic examination and directed biopsy are the mainstay of diagnosis of VAIN. Typically, the lesions are located along the vaginal ridges, are ovoid in shape and slightly raised, and often have surface spicules. VAIN 1 lesions usually are accompanied by a significant amount of koilocytosis indicating their HPV origin (Fig. 16.15). As the lesions progress to the VAIN 2, they have a thicker acetowhite epithelium, a more raised external border, and less iodine uptake (Fig. 16.16). When VAIN 3 occurs, the surface may become papillary and the vascular patterns of punction and mosaic may occur (Fig. 16.17). Early invasion is typified by vascular patterns similar to those of the cervix.

474

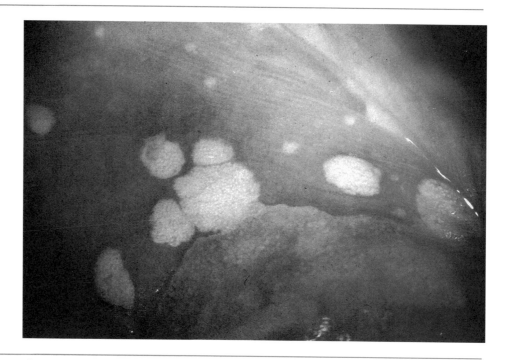

Figure 16.14   Vaginal condylomata in the posterior fornix.

Figure 16.15   HPV/VAIN 1. Note the surface spicules with partial uptake of Lugol's stain.

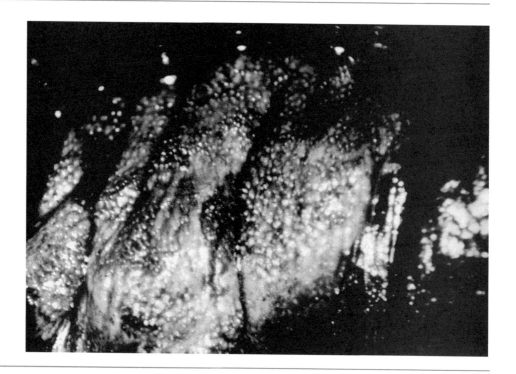

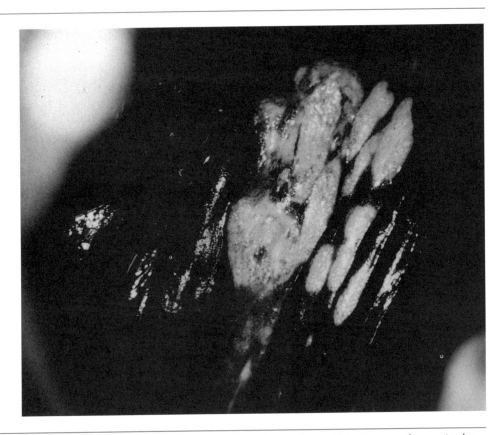

Figure 16.16   VAIN 2. There are multifocal raised, ovoid lesions on the vaginal rugae that are outlined by Lugol's stain.

Figure 16.17   VAIN 3. The lesion is located in the center of HPV spicules with partial uptake of Lugol's stain.

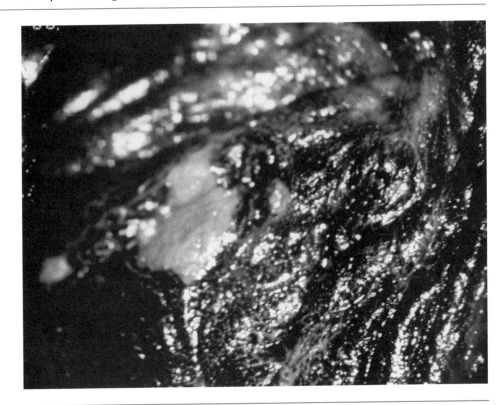

Treatment

Patients with VAIN 1/HPV infection do not require treatment. These lesions will often regress, are often multifocal, and recur quickly when treated with ablative therapy. VAIN 2 lesions are generally treated by laser ablation. VAIN 3 lesions are more likely to harbor an early invasive lesion. Hoffman reported 32 patients who underwent upper vaginectomy for VAIN 3 (80). Occult invasive carcinoma was found in nine patients (28%). It is recommended that in older patients VAIN 3 lesions located in the dimples of the vaginal cuff be excised in order to rule out occult invasive cancer. **VAIN 3 lesions that are adequately sampled to rule out invasive disease can be treated with laser therapy.**

Cryosurgery should not be used in the vagina because the depth of injury cannot be controlled and inadvertent injury to the bladder or rectum may occur. Superficial fulguration with electrosurgical ball cautery may be utilized under colposcopic control to observe the depth of destruction by wiping away the epithelial tissue as it is ablated. Excision is an excellent method for treatment of upper vaginal lesions in a small area. Occasionally, total vaginectomy will be required for a VAIN 3 lesion occupying the entire vagina. It should be accompanied by a split-thickness skin graft. This aggressive treatment for widespread vaginal lesions should not be used for VAIN 2.

The malignant potential of VAIN appears to be less than that of CIN. In a review of 136 cases of carcinoma *in situ* of the vagina over a 30-year period (79), four cases (3%) progressed to invasive vaginal cancer despite the use of various treatment methods.

Vulvar Intraepithelial Disease

Vulvar Dystrophies

In the past, terms such as "leukoplakia," "lichen sclerosis et atrophicus," "primary atrophy," "sclerotic dermatosis," "atrophic and hyperplastic vulvitis," and "kraurosis vulvae" have been used to denote disorders of epithelial growth and differentiation (81). In 1966, Jeffcoate (82) suggested that these terms did not refer to separate disease entities because their macroscopic and microscopic appearances were variable and interchangeable. He assigned the generic term *chronic vulvar dystrophy* to the entire group of lesions.

The International Society for the Study of Vulvar Disease (ISSVD) recommended that the old "dystrophy" terminology be replaced by a new classification under the pathologic heading "nonneoplastic epithelial disorders of skin and mucosa." This classification is shown in Table 16.13. In all cases, diagnosis requires biopsy of suspicious-looking lesions,

---

Table 16.13   Classification of Epithelial Vulvar Diseases

Nonneoplastic epithelial disorders of skin and mucosa
   Lichen sclerosus (lichen sclerosis et atrophicus)
   Squamous hyperplasia (formerly hyperplastic dystrophy)
   Other dermatoses
Mixed nonneoplastic and neoplastic epithelial disorders
Intraepithelial neoplasia
   Squamous intraepithelial neoplasia
      VIN 1
      VIN 2
      VIN 3 (severe dysplasia or carcinoma *in situ*)
   Nonsquamous intraepithelial neoplasia
      Paget's disease
      Tumors of melanocytes, noninvasive
Invasive tumors

From **Committee on Terminology, International Society for the Study of Vulvar Disease.** New nomenclature for vulvar disease. *Int J Gynecol Pathol* 1989;8:83.

which are best detected by careful inspection of the vulva in a bright light aided, if necessary, by a magnifying glass (83).

The malignant potential of these nonneoplastic epithelial disorders is low, particularly now that the lesions with atypia are classified as vulvar intraepithelial neoplasia (VIN). However, patients with lichen sclerosis and concomitant hyperplasia may be at particular risk (84).

Vulvar Intraepithelial Neoplasia

As with the vulvar dystrophies, there has been confusion regarding the nomenclature for VIN. Four major terms have been used: "erythroplasia of Queyrat," "Bowen's disease," "carcinoma *in situ simplex*," and "Paget's disease." In 1976, the ISSVD decreed that the first three lesions were merely gross variants of the same disease process and that all of these entities should be included under the umbrella term "squamous cell carcinoma *in situ*" (stage 0) (81). In 1986, the ISSVD recommended the term "vulvar intraepithelial neoplasia (VIN)" (Table 16.13).

VIN is graded as 1 (mild dysplasia), 2 (moderate dysplasia), or 3 (severe dysplasia or carcinoma *in situ*) on the basis of cellular immaturity, nuclear abnormalities, maturation disturbance, and mitotic activity. In VIN 1, immature cells, cellular disorganization, and mitotic activity occur predominantly in the lower one-third of the epithelium, whereas in VIN 3, immature cells with scanty cytoplasm and severe chromatinic alterations occupy most of the epithelium (Fig. 16.18). Dyskeratotic cells and mitotic figures occur in the superficial layer. The appearance of VIN 2 is intermediate between VIN 1 and VIN 3. Additional cytopathic changes of HPV infection, such as perinuclear halos with displacement of the nuclei by the intracytoplasmic viral protein, thickened cell borders, binucleation, and multinucleation, are common in the superficial layers of VIN, especially in VIN 1 and VIN 2.

Figure 16.18   Carcinoma *in situ* of the vulva (VIN 3). Immature atypical cells are seen throughout epithelium. (From **Fu YS, Woodruff JD.** Pathology. In: **Berek JS, Hacker NF,** eds. *Practical Gynecologic Oncology.* 2nd ed. Baltimore: Williams & Wilkins, 1994:161.)

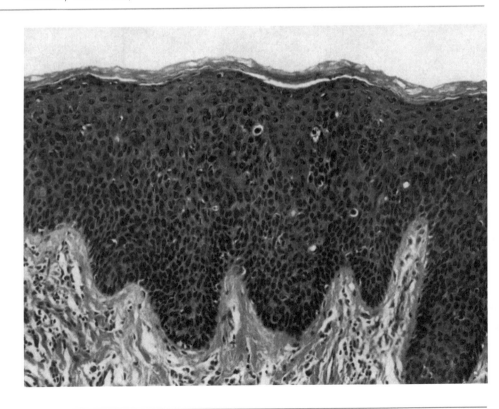

These viral changes are not definitive evidence of neoplasia but are indicative of viral exposure (85). Most vulvar condylomas are associated with HPV types 6 and 11, whereas HPV type 16 is detected in more than 80% of VIN by molecular techniques.

Vulvar intraepithelial neoplasia 3 can be unifocal or multifocal. Typically, multifocal VIN 3 presents with small hyperpigmented lesions on the labia major (Fig. 16.19). Some cases of VIN 3 are more confluent, extending to the posterior fourchette and involving the perineal tissues. The term *bowenoid papulosis* (bowenoid dysplasia) has been used to describe multifocal VIN lesions ranging from grade 1 to grade 3. Clinically, patients with bowenoid papulosis present with multiple small, pigmented papules (40% of cases) that are usually <5 mm in diameter. Most women are in their twenties, and some are pregnant. After childbirth, the lesions may regress spontaneously. However, the term "bowenoid papulosis" is no longer recommended by the ISSVD.

Paget's Disease of the Vulva

Extramammary Paget's disease of the vulva (adenocarcinoma *in situ*) was described (86) 27 years after the description by Sir James Paget of the mammary lesion that now bears his name. Some patients with vulvar Paget's disease have an underlying adenocarcinoma, although the precise frequency is difficult to ascertain.

Most cases of vulvar Paget's disease are intraepithelial. Because these lesions demonstrate apocrine differentiation, the malignant cells are believed to arise from undifferentiated basal cells, which convert into an appendage type of cell during carcinogenesis (Fig. 16.20). The "transformed cells" spread intraepithelially throughout the squamous epithelium and may extend into the appendages. In most patients with an underlying invasive carcinoma of the apocrine sweat gland, Bartholin gland, or anorectum, the malignant cells

Figure 16.19 VIN 3. *A,* A multifocal VIN 3 lesion with multiple small hyperpigmented lesions on the labia major. *B,* VIN 3 with more confluent hyperpigmented areas on the posterior fourchette with extensive perianal involvement. (From **Berek JS, Hacker NF,** eds. *Practical Gynecologic Oncology.* 2nd ed. Baltimore: Williams & Wilkins, 1994:213.)

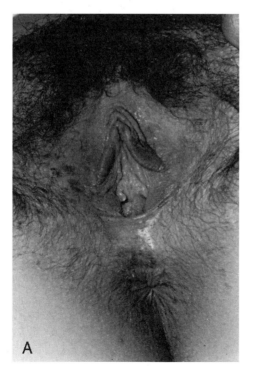 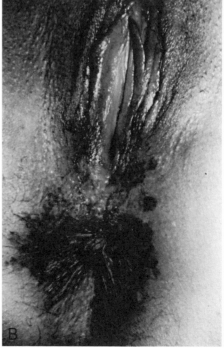

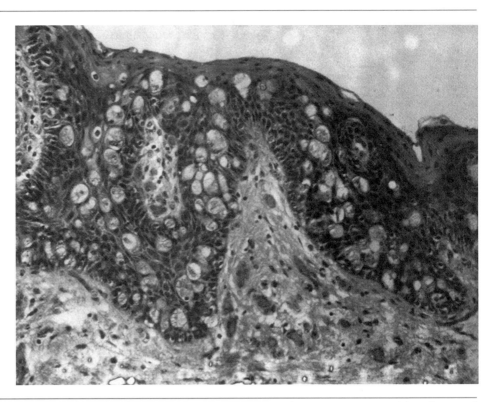

Figure 16.20   Paget's disease of vulva. The epidermis is permeated by abnormal cells with vacuolated cytoplasm and atypical nuclei. This heavy concentration of abnormal cells in the parabasal layers is typical of Paget's disease. (From **Fu YS, Woodruff JD.** Pathology. In: **Berek JS, Hacker NF,** eds. *Practical Gynecologic Oncology.* 2nd ed. Baltimore: Williams & Wilkins, 1994:162.)

are believed to migrate through the dermal ductal structures and reach the epidermis. In such cases, metastasis to the regional lymph nodes and other sites can occur.

Paget's disease must be distinguished from superficial spreading melanoma. All sections should be studied thoroughly using differential staining, particularly *periodic acid-Schiff* (PAS) and *mucicarmine* stains. Mucicarmine has routinely positive results in the cells of Paget's disease and negative results in melanotic lesion.

Clinical Features   Paget's disease of the vulva predominantly affects postmenopausal Caucasian women, and the presenting symptoms are usually pruritus and vulvar soreness. The lesion has an eczematoid appearance macroscopically and usually begins on the hair-bearing portions of the vulva (Fig. 16.21). It may extend to involve the mons pubis, thighs, and buttocks. Extension to involve the mucosa of the rectum, vagina, or urinary tract also has been described (87). The more extensive lesions are usually raised and velvety in appearance.

A second synchronous or metachronous primary neoplasm is associated with extramammary Paget's disease in about 30% of patients (88). Associated carcinomas have been reported in the cervix, colon, bladder, gallbladder, and breast. When the anal mucosa is involved, there usually is an underlying rectal adenocarcinoma (84).

Treatment

VIN   The treatment of VIN has varied from wide excision to the performance of a superficial or "skinning" vulvectomy (90–93). Although the treatment originally recommended for "carcinoma *in situ*" of the vulva was wide excision, fears that the disease frequently was preinvasive led to the widespread use of superficial vulvectomy (92). Because the risk

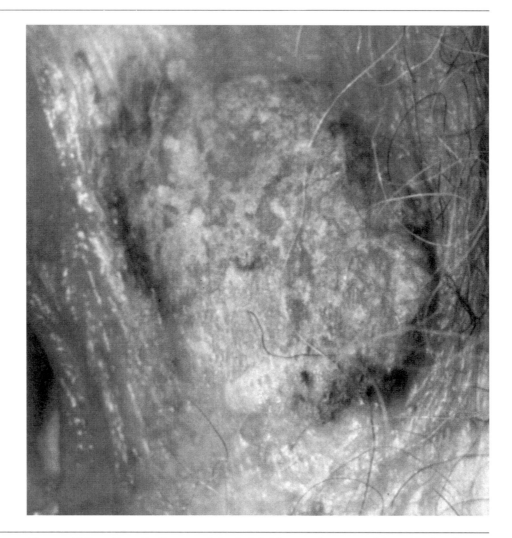

Figure 16.21   Paget's disease of the left labium majus treated by wide local excision. (From **Wilkinson EJ, Stone IK.** *Atlas of Vulvar Disease.* Baltimore: Williams & Wilkins, 1995:87.)

of progression is relatively uncommon, typically 5–10% (90), extensive surgery is not warranted. This is particularly true because many VIN lesions are found in premenopausal women.

The therapeutic alternatives for VIN are 1) simple excision, 2) laser ablation, or 3) superficial vulvectomy with or without split-thickness skin grafting.

Excision of small foci of disease produces excellent results and has the advantage of providing a histopathologic specimen. Although multifocal or extensive lesions may be difficult to treat by this approach, it offers the potential for the most cosmetic result. Repeat excision is often necessary but can typically be accomplished without vulvectomy (91, 93).

The carbon dioxide laser can be used for multifocal lesions but is unnecessary for unifocal disease. The disadvantages are that it can be painful and costly and it does not provide a histopathologic specimen (94).

Superficial vulvectomy is appropriate for extensive and recurrent VIN (93). The goal of the surgery is to extirpate all of the disease while preserving as much of the normal vulvar anatomy as possible. The anterior vulva and the clitoris should be preserved if possible. In

481

some patients, the disease extends up the anus, which also must be resected. An effort should be made to close the vulvar defect primarily, reserving the use of skin grafts for instances in which the vulvar defect cannot be closed because the resection is so extensive. Split-thickness skin grafts can be harvested from the thighs or buttocks, but the latter is more easily concealed (95).

Paget's Disease   **Unlike squamous cell carcinoma *in situ*, in which the histologic extent of disease usually correlates closely with the macroscopic lesion, Paget's disease usually extends well beyond the gross lesion** (96). This extension results in positive surgical margins and frequent local recurrence unless a wide local excision is performed. **Underlying adenocarcinomas are usually clinically apparent, but this finding does not occur invariably; therefore, the underlying dermis should be removed for adequate histologic evaluation.** For this reason, laser therapy is unsatisfactory in treating primary Paget's disease. If underlying invasive carcinoma is present, it should be treated in the same manner as a squamous vulvar cancer. This treatment usually will require radical vulvectomy and at least an ipsilateral inguinal-femoral lymphadenectomy.

Recurrent lesions are almost always *in situ*, although there has been at least one report of an underlying adenocarcinoma in recurrent Paget's disease (83). In general, it is reasonable to treat recurrent lesions with surgical excision.

References

1. **Pund ER, Nieburgs H, Nettles JB, Caldwell JD.** Preinvasive carcinoma of the cervix uteri: seven cases in which it was detected by examination of routine endocervical smears. *Arch Pathol Lab Med* 1947;44:571–7.

2. **Koss LG, Stewart FW, Foote FW, Jordan MJ, Bader GM, Day E.** Some histological aspects of behavior of epidermoid carcinoma *in situ* and related lesions of the uterine cervix. *Cancer* 1963;16:1160–211.

3. **Richart RM.** Natural history of cervical intraepithelial neoplasia. *Clin Obstet Gynecol* 1968; 10:748.

4. **Nasiell K, Roger V, Nasiell M.** Behavior of mild cervical dysplasia during long-term follow-up. *Obstet Gynecol* 1986;5:665–9.

5. **Hatch KD.** *Handbook of Colposcopy. Diagnosis and Treatment of Lower Genital Tract Neoplasia and HPV Infections.* Boston: Little, Brown and Co., 1989:7–19.

6. **Koss LG, Durfee GR.** Unusual patterns of squamous epithelium of the uterine cervix: cytologic and pathologic study of koilocytotic atypia. *Ann N Y Acad Sci* 1956;63:1235–40.

7. **Meisels A, Fortin R, Roy M.** Condylomatous lesions of the cervix. II. Cytologic, colposcopic and histopathologic study. *Acta Cytol* 1977;21:379–90.

8. **Beckmann AM, Myerson D, Daling JR, Kiuiat NB, Fenoglio CM, McDougall JK.** Detection and localization of human papillomavirus DNA in human genital condylomas by *in situ* hydridization with biotinylated probes. *J Med Virol* 1985;16:265–73.

9. **Schneider A, Oltersdorf T, Schneider V, Gissman L.** Distribution pattern of human papilloma virus 16 genome in cervical neoplasia by molecular *in situ* hybridization of tissue sections. *Int J Cancer* 1987;39:717–21.

10. **Crum CP, Mitao M, Levine RU, Silverstein S.** Cervical papilloma viruses segregate within morphologically distinct precancerous lesions. *J Virol* 1985;54:675–81.

11. **Durst M, Kleinheinz A, Hotz M, Gissman L.** The physical state of human papillomavirus type 16 DNA in benign and malignant genital tumors. *J Gen Virol* 1985;66:1515–22.

12. **Munger K, Phelps WC, Bubb V, Howley PM, Schlegal R.** The E6 and E7 genes of the human papillomavirus type 16 together are necessary and sufficient for transformation of primary human keratinocytes. *J Virol* 1989;63:4417–21.

13. **McCance DJ, Kopan R, Fuchs E, Laimins LA.** Human papillomavirus type 16 alters human epithelial cell differentiation *in vitro*. *Proc Natl Acad Sci U S A* 1988;85:7169–73.

14. **Dyson N, Howley PM, Munger K, Harlow E.** The human papillomavirus-16E-oncoprotein is able to bind to the retinoblastoma gene produce. *Science* 1989;243:934–7.

15. **Yee CL, Krishnan-Hewiett I, Baker CC, Schlegal R, Howley PM.** Presences and expression of human papillomavirus sequences in human cervical carcinoma cell lines. *Am J Pathol* 1985; 119:3261–6.

16. **Koutsky LA, Holmes KK, Critchlow CW, Stevens CE, Paavonen J, Becicman AM.** A cohort study of the risk of cervical intraepithelial neoplasia grade 2 or 3 in relation to papillomavirus infection. *N Engl J Med* 1992;327:1272–8.

17. **Lorincz AT, Reid R, Jenson AB, Kurman RT.** Human papillomavirus infection of the cervix: relative risk associations of 15 common anogenital types. *Obstet Gynecol* 1992;79:328–37.

18. **Bauer HM, Ting Y, Greer CE, Chambers JC, Tashiro CJ, Chimera J, et al.** Genital human papillomavirus infection in female university students as determined by a PCR-based method. *JAMA* 1991;265:472–7.

19. **Ley C, Bauer HM, Reingold A, Schiffman MH, Chambers JC, Tashiro CJ, et al.** Determinants of genital papillomavirus infection in young women. *J Natl Cancer Inst* 1991;83:997–1003.

20. **Shiffman MH.** Recent progress in defining the epidemiology of human papillomavirus infection and cervical cancer. *J Natl Cancer Inst* 1992;84:398–9.

21. **National Cancer Institute Workshop.** The 188 Bethesda system for reporting cervical/vaginal cytological diagnoses. *JAMA* 1989;262:931–4.

22. **Kataja V, Syrjanen K, Syrjanen S, Mantyjarui R, Yiskoski M, Sacriicoski S, et al.** Prospective follow-up of genital HPV infections: survival analysis of the HPV typing data. *Eur J Epidemiol* 1990;6:9–14.

23. **Willett GD, Kurman RJ, Reid R, Greenberg M, Jenson AB, Lorincz AT.** Correlation of the histologic appearance of intraepithelial neoplasia of the cervix with human papillomavirus types. Emphasis on the low grade lesions including so-called flat condyloma. *Int J Gynecol Pathol* 1989;8:18–25.

24. **Ismail SM, Colclough AB, Dinnen JS, Eakins D, Evans DMD, Gradwell E, et al.** Reporting cervical intraepithelial neoplasia (CIN): intra- and interpathologist variation and factors associated with disagreement. *Histopathology* 1990;16:371–6.

25. **Sherman ME, Schiffman MH, Erozan YS, Wacholder S, Kurman RJ.** The Bethesda system. A proposal for reporting abnormal cervical smears based on the reproducibility of cytopathologic diagnoses. *Arch Pathol Lab Med* 1992;116:1155–8.

26. **Richart RM, Wright TC.** Controversies in the management of low grade cervical intraepithelial neoplasia. *Cancer* 1993;71:1413–21.

27. **Weitzman GA, Korhonen MO, Reeves KO, Irwin JF, Carter TS, Kaufman RH.** Endocervical brush cytology: an alternative to endocervical curettage? *J Reprod Med* 1988;33–677.

28. **Campion MJ, McCance DJ, Cuzick J, Singer A.** Progressive potential of mild cervical atypia: prospective cytological, colposcopic and virological study. *Lancet* 1986;2:237–40.

29. **Benedet JL, Anderson GH, Boyes DA.** Colposcopic accuracy in the diagnosis of microinvasive and occult invasive carcinoma of the cervix. *Obstet Gynecol* 1985;65:577–62.

30. **Townsend DE, Richart RM.** Diagnostic errors in colposcopy. *Gynecol Oncol* 1981;12:S259–64.

31. **Urcuyo R, Rome RM, Nelson JH.** Some observations on the value of endocervical curettage performed as an integral part of colposcopic examination of patients with abnormal cervical cytology. *Am J Obstet Gynecol* 1977;128:787–92.

32. **Cox JT, Lorincz AT, Schiffman MH, Sherman ME, Cullen A, Kurman RJ.** Human papillomavirus testing by hybrid capture appears to be useful in triaging women with cytologic diagnosis of atypical squamous cells of undetermined significance. *Am J Obstet Gynecol* 1995; 172:946–54.

33. **August N.** Cervicography for evaluating the "atypical" Papanicolaou smear. *J Reprod Med* 1991;36:89.

34. **Jones DED, Creasman WT, Dombroski RA, Lentz SS, Waeltz JL.** Evaluation of the atypical pap smear. *Am J Obstet Gynecol* 1987;157:544–9.

35. **Campion MJ, diPaola FM, Franklin III EW, Stone K, Vellios F.** Cancer Research and Treatment Center, St. Joseph's Hospital of Atlanta: Cervicography: Screening Tool or Triage Strategy. I. Prospective Evaluation in Cervical Screening. Abstract: International Federation of Colposcopy and Cervical Pathology, Rome 1991.

36. **Tawa K, Forsythe A, Cove JK, Saltz A, Peters HW, Watring WG.** A comparison of the Papanicolaou smear and the cervigram: sensitivity, specificity, and cost analysis. *Obstet Gynecol* 1988;71:229–35.

37. **Borst M, Butterworth CE, Baker V, Kay Kendall K, Gore H, Soong SJ, Hatch KO.** HPV screening for women with atypical Pap smears. *J Reprod Med* 1991;36:95–9.

38. **van Oortmarssen GJ, Habbema JDF.** Epidemiological evidence for age-dependent regression of preinvasive cervical cancer. *Br J Cancer* 1991;64:559–65.

39. **Noumoff JS.** Atypia in cervical cytology as a risk factor for intraepithelial neoplasia. *Am J Obstet Gynecol* 1987;156:628–31.

40. **Syrjanen K, Kataja V, Yliskoski M, Chang F, Syrjanen S, Saarikoski S.** National history of cervical human papillomavirus lesions does not substantiate the biologic relevance of the Bethesda system. *Obstet Gynecol* 1992;79:675–82.

41. **Andersen ES, Thorup K, Larsen G.** Results of cryosurgery for cervical intraepithelial neoplasia. *Gynecol Oncol* 1988;30:21–5.

42. **Ostergard DR.** Cryosurgical treatment of cervical intraepithelial neoplasia. *Obstet Gynecol* 1980;56:231–3.

43. **Creasman WT, Weed JC, Curry SL, Johnston WW, Parker RT.** Efficacy of cryosurgical treatment of severe cervical intraepithelial neoplasia. *Obstet Gynecol* 1973;41:501–5.

44. **Benedet JL, Miller DM, Nickerson KG, Anderson GH.** The results of cryosurgical treatment of cervical intraepithelial neoplasia at one, five, and ten years. *Am J Obstet Gynecol* 1987;157:268–73.

45. **Townsend DE.** Cryosurgery for CIN. *Obstet Gynecol Surv* 1979;34:828.

46. **Andersen MC, Hartley RB.** Cervical crypt involvement by intraepithelial neoplasia. *Am J Obstet Gynecol* 1980; 55:546–50.

47. **Wright VC, Riopelle MA.** The geometry of cervical intraepithelial neoplasia as a guide to its eradication. *Cervix* 1986;9:21–6.

48. **Bostofte E, Berget A, Larsen JF, Hjortkjaer Pederson P, Rank F.** Conization by carbon dioxide laser or cold knife in the treatment of cervical intraepithelial neoplasia. *Acta Obstet Gynecol Scand* 1986;65:199–202.

49. **Burke L.** The use of the carbon dioxide laser in the therapy of cervical intraepithelial neoplasia. *Am J Obstet Gynecol* 1982;144:377–40.

50. **Wright VC.** Laser surgery for cervical intraepithelial neoplasia. *Acta Obstet Gynecol Scand* 1984;125(Suppl):17.

51. **Rylander E, Isberg A, Joelsson I.** Laser vaporization of cervical intraepithelial neoplasia: a five-year follow-up. *Acta Obstet Gynecol Scand Suppl* 1984;125:33–6.

52. **Jordan JA, Mylotte MJ, Williams DR.** The treatment of cervical intraepithelial neoplasia by laser vaporization. *Br J Obstet Gynecol* 1985;92:394–8.

53. **Baggish MS, Dorsey JH, Adelson M.** A ten-year experience treating cervical intraepithelial neoplasia with CO_2 laser. *Am J Obstet Gynecol* 1989;161:60–8.

54. **Benedet JL, Miller DM, Nickerson KG.** Results of conservative management of cervical intraepithelial neoplasia. *Obstet Gynecol* 1992;79:10–110.

55. **Larsson G, Gullberg BO, Grundsell H.** A comparison of complications of laser and cold knife conization. *Obstet Gynecol* 1983;62:213–7.

56. **Baggish MS.** A comparison between laser excisional conization and laser vaporization for the treatment of cervical intraepithelial neoplasia. *Am J Obstet Gynecol* 1986;155:39–44.

57. **Bjerre B, Eliasson G, Linell F, Soderberg H, Sjoberg NO.** Conization as only treatment of carcinoma in situ of the uterine cervix. *Am J Obstet Gynecol* 1976;15:143–51.

58. **Kolstad P, Klem V.** Long-term follow-up of 1,121 cases of carcinoma *in situ*. *Obstet Gynecol* 1979;48:125–9.

59. **Jones III HW.** Treatment of cervical intraepithelial neoplasia. *Clin Obstet Gynecol* 1990;33:826–36.

60. **Luesley DM, McCann A, Terry PB, Wade-Evans T, Nicholson HD, Mylotte MJ, et al.** Complications of cone biopsy related to the dimensions of the cone and the influence of prior colposcopic assessment. *Br J Obstet Gynecol* 1985;92:158–62.

61. **Prendiville W, Cullimore J, Norman S.** Large loop excision of the transformation zone (LLETZ). A new method of management for women with cervical intraepithelial neoplasia. *Br J Obstet Gynecol* 1989;96:1054–60.

62. **Whiteley PF, Olah KS.** Treatment of cervical intraepithelial neoplasia: experience with the low-voltage diathermy loop. *Am J Obstet Gynecol* 1990;162:1272–7.

63. **Mor-Yosef S, Lopes A, Pearson S, Monaghan JM.** Loop diathermy cone biopsy. Instruments and methods. *Obstet Gynecol* 1990;75:884–6.

64. **Bigrigg MA, Codling BW, Pearson P, Read MD, Swingler GR.** Colposcopic diagnosis and treatment of cervical dysplasia at a single clinic visit. Experience of low-voltage diathermy loop in 1000 patients. *Lancet* 1990;336:229–31.

65. **Gunasekera PC, Phipps JH, Lewis BV.** Large loop excision of the transformation zone (LLETZ) compared to carbon dioxide laser in the treatment of CIN: a superior mode of treatment. *Br J Obstet Gynecol* 1990;97:995–8.

66. **Howe DT, Vincenti AC.** Is large loop excision of the transformation zone (LLETZ) more accurate than colposcopically directed biopsy in the diagnosis of cervical intraepithelial neoplasia? *Br J Obstet Gynecol* 1991;588–91.

67. **Minucci D, Cinel A, Insacco E.** Diathermic loop treatment for CIN and HPV lesions. A follow-up of 130 cases. *Eur J Gynecol Oncol XII* 1991;5:385–93.

68. **Wright TC, Gagnon S, Richart RM, Ferenczy A.** Treatment of cervical intraepithelial neoplasia using the loop electrosurgical excision procedure. *Obstet Gynecol* 1991;79:173–8.

69. **Luesley DM, Cullimore J, Redman CWE, Lawton FG, Emens JM, Rollason JP, et al.** Loop diathermy excision of the cervical transformation zone in patients with abnormal cervical smears. *BMJ* 1990;300:1690–3.

70. **Chappatte OA, Bryne DL, Raju KS, Nayagam M, Kenny A.** Histological differences between colposcopic-directed biopsy and loop excision of the transformation zone (LETZ): A cause for concern. *Gynecol Oncol* 1991;43:46–50.

71. **Murdoch JB, Grimshaw RN, Monaghan JM.** Loop diathermy excision of the abnormal cervical transformation zone. *Int J Gynecol Cancer* 1991;1:105–11.

72. **Demopoulos RI, Horowitz LF, Vamvakas EC.** Endocervical gland involvement by cervical intraepithelial neoplasia grade 3. *Cancer* 1991;68:1932–36.

73. **Coppleson M.** Management of preclinical carcinoma of the cervix. In: **Jordan JA, Singer A,** eds. *The Cervix Uteri.* London: WB Saunders, 1976:453.

74. **Goff B, Atanasoff P, Brown E, Muntz H, Bell DA, Rice LW.** Endocervical glandular atypia in Papanicolaou smears. *Obstet Gynecol* 1992;79:101–4.

75. **Boone ME, Baak JPA, Kurver JPH, Overdiep AH, Verdonk GW.** Adenocarcinoma *in situ* of the cervix: an underdiagnosed lesion. *Cancer* 1981;48:768–73.

76. **Bertrand M, Lickrish MB, Colgan TJ.** The anatomic distribution of cervical adenocarcinoma *in situ:* implications for treatment. *Am J Obstet Gynecol* 1987;157:21–5.

77. **Muntz HG, Bell DA, Lage JM, Goff BA, Feldman S, Rice LW.** Adenocarcinoma *in situ* of the uterine cervix. *Obstet Gynecol* 1992;80:935–9.

78. **Pyonor EA, Barakat RR, Hoskins WJ.** Management and follow-up of patients with adenocarcinoma *in situ* of the uterine cervix. *Gynecol Oncol* 1995;57:158–64.

79. **Benedet JL, Saunders BH.** Carcinoma *in situ* of the vagina. *Am J Obstet Gynecol* 1984;148:695–9.

80. **Hoffman MS, DeCesare SL, Roberts WS, Fiorica JU, Finan MA, Cavanaugh D.** Upper vaginectomy for *in situ* and occult superficially invasive carcinoma of the vagina. *Am J Obstet Gynecol* 1992;166:30–3.

81. **Gardner HL, Friedrich EG Jr, Kaufman RH, Woodruff JD.** The vulvar dystrophies, atypias, and carcinoma *in situ.* An invitational symposium. *J Reprod Med* 1976;17:131–7.

82. **Jeffcoate TNA.** Chronic vulval dystrophies. *Am J Obstet Gynecol* 1966;95:61–74.

83. **Committee on Terminology, International Society for the Study of Vulvar Disease.** New nomenclature for vulvar disease. *Int J Gynecol Pathol* 1989;8:83.

84. **Rodke G, Friedrich EG, Wilkinson EJ.** Malignant potential of mixed vulvar dystrophy (lichen sclerosis associated with squamous cell hyperplasia). *J Reprod Med* 1988;33:545–50.

85. **Rusk D, Sutton GP, Look KY, Roman A.** Analysis of invasive squamous cell carcinoma of the vulva and vulvar intraepithelial neoplasia for the presence of human papillomaviral DNA. *Obstet Gynecol* 1991;77:918–22.

86. **Dubreuilh W.** Pigmentation of the skin due to demodex folliculorum. *Br J Dermatol* 1901; 13:403.

87. **Lee RA, Dahlin DC.** Paget's disease of the vulva with extension into the urethra, bladder, and ureters: a case report. *Am J Obstet Gynecol* 1981;140:834–6.

88. **Hart WR, Millman JB.** Progression of intraepithelial Paget's disease of the vulva to invasive carcinoma. *Cancer* 1977;40:2333–7.

89. **Stacy D, Burrell MO, Franklin EW III.** Extramammary Paget's disease of the vulva and anus: use of intraoperative frozen-section margins. *Am J Obstet Gynecol* 1986;155:519–23.

90. **Buscema J, Woodruff JD, Parmley T, Genadry R.** Carcinoma *in situ* of the vulva. *Obstet Gynecol* 1980;55:225–30.

91. **Friedrich EG, Wilkinson EJ, Fu YS.** Carcinoma *in situ* of the vulva: a continuing challenge. *Am J Obstet Gyncol* 1980;136:880–43.

92. **Rutledge F, Sinclair M.** Treatment of intraepithelial carcinoma of the vulva by skin excision and graft. *Am J Obstet Gynecol* 1968;102:806–12.

93. **Chafee W, Ferguson K, Wilkinson EJ.** Vulvar intraepithelial neoplasia (VIN); principles of surgical therapy. *Colpo Gynecol Surg* 1988;4:125–30.

94. **Reid R.** Superficial laser vulvectomy III. A new surgical technique for appendage-conserving ablation of refractory condylomas and vulvar intraepithelial neoplasia. *Am J Obstet Gynecol* 1985;152:504–9.

95. **Berek JS, Hacker NF, Lagasse LD.** Reconstructive operations. In: **Knapp RC, Berkowitz RS,** eds. *Gynecologic Oncology.* 2nd ed. Philadelphia: WB Saunders, 1994:420–32.

96. **Gunn RA, Gallager HS.** Vulvar Paget's disease: a topographic study. *Cancer* 1980;46:590–4.

17 Early Pregnancy Loss and Ectopic Pregnancy

Thomas G. Stovall
Marian L. McCord

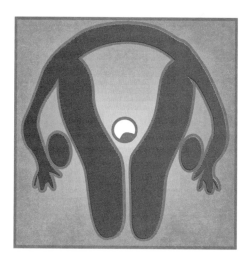

An abnormal gestation is either intrauterine or extrauterine. Extrauterine or ectopic pregnancy occurs when the fertilized ovum becomes implanted in tissue other than the endometrium. Although most ectopic gestations are located in the ampullary segment of the fallopian tube, such pregnancies may also occur in other sites (Table 17.1). Abnormal intrauterine pregnancy often results in pregnancy loss early in gestation. Such abnormalities can be related to a number of factors. With both abnormal intrauterine and extrauterine gestation, early recognition is key to diagnosis and management.

Abnormal Intrauterine Pregnancy

Spontaneous Abortion

Anembryonic gestation, inevitable abortion, incomplete abortion, and completed abortion are types of first trimester abortions. **About 15–20% of known pregnancies terminate in spontaneous abortion. Using serial human chorionic gonadotropin (hCG) measurements to detect early subclinical pregnancy losses, the percentage increases to 30%. About 80% of spontaneous pregnancy losses occur in the first trimester; the incidence decreases with each gestational week.** In a study of 347 patients with a first-trimester pregnancy documented by ultrasound, the overall pregnancy loss was 6.1—4.2% in patients without bleeding and 12.4% in patients with bleeding (1). In women who have had one prior abortion, the rate of spontaneous abortion in a subsequent pregnancy is about 20%; in women who have had three consecutive losses, the rate is 50%. The causes of this condition are varied and most often unknown (Table 17.2). Patients should be reassured that, in most cases, spontaneous abortion will not recur.

Threatened Abortion

Threatened abortion is defined as vaginal bleeding prior to 20 weeks of gestation. It occurs in approximately 30–40% of all pregnancies. The bleeding is usually light and may be associated with mild lower abdominal or cramping pain. It is often not possible to differentiate clinically between threatened abortion, completed abortion, and ectopic preg-

Table 17.1   Definitions of Types of Abnormal Intrauterine and Extrauterine Pregnancies

Extrauterine Pregnancy

Tubal pregnancy	A pregnancy occurring in the fallopian tube — most often these are located in the ampullary portion of the fallopian tube.
Interstitial pregnancy	A pregnancy that implants within the interstitial portion of the fallopian tube.
Abdominal pregnancy	Primary abdominal pregnancy — the first and only implantation occurs on a peritoneal surface. Secondary abdominal pregnancy — implantation originally in the tubal ostia, subsequently aborted, and then reimplanted onto a peritoneal surface.
Cervical pregnancy	Implantation of the developing conceptus in the cervical canal.
Ligamentous pregnancy	A secondary form of ectopic pregnancy in which a primary tubal pregnancy erodes into the mesosalpinx and is located between the leaves of the broad ligament.
Heterotopic pregnancy	A condition in which ectopic and intrauterine pregnancies coexist.
Ovarian pregnancy	A condition in which an ectopic pregnancy implants within the ovarian cortex.

Abnormal Intrauterine Pregnancy

Incomplete abortion	Expulsion of some but not all of the products of conception before 20 completed weeks of gestation.
Complete abortion	Spontaneous expulsion of all fetal and placental tissue from the uterine cavity before 20 weeks of gestation.
Inevitable abortion	Uterine bleeding from a gestation of <20 weeks accompanied by cervical dilation but without expulsion of placental or fetal tissue through the cervix.
Anembryonic gestation	An intrauterine sac without fetal tissue is present at more than 7.5 weeks of gestation.
First trimester fetal death	Death of the fetus in the first 12 weeks of gestation.
Second trimester fetal death	Death of the fetus between 13 and 24 weeks of gestation.
Recurrent spontaneous abortion	The loss of more than three pregnancies before 20 weeks.

Table 17.2   Potential Causes of Spontaneous Pregnancy Loss

Pathologic (blighted) ovum — anembryonic gestation
Embryonic anomalies
Chromosomal anomalies
Increased maternal age
Uterine anomalies
Intrauterine device
Teratogen
Mutagen
Maternal disease
Placental anomalies
Extensive maternal trauma

nancy in an unruptured tube. The differential diagnosis in these patients includes consideration of possible cervical polyps, vaginitis, cervical carcinoma, gestational trophoblastic disease, ectopic pregnancy, trauma, and foreign body. On physical examination, the abdomen is usually not tender and the cervix is closed. Bleeding can be seen coming from the os, and there is no cervical motion or adnexal tenderness. Although most patients experience bleeding at 8–10 weeks of gestation, the actual loss usually occurs before 8 weeks of gestation. Only 3.2% of patients experience a pregnancy loss after 8 weeks of gestation (2).

Evaluation of a threatened abortion should include serial hCG measurements unless the patient has an intrauterine pregnancy documented by ultrasound, eliminating the possibility of an ectopic pregnancy. Endovaginal ultrasonography can detect a gestational sac at an hCG level of 1000–2000 mIU/ml. By 7 weeks of gestation, a fetal pole with fetal cardiac activity can be seen. When a gestational sac is visualized, subsequent loss of the pregnancy occurs in 11.5% of patients. If a yolk sac is present, the loss rate is 8.5%; with an embryo of 5 mm, the loss rate is 7.2%; with an embryo of 6–10 mm, the loss rate is 3.2%; and when the embryo is 10 mm, the loss rate is only 0.5%. The fetal loss rate after 14 weeks of gestation is approximately 2.0% (3). Transvaginal measurement of gestational sac size is useful in differentiating viable from nonviable intrauterine pregnancies. A mean sac diameter $\geq$13 mm without a visible yolk sac or a mean sac diameter $\geq$ 17 mm lacking an embryo predicts nonviability in all cases (4).

There is no effective therapy for a threatened intrauterine pregnancy. Bedrest, although advocated, is not effective. Progesterone or sedatives should not be used. All patients should be counseled and reassured so they understand the situation. Treatment should be given for any vaginal infection.

Inevitable Abortion

With an inevitable abortion, the volume of bleeding is often greater and the cervical os is open and effaced, but no tissue has been passed. Most patients have crampy lower abdominal pain and some have cervical motion or adnexal tenderness. When it is certain that the pregnancy is not viable because the cervical os is dilated or excessive bleeding is present, suction curettage should be performed. Blood type and Rh determination and a complete blood count should be obtained if there is any concern about the amount of bleeding. **Rho(D) immune globulin (RhoGAM) should be given either before or after the uterus is evacuated if the patient's blood is Rh negative.**

Incomplete Abortion

An incomplete abortion is a partial expulsion of the pregnancy tissue. Prior to 6 weeks of gestation, the placenta and fetus are generally passed together, but after this time they are often passed separately. Although most patients have vaginal bleeding, only some have passed tissue. Lower abdominal cramping is invariably present, and the pain may be described as resembling labor. On physical examination, the cervix is dilated and effaced and bleeding is present. Often, clots are admixed with products of conception. If the bleeding is profuse, the patient should be examined promptly for tissue protruding from the cervical os; removal of this tissue with a ring forceps will reduce the bleeding. A vasovagal bradycardia may occur, which will respond to removal of the tissue. All patients with an incomplete abortion should undergo suction curettage as quickly as possible. A complete blood count, maternal blood type, and Rh determination should be obtained; **Rh-negative patients should receive RHo(D) immune globulin.**

If the patient is febrile, broad-spectrum antibiotic therapy should be administered before suction curettage is performed to reduce the incidence of postabortal endometritis and pelvic inflammatory disease, thereby reducing potential deleterious effects on fertility. The antibiotic regimen chosen should be similar to the regimens used for treatment of pelvic inflammatory disease (PID). In patients who do not have clinical signs of infection, prophylactic antibiotic therapy should be instituted: *doxycycline* 100 mg orally twice daily or *tetracycline* 250 mg orally four times daily for 5–7 days is used; another antibiotic of similar spectrum may be used.

Ectopic Pregnancy

Incidence

The most comprehensive data available on ectopic pregnancy rates have been collected by the Centers for Disease Control and Prevention (5). They show a significant increase in the number of ectopic pregnancies in the United States during the past 20 years (Fig. 17.1). In 1989, the latest year for which statistics were published, there were an estimated 88,400 ectopic pregnancies, at a rate of 16 ectopic pregnancies per 1000 reported pregnancies. These numbers represent a fivefold increase compared with the 1970 rates. The highest rates occurred in women aged 35–44 years (27.2/1000 reported pregnancies). When the data are analyzed by race, the risk of ectopic pregnancy among African-Americans and other minorities (20.8/1000) is 1.6 times greater than the risk among whites (13.4/1000). In 1988, 44 deaths were attributed to complications of ectopic pregnancy, which represents 15% of all maternal deaths. The risk of death is higher for African-Americans and other minorities than for whites (6). For both races, teenagers have the highest mortality rates, but the rate for African-American and other minority teenagers is almost five times that for white teenagers. **After an ectopic pregnancy, there is a 7- to 13-fold increase in the risk of a subsequent ectopic pregnancy. The chance that a subsequent pregnancy will be intrauterine is 50–80%, and the chance that the pregnancy will be tubal is 10–25%;**

Figure 17.1 Estimation of the number of ectopic pregnancies (United States, 1970–1989). Dashed lines represent the upper and lower limits of 95% confidence intervals.

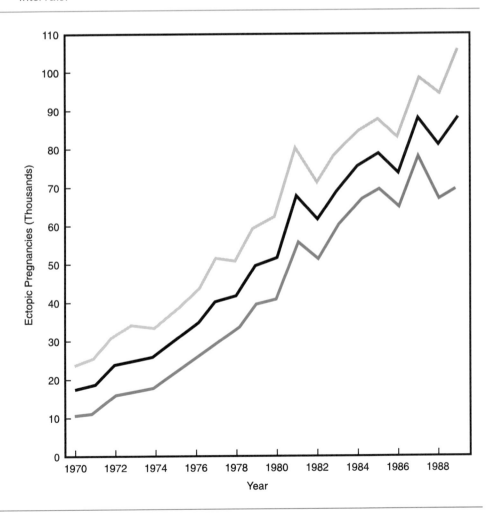

the remaining patients will be infertile (7–9). Many variables make accurate assessment of risk very difficult (e.g., size and location of the ectopic pregnancy, status of the contralateral adnexa, treatment method, and history of infertility).

Etiology and Risk Factors

Tubal damage results from inflammation, infection, and surgery. Inflammation and infection may cause damage without complete tubal obstruction. Complete blockage may result from salpingitis, incomplete tubal ligation, tubal fertility surgery, partial salpingectomy, or congenital midsegment tubal atresia (10–14). Damage to the mucosal portion of the tube or fimbria accounts for about one-half of all tubal pregnancies (15). Tubal diverticula may result in abnormalities that entrap the blastocyst or impede transport (16, 17). Tubal pregnancy may occur in a blocked tube with contralateral tubal patency, with the sperm migrating across the abdomen to fertilize an egg released from the blocked side.

Myoelectrical activity is responsible for propulsive activity in the fallopian tube (16). This activity facilitates movement of the sperm and ova toward each other and propels the zygote toward the uterine cavity. Estrogen increases smooth muscle activity and progesterone decreases muscle tone. Aging results in progressive loss of myoelectrical activity along the fallopian tube, which may explain the increased incidence of tubal pregnancy in perimenopausal women (16). Hormonal control of the muscular activity in the fallopian tube may explain the increased incidence of tubal pregnancy associated with failures of the morning-after pill, minipill, progesterone-containing intrauterine devices (IUDs), and ovulation induction. Blighted ova occur more commonly in tubal conceptions than in intrauterine conceptions, although there is no increase in the incidence of chromosomal abnormalities in ectopic pregnancies (18).

Independent risk factors consistently shown to increase the risk of tubal pregnancy include the following:

1. Previous laparoscopically proven PID

2. Previous tubal pregnancy

3. Current IUD use

4. Previous tubal surgery for infertility

Many other factors, including contraceptive choice, prior surgery, previous pregnancies, and fertility status, also have been identified.

Pelvic Infection

The relationship of PID, tubal obstruction, and ectopic pregnancy is well documented (13, 19). In a study of 415 women with laparoscopically proven PID, the incidence of tubal obstruction increased with successive episodes of PID: 13% after one episode, 35% after two, and 75% after three (19). Furthermore, after one episode of PID, the ratio of ectopic pregnancy to intrauterine pregnancy was one in 24, a sixfold increase over the incidence for women with laparoscopically negative results (1 in 147). In a prospective study of 1204 patients followed until first pregnancy after infection, 47 of 746 (6%) women with laparoscopically documented PID had a tubal gestation, which is significantly higher than the 0.9% incidence in the control group (20).

Chlamydia is an important pathogen causing tubal damage and subsequent tubal pregnancy. Because many cases of chlamydia salpingitis are indolent, cases may go unrecognized or are treated on an outpatient basis. Chlamydia has been cultured from 7 to 30% of patients with tubal pregnancy (7, 21). A strong association between chlamydia infection and tubal pregnancy has been shown with serologic tests for chlamydia (22–25). Conception is three times as likely to be tubal in women with an anti-*chlamydia trachomatis* titer ≥1:64 than in those women whose titer was negative (7, 26).

Contraceptive Use

Inert and copper-containing IUDs prevent both intrauterine and extrauterine pregnancies (27, 28). **Women who conceive with an IUD in place, however, are 0.4–0.8 times more likely to have a tubal pregnancy than those not using contraceptives. However, because IUDs prevent implantation more effectively in the uterus than in the tube, a woman conceiving with an IUD is six to 10 times more likely to have a tubal pregnancy than if she conceives without contraception** (27, 28).

With copper IUDs, 4% of contraceptive failures are tubal pregnancies. Progesterone IUDs are less effective than copper IUDs in preventing tubal pregnancy; 17% of failures result in tubal pregnancy. Furthermore, the rate of ectopic pregnancy in women using progesterone IUDs is higher than in women not using contraceptives: 1.9 per 100 woman-years (vs. 0.5 for copper IUDs) (29). This finding suggests that failures occur for different reasons. Although all IUDs prevent intrauterine implantation, copper IUDs prevent fertilization by cytotoxic and phagocytic effects on the sperm and oocytes. Progesterone-containing IUDs are probably less effective in preventing conception.

Duration of IUD use does not increase the absolute risk of tubal pregnancy (1.2 per 1000 years of exposure), but with increasing use there is an increase in the percentage of pregnancies that are tubal (30). It is unclear whether past use of IUDs increases the risk of tubal pregnancy. Only past use of the Dalkon Shield is associated with a twofold increased risk (31). One study showed that previous use of an IUD for longer than 2 years was associated with a fourfold risk, but this risk was present for only the first year after discontinuation of IUD use (27). However, subsequent studies have found no increased risk of tubal pregnancy following IUD use (30, 32).

The risk of the pregnancy being ectopic with combination oral contraceptive use has been calculated to be 0.5–4% (27, 28, 33). Past use of oral contraceptives does not increase the subsequent risk of ectopic pregnancy (8). Progesterone-only contraceptives, including oral contraceptives (minipill) and subdermal implants (*Norplant*), protect against both intrauterine and ectopic pregnancy when compared with no contraception. If a pregnancy does occur, however, the chance of the pregnancy being ectopic is 4–10% for the minipill (34, 35) and up to 30% if pregnancy occurs while *Norplant* is in place (36, 37). Condom and diaphragm use protects against both intrauterine and ectopic pregnancy, and there is no increased incidence of ectopic pregnancy (30, 33, 38).

Sterilization

The greatest risk for pregnancy, including ectopic pregnancy, occurs in the first 2 years after sterilization (39). Despite a greater proportion of poststerilization failures resulting in ectopic pregnancy, the absolute rate of ectopic pregnancy is decreased. Calculating cumulative lifetime risk of ectopic pregnancy according to method of contraception, sterilized women have a lower cumulative risk of ectopic pregnancy than IUD users or nonusers of contraception, and women using barrier methods or oral contraceptives have the lowest risk (40).

The risk of tubal pregnancy after any sterilization procedure is 5–16% (10, 39, 40). The risk depends on the sterilization technique: about one-half of postelectrocautery failures are ectopic, compared with 12% after nonlaparoscopic, nonelectrocautery procedures (41). Laparoscopic coagulation has a reduced risk of pregnancy compared with mechanical devices, but the risk of ectopic pregnancy is ninefold when a failure does occur (10, 42, 43).

Tubal repair or reconstruction may be performed to correct an obstruction, lyse adhesions, or evacuate an unruptured ectopic pregnancy. Although it is clear that tubal surgery is associ-

492

ated with an increased risk of ectopic pregnancy, it is unclear whether the increased risk results from the surgical procedure or from the underlying problem. A four- to fivefold increased risk is associated with salpingostomy, neosalpingostomy, fimbroplasty, anastomosis, and lysis of complex peritubal and periovarian adhesions (7, 11, 43). After tubal surgery, the overall rate of ectopic pregnancy is 2–7%, and the viable intrauterine pregnancy rate is 50%.

There has been a concern that conservation of the tube at the time of removal of a ectopic pregnancy would increase the risk of recurrent ectopic pregnancy. However, after either tubal removal or conservation, the rates for intrauterine pregnancy (40%) and ectopic pregnancy (12%) have been found to be identical (44). In another study, the incidence of ectopic pregnancy could be predicted by the status of the contralateral tube: normal (7%), abnormal (18%), or absent (25%) (42). In a study of pregnancy outcomes of 1152 patients treated for ectopic pregnancy, preservation of the tube did not increase the incidence of repeat ectopic pregnancy, but it did improve overall fertility rates (45).

Sterilization reversal also increases risk for ectopic pregnancy. The exact risk depends on the method of sterilization, site of tubal occlusion, residual tube length, coexisting disease, and surgical technique. In general, the risk for reanastomosing a cauterized tube is about 15%, and it is less than 3% for reversal of Pomeroy or Fallope ring procedures (46, 47).

Prior Abdominal Surgery

Many patients with ectopic pregnancies have a history of previous abdominal surgery (7, 8, 48). The role of abdominal surgery in ectopic pregnancy is unclear. In one study, there appeared to be no increased risk for cesarean delivery, ovarian surgery, or removal of an unruptured appendix (49). Other studies have shown that ovarian cystectomy or wedge resection increases the risk of ectopic pregnancy, presumably as a result of peritubal scarring (50, 51). Although there is general agreement that an increased risk of ectopic pregnancy is associated with a ruptured appendix (7, 43), one study did not confirm this (49).

Other Causes

Abortion   There is no established association between ectopic pregnancy and spontaneous abortion (7, 9, 52). With recurrent abortion (fewer than two consecutive abortions) the risk is increased two to four times. This may reflect a shared risk factor, such as with luteal phase defect. Uncomplicated elective abortion, regardless of the number of procedures or gestational age at which they were performed, is not associated with increased risk (7, 8, 53, 54). In areas with a high incidence of illegal abortion, the risk is increased 10-fold. Presumably, this increased incidence is secondary to postoperative infection and improperly performed procedures (54).

Infertility   Although the incidence of ectopic pregnancy increases with increasing age and parity, there is also a significant increase in nulliparous women undergoing infertility treatment (7, 8, 44). For nulliparous women, conceptions after at least 1 year of unprotected intercourse are 2.6 times more likely to be tubal (55). Additional risks for infertile women are associated with specific treatments, including reversal of sterilization, tuboplasty, ovulation induction, and *in vitro* fertilization (IVF).

Hormonal alterations characteristic of *clomiphene citrate* and gonadotropin ovulation-induction cycles may predispose tubal implantation. About 1.1–4.6% of conceptions associated with ovulation induction are ectopic pregnancies (8, 55). In many of these patients, the results of hysterosalpingography are normal and there is no evidence of intraoperative tubal pathology. Hyperstimulation, with high estrogen levels, may play a role in tubal pregnancy (56, 57); however, not all studies have shown this relationship (58).

The first pregnancy obtained with *in vitro* fertilization (IVF) was a tubal pregnancy (59). About 2–8% of IVF conceptions are tubal. Tubal factor infertility is associated with a further increased risk of 17% (60–62). Predisposing factors are unclear but may include placement of the embryo high in the uterine cavity, fluid reflux into the tube, and a predisposing tubal factor that prevents the refluxed embryo from returning to the uterine cavity.

Salpingitis Isthmica Nodosa   Salpingitis isthmica nodosa (SIN) is a noninflammatory pathologic condition of the tube in which tubal epithelium extends into the myosalpinx and forms a true diverticulum. The reported prevalence ranges from 1 in 146 to 11 in 100. This condition is found more often in the tubes of women with an ectopic pregnancy than in nonpregnant women (17, 63, 64). Myometrial electrical activity over the diverticula has been found to be abnormal (16). Whether tubal pregnancy is caused by SIN or whether the association is coincidental is unknown.

Endometriosis and Leiomyomata   Endometriosis or leiomyomata can cause tubal obstruction. However, either is not commonly associated with ectopic pregnancy.

Diethylstilbestrol   Women exposed to diethylstilbestrol (DES) *in utero* who subsequently conceive are at increased risk for ectopic pregnancy. In several case-control studies, these women were more than twice as likely to have a tubal pregnancy (65, 66). The Collaborative Diethylstilbestrol-Adenosis Project, which monitored 327 DES-exposed women, found that about 50% had uterine cavity abnormalities (65). In DES-exposed women, the risk of ectopic pregnancy was 13% compared with 4% for women who had a normal uterus. No specific type of defect was related to the risk of ectopic.

Smoking   Current cigarette smoking is associated with a more than twofold risk of tubal pregnancy (28, 51, 67–69). A case-control study showed a dose relationship: current smokers of more than 20 cigarettes a day had a relative risk of 2.5 compared with nonsmokers, whereas smokers of 1 to 10 cigarettes had a risk of 1.3 (68). Alterations of tubal motility, ciliary activity, and blastocyst implantation are all associated with nicotine intake.

Pathology

Chorionic villi, usually found in the lumen, are pathognomic findings of tubal pregnancy. Gross or microscopic evidence of an embryo is seen in two-thirds of cases (70). The unruptured tubal pregnancy is characterized by irregular dilation of the tube, with a blue discoloration caused by hematosalpinx. The ectopic pregnancy may not be readily apparent. Bleeding associated with tubal pregnancies is mainly extraluminal but may be luminal (hematosalpinx) and may extrude from the fimbriated end. A hematoma is frequently seen surrounding the distal segment of the tube. Patients who have tubal pregnancies that spontaneously resolve and those treated with *methotrexate* frequently have an enlargement of the ectopic mass associated with blood clots and extrusion of tissue from the fimbriated end. Hemoperitoneum is nearly always present but is confined to the cul-de-sac unless tubal rupture has occurred. The natural progression of tubal pregnancy is either expulsion from the fimbriated end (tubal abortion), involution of the conceptus, or rupture, usually around the eighth gestational week. Some tubal pregnancies form a chronic inflammatory mass that is associated with involution and reestablishment of menses and thus is difficult to diagnose. Extensive histologic sampling may be required to disclose a few ghost villi.

Histologic findings associated with tubal gestation include evidence of chronic salpingitis and SIN. Inflammation associated with salpingitis causes adhesions as a result of fibrin deposition. Healing and cellular organization lead to permanent scarring between folds of tissue. This scarring may allow transport of sperm but not the passage of the larger blastocyst. About 45% of patients with tubal pregnancies will have pathologic evidence of prior salpingitis (71).

The etiology of SIN is unknown but is speculated to be an adenomyosis-like process or, less likely, inflammation (72, 73). This condition is rare before puberty, indicating a noncongenital origin. Tubal diverticuli are identified in about one-half of patients who have ectopic pregnancies, as opposed to 5% of women who do not have ectopic pregnancies (17).

Histologic findings include the Arias-Sella reaction, which is characterized by localized hyperplasia of endometrial glands that are hypersecretory (74). The cells have enlarged nuclei that are hyperchromatic and irregular. The Arias-Sella reaction is a nonspecific finding that can be seen in patients with intrauterine pregnancies (Fig. 17.2).

Diagnosis

The diagnosis of ectopic pregnancy is complicated by the wide spectrum of clinical presentations, from asymptomatic patients to those who have an acute abdomen and hemodynamic shock. The diagnosis and management of a ruptured ectopic pregnancy is straightforward; the primary goal is achieving hemostasis. If an ectopic pregnancy can be identified prior to rupture or irreparable tubal damage, consideration may be given to optimizing future fertility. With patients presenting earlier in the disease process, the number of those who are asymptomatic or who have minimal symptoms has increased. Therefore, there must be a high degree of suspicion of ectopic pregnancy, especially in areas of high prevalence. History and physical examination will identify patients at risk, improving the probability of detection of ectopic pregnancy prior to rupture.

History

Patients who have an ectopic pregnancy generally have an abnormal menstrual pattern or the perception of a spontaneous pregnancy loss. Pertinent history includes the menstrual history, previous pregnancy, history of infertility, current contraceptive status, risk factor assessment, and current symptoms.

The classic symptom triad of ectopic pregnancy is pain, amenorrhea, and vaginal bleeding. This symptom group is present in only about 50% of patients, however, and

Figure 17.2   The Arias-Stella reaction of the endometrium. The glands are closely packed and hypersecretory with large, hyperchromatic nuclei suggesting malignancy. (From **Berek JS, Hacker NF.** *Practical Gynecologic Oncology.* 2nd ed. Baltimore: Williams & Wilkins, 1994:125.)

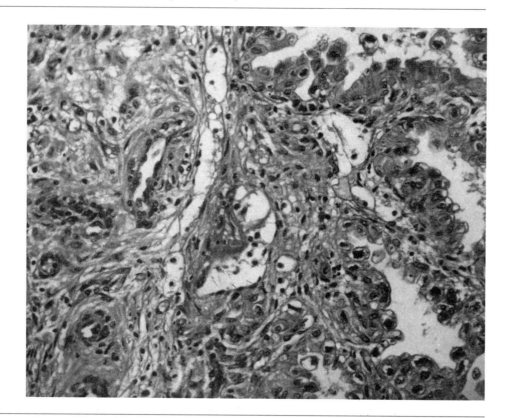

is most typical in patients in whom an ectopic pregnancy has ruptured. Abdominal pain is the most common presenting complaint, but the severity and nature of the pain varies widely. There is no pathognomonic pain that is diagnostic of ectopic pregnancy. Pain may be unilateral or bilateral and may occur in the upper or lower abdomen. The pain may be dull, sharp, or crampy and either continuous or intermittent. With rupture, the patient may experience transient relief of the pain, as stretching of the tubal serosa ceases. Shoulder and back pain, thought to result from hemoperitoneal irritation of the diaphragm, may indicate intra-abdominal hemorrhage.

Physical Examination

The physical examination should include measurements of vital signs and examination of the abdomen and pelvis. Frequently, the findings prior to rupture and hemorrhage are nonspecific, and vital signs are normal. The abdomen may be nontender or mildly tender, with or without rebound. The uterus may be slightly enlarged, with findings similar to a normal pregnancy (75). Cervical motion tenderness may or may not be present. An adnexal mass may be palpable in up to 50% of cases, but the mass varies markedly in size, consistency, and tenderness. A palpable mass may be the corpus luteum and not the ectopic pregnancy. With rupture and intra-abdominal hemorrhage, the patient develops tachycardia followed by hypotension. Bowel sounds are decreased or absent. The abdomen is distended, with marked tenderness and rebound tenderness. Cervical motion tenderness is present. Frequently, the pelvic examination is inadequate because of pain and guarding.

History and physical examination may or may not provide useful diagnostic information. The accuracy of the initial clinical evaluation is less than 50% (76). Additional tests are frequently required to differentiate early viable intrauterine pregnancy or suspected ectopic or abnormal intrauterine pregnancy.

Serial Quantitative Human Chorionic Gonadotropin

Quantitative β-hCG measurements are the diagnostic cornerstone for ectopic pregnancy. The hCG enzyme immunoassay, with a sensitivity of 25 mIU/ml, is an accurate screening test for detection of ectopic pregnancy. The assay is positive in virtually all documented ectopic pregnancies.

Reference Standards   There are three reference standards for β-hCG measurement. The World Health Organization introduced the First International Standard (1st IS) in the 1930s. Testing for hCG and its subunits have improved over the years. The Second International Standard (2nd IS), introduced in 1964, has varying amounts of hCG α and β subunits. A purified preparation of β-hCG is now available. Originally referred to as the First International Reference Preparation (1st IRP), the test standard is now referred to as the Third International Standard (3rd IS). Although each standard has its own scale, as a general rule, the 2nd IS is about one-half of the 3rd IS. For example, if a level is reported as 500 mIU/ml (2nd IS), it is equivalent to a level of 1000 mIU/ml (3rd IS). The assay standard used must be known in order to correctly interpret hCG results (77).

Doubling Time   The hCG level correlates with the gestational age (78). During the first 6 weeks of amenorrhea, the serum hCG level increases exponentially. Thus, during this time period, the doubling time of hCG is relatively constant, regardless of the initial level. After the sixth week of gestation, when the hCG levels are >6000–10,000 mIU/ml, the hCG rise is slower and not constant (79).

The hCG doubling time can differentiate an ectopic pregnancy from an intrauterine pregnancy—a 66% rise in the hCG level over 48 hours (85% confidence level) represents the lower limit of normal values for viable intrauterine pregnancies (80). Approximately 15% of patients with viable intrauterine pregnancies will have a <66% rise in hCG level over 48 hours, and a similar percentage with an ectopic pregnancy will have a >66% rise. If the sampling interval is reduced to 24 hours, the overlap between normal and abnormal pregnancies is even greater. Patients with a normal intrauterine pregnancy usually have a >50% rise in the hCG level over 48 hours when the starting level is less than 2000 mIU/ml. **The hCG pattern that is most predictive of an ectopic pregnancy is one that has reached a plateau (a doubling time of more than 7 days). For falling levels, a half-life of less than 1.4 days is rarely associated with an ectopic pregnancy, whereas a half-life more than 7 days is most predictive of ectopic pregnancy.**

Serial hCG levels are usually required when the initial ultrasound examination is indeterminate (i.e., when there is no evidence of an intrauterine gestation or extrauterine cardiac activity consistent with an ectopic pregnancy). When the hCG level is less than 2000, doubling time predicts viable intrauterine gestation (normal rise) versus nonviability (subnormal rise). With normally rising levels, a second ultrasound is performed when the level is expected (by extrapolation) to reach 2000 mIU/ml. Abnormally rising levels (<2000 mIU/ml) indicate a nonviable pregnancy. The location (i.e., intrauterine vs. extrauterine) must be determined surgically, either by laparoscopy or dilation and curettage. Indeterminate ultrasonography and a hCG >2000 mIU/ml are diagnostic of nonviable gestation, either ectopic pregnancy or a complete abortion. As a general rule, a completed abortion will have a rapidly falling hCG level (50% over 48 hours), whereas levels of an ectopic pregnancy will rise or plateau.

Single hCG Level   A single hCG measurement has limited usefulness because there is considerable overlap of values between normal and abnormal pregnancies at a given gestational age. The ectopic pregnancy site and hCG level do not correlate (81). Also, many patients in whom the diagnosis of ectopic pregnancy is being considered are uncertain about their menstrual dates. A single hCG level may be useful when measured by sensitive enzyme immunoassays which, if negative, exclude a diagnosis of ectopic pregnancy. Measurement of a single level may also be helpful in predicting pregnancy outcome after timed conceptions using advanced reproductive technology. If the hCG level is more than 300 mIU/ml on day 16–18 after artificial insemination, there is an 88% chance of a live birth (82). If the hCG level is less than 300 mIU/ml, the chance of a live birth is only 22%. Also, a single hCG level may facilitate the interpretation of ultrasonography when an intrauterine gestation is not visualized. An hCG level greater than the ultrasound discriminatory zone indicates a possible extrauterine pregnancy. However, determination of serial hCG levels may be needed to differentiate an ectopic pregnancy from a completed abortion. Further tests are required for patients in whom ultrasonography examinations are inconclusive and hCG levels are below the discriminatory zone.

Serum Progesterone

In general, the mean serum progesterone level in patients with ectopic pregnancies is lower than those with normal intrauterine pregnancies (83, 84). However, in studies of more than 5000 patients with first-trimester pregnancies, a spectrum of progesterone levels in patients with both normal and abnormal pregnancies has been found (85–87). Approximately 70% of patients with a viable intrauterine pregnancy have serum progesterone levels >25 ng/ml, whereas only 1.5% of patients with an ectopic pregnancies have serum progesterone levels higher than 25 ng/ml and most of these pregnancies exhibit cardiac activity (85–87).

A serum progesterone level can be used as an ectopic pregnancy screening test for both normal and abnormal pregnancy, particularly in settings in which hCG levels and ultrasonography are not readily available. **A serum progesterone level <5.0 ng/ml is highly suggestive of an abnormal pregnancy, but it is not 100% predictive.** The risk of a normal pregnancy with a serum progesterone level <5.0 ng/ml is approximately 1/1500 (88).

Other Endocrinologic and Protein Markers

In an effort to improve early ectopic pregnancy detection, various endocrinologic and protein markers have been studied. Estradiol levels increase slowly from conception until 6 weeks of gestation and then rise rapidly as placental production of estradiol increases (89).

Estradiol levels are significantly lower in ectopic pregnancies when compared with viable pregnancies. However, there is considerable overlap between normal and abnormal pregnancies, as well as between intrauterine and extrauterine pregnancies (90, 91).

Maternal serum creatine kinase has been studied as a marker for ectopic pregnancy diagnosis (92). Maternal serum creatine kinase levels were significantly higher in all patients with tubal pregnancy when compared to patients who had missed abortions or normal intrauterine pregnancies, but no correlation between the creatine kinase level and the clinical presentation of the patient was found and there was no correlation with the hCG levels.

Schwangerschafts-protein 1 (SP$_1$), also known as pregnancy-associated plasma protein C (PAPP-C) or pregnancy-specific β glycoprotein (PSBS), is produced by the syncytiotrophoblast (90). The main advantage of SP1 levels may be in diagnosis of conception after recent hCG administration. A level of 2 ng/L might be used for the diagnosis of pregnancy; however, it is doubtful that a diagnosis can be established prior to delay of menses. Although the SP level increases late in all patients with a nonviable pregnancy, a single SP level does not have prognostic value (93).

Relaxin is a protein hormone produced solely by the corpus luteum of pregnancy. It appears in the maternal serum at 4–5 weeks of gestation, peaks at about 10 weeks of gestation, and decreases until term (94). Relaxin levels are significantly lower in ectopic pregnancies and spontaneous abortions than in normal intrauterine pregnancies. Prorenin and active renin levels are significantly higher in viable intrauterine pregnancies than in either ectopic pregnancies or spontaneous abortions, with a single level >33 pg/ml excluding the diagnosis of ectopic pregnancy (95). However, the clinical utility of relaxin, prorenin, and renin levels in diagnosing ectopic pregnancy has not yet been determined.

CA125 is a glycoprotein, the origin of which is uncertain during pregnancy. Levels of CA125 rise during the first trimester and return to a nonpregnancy range during the second and third trimesters. After delivery, maternal serum concentrations increase again (96, 97). CA125 levels have been studied in an effort to predict spontaneous abortion. Although a positive correlation has been found between elevated CA125 levels 18–22 days postconception and spontaneous abortion, repeat measurements at 6 weeks of gestation did not correlate with outcome (98). Conflicting results have been reported—one study showed a higher serum CA125 level in normal than in ectopic pregnancies 2–4 weeks after a missed menses, whereas another study found higher CA125 levels for ectopic pregnancies compared with normal pregnancies (99, 100).

Maternal serum α-fetoprotein (AFP) levels are elevated in ectopic pregnancies (101, 102); however, the use of AFP measurements as a screening technique for ectopic pregnancy has not been studied. A combination of AFP with three other markers, β-hCG, progesterone, and estradiol, has a 98.5% specificity and 94.5% accuracy for the prediction of ectopic pregnancy.

C-reactive protein is an acute phase reactant that increases with trauma or infection. This protein is lower in patients with ectopic pregnancy than in patients with an acute infectious process. Thus, when an infectious process is part of the differential diagnosis, measurement of C-reactive protein may be beneficial (103).

Ultrasonography

Improvements in ultrasonography have resulted in the earlier diagnosis of intrauterine and ectopic gestations (104). However, the sensitivity of the β-hCG assay usually allows the diagnosis of pregnancy prior to direct visualization by ultrasonography.

The complete examination should include both transvaginal and transabdominal ultrasonography. Transvaginal ultrasonography is superior to transabdominal ultrasonography in evaluating intrapelvic structures. The closeness of the vaginal probe to the pelvic organs allows use of higher frequencies (5–7 mHz), which improves resolution. The diagnosis of an intrauterine pregnancy can be made 1 week earlier with transvaginal than with transabdominal sonography. The demonstration of an empty uterus, detection of adnexal masses and free peritoneal fluid, and direct signs of ectopic pregnancy are more reliably established with a transvaginal procedure (105–109). Transabdominal ultrasonography permits visualization of both the pelvis and abdominal cavity and should be included as part of the complete ectopic pregnancy evaluation to detect adnexal masses and hemoperitoneum.

The earliest ultrasonographic finding of an intrauterine pregnancy is a small fluid space and the gestational sac, surrounded by a thick echogenic ring, located eccentrically within the endometrial cavity. The earliest normal gestational sac is seen at 5 weeks of gestation with transabdominal ultrasonography and at 4 weeks of gestation with transvaginal ultrasonography (110). As the gestational sac grows, a yolk sac is seen within it, followed by an embryo with cardiac activity.

The appearance of a normal gestational sac may be simulated by intrauterine fluid collection, the pseudogestational sac, which occurs in 8–29% of patients with ectopic pregnancy (111–113). This ultrasonographic lucency, centrally located, probably represents bleeding into the endometrial cavity by the decidual cast. Clots within this lucency may mimic a fetal pole.

Morphologically, identification of the double decidual sac sign (DDSS) is the best known method of ultrasonographically differentiating true sacs from pseudosacs (114). The double sac, believed to be the decidua capsularis and parietalis, is seen as two concentric echogenic rings separated by a hypoechogenic space. Although useful, there are some limitations of sensitivity and specificity—the DDSS sensitivity ranges from 64 to 95% (113). Pseudosacs may occasionally appear as the DDSS; intrauterine sacs of failed pregnancies may appear as pseudosacs.

The appearance of a yolk sac within the gestational sac is superior to the DDSS in proving an intrauterine pregnancy (115). The yolk sac is consistently visible on transabdominal ultrasonography with a gestational sac size of 2.0 cm, and on transvaginal ultrasonography at a gestational sac size of 0.6–0.8 cm (116, 117). Intrauterine sacs <1 cm on transabdominal sonography and <0.6 cm on transvaginal ultrasonography are considered indeterminate. Larger sacs without DDSS or yolk sac represent either a failed intrauterine or ectopic pregnancy.

The presence of cardiac activity within the uterine cavity is definitive evidence of an intrauterine pregnancy. This finding essentially eliminates the diagnosis of ectopic pregnancy, because the incidence of combined intrauterine and extrauterine pregnancy is 1/30,000.

The demonstration of an adnexal gestational sac with a fetal pole and cardiac activity is the most specific but least sensitive sign of ectopic pregnancy, occurring in only 10–17% of cases (103, 118, 119). The recognition of other characteristics of ectopic pregnancy has improved ultrasonographic sensitivity. Adnexal rings (fluid sacs with thick echogenic rings) that have a yolk sac or nonliving embryo are accepted as specific ultrasonographic signs of ectopic pregnancy (120). Adnexal rings are visualized in 22% of ectopic pregnancies using transabdominal ultrasonography and 38% using transvaginal sonography (105). Other studies have identified adnexal rings in 33–50% of ectopic pregnancies (103, 119). The adnexal ring may not always be apparent, because bleeding around the sac results in the appearance of a nonspecific adnexal mass.

Complex or solid adnexal masses are frequently associated with ectopic pregnancy (1, 3, 19); however, the mass may represent a corpus luteum, endometrioma, hydrosalpinx, ovarian neoplasm (e.g., dermoid cyst), or pedunculated fibroid. Free cul-de-sac fluid is frequently associated with ectopic pregnancy and is no longer considered evidence of rupture. The presence of intra-abdominal free fluid should raise concern about tubal rupture (121).

Accurate interpretation of ultrasonography findings requires correlation with the hCG level (discriminatory zone) (112, 117, 120, 122). All viable intrauterine pregnancies can be visualized by transabdominal sonography for serum hCG levels >6500 mIU/ml; none are seen at 6000 mIU/ml. Nonvisualization of an intrauterine gestation >6500 mIU/ml indicates an abnormal (failed intrauterine or ectopic) pregnancy. Intrauterine sacs seen at hCG levels below the discriminatory zone are abnormal and represent either failed intrauterine pregnancies or the pseudogestational sacs of ectopic pregnancy. If there is no definite sign of an intrauterine gestation (the empty uterus sign) and the hCG level is below the discriminatory zone, the differential diagnosis includes considerations:

1. Normal intrauterine pregnancy too early for visualization

2. Abnormal intrauterine gestation

3. Recent abortion

4. Ectopic pregnancy

5. Nonpregnant

The discriminatory zone has been lowered progressively with improvements in ultrasonography resolution. Discriminatory zones for transvaginal ultrasonography have been reported at levels from 1000 to 2000 mIU/ml (112, 117, 120, 122). Discriminatory zones will vary according to the expertise of the examiner and capability of the equipment.

Although the discriminatory zone for intrauterine pregnancy is well established, there is no such zone for ectopic pregnancy. Levels of hCG have not been shown to correlate with the size of ectopic pregnancy. Regardless of how high the hCG level may be, nonvisualization does not exclude ectopic pregnancy. An ectopic pregnancy may be present anywhere in the abdominal cavity, making ultrasonographic visualization difficult.

Doppler Ultrasonography

A Doppler shift occurs whenever the source of an ultrasound beam is moving. The usual sources of Doppler-shifted frequencies are red blood cells. The presence of intravascular blood flow, flow direction, and flow velocity can be determined (123). Pulsed Doppler provides ultrasonographic control over which vessels are sampled. The vascular information is provided both by the shape of the time-velocity waveform (high- or low-resistance type flow) and by its systolic, diastolic, and mean velocities (or Doppler frequency shifts) (124). Color flow Doppler ultrasonography analyzes very low-amplitude signals from an entire ultrasound tomogram; the Doppler shift is then modulated into color. This information is used to gauge generalized tissue vascularity and to guide pulsed Doppler vascular sampling of specific vessels.

The waveform in the uterine arteries in the nongravid state and in the first trimester of pregnancy shows a high-resistance (little or no diastolic flow), low-velocity pattern. Conversely, a high-velocity, low-resistance signal is localized to the area of developing placentation (125–127). This pattern, seen near the endometrium, is associated with normal and abnormal intrauterine pregnancies and is termed *peritrophoblastic flow*. Whereas transvaginal ultrasonography requires a well-developed double decidual sac (or possibly cardiac activity) to localize an intrauterine gestation, the use of Doppler techniques allows detection of an intrauterine pregnancy at an earlier date. The combined use of Doppler and two-dimensional imaging allows the differentiation of pseudogestational sacs and true intrauterine gestational sacs (128) and the differentiation of the empty uterus sign as either the presence of an intrauterine pregnancy (normal and abnormal) or absence of an intrauterine pregnancy (with an increased risk of ectopic pregnancy) (121).

A similar high-velocity, low-impedence flow characterizes ectopic pregnancies. The addition of Doppler to the ultrasonographic evaluation of suspected ectopic pregnancy improves diagnostic sensitivity for individual diagnoses: from 71% to 87% for ectopic pregnancy, from 24% to 59% for failed intrauterine pregnancy, and from 90% to 99% for normal intrauterine pregnancy (120, 121, 128).

Dilation and Curettage

Uterine curettage is performed when the pregnancy has been confirmed to be nonviable and the location of the pregnancy cannot be determined by ultrasonography. The decision to evacuate the uterus in the presence of a positive pregnancy test must be made with caution to avoid the unintentional disruption of a viable intrauterine pregnancy. Although suction curettage traditionally has been performed in the operating room, it can now be accomplished under local anesthesia on an outpatient basis. Endometrial sampling methods (e.g., a Novak curettage or Pipelle endometrial sampling device) are accurate in diagnosing abnormal uterine bleeding, but their reliability for intrauterine pregnancy evacuation has not been studied. These devices might miss intrauterine villi and falsely suggest the diagnosis of ectopic pregnancy.

It is essential to confirm the presence of trophoblastic tissue as rapidly as possible so therapy for the patient with an extrauterine gestation may be instituted. Once tissue is obtained by curettage, it can be added to saline, in which it will float (Fig. 17.3). Decidual tissue does not float. Chorionic villi are usually identified by their characteristic lacy frond ap-

Figure 17.3   When floated in saline, chorionic villi are often readily distinguishable as lacy fronds of tissue. (Reproduced with permission from **Stovall TG, Ling FW.** *Extrauterine Pregnancy: Clinical Diagnosis and Management.* New York: McGraw-Hill, Inc., 1993:186.)

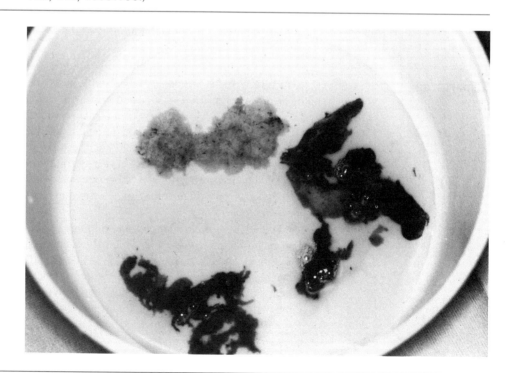

pearance. The sensitivity and specificity of this technique are 95%. Because flotation of curettings is not 100% accurate in differentiating an intrauterine from extrauterine gestation, histologic confirmation or serial β-hCG level measurement are required. A rapid assessment of the presence of chorionic villi may be obtained with frozen section, which avoids the at least 48-hour waiting period for permanent histologic evaluation. Immunocytochemical staining techniques have been used to identify intermediate trophoblasts that are not normally identified by light microscopy (74).

When frozen section is not available, serial hCG levels permit rapid diagnosis. After evacuation of an abnormal intrauterine pregnancy, the hCG level decreases by >15% within 12–24 hours. A borderline fall may represent interassay variability. A repeat level should be obtained in 24–48 hours to confirm the decline. If the uterus is evacuated and the pregnancy is extrauterine, the hCG level will plateau or continue to increase, indicating the presence of extrauterine trophoblastic tissue.

Culdocentesis

Culdocentesis has been used widely as a diagnostic technique for ectopic pregnancy. With the use of hCG testing and transvaginal ultrasound, however, culdocentesis is rarely indicated. The purpose of the procedure is to determine the presence of nonclotting blood, which increases the likelihood of ruptured ectopic pregnancy. After exposing the posterior vaginal fornix with a bivalve vaginal speculum, the posterior lip of the cervix is grasped with a tenaculum. The cul-de-sac is then entered through the posterior vaginal wall with an 18- to 20-gauge spinal needle with a syringe attached. As the cul-de-sac is entered, suction is applied and the intraperitoneal contents are aspirated. If nonclotting blood is obtained, the results are positive. In the presence of serous fluid, results are negative. A lack of fluid return or clotted blood is nondiagnostic.

Historically, if the culdocentesis results were positive, laparotomy was performed for a presumed diagnosis of ruptured tubal pregnancy. However, **the results of culdocentesis do not always correlate with the status of the pregnancy.** Although approximately 70–90% of patients with ectopic pregnancy have a hemoperitoneum demonstrated by culdocentesis, only 50% of patients have a ruptured tube (129). Furthermore, approximately 6% of women with positive culdocentesis results do not have an ectopic gestation at the time of laparotomy. Nondiagnostic taps occur in 10–20% of patients with ectopic pregnancy and, therefore, are not definitive.

Laparoscopy

Laparoscopy is the "gold standard" for the diagnosis of ectopic pregnancy. Generally, the fallopian tubes are easily visualized and evaluated, although the diagnosis of ectopic pregnancy is missed in 3–4% of patients who have very small ectopic gestations. The ectopic gestation is usually seen distorting the normal tubal architecture. With earlier diagnosis, there is an increasing possibility that a small ectopic pregnancy may not be visualized. Pelvic adhesions or previous tubal damage may compromise assessment of the tube. False-positive results occur when tubal dilation or discoloration is misinterpreted as an ectopic pregnancy, in which case the tube can be incised unnecessarily and damaged.

The presenting symptoms and physical findings of patients with an unruptured ectopic pregnancy are similar to those with a normal intrauterine pregnancy (87). History, risk factor assessment, and physical examination are the initial steps in the management of suspected ectopic pregnancy. Patients in a hemodynamically unstable condition should undergo immediate surgical intervention. Patients in a stable condition who are relatively asymptomatic may be assessed as outpatients.

If the diagnosis of ectopic pregnancy can be confirmed without laparoscopy, several potential benefits result. First, both the anesthetic and surgical risks of laparoscopy are avoided and, second, medical therapy becomes a treatment option. Because many ectopic pregnancies occur in histologically normal tubes, resolution without surgery may spare the tube from additional trauma and improve subsequent fertility. An algorithm for the diagnosis of ectopic pregnancy without laparoscopy proved to be 100% accurate in a randomized clinical trial (Fig. 17.4) (130, 131). This screening algorithm combines the use of history and physical examination, serial hCG levels, serum progesterone levels, vaginal ultrasonography, and dilation and curettage. When hCG levels and transvaginal ultrasonography are available in a timely fashion, serum progesterone screening is not required. Serial hCG levels are used to assess pregnancy viability, correlated with transvaginal ultrasonography findings, and measured serially after a suction curettage.

In this algorithm, transvaginal ultrasonography is used as follows:

1. The identification of an intrauterine gestational sac or pregnancy effectively excludes the presence of an extrauterine pregnancy. If the patient has a rising hCG level >2000 mIU/ml and no intrauterine gestational sac is identified, this patient is considered to have an extrauterine pregnancy and can be treated without further testing.

2. Adnexal cardiac activity, when seen, definitively confirms the diagnosis of ectopic pregnancy.

3. A tubal mass as small as 1 cm can be identified and characterized. Masses >3.5–4.0 cm should not be treated with medical therapy.

Suction curettage is used to differentiate nonviable intrauterine pregnancies from ectopic gestations (<50% rise in hCG level over 48 hours, an hCG level <2000 mIU/ml, and an indeterminate sonogram). Performance of this procedure will avoid unnecessary use of *methotrexate* in patients with abnormal intrauterine pregnancy that can only be diagnosed by evacuating the uterus. An unlikely potential problem with suction curettage is missing either an early nonviable intrauterine pregnancy or combined intrauterine and extrauterine pregnancies.

Treatment

Ectopic pregnancy can be treated either medically or surgically. Both methods are effective, and the choice depends on the clinical circumstances, the site of the ectopic pregnancy, and the available resources.

Surgical Treatment

Operative management is the most widely used treatment for ectopic pregnancy. There has been debate about which surgical procedure is best. Salpingo-oophorectomy was once considered appropriate because it was theorized that this technique would eliminate transperitoneal migration of the ovum or zygote, which was thought to predispose to recurrent ectopic pregnancy (132). Ovarian removal results in all ovulations occurring on the side with the remaining normal fallopian tube. Subsequent studies have not confirmed that ipsilateral oophorectomy increases the likelihood of conceiving an intrauterine pregnancy; therefore, this practice is not recommended (133).

Salpingectomy versus Salpingostomy

Linear salpingostomy is currently the procedure of choice when the patient has an unruptured ectopic pregnancy and wishes to retain her potential for future fertility. The products of conception are removed through an incision made into the tube on its antimesenteric border. The procedure can be accomplished with either a needle tip cautery, laser, scalpel, or scissors. It can be done by operative laparoscopic techniques or laparotomy. In a study in which patients treated with either salpingectomy or salpingostomy were

503

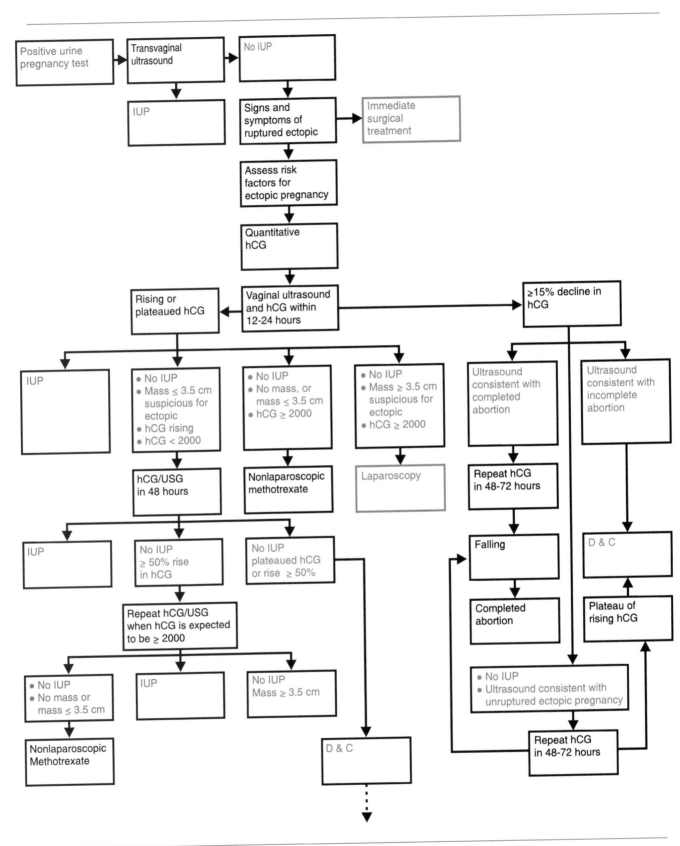

Figure 17.4   Nonlaparoscopic algorithm for diagnosis of ectopic pregnancy.

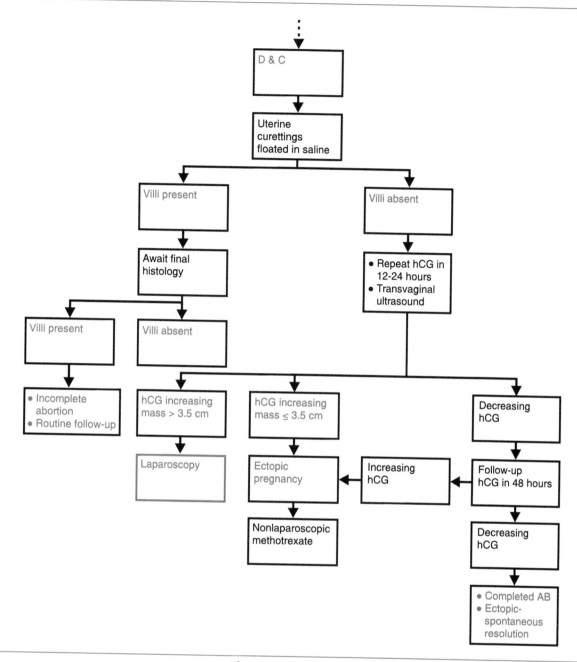

Figure 17.4—*continued*

followed for a period of 3 to approximately 12.5 years, there was no difference in pregnancy rates (134). A history of infertility is the most significant determinant of future fertility, and such patients are probably better served by salpingectomy to decrease their subsequent chance of a recurrent ectopic pregnancy. Linear salpingostomy is as effective as segmental resection with primary reanastomosis, even for ectopic pregnancies occurring in the isthmic tubal segment, and it is technically less difficult and has a shorter operative time (135).

Milking the tube to affect a tubal abortion has been advocated; if the pregnancy is fimbrial, this technique may be effective. However, when milking is compared with linear salpingostomy for ampullary ectopic pregnancies, milking was associated with a twofold increase in the recurrent ectopic pregnancy rate (136).

505

Laparotomy versus Laparoscopy

Salpingostomy, salpingectomy, or segmental resection can be accomplished via laparoscopy or laparotomy. The approach used depends on the hemodynamic stability of the patient, the size and location of the ectopic mass, and the surgeon's expertise. Laparotomy is indicated when the patient becomes hemodynamically unstable, whereas laparoscopy is reserved for patients who are hemodynamically stable. A ruptured ectopic pregnancy does not necessarily require laparotomy. However, if large blood clots are present or the intra-abdominal blood cannot be evacuated in a timely manner, laparotomy should be considered. Cornual or interstitial pregnancies often require laparotomy, although laparoscopic management has been described (137). Laparotomy is chosen for the management of most ovarian and abdominal pregnancies. In some cases, the patient may have extensive abdominal or pelvic adhesive disease, making laparoscopy difficult and laparotomy more feasible.

Laparoscopy has advantages over laparotomy for management of ectopic pregnancy. In a case-control study of 50 patients comparing the use of laparoscopy and laparotomy for ectopic pregnancy management, hospital stay was significantly shorter (1.3 ± 0.8 vs. 3.0 ± 1.1 days), operative time was shorter (78 ± 26 vs. 104 ± 27 minutes) and convalescence was shorter (9 ± 8 vs. 26 ± 16 days) in the laparoscopy group (138). In a randomized study in which 30 patients in each group were compared, patients undergoing laparoscopic management had less estimated blood loss, shorter hospital stay, equivalent tubal pregnancy rates, and similar pregnancy and persistent trophoblast rates (139). In another study, patients were assigned during alternate months to undergo laparoscopic management (n = 26) or laparotomy (n = 37) (140). There were no differences in operative time, although patients undergoing laparoscopy had a significant decrease in blood loss, postoperative hospital stay, narcotic requirement, and time to return to normal activity. Laparoscopic management was associated with significant cost savings when compared with laparotomy ($\$5528 \pm 1586$ vs. $\$6793 \pm 155$). Using a prospective analysis, 105 patients with tubal pregnancy were stratified with regard to age and risk factors and then randomized to undergo either laparoscopic management or laparotomy (141). Seventy-three patients subsequently underwent a "second-look" laparoscopy to assess the degree of adhesion formation. Patients treated by laparotomy had significantly more adhesions at the surgical site than those treated by laparoscopy, but tubal patency rates were similar. Pregnancy rates were not analyzed.

Reproductive Outcome

Reproductive outcome after ectopic pregnancy is usually evaluated by determining tubal patency by hysterosalpingography, the subsequent intrauterine pregnancy rate, and the recurrent ectopic pregnancy rate. Pregnancy rates are similar in patients treated by either laparoscopy or laparotomy. Tubal patency on the ipsilateral side after conservative laparoscopic management is approximately 84%.

In a study of 143 patients followed after undergoing laparoscopic procedures for ectopic pregnancy, the overall intrauterine pregnancy rates for laparoscopic salpingostomy (60%) and laparoscopic salpingectomy (54%) were not significantly different (142). If the patient had evidence of tubal damage, pregnancy rates (42%) were significantly lower than in those women who did not have tubal damage (79%). In another study, the reproductive outcome of 188 patients followed for a mean of 7.2 years (range, 3–15) was reported after conservation by laparotomy for ectopic pregnancy (143). An intrauterine pregnancy occurred in 83 (70%) patients, with a recurrent ectopic pregnancy rate of 13%, suggesting that reproductive outcome after an ectopic pregnancy treated by laparotomy is similar to that of patients undergoing laparoscopic or medical management. Thus, when compared to medical therapy, surgical management appears to have equal reproductive outcome, although a prospective randomized trial has not been reported.

Medical Treatment

The medical management of ectopic pregnancy is most frequently *methotrexate,* although other agents have been studied, including potassium chloride (KCl), hyperosmolar glucose, prostaglandins, and *RU-486*. These agents may be given systemically (intravenous, intramuscular, or oral) or locally (laparoscopic direct injection, transvaginal ultrasound-directed injection, or retrograde salpingography).

Methotrexate   *Methotrexate* is a folic acid analogue that inhibits dehydrofolate reductase and thereby prevents synthesis of DNA. It has been used extensively for the treatment of gestational trophoblastic disease (see Chapter 35). Commonly reported side effects include leukopenia, thrombocytopenia, bone marrow aplasia, ulcerative stomatitis, diarrhea, and hemorrhagic enteritis. Other reported side effects include alopecia, dermatitis, elevated liver enzymes, and pneumonitis (144). However, no significant side effects have been reported at the low doses used for ectopic pregnancy treatment. Minor side effects have been reported with multiple doses; *citrovorum factor* reduces the incidence of these side effects and is generally used when prolonged treatment is required. Importantly, long-term follow-up of women treated with methotrexate for gestational trophoblastic disease shows no increase in congenital malformation, spontaneous abortions, or second tumors after chemotherapy (145). A smaller total dose of *methotrexate* is required and shorter treatment duration is used for ectopic pregnancy than for gestational trophoplastic disease.

Initially, *methotrexate* was used for the treatment of trophoblastic tissue left *in situ* after exploration for an abdominal pregnancy (146). In 1982, Tanaka et al. treated an unruptured interstitial gestation with a 15-day course of intramuscular *methotrexate* (147). The use of *methotrexate* for primary treatment of ectopic pregnancy has been reported in over 300 patients (148–157).

A trial of intramuscular *methotrexate* (1 mg/kg/day) followed by *citrovorum factor* (0.1 mg/kg/day) on alternate days was given to 100 patients with a success rate of 96% (151, 153). This outpatient treatment protocol used *methotrexate/citrovorum factor* given only until the hCG level began to decline. Treatment was given until there was at least a 15% decline between two consecutive daily hCG levels. *Citrovorum factor* is given on the day after the *methotrexate* is administered, even if no further *methotrexate* is indicated. Once *methotrexate* is discontinued, hCG levels are measured weekly until the results are negative. A second course of *methotrexate/citrovorum factor* is given only if there is a plateau or rise in the hCG level. Of the 96 patients successfully treated, 17 required only one *methotrexate/citrovorum factor* dose, and 19 required four doses. Four patients treated with *methotrexate* failed therapy and required surgical treatment for tubal rupture, and each of these cases was different with respect to ectopic pregnancy size, hCG level, and time of rupture. Of five ectopic pregnancies with cardiac activity, four were successfully treated. No conclusions can be drawn regarding risk factors or predictors of ectopic pregnancy rupture.

Single-dose intramuscular *methotrexate* for ectopic pregnancy treatment was administered to 31 patients with an injection of 50 mg/m^2 without *citrovorum factor*. Twenty-nine of 30 patients (96.7%) were successfully treated, and no patients experienced *methotrexate*-related side effects. Some 200 patients have now been treated using the single-dose protocol outlined in Table 17.3. Compared with the multidose protocol, single-dose *methotrexate* is less expensive, patient acceptance is greater because less monitoring is required during treatment, the incidence of side effects is decreased, and the treatment results and prospects for future fertility are comparable.

Initiating Methotrexate   Table 17.4 outlines a checklist that should be followed by the physician before initiating *methotrexate* and lists instructions that are helpful to the patient.

Patient Follow-Up   After intramuscular administration of *methotrexate,* patients are monitored on an outpatient basis. Patients who report severe pain or pain that is prolonged are evaluated by measuring hematocrit levels and performing transvaginal ultrasonography. The ultrasonography findings during follow-up, although not usually helpful, can be

Table 17.3   Single–Dose Methotrexate Protocol for Ectopic Pregnancy

Day	Therapy
0	D&C, hCG
1	CBC, SGOT, BUN, creatinine, blood type and Rh
4	Methotrexate 50 mg/M^2 I.M.
7	hCG

If <15% decline in hCG level between days 4 and 7, give second dose of methotrexate 50 mg/m^2 on day 7.
If >15% decline in hCG level between days 4 and 7, follow weekly until hCG <10 mIU/ml.
In patients not requiring D&C (hCG >2000 mIU/ml and no gestational sac on transvaginal ultrasonography), days 0 and 1 are combined.
D&C, dilation and curettage; hCG, human chorionic gonadotropin; CBC, complete blood count; SGOT, serum glutamic-oxaloacetic transaminase; BUN, blood urea nitrogen; MTX, methotrexate.

Table 17.4   Initiation of Methotrexate: Physician Checklist and Patient Instructions

Physician Checklist:

Obtain hCG level.
Perform transvaginal ultrasound within 48 hours.
Perform endometrial curettage if hCG level <2000 mIU/ml.
Obtain normal liver function (SGOT), normal renal function (BUN, creatinine), and a
    normal CBC (WBC <2000/ml and platelet count >100,000)
Administer Rhogam if patient is Rh-negative.
Identify unruptured ectopic pregnancy <3.5 cm.
Obtain informed consent.
Prescribe FeSO$_4$ 325 mg PO bid if hematocrit <30%.
Schedule follow-up appointment on days 4, 6, and 7.

Patient Instructions:

Refrain from alcohol use, multivitamins containing folic acid, and sexual intercourse
    until hCG level is negative.
Call your physician:
    If you experience prolonged or heavy vaginal bleeding.
    The pain is prolonged or severe (lower abdomen and pelvic pain is normal during the
        first 10–14 days of treatment).
    Use oral contraception or barrier contraceptive methods.

Approximately 4–5% of women experience unsuccessful methotrexate treatment and require surgery.
hCG, human chorionic gonadotropin; SGOT, serum glutamic-oxaloacetic transaminase; BUN, blood urea nitrogen; CBC, complete blood count; WBC, white blood cell.

used to provide reassurance that the tube has not ruptured (158). Cul-de-sac fluid is very common, and the amount of fluid may increase if a tubal abortion occurs. However, it is usually not necessary to intervene surgically unless the patient has a precipitous drop in hematocrit levels or she becomes hemodynamically unstable.

Patients are asked not to become pregnant for at least 2 months after treatment. Hysterosalpingography can be performed, although the procedure is not mandatory.

Candidates for Methotrexate   In order to maximize the safety of treatment and to eliminate the possibility of treating in the presence of a nonviable or early viable intrauterine pregnancy, patients considered candidates for *methotrexate* treatment should include those to whom the following factors apply:

1. An hCG level is present after salpingostomy or salpingotomy

2. A rising or plateaued hCG level is present at least 12–24 hours after suction curettage

3. No intrauterine gestational sac or fluid collection is detected by transvaginal ultrasound, hCG level is <2000 mIU/ml, and an ectopic pregnancy mass ≤3.5 cm is demonstrated

One must interpret the ultrasound finding with caution, because the most unruptured ectopic pregnancies will be accompanied by fluid in the cul-de-sac.

Opponents of *methotrexate* therapy cite potential side effects as the reason not to use it. Most reported side effects have occurred in patients treated with intravenous *methotrexate* with higher doses and for more prolonged treatment courses than now required. When using the single-dose intramuscular regimen, the incidence of side effects is <1% and the failure rate is comparable to conservative laparoscopic surgery. One problem that remains puzzling is the inability to predict treatment failures with *methotrexate*. However, the same is true with conservative surgical procedures; thus, the need to monitor hCG levels following either salpingostomy or *methotrexate* remains. Although surgical management of ectopic pregnancy remains the mainstay of treatment worldwide, *methotrexate* treatment is appropriate in select patient populations.

Reproductive Function   Although there are few data, reproductive function after *methotrexate* treatment can be assessed on the basis of tubal patency and pregnancy outcome. Tubal patency is reported to be 50–100%, with a mean of 71%, after systemic *methotrexate* treatment. In two separate reports of 23 and 62 patients, the tubal patency rate on the ipsilateral side was 81.4% and 82.3%, respectively (154, 159).

Pregnancy outcome after *methotrexate* administration was reported in a group of 14 patients who attempted pregnancy after multiple intramuscular doses. Eleven of these 14 (78.6%) became pregnant; 10 of 11 (90.9%) were intrauterine pregnancies and one (9%) was an extrauterine pregnancy (154). The mean time from first attempting to achieving pregnancy was 2.3 months (range, 1–4). In another study of 49 patients who were attempting pregnancy after completion of single-dose intramuscular *methotrexate*, 39 (80%) became pregnant; 34 (87%) were intrauterine pregnancies and five (13%) were ectopic pregnancies (160). The mean time from attempting to achieving pregnancy was 3.2 ± 1.1 months. In 87 pregnancies after *methotrexate* therapy, the combined intrauterine pregnancy rate was 86% and the ectopic pregnancy rate was 14%.

In a combined series of 527 patients treated by laparoscopic linear salpingostomy or salpingotomy, the intrauterine pregnancy rate was 54% and the recurrent ectopic pregnancy rate was 13% (161). Comparison of laparoscopically treated patients with *methotrexate*-treated patients suggests that the two methods have similar reproductive outcomes.

Other Drugs and Techniques

Salpingocentesis is a technique in which agents such as KCl, *methotrexate*, prostaglandins, or hyperosmolar glucose are injected into the ectopic pregnancy transvaginally using ultrasound guidance, by transcervical tubal cannulization, or by laparoscopy. Agents injected under ultrasound guidance have included *methotrexate* (162–166), KCl (167), combined *methotrexate* and KCl (168), and prostaglandin E_2 (PGE_2) (169). The potential advantages of salpingocentesis include a one-time injection with the potential avoidance of systemic side effects. Reproductive function after this form of treatment has not been reported. Because of the limited experience, this treatment cannot be recommended until there is further study.

Agents injected into the amniotic sac at laparoscopy have included $F_{2\alpha}$ (170) hyperosmolar glucose (171) and *methotrexate* (172). This method has the obvious disadvantage of requiring laparoscopy, but it can be used if laparoscopy has been performed. Other agents reported for the treatment of ectopic pregnancy include *RU-486* (173) and anti-hCG antibody (174).

Types of Ectopic Pregnancy

Spontaneous Resolution

Some ectopic pregnancies resolve by resorption or by tubal abortion, obviating the need for medical or surgical therapy (175–179). The proportion of ectopic pregnancies that resolve spontaneously and the reason they do so while others do not are unknown. There are no specific criteria for patient selection that predict successful outcome after spontaneous resolution. A falling hCG level is the most common indicator used, but ectopic pregnancy rupture can occur even with falling hCG levels.

Persistent Ectopic Pregnancy

Persistent ectopic pregnancy occurs when a patient has undergone conservative surgery (e.g., salpingostomy, fimbrial expression) and viable trophoblastic tissue remains. Histologically, there is no identifiable embryo, the implantation is usually medial to the previous tubal incision, and residual chorionic villi are usually confined to the tubal muscularis. Peritoneal trophoblastic tissue implants may also be responsible for persistence (180–185).

The incidence of persistent ectopic pregnancy has increased with the increased use of surgery that conserves the tubes. Persistence is diagnosed when the hCG levels plateau after conservative surgery. Persistent ectopic gestation is best diagnosed by an initial measurement of serum hCG or progesterone 6 days postoperatively and at 3-day intervals thereafter (183).

Risk factors for persistent ectopic pregnancy are based on the type of surgical procedure, the initial hCG level, the duration of amenorrhea, and the size of the ectopic pregnancy. A slower decline of serum hCG levels has been seen in patients treated with salpingostomy compared with patients treated by salpingectomy. The incidence of persistence after laparoscopic linear salpingostomy ranges from 3–20% (186, 187). It is uncertain whether the incidence of persistent ectopic pregnancy is the same or greater when the procedure is performed by laparoscopy versus laparotomy. In a review of medical records from 157 patients who underwent salpingostomy for intact ampullary ectopic pregnancy, 16 of 103 patients (16%) undergoing laparoscopic salpingostomy were treated for persistent ectopic pregnancy, whereas one of 54 women (2%) who had salpingostomy by laparotomy was treated for persistent ectopic pregnancy (182). Lundorff et al. reported that 23% of women with a preoperative hCG level <3000 mIU/ml developed persistent ectopic pregnancy, whereas only one of 67 with a level >3000 persisted (184). They also noted that 36% of women with an hCG level >1000 mIU/ml on the second postoperative day and 64% of patients with a level >1000 on the seventh postoperative day developed persistence. Amenorrhea of less than 7 weeks' duration and ectopic mass <2 cm have also been reported to increase the risk for persistent ectopic pregnancy (182, 184).

Treatment of persistent ectopic pregnancy can be either surgical or medical; surgical therapy consists of either repeat salpingostomy or, more commonly, salpingectomy. *Methotrexate* offers an alternative to patients who are hemodynamically stable at the time of diagnosis. *Methotrexate* may be the treatment of choice because the persistent trophoblastic tissue may not be confined to the tube and, therefore, not readily identifiable during repeat surgical exploration (187–189).

Chronic Ectopic Pregnancy

Chronic ectopic pregnancy is a condition in which the pregnancy does not completely resorb during expectant management. The condition arises when there is persistence of the chorionic villi with bleeding into the tubal wall, which is distended slowly and does not rupture. It may also arise from chronic bleeding from the fimbriated end of the fallopian tube with subsequent tamponade. In a series of 50 patients with a chronic ectopic pregnancy, pain was present in 86%, vaginal bleeding was present in 68%, and both symptoms were present in 58% (190). Ninety percent of the patients had amenorrhea ranging from 5 to 16 weeks (mean, 9.6 weeks). Most patients develop a pelvic mass that is usually symptomatic. The hCG level is usually low but may be absent, ultrasound may be helpful in the diagnosis, and rarely bowel involvement or ureteral compression or obstruction exists (190, 191).

This condition is treated surgically with removal of the affected tube. Often, the ovary must be removed because there is inflammation with subsequent adhesion development. A hematoma may be present secondary to chronic bleeding.

Nontubal Ectopic Pregnancy

Cervical Pregnancy   The incidence of cervical pregnancy in the United States ranges from 1:2400 to 1:50,000 pregnancies (192). A variety of conditions are thought to predispose to the development of a cervical pregnancy, including previous therapeutic abortion, Asherman's syndrome, previous cesarean delivery, diethylstilbestrol exposure, leiomyomata, and *in vitro* fertilization (192–194).

The diagnostic criteria for cervical pregnancy were established based upon histologic analysis of a hysterectomy specimen (192). Clinical criteria include the following findings (194):

1. The uterus surrounding the distended cervix is smaller.

2. The internal os is not dilated.

3. Curettage of the endometrial cavity is nonproductive of placental tissue.

4. The external os opens earlier than in spontaneous abortion.

Ultrasonographic diagnostic criteria have also been described that are helpful in differentiating a true cervical pregnancy from an ongoing spontaneous abortion (Table 17.5). Magnetic resonance imaging of the pelvis has also been used in this situation (195). Other potential diagnoses that must be differentiated from cervical pregnancy include cervical carcinoma, cervical or prolapsed submucous leiomyomata, trophoblastic tumor, placenta previa, or low-lying placenta.

When a cervical pregnancy is diagnosed before surgery, the preoperative preparation should include blood typing and cross-matching, establishment of intravenous access, and detailed informed consent. This consent should include the possibility of hemorrhage that may require transfusion or hysterectomy. Nonsurgical treatment including intra-amniotic and systemic *methotrexate* administration have been used successfully (196, 197).

The diagnosis may not be suspected until the patient is undergoing suction curettage for a presumed incomplete abortion and hemorrhage occurs. In some cases, bleeding is light, and

---

Table 17.5   Ultrasound Criteria for Cervical Pregnancy

1. Echo-free uterine cavity or the presence of a false gestational sac only.
2. Decidual transformation of the endometrium with dense echo structure.
3. Diffuse uterine wall structure.
4. Hourglass uterine shape.
5. Ballooned cervical canal.
6. Gestational sac in the endocervix.
7. Placental tissue in the cervical canal.
8. Closed internal os.

Reproduced with permission from **Hofmann HMH, Urdl W, Hofler H, Honigl W, Tamussino K.** Cervical pregnancy: case reports and current concepts in diagnosis and treatment. *Arch Gynecol Obstet* 1987;241:63–9.

in others, there is hemorrhage. Various techniques that can be used to control bleeding include uterine packing, lateral cervical suture placement to ligate the lateral cervical vessels, placement of a cerclage, or insertion of an intracervical 30-ml Foley catheter in an attempt to tamponade the bleeding. Alternatively, angiographic artery embolization can be used or, if laparotomy is required, an attempt can be made to ligate the uterine or internal iliac arteries (198–200). When none of these methods is successful, hysterectomy is required.

Ovarian Pregnancy   A pregnancy confined to the ovary represents 0.5–1.0% of all ectopic pregnancies and is the most common type of nontubal ectopic pregnancy. The incidence ranges from one in 40,000 to one in 7000 deliveries (201, 202). The diagnostic criteria were described in 1878 by Spiegelberg (Table 17.6). Unlike tubal gestation, ovarian pregnancy is associated with neither pelvic inflammatory disease nor infertility. The only risk factor associated with the development of an ovarian pregnancy is the current use of an intrauterine device.

Patients have symptoms similar to those of ectopic pregnancies in other sites. Misdiagnosis is common because it is confused with a ruptured corpus luteum in up to 75% (201). As with other types of ectopic pregnancy, an ovarian pregnancy has also been reported after hysterectomy (203). Ultrasonography has made preoperative diagnosis possible in some cases (204).

The treatment of ovarian pregnancy has changed. Whereas oophorectomy has been advocated in the past, ovarian cystectomy has become the preferred treatment (205). It is possible to perform cystectomy using laparoscopic techniques (206, 207). Treatment with *methotrexate* or prostaglandin injection has also been reported (207).

Abdominal Pregnancy   Abdominal pregnancies are classified as primary and secondary. Table 17.7 lists criteria for classifying a primary abdominal pregnancy. Secondary abdominal pregnancies are by far the most common and result from tubal abortion or rupture or, less often, after uterine rupture with subsequent implantation within the abdomen. The incidence of abdominal pregnancy varies from one in 372 to one in 9714 live births (208). Abdominal pregnancy is associated with high morbidity and mortality, with the risk of death seven to eight times greater than from tubal ectopic pregnancy and 90 times greater than from intrauterine pregnancy. There are scattered reports of term abdominal pregnancies. When this occurs, perinatal morbidity and mortality are high, usually as a result of growth restriction and congenital anomalies such as fetal pulmonary hypoplasia, pressure deformities, and facial and limb asymmetry. The incidence of congenital anomalies ranges from 20–40% (209).

Table 17.6   Criteria for Ovarian Pregnancy Diagnosis

1. The fallopian tube on the affected side must be intact.
2. The fetal sac must occupy the position of the ovary.
3. The ovary must be connected to the uterus by the ovarian ligament.
4. Ovarian tissue must be located in the sac wall.

From **Spiegelberg O.** Casusistik der ovarialschwangerschaft. *Arch Gynaecol* 1878;13:73.

Table 17.7   Studdiford's Criteria for Diagnosis of Primary Abdominal Pregnancy

1. Presence of normal tubes and ovaries with no evidence of recent or past pregnancy.
2. No evidence of uteroplacental fistula.
3. The presence of a pregnancy related exclusively to the peritoneal surface and early enough to eliminate the possibility of secondary implantation after primary tubal nidation.

The presentation of patients with an abdominal pregnancy varies and depends on the gestational age. In the first and early second trimester, the symptoms may be the same as with tubal ectopic gestation; in advanced abdominal pregnancy, the clinical presentation is more variable. The patient may complain of painful fetal movement, fetal movements high in the abdomen, or sudden cessation of movements. Physical examination may disclose persistent abnormal fetal lies, abdominal tenderness, a displaced uterine cervix, "easy" palpation of fetal parts, and palpation of the uterus separate from the gestation. The diagnosis may be suspected when there are no uterine contractions after oxytocin infusion. Other diagnostic aids include abdominal x-ray, abdominal ultrasound, computed tomography scanning, and magnetic resonance imaging (210, 211).

Because the pregnancy can continue to term, the potential maternal morbidity and mortality is very high. As a result, surgical intervention is recommended when an abdominal pregnancy is diagnosed. At surgery, the placenta can be removed if its vascular supply can be identified and ligated, but hemorrhage can occur, requiring abdominal packing that is left in place and removed after 24–48 hours. Angiographic arterial embolization has been described (212). If the vascular supply cannot be identified, the cord is ligated near the placental base and the placenta is left in place. Placental involution can be monitored using serial ultrasonography and hCG levels. Potential complications of leaving the placenta in place include bowel obstruction, fistula formation, or sepsis as the tissue degenerates. *Methotrexate* treatment appears to be contraindicated, because a high rate of complications has been reported, including sepsis and death, believed to be a result of rapid tissue necrosis (213).

Interstitial Pregnancy   Interstitial pregnancies represent approximately 1% of ectopic pregnancies. These patients tend to present later in gestation than those with tubal pregnancies. Interstitial pregnancies often are associated with uterine rupture; therefore, they represent a disproportionately large percentage of fatalities from ectopic pregnancy. Treatment is cornual resection by laparotomy, although laparoscopic management has also been described (214).

Interligamentous Pregnancy   Interligamentous pregnancy is a rare form of ectopic pregnancy and occurs in approximately one in every 300 ectopic pregnancies (215). An interligamentous pregnancy usually results from trophoblastic penetration of a tubal pregnancy through the tubal serosa and into the mesosalpinx, with secondary implantation between the leaves of the broad ligament. It can also occur if a uterine fistula develops between the endometrial cavity and the retroperitoneal space. As with an abdominal pregnancy, the placenta may be adherent to the uterus, bladder, and pelvic side walls. If possible, the placenta should be removed; when this is not possible, it can be left *in situ* and allowed to resorb. As in abdominal pregnancy, there are reported cases of live birth with this type ectopic gestation (215).

Heterotropic Pregnancy   Heterotropic pregnancy occurs when there are coexisting intrauterine and ectopic pregnancies. The reported incidence varies widely from one in 100 to one in 30,000 pregnancies (216). Patients who have undergone ovulation induction have a much higher incidence of heterotropic pregnancy than those who have a spontaneous conception. An intrauterine pregnancy is seen during ultrasound examination, and an extrauterine pregnancy may be overlooked easily. Serial hCG levels are often not helpful because the intrauterine pregnancy will cause the hCG level to rise appropriately.

The treatment of the ectopic pregnancy is operative, once the ectopic pregnancy has been removed; intrauterine pregnancy continues in most patients. It may be possible to use nonchemotherapeutic medical treatment such as KCl by transvaginal or laparoscopically directed injection for treatment of the ectopic pregnancy.

Multiple Ectopic Pregnancies   Twin or multiple ectopic gestations occur less frequently than heterotopic gestations and may appear in a variety of locations and combinations. About 250 twin ectopic gestations have been reported (217). Although most reports are confined to twin tubal gestations, ovarian, interstitial, and abdominal twin pregnancies have been reported. Twin and triplet gestations have been reported following partial salpingectomy (218) and after *in vitro* fertilization (219). Management is similar to other types of ectopic pregnancy and is somewhat dependent on the location of the pregnancy.

Pregnancy after Hysterectomy   The most unusual form of ectopic pregnancy is one that occurs after either vaginal or abdominal hysterectomy (220, 221). Such a pregnancy may occur after supracervical hysterectomy, because the patient has a cervical canal that may provide intraperitoneal access. Pregnancy may occur in the perioperative period with implantation of the fertilized ovum in the fallopian tube. Pregnancy after total hysterectomy probably occurs secondary to a vaginal mucosal defect that allows sperm into the abdominal cavity.

References

1. **Hill LM, Guzick D, Fries J, Hixson J.** Fetal loss rate after ultrasonically documented cardiac activity between 6 and 14 weeks menstrual age. *J Clin Ultrasound* 1991;19:221–3.

2. **Simpson JL, Mills JL, Holmes LB, Ober CL, Aarsons J, Jovanovic L, Knopp RH.** Low fetal loss rates after ultrasound-proved viability in early pregnancy. *JAMA* 1987;258:2555–7.

3. **Goldstein SR.** Embryonic death in early pregnancy: a new look at the first trimester. *Obstet Gynecol* 1994;84:294–7.

4. **Tongsong T, Wanapirak C, Srisomboon J, Sirichotiyakul S, Polsrisuthikul T, Pongsatha S.** Transvaginal ultrasound in threatened abortions with empty gestational sacs. *Int J Gynaecol Obstet* 1994;46:297–301.

5. **Goldner TE, Lawson HW, Xia Z, Atrash HK.** Surveillance for ectopic pregnancy—United States, 1970-1989. *MMWR CDC Surveillance Summary* 1993;42:(SS-6);73–85.

6. **National Center for Health Statistics.** *Annual Summary of Births, Marriages, Divorces and Deaths: United States, 1989.* Hyattsville, MD: US Department of Health and Human Services, Public Health Service, 1990;38(13):23.

7. **Diquelou JY, Pia P, Tesquier L, Henry-Suchet J, Gicquel JM, Boyer S.** The role of Chlamydia trachomatis in the infectious etiology of extra-uterine pregnancy. *J Gynecol Obstet Biol Reprod (Paris)* 1988;17:325–32.

8. **Chow WH, Daling JR, Cates W Jr, Greenberg RS.** Epidemiology of ectopic pregnancy. *Epidemiol Rev* 1987;9:70–94.

9. **Levin AA, Schoenbaum SC, Stubblefield PG, Zimicki S, Monson RR, Ryan KJ.** Ectopic pregnancy and prior induced abortion. *Am J Public Health* 1982;72:253–6.

10. **Chi IC, Potts M, Wilkens L.** Rare events associated with tubal sterilizations: an international experience. *Obstet Gynecol Surv* 1986;41:7–19.

11. **Lavy G, Diamond MP, DeCherney AH.** Ectopic pregnancy: its relationship to tubal reconstructive surgery. *Fertil Steril* 1987;47:543–56.

12. **Cartwright PS, Entman SS.** Repeat ipsilateral tubal pregnancy following partial salpingectomy: a case report. *Fertil Steril* 1984;42:647–8.

13. **Richardson DA, Evans MI, Talerman A, Maroulis GB.** Segmental absence of the mid-portion of the fallopian tube. *Fertil Steril* 1982;37:577–9.

14. **Wanerman J, Wulwick R, Brenner S.** Segmental absence of the fallopian tube. *Fertil Steril* 1986;46:525–7.

15. **Weinstein L, Morris MB, Dotters D, Christian CD.** Ectopic pregnancy—a new surgical epidemic. *Obstet Gynecol* 1983;61:698–701.

16. **Pulkkinen MO, Talo A.** Tubal physiologic consideration in ectopic pregnancy. *Clin Obstet Gynecol* 1987;30:164–72.

17. **Persaud V.** Etiology of tubal ectopic pregnancy: radiologic and pathologic studies. *Obstet Gynecol* 1970;36:257–63.

18. **Elias S, LeBeau M, Simpson JL, Martin AO.** Chromosome analysis of ectopic human conceptuses. *Am J Obstet Gynecol* 1981;141:698–703.

19. **Westrom L, Bengtsson LPH, Mardh P-A.** Incidence, trends, and risks of ectopic pregnancy in a population of women. *BMJ* 1981;282:15–8.

20. **Westrom L.** Influence of sexually transmitted diseases on sterility and ectopic pregnancy. *Acta Eur Fertil* 1985;16:21–4.

21. **Berenson A, Hammill H, Martens M, Faro S.** Bacteriologic findings with ectopic pregnancy. *J Reprod Med* 1991;36:118–120.

22. **Coste J, Job-Spira N, Fernandez H, Papiernik E, Spira A.** Risk factors for ectopic pregnancy: a case-control study in France, with special focus on infectious factors. *Am J Epidemiol* 1991;133:839–49.

23. **Svensson L, Mardh P-A, Ahlgren M, Nordenskjold F.** Ectopic pregnancy and antibodies to Chlamydia trachomatis. *Fertil Steril* 1985;44:313–7.

24. **Brunham RC, Binns B, McDowell J, Paraskevas M.** Chlamydia trachomatis infection in women with ectopic pregnancy. *Obstet Gynecol* 1986;67:722–6.

25. **Miettinen A, Heinonen PK, Teisala K, Hakkarainen K, Punnonen R.** Serologic evidence for the role of Chlamydia trachomatis, Neisseria gonorrhoeae, and Mycoplasma hominis in the etiology of tubal factor infertility and ectopic pregnancy. *Sex Transm Dis* 1990;17:10–4.

26. **Chow JM, Yonekura ML, Richwald GA, Greenland S, Sweet RL, Schachter J.** The association between Chlamydia trachomatis and ectopic pregnancy: a matched-pair, case-control study. *JAMA* 1990;263:3164–7.

27. **Ory HW. The Women's Health Study.** Ectopic pregnancy and intrauterine contraceptive devices: new perspectives. *Obstet Gynecol* 1981;57:137–44.

28. **The World Health Organization's Programme of Research, Development and Research Training in Human Reproduction: Task Force on Intrauterine Devices for Fertility Regulation.** A multinational case-control study of ectopic pregnancy. *Clin Reprod Fertil* 1985;3(2):131–43.

29. **Sivin I.** Dose- and age-dependent ectopic pregnancy risks with intrauterine contraception. *Obstet Gynecol* 1991;78:291–8.

30. **Vessey M, Meisler L, Flavel R, Yeates D.** Outcome of pregnancy in women using different methods of contraception. *Br J Obstet Gynaecol* 1979;86:548–56.

31. **Chow WH, Daling JR, Weiss NS, Moore DE, Soderstrom RM, Metch BJ.** IUD use and subsequent tubal ectopic pregnancy. *Am J Public Health* 1986;76:536–9.

32. **Wilson JC.** A prospective New Zealand study of fertility after removal of copper intrauterine contraceptive devices for conception and because of complications: a four-year study. *Am J Obstet Gynecol* 1989;160:391–6.

33. **Franks AL, Beral V, Cates W Jr, Hogue CJR.** Contraception and ectopic pregnancy risk. *Am J Obstet Gynecol* 1990;163:1120–3.

34. **Rantakyla P, Ylostalo P, Jarvinen PA, Vuorjoki A.** Ectopic pregnancies and the use of intrauterine device and low dose progestogen contraception. *Acta Obstet Gynecol Scand* 1977;56:61–2.

35. **Liukko P, Erkkola R, Laakso L.** Ectopic pregnancies during use of low-dose progestogens for oral contraception. *Contraception* 1977;16:575–80.

36. **Sivin I.** International experience with NORPLANT and NORPLANT-2 contraceptives. *Stud Fam Plann* 1988;19:81–94.

37. **Shoupe D, Mishell DR Jr, Bopp BL, Fielding M.** The significance of bleeding patterns in Norplant implant users. *Obstet Gynecol* 1991;77:256–60.

38. **Trussell J, Kost K.** Contraceptive failure in the United States: a critical review of the literature. *Stud Fam Plann* 1987;18:237–83.

39. **Cheng MC, Wong YM, Rochat RW, Ratman SS.** Sterilization failures in Singapore: an examination of ligation techniques and failure rates. *Stud Fam Plann* 1977;8:109–15.

40. **DeStefano F, Peterson HB, Layde PM, Rubin GL.** Risk of ectopic pregnancy following tubal sterilization. *Obstet Gynecol* 1982;60:326–30.

41. **McCausland A.** High rate of ectopic pregnancy following laparoscopic tubal coagulation failures: incidence and etiology. *Am J Obstet Gynecol* 1980;136:97–101.

42. **Langer R, Bukovsky I, Herman A, Sherman D, Sadovsky G, Caspi E.** Conservative surgery for tubal pregnancy. *Fertil Steril* 1982;38:427–30.

43. **Lavy G, DeCherney AH.** The hormonal basis of ectopic pregnancy. *Clin Obstet Gynecol* 1987; 30:217–24.

44. **DeCherney AH, Cholst I, Naftolin F.** Structure and function of the fallopian tubes following exposure to diethylstilbestrol (DES) during gestation. *Fertil Steril* 1981;36:741–5.

45. **Hallatt JG.** Tubal conservation in ectopic pregnancy: a study of 200 cases. *Am J Obstet Gynecol* 1986;154:1216–21.

46. **Lennox CE, Mills JA, James GB.** Reversal of female sterilization: a comparative study. *Contraception* 1987;35:19–27.

47. **Hulka JF, Halme J.** Sterilization reversal: results of 101 attempts. *Am J Obstet Gynecol* 1988; 159:767–74.

48. **Marchbanks PA, Annegers JF, Coulam CB, Strathy JH, Kurland LT.** Risk factors for ectopic pregnancy: a population-based study. *JAMA* 1988;259:1823–7.

49. **Ni H, Daling JR, Chu J, Stergachis A, Voigt LF, Weiss WS.** Previous abdominal surgery and tubal pregnancy. *Obstet Gynecol* 1990;75:919–22.

50. **Trimbos-Kemper T, Trimbos B, van Hall E.** Etiological factors in tubal infertility. *Fertil Steril* 1982;37:384–8.

51. **Weinstein D, Polishuk WZ.** The role of wedge resection of the ovary as a cause for mechanical sterility. *Surg Gynecol Obstet* 1975;141:417–8.

52. **Shoupe D, Mishell DR.** Norplant: subdermal implant system for long-term contraception. *Am J Obstet Gynecol* 1989;160:1286–92.

53. **Burkman RT, Mason KJ, Gold EB.** Ectopic pregnancy and prior induced abortion. *Contraception* 1988;37:21–7.

54. **Kalandidi A, Doulgerakis M, Tzonou A, Hsieh CC, Aravandinos D, Trichopoulos D.** Induced abortions, contraceptive practices, and tobacco smoking as risk factors for ectopic pregnancy in Athens, Greece. *Br J Obstet Gynaecol* 1991;98:207–13.

55. **Marchbanks PA, Coulam CB, Annegers JF.** An association between clomiphene citrate and ectopic pregnancy: a preliminary report. *Fertil Steril* 1985;44:268–70.

56. **McBain JC, Evans JH, Pepperell RJ, Robinson HP, Smith MA, Brown JB.** An unexpectedly high rate of ectopic pregnancy following the induction of ovulation with human pituitary and chorionic gonadotropin. *Br J Obstet Gynaecol* 1980;87:5–9.

57. **Gemzell C, Guillome J, Wang CF.** Ectopic pregnancy following treatment with human gonadotropins. *Am J Obstet Gynecol* 1982;143:761–5.

58. **Oelsner G, Blankstein J, Menashe Y, tur-Kaspa I, Ben-Rafael Z, Blankenstein J, Serr DM, Mashiach S.** The role of gonadotropins in the etiology of ectopic pregnancy. *Fertil Steril* 1989;52:514–6.

59. **Steptoe PC, Edwards RG.** Reimplantation of a human embryo with subsequent tubal pregnancy. *Lancet* 1976;1:880–2.

60. **Carson SL, Dickey RP, Gocial B, Batzer FR, Eisenberg E, Huppert L, Maislin G.** Outcome in 242 in vitro fertilization-embryo replacement or gamete intrafallopian transfer-induced pregnancies. *Fertil Steril* 1989;51:644–50.

61. **Herman A, Ron-El R, Golan A, Weinraub Z, Bukovsky I, Caspi E.** The role of tubal pathology and other parameters in ectopic pregnancies occurring in in vitro fertilization and embryo transfer. *Fertil Steril* 1990;54:864–8.

62. **Dor J, Seidman DS, Levron D, Ben-Rafael Z, BenShlomo I, Masiach S.** The incidence of combined intrauterine and extrauterine pregnancy after in vitro fertilization and embryo transfer. *Fertil Steril* 1991;55:833–4.

63. **Dubuisson JB, Aubriot FX, Cardone V, Vacher-Lavenu MC.** Tubal causes of ectopic pregnancy. *Fertil Steril* 1986;46:970–2.

64. **Homm RJ, Holtz G, Garvin AJ.** Isthmic ectopic pregnancy and salpingitis isthmica nodosa. *Fertil Steril* 1987;48:756–60.

65. **Barnes AB, Colton T, Gundersen J, Noller KL, Tilley BC, Strama T, Townsend DE, Hatab P, O'Brien PC.** Fertility and outcome of pregnancy in women exposed in utero to diethylstilbestrol. *N Engl J Med* 1980;302:609–13.

66. **Herbst AL, Hubby MM, Blough RR, Azizi F.** A comparison of pregnancy experience in DES-exposed and DES-unexposed daughters. *J Reprod Med* 1980;24:62–9.

67. **Kullander S, Kaellen B.** A prospective study of smoking and pregnancy. *Acta Obstet Gynecol Scand* 1971;50:83–94.

68. **Coste J, Job-Spira N, Fernandez H.** Increased risk of ectopic pregnancy with maternal cigarette smoking. *Am J Public Health* 1991;81:199–201.

69. **Handler A, Davis F, Ferre C, Yeko T.** The relationship of smoking and ectopic pregnancy. *Am J Public Health* 1989;79:1239–42.

70. **Niles JH, Clark JFJ.** Pathogenesis of tubal pregnancy. *Am J Obstet Gynecol* 1969;105:1230–4.

71. **Westrom L.** Effect of acute pelvic inflammatory disease on fertility. *Am J Obstet Gynecol* 1975;121:707–13.

72. **Benjamin CL, Beaver DC.** Pathogenesis of salpingitis isthmica nodosa. *Am J Clin Pathol* 1951;21:212–22.

73. **Wrork DH, Broders AC.** Adenomyosis of the fallopian tube. *Am J Obstet Gynecol* 1942; 44:412–32.

74. **Kurman RJ, Main CS, Chen HC.** Intermediate trophoblast: a distinctive form of trophoblast with specific morphological, biochemical, and functional features. *Placenta* 1984;5:349–69.

75. **Stabile I, Grudzinskas JG.** Ectopic pregnancy: a review of incidence, etiology, and diagnostic aspects. *Obstet Gynecol Surv* 1990;45:335–47.

76. **Tuomivaara L, Kauppila A, Puolakka J.** Ectopic pregnancy—an analysis of the etiology, diagnosis and treatment in 552 cases. *Arch Gynecol* 1986;237:135–47.

77. **Storring PL, Gaines-Das RE, Bangham DR.** International reference preparation of human chorionic gonadotrophin for immunoassay: potency estimates in various bioassays and protein binding assay systems; and international reference preparations of the alpha and beta subunits of human chorionic gonadotrophin for immunoassay. *J Endocrinol* 1980;84:295–310.

78. **Marshall JR, Hammond CB, Ross GT, Jacobson A, Rayford P.** Plasma and urinary chorionic gonadotropin during early human pregnancy. *Obstet Gynecol* 1968;32:760–4.

79. **Daus K, Mundy D, Graves W, Slade BA.** Ectopic pregnancy: what to do during the 20-day window. *J Reprod Med* 1989;34:162–6.

80. **Kadar N, Caldwell BV, Romero R.** A method of screening for ectopic pregnancy and its indications. *Obstet Gynecol* 1981;58:162–5.

81. **Cartwright PS, Moore RA, Dao AH, Wong SW, Anderson JR.** Serum beta-human chorionic gonadotropin levels relate poorly with the size of a tubal pregnancy. *Fertil Steril* 1987; 48:679–80.

82. **Pearlstone AC, Oei ML, Wu TCJ.** The predictive value of a single, early human chorionic gonadotropin measurement and the influence of maternal age on pregnancy outcome in an infertile population. *Fertil Steril* 1992;57:302–4.

83. **Milwidsky A, Adoni A, Segal S, Palti Z.** Chorionic gonadotropin and progesterone levels in ectopic pregnancy. *Obstet Gynecol* 1977;50:145–7.

84. **Radwanska E, Frankenberg J, Allen EI.** Plasma progesterone levels in normal and abnormal early human pregnancy. *Fertil Steril* 1978;30:398–402.

85. **Stovall TG, Ling FW, Andersen RN, Buster JE.** Improved sensitivity and specificity of a single measurement of serum progesterone over serial quantitative beta-human chorionic gonadotrophin in screening for ectopic pregnancy. *Hum Reprod* 1992;7:723–5.

86. **Stovall TG, Ling FW, Cope BJ, Buster JE.** Preventing ruptured ectopic pregnancy with a single serum progesterone. *Am J Obstet Gynecol* 1989;160:1425–31.

87. **Stovall TG, Kellerman AL, Ling FW, Buster JE.** Emergency department diagnosis of ectopic pregnancy. *Ann Emerg Med* 1990;19:1098–1103.

88. **Cowan BD, Vandermolen DT, Long CA, Whitworth NS.** Receiver operator characteristics, efficiency analysis, and predictive value of serum progesterone concentration as a test for abnormal gestations. *Am J Obstet Gynecol* 1992;166:1729–34.

89. **Barnes ER, Oelsner G, Benveniste R, Romero R, DeCherney AH.** Progesterone, estradiol, and alpha-human chorionic gonadotropin secretion in patients with ectopic pregnancy. *J Clin Endocrinol Metab* 1986;62:529–31.

90. **Witt BR, Wolf GC, Wainwright CJ, Johnston PD, Thorneycroft IH.** Relaxin, CA125, progesterone, estradiol, Schwangerschaft protein, and human chorionic gonadotropin as predictors of outcome in threatened and non-threatened pregnancies. *Fertil Steril* 1990;53: 1029–36.

91. **Guillaume J, Benjamin F, Sicuranza BJ, Deutsch S, Seltzer VL, Tores W.** Serum estradiol as an aid in the diagnosis of ectopic pregnancy. *Obstet Gynecol* 1990;76:1126–9.

92. **Lavie O, Beller U, Neuman M, Ben-Chetrit A, Gottcshalk-Sabag S, Diamant YZ.** Maternal serum creatine kinase: a possible predictor of tubal pregnancy. *Am J Obstet Gynecol* 1993;169:1149–50.

93. **Ho PC, Chan SYW, Tang GWK.** Diagnosis of early pregnancy by enzyme immunoassay of Schwangerschafts-protein 1. *Fertil Steril* 1988;49:76–80.

94. **Bell RJ, Eddie LW, Lester AR, Wood EC, Johnston PD, Niall HD.** Relaxin in human pregnancy serum measured with an homologous radioimmunoassay. *Obstet Gynecol* 1987;69: 585–9.

95. **Meunier K, Mignot TM, Maria B, Guichard A, Zorn JR, Cedard L.** Predictive value of the active renin assay for the diagnosis of ectopic pregnancy. *Fertil Steril* 1991;55:432–5.

96. **Niloff JM, Knapp RC, Schaetzl E, Reynolds C, Bast RC.** CA125 antigen levels in obstetric and gynecologic patients. *Obstet Gynecol* 1984;64:703–7.

97. **Kobayashi F, Sagawa N, Nakamura K, Nonogaki M, Ban C, Fujii S, Mori T.** Mechanism and clinical significance of elevated CA125 levels in the sera of pregnant women. *Am J Obstet Gynecol* 1989;160:563–6.

98. **Check JH, Nowroozi K, Winkel CA, Johnson T, Seefried L.** Serum CA125 levels in early pregnancy and subsequent spontaneous abortion. *Obstet Gynecol* 1990;75:742–4.

99. **Brumsted JR, Nakajima ST, Badger G, Riddick DH, Gibson M.** Serum concentration of CA125 during the first trimester of normal and abnormal pregnancies. *J Reprod Med* 1990; 35:499–502.

100. **Sadovsky Y, Pineda J, Collins JL.** Serum CA125 levels in women with ectopic and intrauterine pregnancies. *J Reprod Med* 1991;36:875–8.

101. **Cederqvist LL, Killackey MA, Abdel-Latif N, Gupta R, Saxena BB.** Alpha-fetoprotein and ectopic pregnancy. *BMJ* 1983;286:1247–8.

102. **Grosskinsky CM, Hage ML, Tyrey L, Christakos AC, Hughes CL.** hCG, progesterone, alpha-fetoprotein, and estradiol in the identification of ectopic pregnancy. *Obstet Gynecol* 1993;81:705–9.

103. **Theron GB, Shepherd EGS, Strachan AF.** C-reactive protein levels in ectopic pregnancy, pelvic infection and carcinoma of the cervix. *S Afr Med J* 1986;69:681–2.

104. **Cacciatore B.** Can the status of tubal pregnancy be predicted with transvaginal sonography? A prospective comparison of sonographic, surgical, and serum hCG findings. *Radiology* 1990;177:481–4.

105. **Thorsen MK, Lawson TL, Aiman EJ, Miller DP, McAsey ME, Erickson SJ, Quiroz F, Perret RS.** Diagnosis of ectopic pregnancy: endovaginal vs transabdominal sonography. *Am J Roentgenol* 1990;155:307–10.

106. **Bateman BG, Nunley WC Jr, Kolp LA, Kitchin JD III, Felder R.** Vaginal sonography findings and hCG dynamics of early intrauterine and tubal pregnancies. *Obstet Gynecol* 1990;75:421–7.

107. **Cacciatore B, Stenman UH, Ylostalo P.** Comparison of abdominal and vaginal sonography in suspected ectopic pregnancy. *Obstet Gynecol* 1989;73:770–4.

108. **Fleischer AC, Pennell RG, McKee MS, Worrell JA, Keffe B, Herbert CM, Hill GA, Cartwright PS, Kepple DM.** Ectopic pregnancy: features at transvaginal sonography. *Radiology* 1990;174:375–8.

109. **Timor-Tritsch IE, Yeh MN, Peisner DB, Lesser KD, Slavik TA.** The use of transvaginal ultrasonography in the diagnosis of ectopic pregnancy. *Am J Obstet Gynecol* 1989;161: 157–61.

110. **Bree RL, Marn CS.** Transvaginal sonography in the first trimester: embryology, anatomy, and hCG correlation. *Semin Ultrasound CT MR* 1990;11:12–21.

111. **Cacciatore B, Ylostalo P, Stenman UH, Widholm O.** Suspected ectopic pregnancy: ultrasound findings and hCG levels assessed by an immunofluorometric assay. *Br J Obstet Gynaecol* 1988;95:497–502.

112. **Abramovici H, Auslender R, Lewin A, Faktor JH.** Gestational-pseudogestational sac: a new ultrasonic criterion for differential diagnosis. *Am J Obstet Gynecol* 1983;145:377–9.

113. **Nyberg DA, Filly RA, Laing FC, Mack LA, Zarutskie PW.** Ectopic pregnancy, diagnosis by sonography correlated with quantitative HCG levels. *J Ultrasound Med* 1987;6:145–50.

114. **Bradley WG, Fiske CE, Filly RA.** The double sac sign of early intrauterine pregnancy: use in exclusion of ectopic pregnancy. *Radiology* 1982;143:223–6.

115. **Nyberg DA, Mack LA, Harvey D, Wang K.** Value of the yolk sac in evaluating early pregnancies. *J Ultrasound Med* 1988;7:129–35.

116. **Jain KA, Hamper UM, Sanders RC.** Comparison of transvaginal and transabdominal sonography in the detection of early pregnancy and its complications. *Am J Roentgenol* 1988;151:1139–43.

117. **Bree RL, Edwards M, Bohm VM, Beyer S, Roberts J, Mendelson EB.** Transvaginal sonography in the evaluation of normal early pregnancy: correlation with HCG level. *Am J Roentgenol* 1989;53:75–9.

118. **Nyberg DA, Hughes MP, Mack LA, Wang KY.** Extrauterine findings of ectopic pregnancy at transvaginal US: importance of echogenic fluid. *Radiology* 1991;178:823–6.

119. **Rottem S, Thaler I, Levron J, Peretz BA, Itskovitz J, Brandes JM.** Criteria for transvaginal sonographic diagnosis of ectopic pregnancy. *J Clin Ultrasound* 1990;18:274–9.

120. **Nyberg DA, Mack LA, Laing FC, Jeffrey RB.** Early pregnancy complications: endovaginal sonographic findings correlated with human chorionic gonadotropin levels. *Radiology* 1988;167:619–22.

121. **Emerson DS, Cartier MS, Altieri LA, Felker RE, Smith WC, Stovall TG, Gray LA.** Diagnostic efficacy of endovaginal color Doppler flow imaging in an ectopic pregnancy screening program. *Radiology* 1992;183:413–20.

122. **Bernaschek G, Rudelstorfer R, Csaicsich P.** Vaginal sonography versus serum human chorionic gonadotropin in early detection of pregnancy. *Am J Obstet Gynecol* 1988;158:608–12.

123. **Diamond MP, DeCherney AH.** *Ectopic Pregnancy.* Philadelphia: WB Saunders Co., 1991:163.

124. **Menard A, Crequat J, Mandelbrot L, Hanny JP, Madelenat P.** Treatment of unruptured tubal pregnancy by local injection of methotrexate under transvaginal sonographic control. *Fertil Steril* 1990;54:47–50.

125. **Campbell S, Pearce JM, Hackett G, Cohen-Overbeek T, Hernandez C.** Qualitative assessment of uteroplacental blood flow: early screening test for high-risk pregnancies. *Obstet Gynecol* 1986;68:649–53.

126. **McCowan LM, Ritchie K, Mo LY, Bascom PA, Sherret H.** Uterine artery flow velocity waveforms in normal and growth-retarded pregnancies. *Am J Obstet Gynecol* 1988;158:499–504.

127. **Taylor KJ, Ramos IM, Feyock AL, Snower DP, Carter D, Shapiro BS, Meyer WR, DeCherney AH.** Ectopic pregnancy: duplex Doppler evaluation. *Radiology* 1989;173:93–7.

128. **Dillon EH, Feyock AL, Taylor KJW.** Pseudogestational sacs: doppler US differentiation from normal or abnormal intrauterine pregnancies. *Radiology* 1990;176:359–64.

129. **Vermesh M, Graczykowski JW, Sauer MV.** Reevaluation of the role of culdocentesis in the management of ectopic pregnancy. *Am J Obstet Gynecol* 1990;162:411–3.

130. **Stovall TG, Ling FW, Carson SA, Buster JE.** Serum progesterone and uterine curettage in the differential diagnosis of ectopic pregnancy. *Fertil Steril* 1992;57:456–8.

131. **Stovall TG, Ling FW.** Ectopic pregnancy: diagnostic and therapeutic algorithms minimizing surgical intervention. *J Reprod Med* 1993;38:807–12.

132. **Jeffcoate TN.** Salpingectomy or salpingo-oophorectomy. *J Obstet Gynaecol Br Emp* 1955;62:214–5.

133. **Schenker JG, Eyal F, Polishuk WZ.** Fertility after tubal surgery. *Surg Gynecol Obstet* 1972;135:74–6.

134. **Ory SJ, Nnadi E, Herrmann R, O'Brien PS, Melton LJ.** Fertility after ectopic pregnancy. *Fertil Steril* 1993;60:231–5.

135. **Timonen S, Nieminen U.** Tubal pregnancy: choice of operative methods of treatment. *Acta Obstet Gynecol Scand* 1967;46:327–39.

136. **Smith HO, Toledo AA, Thompson JD.** Conservative surgical management of isthmic ectopic pregnancies. *Am J Obstet Gynecol* 1987;157:604–10.

137. **Hill GA, Segars JH Jr, Herbert CM III.** Laparoscopic management of interstitial pregnancy. *J Gynecol Surg* 1989;5:209–12.

138. **Brumsted J, Kessler C, Gibson C, Nakajima S, Riddick DH, Gibson M.** A comparison of laparoscopy and laparotomy for the treatment of ectopic pregnancy. *Obstet Gynecol* 1988;71:889–92.

139. **Vermesh M, Silva PD, Rosen GF, Stein AL, Fossum GT, Sauer MV.** Management of unruptured ectopic gestation by linear salpingostomy: a prospective, randomized clinical trial of laparoscopy versus laparotomy. *Obstet Gynecol* 1989;73:400–4.

140. **Murphy AA, Nager CW, Wujek JJ, Kettel LM, Torp VA, Chin HG.** Operative laparoscopy versus laparotomy for the management of ectopic pregnancy: a prospective trial. *Fertil Steril* 1992;57:1180–5.

141. **Lundorff P, Hahlin M, Kallfelt B, Thorburn J, Lindblom B.** Adhesion formation after laparoscopic surgery in tubal pregnancy: a randomized trial versus laparotomy. *Fertil Steril* 1991;55:911–5.

142. **Silva PD, Schaper AM, Rooney B.** Reproductive outcome after 143 laparoscopic procedures for ectopic pregnancy. *Obstet Gynecol* 1993;81:710–15.

143. **Langer R, Raziel A, Ron-El R, Golan A, Bukovsky I, Caspi E.** Reproductive outcome after conservative surgery for unruptured tubal pregnancies—a 15-year experience. *Fertil Steril* 1990;53:227–31.

144. **Berkowitz RS, Goldstein DP, Jones MA, Marean AR, Berstein MR.** Methotrexate with citrovorum factor rescue: reduced chemotherapy toxicity in the management of gestational trophoblastic neoplasms. *Cancer* 1980;45:423–6.

145. **Rustin GJS, Rustin F, Dent J, Booth M, Salt S, Bagshawe KD.** No increase in second tumors after cytotoxic chemotherapy for gestational trophoblastic tumors. *N Engl J Med* 1983;308:473–6.

146. **St. Clair JT, Whealer DA, Fish SA.** Methotrexate in abdominal pregnancy. *JAMA* 1969;208:529–31.

147. **Tanaka T, Hayashi H, Kutsuzawa T, Fujimoto S, Ichinoe K.** Treatment of interstitial ectopic pregnancy with methotrexate: report of a successful case. *Fertil Steril* 1982;37:851–2.

148. **Ory SJ, Villanueva AL, Sand PK, Tamura RK.** Conservative treatment of ectopic pregnancy with methotrexate. *Am J Obstet Gynecol* 1986;154:1299–306.

149. **Ichinoe K, Wake N, Shinkai N, Shiinaa Y, Miyazaki Y, Tanaka T.** Nonsurgical therapy to preserve oviduct function in patients with tubal pregnancies. *Am J Obstet Gynecol* 1987;156:484–7.

150. **Sauer MV, Gorrill MJ, Rodi IA, Yeko TR, Greenberg LH, Bustillo M, Gunning JE, Buster JE.** Nonsurgical management of unruptured ectopic pregnancy: an extended clinical trial. *Fertil Steril* 1987;48:752–5.

151. **Stovall TG, Ling FW, Buster JE.** Outpatient chemotherapy of unruptured ectopic pregnancy. *Fertil Steril* 1989;51:435–8.

152. **Stovall TG, Ling FW, Gray LA, Carson SA, Buster JE.** Methotrexate treatment of unruptured ectopic pregnancy: a report of 100 cases. *Obstet Gynecol* 1991;77:749–53.

153. **Stovall TG, Ling FW, Gray LA.** Single-dose methotrexate for treatment of ectopic pregnancy. *Obstet Gynecol* 1991;77:754–7.

154. **Stovall TG, Ling FW.** Single-dose methotrexate: an expanded clinical trial. *Am J Obstet Gynecol* 1993;170:1840–1.

155. **Hoppe D, Bekkar BE, Nager CW.** Single-dose system methotrexate for the treatment of persistent ectopic pregnancy after conservative surgery. *Obstet Gynecol* 1994;83:51–4.

156. **Schafer D, Kryss J, Pfuhl JP, Baumann R.** Systemic treatment of ectopic pregnancy with single-dose methotrexate. *J Am Assoc Gynecol Laparosc* 1994;1:213–8.

157. **Henry MA, Gentry WL.** Single injection of methotrexate for treatment of ectopic pregnancies. *Am J Obstet Gynecol* 1994;171:1584–7.

158. **Brown DL, Felker RE, Stovall TG, Emerson DS, Ling FW.** Serial endovaginal sonography of ectopic pregnancies treated with methotrexate. *Obstet Gynecol* 1991;77:406–9.

159. **Kooi S, Kick HCLV.** Treatment of tubal pregnancy by local injection of methotrexate after adrenaline injection into the mesosalpinx: a report of 25 patients. *Fertil Steril* 1990;54:580–4.

160. **Stovall TG, Ling FW, Buster JE.** Reproductive performance after methotrexate treatment of ectopic pregnancy. *Am J Obstet Gynecol* 1990;162:1620–4.

161. **Vermesh M.** Conservative management of ectopic gestation. *Fertil Steril* 1990;53:382–7.

162. **Menard A, Crequat J, Mandelbrot L, Hanny J, Madelenat P.** Treatment of unruptured tubal pregnancy by local injection of methotrexate under transvaginal sonographic control. *Fertil Steril* 1990;54:47–50.

163. **Shalev E, Peleg D, Bustan M, Romano S, Tsabari A.** Limited role for intratubal methotrexate treatment of ectopic pregnancy. *Fertil Steril* 1995;63:20–4.

164. **Tulandi T, Atri M, Bret P, Falcone T, Khalife S.** Transvaginal intratubal methotrexate treatment of ectopic pregnancy. *Fertil Steril* 1992;58:98–100.

165. **Fernandez H, Benifla JL, Lelaidier C, Baton C, Frydman R.** Methotrexate treatment of ectopic pregnancy: 100 cases treated by primary transvaginal injection under sonographic control. *Fertil Steril* 1993;59:773–7.

166. **Fernandez H, Pauthier S, Daimerc S, Lelaidier C, Olivennes F, Ville Y, Frydman R.** Ultrasound-guided injection of methotrexate versus laparoscopic salpingotomy in ectopic pregnancy. *Fertil Steril* 1995;63:25–9.

167. **Oelsner G, Admon D, Shalev E, Shalev Y, Kukia E, Mashiach S.** A new approach for the treatment of interstitial pregnancy. *Fertil Steril* 1993;59:924–5.

168. **Aboulghar MA, Mansour RT, Serour GI.** Transvaginal injection of potassium chloride and methotrexate for the treatment of tubal pregnancy with a live fetus. *Hum Reprod* 1990;5:887–8.

169. **Feichtinger W, Kemeter P.** Treatment of unruptured ectopic pregnancy by needling of sac and injection of methotrexate or PGE_2 under transvaginal sonography control. *Arch Gynecol Obstet* 1989;246:85–9.

170. **Hagstrom HG, Hahlin M, Sjöblom P, Lindblom B.** Prediction of persistent trophoblastic activity after local prostaglandin $F_{2\alpha}$ injection for ectopic pregnancy. *Hum Reprod* 1994;9: 1170–4.

171. **Laatikainen T, Tuomivaara L, Kauppila K.** Comparison of a local injection of hyperosmolar glucose solution with salpingostomy for the conservative treatment of tubal pregnancy. *Fertil Steril* 1993;60:80–4.

172. **Kojima E, Abe Y, Morita M, Ito M, Hirakawa S, Momose K.** The treatment of unruptured tubal pregnancy with intratubal methotrexate injection under laparoscopic control. *Obstet Gynecol* 1990;75:723–5.

173. **Kenigsberg D, Porte J, Hull M, Spitz IM.** Medical treatment of residual ectopic pregnancy: RU 486 and methotrexate. *Fertil Steril* 1987;47:702–3.

174. **Frydman R, Fernandez H, Troalen F, Ghillani P, Rainhorn JD, Bellet D.** Phase I clinical trial of monoclonal anti-human chorionic gonadotropin antibody in women with an ectopic pregnancy. *Fertil Steril* 1989;52:734–8.

175. **Garcia AJ, Aubert JM, Sama J, Josimovich JB.** Expectant management of presumed ectopic pregnancies. *Fertil Steril* 1987;48:395–400.

176. **Carson SA, Stovall TG, Ling FW, Buster JE.** Low human chorionic somatomammotropin fails to predict spontaneous resolution of unruptured ectopic pregnancies. *Fertil Steril* 1991;55:629–30.

177. **Fernandez H, Rainhorn JD, Papiernik E, Bellet D, Frydman R.** Spontaneous resolution of ectopic pregnancy. *Obstet Gynecol* 1988;71:171–4.

178. **Gretz E, Quagliarello J.** Declining serum concentrations of the beta-subunit of human chorionic gonadotropin and ruptured ectopic pregnancy. *Am J Obstet Gynecol* 1987;156:940–1.

179. **Makinen JI, Kivijarvi AK, Irjala KMA.** Success of non-surgical management of ectopic pregnancy. *Lancet* 1990;335:1099.

180. **Seifer DB, Gutmann JN, Doyle MB, Jones EE, Diamond MP, DeCherney AH.** Persistent ectopic pregnancy following laparoscopic linear salpingostomy. *Obstet Gynecol* 1990;76:1121–5.

181. **Pouly JL, Mahnes H, Mage G, Canis M, Bruhat MA.** Conservative laparoscopic treatment of 321 ectopic pregnancies. *Fertil Steril* 1986;46:1093–7.

182. **Seifer DB, Gutmann JN, Grant WD, Kamps CA, DeCherney AH.** Comparison of persistent ectopic pregnancy after laparoscopic salpingostomy versus salpingostomy at laparotomy for ectopic pregnancy. *Obstet Gynecol* 1993;81:378–82.

183. **Vermesh M, Silva PD, Sauer MV, Vargyas JM, Lobo RA.** Persistent tubal ectopic gestation: patterns of circulating Beta-human chorionic gonadotropin and progesterone, and management options. *Fertil Steril* 1988;50:584–8.

184. **Lundorff P, Hahlin M, Sjoblom P, Lindblom B.** Persistent trophoblast after conservative treatment of tubal pregnancy: prediction and detection. *Obstet Gynecol* 1991;77:129–33.

185. **Cartwright PS.** Peritoneal trophoblastic implants after surgical management of tubal pregnancy. *J Reprod Med* 1991;36:523–4.

186. **Foulot H, Chapron C, Morice Ph, Mouly M, Aubriot FX, Dubuisson JB.** Failure of laparoscopic treatment for peritoneal trophoblastic implants. *Hum Reprod* 1994;9:92–3.

187. **Higgins KA, Schwartz MB.** Treatment of persistent trophoblastic tissue after salpingostomy with methotrexate. *Fertil Steril* 1986;45:427–8.

188. **Rose PG, Cohen SM.** Methotrexate therapy for persistent ectopic pregnancy after conservative laparoscopic management. *Obstet Gynecol* 1990;76:947–9.

189. **Bengtsson G, Bryman I, Thorburn J, Lindblom B.** Low-dose oral methotrexate as second-line therapy for persistent trophoblast after conservative treatment of ectopic pregnancy. *Obstet Gynecol* 1992;79:589–91.

190. **Cole T, Corlett RC Jr.** Chronic ectopic pregnancy. *Obstet Gynecol* 1982;59:63–8.

191. **Rogers WF, Shaub M, Wilson R.** Chronic ectopic pregnancy: ultrasonic diagnosis. *J Clin Ultrasound* 1977;5:257–60.

192. **Parente JT, Ou CS, Levy J, Legatt E.** Cervical pregnancy analysis: a review and report of five cases. *Obstet Gynecol* 1983;62:79–82.

193. **Weyerman PC, Verhoeven ATM, Alberda AT.** Cervical pregnancy after in vitro fertilization and embryo transfer. *Am J Obstet Gynecol* 1989;161:1145–64.

194. **Hofmann HMH, Urdl W, Hofler H, Honigl W, Tamussino K.** Cervical pregnancy: case reports and current concepts in diagnosis and treatment. *Arch Gynecol Obstet* 1987;241:63–9.

195. **Bader-Armstrong B, Shah Y, Rubens D.** Use of ultrasound and magnetic resonance imaging in the diagnosis of cervical pregnancy. *J Clin Ultrasound* 1989;17:283–6.

196. **Stovall TG, Ling FW, Smith WC, Felker R, Rasco BJ, Buster JE.** Successful nonsurgical treatment of cervical pregnancy with methotrexate. *Fertil Steril* 1988;50:672–4.

197. **Oyer R, Tarakjian D, Lev-Toaff A, Friedman A, Chatwani A.** Treatment of cervical pregnancy with methotrexate. *Obstet Gynecol* 1988;71:469–71.

198. **Bernstein D, Holzinger M, Ovadia J, Frishman B.** Conservative treatment of cervical pregnancy. *Obstet Gynecol* 1981;58:741–2.

199. **Wharton KR, Gore B.** Cervical pregnancy managed by placement of a Shirodkar cerclage before evacuation: a case report. *J Reprod Med* 1988;33:227–9.

200. **Nolan TE, Chandler PE, Hess LW, Morrison JC.** Cervical pregnancy managed without hysterectomy: a case report. *J Reprod Med* 1989;34:241–3.

201. **Hallatt JG.** Primary ovarian pregnancy: a report of twenty-five cases. *Am J Obstet Gynecol* 1982;143:55–60.

202. **Grimes HG, Nosal RA, Gallagher JC.** Ovarian pregnancy: a series of 24 cases. *Obstet Gynecol* 1983;61:174–80.

203. **Malinger G, Achiron R, Treschan O, Zakut H.** Case report: ovarian pregnancy-ultrasonographic diagnosis. *Acta Obstet Gynecol Scand* 1988;67:561–3.

204. **DeVries K, Atad J, Arodi J, Shmilovici J, Abramovici H.** Primary ovarian pregnancy: a conservative surgical approach by wedge resection. *Int J Fertil* 1981;26:293–4.

205. **Van Coevering RJ, Fisher JE.** Laparoscopic management of ovarian pregnancy: a case report. *J Reprod Med* 1988;33:774–6.

206. **Russell JB, Cutler LR.** Transvaginal ultrasonographic detection of primary ovarian pregnancy with laparoscopic removal: a case report. *Fertil Steril* 1989;51:1055–6.

207. **Koike H, Chuganji Y, Watanabe H, Kaneko M, Noda S, Mori N.** Conservative treatment of ovarian pregnancy by local prostaglandin $F_{2\alpha}$ injection, (Letter). *Am J Obstet Gynecol* 1990;163:696.

208. **Atrash HK, Friede A, Hogue CJR.** Abdominal pregnancy in the United States: frequency and maternal mortality. *Obstet Gynecol* 1987;69:333–7.

209. **Rahman MS, Al-Suleiman SA, Rahman J, Al-Sibai MH.** Advanced abdominal pregnancy-observations in 10 cases. *Obstet Gynecol* 1982;59:366–72.

210. **Stanley JH, Horger EO III, Fagan CJ, Andriole JG, Fleischer AC.** Sonographic findings in abdominal pregnancy. *Am J Roentgenol* 1986;147:1043–6.

211. **Harris MB, Angtuaco T, Frazer CN, Mattison DR.** Diagnosis of a viable abdominal pregnancy by magnetic resonance imaging. *Am J Obstet Gynecol* 1988;159:150–1.

212. **Martin JN Jr, Ridgway LE III, Connors JJ, Sessums JK, Martin RW, Morrison JC.** Angiographic arterial embolization and computed tomography-directed drainage for the management of hemorrhage and infection with abdominal pregnancy. *Obstet Gynecol* 1990;76:941–5.

213. **Martin JN Jr, Sessums JK, Martin RW, Pryor JA, Morrison JC.** Abdominal pregnancy: current concepts of management. *Obstet Gynecol* 1988;71:549–57.

214. **Pasic R, Wolfe WM.** Laparoscopic diagnosis and treatment of interstitial ectopic pregnancy: a case report. *Am J Obstet Gynecol* 1990;163:587–8.

215. **Vierhout ME, Wallenburg HCS.** Intraligamentary pregnancy resulting in a live infant. *Am J Obstet Gynecol* 1985;152:878–9.

216. **Reece EA, Petrie RH, Sirmans MF, Finster M, Todd WD.** Combined intrauterine and extrauterine gestations: a review. *Am J Obstet Gynecol* 1983;146:323–30.

217. **Olsen ME.** Bilateral twin ectopic gestations with intraligamentous and interstitial components: a case report. *J Reprod Med* 1994;39:118–20.

218. **Adair CD, Benrubi GI, Sanchez-Ramos L, Rhatigan R.** Bilateral tubal ectopic pregnancies after bilateral partial salpingectomy: a case report. *J Reprod Med* 1994;39:131–3.

219. **Goffner L, Bluth MJ, Fruauff A, Losada RA.** Ectopic gestation associated with intrauterine triplet pregnancy after in vitro fertilization. *J Ultrasound Med* 1993;12:63–4.

220. **Jackson P, Barrowclough IW, France JT, Phillips LI.** A successful pregnancy following total hysterectomy. *Br J Obstet Gynaecol* 1980;87:353–5.

221. **Nehra PC, Loginsky SJ.** Pregnancy after vaginal hysterectomy. *Obstet Gynecol* 1984;64:735–7.

18 Benign Breast Disease

Armando E. Giuliano

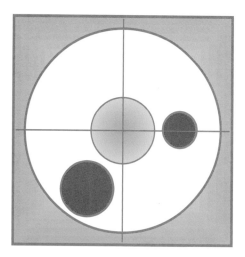

Understanding of the diagnosis and management of common benign breast conditions, particularly those that mimic malignancy, and an appreciation of treatment options are essential for the practicing gynecologist.

Detection

Physical Examination

Breast tumors, particularly cancerous ones, usually are asymptomatic and are discovered only by physical examination or screening mammography. The breast changes slightly during the menstrual cycle. During the premenstrual phase, most women have increased innocuous nodularity and mild engorgement of the breast. Rarely, this can obscure an underlying lesion and make examination difficult. Findings should be carefully documented in the medical record to serve as a baseline for future reference.

Inspection

Inspection is done initially while the patient is seated comfortably with her arms relaxed at her sides. The breasts are compared for symmetry, contour, and skin appearance. Edema or erythema is identified easily, and skin dimpling or nipple retraction is demonstrated by having the patient raise her arms above her head and then press her hands on her hips, thereby contracting the pectoralis muscles (Fig. 18.1). Palpable and even nonpalpable tumors that distort Cooper's ligaments may lead to skin dimpling with these maneuvers.

Palpation

While the patient is seated, each breast should be palpated methodically. Some physicians recommend palpating the breast in long strips, but the exact palpation technique used is probably not as important as the thoroughness of its application over the entire breast. One very effective method is to palpate the breast in enlarging concentric circles until the entire breast has been covered. A pendulous breast can be palpated by placing one hand between the breast and the chest wall and gently palpating the breast between both examin-

525

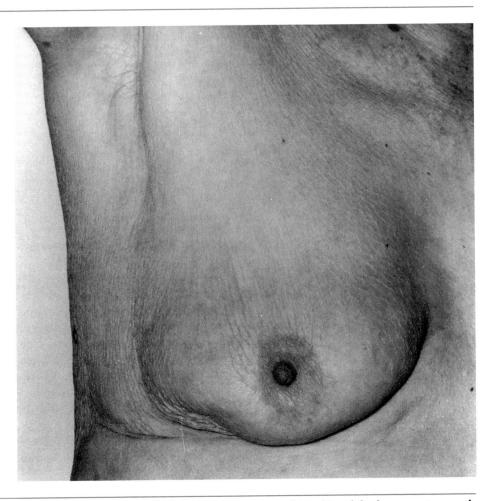

Figure 18.1   Raising the arm reveals retraction of the skin of the lower outer quadrant caused by a small palpable carcinoma. (Reproduced with permission from **Giuliano AE.** Breast disease. In: **Berek JS, Hacker NF,** eds. *Practical Gynecologic Oncology.* 2nd ed. Baltimore: Williams & Wilkins, 1994:482.)

ing hands. The axillary and supraclavicular areas should be palpated for enlarged lymph nodes. The entire axilla, the upper outer quadrant of the breast, and the axillary tail of Spence are palpated for possible masses.

While the patient is supine with one arm over her head, the ipsilateral breast is again methodically palpated from the clavicle to the costal margin. If the breast is large, a pillow or towel should be placed beneath the scapula to elevate the side being examined; otherwise the breast tends to fall to the side, making palpation of the lateral hemisphere more difficult.

The major features to be identified on palpation of the breast are tenderness, nodularity, and dominant masses. Most premenopausal patients have normally nodular breast parenchyma. The nodularity is diffuse but predominantly in the upper outer quadrants where there is more breast tissue. These benign parenchymal nodules are small, similar in size, and indistinct. By comparison, breast cancer is usually a nontender, firm mass with irregular margins. This mass feels distinctly different from the surrounding nodularity. A malignant mass may be fixed to the skin or to the underlying fascia.

**Breast
Self-Examination**

Self-examination of the breast increases early detection of cancer and may improve the survival of patients with breast carcinoma (1). In fact, most breast cancers are palpated first by the patient rather than by the physician. Although young women have a low incidence of breast cancer, it is important to teach self-examination early so that it becomes habitual. Organizations such as the American Cancer Society sponsor courses in breast self-examination. Reassurance, support, and patient education may encourage women to overcome psychological barriers to routine breast self-examination.

The woman should inspect her breasts while standing or sitting before a mirror, looking for any asymmetry, skin dimpling, or nipple retraction. Elevating her arms over her head or pressing her hands against her hips to contract the pectoralis muscles will highlight any skin dimpling. While standing or sitting, she should carefully palpate her breasts with the fingers of the opposite hand. This may be performed while showering, because soap and water may increase the sensitivity of palpation. Finally, she should lie down and again palpate each quadrant of the breast, as well as the axilla.

Premenopausal women should examine their breasts monthly during the week after menses. All women should be instructed to report any abnormalities or changes to their physician. If the physician cannot confirm the patient's findings, the examination should be repeated in 1 month or after her next menstrual period.

Breast Imaging

Mammography and ultrasonography are the most reliable and common imaging techniques for early detection of breast lesions. Thermography is not useful and should be abandoned because it cannot reliably differentiate benign and malignant breast disease and it has an unacceptably high rate of false-positive findings (2). Magnetic resonance imaging (MRI) may be valuable for assessing breast lesions of an indeterminate nature based on clinical and mammographic examination or in patients with implants.

Mammography

Slowly growing breast cancers can be identified by mammography at least 2 years before the mass reaches a size detectable by palpation (3, 4). In fact, mammography is the only reproducible method of detecting nonpalpable breast cancer. However, its accurate use requires state-of-the-art equipment and a skilled radiologist. Vigorous compression of the breast is necessary to obtain good images, and patients should be forewarned that breast compression is uncomfortable.

In breast cancer, the most common diagnostic mammographic abnormalities are clustered pleomorphic microcalcifications (5). Typically, 5–8 or more calcifications are aggregated in one part of the breast. These calcifications may be associated with a mammographic mass density, or a mass density may appear without evidence of calcifications. Such a density usually has irregular or ill-defined borders and may lead to architectural distortion, which may be subtle and difficult to detect in a dense breast. Other mammographic findings suggesting breast cancer are a mass, architectural distortion, and skin thickening or retraction.

There are several indications for mammography:

1. To screen, at regular intervals, women who are at high risk for developing breast cancer. About one-third of the abnormalities detected on screening mammography prove malignant when biopsy is performed (6).

2. To evaluate a questionable or ill-defined breast mass or other suspicious change in the breast.

3. To evaluate each breast initially and at yearly intervals to diagnose a potentially curable breast cancer before it has been diagnosed clinically.

4. To search for occult breast cancer in a patient with metastatic disease in axillary nodes or elsewhere from an unknown primary origin.

527

5. To screen for unsuspected cancer prior to cosmetic operations or biopsy of a mass.

6. To monitor breast cancer patients who have been treated with a breast-conserving operation and radiation.

Biopsy must be performed on patients with a dominant or suspicious mass despite mammographic findings. Mammography should be performed before biopsy so other suspicious areas can be noted and the contralateral breast can be checked (Fig. 18.2). **Mammography is never a substitute for biopsy because it may not reveal clinical cancer** (especially that occurring in the dense breast tissue of young women with fibrocystic changes). In fact, the sensitivity of mammography varies from approximately 60 to 90%, depending on the patient's age (breast density) and the size, location, and mammographic appearance of the tumor.

Mammography is less sensitive in young women with dense breast tissue than in older women, who tend to have fatty breasts in which mammography can detect at least 90% of malignancies. Small tumors, particularly those without calcifications, are more difficult to detect, especially in women with dense breasts. The specificity of mammography is about 30–40% for nonpalpable mammographic abnormalities and 85–90% for clinically evident malignancies (7).

Xeromammography has been used effectively for the past 20 years and produces excellent images. However, it results in a higher dose of radiation to the breast than screen-film tech-

Figure 18.2   Bilateral mammography shows the extent of breast carcinoma, illustrating the importance of bilateral mammography in the workup of a clinically apparent mass. (Reproduced with permission from **Giuliano AE.** Breast disease. In: **Berek JS, Hacker NF,** eds. *Practical Gynecologic Oncology.* 2nd ed. Baltimore: Williams & Wilkins, 1994:484.)

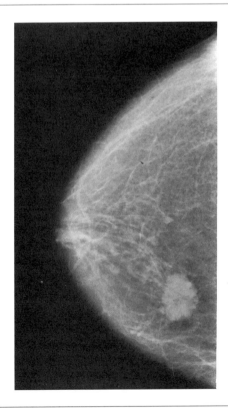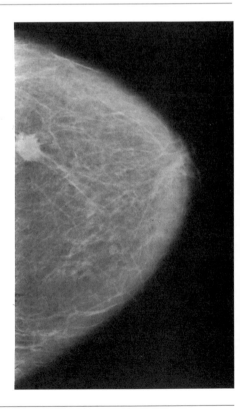

niques (8). For this reason, xeromammography is being used less frequently and will probably be abandoned. Screen-film mammography can produce images of as high quality as those seen with xeromammography. With a good technique and well-maintained modern equipment, screen-film mammography delivers only 0.02–0.03 cGy to the midbreast, with a total skin dose of 0.2–0.3 cGy (9).

Ultrasonography

Both handheld and automated breast ultrasonography are popular imaging techniques. Although early reports suggested cancer-detection rates nearly as high as those achieved with x-ray mammography, repeat studies have failed to show any value for ultrasonography as a screening technique (10). Ultrasonography cannot detect microcalcifications, and it is not as useful as mammography in fatty breasts. Ultrasonography may be useful in identifying noncalcified cancers in the dense breast tissue of premenopausal women, but it is usually used to distinguish a benign cyst from a solid tumor.

Handheld or real-time ultrasonography is 95–100% accurate in differentiating solid masses from cysts (11). However, this is of limited clinical value because a dominant mass should be studied by biopsy, and a cystic mass can be studied by needle aspiration, which is far less expensive than ultrasonography. The primary role of handheld ultrasonography is in the evaluation of a benign-appearing, nonpalpable density identified by mammography. If such a lesion proves to be a simple cyst, no further workup is necessary. Rarely, ultrasonography may identify a small cancer within a cyst—an intracystic carcinoma. These "complex cysts" warrant surgical biopsy. However, ultrasound is far less reliable than mammography in detecting cancer (12).

Magnetic Resonance Imaging

MRI is increasing in popularity as a means of imaging the breast (13). It tends to be highly sensitive but not very specific, leading to biopsies of many benign lesions. Image enhancement with gadolinium chelate can discriminate between benign and malignant lesions with varying degrees of accuracy.

Several roles have been proposed for breast MRI. Its lack of radiation exposure makes MRI ideal for mass screening of healthy women, although such widespread use is probably too costly. There may be a role for MRI in evaluation of focal, asymmetric areas detected mammographically. Focal asymmetry is usually benign but can be malignant, and MRI may help identify patients in whom focal asymmetric areas should be biopsied. Usually, a scar can easily be distinguished from recurrent tumor based on the evaluation and diminution of the scar over time. Some scars, however, do not diminish rapidly and are confused with cancer or, more commonly, with recurrent cancer after breast-conserving operation and radiation. Ideally, such cases are evaluated with MRI, sometimes obviating the need for biopsy. MRI is extremely useful in identifying silicone released by a ruptured breast implant in patients with augmented breasts (Fig. 18.3). In patients with implants, MRI with gadolinium may be performed to detect breast cancer, even if free silicone is not suspected.

The International Cooperative Magnetic Resonance Mammography Study that is currently under way will help identify the advantages and limitations of MRI. At present, MRI should be considered only after conventional imaging is performed; it should not be used as a screening tool or a substitute for mammography or biopsy.

Screening

Because about 35–50% of early breast cancers can be discovered only by mammography and about 20% can be detected only by palpation, a number of programs have used physical and mammographic breast examination for mass screening of asymptomatic women. Such programs frequently identify about 10 cancers per 1000 women older than 50 years of age and about two cancers per 1000 women under 50 years of age (14). About 80% of these women have negative axillary lymph nodes at the time of surgery, whereas in the

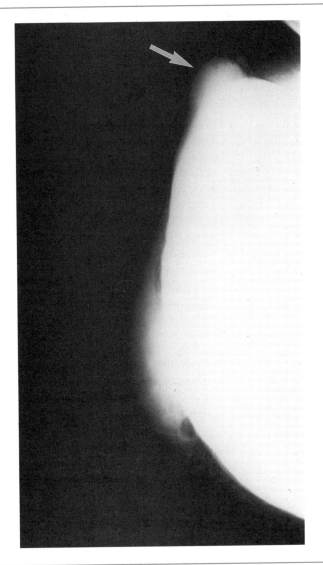

Figure 18.3   Mammography shows implant and extracapsular free silicone (arrow).

course of usual medical practice, only 45% of patients have uninvolved axillary nodes. Detecting breast cancer before it has spread to the axillary nodes greatly increases the chance of survival: about 85% of such women will survive at least 5 years (15, 16).

Mammography's lack of sensitivity in dense breast tissue has lead to questions concerning its screening value in women 40–50 years of age. In February 1993, the National Cancer Institute held an international workshop on screening for breast cancer (3). The purpose of this workshop was to undertake a critical review of recent clinical screening trials. The participants examined only randomized studies and focused on clinical evidence related to the efficacy of breast cancer screening in various age groups. Of the eight randomized trials identified, only the Health Insurance Plan (HIP) project demonstrated a beneficial effect of screening for women between 40 and 49 years of age. This benefit was seen 10–18 years after entry into the study and resulted in a 25% decrease in deaths from breast cancer. Several Swedish trials showed a 13% decrease in breast cancer mortality for women in this age group after 12 years of follow-up; however, this decrease was not statistically significant (17–19). In a meta-analysis of five randomized trials, the breast cancer rates were independent of screening in women aged 40–49 years (20). The beneficial effect of screening in women aged 50–69 years was confirmed by all clinical trials. The efficacy of screening in women older than 70 years of age was inconclusive because of the small sample size.

According to the National Cancer Institute, the American Cancer Society, and the American College of Radiology, annual physical examination and mammography should be performed for women older than 50 years of age. There is no consensus on screening for women younger than 50 years of age (21, 22). **The American College of Radiology, the American Cancer Society, and the American College of Obstetricians and Gynecologists continue to recommend a screening mammogram to begin by 40 years of age and then every 1–2 years until 50 years of age, after which screening should be performed every year** (23). These recommendations seem reasonable but may be too costly. The value of mammography in women aged 40–50 years will remain controversial because of the difficulty in showing a beneficial effect among patients in whom the disease has a low incidence. It is unlikely, however, that mammography is harmful to these patients, and each should be given the option of routine screening, especially those who are at higher risk (24). Screening of women older than 70 years of age should be performed after consideration of the patient's comorbid conditions and her overall state of health.

Breast Biopsy

The diagnosis of breast cancer depends ultimately on examination of tissue removed by biopsy. Because cancer is found in the minority of patients who require biopsy for diagnosis of a breast mass, treatment should never be undertaken without an unequivocal histological diagnosis of cancer.

The safest course is biopsy examination of all dominant masses found on physical examination and, in the absence of a mass, of suspicious lesions demonstrated by mammography. About 30% of lesions suspected to be cancer prove on biopsy to be benign, and about 15% of lesions believed to be benign prove to be malignant (6, 25). Dominant masses or suspicious nonpalpable mammographic findings must be biopsied. A breast mass should not be followed without histologic diagnosis, except perhaps in premenopausal women with a nonsuspicious mass presumed to be fibrocystic disease. However, an apparently fibrocystic lesion that does not completely resolve within several menstrual cycles should be biopsied. Any mass in a postmenopausal woman who is not taking estrogen replacement should be presumed to be malignant. Figures 18.4 and 18.5 present algorithms for management of breast masses in premenopausal and postmenopausal patients.

If the presence of breast cancer is strongly suggested by physical examination, the diagnosis can be confirmed by fine-needle cytology or core biopsy, and the patient may be counseled regarding treatment. The results of physical examination and mammography without biopsy should not be used to determine treatment. **The most reasonable approach to the diagnosis and treatment of breast cancer is outpatient biopsy (either needle or excision) followed by definitive surgery at a later date.** This two-step approach allows patients to adjust to the diagnosis of cancer, carefully consider alternative forms of therapy, and seek a second opinion if they wish. Studies have shown no adverse effect from the 1- to 2-week delay associated with the two-step procedure. However, the two-step procedure should be reexamined in view of the increasing popularity of lumpectomy. Suspicious lesions may be best excised as the definitive lumpectomy specimen even if biopsy has not shown malignancy. The lumpectomy is, in essence, a biopsy that ensures a rim of normal tissue around the mass. It is better performed with the mass in place than after a prior excisional biopsy.

The estrogen and progesterone receptor status of the tumor should be determined at the time of initial biopsy. This may be performed either quantitatively on fresh tissue or on paraffin-fixed tissue by immunohistochemistry (26).

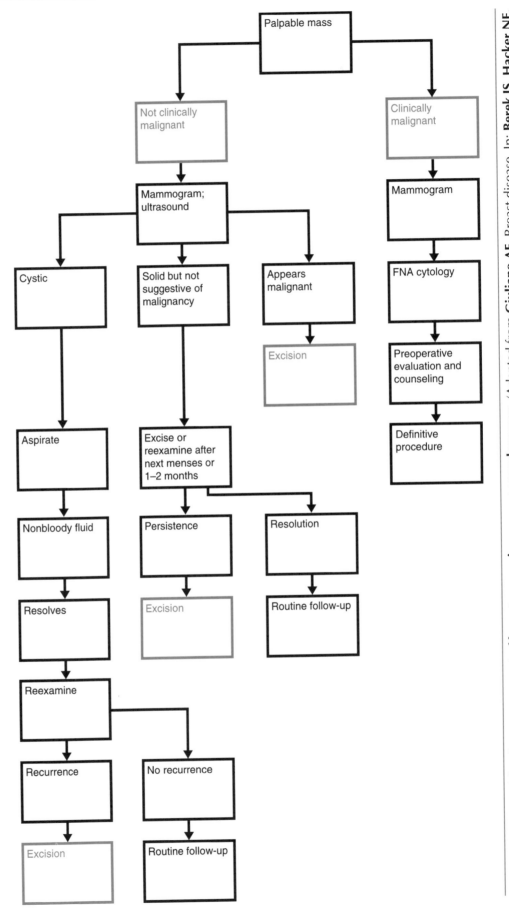

Figure 18.4   Algorithm for management of breast masses in premenopausal women. (Adapted from **Giuliano AE.** Breast disease. In: **Berek JS, Hacker NF,** eds. *Practical Gynecologic Oncology.* 2nd ed. Baltimore: Williams & Wilkins, 1994:492.)

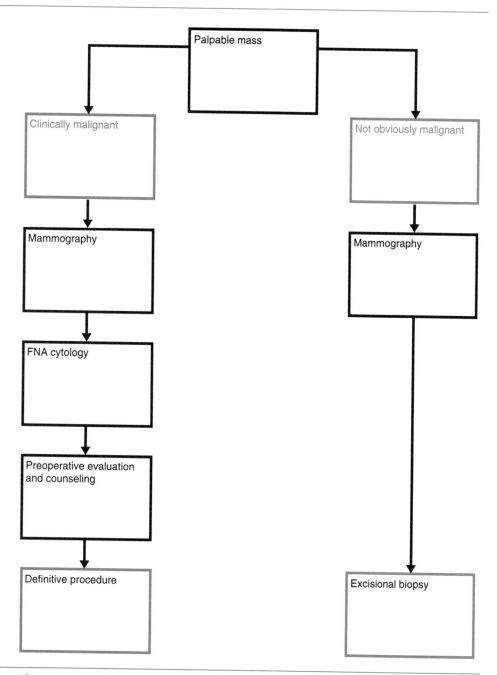

Figure 18.5   Algorithm for management of breast masses in postmenopausal women. (Adapted from **Giuliano AE.** Breast disease. In: **Berek JS, Hacker NF,** eds. *Practical Gynecologic Oncology.* 2nd ed. Baltimore: Williams & Wilkins, 1994:493.)

Needle Biopsy

Needle biopsy is performed by aspirating tumor cells (fine-needle aspiration cytology) or by obtaining a small core of tissue with a Vim-Silverman or other special needle (27). Large-needle (core-needle) biopsy removes a core of tissue with a large cutting needle (28). As in the case of any needle biopsy, the main drawback is false-negative findings caused by improper positioning of the needle.

Fine-needle aspiration cytology is a useful technique whereby cells from a breast tumor are aspirated with a small (usually 22-gauge) needle and examined by a pathologist. This technique can be performed easily with no morbidity and is much less expensive than excisional or open biopsy. However, it requires the availability of a pathologist skilled in the cytologic diagnosis of breast cancer to interpret the results and it is subject to sampling problems, particularly when lesions are deep. The incidence of false-positive diagnoses is only about 1–2%, but the rate of the false-negative diagnoses is as high as 10% in some series (29). Most experienced clinicians will not leave a dominant mass in the breast even when fine-needle aspiration cytology results are negative. Some clinicians will follow a mass when results of the clinical diagnosis, breast imaging studies, and cytologic studies are all in agreement. However, occasionally a malignancy will be diagnosed later.

Open biopsy with local anesthesia as a separate procedure prior to deciding on definitive treatment is the most reliable means of diagnosis and is required when the results of needle biopsy are nondiagnostic or equivocal.

Other Cytologic Assessment

Cytologic examination of nipple discharge or cyst fluid is rarely performed. Mammography (or ductography) and breast biopsy may be performed when nipple discharge or cyst fluid is bloody or cytologically questionable. However, excision and examination of the involved ductal system is the preferred method of diagnosis and cytology should not be relied on for diagnosis.

Benign Breast Conditions

Fibrocystic Changes

Fibrocystic change, the most common lesion of the breast, is an imprecise term that covers a spectrum of clinical signs and symptoms and histologic changes (27, 28). It is common in women 30–50 years of age but rare in postmenopausal women not taking hormone replacement therapy. The presence of estrogen seems necessary for the clinical symptoms to occur. In essence, a diagnosis of fibrocystic change is of little clinical significance as long as malignancy is excluded. These lesions are always associated with benign changes in the breast epithelium, some of which are so common that they are probably innocuous variants of normal breast histology (29).

Clinical Findings

Fibrocystic changes may produce an asymptomatic mass but more often are accompanied by pain or tenderness and sometimes nipple discharge. In many cases, discomfort coincides with the premenstrual phase of the cycle, when the cysts tend to enlarge. Fluctuation in size and rapid appearance or disappearance of a breast mass are common. Multiple or bilateral masses appear frequently, and many patients will give a history of a transient mass in the breast or cyclic breast pain. Cyclic breast pain is the most common symptom of fibrocystic changes.

Differential Diagnosis

Pain, fluctuation in size, and multiplicity of lesions are the features most helpful for differentiation from carcinoma. If a dominant mass is present, however, the diagnosis of cancer should be suspected until it is disproven by biopsy. Final diagnosis of the mass usually depends on biopsy. Mammography may be helpful, but there are no mammographic signs diagnostic of fibrocystic change. Ultrasonography is useful in differentiating a cystic from a solid mass. The finding of a simple cyst rules out carcinoma.

Diagnosis Tests

Because a fibrocystic mass is frequently indistinguishable from carcinoma on the basis of clinical findings, suspicious lesions should be biopsied. Microscopic findings include cysts (gross and microscopic), papillomatosis, adenosis, fibrosis, and ductal epithelial hyperplasia (30).

When the diagnosis of fibrocystic change has been established by previous biopsy or is practically certain because the history is classic, aspiration of a discrete mass suggestive of a cyst is indicated. Aspiration may be performed with ultrasound guidance, but this usually is not necessary (31). The patient is reexamined at intervals thereafter. If no fluid is obtained or if fluid is bloody, if a mass persists after aspiration, or if at any time during follow-up a persistent mass is noted, biopsy should be performed. Even if a needle biopsy is performed and results are negative for malignancy, a suspicious mass that does not resolve over several months should be excised. Surgery should be conservative, because the primary objective is to exclude cancer. Simple mastectomy or extensive removal of breast tissue is rarely, if ever, indicated for fibrocystic disease. Most patients do not require treatment.

Breast pain associated with generalized fibrocystic changes is best treated by avoiding trauma and by wearing (night and day) a brassiere that gives good support and protection (32). Hormone therapy is not advisable because it does not relieve symptoms and has undesirable side effects. *Danazol* (100–200 mg twice daily orally), a synthetic androgen, has been used for patients with severe pain (33). This treatment suppresses pituitary gonadotropins, and its androgenic effects (acne, edema, hirsutism) are usually intolerable; therefore, it probably should not be used.

The role of caffeine consumption in the development and treatment of fibrocystic change is controversial. Some studies suggest that eliminating caffeine from the diet is associated with improvement (34). Many patients are aware of these studies and report relief of symptoms after discontinuing intake of coffee, tea, and chocolate. Similarly, many women find vitamin E (400 IU daily) helpful. However, observations about these effects have been difficult to confirm and are anecdotal. Exacerbations of pain, tenderness, and cyst formation may occur at any time until menopause, when symptoms usually subside unless patients are taking estrogen. A patient with fibrocystic changes should be advised to examine her own breasts each month just after menstruation and to inform her physician if a mass appears.

Fibrocystic Change and Cancer

Fibrocystic change is not associated with an increased risk of breast cancer unless there is histologic evidence of epithelial proliferative changes with or without atypia. The common coincidence of fibrocystic disease and malignancy in the same breast reflects the fact that one in every nine women will develop breast cancer and as many as 80% of biopsies show fibrocystic changes. Page and Dupont (35) evaluated the relationship between fibrocystic change and breast cancer in 10,366 women who underwent biopsy from 1950 until 1968 and were followed for a median of 17 years. Approximately 70% of the biopsies showed nonproliferative breast disease, whereas 30% showed proliferative breast disease. Cytologic atypia was present in 3.6% of cases. Women with nonproliferative disease had no increased risk of breast cancer, whereas women with proliferative breast disease and no atypical hyperplasia had a twofold higher breast cancer risk. **Patients whose biopsies showed atypical hyperplasia had an approximately fivefold higher risk than women with nonproliferative disease.** A family history of breast cancer added little risk for women with nonproliferative disease, but family history plus atypia increased breast cancer risk 11-fold. The presence of cysts alone did not increase the risk of breast cancer, but cysts combined with a family history of breast cancer increased the risk about three-fold. Others have shown similar results (28, 36). Women with these risk factors (family history and proliferative breast disease) should be followed carefully with physical examination and mammography.

Benign Tumors

Fibroadenoma

Fibroadenomas are the most common benign tumors of the breast. They usually occur in young women (aged 20–35 years) and may occur in teenagers (37). Before 25 years of age, fibroadenomas are more common than cysts. They rarely occur after menopause, although occasionally they are found, often calcified, in postmenopausal women. For this reason, it is postulated that fibroadenomas are responsive to estrogen stimulation. Although the presence of a fibroadenoma does not increase the risk of breast carcinoma, this subject still generates controversy (38).

On gross examination, fibroadenomas appear encapsulated and sharply delineated from the surrounding breast parenchyma. Microscopically, they have an epithelial and a stromal component. In longstanding lesions and in postmenopausal patients, calcifications may be observed within the stroma. Fibroadenomas may appear in multiples. Clinically, a young patient usually notices a mass while showering or dressing. Most masses are 2–3 cm in diameter when detected, but they can become extremely large (i.e., the giant fibroadenoma). On physical examination, they are firm, smooth, and rubbery. They do not elicit an inflammatory reaction, are freely mobile, and cause no dimpling of the skin or nipple retraction. They are often bilobed, and a groove can be palpated on examination. Mammographically, they have typical benign-appearing features with smooth, clearly defined margins.

A suspected fibroadenoma should be confirmed by either excisional biopsy or fine-needle aspiration cytology. Complete excision of a fibroadenoma with the local anesthesia can be used to treat the lesion and confirm the absence of malignancy. However, a young woman with a clinical fibroadenoma can undergo needle cytology and observation of the mass (39). Rarely will they increase to more than 2–3 cm in size. Large or growing fibroadenomas must be excised.

Cystosarcoma Phyllodes

Cystosarcoma phyllodes, which are perhaps best referred to as "phyllodes tumors," may occur at any age but tend to be more common in women who are in their forties and fifties (40). These lesions are rarely bilateral and usually appear as isolated masses that are difficult to distinguish clinically from a fibroadenoma. Patients often relate a long history of a previously stable nodule that suddenly increased in size. Size is not a diagnostic criterion, although cystosarcomas tend to be larger than fibroadenomas, probably because of their rapid growth. There are no good clinical criteria by which to distinguish a cystosarcoma from a fibroadenoma.

The histologic distinction between fibroadenoma, "benign" cystosarcoma, and malignant cystosarcoma can be very difficult (41). Tumors judged by the pathologist to be benign tend to recur locally in 15–40% of patients. Malignant cystosarcomas tend to recur locally and can metastasize to the lung. The stromal component of the tumor is malignant and metastasizes, behaving like a sarcoma. Axillary involvement is extremely unusual. Often, the appearance of metastases is the first sign that a cystosarcoma is malignant.

Treatment is wide local excision (41, 42). Massive tumors, or large tumors in relatively small breasts, may require mastectomy; otherwise, mastectomy should be avoided and axillary lymph node dissection is not indicated. Typically, a patient will undergo excisional biopsy of a mass believed to be fibroadenoma, but histologic examination will reveal cys-

536

tosarcoma phyllodes. When the pathologic diagnosis is cystosarcoma, complete reexcision of the area should be undertaken so that the prior biopsy site and any residual tumor are removed. The value of radiation therapy is not known and this modality probably should be avoided. True soft-tissue sarcomas of the breast are rare (43).

Breast Conditions Requiring Evaluation

Nipple Discharge

In order of increasing frequency, the following are the most common causes of nipple discharge in nonlactating women: carcinoma, intraductal papilloma, and fibrocystic change with ectasia of the ducts. The important characteristics of the discharge and other factors to be evaluated by history and physical examination are as follows (44):

1. Nature of discharge (serous, bloody, or milky)

2. Association with a mass

3. Unilateral or bilateral

4. Single or multiple ducts

5. Discharge that is spontaneous (persistent or intermittent) or expressed by pressure at a single site or on entire breast

6. Relation to menses

7. Premenopausal or postmenopausal

8. Hormonal medication (contraceptive pills or estrogen)

Unilateral, spontaneous, bloody, or serosanguineous discharge from a single duct is usually caused by an intraductal papilloma or rarely by an intraductal cancer. In either case, a mass may not be palpable. The involved duct may be identified by pressure at different sites around the nipple and at the margin of the areola. Bloody discharge is more suggestive of cancer but is usually caused by a benign papilloma in the duct. Cytologic examination is usually of no value but may identify malignant cells. Negative findings do not rule out cancer, which is more likely in women older than 50 years of age. In any case, the involved duct—and a mass, if present,—should be excised (45). Although ductography may identify a filling defect prior to excision of the duct system, this study is of little value.

In premenopausal women, spontaneous multiple-duct discharge, unilateral or bilateral, most marked just before menstruation, is often caused by fibrocystic change. Discharge may be green or brownish. Papillomatosis and ductal ectasia are usually seen on biopsy. If a mass is present, it should be removed. Milky discharge from multiple ducts in nonlactating women presumably reflects increased secretion of pituitary prolactin; serum prolactin and thyroid-stimulating hormone levels should be obtained to search for a pituitary tumor or hypothyroidism. Hypothyroidism may cause galactorrhea. Alternatively, phenothiazines may cause milky discharge that disappears when medication is discontinued. Oral contraceptive agents may cause clear, serous, or milky discharge from multiple ducts or, less often, from a single duct. The discharge is more evident just before menstruation and disappears when the medication is stopped. If discharge does not stop and is from a single duct, surgical exploration should be performed.

When localization is not possible and no mass is palpable, the patient should be reexamined every week for 1 month. When unilateral discharge persists, even without definite localization or tumor, surgical exploration must be considered. The alternative is careful follow-up at intervals of 1–3 months. Mammography should be performed. Chronic unilateral nipple discharge, especially if it is bloody, is an indication for resection of the involved ducts. Purulent discharge may originate in a subareolar abscess and requires excision of the abscess and related lactiferous sinus (46).

Fat Necrosis

Fat necrosis of the breast is rare but clinically important because it produces a mass, often accompanied by skin or nipple retraction, which is indistinguishable from carcinoma. Trauma is presumed to be the cause, although only about one-half of patients have a history of injury to the breast. Ecchymosis is occasionally seen near the tumor. Tenderness may or may not be present. If untreated, the mass associated with fat necrosis gradually disappears. As a rule, the safest course is needle or excisional biopsy of the entire mass to rule out carcinoma. Fat necrosis is common after segmental resection and radiation therapy.

Breast Abscess

Infection in the breast is rare unless the patient is lactating. During lactation, an area of redness, tenderness, and induration frequently develops in the breast. The organism most commonly found in these abscesses is *Staphylococcus aureus* (47). In its early stages, the infection can often be reversed while nursing is continued from that breast by administering an antibiotic such as *dicloxacillin* or *oxacillin,* 250 mg four times daily for 7–10 days. If the lesion progresses to a localized mass with local and systemic signs of infection, an abscess is present and should be drained, and nursing should be discontinued.

Rarely, an infection or abscess may develop in young or middle-aged women who are not lactating (48). These infections tend to recur after incision and drainage, unless excision of the involved lactiferous duct(s) at the base of the nipple is undertaken during a quiescent interval. Because inflammatory carcinoma must always be considered in the presence of erythema of the breast, findings suggestive of abscesses are an indication for incision and biopsy of any indurated tissue. Patients should not undergo prolonged treatment for an apparent infection unless biopsy has eliminated the possibility of inflammatory carcinoma.

Disorders of the Augmented Breast

Estimates indicate that nearly 4 million American women have undergone augmentation mammoplasty. Breast implants are usually placed under the pectoralis muscle or, less desirably, in the subcutaneous tissue of the breast. Most implants are made of an outer silicone shell filled with a silicone gel or saline.

The complications of breast implantation are not insignificant. About 15–25% of patients develop capsule contraction or scarring around the implant, leading to a firmness and distortion of the breast that can be painful and sometimes requires removal of the implant and capsule. Implant rupture may occur in as many as 5–10% of women, and bleeding of gel through the capsule is even more common (49). In April 1992, the Food and Drug Administration (FDA) concluded that the safety and effectiveness of silicone gel breast implants had not been established and called for additional preclinical and clinical studies (50). The FDA advised symptomatic women with ruptured implants to discuss the need for surgical removal with their physicians. When there is no evidence of associated symptoms or rupture, implant removal is generally not indicated, because the risks of removal are probably greater than those of retention.

A suggested association between silicone gel and autoimmune disease has been poorly documented (51, 52). There are no clinical data proving an increased incidence of connective tissue disorders in patients with silicone gel breast implants, and a retrospective cohort study from the Mayo Clinic showed no increased incidence of autoimmune disorders among women with silicone implants (53). Even so, patients who have symptoms suggestive of an autoimmune disorder should discuss with their physician the risks and benefits of implant removal.

Any association between implants and an increased incidence of breast cancer is unlikely (54). However, breast cancer may develop in any patient with a silicone gel prosthesis.

References

1. **Baines CJ.** Breast self-examination. *Cancer* 1989;64:2661–3.

2. **Moskowitz M, Milbrath J, Gartside P, Zermeno A, Mandel D.** Lack of efficacy in thermography as a screening tool for minimal and stage I breast cancer. *N Engl J Med* 1976;295:249–52.

3. **Fletcher SW, Black W, Harris R, Rimer BK, Shapiro S.** Report of the International Workshop on Screening for Breast Cancer. *J Natl Cancer Inst* 1993;85:1644–56.

4. **Walter SD, Day NE.** Estimation of the duration of a pre-clinical disease state using screening data. *Am J Epidemiol* 1983;118:865–86.

5. **Sickles EA.** Mammographic features of 300 consecutive nonpalpable breast cancers. *Am J Roentgenol* 1986;146:661–3.

6. **Bassett LW, Liu TH, Giuliano AE, Gold RH.** The prevalence of carcinoma in palpable vs. impalpable, mammographically detected lesions. *Am J Roentgenol* 1991;157:21–4.

7. **Sickles EA, Ominsky SH, Sollitto RA, Galvin HG.** Medical audit of a rapid-throughput mammography screening practice: methodology and results of 27,114 examinations. *Radiology* 1990;175:323–7.

8. **Feig SA, Ehrlich SM.** Estimation of radiation risks from screening mammography: recent trends and comparison with expected benefits. *Radiology* 1990;174:638–47.

9. **Dershaw DD, Masterson ME, Malik S, Cruz NM.** Mammography using an ultrahigh-strip-density, stationary, focused grid. *Radiology* 1985;156:541–4.

10. **McLelland R.** Challenges and progress with mammography. *Cancer* 1989;64:2664–6.

11. **Sickles EA, Filly RA, Callen PW.** Benign breast lesions: ultrasound detection and diagnosis. *Radiology* 1984;151:467–70.

12. **Egan R, Egan KL.** Detection of breast cancer: comparison of water-bath whole breast sonography, mammography and physical examination. *Am J Roentgenol* 1985;145:1–8.

13. **Brenner RJ.** Breast MR imaging. *MRI Clin North Am* 1994;2:705.

14. **Tabar L, Fagerberg CJ, Gad A, Baldetorp L, Holmberg LH, Grontoft O, et al.** Reduction in mortality from breast cancer after mass screening with mammography. Randomised trial from the Breast Cancer Screening Working Group of the Swedish National Board of Health and Welfare. *Lancet* 1985;1:829–32.

15. **Shapiro S, Venet W, Strax P, Venet L, Roeser R.** Ten- to fourteen-year effect of screening on breast cancer mortality. *J Natl Cancer Inst* 1982;69:349–55.

16. **Hurley SF, Kaldor JM.** The benefits and risks of mammographic screening for breast cancer. *Epidemiol Rev* 1992;14:101–30.

17. **Pertschuk LP, Eisenberg KB, Carter AC, Feldman JG.** Immunohistochemical localization of estrogen receptors in breast cancer with monoclonal antibodies. Correlation with biochemistry and clinical endocrine response. *Cancer* 1985;55:1513–8.

18. **Leis HP Jr.** Concepts regarding breast biopsies. *Breast Disease* 1991;4:223.

19. **Parker SH.** Percutaneous large core breast biopsy. *Cancer* 1994;74:256–62.

20. **Kopans DB.** Screening for breast cancer and mortality reduction among women 40–49 years of age. *Cancer* 1994;74:311–22.

21. **Miller AB.** Mammography screening guidelines for women 40 to 49 and over 65 years old. *Ann Epidemiol* 1994;4:96–101.

22. **Smart CR.** Highlights of the evidence of benefit for women aged 40–49 years from the 14-year follow-up of the Breast Cancer Detection Demonstration Project. *Cancer* 1994;74:296–300.

23. **Dodd GD.** American Cancer Society guidelines on screening for breast cancer. An overview. *Cancer* 1992;7:1885–7.

24. **Chalmers TC.** Screening for breast cancer: what should national health policy be? *J Natl Cancer Inst* 1993;85:1619–21.

25. **Miller AB, Bulbrook RD.** Screening, detection and diagnosis of breast cancer. *Lancet* 1982;1:1109.

26. **Vetrani A, Fulciniti F, Di Benedetto G, Zeppa P, Troncone G, Boscaino A, et al.** Fine-needle aspiration biopsies of breast masses: an additional experience with 1153 cases (1985-1988) and a metaanalysis. *Cancer* 1992;69:736–40.

27. **Giuliano AE.** Fibrocystic disease of the breast. In: **Cameron J,** ed. *Current Problems in Surgery.* St Louis: CV Mosby, 1986.

28. **McDivitt RW, Stevens JA, Lee NC, Wingo PA, Rubin GL, Gersell D.** Histologic types of benign breast disease and the risk for breast cancer. The Cancer and Steroid Hormone Study Group. *Cancer* 1992;69:1408–14.

29. **Bland KI, Love N.** Evaluation of common breast masses. *Postgrad Med* 1002;92:95–7.

30. **Azzopardi JG.** Terminology of benign diseases and the benign epithelial hyperplasias. In: **Azzopardi JG,** ed. *Problems in Breast Pathology.* Philadelphia: WB Saunders, 1979:23.

31. **Meyer JE, Christian RL, Frenna TH, Sonnenfeld MR, Waitzkin ED, Shaffer K.** Image-guided aspiration of solitary occult breast cysts. *Arch Surg* 1992;127:433–5.

32. **Maddox PR, Mansel RE.** Management of breast pain and nodularity. *World J Surg* 1989;13:699–705.

33. **Gateley CA, Miers M, Mansell RE, Hughes LE.** Drug treatments for mastalgia: 17 years experience in the Cardiff Mastalgia Clinic. *J Royal Soc Med* 1992;85:12.

34. **Lawson DH, Jick H, Rothman KJ.** Coffee and tea consumption and breast disease. *Surgery* 1981;90:801–3.

35. **Page DL, Dupont WD.** Anatomic markers of human premalignancy and risk of breast cancer. *Cancer* 1990;66:1326–35.

36. **London SJ, Connolly JL, Schnitt SJ, Colditz GA.** A prospective study of benign breast disease and the risk of breast cancer. *JAMA* 1992;267:941–4.

37. **Dent DM, Cant PJ.** Fibroadenoma. *World J Surg* 1989;13:701–10.

38. **Dupont WD, Page DL, Parl FF, Venecak-Jones CL, Plummer WD, Rados MS, et al.** Long-term risk of breast cancer in women with fibroadenoma. *N Engl J Med* 1994;331:10–5.

39. **Hindle WH, Alonzo LJ.** Conservative management of breast fibroadenomas. *Am J Obstet Gynecol* 1991;164:1647–50.

40. **Chua CL, Thomas A.** Cystosarcoma phyllodes tumors. *Surg Gynecol Obstet* 1988;166:302–6.

41. **Hart J, Layfield LJ, Trumbull WE, Brayton D, Barker WF, Giuliano AE.** Practical aspects in the diagnosis and management of cystosarcoma phyllodes. *Arch Surg* 1988;123:1079–83.

42. **Zurrida S, Bartoli C, Galimberti V, Squicciarini P, Delledonne V, Veronessi P, et al.** Which therapy for unexpected phyllode tumour of the breast? *Eur J Cancer* 1992;28:654–7.

43. **Naruns PL, Giuliano AE.** Sarcomas of the breast. In: **Eilber FR, Morton DL, Sondak VK, Economou JS,** eds. *The Soft Tissue Sarcomas.* New York: Grune & Stratton, 1987:169–82.

44. **Leis HP Jr.** Management of nipple discharge. *World J Surg* 1989;13:736–42.

45. **Gulay H, Bora S, Kilicturgay S, Hamaloglu E, Goksel HA.** Management of nipple discharge. *J Am Coll Surg* 1994;178:471–4.

46. **Dixon JM.** Outpatient treatment of non-lactational breast abscesses. *Br J Surg* 1992;79:56–7.

47. **Thomsen AC, Espersen T, Maigaard S.** Course and treatment of milk stasis, noninfectious inflammation of the breast, and infectious mastitis in nursing women. *Am J Obstet Gynecol* 1984;149:492–5.

48. **Edmiston CE Jr, Walker AP, Krepel CJ, Gohr C.** The nonpuerperal breast infection: aerobic and anaerobic microbial recovery from acute and chronic disease. *J Infect Dis* 1990;162:695–9.

49. **Nemecek JA, Young VL.** How safe are silicone breast implants? *South Med J* 1993;86:932–44.

50. **Kessler DA.** The basis of the FDA's decision on breast implants. *N Engl J Med* 1992;326:1713–5.

51. **Sanchez-Guerrero J, Schur PH, Sergent JS, Liang MH.** Silicone breast implants and rheumatic disease. Clinical, immunologic, and epidemiologic studies. *Arthritis Rheum* 1994;37:158–68.

52. **Duffy MJ, Woods JE.** Health risks of failed silicone gel breast implants: a 30-year clinical experience. *Plast Reconstr Surg* 1994;94:295–9.

53. **Gabriel SE, O'Fallon WM, Kurland LT, Beard CM, Woods JE, Melton LJ 3rd.** Risk of connective tissue diseases and other disorders after breast implantation. *N Engl J Med* 1994; 330:1697–702.

54. **Bryant H, Brasher P.** Breast implants and breast cancer—reanalysis of a linkage study. *N Engl J Med* 1995;332:1535–9.

19 Preoperative Evaluation and Postoperative Management

Daniel L. Clarke-Pearson
George Olt
Gustavo Rodriguez
Matthew Boente

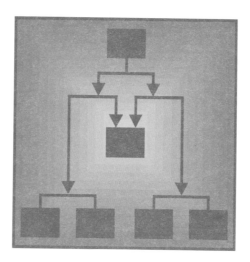

The successful outcome of gynecologic surgery is based on thorough evaluation, preoperative preparation, and careful postoperative management of the patient. Approaches to the general perioperative management of patients undergoing major gynecologic surgery with specific medical problems that could complicate the surgical outcome are presented.

Medical History and Physical Examination

The hazards of undertaking surgery without a thorough understanding of a patient's medical history and performing a complete physical examination cannot be overstated. The preoperative medical history should include any significant past medical illnesses that might be aggravated by surgery or that might complicate anesthesia or surgical recovery.

1. **Inquiry should be made regarding medications currently being taken as well as those discontinued within the previous months prior to surgery.** This inquiry should include notation of nonprescription drugs being taken and the use of oral contraceptives, which many patients consider a routine part of their living rather than a medication. Specific instructions must be given to the patient regarding the need to discontinue any medications prior to surgery (e.g., *aspirin* or oral contraceptives) as well as those medications that should be continued (e.g., cardiac or antihypertensive medications).

2. **The patient should be questioned regarding known allergies to medications (e.g., sulfa and *penicillin*), foods, or environmental agents.** A history of sensitivity to shellfish may be the only clue of an iodine sensitivity, which may be significant because iodinated intravenous contrast material is used for intravenous

pyelography, enhanced computed tomography (CT) scanning, and venography/arteriography. A history of hypersensitivity to intravenously administered iodine-containing compounds or shellfish should be clearly noted, and the patient should not undergo further exposure to iodine-containing compounds unless such exposure is absolutely mandatory. When intravenous contrast material must be used, corticosteroid preparation may prevent life-threatening anaphylactic reactions.

3. **Previous surgical procedures, and the patient's course following those surgical procedures, should be reviewed to identify complications of previous operations that might be avoided.** Reactions and response to anesthetic techniques should be evaluated with the anesthesiologist in charge. The patient should be asked about specific complications, such as excessive bleeding, wound infection, deep vein thrombosis, peritonitis, or bowel obstruction. A history of pelvic surgery should alert the gynecologist to the possibility of distorted surgical anatomy and possible preexisting injury to adjacent organ systems such as small bowel adhesions in the pelvis or ureteral stenosis from previous periureteral scarring. Intravenous pyelography (IVP) may be helpful in such cases to establish ureteral anatomy and patency and to identify any preexisting abnormality. Many patients may not be entirely clear about the extent of the previous surgical procedure or the details of intraoperative findings. Therefore, operative notes from previous pelvic operations should be obtained and reviewed to determine the details of the prior surgical procedure and surgical findings. This is particularly important in patients who have had surgery for pelvic inflammatory disease, pelvic abscess, endometriosis, or pelvic malignancy.

4. **Family history may identify familial traits that might complicate planned surgery.** A family history of excessive intraoperative or postoperative bleeding, malignant hyperthermia, and other potentially inherited conditions should be sought. General review of systems should also be included in the questioning, in an effort to identify any coexisting medical or surgical conditions. Inquiry about gastrointestinal and urologic function is particularly important prior to undertaking pelvic surgery, and many gynecologic diseases also involve adjacent nongynecologic viscera.

5. **Although many women undergoing gynecologic surgical procedures are otherwise healthy, with pathology identified only on pelvic examination, other major organ systems should not be neglected in the physical examination.** Identification of abnormalities such as a heart murmur or pulmonary compromise should lead the surgeon to obtain additional testing and consultation in order to minimize intraoperative and postoperative complications.

Laboratory Evaluation

The selection of appropriate preoperative laboratory studies will depend on the extent of the anticipated surgical procedure and the patient's medical status.

1. For patients undergoing general anesthesia, a blood count including hematocrit, white cell count, and platelet count should be obtained routinely.

2. Serum chemistries and liver function testing results are rarely abnormal in the asymptomatic patient who has no significant medical history and who is not taking medications.

3. Coagulation studies are of little value unless the patient has a significant medical history (1).

4. In women under 40 years of age, a chest x-ray and electrocardiography are of very low yield in identifying asymptomatic cardiopulmonary disease and thus may not be necessary (2, 3). However, women over 40 years of age and those undergoing major gynecologic surgical procedures should have a chest x-ray, electrocardiography, and serum electrolyte analysis preoperatively. Even if the results of these studies are normal, they will serve as baseline data for comparison to other studies that may be required in the evaluation of a postoperative complication.

Radiographic evaluation of adjacent organ systems should be undertaken in individual cases as follows:

1. Intravenous pyelography is helpful to delineate ureteral patency and course, especially in the presence of a pelvic mass, gynecologic cancer, or congenital müllerian anomaly. **However, an IVP is not of significant value in the evaluation of most patients undergoing pelvic surgery** (4).

2. A barium enema or upper gastrointestinal series with small bowel assessment may be of significant value in evaluating some patients before undergoing pelvic surgery. Because of the proximity of the female genital tract to the lower gastrointestinal tract, the rectum and sigmoid colon may be involved with benign (endometriosis or pelvic inflammatory disease) or malignant gynecologic conditions. Conversely, a pelvic mass could have a gastrointestinal origin such as a diverticular abscess or a mass of inflamed small intestines (Crohn's disease). Clearly, any patient with gastrointestinal symptoms should be further evaluated with contrast radiography as well as proctosigmoidoscopy, flexible sigmoidoscopy, or colonoscopy.

3. Other imaging studies, including ultrasound, CT scanning, or magnetic resonance imaging (MRI), are useful only in selected patients.

Preoperative Discussion and Informed Consent

The verbal and nonverbal rapport and trust that exist between the patient and her gynecologist begin on the initial office visit and should be built on during each subsequent visit. During the initial discussion, the physician should explain in sufficient detail to the patient the findings of examination, the results of testing, the natural history of the disease process, and the goals of the surgical procedure. Because most gynecologic surgery is elective, the gynecologist has the opportunity to evaluate the patient from a medical point of view, as well as to allow the patient to develop psychological coping mechanisms and to answer questions that may not have been discussed initially. The surgeon should be available to discuss in person or by phone any questions that arise before actual hospital admission.

The goals of the preoperative discussion should serve to allay the patient's anxiety and fears and to answer any questions. The discussion should serve to expand further on issues relative to the surgery, its expected outcome, and risks and is the basis for obtaining the signed informed consent (5). Informed consent is an educational process for the patient and her family and fulfills the physician's need to convey information in understandable terms. The following items should be discussed and, after each item, the patient and family should be invited to ask questions.

1. The nature and extent of the disease process.

2. The extent of the actual operation proposed and the potential modifications of the operation, depending on intraoperative findings.

3. The anticipated benefits of the operation, with a conservative estimate of successful outcome.

4. The risks and potential complications of the surgery.

5. Alternative methods of therapy and the risks and results of those alternative methods of therapy.

6. The results likely if the patient is not treated.

A discussion of the nature and the extent of the disease process should include an explanation in lay terms of the significance of the disease. Is it life-threatening, or will it likely result in significant disability or dysfunction? To what extent does the disease process alter the patient's daily living? If untreated, could the disease spontaneously resolve, or could it potentially worsen? What is the time course and natural history of the disease?

The goals of surgery should be discussed in detail. Some gynecologic surgical procedures are performed purely for diagnostic purposes (e.g., dilation and curettage, cold knife conization, a diagnostic laparoscopy, or staging laparotomy), while most are clearly aimed at correcting an anatomic defect or a specific disease process. The extent of the surgery should be outlined, including which organs will be removed. Most patients like to be informed regarding the type of surgical incision and the estimated duration of anesthesia.

The expected outcome of the surgical procedure should be explained. If the procedure is being performed for diagnostic purposes, the outcome will depend on surgical or pathologic findings that are not known before surgery. When treating anatomic deformity or disease, the expected success of the operation should be discussed, as well as the potential for failure of the operation. This discussion should include the probability of failure (i.e., failure of tubal sterilization or the possibility that stress urinary incontinence may not be alleviated). When treating cancer, the possibility of finding more advanced disease and the potential need for adjunctive therapy (e.g., postoperative radiation therapy or chemotherapy) should be mentioned. Other issues of importance to the patient include discussion of loss of fertility or loss of ovarian function. These issues should be raised by the physician to ensure that the patient adequately understands the pathophysiology that may result from the surgery and to allow her to express her feelings regarding these emotionally charged issues.

The risks and potential complications of the surgical procedure should be discussed with the patient, including the most frequent complications of the particular surgical procedure. For most major gynecologic surgery, the risks include intraoperative and postoperative hemorrhage, postoperative infection, venous thrombosis, and injury to adjacent viscera. If the patient has a preexisting medical problem, what additional risks might be encountered? Unanticipated findings at the time of surgery should also be mentioned. For example, if the ovaries are found unexpectedly to be diseased, it may be the best surgical judgment that they should be removed.

The usual postoperative course should be discussed in enough detail to allow the patient to understand what to expect in the days following surgery. Information regarding the need for a suprapubic catheter or prolonged central venous monitoring helps the patient accept her postoperative course and avoids surprises to the patient that may be very disconcerting. The expected duration of the recovery period, both in and out of the hospital, should be noted.

Alternative methods of therapy should be mentioned as part of the preoperative discussion. Other medical management or surgical approaches should be discussed, along with their potential benefits and complications. Finally, the patient should have an understanding of the outcome of the disease if nothing is done. Following this discussion, it should be clear to the patient why the proposed surgery is the appropriate next step in her care. The preoperative discussion and signing of the consent form should include witnesses—a family member and another member of the health care team. The informed consent discussion detailing the information given to the patient should be documented in the patient's chart.

The anesthesiologist responsible for the surgical procedure should also have the opportunity to examine the patient, review her laboratory findings, and discuss the proposed anesthetic method with the patient. In many institutions, the consent to the administration of anesthetic is included in the surgical consent form, whereas in other institutions, it is a separate form that should be obtained by the anesthesiologist after appropriate preoperative discussion.

General Considerations

Nutrition

In general, patients undergoing elective gynecologic surgery have adequate nutritional stores and, for the most part, do not require nutritional support. However, all patients should have an adequate nutritional assessment, especially those undergoing gynecologic cancer surgery or other major gynecologic procedures in which the postoperative recovery is expected to be prolonged, because physicians often fail to recognize malnutrition in the perioperative setting (6). Protein calorie malnutrition is associated with delayed wound healing, an increased risk of infection, and increased mortality.

Surgery increases the nutritional requirements of patients for several reasons. First, there is a period of time following surgery during which oral intake is not allowed or is very limited. In addition, the operation itself causes increased protein catabolism, increased energy requirements, and a negative nitrogen balance. If the surgery is uncomplicated and the patient is without food for less than 7 days, this response is limited and patients usually recover without the need for nutritional support. If there are complications such as infection or prolonged return of bowel function secondary to single or multiple enterectomy, the negative nitrogen balance may be severe and nutritional support may be required.

All patients should undergo nutritional assessment preoperatively as well as at regular intervals postoperatively until they have successfully returned to a regular diet. Although there is no single test to determine an adequate nutritional state, decisions regarding the need for nutritional support should be made based on the patient's prior nutritional state, the anticipated length of time in which the patient will not be able to eat, the severity of surgery, and the likelihood of complications and thus negative nitrogen balance. The goal of nutritional support is to minimize the length of time a negative nitrogen balance exists and to maintain the patient's nutritional status until they can eat again. Approximately 30–50% of surgical patients are moderately or severely malnourished as a consequence of their diagnosis or possibly from the therapeutic modality used to treat their disease (7–9). Nutritional assessment should determine whether the cause of the malnutrition is increased enteral loss (malabsorption, intestinal fistula) or if it is secondary to decreased oral intake or possibly increased nutritional requirements as a result of hypermetabolism (sepsis, malignancy) or a combination of these factors. Severe malnutrition, if not corrected, can further complicate the postoperative problem by causing altered immune function, chronic anemia, impaired wound healing, and eventually, multiple organ system failure and death.

A careful history and physical examination are the most useful, reliable, and cost-effective methods of assessing the nutritional status of a patient. In particular, information about recent weight loss as well as the patient's dietary history, including alcohol use, are quite

547

helpful in assessing the patient's nutritional status. Patients who have lost less than 6% of their ideal body weight do not need preoperative nutritional intervention. **Patients who have lost more than 12% of their ideal body weight, however, should be considered for preoperative intervention;** those who have lost between 6 and 12% should undergo further studies with serum protein measurements as well as measurement of various anthropometric, biochemical, immunologic, and body composition parameters.

Anthropometric measurements of skin-fold thickness and arm-muscle circumference provide an estimate of total body fat and lean muscle mass. Unfortunately, these measurements have not been reproducible and traditionally have been poor predictors of nutritional status and clinical outcome (10, 11).

Recently, isotope dilution techniques have been used to determine the ratios of exchangeable sodium and potassium, which can determine body cell mass and thus give another parameter for chronic malnutrition. Whole body counters that can measure radioactive intracellular calcium can also be used to determine skeletal muscle mass. More recently, gamma neutron activation has been used to measure total body nitrogen, which is currently considered the state-of-the-art method for the determination of total body protein (12, 13). Practically, however, the degree of malnutrition is usually estimated based on serum concentrations of albumin, transferrin, prealbumin, and retinal binding protein (RBP). The levels of these serum proteins is greatly influenced by the patient's level of hydration. Prealbumin and RBP have the shortest half-lives, and levels are depressed very early in comparison with serum transferrin and albumin which have half-lives of 8 and 20 days, respectively (14).

Although a number of conditions result in anergy to recall skin testing, such testing can be used to determine the amount of visceral protein depletion. Determining the status of cell-mediated immunity and reversing this status if it is lost preoperatively may help reduce postoperative morbidity and mortality. However, improvements in body weight and other traditional nutritional parameters usually are seen long before the reversal of skin test and anergy.

No single test accurately predicts the outcome in malnourished surgical patients. Because of this, a number of formulas incorporating a variety of nutritional indices have been proposed to assess the perioperative risk secondary to malnutrition. Mullen and co-workers have prospectively evaluated a model that incorporates albumin (ALB), triceps skin-fold thickness (TSF), transferrin (TFN), and delayed hypersensitivity (DH). By a step-wise regression analysis, a linear predictive model called the prognostic nutritional index (PNI) was developed to relate these factors. It is calculated as follows:

$$\textbf{PNI (\%)} = \textbf{158} - \textbf{16.6 (ALB)} - \textbf{0.78 (TSF)} - \textbf{0.20 (TFN)} - \textbf{5.8 (DH)}$$

This model was tested on 100 patients undergoing elective surgery and was shown to be valid (15).

Calculation of Caloric Requirements

The most precise method for calculating a patient's daily caloric requirements is indirect calorimetry. This method is very costly, however, and is not routinely used clinically. Caloric requirements can be calculated based on the Harrison-Benedict formula for basal energy expenditure:

$$\textbf{Basal energy expenditure (Kcal)} =$$
$$\textbf{655} + [\textbf{9.6} \times \textbf{wt (kg)}] + [\textbf{1.7} \times \textbf{ht (cms)}] - [\textbf{4.7} \times \textbf{age (years)}]$$

1. **The daily caloric requirements can then be met by providing 1000 calories more than the patient's basal energy expenditure.** Alternatively, daily caloric

requirements can be met by giving the patient 35 kcal/kg/day for maintenance and 45 kcal/kg/day for anabolic states. Daily nitrogen requirements may be met by providing 1 g of nitrogen (6.25 g of protein) for every 125–150 calories.

2. **The maximal rate of glucose oxygenation in adults is approximately 7 g/kg/day.** Patients with very high caloric requirements or diabetes mellitus should receive calories in excess of this in the form of lipids. Insulin should be used to maintain serum glucose concentration between 150 and 250 mg/dl, and it may be added directly to the TPN solution. Glucose administration in excess of the caloric requirements can lead to fatty infiltration of the liver and other metabolic complications.

3. **Lipid in a 10–20% emulsion can be given as further caloric supplement.** More calories can be given in the form of free fatty acids, which are the major source of energy for most peripheral tissues. When lipids are used as a major source of calories, a minimum of 50–150 g/per/day of glucose should also be given to provide a substrate for the central nervous system. Most patients can tolerate up to 2 g of fat/kg/day, and daily dosages should not exceed 4 g of fat/kg/day. These lipid emulsions are isotonic and can be delivered simultaneously with the protein and carbohydrate mixture in a 3-l bag over a 24-hour infusion. In general, 30–50% of nonprotein calories should be supplied in lipid form. Serum triglyceride levels should be monitored to ensure that the patient can metabolize the fat.

4. **In addition to calories and protein, nutritional support should be maintained in terms of electrolytes, vitamins, and trace elements.** Daily maintenance requirements for electrolytes are as follows: sodium, 60–120 mEq; chloride, 60–120 mEq; magnesium, 8–10 mEg; calcium, 200–400 mg; and phosphorous, 300–400 mg. A number of vitamins and trace elements must also be supplied to ensure that the patient is eumetabolic.

Route of Administration

After the decision has been made that nutritional support is required, the appropriate route of administration must be determined. Enteral nutrition should be considered primarily because it is easy to deliver, associated with the fewest complications, and relatively inexpensive. Contraindications to this route of delivery include intestinal obstruction, gastrointestinal bleeding, and diarrhea. Many different types are commercially available and can be chosen based on their caloric content, fat content, protein content, osmolality, viscosity, and price. Depending on the patient's problem, the route of delivery may be through a Dubhoff feeding tube, a gastrostomy tube, or a feeding jejunostomy tube.

Total parenteral nutrition (TPN) must be delivered through a central vein and has gained wide acceptance as a means of providing nutritional support for surgically ill patients. It must be delivered through a subclavian or internal jugular vein, and the catheter must be placed using meticulous sterile surgical technique. Proper daily care is required to avoid infectious complications and a eumetabolic state may be obtained if multivitamins (including folate and B_{12}), and trace metals (cobalt, iodine, manganese, and zinc) are used to supplement the 2- to 3-l/day TPN solution. Essential fatty acids are supplied weekly and iron may be added if hyperalimentation is prolonged and bone marrow stores have become depleted. Appropriate adjustments in the contents of the TPN are required for patients with liver, renal, or cardiac dysfunction. When managed by an experienced team, the most frequent complication, infection, can be reduced to a very reasonable level (5–10%) (16).

Postoperative Outcome

A number of retrospective clinical studies, mostly from the general surgical literature, have demonstrated that nutritional support improves postoperative outcome in a variety of categories, including surgical complications, sepsis, wound infections, and mortality. A number of prospective randomized trials, however, have failed to demonstrate that preoperative TPN improved clinical outcome (17–21). Recently, a multi-institutional, prospective, randomized trial evaluating TPN use in the Veterans Affairs Total Parenteral Nutrition Cooperative Study Group was reported (21). The study reported a series of 395 malnourished patients who were randomly assigned to receive TPN for 7–15 days before surgery and 3 days postoperatively (treatment arm) or no perioperative TPN (control arm). The patients were then followed for 90 days after the surgery and were evaluated in terms of morbidity and mortality. Major complications during the first 30 days, as well as the overall 90-day mortality rates, were then analyzed and were similar in both the treated and control arms. However, in a small group of patients with extremely severe malnutrition, the incidence of noninfectious complications was significantly less common in the group given TPN. The study defined severe malnutrition as a nutritional risk index score of less than 83. The authors of that study concluded that preoperative TPN should be limited to patients who were severely malnourished unless there were other specific indications. More recently, studies have shown that when severe malnutrition does exist, a 10-day preoperative course of parenteral nutrition prior to surgery would save approximately $1720 (U.S.) per patient (22).

When only mild or moderate malnutrition exists preoperatively, or when the patient is nutritionally normal biochemically but the proposed surgery is likely to require a prolonged catabolic period of more than 7–10 days, then TPN should be instituted in the early postoperative period as soon as the patient is hemodynamically stable. This type of management should be strongly considered in patients undergoing pelvic exenterations, urinary diversions, or multiple enterectomies (23).

In summary, clinical trials have demonstrated that TPN can improve nutritional status as measured by biochemical assays, immune function, and nitrogen balance. The effect of TPN on clinical outcome, however, is less well established. Despite what would seem reasonable based on common sense as well as preoperative nutritional parameters, the data do not support TPN for mild to moderately malnourished patients. With severe malnutrition, preoperative TPN would seem to be beneficial and should be instituted.

Fluid and Electrolytes

In the average woman, total water constitutes approximately 50–55% of body weight. Two-thirds of this water is contained in the intracellular compartment. One-third is contained in the extracellular compartment, of which one-fourth is contained in plasma, and the remaining three-quarters is in the interstitium.

Osmolarity, or tonicity, is a property derived from the number of particles in a solution. Sodium and chloride are the primary electrolytes contributing to the osmolarity of the extracellular fluid compartment. Potassium and, to a lesser extent, magnesium and phosphate are the major intracellular electrolytes. Water flows freely between the intracellular and the extracellular spaces to maintain osmotic neutrality throughout the body. Any shifts in osmolarity in any fluid spaces within the body are accompanied by corresponding shifts in free water from spaces of lower to higher osmolarity, thus maintaining equilibrium.

The daily fluid maintenance requirement for the average adult is approximately 30 ml/kg/day, or 2000–3000 ml/day (24). This is offset partially by insensible losses of 1200 ml/day. which includes losses from the lungs (600 ml), skin (400 ml), and gastrointestinal tract (200 ml). Urinary output from the kidney will provide the remainder of the fluid loss, and this output will vary depending on total body intake of water and sodium. Approximately 600–800 mOsm of solute are excreted by the kidney per day. Healthy kidneys can concentrate urine up to approximately 1200 mOsm and, therefore, the minimum output can range between 500 and 700 ml/day. The maximal urinary output of the kidney can be as high as 20 l/day, as seen in patients with diabetes insipidus. In healthy patients, the kidney adjusts urine output commensurate with the daily fluid intake.

The major extracellular buffer used in acid-base balance is the bicarbonate-carbonic acid system: $CO_2 + H_2O \leftrightarrow H_2CO_3 \leftrightarrow H^+ + HCO_3^-$ (25). Typically, the body will maintain a bicarbonate to carbonic acid ratio of 20:1 in order to maintain an extracellular pH of 7.4. Both the lung and kidney play integral roles in the maintenance of normal extracellular pH via retention or excretion of carbon dioxide and bicarbonate. Under conditions of alkalosis, minute ventilation decreases and renal excretion of bicarbonate increases to restore the normal bicarbonate to carbonic acid ratio. The opposite occurs with acidosis.

Ultimately, the kidney plays the most important role in fluid and electrolyte balance through excretion and retention of water and solute. Circulating antidiuretic hormone and aldosterone help modulate the process. Serum osmolarity affects hypothalamic release of antidiuretic hormone, and aldosterone secretion is responsive to renal perfusion. Under states of dehydration or hypovolemia, serum antidiuretic hormone levels increase, leading to increased resorption of water in the distal tubule of the kidney. In addition, increased aldosterone release promotes increased renal sodium and water retention. The opposite occurs in states of fluid excess. As a result, individuals with normal renal function and circulating antidiuretic hormone and aldosterone levels maintain normal serum osmolarity and electrolyte composition despite daily fluctuation of fluid and electrolyte intake.

Various disease states can alter the normal fluid and electrolyte homeostatic mechanisms, making perioperative fluid and electrolyte management more difficult. Patients with intrinsic renal disease are unable to excrete solute and to maintain acid-base balance. In patients undergoing the stress of chronic starvation or severe illness, there may be an inappropriately high level of circulating antidiuretic hormone and aldosterone, resulting in fluid and sodium retention. With severe cardiac disease, secondary renal hypoperfusion can lead to increased aldosterone synthesis and, therefore, increased sodium and water retention by the kidney. Finally, patients with severe diabetes can have significant osmotic diuresis as well as acid-base dysfunction secondary to circulating ketoacids. Correction and optimization of renal, cardiac, or endocrinologic disorders preoperatively are imperative and will often rectify fluid and electrolyte abnormalities.

Fluid and electrolyte management in the preoperative and perioperative periods requires knowledge of the daily fluid and electrolyte requirements for maintenance, replacement of ongoing fluid and electrolyte losses, as well as correction of any existing abnormalities.

Fluid and Electrolyte Maintenance Requirements

The normal daily fluid requirement in the average adult is 2000–3000 ml. The body adjusts to higher and lower volumes of intake by changes in plasma tonicity. Alterations in plasma tonicity induce adjustments in circulating antidiuretic hormone levels, which ultimately regulate the amount of water retained in the distal tubule of the kidney. In the preoperative and the early postoperative periods, it is usually only necessary to replace sodium and potassium. Chloride is automatically replaced, concomitant with sodium and potassium because chloride is the usual anion used to balance sodium and potassium in electrolyte solutions. There are various commercially available solutions containing 40 mmol of sodium chloride, with smaller amounts of potassium, calcium, and magnesium designed to meet the requirements of a patient who is receiving 3 l of intravenous fluids per day. The daily requirement, however, can be met by any combination of intravenous fluids. For example, 2 l of D5/0.45 normal saline (7 mEq sodium chloride each), supplemented with 20 mEq of potassium chloride, followed by 1 l of D5W with 20 mEq of potassium chloride, would suffice.

Fluid and Electrolyte Replacement

Fluid and electrolyte losses beyond the daily average must be replaced by appropriate solutions. The choice of solutions for replacement depends on the composition of the fluids lost. Often, it is difficult to measure free water loss, particularly in patients who have high losses from the lungs, skin, or the gastrointestinal tract. Procurement of daily weights in these patients can be very useful. Up to 300 g of weight loss daily can be attributable to weight loss from catabolism of protein and fat in the patient who is taking nothing by mouth (24). Anything beyond this, however, would be due to fluid loss and should be replaced accordingly.

Patients with a high fever can have increased pulmonary and skin loss of free water, sometimes in excess of 2–3 l/day. These losses should be replaced with free water in the form of D5W. Perspiration typically has one-third the osmolarity of plasma and can be replaced with D5W or, if excessive, with D5/0.25 normal saline.

The patient with acute blood loss needs replacement with appropriate isotonic fluid or blood or both. There is a wide range of plasma volume expanders, including albumin, dextran, and hetastarch solutions, that contain large molecular weight particles ($>50,000$ molecular weight). These particles are slow to exit the intravascular space, and about one-half of the particles remain after 24 hours. These solutions are expensive, however, and for most cases, simple replacement with 0.9 normal saline or lactated Ringer's solution will suffice. One-third of the volume of lactated Ringer's solution or normal saline will typically remain in the intravascular space, and the remainder goes to the interstitium.

Appropriate replacement of gastrointestinal fluid loss depends on the source of fluid loss in the gastrointestinal tract. Gastrointestinal secretions beyond the stomach and up to the colon are typically isotonic with plasma, with similar amounts of sodium, slightly lower amounts of chloride, slightly alkaline pH, more potassium, in the range of 10–20 mEq/l. Under normal conditions, stool is hypotonic. However, under conditions of increased flow (i.e., severe diarrhea), stool contents are isotonic with a composition similar to that of the small bowel. Gastric contents are typically hypotonic, with one-third the sodium of plasma, increased amounts of hydrogen ion, and low pH.

In patients with gastric outlet obstruction, nausea, and vomiting, or who undergo nasogastric suction, appropriate replacement of gastric secretions can be provided with a solution such as D5/0.45 normal saline with 20 mEq/l of potassium. Potassium supplementation is particularly important to prevent hypokalemia in these patients, whose kidneys attempt to conserve hydrogen ion in the distal tubule of the kidney in exchange for potassium ion.

In patients with bowel obstruction, 1–3 l of fluid can be sequestered daily in the gastrointestinal tract. This fluid should be replaced with isotonic saline or lactated Ringer's solution. Similarly, patients with enterocutaneous fistulas or new ileostomies should receive replacement with isotonic fluids.

Correction of Existing Fluid and Electrolyte Abnormalities

Patients who have fluid or electrolyte abnormalities preoperatively can pose a diagnostic challenge. The correct diagnosis and therapy is contingent on a correct assessment of total body fluid and electrolyte status. The management of hyponatremia, for example, may be either fluid restriction or fluid replacement. The choice of treatment depends on whether there is overall extracellular fluid excess and normal body sodium stores or decreased overall total body sodium stores and extracellular fluid. A detailed history is necessary to disclose any underlying medical illness and to assess the amount and duration of any abnormal fluid losses or intake. Initial evaluation should include an assessment of hemodynamic, clinical, and urinary parameters in order to determine the overall level of hydration as well as the fluid status of the extracellular fluid compartment. The patient who has good skin turgor, moist mucosa, stable vital signs, and good urinary output is well hydrated. Nonpitting edema is indicative of extracellular fluid excess, whereas patients with orthostasis, sunken eyes, parched mouth, and decreased skin turgor clearly have extracellular volume contraction. A patient's overall extracellular fluid status does not always reflect the hydration status of the intravascular compartment, however. A patient can have increased interstitial fluid and yet be intravascularly dry, requiring replacement with isotonic fluid.

Laboratory workup for patients who may have preexisting fluid problems should include blood hematocrit, serum chemistry, glucose, blood urea nitrogen (BUN) and creatinine, urine osmolality, and urine electrolyte levels. Serum osmolality is mainly a function of the concentration of sodium and is given by the following equation:

$$2 \times Na^+ + \frac{glucose\ (mg/dl)}{18} + \frac{BUN\ (mg/dl)}{2.8}$$

Normal serum osmolarity is typically 290–300 mOsm. Blood hematocrit will rise or fall inversely at a rate of 1%/500 ml alteration of extracellular fluid volume. The BUN to creatinine ratio is typically 10:1 but will rise to a ratio of greater than 20:1 under conditions of extracellular fluid contraction. Under conditions of extracellular fluid deficit, urine osmolality will typically be high (>400 mOsm), whereas urine sodium concentration is low (<15 mEq/l) indicative of an attempt by the kidney to conserve sodium. Under conditions of extracellular fluid excess or in cases of renal disease in which the kidney has impaired ability to retain sodium and water, urine osmolality will be low and urine sodium will be high (>30 mEq/l). Finally, changes in sodium can give insight into the degree of extracellular fluid excess or deficit. In the average person, the serum sodium rises by 3 mmol/l for every liter of water deficit, and falls by 3 mmol/l for each liter of water excess. One must, however, be careful in making these estimates, because patients with prolonged water and electrolyte loss can have low serum sodium levels and marked water deficits.

Specific Electrolyte Disorders

Hyponatremia **Because sodium is the major extracellular cation, shifts in serum sodium are usually inversely correlated with the hydration state of the extracellular fluid compartment.** The pathophysiology of hyponatremia, then, is usually expansion of body fluids leading to excess total body water (25). Symptomatic hyponatremia usually does not occur until the serum sodium is below 120–125 mEq/l. The severity of the symptoms (nausea, vomiting, lethargy, seizures) is related more to the rate of change of serum sodium than to the actual serum sodium level.

Hyponatremia in the form of extracellular fluid excess can be seen in patients with renal or cardiac failure as well as in conditions such as nephrotic syndrome, in which total body salt and water are increased, with a relatively greater increase in the latter. Administration of hypertonic saline to correct the hyponatremia would be inappropriate in this setting. The treatment should include, in addition to correcting the underlying disease process, water restriction with diuretic therapy.

Inappropriate secretion of antidiuretic hormone (ADH) can occur with head trauma, pulmonary or cerebral tumors, and states of stress. The abnormally elevated ADH results in excess water retention. Treatment includes water restriction and, if possible, correction of the underlying cause. Demeclocycline has been shown to be effective in this disorder via its action in the kidney.

Inappropriate replacement of body salt losses with water alone will result in hyponatremia. This will typically occur in patients who are losing large amounts of electrolytes secondary to vomiting, nasogastric suction, diarrhea, or gastrointestinal fistulas, who received replacement with hypotonic solutions. Simple replacement with isotonic fluids and potassium will usually correct the abnormality. Rarely, rapid correction of the hyponatremia is necessary, in which case hypertonic saline (3%) can be administered. Hypertonic saline should be administered very cautiously in order to avoid a rapid shift in serum sodium, which will induce central nervous system dysfunction.

Hypernatremia **Hypernatremia is an uncommon condition that can be life-threatening if severe (serum sodium >160 mEq/l).** The pathophysiology is extracellular fluid deficit. The resultant hyperosmolar state leads to decreased water volume in cells in the central nervous system, which, if severe, can cause disorientation, seizures, intracranial bleeding, and death. The causes include excessive extrarenal water loss, which can occur in patients who have a high fever, have undergone tracheostomy in a dry environment, or have extensive thermal injuries; who have diabetes insipidus, either central or nephrogenic; and who have iatrogenic salt loading. The treatment involves correction of the underlying cause (correction of fever, humidification of the tracheostomy, pitressin for control of central diabetes insipidus) and replacement with free water either by the oral route or intravenously with D5W. As with severe hyponatremia, marked hypernatremia should be corrected slowly.

Hypokalemia   Hypokalemia may be encountered preoperatively in patients with significant gastrointestinal fluid loss (prolonged emesis, diarrhea, nasogastric suction, intestinal fistulas) and marked urinary potassium loss secondary to renal tubular disorders (renal tubular acidosis, acute tubular necrosis, hyperaldosteronism, prolonged diuretic use). It can also arise from prolonged administration of potassium-free parenteral fluids in patients who are restricted from ingesting anything by mouth. The symptoms associated with hypokalemia include neuromuscular disturbances, ranging from muscle weakness to flaccid paralysis, and cardiovascular abnormalities, including hypotension, bradycardia, arrhythmias, and enhancement of digitalis toxicity. These symptoms rarely occur unless the serum potassium is <3 mEq/l. The treatment is potassium replacement. Oral therapy is preferable in patients who are on an oral diet. If necessary, potassium replacement can be given intravenously in doses that should not exceed 10 mEq/hr.

Hyperkalemia   Hyperkalemia is encountered infrequently in preoperative patients. It is usually associated with renal impairment but can also be seen in patients with adrenal insufficiency, with the use of potassium-sparing diuretics, and with marked tissue breakdown such as that occurring in patients with crush injuries, massive gastrointestinal bleeding, or hemolysis. The clinical manifestations are mainly cardiovascular. Marked hyperkalemia (potassium >7 mEq/l) can result in bradycardia, ventricular fibrillation, and cardiac arrest. The treatment chosen depends on the severity of the hyperkalemia and whether there are associated cardiac abnormalities as seen with electrocardiography. Calcium gluconate (10 ml of a 10% solution) given intravenously can offset the toxic effects of hyperkalemia on the heart. One ampule each of sodium bicarbonate and D50, with or without insulin, will cause a rapid shift of potassium into cells. Longer-term, cation exchange resins such as Kay exalate, taken either orally or by enema, will bind and decrease total body potassium. Hemodialysis is reserved for emergent conditions in which other measures are not sufficient or have failed.

Postoperative Fluid and Electrolyte Management

Several hormonal and physiologic alterations in the postoperative period may complicate fluid and electrolyte management. The stress of surgery induces an inappropriately high level of circulating ADH. Circulating aldosterone levels are also increased, especially if sustained episodes of hypotension have occurred either intraoperatively or postoperatively. The elevated levels of circulating ADH and aldosterone make the postoperative patient prone to sodium and water retention.

Total body fluid volume may be altered significantly postoperatively. First, 1 ml of free water is released for each gram of fat or tissue that is catabolized and, in the postoperative period, several hundred milliliters of free water is released daily from tissue breakdown, particularly in the patient who has undergone extensive intra-abdominal dissection and who is restricted from ingesting food and fluids by mouth. This free water is often retained, in response to the altered levels of ADH and aldosterone. Second, fluid retention is further enhanced by "third spacing" or sequestration of fluid in the surgical field. The development of an ileus may result in an additional 1–3 l of fluid per day being sequestered in the bowel lumen, bowel wall, and peritoneal cavity.

In contrast to renal sodium homeostasis, the kidney lacks the capacity for retention of potassium. In the postoperative period, the kidneys will continue to excrete a minimum of 30–60 mEq/l of potassium daily, irrespective of the serum potassium level and total body potassium stores (25). If this potassium loss is not replaced, hypokalemia may develop. Tissue damage and catabolism during the first postoperative day usually result in the release of sufficient intracellular potassium to meet the daily requirements. However, beyond the first postoperative day, potassium supplementation is necessary.

Correct maintenance of fluid and electrolyte balance in the postoperative period starts with the preoperative assessment, with emphasis on establishing normal fluid and electrolyte parameters prior to surgery. Postoperatively, close monitoring of daily weight, urine output, serum hematocrit, serum electrolytes, and hemodynamic parameters will yield the necessary information to make correct adjustments in crystalloid replacement. The normal daily fluid and electrolyte requirements must be met, and any unusual fluid and electrolyte losses, such as from the gastrointestinal tract, lungs, or skin, must be replaced. After the first few postoperative days, third-space fluid begins to mobilize back into the intravascular space and ADH and aldosterone levels revert to normal. The excess fluid retained perioperatively is thus mobilized and excreted through the kidneys, and exogenous fluid requirements decrease. The patient with inadequate cardiovascular or renal reserve is prone to fluid overload during this time of third-space reabsorption, especially if intravenous fluids are not appropriately reduced.

The most common fluid and electrolyte disorder in the postoperative period is fluid overload. The fluid excess can occur concomitant with normal or decreased serum sodium. Large amounts of isotonic fluids are usually infused intraoperatively and postoperatively to maintain blood pressure and urine output. Because the infused fluid is often isotonic with plasma, it will remain in the extracellular space. Under such conditions, serum sodium will remain within normal levels. Fluid excess with hypotonicity (decreased serum sodium) can occur if large amounts of isotonic fluid losses (e.g., blood and gastrointestinal tract) are inappropriately replaced with hypotonic fluids. Again, the predisposition toward retention of free water in the immediate postoperative period compounds the problem. An increase in body weight occurs concomitant with the fluid expansion. In the patient who is not allowed anything by mouth, catabolism should induce a daily weight loss as great as 300 g/day. Clearly, the patient who is gaining weight in excess of 150 g/day is in a state of fluid expansion. Simple fluid restriction will correct the abnormality. When necessary, diuretics can be used to increase urinary water excretion.

States of fluid dehydration are uncommon but will occur in patients who have large daily fluid losses that are not replaced. Gastrointestinal losses should be replaced with the appropriate fluids. Patients with high fevers should be given appropriate free water replacement, because up to 2 l/day of free water can be lost through perspiration and hyperventilation. Although these increased losses are difficult to monitor, a reliable estimate can be obtained by monitoring body weight.

Postoperative Acid-Base Disorders

A variety of metabolic, respiratory, and electrolyte abnormalities in the postoperative period can result in an imbalance in normal acid-base homeostasis, leading to alkalosis or acidosis. Changes in the respiratory rate will directly affect the amount of carbon dioxide that is exhaled. Respiratory acidosis will result from carbon dioxide retention in patients who have hypoventilation from central nervous system depression, which can occur under conditions of oversedation from narcotics, particularly in the presence of concurrent severe chronic obstructive pulmonary disease. Respiratory alkalosis will result from hyperventilation caused by excitation of the central nervous system from drugs, pain, or excess ventilator support. Numerous metabolic derangements can result in alkalosis or acidosis, and these are discussed further in this section. Proper fluid and electrolyte replacement as well as maintenance of adequate tissue perfusion will help prevent most acid-base disorders that occur in the postoperative period.

555

Alkalosis   The most common acid-base disorder encountered in the postoperative period is alkalosis (25). Alkalosis is usually of no clinical significance and resolves spontaneously. Several etiologic factors may include hyperventilation associated with pain; posttraumatic transient hyperaldosteronism, which results in decreased renal bicarbonate excretion; nasogastric suction, which removes hydrogen ions; infusion of bicarbonate during blood transfusions in the form of citrate, which is converted to bicarbonates; administration of exogenous alkali; and use of diuretics. Alkalosis can usually be easily corrected with removal of the inciting cause, as well as with correction of extracellular fluid and potassium deficits (Table 19.1). Full correction can usually be safely achieved over 1–2 days.

Marked alkalosis, with serum pH higher than 7.55, can result in serious cardiac arrhythmias or central nervous system seizures. Myocardial excitability will be particularly pronounced with concurrent hypokalemia. Under such conditions, fluid and electrolyte replacement may not be sufficient to correct the alkalosis rapidly. *Acetazolamide* (250–500 mg), orally or intravenously, can be given 2–4 times daily to induce renal bicarbonate diuresis. Treatment with an acidifying agent is rarely necessary and should be reserved for acutely symptomatic patients (i.e., those with cardiac or central nervous system dysfunction) or for patients with advanced renal disease. Under such conditions, HCl (5–10 mEq/hr of a 100-mmol solution) can be given via a central intravenous line. *Ammonium chloride* can also be given orally or intravenously but should not be given to patients with hepatic disease.

Acidosis   Metabolic acidosis is less common than alkalosis in the postoperative period, but acidosis can potentially be serious because of its effect on the cardiovascular system. Under conditions of acidosis, there are decreased myocardial contractility, a propensity for vasodilation of the peripheral vasculature leading to hypotension, and refractoriness of the fibrillating heart to defibrillation (25). These effects promote decompensation of the cardiovascular system and can hinder attempts at resuscitation.

Metabolic acidosis results from a decrease in serum bicarbonate levels caused by the consumption and replacement of bicarbonate by circulating acids or the replacement by other anions such as chloride. The proper workup includes a measurement of the anion gap:

$$\text{Anion gap} = [Na^+ + K^+] - [Cl^- + HCO_3^-] = 10\text{–}14 \text{ mEq/l (normal)}$$

The anion gap is composed of circulating protein, sulfate, phosphate, citrate, and lactate (26).

With metabolic acidosis, the anion gap can be increased or normal. An increase in circulating acids will consume and replace bicarbonate ion, thus increasing the anion gap. The causes include an increase in circulating lactic acid secondary to anaerobic glycolysis, such

Table 19.1   Causes of Metabolic Alkalosis

Disorder	*Source of Alkali*	*Cause of Renal HCO Retention*
Gastric alkalosis Nasogastric suction Vomiting	Gastric mucosa	↓ECF, ↓K
Renal alkalosis Diuretics	Renal epithelium	↓ECF, ↓K
Respiratory acidosis and diuretics		↓ECF, ↓K, ↑PCO₂
Exogenous base	NaHCO₃, Na citrate, Na lactate	Coexisting disorder of ECF, K, PaCO₂

↓ECF, extracellular fluid depletion; ↓K, potassium depletion; ↑PCO₂, carbon dioxide retention.

as that seen under conditions of poor tissue perfusion; increased ketoacids, as with cases of severe diabetes or starvation; exogenous toxins; and renal dysfunction, which leads to increased circulating sulfates and phosphates (27). The diagnosis can be established via a thorough history and measurement of serum lactate (normal <2 mmol/l), serum glucose, and renal function parameters. Metabolic acidosis in the face of a normal anion gap is usually the result of an imbalance of the ions chloride and bicarbonate, which occurs under conditions leading to excess chloride and decreased bicarbonate. Hyperchloremic acidosis can be seen in patients who have undergone saline loading. Bicarbonate loss will be seen in patients with small bowel fistula, new ileostomies, severe diarrhea, or renal tubular acidosis. Finally, in patients with marked extracellular volume expansion, which often occurs postoperatively, the relative decrease in serum sodium and bicarbonate will result in a mild acidosis. A summary of the various causes of metabolic acidosis is shown in Table 19.2.

The treatment of metabolic acidosis depends on the cause. In patients with lactic acidosis, restoration of tissue perfusion is imperative. This can be accomplished through cardiovascular and pulmonary support as needed, oxygen therapy, and aggressive treatment of systemic infection wherever appropriate. Ketosis from diabetes can be corrected gradually with insulin therapy. Ketosis resulting from chronic starvation or from lack of caloric support postoperatively can be corrected with nutrition. In patients with normal anion gap acidosis, bicarbonate losses from the gastrointestinal tract should be replaced, excess chloride administration can be curtailed, and where necessary, a loop diuretic can be used to induce renal clearance of chloride. Dilutional acidosis can be corrected with mild fluid restriction.

Bicarbonates should not be given unless serum pH is lower than 7.2 or severe cardiac complications secondary to acidosis. Furthermore, close monitoring of serum potassium levels is mandatory. Under states of acidosis, potassium will exit the cell and enter the circulation. The patient with a normal potassium concentration and metabolic acidosis is actually intracellularly potassium depleted. Treatment of the acidosis without potassium replacement will result in severe hypokalemia with its associated risks. A summary of the various acid-base abnormalities and associated therapies is shown in Table 19.3.

Perioperative Pain Management

Although satisfactory analgesia is easily achievable with currently available methods, patients continue to suffer unnecessarily from postoperative pain. Studies have consistently shown that 30–40% of patients suffer moderate to severe pain in the postoperative period (28). There are several reasons for the existing inadequacies in pain management. First, patient expectations of pain relief are low and they are not aware of the extent of analgesia that they should expect. In a study of the perceptions of pain relief after surgery, 86% of patients had moderate to severe pain after surgery, but 70% felt that the pain was as severe as they had expected (29). In a similar study, more than 80% of patients were satisfied with their postoperative analgesia, but most patients reported significant pain (30). Second,

Table 19.2   Causes of Metabolic Acidosis

	Normal Anion Gap	
High Anion Gap	*Hyperkalemic*	*Hypokalemic*
Uremia	Hyporeninism	Diarrhea
Ketoacidosis	Primary adrenal failure	Renal tubular acidosis
Lactic acidosis	NH_2Cl	Ileal and sigmoid bladders
Aspirin	Sulfur poisoning	Hyperalimentation
Paraldehyde	Early chronic renal failure	
Methanol	Obstructive uropathy	
Ethylene glycol		
Methyl malonic aciduria		

From **Narins RG, Lazarus MJ.:** Renal system. In: **Vandam LD.** ed. *To Make the Patient Ready for Anesthesia: Medical Care of the Surgical Patient.* 2nd ed. Menlo Park, CA: Addison-Wesley Publishing Co., 1984:67–114.

Table 19.3   Acid-Base Disorders and Their Treatment

Primary Disorder	Defect	Common Causes	Compensation	Treatment
Respiratory acidosis	Carbon dioxide (hypoventilation)	Central nervous system depression Airway and lung impairment	Renal excretion of acid salts Bicarbonate retention Chloride shift into red cells	Restoration ventilation Control of excess dioxide production
Respiratory alkalosis	Hyperventilation	Central nervous excitation system Excess ventilator support	Renal excretion of sodium, potassium bicarbonate Absorption of hydrogen and chloride ions Lactate release from red cells	Correction hyperventilation
Metabolic acidosis	Excess loss of base Increased nonvolatile acids	Excess chloride versus sodium Increased bicarbonate loss Lactic, ketoacidosis Uremia Dilutation acidosis	Respiratory alkalosis Renal excretion of hydrogen and chloride ions Resorption of potassium bicarbonate	Increase sodium load Waste Give bicarbonate for pH <7.2 Restore buffers, protein, hemoglobin
Metabolic acidosis	Excess loss of chloride and potassium Increased bicarbonate	Gastrointestinal losses of chloride Excess intake of bicarbonate Diuretics Hypokalemia Extracellular fluid volume contraction	Respiratory acidosis May be hypoxia Renal excretion of bicarbonate and potassium Absorption of hydrogen and chloride ions	Increased chloride content Potassium replacement Acetazolamide (Diamox) to waste bicarbonate Vigorous volume replacement Occasional 0.1 N HCl as needed

there is a lack of formal physician training in pain management. This lack is epitomized by the commonly written order prescribing a range of narcotic to be given intramuscularly every 3–4 hours as needed, leaving pain management decisions to the nursing staff, with no attempt to titrate the dose of the prescribed narcotic commensurate with individual patient requirements (31). Third, attitudes continue to be influenced by the common misconception that the use of narcotics in the postoperative period can result in opioid dependence. In one review, 20% of nurses responding to a staff questionnaire expressed concern that use of opioid analgesics in the postoperative period could cause addiction (29). Studies have confirmed that nurses will administer less than one-quarter of the total dose of narcotic that is prescribed on an "as-needed" basis (30, 32).

The *minimum effective analgesic concentration (MEAC)* **refers to the serum concentration of a drug below which very little analgesia is achieved** (28). At the MEAC, receptor and plasma concentrations of a drug are in equilibrium (33). Steady-state drug concentrations above the MEAC are difficult to achieve with intramuscular depot injection. In one study, patients receiving intramuscular injections with meperidine hydrochloride *(Demerol)* every 4 hours, experienced marked intra- and interpatient variations in narcotic drug peak concentrations as well as in the time required to reach these peaks. As a result, serum concentrations of drug were above the MEAC an average of only 35% of each 4-hour dosing interval. Variable pain control following intermittent intramuscular injections was the result of inadequate, highly variable, and unpredictable blood concentrations (34). Adequate analgesia can be achieved through intramuscular or subcutaneous modes of administration, but unpredictable absorption can make titration difficult. Small intravenous boluses can be more easily titrated but may be shorter acting, requiring more frequent injections and thus intensive nursing care, whereas larger intravenous boluses may be associated with a higher incidence of central nervous system and respiratory depression. The *patient-controlled analgesia (PCA) technique,* which allows patients to self-administer small doses of narcotic on demand, allows titration of measured boluses of narcotic as needed to relieve pain and can provide a more thorough analgesia with maintenance of steady-state drug concentrations above the MEAC.

Irrespective of the route of administration, analgesics must be front-loaded in order to provide prompt analgesia from the start. Without front-loading, attainment of the MEAC will not occur for at least three elimination half-lives of the narcotic agent that is used. After front-loading, additional small boluses of narcotic can be administered until analgesia is achieved. From the total dose of drug required to achieve analgesia, maintenance drug dosages can then be determined and administered either as a continuous infusion or on a scheduled basis so that the dose of drug administered offsets the amount that is cleared (Table 19.4). Thereafter, prescribed doses of narcotic can be further adjusted as needed.

Patient-Controlled Analgesia

Patient-controlled analgesia (PCA) devices are electronically controlled infusion pumps that deliver a preset dose of narcotic into a patient's indwelling intravenous catheter upon patient request (35–37). The devices all contain delay intervals or lockout times during

Table 19.4   Guidelines for Front-Loading IV Analgesics* for Relief of Perioperative Pain

Drug	Total Front-Loaded Dose	Increments	Cautions
Morphine	0.08–0.12 mg/kg	0.03 mg/kg q 10 h	Histaminergic effects; nausea; biliary colic; reduce dose for elderly
Meperidine	1.0–1.5 mg/kg	0.30 mg/kg/q 10 h	Reduce dose or change drug for impaired renal function
Codeine	0.5–1.0 mg/kg	1/3 total q 15 h	Nausea
Methadone	0.08–0.12 mg/kg	0.03 mg/kg q 15 h	Do not administer maintenance dose after analgesia
Levorphanol	10.02 mg/kg	50–75 ug/kg q 15 h	Similar to methadone
Hydromorphone sulfate	0.02 mg/kg	25–50 ug/kg q 10 h	Similar to morphine
Pentazocine	0.5–1.0 mg/kg	1/2 total q 15 h	Psychomimetic effects; may cause withdrawal in narcotic-dependent patients
Nalbuphine	0.08–0.15 mg/kg	0.03 mg/kg q 10 h	Less psychomimetic effect than pentazocine; sedation
Butorphanol	0.01–0.04 mg/kg	0.01 mg/kg q 10 h	Sedation; psychomimetic effects like nalbuphine
Buprenorphine	Up to 0.2 mg/kg	1/4 total q 10 h	Long-acting like methadone, levorphanol; may precipitate withdrawal in narcotic-dependent patients; safe to give subcutaneous maintenance after analgesia—different from methadone

*A scheme for front-loading the opioids most commonly used in postoperative pain treatment.

559

which patient demands for more narcotic are not met. These devices eliminate the delay between the onset of pain and the administration of analgesic agents, a common problem on busy hospital wards inherent with on-demand analgesic orders. Patient-controlled analgesia has enjoyed excellent patient acceptance. Compared with conventional intramuscular injections, serum narcotic levels have significantly lower variability in patients using PCA (38). Patients have been shown to have improved analgesia (38, 39, 49), a lower incidence of postoperative pulmonary complications (38, 39), and less confusion (38). Furthermore, the total dose of narcotic used has been lower with PCA than with conventional intramuscular depot injection (39, 41, 43).

Carefully supervised regimens using continuous infusions (42), on-demand intramuscular therapy (44, 45), or fixed dosage schedules (every-4-hour dosing) with on-demand supplementation (46) can have analgesic efficacy comparable with PCA. Nonetheless, the type of close supervision required to achieve adequate on-demand analgesia without PCA is difficult to achieve. Continuous infusion regimens eliminate the delay inherent to on-demand regimens but have been associated with an increased risk of oversedation and apnea (33, 47). Use of PCA shortens the time between the onset of pain and the administration of pain medication, provides more continuous access to analgesics, and allows for an overall steadier state of pain control.

Intraspinal Analgesia

Intraspinal anesthetics and narcotics administered either in the epidural space or intrathecally are among the most potent analgesic agents available; the efficacy of these agents is greater than that provided by intravenous PCA techniques (48). These drugs can be administered in one of several ways, including a single-shot dose given by epidural or intrathecal injection, intermittent injection given either on schedule or on demand, and continuous infusions (28).

Because of the risk of central nervous system infections and headaches, intrathecal administration is usually limited to a single dose (49). Duration of action for a single dose is increased via the intrathecal route as compared with epidural administration as a result of the high concentrations of drug attained in the cerebrospinal fluid. However, the risk of central nervous system and respiratory depression, as well as systemic hypotension, is also increased. Even low doses of intrathecal morphine have been associated with a high risk of complications. Therefore, some investigators have warned against the use of intrathecal spinal analgesia outside the intensive care setting (50).

Epidural administration is the preferred approach and provides extended (>24 hours) pain control in the postoperative period. Relative contraindications are the presence of coagulopathy, sepsis, and hypotension. Both anesthetic and narcotic agents have been used with excellent efficacy. Among the anesthetic agents, *bupivacaine* has been the most popular, providing excellent analgesia with no motor blockade and minimal toxicity (49). Epidural analgesia is best suited for pain control in the lower abdomen and extremities. One potential adverse effect is that of sympathetic blockade, precluding the use of this method for attainment of high blocks. Other adverse effects include urinary retention and hypotension, as well as central nervous system and cardiac depression. In contrast to anesthetic agents, opioids offer excellent analgesia without accompanying sympathetic blockade. Epidural opioids tend to have a much longer duration of action, and hypotension is a rare complication. Compared with epidural anesthetics, however, there is a higher incidence of nausea and vomiting, respiratory depression, and pruritus (50). Initial studies of the use of epidural *clonidine* have shown encouraging results. In one study, epidural *clonidine* (1 μg/kg) plus *sufentanil* (25 μg) afforded greater pain relief than the use of *sufentanil* (50 μg) alone (51).

Compared with analgesics administered intramuscularly or intravenously, epidural analgesia has been shown to be associated with improved pulmonary function postoperatively, a lower incidence of postoperative pulmonary complications, a decrease in postoperative venous thromboembolic complications (most likely secondary to earlier ambulation), fewer adverse gastrointestinal side effects, a lower incidence of central nervous system depression, and shorter convalescence. Severe respiratory depression is the most serious potential complication, seen in fewer than 1% of patients. A lower incidence of respiratory depression is seen with the more lipophilic drugs such as *fentanyl,* which is quickly absorbed within the spinal cord and is therefore less likely to diffuse to the central nervous system respiratory control centers. Pruritus, nausea, and urinary retention are common but can be easily managed and are usually of little clinical significance (49). Cost is perhaps the main and most limiting drawback of epidural analgesia.

Close monitoring by nursing staff is required for safe administration of epidural analgesia. However, an intensive care setting is not necessary. Epidural analgesics can be administered safely in a hospital ward setting under close nursing supervision using respiratory monitoring with hourly ventilatory checks during the first 8 hours of epidural analgesia (28).

Nonsteroidal Anti-Inflammatory Drugs (NSAIDs)

The nonsteroidal anti-inflammatory agent *ketorolac* is a safe and potent drug that can ameliorate postoperative pain to a degree comparable to that of *morphine* and other commonly prescribed opiates, and it is less costly (52). NSAIDs are becoming increasingly popular for the treatment of pain in the postoperative setting for patients undergoing major and minor surgical procedures. *Ketorolac* has a slightly slower onset of activity than *fentanyl* (53) but has an analgesic potency comparable to *morphine* (54). The advantages of NSAIDs over opioids include absence of respiratory depression, lack of abuse potential, decreased sedative effects, decreased nausea, early return of bowel function, and faster recovery (53–58). Because of these advantages, many advocate NSAIDs over opioids for perioperative pain management.

Potential adverse effects associated with the use of NSAIDs include an increased risk of renal ischemia (particularly in patients suffering from acute hypovolemia) as well as medical diseases including atherosclerotic heart disease, congestive heart failure, cirrhosis, renal insufficiency, diabetes, and concurrent diuretic therapy. Although NSAIDs cause a modest increase in bleeding time, this does not appear to be clinically significant. Controlled perspective studies have not demonstrated a significant increase in blood loss in patients who receive NSAIDs perioperatively (56). These agents should be used with extreme care, if at all, in patients with asthma because 5–10% of adult patients with asthma are sensitive to *aspirin* and other NSAID preparations. *Ketorolac* is active when administered both intravenously and orally, making it easy to administer in the perioperative setting for patients undergoing minor procedures.

Antibiotic Prophylaxis

Gynecologic operations that carry a significant risk of postoperative infection include vaginal hysterectomy, abdominal hysterectomy, surgical treatment of pelvic abscess or inflammation, selected cases of pregnancy termination, and radical surgery for gynecologic cancers. Most other gynecologic procedures are considered "clean" and have a low risk (<5%) of postoperative wound infection (59). Included in these are procedures confined to the abdomen, Retzius' space, perineum, and vagina.

Pathogens that can contaminate during gynecologic surgery are organisms indigenous to the vaginal tract, including Gram-positive and Gram-negative aerobes and anaerobes (Table 19.5). The primary pathogenic bacteria include the coliforms, streptococci, fusobacteria, and bacteroides.

The following are proposed guidelines for antibiotic prophylaxis in gynecologic procedures (60):

1. The procedure should carry a significant risk of postoperative infection.

2. The surgery should involve considerable bacterial contamination.

561

Table 19.5   Bacteria Indigenous to the Lower Genital Tract

Lactobacillus	Enterobacter agglomerans
Diphtheroids	Klebsiella pneumoniae
Staphylococcus aureus	Proteus mirabilis
Staphylococcus epidermidis	Proteus vulgaris
Streptococcus agalactiae	Morganella morganii
Streptococcus faecalis	Citrobacter diversus
Alpha-hemolytic streptococci	
Group D streptococci	Bacteroides species
Peptostreptococci	B. bivius
Peptococcus	B. disiens
Clostridium	B. fragilis
Gaffky ancerobia	B. melaninogenicus
Escherichia coli	
Fusobacterium	
Enterobacter cloacae	

3. The antibiotic chosen for prophylaxis should be effective against most contaminating organisms.

4. The antibiotic should be present in the tissues at the time of contamination.

5. The shortest possible course of antibiotic prophylaxis should be given.

6. The prophylactic antibiotic chosen should not be one considered for treatment if a postoperative infection occurs.

7. The risk of complications from the prophylactic antibiotic should be low.

The existing literature uniformly supports the use of the prophylactic antibiotics for vaginal hysterectomy; however, the use of prophylactic antibiotics for patients who undergo abdominal hysterectomy is controversial. A review of the placebo-controlled trials in the literature regarding antibiotic prophylaxis in vaginal and abdominal hysterectomy included 48 studies of 5524 patients who underwent vaginal hysterectomy and 30 studies of 3752 patients who underwent abdominal hysterectomy (61). In vaginal hysterectomy, prophylactic antibiotics decreased febrile morbidity from 40% in control patients to 15% in treated patients and lowered the pelvic infection rate from 25% in control patients to 5% in treated patients. The benefits of antibiotic prophylaxis were less pronounced with abdominal hysterectomy; antibiotic prophylaxis reduced febrile morbidity from 28% in control patients to 16% in treated patients, pelvic infections from 10% to 5%, and wound infections from 8% to 3%. **Therefore, antibiotic prophylaxis should be used in all patients who undergo vaginal hysterectomy as well as in selected high-risk patients who undergo abdominal hysterectomy.** Factors that have been identified as placing patients at high risk for posthysterectomy infection have included low socioeconomic status, duration of surgery longer than 2 hours, presence of malignancy, and increased number of surgical procedures performed. Obesity, menopausal status, and estimated blood loss have not been shown to be risk factors for postoperative infection when evaluated by multivariate analysis (62, 63).

The antibiotic chosen for prophylaxis for gynecologic surgery should have activity against the broad range of vaginal organisms. The first- and second-generation cephalosporins are well suited for this purpose because of their activity against Gram-positive, Gram-negative, and anaerobic organisms. Most classes of antibiotics (including *penicillin, tetracycline, sulfonamide,* broad-spectrum *penicillin,* and cephalosporins) and anaerobic drugs (*clindamycin/metronidazole*) have been shown to be as effective as prophylactic antibiotics, but none has been demonstrated to be consistently more effective than first-generation cephalosporins (67–70).

The timing of administration of the prophylactic antibiotic agent is important. Antibiotics given for prophylaxis are most active if present in tissues prior to contamination with an inoculum of bacteria (71). For patients who undergo hysterectomy, the antibiotic should be present in the tissues prior to the opening of the vaginal cuff, at which time vaginal organisms gain access to the pelvic cavity. Infusion of an antibiotic within 30 minutes of surgery is ideal for this purpose. For long surgical procedures, particularly when there is a large blood loss or when an antibiotic agent with short half-life is used, a second antibiotic dose should be given intraoperatively.

Many prospective studies have documented that short courses of prophylactic antibiotics (24 hours or shorter) are as efficacious as longer ones. Moreover, several clinical trials have found that one perioperative dose of prophylactic antibiotic is sufficient (67, 68, 72–75). The use of one dose of prophylactic antibiotic has many advantages, including decreased cost, decreased toxicity, minimal alteration of host flora, and decreased induction of resistant pathogens.

Despite the advantages of using prophylactic antibiotics, the importance of good surgical technique must be emphasized—delicate handling of tissues, good hemostasis, adequate drainage, and avoidance of unnecessarily large pedicles of tissue in ligatures.

Postoperative Surgical Infections

Infections are a major source of morbidity in the postoperative period. Risk factors for infectious morbidity include a lack of perioperative antibiotic prophylaxis, contamination of the surgical field from infected tissues or from spillage of large bowel contents, an immunocompromised host, poor nutrition, chronic and debilitating severe illness, poor surgical technique, and preexisting focal or systemic infection. Sources of postoperative infection can include the lung, urinary tract, surgical site, pelvic side wall, vaginal cuff, abdominal wound, and sites of indwelling intravenous catheters. Early identification and treatment of any infections will result in the best outcome from these potentially serious complications.

Although infectious morbidity is an inevitable complication of surgery, the incidence of infections can be decreased by the appropriate use of simple preventive measures. In cases that involve transection of the large bowel, spillage of fecal contents also inevitably occurs. A thorough preoperative mechanical and antibiotic bowel preparation in combination with systemic antibiotic prophylaxis will help decrease the incidence of postoperative pelvic and abdominal infections in these patients. The surgeon can further decrease the risk of postoperative infections by using meticulous surgical technique. Blood and necrotic tissue are excellent media for the growth of aerobic and anaerobic organisms. In cases in which there is higher-than-usual potential for serum and blood to collect in spaces that have been contaminated by bacterial spill, closed-suction drainage may reduce the risk of infection. Antibiotic therapy, rather than prophylaxis, should be initiated at surgery in patients who have frank intra-abdominal infection or pus.

Elective surgical procedures should be postponed in patients who have an infection preoperatively. In an epidemiologic study conducted by the Centers for Disease Control and Prevention, the incidence of nosocomial surgical infections ranged from 4.3% in community hospitals to 7% in municipal hospitals (76). Urinary tract infections accounted for approximately 40% of these nosocomial infections. Infections of the skin and wound accounted for approximately one-third of the infections, and respiratory tract infections accounted for approximately 16%. In patients who had any type of infection prior to surgery, the risk of infection at the surgical wound site was increased fourfold. Rates of infection were higher in older patients, in patients with increased length of surgery, and in those with increased length of hospital stay prior to surgery. The relative risk was three times higher in patients with a community-acquired infection prior to surgery. These community-acquired infections included infections of the urinary and respiratory tract.

The standard definition of febrile morbidity for surgical patients has been the presence of a temperature higher than or equal to 100.4°F (38°C) on two occasions at least

4 hours apart in the postoperative period, excluding the first 24 hours. Febrile morbidity has been estimated to occur in as many as one-half of patients. It often occurs within the first 2 postoperative days and is self-limited, resolving without therapy (78). Although fever is a sign of infection, the diagnosis of infection is based on the combination of fever and clinical and laboratory evidence of an infected focus.

The assessment of febrile surgical patients should include a review of the patient's history with regard to risk factors. Both the history and the physical examination should focus on the potential sites of infection (Table 19.6). The examination should include inspection of the pharynx, a thorough pulmonary examination, palpation of the kidneys and the costovertebral angles for tenderness, inspection and palpation of the abdominal incision, examination of sites of intravenous catheters, and an examination of the extremities for evidence of deep venous thrombosis or thrombophlebitis. In gynecologic patients, appropriate workup may also include inspection and palpation of the vaginal cuff for signs of induration, tenderness, or purulent drainage. A pelvic examination should also be performed in order to identify a mass consistent with a pelvic hematoma or abscess and to look for signs of pelvic cellulitis.

The laboratory and radiologic evaluation may include complete and differential white blood cell counts, a catheterized urinalysis and culture, and a chest x-ray for patients with signs and symptoms localizing to the lung. Blood cultures can also be obtained but will most likely be of little yield unless the patient has a high fever ($>102°F$). In patients with costovertebral angle tenderness, IVP may be indicated to rule out the presence of ureteral damage or obstruction from surgery, particularly in the absence of laboratory evidence of urinary tract infection. Patients who have persistent fevers without a clear localizing source should undergo CT scanning of the abdomen and pelvis to rule out the presence of an intra-abdominal abscess. Finally, in patients who have had gastrointestinal surgery, a barium enema or upper gastrointestinal series with small bowel follow-through may be indicated late in the course of the first postoperative week if fever persists to rule out an anastomotic leak or fistula.

Urinary Tract Infections

Historically, the urinary tract has been the most common site of infection in surgical patients (76). However, the incidence reported in the more recent gynecologic literature has been less than 4% (78, 79). This decrease in urinary tract infections is most likely the result of increased perioperative use of prophylactic antibiotics. The incidence of postoperative urinary tract infection in gynecologic surgical patients not receiving prophylactic antibiotics has been confirmed to be as high as 40% (80), and even a single dose of

Table 19.6   Posthysterectomy Infections

Operative Site	Nonoperative Site
Vaginal cuff	Urinary tract
Pelvic cellulitis	Asymptomatic bacteriuria
pelvic abscess	Cystitis
Supervaginal, extraperitoneal	Pyelonephritis
Intraperitoneal	Respiratory
Adnexa	Atelectasis
Cellulitis	Pneumonia
Abscess	Vascular
Abdominal incision	Phlebitis
Cellulitis	Septic pelvic thrombophlebitis
Simple	
Progressive bacterial synergistic	
Necrotizing fasciitis	
Myonecrosis	

perioperative prophylactic antibiotic has been shown to decrease the incidence of postoperative urinary tract infection from 35% to 4% (81).

Symptoms of a urinary tract infection may include urinary frequency, urgency, and dysuria. In patients with pyelonephritis, other symptoms include headache, malaise, nausea, and vomiting. A urinary tract infection is diagnosed on the basis of microbiology and has been defined as the growth of $>10^5$ organisms/ml urine cultured. Most infections are caused by coliform bacteria, with *Escherichia coli* being the most frequent pathogen. Other pathogens include *Klebsiella, Proteus,* and *Enterobacter* species. *Staphylococcus* organisms are the causative bacteria in fewer than 10% of cases.

Despite the high incidence of urinary tract infections in the postoperative period, few of these infections are serious. Most are confined to the lower urinary tract. Pyelonephritis is a rare complication (82). Catheterization of the urinary tract, either intermittently or continuously with the use of an indwelling catheter, has been implicated as a main cause of urinary tract contamination (83). In fact, more than 1 million catheter-associated urinary tract infections occur yearly in the U.S., and catheter-associated bacteria remains the most common etiology of Gram-negative bacteremia in hospitalized patients. Bacteria adhere to the surface of urinary catheters and grow within bile films, which appear to protect embedded bacteria from antibiotics, making treatment less effective. Therefore, the use of urinary tract catheters should be minimized. An indwelling catheter should be either removed or replaced in patients undergoing treatment for catheter-related infections.

The treatment of urinary tract infection includes hydration and antibiotic therapy. Commonly prescribed and effective antibiotics include *penicillin, sulfonamide, cephalosporins, fluoroquinolones,* and *nitrofurantoin*. The choice of antibiotic should be based on knowledge of the susceptibility of organisms cultured at a particular institution. In some institutions, for example, more than 40% of *Escherichia coli* strains are resistant to *ampicillin*. For uncomplicated urinary tract infections, an antibiotic that has good activity against *E. coli* should be given in the interim while awaiting the urine culture and sensitivity data. Patients who have a history of recurrent urinary tract infections, those with chronic indwelling catheters (Foley catheters or ureteral stents), and those who have urinary conduits should be treated with antibiotics that will be effective against the less common urinary pathogens such as *Klebsiella* and *Pseudomonas*. Chronic use of the *fluoroquinolones* for prophylaxis is not advised, because these agents are notorious for inducing antibiotic-resistant strains of bacteria.

Pulmonary Infections

The respiratory tract is an uncommon site for infectious complications in gynecologic surgical patients. Hemsell noted only six cases of pneumonia in more than 4000 women who underwent elective hysterectomy (78). This low incidence is probably a reflection of the young age and good health status of gynecologic patients in general. In acute care facilities, pneumonia is a frequent hospital-acquired infection, particularly in elderly patients (84). Risk factors include extensive or prolonged atelectasis, preexistent chronic obstructive pulmonary disease, severe or debilitating illness, central neurologic disease causing an inability to clear oropharyngeal secretions effectively, and nasogastric suction (84). In surgical patients, early ambulation and aggressive management of atelectasis are the most important preventive measures. The role of prophylactic antibiotics remains unclear.

A significant proportion (40–50%) of hospital-acquired pneumonias are caused by Gram-negative organisms. These organisms gain access to the respiratory tract from the oral pharynx. Gram-negative colonization of the oral pharynx has been shown to be increased in patients in acute care facilities and has been associated with the presence of nasogastric tubes, preexisting respiratory disease, mechanical ventilation, tracheal intubation, and paralytic ileus, which is associated with microbial overgrowth in the stomach (85). Interestingly, the use of antimicrobial drugs seems to significantly increase the frequency of colonization of the oral pharynx with Gram-negative bacteria.

A thorough lung examination should be included in the assessment of all febrile surgical patients. In the absence of significant lung findings, a chest x-ray is probably of little benefit in patients at low risk for postoperative pulmonary complications. In patients with pulmonary findings or with risk factors for pulmonary complications, a chest x-ray should be obtained. A sputum sample should also be obtained for Gram stain and culture. The treatment should include postural drainage, aggressive pulmonary toilet, and antibiotics. The antibiotic chosen should be effective against both Gram-positive and Gram-negative organisms, and in patients who are receiving assisted ventilation, the antibiotic spectrum should include drugs that are active against *Pseudomonas* organisms.

Phlebitis

Intravenous catheter-related infections are common; the reported incidence is from 25 to 35% (86). The intravenous site should be inspected daily and the catheter should be removed if there is any associated pain, redness, or induration. Unfortunately, phlebitis can occur even with close surveillance of the intravenous site. In one study, more than 50% of the cases of phlebitis became evident more than 12 hours after discontinuation of intravenous catheters (87). In addition, fewer than one-third of patients had symptoms related to the intravenous catheter site 24 hours prior to the diagnosis of phlebitis.

Intravenous catheters should be inserted using sterile technique, and they should be changed frequently. The institution of intravenous therapy teams has decreased the incidence of phlebitis by as much as 50% (86). This decrease is related not so much to surveillance of the intravenous catheter site as it is to frequent changing of intravenous catheters. The incidence of catheter-related phlebitis increases significantly after 72 hours. Therefore, intravenous catheters should be changed at least every 3 days.

The diagnosis of phlebitis can be made based on the presence of fever, pain, redness, induration, or a palpable venous cord. Occasionally, suppuration will be present. Phlebitis is usually self-limited and resolves within 3–4 days. The treatment includes application of warm, moist compresses and prompt removal of any catheters from the infected vein. Antibiotic therapy with antistaphylococcal agents should be instituted for catheter-related sepsis. Excision or drainage of an infected vein is rarely necessary.

Wound Infections

The results of a prospective study of more than 62,000 wounds were revealing in regard to the epidemiology of wound infections (88). The wound infection rate varied markedly, depending on the extent of contamination of the surgical field. The wound infection rate for clean surgical cases (infection not present in the surgical field, no break in aseptic technique, no viscus entered) was lower than 2%, whereas the incidence of wound infections with dirty, infected cases was 40% or higher. Preoperative showers with *hexachlorophene* slightly lowered the infection rate for clean wounds, whereas preoperative shaving of the wound site with a razor increased the infection rate. A 5-minute wound preparation immediately before surgery was as effective as preparation 10 minutes before surgery. The wound infection rate increased with the duration of preoperative hospital stay as well as with the duration of surgery. In addition, incidental appendectomy increased the risk of wound infection in patients undergoing clean surgical procedures. The study concluded that the incidence of wound infections could be decreased by short preoperative hospital stays, hexachlorophene showers prior to surgery, minimizing shaving of the wound site, use of meticulous surgical technique, decreasing operative time as much as possible, bringing drains out through sites other than the wound, and dissemination of information to surgeons regarding their wound infection rates. A program instituting these conclusions led to a fall in the clean wound infection rate from 2.5 to 0.6% over an 8-year period. The wound infection rate in most gynecologic services has been lower than 5%, reflective of the "clean" nature of most gynecologic operations.

The symptoms of wound infection often occur late in the postoperative period, usually after the fourth postoperative day, and may include the presence of fever, erythema, tenderness, induration, and purulent drainage. The management is mostly mechanical and involves opening the infected portion of the wound above the fascia, with cleansing and debridement of the wound edges as necessary. Wound care, consisting of debridement and dressing changes 2–3 times daily with mesh gauze, will promote growth of granulation tissue, with gradual filling in of the wound defect by secondary intention. Packing wounds with dry rather than wet gauze provides better debridement of the wound edges upon its removal. Clean, granulating wounds can often be secondarily closed with good success, shortening the time required for complete wound healing.

The technique of delayed primary wound closure can be used in contaminated surgical cases to lower the incidence of wound infection. Briefly, this technique involves leaving the wound open above the fascia at the time of the initial surgical procedure. Vertical interrupted mattress sutures though the skin and subcutaneous layers are placed 3 cm apart but are not tied. Wound care is instituted immediately after surgery and continued until the wound is noted to be granulating well. Sutures may then be tied and the skin edges further approximated using staples. Using this technique of delayed primary wound closure, the overall wound infection rate has been shown to be decreased from 23 to 2.1% in high-risk patients (89).

Pelvic Cellulitis

Vaginal cuff cellulitis is present to some extent in most patients who have undergone hysterectomy. It is characterized by erythema, induration, and tenderness at the vaginal cuff. Occasionally, a purulent discharge from the apex of the vagina may also be present. The cellulitis is often self-limited and does not require any treatment. Fever, leukocytosis, and pain localized to the pelvis may accompany severe cuff cellulitis and most often signifies extension of the cellulitis to adjacent pelvic tissues. In such cases, broad-spectrum antibiotic therapy should be instituted with coverage for Gram-negative, Gram-positive, and anaerobic organisms. If purulence at the vaginal cuff is excessive or if there is a fluxuant or a mass noted at the vaginal cuff, the vaginal cuff should be gently probed and opened with a blunt instrument. The cuff can then be left open for dependent drainage or, alternatively, a drain can be placed into the lower pelvis through the cuff and removed when drainage, fever, and symptoms in the lower pelvic region have resolved.

Intra-abdominal and Pelvic Abscess

The development of an abscess in the surgical field or elsewhere in the abdominal cavity is an uncommon complication after a gynecologic surgery. It is most likely to occur in contaminated cases in which the surgical site is not adequately drained or as a secondary complication of hematomas. The causative pathogens in patients who have intra-abdominal abscess are usually polymicrobial in nature. The aerobes most commonly identified include *Escherichia coli, Klebsiella, Streptococcus, Proteus,* and *Enterobacter.* Anaerobic isolates are also common, usually from the *Bacteroides* group. These pathogens are mainly from the vaginal tract but also can be derived from the gastrointestinal tract, particularly when the colon has been entered at the time of surgery.

Intra-abdominal abscess is sometimes difficult to diagnose. The evolving clinical picture is often one of persistent febrile episodes with a rising white blood cell count. Findings on abdominal examination may be equivocal. If an abscess is located deep in the pelvis, it may be palpable by pelvic or rectal examination. For abscesses above the pelvis, diagnosis will depend on radiologic confirmation.

Ultrasound can occasionally delineate fluid collections in the upper abdomen as well as in the pelvis. However, bowel gas interference makes visualization of fluid collections or abscesses in the midabdomen difficult to distinguish. CT scanning is therefore much more sensitive and specific for diagnosing intra-abdominal abscesses and is often the radiologic procedure of choice. Occasionally, if conventional radiologic methods fail to identify an abscess and the index of suspicion for an abscess remains high, labeled leukocyte scanning may be useful for locating the infected focus.

Standard therapy for intra-abdominal abscess is surgical evacuation and drainage combined with appropriate parenteral administration of antibiotics. Abscesses located low in the pelvis, particularly in the area of the vaginal cuff, can often be reached through a vaginal approach. In many patients, the ability to drain an abscess by placement of a drain percutaneously under CT guidance has obviated the need for surgical exploration. With CT guidance, a pigtail catheter is placed into an abscess cavity and is left in place until drainage decreases. Gram stain and anaerobic and aerobic cultures should be obtained to guide antibiotic selection. The "gold standard" of initial antibiotic therapy has been the combination of *ampicillin, gentamicin,* and *clindamycin.* Adequate treatment can also be achieved with currently available broad-spectrum single agents (including the broad-spectrum *penicillin*), second- and third-generation cephalosporins, and the *sulbactam/clavulanic acid*-containing preparations (90–93).

Necrotizing Fasciitis

Necrotizing fasciitis is an uncommon infectious disorder; approximately 1000 cases occur annually in the U.S. (94). The disorder is characterized by a rapidly progressive bacterial infection involving the subcutaneous tissues and fascia while characteristically sparing underlying muscle. Systemic toxicity is a frequent feature of this disease, as manifest by the presence of dehydration, septic shock, disseminated intravascular coagulation, and multiorgan system failure.

The pathogenesis of necrotizing fasciitis involves a polymicrobial infection of the dermis and subcutaneous tissue. Hemolytic streptococcus was initially believed to be the primary pathogen responsible for the infection in necrotizing fasciitis (95). However, it is now evident that numerous other organisms are often cultured in addition to streptococcus, including other Gram-positive organisms, coliforms, and anaerobes (95–100). Bacterial enzymes such as hyaluronidase and lipase released in the subcutaneous space destroy the fascia and adipose tissue and induce a liquefactive necrosis. In addition, noninflammatory intravascular coagulation or thrombosis subsequently occurs. Intravascular coagulation results in ischemia and necrosis of the subcutaneous tissues and skin (96, 97). Late in the course of the infection, destruction of the superficial nerves produces anesthesia in the involved skin. The release of bacteria and bacterial toxins into the systemic circulation can cause septic shock, acid-base disturbances, and multiorgan impairment.

The diagnostic criteria for necrotizing fasciitis include extensive necrosis of the superficial fascia and subcutaneous tissue with peripheral undermining of the normal skin, a moderate to severe systemic toxic reaction, the absence of muscle involvement, the absence of *clostridia* in wound and blood culture, the absence of major vascular occlusion, intensive leukocytic infiltration, and necrosis of subcutaneous tissue (101).

Most patients with necrotizing fasciitis suffer pain, which in the early stages of the disease is often disproportionately greater than that expected from the degree of cellulitis present. Late in the course of the infection, the involved skin may actually be anesthetized secondary to necrosis of superficial nerves. Temperature abnormalities, both hyperthermia and hypothermia, are common concomitant with the release of bacterial toxins as well as with bacterial sepsis, which is present in up to 40% of patients (99). The involved skin is initially tender, erythematous, and warm. Edema develops and the erythema spreads diffusely, fading into normal skin, characteristically without distinct margins or induration. Subcutaneous microvascular thrombosis induces ischemia in the skin, which becomes cyanotic and blistered. Eventually, as necrosis develops, the skin becomes gangrenous and may slough spontaneously. Most patients will have leukocytosis and acid-base abnormalities. Finally, subcutaneous gas may develop, which can be identified by palpation and by x-ray. The finding of subcutaneous gas by x-ray is often indicative of clostridial infection, although it is not a specific finding and may be caused by other organisms. These organisms include *Enterobacter, Pseudomonas,* anaerobic streptococci, and *Bacteroides* (102), which, unlike clostridial infections, spare the muscles underlying the affected area. A tissue biopsy specimen for Gram stain and aerobic and anaerobic culture should be obtained from the necrotic center of the lesion in order to identify the etiologic organisms (97). Although necrotizing fasciitis is often diagnosed during surgery, a high index of suspicion as well as liberal use of frozen-section biopsy can often provide an early lifesaving diagnosis and minimize morbidity (103).

Predisposing risk factors for necrotizing fasciitis include diabetes mellitus, alcoholism, an immunocompromised state, hypertension, peripheral vascular disease, intravenous drug abuse, and obesity (94, 96, 99, 100, 102, 104, 106). The most frequent site of infection has been in the extremities (97), but the infection can occur anywhere in the subcutaneous tissues, including the head and neck, trunk, and perineum. Necrotizing fasciitis has been known to occur after trauma, surgery, burns, and lacerations; as a secondary complication in perirectal infections or Bartholin duct abscesses; and *de novo* (94–97, 103, 106–108). Increased age, delay in diagnosis, inadequate debridement during initial surgery, extent of disease on initial presentation, and the presence of diabetes mellitus are all factors that have been associated with an increased likelihood of mortality from necrotizing fasciitis (94, 99, 109). Clearly, early diagnosis and aggressive management of this lethal disease have led to improved survival. In an earlier series, the mortality rate was consistently higher than 30%; in more recent series, the mortality rate has decreased to less than 10% (102, 110, 111).

Successful management of necrotizing fasciitis involves early recognition, immediate initiation of resuscitative measures (including correction of fluid, acid-base, electrolyte, and hematologic abnormalities), aggressive surgical debridement and redebridement as necessary, and broad-spectrum antibiotic therapy. Many patients will benefit from central venous monitoring, as well as from high caloric nutritional support.

During surgery, the incision should be made through the infected tissue down to the fascia. An ability to undermine the skin and subcutaneous tissues with digital palpation often will confirm the diagnosis. Multiple incisions can be made sequentially toward the periphery of the affected tissue until well-vascularized, healthy, resistant tissue is reached at all margins. The remaining affected tissue must be excised. The wound can then be packed and sequentially debrided on a daily basis as necessary until healthy tissue is displayed at all margins.

Hyperbaric oxygen therapy may be of some benefit, particularly in patients for whom culture results are positive for anaerobic organisms. In one retrospective nonrandomized study (94), the addition of hyperbaric oxygen therapy to surgical debridement and antimicrobial therapy appeared to significantly decrease both wound morbidity, as measured by the required number of debridements, and overall mortality in patients with necrotizing fasciitis. The demonstrated benefit of hyperbaric therapy in this study was remarkable, given that patients receiving hyperbaric oxygen were sicker, with a higher incidence of diabetes mellitus, leukocytosis, and shock.

After the initial resuscitative efforts and surgical debridement, the primary concern is the management of the open wound. Allograft and xenograft skin can be used to cover open wounds, thus decreasing heat and evaporative water loss. Interestingly, temporary biologic closure of open wounds also seems to decrease bacterial growth (112). Amniotic membranes have also been shown to be an effective wound covering in patients with necrotizing fasciitis (104). Finally, skin flaps can be mobilized to help cover open wounds once the wound infections have resolved and granulation has begun.

Gastrointestinal Preparation

Preparation of the lower gastrointestinal tract prior to elective gynecologic surgery has several goals. In most gynecologic surgery, when the gastrointestinal tract is not entered, mechanical preparation of the bowel reduces gastrointestinal contents and thus allows more room in the abdomen and pelvis, facilitating the surgical procedure. If a rectosigmoid colon enterotomy occurs, the mechanical bowel preparation eliminates formed stool and reduces the risk of bacterial contamination, thus reducing infectious complications. Mechanical bowel preparation may be accomplished by several methods (Table 19.7). The traditional use of laxatives and enemas requires at least 12–24 hours and generally causes moderate abdominal distention and crampy pain. In addition, nursing supervision of enema administration and the need for intravenous fluid replacement makes this regimen relatively expensive. Randomized trials comparing traditional mechanical bowel preparation with oral gut lavage (GoLYTELY) have found that the use of approximately 4 liters of GoLYTELY (administered until the rectal effluent is clear) provides more complete, faster, and more comfortable bowel preparation (113). Furthermore, the fluid loss following gut lavage with GoLYTELY appears to be clinically insignificant. Gut lavage can usually be performed at home the day prior to scheduled surgery. Rarely, if the patient cannot drink the 4 liters, the GoLYTELY may be administered through a small-caliber nasogastric tube.

High infection rates after colonic surgery have lead to investigation of methods aimed at reducing these significant complications. Although mechanical bowel preparation is an essential part of all colonic surgery preparation regimens, it does not reduce the infection rate satisfactorily. Reduction of the number of pathogenic flora in the colon is the primary strategy to reduce infection after colonic surgery. The colon has the greatest concentration of bacteria in the body, including both aerobes and anaerobes. Anaerobes outnumber aerobes by 1000:1. After reducing the bacterial load by mechanical preparation, the addition of antibiotics to the colon can further reduce the bacterial count. Of the many trials reported, the most widely accepted regimen combines *erythromycin* base and *neomycin* administered orally (Table 19.7) (114–116). Many surgeons substitute *metronidazole* for the *erythromycin;* there is no significant difference in infection rates, but some patients tolerate *metronidazole* better than *erythromycin.* The use of oral antibiotics 24 hours prior to colonic resection has reduced the infection rate from approximately 40% to 5–10% in randomized trials. Because these oral antibiotics are poorly absorbed and many do little to reduce infection from vaginal contamination, an intravenous antibiotic (first-generation *cephalosporin*) can be added to the preoperative regimen. Antibiotic bowel prophylaxis should be used for patients who are likely to undergo colorectal surgery (pelvic exenteration, ovarian cancer debulking) and those who are at high risk for rectal injury (such as severe cases of endometriosis or pelvic inflammatory disease).

Table 19.7   Bowel Preparation Regimens to Begin Day Prior to Surgery

Time	Mechanical Prep	Antibiotic Prep
Preoperative day 2 pm	Clear liquid diet	
Preoperative day 1 Noon	Clear liquid diet *Magnesium citrate* (240 cc po), or *GoLYTELY* (4 l po over 3 hrs)	
1 pm		*Erythromycin* base 500 mg po, plus *Neomycin* 1 gm po *Metronidazole* 500mg po may be substituted
2 pm		Repeat po antibiotics
8 pm	Enemas until clear IV D5/0.5 NS + 20 mEq KCL at 125 cc/hr (optional)	
11 pm		Repeat po antibiotics
Operative day 12 midnight am	Nothing by mouth Surgery	Prophylactic IV antibiotics

Postoperative Gastrointestinal Complications

Ileus

Following abdominal or pelvic surgery, most patients will experience some degree of intestinal ileus. The exact mechanism by which this arrest and disorganization of gastrointestinal motility occurs is unknown, but it appears to be associated with the opening of the peritoneal cavity and is aggravated by manipulation of the intestinal tract and prolonged surgical procedures. Infection, peritonitis, and electrolyte disturbances may also result in ileus. For most patients undergoing common gynecologic operations, the degree of ileus is minimal and gastrointestinal function returns relatively rapidly, allowing the resumption of oral intake within a few days of surgery. Patients who have persistently diminished bowel sounds, abdominal distention, and nausea and vomiting require further evaluation and more aggressive management.

Ileus is usually manifest by abdominal distention and should be evaluated initially by physical examination. Pertinent points of the abdominal examination include assessment of the quality of bowel sounds and palpation searching for tenderness or rebound. The possibility that the patient's signs and symptoms may be associated with a more serious intestinal obstruction or other intestinal complication must be considered. Pelvic examination should be performed to evaluate the possibility of a pelvic abscess or hematoma that may contribute to the ileus. Abdominal x-ray to evaluate the abdomen in the flat (supine) position as well as in the upright position usually will aid in the diagnosis of an ileus. The most common radiographic findings include dilated loops of small and large bowel as well as air-fluid levels in the upright position. Sometimes, massive dilation of the colon or stomach may be noted. The remote possibility of distal colonic obstruction suggested by a dilated cecum should be excluded by rectal examination, proctosigmoidoscopy, or barium enema. In the postoperative gynecology patient, especially in the upright position, the flat plate of the abdomen may also show evidence of free air. This is a common finding following surgery, which lasts 7–10 days in some instances and is not indicative of a perforated viscus in most patients.

The initial management of a postoperative ileus is aimed at gastrointestinal tract decompression and maintenance of appropriate intravenous replacement fluids and electrolytes.

1. **A nasogastric tube should evacuate the stomach of its fluid and gaseous contents.** Prolonged nasogastric suction continues to remove swallowed air, which is the most common source of air in the small bowel. Some clinicians prefer to use a longer small intestinal tube (Cantor or Miller-Abbott tube) (117). This tube, which usually has a mercury-filled bag on its distal tip, may be propelled by peristalsis through the pylorus and into the small bowel, thus allowing a better evacuation of the small bowel. The disadvantage of "long tubes" is that they take a longer time to become positioned and may not enter the small bowel as a result of the decreased intestinal motility associated with ileus.

2. **Fluid and electrolyte replacement must be adequate to keep the patient well perfused.** Significant amounts of third-space fluid loss occur in the bowel wall, the bowel lumen, and the peritoneal cavity during the acute episode. Gastrointestinal fluid losses from the stomach may lead to a metabolic alkalosis and depletion of other electrolytes as well. Careful monitoring of serum chemistries and appropriate replacement are necessary.

3. **Most cases of severe ileus will begin to improve over a period of several days.** In general, this is recognized by reduction in the abdominal distention, return of normal bowel sounds, and passage of flatus or stool. Follow-up abdominal x-rays should be obtained as necessary for further monitoring.

4. **When the gastrointestinal tract function appears to have returned to normal, the nasogastric tube may be removed and a liquid diet may be instituted.**

571

5. **If a patient shows no evidence of improvement during the first 48–72 hours of medical management, other causes of ileus should be sought.** Such cases may include ureteral injury, peritonitis from pelvic infection, unrecognized gastrointestinal tract injury with peritoneal spill, or fluid and electrolyte abnormalities such as hypokalemia. In the evaluation of persistent ileus, the use of water-soluble upper gastrointestinal contrast studies may assist in the resolution of the ileus, but prospective randomized data regarding this maneuver are lacking.

Small Bowel Obstruction

Obstruction of the small bowel following major gynecologic surgery occurs in approximately 1–2% of patients (118). The most common cause of small bowel obstruction is adhesions to the operative site. If the small bowel becomes adherent in a twisted position, partial or complete obstruction may result from distention, ileus, or bowel wall edema. Less common causes of postoperative small bowel obstruction include entrapment of the small bowel into an incisional hernia and an unrecognized defect in the small bowel or large bowel mesentery. **Early in its clinical course, a postoperative small bowel obstruction may exhibit signs and symptoms identical to those of ileus. Initial conservative management as outlined for the treatment of ileus is appropriate.** Because of the potential for mesenteric vascular occlusion and resulting ischemia or perforation, worsening symptoms of abdominal pain, progressive distention, fever, leukocytosis, or acidosis should be evaluated carefully because immediate surgery may be required.

In most cases of small bowel obstruction following gynecologic surgery, the obstruction is only partial and the symptoms usually resolve with conservative management.

1. **Further evaluation after several days of conservative management may be necessary.** Evaluation of the gastrointestinal tract with barium enema and an upper gastrointestinal series with small bowel follow-through are appropriate. In most cases, complete obstruction is not documented, although a narrowing or tethering of the segment of small bowel may indicate the site of the problem.

2. **Further conservative management with nasogastric decompression and intravenous fluid replacement may allow time for bowel wall edema or torsion of the mesentery to resolve.**

3. **If resolution is prolonged and the patient's nutritional status is marginal, the use of total parenteral nutrition may be necessary.**

4. **Conservative medical management of postoperative small bowel obstruction usually results in complete resolution.** However, if persistent evidence of small bowel obstruction remains after full evaluation and an adequate trial of medical management, exploratory laparotomy may be necessary to surgically evaluate and manage the obstruction. In most cases, lysis of adhesions is all that is required, although a segment of small bowel that is badly damaged or extensively sclerosed from adhesions may require resection and reanastomosis.

Colonic Obstruction

Postoperative colonic obstruction following surgery for most gynecologic conditions is exceedingly rare. It is almost always associated with a pelvic malignancy, which in most cases will have been known at the time of the initial operation. Advanced ovarian carcinoma is the most common cause of colonic obstruction in postoperative gynecologic surgery patients and is caused by extrinsic impingement on the colon by the pelvic malignancy. Intrinsic colonic lesions may be undetected, especially in a patient with some other benign gynecologic condition. When colonic obstruction is manifest by abdominal distention and abdominal radiographs reveal a dilated colon and enlarging cecum, further evaluation of the large bowel is required by barium enema or colonoscopy. **Dilation of the ce-**

cum to more than 10–12 cm in diameter as viewed by abdominal x-ray requires immediate evaluation and surgical decompression by performing a colectomy or colostomy. Surgery should be performed as soon as the obstruction is documented. Conservative management of colonic obstruction is not appropriate, because the complication of colonic perforation has an exceedingly high mortality rate.

Diarrhea

Episodes of diarrhea often occur following abdominal and pelvic surgery as the gastrointestinal tract returns to its normal function and motility. However, prolonged and multiple episodes may represent a pathologic process such as impending small bowel obstruction, colonic obstruction, or pseudomembranous colitis. Excessive amounts of diarrhea should be evaluated by abdominal x-rays and stool samples tested for the presence of ova and parasites, bacterial culture, and *Clostridium difficile* toxin. Proctoscopy and colonoscopy may also be advisable in severe cases. Evidence of intestinal obstruction should be managed as outlined previously. Infectious causes of diarrhea should be managed with the appropriate antibiotics as well as fluid and electrolyte replacement. *Clostridium difficile*-associated pseudomembranous colitis may result from exposure to any antibiotic. Discontinuation of these antibiotics (unless they are needed for another severe infection) is advisable, along with the institution of appropriate therapy. Because of the expense of vancomycin, we usually institute therapy with metronidazole. Therapy should be continued until the diarrhea abates, and several weeks of oral therapy may be required in order to obtain complete resolution of the pseudomembranous colitis.

Fistula

Gastrointestinal fistulas are relatively rare following gynecologic surgery. They are most often associated with malignancy, prior radiation therapy, or surgical injury to the large or small bowel that was improperly repaired or unrecognized. Signs and symptoms of gastrointestinal fistula are often similar to those of small bowel obstruction or ileus, except that a fever is usually a more prominent component of the patient's symptoms. When fever is associated with gastrointestinal dysfunction postoperatively, evaluation should include early assessment of the gastrointestinal tract for its continuity. When fistula is suspected, the use of water-soluble gastrointestinal contrast material is advised to avoid the complication of barium peritonitis. Evaluation with abdominal pelvic CT scan may also assist in identification of a fistula and associated abscess. Recognition of an intraperitoneal gastrointestinal leak or fistula formation usually requires immediate surgery unless the fistula has drained spontaneously through the abdominal wall or vaginal cuff.

An *enterocutaneous fistula* arising from the small bowel and draining spontaneously through the abdominal incision may be managed successfully with medical therapy. Therapy should include nasogastric decompression, replacement of intravenous fluids as well as total parenteral nutrition, and appropriate antibiotics to treat an associated mixed bacterial infection. If the infection is under control and there are no other signs of peritonitis, the surgeon may consider allowing potential resolution of the fistula over a period of up to 2 weeks. Some authors have suggested the use of *somatostatin* to decrease intestinal tract secretion and allow earlier healing of the fistula. In some cases, the fistula will close spontaneously with this mode of management. If the enterocutaneous fistula does not close with conservative medical management, surgical correction with resection, bypass, or reanastomosis will be necessary.

A *rectovaginal fistula* that occurs following gynecologic surgery is usually the result of surgical trauma that may have been aggravated by the presence of extensive adhesions in the rectovaginal septum associated with endometriosis, pelvic inflammatory disease, or pelvic malignancy. A small rectovaginal fistula may be managed with a conservative medical approach, in the hope that decreasing the fecal stream will allow closure of the fistula. A small fistula that allows continence except for an occasional leak of flatus may be managed conservatively until the inflammatory process in the pelvis resolves. At that point, usually several months later, correction of the fistula is appropriate. Large rectovaginal fistulas that have no hope of closing spontaneously are best managed by performing an initial diverting colostomy followed by repair of the fistula after inflammation has resolved. After the fistula closure is healed and deemed successful, the colostomy can be closed.

Thromboembolism Prophylaxis

Risk Factors

Deep venous thrombosis and pulmonary embolism, although largely preventable, are significant complications in postoperative patients. The magnitude of this problem is relevant to the gynecologist, because 40% of all deaths following gynecologic surgery are directly attributed to pulmonary emboli (119). Pulmonary embolism is also the second leading cause of death in women who undergo a legally induced abortion (120) and the most frequent cause of postoperative death in patients with uterine (121) or cervical carcinoma (122).

The causal factors of venous thrombosis were first proposed by Virchow in 1858 and include the following: a hypercoagulable state, venous stasis, and vessel intima injury. Two prospective studies have evaluated risk factors associated with the postoperative occurrence of deep venous thrombosis in patients undergoing gynecology surgery. Using logistic regression analysis, the risk factors of 124 patients undergoing vaginal and abdominal surgery for benign gynecologic disease were studied (123). The five factors identified to be associated with postoperative deep venous thrombosis included increasing age, presence of varicose veins, being overweight, prolonged euglobulin lysis time, and presence of or action of serum fibrin-related antigen. The risk factors associated with venous thromboembolic complications were also assessed in 411 patients undergoing major abdominal and pelvic surgery (124). Of these patients, 84% had gynecologic malignancies. Preoperative risk factors identified in this study include advanced age; nonwhite race; increasing stage of malignancy; history of deep venous thrombosis, lower extremity edema or venous stasis changes; presence of varicose veins; being overweight; and a history of radiation therapy. Intraoperative factors associated with postoperative deep venous thrombosis included increased anesthesia time, increased blood loss, and the need for transfusion in the operating room. The recognition of these factors should allow the clinician to stratify patients into low-risk, medium-risk, and high-risk groups.

Prophylactic Methods

During the past two decades, a number of prophylactic methods have undergone clinical trials showing significant reduction in the incidence of deep venous thrombosis, and a few studies have been completed that have demonstrated a reduction in fatal pulmonary emboli. The ideal prophylactic method would be effective, free of significant side effects, well accepted by the patient and nursing staff, widely applicable to most patient groups, and inexpensive.

Low-Dose Heparin

The use of small doses of subcutaneously administered *heparin* for the prevention of deep venous thrombosis and pulmonary embolism is the most widely studied of all prophylactic methods. More than 25 controlled trials have demonstrated that *heparin* given subcutaneously 2 hours preoperatively and every 8–12 hours postoperatively is effective in reducing the incidence of deep venous thrombosis. The value of low-dose *heparin* in preventing fatal pulmonary emboli was established by a randomized, controlled, multicenter international trial, which demonstrated a reduction in fatal postoperative pulmonary emboli in general surgery patients receiving low-dose *heparin* every 8 hours postoperatively (125). Trials of low-dose *heparin* in gynecologic surgery patients are limited, and a clear consensus regarding the value of low-dose *heparin* in all groups of patients has not been established, because of differences in patient selection and length of follow-up. Three randomized controlled studies used the same regimen of low-dose *heparin* administration: 5000 units subcutaneously 2 hours preoperatively and every 12 hours for 7 days postoperatively. Two trials were conducted in patients with benign gynecologic conditions (98%);

all patients were older than 40 years of age, and follow-up was discontinued at the time of discharge from hospital (126, 127). One trial showed a 23% incidence of deep venous thrombosis in the control group, as compared with a 6% incidence of deep venous thrombosis in the patients treated with low-dose *heparin* (127). This difference was statistically significant (P<0.05). Although this was a randomized trial, the control group contained a larger number of patients with malignancy and, when the cancer patients were excluded from the trial analysis, there was no significant value to the use of low-dose *heparin* in patients with benign conditions. In the other study, the nontreated control group had a 29% incidence of deep venous thrombosis compared with a 3.6% incidence in the group treated with low-dose *heparin* (P<0.001) (126). A third trial evaluated a larger group of patients receiving treatment in gynecologic oncology unit, only 16% of whom had benign gynecologic conditions; follow-up included the first 6 weeks postoperatively (128). In this trial, there was no difference in the incidence of thromboembolic complications between the control group (12.4%) and the group treated with low-dose *heparin* (14.8%) (128).

In a subsequent trial (129), two more intense *heparin* regimens were evaluated in high-risk gynecologic oncology patients. *Heparin* was given either in a regimen of 5000 units subcutaneously 2 hours preoperatively and every 8 hours postoperatively or 5000 units subcutaneously every 8 hours preoperatively (a minimum of three preoperative doses) and every 8 hours postoperatively. Both of these prophylaxis regimens were effective in significantly reducing the incidence of postoperative deep venous thrombosis.

Although low-dose *heparin* is considered to have no measurable effect on coagulation, most large series have noted an increase in the bleeding complication rate, especially a higher incidence of wound hematoma. Up to 10–15% of otherwise healthy patients develop a prolonged activated partial thromboplastin time (APTT) after 5000 units of *heparin* is given subcutaneously (130). The transient state of anticoagulation in these patients has also been noted in one carefully monitored trial of low-dose *heparin*. Major bleeding complications were encountered postoperatively in these patients. The estimated blood loss increased from about 250 to 400 ml in patients treated with low-dose *heparin* who were undergoing inguinal or pelvic lymphadenectomy (131). Retrospective studies have suggested that low-dose *heparin* contributed to an increased occurrence of lymphocysts (132, 133), and a prospective study demonstrated a twofold increase in retroperitoneal lymph drainage volume in patients treated with low-dose *heparin* (130). Although relatively rare, thrombocytopenia is associated with low-dose *heparin* use and has been found in 6% of patients after gynecologic surgery (130). Activated thromboplastin time and platelet count should be periodically assessed postoperatively to identify the 22% of patients who have either prolonged APTT or thrombocytopenia and who are most prone to develop major clinical hemorrhagic complications.

Mechanical Methods

Stasis in the veins of the legs has been clearly demonstrated while the patient is undergoing surgery and continues postoperatively for varying lengths of time. Stasis occurring in the capacitance veins of the calf during surgery, plus the hypercoagulable state induced by surgery, are the prime factors contributing to the development of acute postoperative deep venous thrombosis. Prospective studies of the natural history of postoperative venous thrombosis have shown that the calf veins are the predominant site of thrombi and that most thrombi develop within 24 hours of surgery (134). Reduction of venous stasis in the perioperative period by various methods has been less extensively investigated than pharmacologic methods such as low-dose *heparin*. However, mechanical prophylactic methods may play an important role in the prevention of postoperative deep vein thrombosis.

Although probably of only modest benefit, reduction of stasis by short preoperative hospital stays and early postoperative ambulation should be encouraged for all patients. A 20° elevation of the foot of the bed, raising the calf above heart level, allows gravity to drain the calf veins and should further reduce stasis. More active forms of mechanical prophylaxis include elastic gradient compression stockings and external pneumatic leg compression.

Elastic Stockings   In a survey of general surgeons in the U.S., gradient elastic stockings were second only to low-dose heparin as the prophylactic method of choice in high-risk and moderate high-risk surgical patients (135). The simplicity of elastic stockings and the absence of significant side effects are probably the two most important reasons that they are often included in routine postoperative care. Controlled studies of gradient elastic stockings are limited but do suggest modest benefit when they are carefully fitted (136). Poorly fitted stockings may be hazardous to some patients who develop a tourniquet effect at the knee or midthigh (120). Variations in human anatomy do not allow perfect fit of all patients to available stocking sizes.

External Pneumatic Compression   The largest body of literature dealing with the reduction of postoperative venous stasis deals with intermittent external compression of the leg by pneumatically inflated sleeves placed around the calf or leg during intraoperative and postoperative periods. Various pneumatic compression devices and leg sleeve designs are available, and the current literature has not demonstrated superiority of one system over another. Single-chambered calf compression devices have been studied most extensively and appear to significantly reduce the incidence of deep venous thrombosis on a level similar to that of low-dose *heparin*. In addition to increasing venous flow and pulsatile emptying of the calf veins, external pneumatic compression also appears to augment endogenous fibrinolysis, which may result in lysis of very early thrombi before they become clinically significant (137).

The duration of postoperative external pneumatic compression has differed in various trials. Because most deep venous thrombosis occurs intraoperatively and in the first 72 hours postoperatively (134), this interval should be a minimum length for external pneumatic compression. External pneumatic compression may be effective only when used in the operating room or in the operating room and for the first 24 hours postoperatively (138, 139).

External pneumatic compression used in patients undergoing major surgery for gynecologic malignancy has been found to reduce the incidence of postoperative venous thromboembolic complications by nearly threefold (140). Calf compression was applied intraoperatively and for the first 5 postoperative days. In a subsequent trial of similar patients that was designed to evaluate whether external pneumatic compression might achieve similar benefits when used only intraoperatively and for the first 24 hours postoperatively, there was no reduction of deep venous thrombosis when compared with the control group (141). Patients with gynecologic malignancies may remain at risk because of stasis and hypercoagulable states for a longer period than general surgical patients; if compression is to be effective, it must be used for a least 5 days postoperatively.

External pneumatic leg compression has no significant side effects or risks, although patient tolerance has been cited as a drawback to its use. However, we have had only two patients of nearly 300 treated with external pneumatic compression request removal because of discomfort. The equipment is easily managed by the nursing staff, and although the initial capital outlay for external pneumatic compressors may seem large, the cost per patient is slightly less than that of low-dose *heparin* given for 7 days postoperatively (142).

Management of Postoperative Deep Venous Thrombosis and Pulmonary Embolism

Because pulmonary embolism is the leading cause of deaths following gynecologic surgical procedures, identification of high-risk patients and the use of prophylactic venous thromboembolism regimens is an essential part of management (119, 121, 122). In addition, the early recognition of deep vein thrombosis and pulmonary embolism and immediate treatment are critical. Most pulmonary emboli arise from the deep venous system of the leg, although following gynecologic surgery, the pelvic veins are a known source of fatal pulmonary emboli as well.

576

The signs and symptoms of deep vein thrombosis of the lower extremities include pain, edema, erythema, and prominent vascular pattern of the superficial veins. These signs and symptoms are relatively nonspecific; 50–80% of patients with these symptoms will not actually have deep vein thrombosis (143). Conversely, approximately 80% of patients with symptomatic pulmonary emboli have no signs or symptoms of thrombosis in the lower extremities (144). Because of the lack of specificity when signs and symptoms are recognized, additional diagnostic tests should be performed to establish the diagnosis of deep vein thrombosis.

Venogram   Although venography has been the "gold standard" for diagnosis of deep vein thrombosis, other diagnostic studies are accurate when performed by a skilled technologist and, in most patients, may replace the need for routine contrast venography. Venography is moderately uncomfortable, requires the injection of a contrast material that may cause allergic reaction or renal injury, and may result in phlebitis in approximately 5% of patients (145). Fortunately, newer diagnostic tests have been developed that are less invasive yet have a high accuracy rate in most patients.

Impedance Plethysmography   **Impedance plethysmography is a noninvasive study that measures the change in electrical impedance of the lower extremities when venous blood flow and volume are altered by an occlusive cuff on the thigh.** This study may be performed at the patient's bedside and repeated as often as necessary without any risk to the patient. Correlation with venography in symptomatic patients approaches 95% (146, 147). The test is effective in the identification of deep venous thrombi in the popliteal, femoral, and external iliac segments. It is less accurate (30%) in identifying calf vein thrombosis and does not identify thrombi occurring in the internal iliac venous system. False-positive results are primarily due to extrinsic venous compression. In gynecology, this might include a large pelvic mass compressing the external iliac or common iliac vein.

Doppler Ultrasound   Doppler ultrasound has been used for the diagnosis of deep vein thrombosis, although its accuracy is slightly less than that of impedance plethysmography. The reason for this is the variable interpretation of audible venous flow patterns, which may be somewhat subjective (148). B-mode duplex Doppler imaging has been found to be effective in the diagnosis of symptomatic venous thrombosis, especially when it arises in the proximal lower extremity. With duplex Doppler imaging, the femoral vein can be visualized and clots may be seen directly (149). Compression of the vein with the ultrasound probe tip allows assessment of venous collapsibility; the presence of a thrombus diminishes vein wall collapsibility. Doppler imaging is less accurate when evaluating the calf venous system and the pelvic veins.

Magnetic Resonance Imaging   Magnetic resonance imaging can identify thrombi in the deep venous system (150). The primary drawback to MRI is the time involved in examining the lower extremity and pelvis as well as the expense of this technology.

Deep Venous Thrombosis   **The treatment of postoperative deep venous thrombosis requires the immediate institution of anticoagulant therapy.**

1. *Heparin* should be initiated: a bolus of 5000 units intravenously, followed by a continuous intravenous infusion of 1000 units per hour.

2. Approximately 4 hours after initiation of *heparin* therapy, an APTT should be obtained to assess the adequacy of the anticoagulant effect. Prolongation of the APTT to 1.5–2.0 times the control level achieves appropriate anticoagulant therapy. The goals of anticoagulant therapy include the prevention of clot propagation or embolization and prevention of rethrombosis in high-risk patients; the risks are bleeding and related complications (151).

3. Oral maintenance therapy using sodium warfarin *(Coumadin)* is advised for at least 3 months. Standard treatment regimens have called for the use of intra-

venous *heparin* for 10 days, followed by continuation of *Coumadin* for 3 months (152).

A randomized trial evaluated a 10-day regimen of *heparin* compared with a 5-day regimen of *heparin* and found the 5-day regimen to be equally effective in treating the acute thrombosis and preventing rethrombosis (153). **Therefore, it is recommended that intravenous *heparin* administration be maintained for 5 days and that oral administration of *Coumadin* be initiated during that time. The goals of *Coumadin* therapy are to achieve an oral dose of medication that will prolong the prothrombin time (PT) values to approximately 1.5 times the control value.** Initially, PT values should be obtained on a daily basis until a stable dose of *Coumadin* is established. Thereafter, the PT is checked every 1–2 weeks for the 3 months of therapy. Anticoagulant therapy may be discontinued in 3 months if the cause of the deep vein thrombosis episode (i.e., an acute surgical event or trauma) has been eliminated.

The major postoperative hazard of anticoagulant therapy is an increased risk of bleeding complications. Therefore, it is important that APTT, PT, platelet count, and hematocrit levels be followed carefully and that the anticoagulant does not incur a hypocoagulable state. *Heparin*-induced thrombocytopenia is a rare complication and has been reported in association with the use of both low-dose prophylactic *heparin* and standard anticoagulant doses (154). Therefore, periodic checks of platelet counts are advised while the patient is taking *heparin* therapy. Thrombolytic therapy (*streptokinase* or *urokinase*) has been advocated for the treatment of acute deep vein thrombosis. However, the risk of bleeding complications in a surgical site contraindicate thrombolytic therapy in postoperative patients.

Pulmonary Embolism   **Many of the signs and symptoms of pulmonary embolism are associated with other, more commonly occurring pulmonary complications following surgery. The classic findings of pleuritic chest pain, hemoptysis, shortness of breath, tachycardia, and tachypnea should alert the physician to the possibility of a pulmonary embolism. Many times, however, the signs are much more subtle and may be suggested only by a persistent tachycardia or a slight elevation in the respiratory rate. Patients suspected of pulmonary embolism should be evaluated initially by chest x-ray, electrocardiography, and arterial blood gas assessment. Any evidence of abnormality should be further evaluated by ventilation-perfusion lung scan, searching for evidence of decreased perfusions in areas of adequate ventilation.** Unfortunately, a high percentage of lung scans may be interpreted as "indeterminate." In this setting, careful clinical evaluation and judgment are required to decide whether pulmonary arteriography should be obtained to document or exclude the presence of a pulmonary embolism.

The treatment of pulmonary embolism is as follows:

1. Immediate anticoagulant therapy, identical to that outlined for the treatment of deep vein thrombosis, should be initiated.

2. Respiratory support, including oxygen and bronchodilators and an intensive care setting, may be necessary.

3. Although massive pulmonary emboli are usually quickly fatal, pulmonary embolectomy has been performed successfully on rare occasions.

4. Pulmonary artery catheterization with the administration of thrombolytic agents bears further evaluation and may be important in patients with massive pulmonary embolism.

5. A vena cava interruption may be necessary in situations in which anticoagulant therapy is ineffective in the prevention of rethrombosis and repeated emboliza-

tion from the lower extremities or pelvis. A vena cava umbrella or filter may be situated percutaneously or a large clip can be used to obstruct the vena cava above the level of the thrombosis. In most cases, however, anticoagulant therapy is sufficient to prevent repeat thrombosis and embolism and to allow the patient's own endogenous thrombolytic mechanisms to lyse the pulmonary embolus.

Management of Medical Problems

Endocrine Disease

The three most frequent endocrine disorders that occur in patients undergoing gynecologic surgery are diabetes mellitus, thyroid disease, and adrenal abnormalities. The pathophysiology of these disorders aids in understanding the effects that surgery has on patients with these problems.

Diabetes Mellitus

It is estimated that approximately six million people in the U.S. (2.5% of the population) have diabetes mellitus (DM) and that about one-half of these individuals will undergo surgery at some point in their lives. Approximately 75% of individuals with DM will have surgery after 50 years of age. Many of these procedures are a direct result of the complications of DM: retinopathy, nephropathy, large- and small-vessel occlusive disease, and coronary artery disease. It is the direct effect of DM on the end organs that determines the risk of surgery rather than the type or duration or the control of the condition itself. Diabetes mellitus is a complicated medical disorder of glucose metabolism that is related to a lack of production or resistance to insulin. Patients with DM experience exaggerated hyperglycemia during surgery. This hyperglycemia is multifactorial in origin and is secondary to increased catecholamine production, which inhibits pancreatic release of insulin in increased insulin resistance at the end organs. Elevations instrumental in hormones, such as cortisol, growth hormone, and glucagon, also enhance gluconeogenesis and glycogenolysis. Goals of the preoperative assessment and perioperative management are to ensure metabolic homeostasis and to anticipate problems arising from preexisting complications.

Preoperative Risk Assessment   Large- and small-vessel arterial occlusive disease is the single most important risk factor in the preoperative setting. A careful history and physical examination should be performed to determine the presence or absence of coronary artery or cerebral vascular disease. Assessment of end-organ disease in the retina, kidney, and carotid arteries or evidence of peripheral vascular disease by the presence of foot ulcers should alert the clinician to the presence of small- or large-vessel disease. When extended surgery is possible, as with surgery for gynecologic cancer, exercise stress testing or dipyridamole-thallium imaging should be considered to rule out occult coronary artery disease. Diabetic nephropathy should be documented carefully preoperatively. Imaging studies using contrast dye should be avoided and alternative testing should be performed to reduce the incidence of acute tubular necrosis. If a contrast study must be performed, adequate hydration both before and after the procedure is essential.

Preoperative evaluation should include examination of the skin and urine sediment to detect asymptomatic infection. There is a known predisposition for patients with DM to have Gram-negative and staphylococcal pneumonia as well as an increased incidence of Gram-negative and group B streptococcal sepsis (155). Additionally, 7% of individuals with diabetes will have a postoperative Gram-negative sepsis, a rate approximately seven times higher than in a nondiabetic population. The most common organism cultured in these situations is *Escherichia coli,* and it is well documented that these complications occur more often in patients with poor glucose control (156, 157). Diabetics have an increased risk of wound dehiscence, wound infection, decreased amounts of collagen formation, fibroblast growth, and capillary regrowth, presumably secondary to the pathophysiology of small-vessel disease (158–160).

Autonomic neuropathy has been documented in patients with DM, and these autonomic impairments explained intraoperative hypotension, cardiac arrhythmias, and sudden death as well as abnormal motility of the esophagus, stomach, and small intestine (161). Peripheral sensory and motor neuropathies may or may not be present. The presence of any of these manifestations should prompt a close monitoring of the affected organ system in the perioperative period.

Perioperative hyperglycemia (>250 mg/dl) is associated with increased susceptibility to infection and poor wound healing. Extreme hyperglycemia predisposes patients to metabolic acidosis, and surgery should be cancelled until normal acid-base balance has been documented. *Hyperosmolar hyperglycemic nonketotic states* must be recognized before surgery. Electrolyte disturbances, especially those related to sodium and potassium, should be corrected preoperatively. Hypoglycemia should be avoided at all costs during the perioperative period. Patients with noninsulin-dependent diabetes (Type II) whose condition is controlled with oral hypoglycemic agents or diet are best treated with intravenous fluids containing no dextrose and should not be given *insulin* during the perioperative period. Oral administration of hypoglycemic agents should be discontinued approximately 24 hours prior to the surgery and hyperglycemic episodes in the perioperative period are treated with regular insulin only for blood sugar levels in excess of 250 mg/dl. Longer-lasting agents such as *chlorpropamide* should be discontinued approximately 36 hours before surgery.

Insulin-dependent or type I diabetes poses a more difficult problem. Preoperatively, the goals include avoiding ketoacidosis and hypoglycemia as well as, but to a lesser extent, hyperglycemia. Traditionally, approximately one-third to one-half of the patient's usual daily dose of *NPH insulin* (intermittent acting) is given subcutaneously the morning of surgery. An infusion of 5% dextrose is then given intraoperatively and additional regular *insulin* can be administered as necessary in the operating room and every 6 hours afterward if necessary (155). Alternatively, a continuous infusion of *insulin* and glucose in a fixed ratio has been advocated (156, 157). The patient is much more prone to significant hypoglycemia, however, when a continuous infusion of *insulin* is given. Because of the severe implications associated with intraoperative hypoglycemia unless minute-to-minute intraoperative monitoring of serum glucose can be performed, this method may pose risks and has not been shown to improve the surgical outcome or lessen morbidity.

Postoperative monitoring of patients with DM includes careful monitoring of serum glucose levels approximately every 6 hours until the patient is eating and stable on preoperative regimens. The serum glucose level should be maintained at less than 250 mg/dl, and regular *insulin* should be given on a sliding scale in carefully defined increments of the glucose level. It is essential to prevent the development of severe hypoglycemia or hyperglycemia and the associated complications of diabetic ketoacidosis or a hyperosmolar state. Compulsive perioperative management may obviate some of the infectious and wound healing complications that are more common in these patients (158).

Hyperthyroidism

A history of hyperthyroidism, the use of thyroid replacement therapy, antithyroid medications, or prior thyroid surgery or radioactive iodine therapy should alert the clinician to possible thyroid dysfunction. Diffuse toxic goiter, or Grave's disease, is the most common cause of hyperthyroidism. If the physical examination suggests recent weight loss, tachycardia, or proptosis or myxedema, a more thorough laboratory investigation should be performed to rule out hyperthyroidism. If a palpable abnormality in the thyroid, a diffuse enlargement of the gland, or an asymmetrical gland is noted, the patient should undergo thyroid function tests. Total thyroxin, free T_3, free thyroxin (T_4), and thyroid-stimulating hormone (TSH) tests are useful to confirm underlying thyroid condition.

Because all patients with hyperthyroidism are at risk for a thyroid storm, elective surgery should be cancelled until the patient has been treated adequately with antithyroid agents.

In completely elective situations, the euthyroid state should be maintained for approximately 3 months before a surgical procedure. When surgery is urgent, beta blockers such as *propranolol, atenolol,* or *nadolol* can be used to control sympathomimetic symptoms such as palpitations, diaphoresis, and anxiety. Antithyroid medications such as *propylthiouracil* or radioactive iodine do not render patients euthyroid quickly enough for urgent or emergent surgery. In urgent but not emergent situations, *propylthiouracil* (100–200 mg every 6 hours) along with a beta blocker can be implemented approximately 2 weeks before surgery and, if the patient is carefully monitored postoperatively for signs of increasing hyperthyroidism, optimal results may be achieved (160).

If the patient's condition has been slowly controlled over several months, surgery may be undertaken safely, and no special perioperative monitoring is necessary. Antithyroid and sympatholytic medications can be administered postoperatively when the patient resumes oral intake. However, when performing surgery under urgent or emergent settings, patients should be carefully monitored for tachycardia, arrhythmias, and hypertension. The use of *atropine, cyclopropane,* and *methoxyflurane* should be avoided to avoid exacerbating the symptoms of hyperthyroidism (161). If tachycardia or hypertension develops, prompt administration of a beta blocker can control these symptoms. When the patient has recovered from the acute morbidity of surgery, definitive therapy with an antithyroid agent should be considered. The development of hemodynamic instability, tachycardia, cardiac arrhythmias, hyperpyrexia, diarrhea, or congestive heart failure should alert the physician to an impending thyroid storm and the patient should be immediately transferred to an intensive care unit where the symptoms can be controlled with appropriate beta blockers and antithyroid medications. This condition should be considered a medical emergency necessitating immediate consultation with a medical endocrinologist. An aggressive search should be undertaken for an underlying infection because it can be the nidus of thyroid instability.

Hypothyroidism

Based on elevated TSH levels or low T_4 levels, the prevalence of hypothyroidism is 0.5–0.8% in the adult population. Up to 50% of these cases are caused by prior antithyroid therapy (radioactive iodine or thyroidectomy) for hyperthyroidism. A meticulous history and physical examination should be performed prior to surgery because hypothyroidism can develop insidiously over several weeks to years. Lethargy, an intolerance to cold, lassitude, weight gain, fluid retention, constipation, dry skin, hoarseness, periorbital edema, and brittle hair can be signs of inadequate thyroid function. Physical examination may reveal an increased relaxation phase of the deep tendon reflexes, cardiomegaly, pleural or pericardial effusions, and peripheral edema. Rarely, severe hypothyroidism can cause ascites or a myxedematous coma. As in hyperthyroidism, thyroid function tests are necessary to establish the definitive diagnosis. An abnormal TSH level is the best way to identify most hypothyroid patients, although in the postoperative setting, surgery and general anesthesia may cause a temporary elevation of TSH.

The pathophysiologic effects of hypothyroidism involve almost every organ system. In the past, hypothyroidism was considered a contraindication to surgery in all situations except emergent surgery, although several series have now shown that elective surgery can be carried out safely in patients with mild to moderate hypothyroidism. Patients with hypothyroidism have the same rate of postoperative complications when compared with euthyroid patients (162, 163).

When total elective surgery is planned for hypothyroid patients, surgery should be cancelled and thyroid replacement therapy should be administered: 0.025 mg of *thyroxin* daily, doubled every 2 weeks until the patient is taking a dose of 0.15 mg daily. TSH levels will eventually determine the daily dose. Despite the presence of normal thyroid function study results, physiologic abnormalities will take months to resolve. In patients with mild to moderate hypothyroidism who must undergo urgent surgery, thyroid replacement can begin in the postoperative period as soon as the patient is able to eat. Close postoperative observation should be performed routinely. Cardiac monitoring is not necessary but may be useful in patients with preexisting heart disease. In severely myxedematous patients in whom surgery cannot be avoided, *thyroxin* (0.3–0.5 mg) given intravenously will saturate the carrier protein-binding sites. Standard replacement doses can then be given until the thyroid function tests and TSH determine the optimal dose. In these patients, additional measures are usually necessary because of the severe hypothyroid state. With major abdominal surgery, free water restriction, ventilatory support, diuretics, and nasogastric suction are usually necessary until the patient's condition is stabilized after surgery. In addition, hydrocortisone should be given intravenously (100–300 mg every 8 hours) to avoid the possibility of decreased adrenal reserve.

Adrenal Insufficiency and Exogenous Steroid Use

The physician should ascertain whether a patient has used exogenous steroids for asthma, malignant conditions, arthritis, or irritable bowel syndrome. The type of steroid use, the route, the dose, and the temporal relationship to the timing of the surgical procedure must be determined. High doses of exogenous steroids for prolonged periods can cause circulatory collapse, and they have adverse effects on wound healing and immunocompetence.

The daily replacement dose of cortisol is approximately 5–7.5 mg of *prednisone*. Suppression of the hypothalamic-pituitary-adrenal axis for more than a few weeks may produce relative adrenal insufficiency. When systemic steroids are used for longer periods, adrenal insufficiency may develop for up to 1 year (164). A number of biochemical tests have been recommended to preoperatively evaluate the function of the adrenal gland. The easiest and safest test is the *cosyntropin stimulation test. Cosyntropin,* a synthetic analog of adrenocorticotropic hormone, is given in a dose of 25 units after measuring cortisol before and 60 minutes after the injection. Normal adrenal function is defined as an absolute rise of 7 μg, a value greater than 18 μg, or doubling of the baseline value (165). If the history regarding exogenous steroid use is unclear, then the cosyntropin stimulation test should be performed preoperatively.

Additionally, the type of steroids, the duration and doses used, and the planned operative procedure affect management. Empiric coverage with a "stress" dose of *hydrocortisone* is recommended every 8 hours. With major procedures, a dose of 100–300 mg should be given intravenously with preoperative medications, and the patient should receive additional doses every 8 hours until postoperative stabilization has occurred. Minor ambulatory procedures may require only one dose of hydrocortisone preoperatively and an additional dose 8 hours later. For major diagnostic tests such as CT-guided biopsies or other invasive radiologic procedures, a single dose of hydrocortisone should be given before the procedure and repeated 8 hours later.

Administration of high-dose steroids should be stopped as soon as possible postoperatively, because it can inhibit wound healing and promote infection. Hypertension and glucose intolerance also can develop. It is safe to abruptly discontinue steroid use after a few days of therapy. When a prolonged or involved procedure is performed and longer steroid use is necessary, careful tapering will be required. The recommended approach is to halve the dose of *hydrocortisone* on a daily basis until a dose of 25 mg is reached. Eliminating one daily dose each day until the drug has been stopped is the safest method of withdrawal. Addison's disease is uncommon; it should be considered in the differential diagnosis of perioperative hypotension. In addition to blood and isotonic fluid replacement, a "stress" dose of steroids should be given if adrenal insufficiency is suspected and sepsis and hypovolemia have been excluded.

Cardiovascular Diseases

The incidence of perioperative cardiovascular complications has decreased markedly as a result of improvements in preoperative detection of high-risk patients, preoperative preparation, and surgical and anesthetic techniques (166).

Preoperative Evaluation

The goal of a preoperative cardiac evaluation is to determine the presence of heart disease, its severity, and the potential risk to the patient during the perioperative period. Every patient should be questioned about symptoms of cardiac disease including chest pain, dyspnea on exertion, peripheral edema, wheezing, syncope, claudication, or palpitations. Patients with a history of cardiac disease should be evaluated for worsening of symptoms, which indicates progressive or poorly controlled disease. Records of previous treatment should be obtained. Prescriptions for antihypertensive, anticoagulant, antiarrhythmic, antilipid, or antianginal medications may be the only indication of prior cardiovascular problems. In patients without known heart disease, the presence of diabetes, hyperlipidemia, hypertension, tobacco use, or a family history of heart disease identifies a group of patients at higher risk for heart disease who should be more carefully screened.

On physical examination, the presence of findings such as hypertension, jugular venous distension, laterally displaced point of maximal impulse, irregular pulse, third heart sound, pulmonary rates, heart murmurs, peripheral edema, or vascular bruits should prompt a more complete evaluation. Laboratory evaluation of patients with known or suspected heart disease should include a blood count and serum chemistry analysis. Anemia is poorly tolerated by patients with heart disease, and serum sodium and potassium levels are particularly important in patients taking diuretics and digitalis. Blood urea nitrogen and creatinine values provide information on renal function and hydration status. Assessment of blood glucose levels may detect undiagnosed diabetes. Chest x-ray and electrocardiography are mandatory as part of the preoperative evaluation, and the results may be particularly helpful when compared with those of previous studies.

Coronary Artery Disease

Coronary artery disease is a major risk for cardiac patients undergoing abdominal surgery. In an adult population, the incidence of myocardial infarction following surgery is approximately 0.15% (167) (Table 19.8). In patients who have had a prior myocardial infarction, however, most studies report a reinfarction rate of about 5% (167–169). The risk of reinfarction is inversely proportional to the length of time between infarction and surgery. At 3 months or less, the risk of reinfarction is approximately 30%, and from 3–6 months, the rate falls to 12%. Six months after myocardial infarction, the risk of death as

Table 19.8   Risk Factors for Postoperative Myocardial Infarction

Independent Risk Factors	*Points*
1. Jugular venous distension or S_3 gallop immediately preoperatively	11
2. Myocardial infarction in preceding 6 months	10
3. Presence of premature atrial contractions on preoperative ECG or any rhythm other than sinus	7
4. More than 5 premature ventricular contractions per minute preoperatively	7
5. Evidence of significant aortic valvular stenosis	3
6. Age older than 70 years	5
7. Emergency operation	4
8. Intraperitoneal operation	3
9. Poor general medical condition PO$_2$ <60 or PCO$_2$ 50 mm Hg K<3.0 or HCO$_3$ <20 mEq/l BUN >50 or creatinine >3.0 mg/dl Liver disease or debilitated patient	3

ECG, electrocardiogram.

583

a result of perioperative infarction is similar to that for patients who have no history of ischemic heart disease. Fortunately, careful perioperative management can lower the reinfarction rate even in patients with recent infarctions (170). Perioperative myocardial infarction is associated with a 50% mortality rate (169, 171).

Because of the high mortality and morbidity associated with perioperative myocardial infarction, much effort has been made to predict perioperative cardiac risk. A prospective evaluation of preoperative cardiac risk factors using a multivariate analysis identified independent cardiac risk factors, which are presented in Table 19.9 (172). Using these factors, a *cardiac risk index* has been created that places a patient in one of four risk classes (Table 19.9). Unstable angina, probably because it is relatively uncommon, did not appear as a risk factor, although many believe that patients with unstable angina should be considered at extremely high risk of perioperative cardiac mortality and should undergo coronary artery revascularization prior to any elective gynecologic surgery.

In 1600 patients who had coronary artery disease and left ventricular function defined by angiography and who subsequently underwent major noncardiac surgical procedures, multivariate analysis of potential risk factors revealed only dyspnea on exertion and left ventricular wall motion scores were independently predictive of perioperative cardiac mortality (173). A history of previous myocardial infarction was not an independent risk factor, implying that the degree of left ventricular wall dysfunction was more critical than the less objective information provided by a history of infarction. However, preoperative angiography is an invasive procedure that is less feasible than clinical evaluation of risk.

In an effort to quantitate preoperative cardiac risk, several tests have been used to assess cardiovascular function. *Exercise stress testing* prior to surgery can identify patients who have ischemic heart disease not present at rest. These patients have been shown to be at increased risk of developing cardiac complications in the perioperative period (174). In a study of patients undergoing peripheral vascular surgery, a high-risk group of patients was identified who had ischemic electrocardiographic changes when they exercised to less than 75% of their maximal predicted heart rate (175). In this group, the incidence of perioperative myocardial infarction was 25% and the overall cardiac mortality rate was 18.5%. Conversely, no perioperative infarctions occurred in patients who were able to exercise to more than 75% of their maximal predicted heart rate and who had no electrocardiographic evidence of ischemia. However, the prognostic value of stress testing was not supported in another prospective study that found that only an abnormal preoperative resting electrocardiogram was an independent risk factor (174). The exercise stress test must be selectively applied to a high-risk population because its predictive value is dependent on the prevalence of the disease. Therefore, it is not prudent to screen all patients preoperatively; it is preferable to rely on a careful history to identify a group with symptoms of cardiac disease for whom the test would be most predictive.

Exercise stress testing is limited in some patients who cannot exercise because of musculoskeletal disease, pulmonary disease, or severe cardiac disease. *Dipyridamole-thallium*

Table 19.9   Risk Classes for Postoperative Myocardial Infarction

Total Class	Score	Patients	Patients with life-threatening Complications* or Death
I	0–5	537	5 (1%)
II	6–12	316	21 (7%)
III	13–25	130	18 (14%)
IV	>26	18	14 (78%)

Modified from **Goldman L.** Multifactorial index of cardiac risk in noncardiac surgical procedures. *N Engl J Med* 1977;297:845–50.
*Life-threatening complications are documented intraoperative or postoperative myocardial infarction, pulmonary edema, or ventricular tachycardia without progression to cardiac death.

scanning may be used to overcome the limitations of exercise stress testing. This study has a high degree of sensitivity and specificity, and it relies on the ability of dipyridamole to dilate normal coronary arteries but not stenotic vessels. Normally perfused myocardium readily takes up thallium when it is given intravenously. Conversely, hypoperfused myocardium does not demonstrate good uptake of thallium when scanned 5 minutes after injection. Reperfusion and uptake of thallium 3 hours after injection identify viable but high-risk myocardium. Old infarctions are identified as areas without uptake. Several studies have shown a risk of perioperative myocardial infarction in patients with areas of reperfusion of thallium uptake ranging from 20 to 33% (176–178). The dipyridamole-thallium scan is applicable for patients who are unable to exercise because it uses a medically induced "stress."

The resting *gated blood pool (MUGA)* study provides another test to evaluate cardiac risk in patients who are unable to exercise. Although this test does not directly evaluate coronary artery disease, it has been shown to correlate with perioperative cardiac risk. In a study of 100 preoperative patients with resting MUGA scans, the incidence of postoperative myocardial infarction was 19% if the ejection fraction was higher than 35% but increased to 75% with ejection fractions lower than 35% (179).

It is rare for patients who are younger than 50 years of age and who do not have diabetes, hypertension, hypercholesterolemia, or coronary artery disease to suffer a perioperative myocardial infarction. However, patients with coronary artery disease are at increased risk of myocardial infarction in the postoperative period. Prevention, early recognition, and treatment are important because myocardial infarctions that occur in the postoperative period, with mortality rates of approximately 50%, are more highly lethal than those that are not associated with surgery.

Nearly two-thirds of postoperative myocardial infarctions occur during the first 3 days postoperatively. Although the pathophysiologic factors are complex, the causes of postoperative myocardial ischemia and infarction are related to decreased myocardial oxygen supply coupled with increased myocardial oxygen requirements. In postoperative patients, conditions that decrease oxygen supply to the myocardium include tachycardia, increased preload, hypotension, anemia, and hypoxia (180). Conditions that increase myocardial oxygen consumption are tachycardia, increased preload, increased afterload, and increased contractility. Of all these factors, tachycardia and increased preload are the most important causes of ischemia because both conditions decrease oxygen supply to the myocardium while simultaneously increasing myocardial oxygen demand. Tachycardia decreases the diastolic time, which, when the coronary arteries are perfused, decreases the volume of oxygen available to the myocardium. Increased preload increases the pressure exerted by the myocardial wall on the arterioles within it, thus decreasing myocardial blood flow.

Other factors associated with perioperative cardiac ischemia include physiologic responses to the stress of intubation, intravenous or intra-arterial line placement, emergence from anesthesia, pain, and anxiety. This stress results in catecholamine stimulation of the cardiovascular system, resulting in increased heart rate, blood pressure, and contractility, which may induce or worsen myocardial ischemia. Loss of intravascular volume because of "third-spacing" of fluids or postoperative hemorrhage can also induce ischemia.

Postoperative myocardial infarction is often difficult to diagnose. Chest pain, which is present in 90% of nonsurgical patients with myocardial infarction, may be present in only 50% of patients with postoperative infarction, because of the masking of myocardial pain by coexisting surgical pain and the use of analgesia (170, 181). Thus, maintenance of a high level of suspicion for postoperative infarction is extremely important in patients with coronary artery disease. The presence of arrhythmia, congestive heart failure, hypotension, dyspnea, or elevations of pulmonary artery pressure may indicate infarction and should prompt a thorough cardiac investigation and electrocardiographic monitoring. Measurement of creatine phosphokinase myocardial band (CPK-MB) isoenzyme levels is the most sensitive and specific indicator of myocardial infarction, and assessments should be obtained for all patients suspected of postoperative infarction.

Despite the high incidence of silent myocardial infarction, routinely obtaining postoperative electrocardiograms (ECGs) for all patients with cardiovascular disease is controversial. Many patients will exhibit P-wave changes that spontaneously resolve and do not represent ischemia or infarction. Conversely, patients with proven myocardial infarctions may show few, if any, ECG abnormalities. If routine screening of asymptomatic patients is desired, ECGs should be obtained at 24 hours following surgery because it has been shown that significant ECG changes that occur immediately postoperatively will persist for 24 hours (182). It is prudent to continue serial ECG assessments for at least 3 days postoperatively.

Postoperative management of patients with coronary artery disease is based on maximizing delivery of oxygen to the myocardium as well as decreasing myocardial oxygen utilization. Most patients benefit from supplemental oxygen in the postoperative period, although special care should be exercised in patients with chronic obstructive pulmonary disease. Oxygenation can be easily monitored by pulse oximetry. Anemia is detrimental because of loss of oxygen-carrying capacity as well as resultant tachycardia and should, therefore, be carefully corrected in high-risk patients.

Patients with coronary artery disease may benefit from pharmacologic control of hyperadrenergic states that result from increased postoperative catecholamine production. Beta blockers decrease heart rate, myocardial contractility, and systemic blood pressure, all of which are increased by adrenergic stimulation. Perioperative beta blockade has been shown to significantly reduce arrhythmias and myocardial infarctions (183). For patients receiving beta-blockade therapy prior to surgery, that therapy should be continued in the perioperative period because abrupt withdrawal results in a rebound hyperadrenergic state.

Labetalol, a mixed alpha- and beta-receptor blocker, may be useful in treating patients with coronary artery disease who are also hypertensive because reflex tachycardia is limited. Additionally, labetalol has been shown to have antiarrhythmic effects (184). In patients with asthma, which can be exacerbated by sympathomimetic beta blockers, the use of osmolal is advantageous because it is a cardioselective beta blocker without intrinsic sympathomimetic activity and thus should not cause bronchoconstriction.

Although prophylactic nitrates have been used in the perioperative period for many years, this practice remains controversial. *Nitroglycerin* enhances blood flow to ischemic areas, increases collateral flow, increases myocardial oxygenation, and reduces angina (185–188). The route of administration, dosage, and duration of therapy are controversial; thus, perioperative treatment with nitrates should be initiated in consultation with a cardiologist.

Nifedipine, a calcium channel blocker, may be given sublingually in the postoperative period. It lowers blood pressure by selectively dilating arteries; blood pressure begins to decrease in 5 minutes and plateaus in 30 minutes (189). The ultimate fall in blood pressure is related to the degree of hypertension initially present because vasodilation is more profound in patients with hypertension (190). Care must be taken when giving this drug because ischemia and myocardial infarction have been reported following hypotension associated with the use of nifedipine (191).

Congestive Heart Failure   Patients with congestive heart failure (CHF) face a substantially increased risk of myocardial infarction during surgery (172, 192). The postoperative development of pulmonary edema is a grave prognostic sign and results in death in a high percentage of patients (193). Because patients with heart failure at the time of surgery are significantly more likely to develop pulmonary edema perioperatively, every effort should be made to diagnose and treat CHF before surgery (167). The signs and symptoms of CHF are listed in Table 19.10

Table 19.10   Signs and Symptoms of Congestive Heart Failure

1. Presence of an S_3 gallop
2. Jugular venous distension
3. Lateral shift of the point of maximal impulse
4. Lower extremity edema
5. Basilar rales
6. Increased voltage on electrocardiogram
7. Evidence of pulmonary edema or cardiac enlargement on chest x-ray
8. Tachycardia

---

and should be sought on preoperative history and physical examination. Patients who are able to perform usual daily activities without developing CHF are at limited risk of perioperative heart failure.

To prevent severe postoperative complications, congestive heart failure must be corrected preoperatively. Treatment usually relies on aggressive diuretic therapy, although care must be taken to prevent dehydration, which may result in hypotension during the induction of anesthesia. Hypokalemia can result from diuretic therapy and is especially deleterious to patients who are also taking digitalis. In addition to diuretics and *digitalis,* treatment often includes the use of preload and afterload reducers. Optimal use of these drugs and correction of CHF may be aided by consultation with a cardiologist. In general, it is preferable to continue the usual regimen of cardioactive drugs throughout the perioperative period. **In patients with severe or intractable CHF, the perioperative measurement of left ventricular filling (wedge) pressure with a pulmonary artery catheter (Swan-Ganz) may be extremely helpful to guide perioperative fluid management.**

Postoperative CHF results most frequently from excessive administration of intravenous fluids and blood products. Other common postoperative causes are myocardial infarction, systemic infection, pulmonary embolism, and cardiac arrhythmias.

The cause of postoperative heart failure must be diagnosed because, to be successful, treatment should be directed simultaneously to the underlying cause.

Postoperative diagnosis of CHF is often more difficult than preoperative diagnosis because the signs and symptoms of CHF (Table 19.10) are not specific and may result from other causes. The most reliable method of detecting CHF is chest radiography, in which the presence of cardiomegaly or evidence of pulmonary edema is a helpful diagnostic feature.

Acute postoperative CHF frequently manifests as pulmonary edema. Treatment of pulmonary edema may include the use of intravenous *furosemide,* supplemental oxygen, intravenous *morphine* sulfate, and elevation of the head of the bed. Intravenous *aminophylline* may be useful if cardiogenic asthma is present. Electrocardiography, in addition to laboratory evaluation, including arterial blood gas, serum electrolyte, and renal function chemistry measurements, should be obtained expediently. If the patient does not improve rapidly, she should be transferred to an intensive care unit.

Arrhythmias

Nearly all arrhythmias found in otherwise healthy patients are asymptomatic and of limited consequence. In patients with underlying cardiac disease, however, even brief episodes of arrhythmias may result in significant cardiac morbidity and mortality. Preoperative evaluation of arrhythmias by a cardiologist and anesthesiologist is important because many anesthetic agents as well as surgical stress contribute to the development or worsening of arrhythmias. In patients undergoing continuous cardiographic monitoring during surgery, a 60% incidence of arrhythmias, excluding sinus tachycardia, has been reported (194). Patients with heart disease have an increased risk of arrhythmias, most commonly ventricular arrhythmias (195, 196). Conversely, patients without cardiac disease are more likely to develop supraventricular arrhythmias during surgery (192). Patients taking antiarrhythmic medications prior to surgery should continue taking those drugs during the perioperative period. Initiation of antiarrhythmic medications is rarely indicated preoperatively, but patients in whom arrhythmias are detected prior to surgery should receive cardiology consultation.

Patients with first-degree atrioventricular (AV) block or asymptomatic Mobitz I (Wenckebach) second-degree AV block require no preoperative therapy. Conversely, a pacemaker should be permanently implanted in patients with symptomatic Mobitz II second- or third-degree AV block before elective surgery (97, 198). In emergency situations, a pacing pulmonary artery catheter can be used. Prior to performing surgery on patients with a permanent pacemaker, the type and location of the pacemaker should be determined because electrocautery units may interfere with demand-type pacemakers (199). When performing gynecologic surgery on patients with pacemakers, it is preferable to place the electrocautery unit ground plate on the leg to minimize interference. In patients with a demand pacemaker in place, the pacemaker should be converted preoperatively to the fixed-rate mode.

Surgery is not contraindicated in patients with bundle branch blocks or hemiblocks. Complete heart block rarely develops during noncardiac surgical procedures in patients with conduction system disease (200–202). However, the presence of a left bundle branch block may indicate the presence of aortic stenosis, which can increase surgical mortality if it is severe.

Valvular Heart Disease

Although there are many forms of valvular heart disease, primarily two types—aortic and mitral stenosis—are associated with significantly increased operative risk (203). Patients with significant aortic stenosis appear to be at greatest risk, which is further increased if atrial fibrillation, congestive heart failure, or coronary artery disease is also present. Significant stenosis of aortic or mitral valves should be repaired prior to elective gynecologic surgery.

Severe valvular heart disease is usually evident during physical examination. Common findings in such patients are listed in Table 19.11. The classic history presented by patients with severe aortic stenosis includes exercise dyspnea, angina, and syncope, whereas the symptoms of mitral stenosis are paroxysmal and effort dyspnea, hemoptysis, and orthopnea. Most patients have a remote history of rheumatic fever. Severe stenosis of either valve is considered to be a valvular area of less than 1 cm^2, and diagnosis can be confirmed by echocardiography or cardiac catheterization.

Table 19.11   Signs and Symptoms of Valvular Heart Disease

Aortic Stenosis

1. Systolic murmur at right sternal border, which radiates into carotids
2. Decreased systolic blood pressure
3. Apical heave
4. Chest x-ray with calcified aortic ring, left ventricular enlargement
5. Electrocardiogram with high R waves, depressed T waves in lead I and precordial leads

Mitral Stenosis

1. Precordial heave
2. Diastolic murmur at apex
3. Mitral opening snap
4. Suffused face and lips
5. Chest x-ray with left atrial dilation
6. Electrocardiogram with large P waves and right axis deviation

Patients with any valvular abnormality should receive prophylactic antibiotics immediately preoperatively to prevent subacute bacterial endocarditis. Table 19.12 outlines the American Heart Association recommendations for antibiotic valvular prophylaxis.

Sinus tachycardias and other tachyarrhythmias are poorly tolerated by patients with aortic and mitral stenosis. In patients with aortic stenosis, sufficient digitalization should be provided to correct preoperative tachyarrhythmias and *propranolol* may be used to control sinus tachycardia. Patients with mitral valve stenosis often have atrial fibrillation and, if present, digitalis should be used to reduce rapid ventricular response.

Patients with mechanical heart valves usually tolerate surgery well (204). Management of these patients requires antibiotic prophylaxis (Table 19.12) and discontinuation of anticoagulant therapy during the perioperative period. Usually, *coumadin* is withheld several days prior to surgery and anticoagulation is obtained by intravenous administration of *heparin* (205). The *heparin* is discontinued 6–8 hours prior to surgery and resumed a few days postoperatively (206). The patient is returned to oral coumadin maintenance therapy. Alternatively, *coumadin* can be stopped 1–3 days preoperatively and restarted several days postoperatively. Both methods of management have essentially no risk of thromboembolic complications and bleeding complication rates of approximately 15%.

In the postoperative period, patients with mitral stenosis should be carefully monitored for pulmonary edema, because they may not be able to compensate for the amount of intravenous fluid administered during surgery. Patients with mitral stenosis also frequently have pulmonary hypertension and decreased airway compliance. Therefore, they may require more pulmonary support and therapy postoperatively, including prolonged mechanical ventilation.

For patients with significant aortic stenosis, it is imperative that a sinus rhythm be maintained during the postoperative period. Even sinus tachycardia can be deleterious because it shortens the diastolic time. Bradycardia less than 45 beats per minute should be treated with atropine. Supraventricular dysrhythmias may be controlled with *verapamil* or direct current cardioversion. Particular attention should be provided to the maintenance of proper fluid status, *digoxin* levels, electrolyte levels, and blood replacement.

Hypertension

Patients with a history of hypertension alone have no increased perioperative risk of cardiac morbidity or mortality (167). However, patients with hypertension and heart disease have a 13% perioperative mortality rate (203). Therefore, the preoperative evaluation of patients with hypertension should emphasize diagnosis of target organ damage. Laboratory studies should include an ECG, chest x-ray, blood count, urinalysis, serum electrolyte as-

---

Table 19.12   Recommendations for Prophylaxis of Bacterial Endocarditis

Standard Regimen:

Ampicillin	2 g, 30 minutes to 1 hour bid, and
Gentamicin	1.5 mg/kg IM or IV, 30 minutes to 1 hour before.

Penicillin-Allergic Patients:

Vancomycin	1 g IV slowly over 1 hour, and
Gentamicin	1.5 mg/kg IM or IV 1 hour before;
	may be repeated once in 12 hours.

Oral Regimen for Minor Procedures in Low-Risk Patients:

Amoxicillin	3 g po, 1 hour before and 1.5 q 6 hours later.

IM, intramuscularly; IV, intravenously.

sessment, and measurement of creatinine levels. Patients with evidence of coexistent heart disease should undergo cardiac evaluation.

Patients with diastolic pressures higher than 110 mm Hg or systolic pressures higher than 180 mm Hg should receive medication to control their hypertension prior to surgery. During surgery, patients with chronic hypertension tend to have increased fluctuations in blood pressure (207). Chronically hypertensive patients are very susceptible to intraoperative hypotension because of an impaired autoregulation of blood flow to the brain and, therefore, require a higher mean arterial pressure to maintain adequate perfusion (208). Hypertensive patients who also complain of sweating, palpitations, and headaches should be evaluated for coexisting pheochromocytoma because this disease is associated with greatly increased perioperative mortality (209).

The treatment of early postoperative hypertension is usually limited to drugs that can be given parenterally because absorption by the gastrointestinal mucosa may be diminished and transdermal absorption may be erratic in patients who are cold and are rewarming. Despite these difficulties, it is generally best to maintain administration of antihypertensive medication postoperatively if blood pressure is elevated. Patients receiving preoperative beta blocker agents should be maintained on parenteral therapy to prevent rebound tachycardia, hypercontractility, and hypertension. A list of commonly used parenteral antihypertensive drugs is given in Table 19.13.

Hemodynamic Monitoring

Hemodynamic monitoring has become integral to the perioperative management of patients with cardiovascular and pulmonary disease. The major impetus for this advancement resided in the need for the quantitative estimate of cardiac function, resulting in the development of bedside pulmonary artery catheterization. The impact of monitoring of cardiac function is demonstrated by the significant reduction of myocardial infarctions in high-risk patients who are aggressively monitored for 72–96 hours postoperatively (170).

Before the development of the pulmonary artery catheter, central venous pressure (CVP) measurement was used to assess intravascular volume status and cardiac function. To measure the CVP, a catheter is placed into the central venous system, most frequently the superior vena cava. A water manometer or a calibrated pressure transducer is connected to the CVP line, thus allowing an estimation of right atrial pressure to be obtained. Right atrial pressure is determined by the balance between cardiac output and venous return. Cardiac output is determined by heart rate, myocardial contractility, preload, and afterload.

Table 19.13 Common Parenteral Antihypertensives

Drug	Route	Initial Dose	Onset	Duration	Side Effects
Nitroprusside	IV drip	0.5 ug/min	Immediate	2–5 minutes	Tachycardia, nausea
Labetalol	IV infusion	20 mg	5–10 minutes	4 hours	Bronchospasm, dizziness, nausea
Esmolol	IV infusion	50 ug/min	2 hours	9 minutes	Headache, somnolence, dizziness, hypotension
Nifedipine	Sublingual	10 mg	5 minutes	2 minutes	Hypotension, headache, dizziness, nausea, peripheral edema
Verapamil	IV	5–10 mg	3–5 minutes	2–5 hours	Nausea, headache, hypotension, dizziness, pulmonary edema

IV, intravenous.

Thus, if the pulmonary vascularity and left ventricular function are normal, the CVP accurately reflects the left ventricular end-diastolic pressure (LVEDP). The LVEDP reflects cardiac output or systemic perfusion and has been considered the standard estimator of left ventricular pump function. Venous return is determined primarily by the mean systemic pressure, which propels blood toward the heart, balanced against resistance to venous return, which acts in the opposite direction. Thus, if right ventricular function is normal, the CVP accurately reflects intravascular volume.

Left and right ventricular function is frequently abnormal or discordant and, therefore, the relationship of CVP to cardiac function to intravascular volume is not maintained. When this occurs, measurement of pulmonary artery occlusion pressures is required to accurately assess volume status and cardiovascular function. The use of a pulmonary artery catheter also allows detection of changes in cardiovascular function with more sensitivity and rapidity than clinical observation.

The *balloon-tipped pulmonary artery catheter* (*Swan-Ganz catheter*) can provide measurement of pulmonary artery and pulmonary artery occlusion pressures (210). The catheter can measure cardiac output, be used to perform intracavitary electrocardiography, and provide temporary cardiac pacing.

The standard pulmonary artery occlusion catheter is a 7 French, radiopaque, flexible, polyvinyl chloride, 4-lumen catheter with a 1.5-ml latex balloon at its distal tip. Most often, a right internal jugular cannulation is used for placement of the catheter because this site provides the most direct access into the right atrium. After the catheter is placed into the right atrium, the balloon is inflated and the catheter is "pulled" by blood flow through the right ventricle into the pulmonary artery. The position of the catheter can be identified and followed by the various pressure wave forms generated by the right atrium, right ventricle, and pulmonary artery. As the catheter passes through increasingly smaller branches, the inflated balloon eventually occludes the pulmonary artery. **The distal lumen of the catheter, which is beyond the balloon, measures left atrial pressure (LAP) and, in the absence of mitral valvular disease, LAP approximates LVEDP. Thus, pulmonary capillary wedge pressure (PCWP) equals the LAP, which equals LVEDP and is normal at 8–12 mm Hg.** Additionally, because the standard pulmonary artery catheter has an incorporated thermistor, thermodilution studies can be performed to determine cardiac output. This thermodilution method is performed by injecting cold 5% dextrose in water through the proximal port of the catheter, which cools the blood entering the right atrium. The change in temperature measured at the more distal thermistor (4 cm from the catheter tip) generates a curve proportional to cardiac output. Knowledge of the cardiac output is helpful in establishing cardiovascular diagnoses. For example, a patient with hypotension, low to normal wedge pressure, and a cardiac output of 3 l/min is most likely hypovolemic. Conversely, the same patient with a cardiac output of 8 l/min is probably septic with resultant low systemic vascular resistance.

Despite the great benefit in critically ill patients, the use of pulmonary artery catheters is associated with a small but significant complication rate. The complications can be grouped into those occurring during venous cannulation and those resulting from the catheter or its placement. The most common problems encountered during venous access are cannulation of the carotid or subclavian artery and introduction of a pneumothorax. Problems resulting from the catheter itself include dysrhythmias, sepsis, and disruption of the pulmonary artery. Pulmonary artery catheters should be placed under the supervision of experienced personnel in a setting in which complications can be rapidly diagnosed and treated.

Hematologic Disorders

Hematologic disorders, although infrequent in gynecology patients, can dramatically increase surgical morbidity and mortality and therefore should be considered routinely preoperatively. The following hematologic problems should be considered during the preoperative evaluation: anemia and transfusion, disorders of platelets and bleeding, disorders of coagulation, and disorders of white blood cells and immunity.

Anemia

The presence of moderate anemia in itself should not be a contraindication to surgery because it can be rectified readily by transfusion. If possible, however, surgery should be postponed until the cause of the anemia can be identified and the anemia can be corrected without resorting to the potential risks and expense of blood transfusion. Current anesthetic and surgical practice usually mandates a hemoglobin of ≥10 g/dl or a hematocrit ≥30%. Rather than strictly adhering to these levels, it is important to individualize application of these guidelines. First, more precisely, it is the circulating blood volume that provides oxygen-carrying capacity and tissue oxygenation. Although in most individuals this capacity is accurately reflected by hemoglobin or hematocrit values, in certain situations it may not. If a recent blood loss has occurred, the hematocrit level may remain normal although the blood volume is very low until the lost volume is replaced with extracellular fluid, which then results in a drop in hematocrit levels. Conversely, overly hydrated patients may exhibit low hematocrit or hemoglobin levels but may have a normal red cell mass.

The patient's general physical condition determines her ability to tolerate anemia. The effects of anemia depend on the oxygen requirement of the patient, the rate at which the red cell mass decreases, the magnitude of the anemia, and the ability of compensatory physiologic mechanisms (211). To maintain the same cardiac output, a patient with a hemoglobin of 10 g/dl requires twice as much coronary blood flow as a patient with a hemoglobin of 14 g/dl (212). A patient with ischemic heart disease will not tolerate anemia as well as a healthy young patient. Therefore, the presence of cardiac, pulmonary, or other serious illness justifies a more conservative approach to the management of anemia. Conversely, patients with longstanding anemia may have normal blood volume levels and tolerate surgical procedures well. There is no evidence that mild to moderate anemia increases perioperative morbidity or mortality (213).

If large perioperative blood losses are anticipated, patients with normal hematocrit levels are generally able to store at least three units of autologous blood preoperatively (214). Additionally, the use of *recombinant human erythropoietin* therapy may increase the amount of blood an autologous donor may store without developing anemia (215). Planning for intraoperative red cell recovery and reuse can also be useful in eliminating or reducing the need for homologous transfusions in selected patients.

Platelet and Coagulation Disorders

Surgical hemostasis is provided by platelet adhesion to an injured vessel, which plugs the opening as the coagulation cascade is activated simultaneously, which leads to the formation of a stabilizing fibrin clot. Thus, the presence of both functioning platelets and coagulation factors is necessary to prevent excessive surgical bleeding. Platelet disorders are more commonly encountered in preoperative patients than are coagulation factor abnormalities.

Platelets may be deficient in both number and function. The normal peripheral blood platelet count is 150,000–400,000/mm^3, and the normal life span of a platelet is approximately 10 days. Although there is no clear-cut correlation between the degree of thrombocytopenia and the presence or amount of bleeding, several generalizations can be made. If the platelet count is higher than 100,000/mm^3 and the platelets are functioning normally, there is little chance of bleeding during surgical procedures. Patients with a platelet counts higher than 75,000/mm^3 almost always have normal bleeding times and a platelet count higher than 50,000/mm^3 is probably adequate. A platelet count lower than 20,000/mm^3 will often be associated with severe and spontaneous bleeding. Platelet counts higher than 1,000,000/mm^3 are often paradoxically associated with bleeding.

If the patient's platelet count is lower than 100,000 mm^3, an assessment of bleeding time should be obtained. If the bleeding time is abnormal and surgery must be performed, an attempt should be made to raise the platelet count by administering platelet transfusions immediately prior to surgery. In patients with immune destruction of platelets, human leukocyte antigen (HLA) donor specific platelets may be required to prevent rapid destruction of transfused platelets. If surgery can be postponed, a hematology consultation should be obtained to identify and treat the cause of the platelet abnormality.

Abnormally low platelet counts result from either decreased production or increased consumption of platelets. Although there are numerous causes of thrombocytopenia, most are exceedingly uncommon. Decreased platelet production may be drug induced and has been most often associated with the use of thiazide diuretics or ethanol, although many other drugs have been implicated sporadically. Drugs may also cause immunologic thrombocytopenia by inducing the formation of cross-reacting antibodies, which increase platelet destruction. Numerous drugs have been reported in this context, but this mechanism has been demonstrated convincingly with the use of *quinine* and *sulfonamide* (216). Frequently, patients receiving cytotoxic chemotherapy or radiation therapy for the treatment of malignancies are thrombocytopenic.

Diseases that are characterized by decreased platelet production include B_{12} and folate deficiencies, aplastic anemia, myeloproliferative disorders, renal failure, and viral infections. Inherited congenital thrombocytopenia is extremely rare. Much more commonly, thrombocytopenia results from immune destruction of platelets by diseases such as idiopathic thrombocytopenia purpura and collagen vascular disorders. Thrombocytopenia is caused by increased consumption of platelets in patients with disseminated intravascular coagulation (DIC). In a preoperative population, DIC nearly always is associated with the presence of malignancy or sepsis.

Platelet dysfunction may be inherited, but it is much more likely to be acquired. Commonly prescribed drugs such as *aspirin, amitriptyline,* and NSAIDs may cause decreased platelet function and number. Large doses of *penicillin* and *carbenicillin* have been shown to increase bleeding times (217). In patients who have prolonged bleeding times because of drug therapy, those drugs should be withheld for 7–10 days before surgery. Uremia and liver disease are also common causes of poorly functioning platelets. The major inherited congenital disorder of platelet dysfunction is von Willebrand's disease. Although it is the second most common inherited coagulation disorder, it is extremely rare in a preoperative population.

Whereas an abnormal platelet number is easily diagnosed by a blood count, platelet dysfunction is most often diagnosed by history and physical examination (218). The signs and symptoms of platelet abnormalities are easy bruisability, petechiae, bleeding from mucous membranes, or prolonged bleeding from minor cuts or wounds. A bleeding time will demonstrate clinically important platelet abnormalities. Further laboratory investigation is warranted in patients with abnormal bleeding times and should be obtained in conjunction with a hematology consultation. The preoperative evaluation must first determine the cause of the platelet abnormality so corrective treatment can be initiated. Elective surgery should be postponed until therapy has been instituted. Even for patients in whom surgery must be performed expediently, the evaluation is helpful in predicting the magnitude of perioperative problems that may be encountered.

Disorders of coagulation factors are most often diagnosed by a thorough history and physical examination. Episodes of excessive bleeding following dental procedures, minor surgery, or childbirth, excessive bleeding during menses, and a family history of a bleeding diathesis may be indicators of a coagulation disorder. Inherited coagulation disorders are very uncommon, but of these rare disorders, factor VIII deficiency (hemophilia), factor IX deficiency (Christmas disease), and von Willebrand's syndrome occur most frequently. There are few commonly prescribed drugs that affect coagulation factors, with the exceptions being coumadin and heparin. Disease states that may be associated with decreased coagulation factor levels are primarily liver disease, vitamin K deficiency (secondary to obstructive biliary disease, intestinal malabsorption, or antibiotic reduction of bowel flora), and DIC.

The use of preoperative laboratory screening for coagulation deficiencies is controversial. Routine screening in patients without historical evidence of a bleeding problem is not warranted (219). However, patients who are seriously ill or who will be undergoing extensive surgical procedures should undergo testing preoperatively to determine prothrombin time, partial thromboplastin time, fibrinogen level, and platelet count.

White Cells and Immune Function

Abnormally high or low white blood cell counts are not an absolute contraindication to surgery. However, they should be considered relative to the need for surgery. Evaluation of an elevated or decreased white blood cell count should be undertaken prior to elective surgery. Clearly, patients with absolute granulocyte counts lower than 1000 mm^3 are at increased risk of severe infection and perioperative morbidity and mortality and should only undergo surgery for life-threatening indications (220).

Blood Component Replacement

Nearly all postoperative hematologic problems are related to perioperative bleeding and blood component replacement. Two-thirds of all blood transfused in the U.S. is administered to surgical patients (221). Although the primary cause of postoperative bleeding—lack of surgical hemostasis—is well known to gynecologic surgeons, other less well-appreciated, nonmechanical factors may compound the problem.

Many patients who are massively transfused (>1 blood volume) develop coagulopathy. This coagulopathy has been attributed to dilution of platelets and labile coagulation factors by the use of platelet- and factor-poor packed red blood cells (PRBCs), fibrinolysis, or DIC. Acceptance of these theories has frequently resulted in the use of dogmatic schemes of replacement of fresh-frozen plasma (FFP) and platelets, depending on the number of units of PRBCs given. However, it is preferable to use both clinical and laboratory evaluations to individualize blood replacement rather than adhere to a set replacement recipe.

Studies of soldiers receiving massive transfusions revealed that for those in whom thrombocytopenia developed following red blood cell replacement, bleeding diatheses that responded to infusion of fresh blood but not FFP also developed (222). The investigators concluded that dilutional thrombocytopenia is a major cause of posttransfusion bleeding. However, more recently in a prospective, randomized, double-blind study, prophylactic platelet administration during massive transfusion was not helpful (223). Although it seems that these studies are contradictory, they demonstrate the need for obtaining platelet counts during transfusion of large amounts of blood. If clinical evidence of excessive bleeding exists and the platelet count is lower than 100,000/mm^3, platelets should be transfused because they are consumed during surgery and higher levels are required to maintain hemostasis following surgery.

Packed red blood cells, which may have been stored for several weeks, are used for most postoperative transfusions. Most clotting factors are stable for long periods, with the exception of factors V and VIII, which decrease to 15% and 50% of normal, respectively. Despite this loss, factors V and VIII rarely decrease below the levels required for hemostasis. In 1985, the National Institutes of Health consensus conference on the use of FFP concluded that there was little or no scientific evidence to support the use of FFP for bleeding diatheses following multiple blood transfusions. FFP should be given, however, if there is clinical bleeding, platelet count higher than 100,000/mm^3, and a partial thromboplastin time higher than 1.5 times control.

It appears that the volume of blood transfused does not correlate with the occurrence of a postoperative bleeding diatheses. Instead, it has been shown that the magnitude of abnormalities in coagulation testing correlates with the duration of hypovolemic shock (224). Patients in hypovolemic shock frequently develop DIC, which may compound the bleeding. Thus, most of the problems associated with massive transfusion are the result of inadequate replacement administered too late.

Donor blood is prevented from coagulating by the addition of citrate, which chelates calcium, thus blocking calcium-dependent steps in the coagulation cascade. Therefore, hypocalcemia following transfusion of large amounts of stored blood that contain excess citrate is a theoretic danger. It has been shown that at high transfusion rates, ionized calcium levels will transiently fall but will return toward baseline levels at the completion of transfusion (225). Citrate is metabolized at the equivalent rate of 20 units of blood administered per hour, and therefore, routine supplemental calcium is not warranted. However, hypothermia, liver disease, and hyperventilation slow the metabolism of citrate, requiring close monitoring of ionized calcium levels when these conditions prevail.

As donor blood is stored, potassium leaches from the red cells and plasma levels may reach as high as 30 mEq/l. Despite this large potassium load, serum potassium levels are rarely elevated, even in patients receiving massive transfusions. Patients often are hypokalemic as a result of the metabolic alkalosis that follows transfusion, which is caused by the hepatic metabolism of citrate to bicarbonate.

Pulmonary Disease

In patients undergoing abdominal surgery, several pulmonary physiologic changes manifest secondary to immobilization, anesthetic irritation of the airways, and the splinting of breathing that inevitably occurs secondary to incisional pain. Pulmonary physiologic changes include a decrease in the functional residual capacity (FRC) and vital capacity (VC), an increase in ventilation perfusion mismatching, and impaired mucociliary clearance of secretions from the tracheobronchial tree. These changes result in transient hypoxemia and atelectasis that, if left untreated, can progress to pneumonia in the postoperative period (226–228). Postoperative pulmonary dysfunction is more pronounced in patients with advanced age, preexisting lung disease, obesity, a significant history of smoking, and upper abdominal surgery (226).

Most postoperative pulmonary complications occur in patients who have preexisting pulmonary disease. In these patients, the incidence of pulmonary complications is higher than 70%, as compared to the low incidence (2–5%) in individuals with healthy lungs (226, 229). The risk of postoperative pulmonary complications is lower in patients undergoing lower abdominal surgery as compared with upper abdominal surgery and in those undergoing nonthoracic, nonabdominal surgery as compared with abdominal operation. The presence of chronic obstructive pulmonary disease markedly increases the risk for all patients (226, 230).

Preoperative spirometry is of unproven value in patients undergoing abdominal surgery in whom the risk of postoperative pulmonary complications is low (231, 232). In high-risk patients, preoperative spirometry should be performed with and without bronchodilators in order to identify patients who may benefit from preoperative treatment with inhaled $beta_2$ agonists and steroids. These patients include those with a history of chronic cough or dyspnea, evidence of pulmonary abnormalities by either physical examination or chest x-ray, and a history of chronic obstructive pulmonary disease, as well as patients with a significant history of smoking. In addition to the preoperative spirometric evaluation, an arterial blood gas assessment should be performed. The spirometric abnormalities most often associated with postoperative atelectasis and pneumonia are shown in Table 19.14.

Young, healthy patients rarely have abnormal chest x-rays. Therefore, chest x-rays should not be performed routinely in these patients. Most patients with abnormal chest x-rays have history or physical examination findings suggestive of pulmonary disease (233). Chest x-rays should be limited to patients older than 40 years of age, patients with a history of

Table 19.14   Predictors of Postoperative Pulmonary Complications*

Parameter	Value
Maximal breathing capacity	<50% predicted
FEV_1	<1 l
FVC	<70% predicted
FEV_1/FVC	<65% predicted
PaO_2	>45 mm Hg
$PaCO_2$	<60 mm Hg

FEV, forced expiration volume; FVC, forced vital capacity.
*Complication defined as atelectasis or pneumonia.
From **Blosser SA, Rock P.** Asthma and chronic obstructive lung disease. In: **Breslow MJ, Miller CJ, Rogers MC,** eds. *Perioperative Management.* St. Louis: CV Mosby, 1990: 259–80.

smoking, patients with a history of pulmonary disease, and patients who have evidence of cardiopulmonary disease.

Asthma

Bronchial asthma affects 5% of the U.S. population (234). It is a disease that is characterized by a history of episodic wheezing, physiologic evidence of reversible obstruction of the airways either spontaneously or following bronchodilator therapy, and pathologic evidence of inflammatory changes in the bronchial mucosa. Asthma is not a disease of airway physiology in which hypertrophy and increased contractility of bronchial smooth muscle is the dominant lesion; rather, it is an inflammatory disease affecting the airways that secondarily results in epithelial damage, leukocytic infiltration, and increased sensitivity of the airways to a number of different stimuli. The treatment of asthma is directed toward relaxing the airways and alleviating inflammation with corticosteroids.

Despite advances in pharmacologic management, morbidity and mortality from asthma have been increasing in recent years (235). This most likely has been the result of underdiagnosis and undertreatment of this disease (236). Multiple stimuli have been noted to precipitate or exacerbate asthma, including environmental allergens or pollutants, respiratory tract infections, exercise, cold air, emotional stress, beta-adrenergic blockers, and *aspirin* (227). Management of asthma includes removal of the inciting stimuli as well as use of appropriate pharmacologic therapy.

The severity of clinical asthma correlates with measurements of the severity of the inflammatory response in the lung (234). Some investigators have referred to asthma as a chronic eosinophilic bronchitis (236). Numerous mediators, including interleukin-3, interleukin-5, granulocyte-macrophage colony-stimulating factors, tumor necrosis factor α, and interferon-γ, are released in the lungs by eosinophils, macrophages, and T cells. The mediators induce microvascular leakage, bronchoconstriction, and epithelial damage, which block the distal airways. The optimal therapy for asthma involves not only managing the acute symptoms but also long-term management of the inflammatory component of the disease.

Pharmacotherapy of Asthma   The recognition of asthma as an inflammatory condition that should be treated with anti-inflammatory agents has led to the use of corticosteroids for treatment. Because corticosteroids inhibit mediator release from eosinophils and macrophages, inhibit the late response to allergens, and reduce hyperresponsiveness of the bronchioles, they have become the first-line therapy for chronic asthma (236). Inhaled steroids have greatly reduced the steroid dose required to achieve optimal results. The steroid effect is dose related, but many patients with asthma can achieve control using low-dose inhaled steroids (<1000 g/day). Onset of action is slow (several hours) and up to 3 months of steroid therapy may be required for optimal improvement of bronchial hyperresponsiveness. Even with acute exacerbation of asthma, steroid treatment can enhance the beneficial effect of beta-adrenergic treatment.

During acute exacerbations of asthma, a short course of oral steroids may be necessary, in addition to inhaled steroids. For adults with chronic asthma, however, only a minority will require chronic oral steroid therapy. Patients taking oral steroids should receive intravenous steroid support perioperatively.

Until recently, beta$_2$-adrenergic agonists were considered the first-line drugs for asthma. These drugs, inhaled four to six times daily, rapidly relax smooth muscle in the airways and are effective for up to 6 hours. Studies of beta$_2$ agonists in chronic asthma, however, have failed to show any influence of these agents on the inflammatory component of asthma. Furthermore, it has been suggested that the long-term use of this class of drugs can lead to a worsening of asthma (236). Thus, beta$_2$ agonists are now recommended for use for short-term relief of bronchospasm or as first-line treatment for patients with very infrequent symptoms or symptoms provoked solely by exercise (237).

Methylxanthines, such as *theophylline,* have been relegated to third-line status in the management of asthma. It is doubtful whether these drugs have any additional benefit in patients who are using maximal inhaler therapy. The xanthines are limited by their narrow therapeutic window. It is necessary to achieve a serum concentration of at least 10 g/ml, but at levels higher than 20 g/ml, significant toxicity develops, including nausea, tremor, and central nervous system excitation. Xanthines have a limited anti-inflammatory effect and no effect on bronchial hyperresponsiveness or eosinophilic degranulation. In addition, plasma concentrations can be altered by drugs or environmental factors, requiring an adjustment in the *theophylline* dose. Smoking and *phenobarbital* use, for example, increase clearance of *theophylline* by the liver, whereas clearance of *theophylline* is decreased with hepatic disease and cardiac failure or with the concomitant use of certain drugs, including *ciprofloxacin, cimetidine, erythromycin,* and *troleandomycin.*

Anticholinergic agents are weak bronchodilators that work via inhibition of muscarinic receptors in the smooth muscle of the airways. The quaternary derivatives such as ipratropium bromide (*Atrovent*) are available in an inhaled form that is not absorbed systemically. Anticholinergic drugs may provide additional benefit in conjunction with standard steroid and bronchodilator therapy but should not be used as single-agent therapy because they do not inhibit mast cell degranulation, do not have any effect on the late response to allergens, and do not have an anti-inflammatory effect.

Cromolyn sodium is highly active in the treatment of seasonal allergic asthma in children and young adults. It is usually not as effective in older patients or in patients in whom asthma is not allergic in nature (237). The drug is taken by inhalation but has a relatively short duration of action (3–4 hours). It has a mild anti-inflammatory effect but is less effective than inhaled cortical steroids, and its role as a single agent is limited.

Perioperative Management of Asthma   In patients with asthma, elective surgery should be postponed whenever possible until pulmonary function and pharmacotherapeutic management are optimized. For mild asthma, this may simply require the use of inhaled beta-adrenergic agonists preoperatively. For chronic asthma, optimization of steroid therapy will greatly decrease alveolar inflammation and bronchiolar hyperresponsiveness. Inhaled beta$_2$ agonists should be added to therapy as needed for further control of asthma. Each drug prescribed should be used in maximal dosage before adding an additional agent. For patients undergoing emergent surgery who have significant bronchoconstriction, a multimodal approach should be instituted, including aggressive bronchodilator inhalation therapy, intravenous methylxanthine administration, as well as steroid therapy. Ideally, steroid therapy can be instituted 3–6 days preoperatively. In all patients with asthma, pharmacotherapeutic response can be monitored with pulmonary function testing as demonstrated by an improvement in the peak expiratory flow rate (237).

Chronic Obstructive Pulmonary Disease

The greatest risk factor for the development of postoperative pulmonary complications is the presence of underlying chronic obstructive pulmonary disease (COPD). The term COPD has been used to encompass both chronic bronchitis and emphysema, disease entities that often occur in tandem. Cigarette smoke is implicated in the pathogenesis of both, and any treatment plan must include cessation of smoking (238). Chronic bronchitis is defined as the presence of productive cough on most days for at least 3 months per year and for at least 2 successive years (227). It is characterized by chronic airway inflammation and excessive mucus production. The histologic changes of emphysema include destruction of alveolar septa and distension of airspaces distal to terminal alveoli. The destruction of alveolar septa is most likely caused by serine elastase, released by neutrophils exposed to cigarette smoke (238). The destruction of alveoli results in air trapping, loss of pulmonary elastic recoil, collapse of the airways in expiration, increased work of breathing, significant ventilation-perfusion mismatching, and an ineffective cough (234). The impaired ability to cough effectively and clear secretions predisposes patients with COPD to atelectasis and pneumonia in the postoperative period.

The severity of obstructive disease can be quantitated with pulmonary function testing (226, 229, 239). Typically, patients with COPD will demonstrate impaired expiratory air flow, manifest by diminished forced expiratory volume (FEV_1), forced vital capacity (FVC), FEV_1/FVC, and maximal expiratory flow rate (MEFR). Arterial blood gas measurement may show varying degrees of hypoxemia and hypercapnia and can be used for prognostic purposes; PaO_2 levels lower than 70 mm Hg and $PaCO_2$ levels higher than 45 mm Hg are associated with an increase in the risk of postoperative pulmonary complications and the need for mechanical ventilation postoperatively (240).

In one study, patients with abnormal pulmonary function tests had a 70% incidence of postoperative pulmonary complications, as compared with a 3% incidence of complications in patients who had normal spirography results (229). In patients considered to be at high risk, the incidence of complications was highest in those undergoing abdominal surgery (92%) or thoracic surgery (78%) and lowest in those undergoing surgery outside the abdomen (26%).

Although *theophylline* was considered for decades to be the first-line treatment for acute exacerbations and maintenance therapy of COPD, recent evidence suggests that *theophylline* offers little benefit to maximally dosed inhaler therapy with beta$_2$-adrenergic agonists, anticholinergic receptor antagonists, and inhaled steroids. The inhaled agents are more effective than *theophylline,* are essentially devoid of significant adverse effects, and do not require serum level monitoring (226).

In patients with severe disease, maximum improvement in airflow limitation can be achieved with a therapeutic trial of high-dose oral corticosteroids followed by a 2-week trial of high-dose inhaled steroid (*beclomethasone* 1.5 mg/day or the equivalent) in addition to inhaled bronchodilator therapy. Inhaled steroids, in particular, address the inflammatory component of COPD.

In gynecologic surgical patients, the risks of postoperative pulmonary complications is confined mainly to patients with a history of heavy smoking and patients with COPD. In these patients, prophylactic measures should be instituted preoperatively and continued postoperatively to minimize the incidence of atelectasis and pneumonia. Several studies have suggested that preoperative pulmonary preparation of patients with preexisting lung disease can decrease significantly the incidence of postoperative pulmonary complications by 50–70% (241–245).

The preoperative preparation of the patient at risk for postoperative pulmonary complications should include cessation of smoking for as long as possible preoperatively. Whereas 2–3 days of smoking abstinence are sufficient for carboxyhemoglobin levels to return to normal (246), 2 months of smoking abstinence is required to significantly lower the risk of postoperative pulmonary complications (247). Longer periods of abstinence can thus be considered in patients undergoing elective surgery. In patients with severe COPD, oral and inhaled steroid therapy can be initiated 1–2 weeks preoperatively. Steroid therapy initiated preoperatively should be maintained throughout the perioperative period and then tapered postoperatively. Beta-adrenergic agonist therapy can be initiated at least 72 hours preoperatively and is beneficial in patients who have demonstrated either clinical or spirometric improvement on bronchodilators. Patients with a suppurative cough and a positive sputum culture should undergo a full course of antibiotic therapy prior to surgery. The antibiotic used should cover the most likely etiologic organisms, *Streptococcus pneumoniae* and *Haemophilus influenzae*. In any patient with acute upper respiratory infection, surgery should be delayed if possible. Instruction in deep breathing maneuvers and chest physical therapy are easily instituted and these measures can be started the evening before surgery (247).

Postoperative Pulmonary Management

Atelectasis   Atelectasis accounts for more than 90% of all postoperative pulmonary complications. The pathophysiology involves a collapse of the alveoli resulting in ventilation-perfusion mismatching, intrapulmonary venous shunting, and a subsequent drop in the PaO_2. Collapsed alveoli are susceptible to superimposed infection and, if managed improperly, atelectasis will progress to pneumonia. Patients with atelectasis have a decreased functional residual capacity (FRC) as well as decreased lung compliance, resulting in increased work during breathing. Despite the decrease in PaO_2, the PCO_2 remains unaffected unless atelectatic changes progress to large volumes of the lung or there is preexisting lung disease.

Physical findings associated with atelectasis may include a low-grade fever. Auscultation of the chest may reveal decreased breath sounds at the bases or dry rates upon inspiration. Percussion of the posterior thorax may suggest elevation of the diaphragm. Radiologic findings include the presence of horizontal lines or plates noted on the posteroanterior chest X-rays, occasionally with adjacent areas containing hyperinflation. These changes are most pronounced during the first 3 postoperative days.

Therapy for atelectasis should be aimed at expanding the alveoli and increasing the functional residual capacity. The most important maneuvers are those that promote maximal inspiratory pressure, which is maintained for as long as possible. This exercise promotes not only an expansion of the alveoli but also secretion of surfactant, which stabilizes alveoli. It can be achieved with aggressive supervised use of incentive spirometry, deep breathing exercises, coughing, and in some cases, the use of positive expiratory pressure with a mask (continuous positive airway pressure). Oversedation should be avoided, and patients should be encouraged to ambulate and change positions frequently. Fiberoptic bronchoscopy for removal of mucopurulent plugs should be reserved for patients who fail to improve with the usual measures.

Cardiogenic (High-Pressure) Pulmonary Edema   Cardiogenic pulmonary edema can result from myocardial ischemia, myocardial infarction, or from intravascular volume overload, particularly in patients who have low cardiac reserve or renal failure. The process usually begins with an increase in the fluid in the alveolar septa and bronchial vascular cuffs, ultimately seeping into the alveoli. Complete filling of the alveoli impairs secretion and production of surfactant. Concomitant with alveolar flooding, there is a decrease in lung compliance, impairment of the oxygen diffusion capacity, and an increase in the arteriolar-alveolar oxygen gradient. Ventilation-perfusion mismatching in the lung results in a decrease in the PaO_2, resulting eventually in decreased oxygenation of the tissues and impairment of cardiac contractility.

Symptoms may include tachypnea, dyspnea, wheezing, and use of the accessory muscles of respiration. Clinical signs may include distention of the jugular veins, peripheral edema, rales upon auscultation of the lungs, and an enlarged heart. Radiographic findings may include the presence of bronchiolar cuffing as well as increased interstitial fluid markings extending to the periphery of the lung. The diagnosis can be further confirmed with the use of central hemodynamic monitoring, which will denote an elevated central venous pressure and, more specifically, an elevation in the pulmonary capillary wedge pressure.

The patient's volume status should be evaluated thoroughly. In addition, myocardial ischemia or infarction should be ruled out by performing ECG and analyzing cardiac enzyme levels. The management of cardiogenic pulmonary edema includes oxygen support, aggressive diuresis, and afterload reduction to increase the cardiac output. In the absence of myocardial infarction, an inotropic agent may be used. Mechanical ventilation should be reserved for cases of acute respiratory failure.

Noncardiogenic Pulmonary Edema (Adult Respiratory Distress Syndrome)   In contrast to cardiogenic pulmonary edema, in which alveolar flooding is a result of an increase in the hydrostatic pressure of the pulmonary capillaries, alveolar flooding in patients with adult respiratory distress syndrome (ARDS) is the result of an increase in pulmonary capillary permeability. The primary pathophysiologic process is one of damage to the capillary side of the alveolar-capillary membrane (248). This damage results in rapid movement of fluid from the capillaries to the pulmonary interstitial space and, thereafter, to the alveoli. Lung compliance decreases and oxygen diffusion capacity is impaired, resulting in hypoxemia. If not managed aggressively, respiratory failure may result.

There are a number of causes as well as several distinct states of ARDS. The causes of ARDS include shock, sepsis, massive nonlung trauma (as from fractures or burns), multiple red blood cell transfusions, aspiration injury, inhalation injury, pneumonia, pancreatitis, DIC, and fat emboli (248). Irrespective of the cause, which should be identified and treated if possible, the evolving clinical picture and management are very similar.

Clinically, ARDS passes through several stages. Initially, patients develop tachypnea and dyspnea with no remarkable findings on clinical evaluation or on chest x-ray. As lung compliance becomes impaired, functional residual capacity, tidal volume, and vital capacity decrease. The PaO_2 decreases and, characteristically, increases only marginally with oxygen supplementation. Attempts to manage and treat the cause can include aggressive efforts toward hemodynamic and circulatory resuscitation in patients with shock, broad-spectrum antibiotic therapy in patients who are septic, and replacement with cryoprecipitate or FFP in patients who have DIC. An attempt should be made to maintain the arterial oxygen above 90%. This may be achievable initially by administering oxygen by mask. For patients with severe hypoxemia, endotracheal intubation with positive-pressure ventilation should be instituted.

Hemodynamic monitoring is invaluable and should be initiated early in the course of the disease process. Patients with any evidence of fluid overload should receive aggressive diuresis, whereas others may require fluid resuscitation for maintenance of tissue perfusion while the pulmonary-capillary wedge pressure is maintained below 15 mm Hg. Other measures for general care should include the placement of a nasogastric tube, gastric acid suppression with H^2 blockers, and administration of steroids in patients with the fat emboli syndrome.

With aggressive management, particularly if the inciting cause is identified and treated, ARDS can be reversed during the first 48 hours with few sequelae. After the first 48 hours, however, progression of the ARDS will cause lung damage that may leave residual pulmonary fibrosis. With progression beyond 10 days, multiorgan system failure occurs and mortality is higher than 80% (33). Guidelines for initial ventilatory support can include a respiratory rate higher than 40 per minute, arterial PO_2 lower than 70 mm Hg, PCO_2 higher than 55 mm Hg, or arterial pH lower than 7.30 (248).

600

Renal Disease

The need for surgical intervention in patients with renal impairment has resulted in the development of a very specialized medical approach to their care. Special precautions are necessary to compensate for the kidney's impaired ability to regulate fluid and electrolytes and excrete metabolic waste products. Equally important are the unique problems that develop in patients with chronic renal impairment, including an increased risk of sepsis, coagulation defects, impaired immune function and wound healing, and a propensity to develop specific acid-based abnormalities. Special consideration must be given to a variety of different medications, anesthetic agents, and numerous hematologic and nutritional factors that are important in the successful surgical care of patients with renal insufficiency.

Management of fluid levels and cardiovascular hemodynamics in patients with acute or chronic renal impairment is paramount. Intervascular fluid volume changes that lead to hypertension or hypotension are very common in these patients and are often difficult to manage secondary to autonomic dysfunction, acidosis, and other problems that are inherent to the underlying kidney disease. Patients undergoing dialysis for whom major abdominal or pelvic surgery is complicated should be treated using a Swan-Ganz catheter interoperatively and postoperatively. The results of physical examination and central venous pressure monitoring correlate poorly with left cardiac filling pressures. Swan-Ganz catheter measurements will help guide fluid replacement and avoid volume overload. Invasive hemodynamic monitoring should be continued as needed throughout the first postoperative week because "third-spacing" will occur during this period of time.

Although prompt postoperative dialysis is necessary to avoid problems associated with fluid overload and hyperkalemia, dialysis alone is not effective in correcting bleeding time and should not be the first-line approach unless additional indications for dialysis exist. A variety of methods to correct the bleeding time are listed in Table 19.15. Dialysis-dependent patients should undergo dialysis approximately 24 hours following surgery. A short-lived but rather significant fall in the number of platelets occurs during dialysis, and *heparin* is used in hemodialysis equipment to prevent clotting. If possible, dialysis should be avoided in the first 12–24 hours following surgery because of these problems. Although ischemic heart disease is the most common cause of death in patients with renal insufficiency, it is not a major cause of mortality (263). A large percentage of perioperative deaths of patients with renal insufficiency are associated with hyperkalemia that is controlled most effectively by dialysis (264).

Patients with chronic renal failure are at an increased risk for postoperative infections resulting from abnormalities in neutrophil and monocyte function (265). Appropriate preoperative antibiotic prophylaxis and an accurate assessment of nutritional status will lower the incidence of postoperative infectious complications.

The major hematologic concern in patients with chronic renal insufficiency is the increased incidence of bleeding. These bleeding problems are secondary to abnormal bleeding times and, in particular, disorders of platelet function related to a decreased amount of factor

Table 19.15   Correction of Abnormal Bleeding Times in Patients with Chronic Renal Insufficiency

Treatment	Dosage
Cryoprecipitate	4–8 units until correction of PTT is demonstrated across
Desmopressin	0.3 mg/kg q 12 and 6 hours prior to surgery
Packed red blood cells	Transfused to a hematocrit >30%
Conjugated estrogens	0.6 mg/kg/day 5 days prior to surgery

PTT, partial thromboplastin time.

VIII/von Willebrand antigen in the serum of uremic patients. Anemia, which is common in patients with renal insufficiency, can contribute to prolonged bleeding times through rheologic mechanisms (266). Abnormalities in arachidonic acid metabolism, acquired platelet storage pool deficiency, and disturbed regulation of platelet calcium content all account for an increased tendency for uremic patients to have significant bleeding during surgery (267). Therefore, the bleeding time should be routinely checked preoperatively in these patients and abnormalities should be corrected before surgery.

Normal renal function is essential for maintenance of acid-base balance in the body. Patients with renal insufficiency can have a normal anion gap or an elevated anion gap acidosis. When mild renal insufficiency develops, a normal anion gap can be seen, whereas in more significant and severe renal dysfunction, an elevated anion gap acidosis occurs. If the patient is acidotic and dialysis is not otherwise indicated, correction of the blood pH to 7.25 is indicated prior to surgery. Sodium bicarbonate should be administered according to the following formula:

$$\text{expected } HCO_3 - \text{observed } HCO_3 \times 50\% \text{ body weight}$$

It is also important to exclude other causes of elevated anion gap acidosis, e.g., ketoacidosis secondary to diabetes, lactic acidosis secondary to infection, or in rare instances, poisoning with ethylene glycol, methanol, or *aspirin*.

Impaired kidney function causes phosphate retention by the kidney and impaired vitamin D metabolism. Therefore, hypocalcemia is common in patients with renal insufficiency but tetany or other signs of hypocalcemia are relatively uncommon because metabolic acidosis raises the level of ionized calcium. Oral phosphate binders such as aluminum hydroxide (1–2 g per meal) and dietary phosphate restriction (1 g/day) is the usual treatment for hypocalcemia-hyperphosphatemia in patients with renal sufficiency. In chronic situations, because of central nervous system toxicity associated with elevated aluminum levels, it is preferable to treat hypocalcemia-hyperphosphatemia with large doses of calcium carbonate (6–12 g of elemental calcium per day) rather with than the standard aluminum-containing antacids (268).

Approximately 20% of patients with renal insufficiency will exhibit clinical evidence of protein calorie malnutrition. Vitamin deficiencies, most notably with water-soluble vitamins, also occur with dialysis. Nutritional disturbances in patients with chronic renal insufficiency arise secondary to deficiencies in protein intake, and studies have shown that the kidney in patients with chronic renal insufficiency is hyperfiltrating (269). Low-protein diets are effective in preventing end-stage renal failure. Ample caloric intake (usually 30 kcal/kg) is necessary to prevent protein breakdown necessary for caloric supplementation. Postoperatively, both protein and caloric intake may need to be dramatically increased to meet catabolic demands in surgical patients. As much as 1.5 g/kg of protein and 45 kcal/kg calories may be needed (269).

Wound healing is impaired in patients with chronic renal failure, and wound dehiscence and evisceration are potential problems. Wound healing is most appropriately aided by nutritional assessment preoperatively and maintenance of adequate caloric and protein intake in the perioperative setting. Antibiotic prophylaxis should be used in these patients, and uremia should be treated with dialysis as indicated. A running mass-closure of the midline vertical incision with continuous running monofilament sutures should be used to further lower the risk of wound dehiscence and evisceration (270).

Patients with chronic renal disease have an altered ability to excrete drugs and are prone to significant metabolic derangements secondary to the altered bioavailability of many commonly used medications. Because of this, as well as the effect of dialysis on drug pharmacokinetics, the gynecologic surgeon and nephrologist must be aware of the lowered metabolism and bioavailability of narcotics, barbiturates, muscle relaxants, antibiotics, and other drugs that require renal clearance. Of particular note is the inability of patients with renal insufficiency to clear the neuromuscular blockade caused by *pancuronium* (271). Care must be taken with *d-tubocurarine,* especially if repeated doses are given (272). *Vecuronium* and *atracurium* have been safely used in patients with renal failure and apparently do not require renal elimination (273, 274). One final note is that *succinylcholine* has been reported to cause significant hyperkalemic responses in patients with renal failure (275). *Succinylcholine* can be used safely in patients with chronic renal insufficiency. Careful monitoring of the serum potassium level is necessary.

Perioperative acute renal failure in previously normal patients may be divided into cases caused by decreased renal perfusion, those caused by nephrotoxins, or those perhaps caused by both. Patients with impaired cardiac function, intravascular volume depletion, sepsis, or hypotension fall under the first category. Nephrotoxic medications such as immunoglycosides, chemotherapeutic agents such as *cisplatin,* or iodinated contrast agents fall under the second category (276–278). The risk of renal impairment becomes cumulative if more than one of these factors exist at the same time and especially if a variety of factors are associated with intervascular volume depletion (279). Several measures should be used to avoid acute renal failure. All nephrotoxic drugs should be discontinued when possible and, when not practical, strict attention should be paid to the pharmacokinetic characteristics of each drug as well as to the regular measurements of the serum creatinine. Patients with diabetes should be given reduced doses of radiocontrast agents and should be well hydrated, because they are particularly susceptible to renal injury from these materials (280). Volume repletion is essential to lower the incidence of renal impairment (281).

Liver Disease

Management of perioperative problems in gynecologic patients with liver disease requires a comprehensive understanding of normal liver physiology and the pathophysiology underlying diseases of the liver that may complicate surgery or recovery. Patients with liver disease often have numerous complicated problems involving nutrition, coagulation, electrolytes, wound healing, encephalopathy, and infection.

History and Physical Examination

Patients with a history of alcohol abuse, drug use, hepatitis, jaundice, or blood product exposure or a family member with liver disease should undergo biochemical evaluation. During the physical examination, note should be made of any jaundice, signs of muscle wasting, ascites, right upper quadrant tenderness, or hepatomegaly.

Laboratory Testing

The biochemical profile (alkaline phosphatase, calcium, lactic acid dehydrogenase, bilirubin, serum glutamic-oxaloacetic transaminase, cholesterol, uric acid, phosphorous, albumin, total protein, and glucose) has not been shown to be useful for routine preoperative evaluation (249). Mild abnormalities lead to further extensive testing requiring consultation, delays in surgery, and increased cost without net benefit. A possible exception is selected use of biochemical testing when the history or physical examination reveals abnormalities. Patients with known liver disease should undergo albumin and bilirubin testing using the Child's risk classification (Table 19.16). This system was originally designed to predict mortality following portosystemic shunt surgery and divides patients into three classes of severity based on five easily assessed clinical parameters. Measurement of prothrombin time may also be helpful in patients with significant histories of liver disease. If a history of hepatitis is ascertained, the patient should be tested with serum aminotransferase, alkaline phosphatase, bilirubin, and albumin. Consideration should also be given to serologic documentation of hepatitis if the patient's history of risk factors is significant. If a patient has a known malignancy, there may be some benefit from biochemical testing of the liver as a screen for metastatic disease, although this has not been proven conclusively.

Table 19.16   Child's Classification of Liver Dysfunction

| Parameter | Child Classification | | |
	A	B	C
Bilirubin	<2.0	2.0–3.0	>3.0
Albumin	>3.5	3.0–3.5	<3.0
Ascites	None	Easily controlled	Poorly controlled
Encephalopathy	None	Mild	Advanced
Nutritional status	Excellent	Good	Poor

Anesthesia

With few exceptions, most anesthetic agents, including those administered by epidural or spinal routes, reduce hepatic blood flow and decrease oxygenation of the liver. *Halothane, enflurane,* and *isoflurane* result in a decreased cardiac output secondary to a decrease in preload from the vasodilation that occurs peripherally. Spinal and epidural anesthetics reduce preload to the heart and cardiac output by peripheral vasodilation. Other perioperative factors—hemorrhage, intraoperative hypotension, hypercarbia, congestive heart failure, and intermittent positive pressure ventilation, especially in critically ill patients—lead to decreased hepatic perfusion and hypoxia (250).

Drug Metabolism

Patients with altered liver function should be carefully monitored because of the prolonged action of many medications used during surgery. In addition to impaired metabolism, hypoalbuminemia causes decreases in drug binding, which alters serum levels and biliary clearance rates. The degree of hepatic metabolism varies greatly, depending on the type of medication being considered. For inhalational anesthetics, *isoflurane* is preferred because it undergoes minimal hepatic metabolism in comparison with *halothane* or *enflurane.* Narcotics, induction agents, sedatives, and neuromuscular blocking agents all undergo abnormal metabolism in patients with decompensated liver disease. *Diazepam, meperidine,* and *phenobarbital* cause prolonged depression of consciousness and may precipitate hepatic encephalopathy because of their altered rates of clearance. *Sufentanyl* and *oxazepam,* which are not affected by altered liver function, are the preferred narcotics and benzodiazepines for patients with altered liver function. Muscle relaxants, such as *D-tubocurarine, pancuronium,* and *vecuronium,* cause prolonged neuromuscular blockade in patients with impaired liver function and are not ideal drugs to use in this situation. *Atracurim* is the preferred muscle relaxant for patients abnormal hepatic function. *Succinylcholine* metabolism is greatly prolonged in patients with hepatic dysfunction and must be used with great caution.

Determination of Operative Risk

Although it is well known that acute hepatobiliary damage results in increased morbidity and mortality in the surgical patient, estimating the operative risk in patients with hepatic dysfunction is troublesome because it is often difficult to determine which patients are at risk based on the history and physical examination. The most accurate method for risk assessment of surgery in patients with hepatic dysfunction is made using Child's classification (Table 19.16). Using this system, accurate assessment of morbidity and mortality can be directly related to the degree of liver dysfunction (251). The Child's classification has been shown to be useful for patients undergoing a variety of different types of abdominal surgery. Operative mortalities of 10%, 31%, and 76% have been reported for each of the three Child's classifications, respectively (252). The major cause of perioperative death was sepsis. This classification correlated significantly with postoperative complications such as bleeding, renal failure, wound dehiscence, and sepsis.

Acute Viral Hepatitis

Acute viral hepatitis poses an increased risk of operative complications and perioperative mortality and, therefore, elective surgery is contraindicated (253). Elective surgery should be delayed for approximately 1 month after the results of all biochemical tests have returned to normal (254). In patients with ectopic pregnancy, hemorrhage, or bowel obstruction secondary to malignancy, however, surgical intervention must take place before normalization of serum transaminase (253). In these "urgent" situations, the perioperative morbidity (12%) and mortality (9.5%) are much higher than when they are performed under ideal situations (254).

Chronic Hepatitis

Chronic hepatitis refers to a group of disorders characterized by inflammation of the liver for at least 3–6 months. The disease is divided by morphologic and clinical criteria into chronic persistent hepatitis and chronic active hepatitis. A liver biopsy is usually required to establish the extent and type of injury. The surgical risk in these patients correlates most closely with the disease severity. The risk of surgery in patients with asymptomatic or mild disease is minimal, in contrast to a significant risk for those patients who have symptomatic chronic active hepatitis (255). Elective surgery is contraindicated in symptomatic patients and nonelective surgery is associated with significant morbidity (254). In the nonelective situation, patients taking chronic corticosteroid therapy should be given appropriate "stress" coverage with a higher dose of corticosteroids during the perioperative period. Preoperatively, patients who are not taking steroids should receive *prednisone* and *azathioprine,* which have been shown to reduce the perioperative risk of complications and may result in remission in up to 80% of patients (256). More recently, a controlled randomized trial of prednisone and interferon-α has documented regression of the hepatitis B core antigen (HbcAg) and hepatitis B viral DNA replication in approximately 30% of patients (257). Consideration should be given to this regimen for patients in whom surgery cannot be avoided.

Asymptomatic carriers of the hepatitis B virus (individuals who test positive for the hepatitis B surface antigen) are not at increased risk for postoperative complications in the absence of elevated aminotransferase levels and liver inflammation. There is, however, a significant risk to the health care professional when operating on these individuals, and hepatitis B immune globulin should be administered immediately to unvaccinated medical personnel who sustain accidental needle sticks. A vaccination series should then be initiated in the early postoperative period. All medical personnel, particularly those in the surgical subspecialties, should receive a full course of recombinant hepatitis B vaccine as recommended by the Immunizations Practices Advisory Committee (258).

Alcoholic Liver Disease

Alcoholic liver disease encompasses a spectrum of diseases including fatty liver, acute alcoholic hepatitis, and cirrhosis. Elective surgery is not contraindicated in patients with fatty liver because liver function is preserved. If nutritional deficiencies are discovered, they should be corrected prior to elective surgery. Acute alcoholic hepatitis is characterized on biopsy by hepatocyte edema, polymorphonuclear leukocyte infiltration, necrosis, and the presence of Mallory bodies. Elective surgery in these patients is contraindicated (259). Abstinence from alcohol for approximately 6–12 weeks along with the clinical resolution of the biochemical abnormalities are recommended before surgery is considered. Severe alcoholic hepatitis may persist for several months, despite abstinence, and if any question of continued activity exists, a liver biopsy should be repeated (260).

Cirrhosis

Cirrhosis is an irreversible liver lesion characterized histologically by parenchymal necrosis, nodular degeneration, fibrosis, and a disorganization of hepatic lobular architecture. The most serious complication of cirrhosis is portal venous hypertension that ultimately leads to bleeding from esophageal varices, ascites, and hepatic encephalopathy. Conventional liver biochemical test results correlate poorly with the degree of liver impairment in patients with cirrhosis. Hepatic dysfunction, however, may be somewhat quantitated by low albumin levels and prolonged prothrombin times.

Surgical risk is clearly increased in patients with cirrhosis, although it is substantially greater in emergency surgery than in elective surgery. Perioperative mortality correlates with the severity of cirrhosis and can be estimated through the use of a Child's classification (Table 19.16). Surgery in patients with a Child class A cirrhosis can usually be performed without significant risk, whereas surgery in patients with Child's class B or C poses a major risk and requires careful preoperative consideration (261). Meticulous preoperative preparation may improve the surgical outcome (262).

References

1. **Rohrer MJ, Michelotti MC, Nahrwold DL.** A prospective evaluation of the efficacy of preoperative coagulation testing. *Ann Surg* 1989;208:554–7.

2. **Lamers RJ, van Engelshoven JM, Pfaff A.** Once again, the routine preoperative thorax photo. *Ned Tijdschr Geneeskd* 1989;133:2288–91.

3. **Loder RE.** Routine preoperative chest radiography. *Anesthesiology* 1987;66:195–8.

4. **Piscitelli JT, Simel DL, Addison WA.** Who should have intravenous pyelograms before hysterectomy for benign disease? *Obstet Gynecol* 1987;69:541–5.

5. **Easley HA, Hammond CB.** Informed consent in obstetrics and gynecology. *Postgrad Obstet Gynecol* 1986;10:1–12.

6. **Roubenoff R, Roubenoff RA, Preto J, Balke CW.** Malnutrition among hospitalized patients: a problem of physician awareness. *Arch Intern Med* 1987;147:1462–5.

7. **Butterworth CE Jr, Weinsier RL.** Malnutrition in hospitalized patients: assessment and treatment. In: **Goodhart RS, Shils ME,** eds. *Modern Nutrition in Health and Disease*. 6th ed. Philadelphia: Lea & Febiger, 1980.

8. **Bistrian BR, Blackburn GL, Hallowell E, Heddle R.** Protein status of general surgical patients. *JAMA* 1974;230:858–60.

9. **Hill GL, Blackett RL, Pickford I, Burkinshaw L, Young GA, Warren JV, et al.** Malnutrition in surgical patients: an unrecognized problem. *Lancet* 1977;1:689–92.

10. **Bozzetti F, Migliavacca S, Gallus G, Radaelli G, Scotti A, Bonalumi MG, et al.** "Nutritional" markers as prognostic indicators of postoperative sepsis in cancer patients. *JPEN* 1985;9:464–7.

11. **Blackburn GL, Bistrian BR, Maini BS, Schlamm HT, Smith MF.** Nutritional and metabolic assessment of the hospitalized patient. *JPEN* 1977;1:11–22.

12. **Shizgal HM, Spanier AH, Kurtz RS.** Effect of parenteral nutrition on body composition in the critically ill patient. *Am J Surg* 1976;131:156–61.

13. **Hill GL, Beddoe AH.** In vivo neutron activation in metabolic and nutritional studies. *J Clin Surg* 1982;1:270.

14. **Bistrian BR.** Nutritional assessment of the hospitalized patient: a practical approach. In: **Wright RA, Heymsfield SN,** eds. *Nutritional Assessment*. Boston: Blackwell Scientific Publications, Inc., 1984:183.

15. **Mullen JL, Buzby GP, Matthews DC, Smale BF, Rosato EF.** Reduction of operative morbidity and mortality by combined preoperative and postoperative nutritional support. *Ann Surg* 1980;192:604–13.

16. **Heymsfield SB, Horowitz J, Lawson DH.** Enteral hyperalimentation. In: **Berk JE,** ed. *Developments in Digestive Diseases*. Vol. 3. Philadelphia: Lea & Febiger, 1980:59–83.

17. **Holter AR, Rosen HM, Fisher JE.** The effects of hyperalimentation on major surgery in patients with malignant disease: a prospective study. *Acta Chir Scand* 1975;466(Suppl):86–90.

18. **Sako K, Lore JM, Kaufman S, Razack MS, Bakmajian V, Reese P.** Parenteral hyperalimentation in surgical patients with head and neck cancer: a randomized study. *J Surg Oncol* 1981;16:391–402.

19. **Thompson BR, Julian TB, Stremple JF.** Perioperative total parenteral nutrition in patients with gastrointestinal cancer. *J Surg Res* 1981;30:497–501.

20. **Bellantone R, Doglietto G, Bossola M, Pacelli F, Negro F, Sofo L, et al.** Preoperative parenteral nutrition of malnourished surgical patients. *Acta Chir Scand* 1988;154:249–51.

21. **Veterans Affairs.** Total parenteral nutrition cooperative study group. Preoperative total parenteral nutrition in surgical patients. *N Engl J Med* 1991;352:525–32.

22. **Twomey PL, Patching SC.** Cost-effectiveness of nutritional support. *JPEN* 1985;9:3–10.

23. **Soper JT, Berchuck A, Creasman WT, Clarke-Pearson DL.** Pelvic exenteration: factors associated with major surgical morbidity. *Gynecol Oncol* 1989;35:93–8.

24. **Pestana C.** *Fluids and Electrolytes in the Surgical Patient.* 4th ed. Baltimore: Williams & Wilkins, 1989.

25. **Miller TA, Duke JH.** Fluid and electrolyte management. In: **Dudrick SJ, Baue AE, Eiseman B, MacLean LD, Rowe MI, Sheldon GF,** eds. *Manual of Preoperative and Postoperative Care.* Philadelphia: WB Saunders Co., 1983:38–67.

26. **Narins RG, Lazarus MJ.** Renal systems. In: **Vandam LD,** ed. *To Make the Patient Ready for Anesthesia: Medical Care of the Surgical Patient.* 2nd ed. Stoneham, MA: Butterworth, 1984: 67–114.

27. **Demling RH, Wilson RF.** Fluids, electrolytes, and acid-base balance. In: **Demling RH, Wilson RF,** eds. *Decision Making in Surgical Critical Care. Philadelphia:* BC Decker Inc, 1988:114–57.

28. **Edwards TW.** Optimizing opioid treatment of postoperative pain. *J Pain Symptom Man* 1990; 5:S24–6.

29. **Kuhn S, Cooke K, Collins M, Jones JM, Mucklow JC.** Perceptions of pain relief after surgery. *BMJ* 1990;300:1687–90.

30. **Donovan M, Dillon P, McGuire L.** Incidence and characteristics of pain in a sample of medical-surgical patients. *Pain* 1987;30:69–73.

31. **Oden V.** Acute postoperative pain: incidence, severity, and the itiology of inadequate treatment. *Anesth Clin North Am* 1989;7:1–5.

32. **Marks RM, Sachar EJ.** Undertreatment of medical inpatients with narcotic analgesics. *Ann Intern Med* 1973;78:173–8.

33. **Smith G.** Management of postoperative pain. *Can J Anaesth* 1989;36:S1–10.

34. **Austin KL, Stapleton JV, Mather LE.** Multiple intramuscular injections: a major source of variability in analgesic response to meperidine. *Pain* 1980;8:47–51.

35. **Forest WH Jr, Smethurst PWR, Kienitz ME.** Self administration of intravenous analgesics. *Anesthesiology* 1970;33:363–6.

36. **Keeri-Szanto M.** Apparatus for demand analgesia. *Can Anaesth Soc J* 1971;18:581–6.

37. **Sechzer PH.** Studies in pain with the analgesic-demand system. *Anesth Analg* 1971;50:1–10.

38. **Egbert Am, Parks LH, Short LM, Burnett ML.** Randomized trial of postoperative patient-controlled analgesia vs intramuscular narcotics in frail elderly men. *Arch Intern Med* 1990;150: 1897–901.

39. **Lange MP, Dahn MS, Jacobs LA.** Patient-controlled analgesia versus intermittent analgesia dosing. *Heart Lung* 1988;17:495–9.

40. **De Conno F, Ripamonti C, Gamba A, Prada A, Ventafridda V.** Treatment of postoperative pain: comparison between administration at fixed hours and "on demand" with intramuscular analgesics. *Eur J Surg Oncol* 1989;15:242–6.

41. **Rose PG, Piver MS, Batista E, Lau T.** Patient-controlled analgesia in gynecologic oncology: a comparative analysis. *J Reprod Med* 1989;34:651–6.

42. **Zacharias M, Pfeifer MV, Herbison P.** Comparison of two methods of intravenous administration of morphine for post-operative pain relief. *Anaesth Intensive Care* 1990;18:205–9.

43. **White PF.** Patient-controlled analgesia: an update on its use in the treatment of postoperative pain. *Anesth Clin North Am* 1989;7:63–70.

44. **Ellis R, Haines D, Shah R, Cotton BR, Smith G.** Pain relief after abdominal surgery: comparison of IM morphine, sublingual buprenorphine, and self-administered IV pethidine. *Br J Anaesth* 1982;54:421–6.

45. **Welchew FA.** On-demand analgesia: a double-blind comparison of on-demand intravenous fentanyl with regular intramuscular morphine. *Anaesthesia* 1983;38:18–24.

46. **Dahl JB, Daugaard JJ, Larsen HV, Mouridsen P, Nielsen TH, Kristoffersen E.** Patient-controlled analgesia: a controlled trial. *Acta Anaesth Scand* 1987;31:744–7.

47. **White PF.** Mishpas with patient-controlled analgesia (PCA). *Anesthesiology* 1987;66:81–6.

48. **Rapp SE, Ready LB, Greer BE.** Postoperative pain management in gynecologic oncology patients utilizing epidural opiate analgesia and patient-controlled analgesia. *Gynecol Oncol* 1989;35:341–8.

49. **Lutz LJ, Lamer TJ.** Management of postoperative pain: review of current techniques and methods. *Mayo Clin Proc* 1990;65:584–90.

50. **Dodson ME.** Postoperative pain relief. In: **Nunn JF, Utting JE, Brown BR Jr,** eds. *General Anesthesia.* 5th ed. Stoneham, MA: Butterworth, 1989:1123–40.

51. **Vercauteren M, Lauwers E, Meert T, De Hert S, Adriaensen H.** Comparison of epidural sufentanil plus clonidine with sufentanil alone for postoperative pain relief. *Anaesthesiology* 1990;45:531–4.

52. **Trotter JP, Reinhart SP, Katz RM, Glazier HS.** Economic assessment of ketorolac versus narcotic analgesics in postoperative pain management. *Clin Ther* 1993;15:938–48.

53. **Wong DH, Weber EC, Schell MJ, Wong AB, Anderson CT, Barker SJ.** Factors associated with postoperative pulmonary complications in patients with severe chronic obstructive pulmonary disease. *Anesth Analg* 1995;80:276–84.

54. **DeAndrade JR, Maslanka M, Maneatis T, Bynum L, Burchmore M.** The use of ketorolac in the management of postoperative pain. *Orthopedics* 1994;7:57–166.

55. **Mather LE.** Do the pharmacodynamics of the nonsteroidal anti-inflammatory drugs suggest a role in the management of postoperative pain? *Drugs* 1992;44(Suppl 5):1–12.

56. **Kinney JM, Long CL, Gump FE, Duke JH.** Tissue composition of weight loss in surgical patients. I. Elective operation. *Ann Surg* 1968;168:459–74.

57. **Ready LB.** Acute postoperative pain. In: **Miller RD,** ed. *Anesthesia.* Vol. II, 4th ed. New York: Churchill-Livingstone, 1994:2327–34.

58. **Stahlgren LR, Trierweiler M, Tommeraasen M, Mehlisch D, Otterson W, Maneatis T, et al.** Comparison of ketorolac and meperidine in patients with postoperative pain—impact no health care utilization. *Clin Ther* 1993;15:571–80.

59. **Flynn NM.** Reducing the risk of infection in surgical patients. In: **Bolt RJ,** ed. *Medical Evaluation of the Surgical Patient.* Mt. Kisco, NY: Rutura Publishing Co., 1987:195–240.

60. **Ledger WJ, Gee C, Lewis WP.** Guidelines for antibiotic prophylaxis in gynecology. *Am J Obstet Gynecol* 1975;121:1038–45.

61. **Hirsch HA.** Prophylactic antibiotics in obstetrics and gynecology. *Am J Med* 1985;78:170–6.

62. **Shapiro M, Munoz A, Tager IB, Schoenbaum SC, Polk BF, et al.** Risk factors for infection at the operative site after abdominal of vaginal hysterectomy. *N Engl J Med* 1982;307:1661–6.

63. **Haley RW, Culver DH, Morgan WM, White JW, Emori G, Hooton TM.** Identifying patients at high risk of surgical wound infection. A simple multivariate index of patient susceptibility and wound contamination. *Am J Epidemiol* 1985;121:206–15.

64. **Roy S, Wilkins J, Galaif E, Azen C.** Comparative efficacy and safety of cefmetazole or cefoxitin in the prevention of postoperative infection following vaginal and abdominal hysterectomy. *J Antimicrob Chemother* 1989;23:109–17.

65. **Trimbos JB, van Lindert AC, Heintz APM, Mattic H, Smit I.** Piperacillin for prophylaxis in gynecological surgery. *Eur J Obstet Gynecol Reprod Biol* 1989;30:141–9.

66. **Davey PG, Duncan ID, Edward D, Scott AC.** Cost-benefit analysis of cephradine and mezlocillin prophylaxis for abdominal and vaginal hysterectomy. *Br J Obstet Gynaecol* 1988;95:1170–7.

67. **Munck JM, Jensen HK.** Preoperative clindamycin treatment and vaginal drainage in hysterectomy. *Acta Obstet Gynecol Scand* 1989;68:241–5.

68. **Gerber B, Wilken H.** Effectiveness of perioperative preventive use of antibiotics with metroidazone or doxycycline in vaginal hysterectomy. *Zentralbl Gynakol* 1989;111:1542–8.

69. **Friese S, Willems FT, Loriaux Sm, Meewis JM.** Prophylaxis in gynaecological surgery: a prospective randomized comparison between single dose prophylaxis with amoxycillin/clavu-

lanate and the combination of cefuroxime and metronidazole. *J Antimicrob Chemother* 1989; 24:213–6.

70. **Chodak GW.** Use of systemic antibiotics for prophylaxis in surgery. *Arch Surg* 1977;112: 326–34.

71. **Burke JF.** The effective period of preventive antibiotic action in experimental incisions and dermal lesions. *Surgery* 1961;50:161–8.

72. **Hemsell DL, Martin JN Jr, Pastorek JG II, Nobles BJ, Hemsell PG, Helman N, et al.** Single-dose antimicrobial prophylaxis at abdominal hysterectomy. Cefamandole vs cefotaxime. *J Reprod Med* 1988;33:939–44.

73. **Hemsell DL, Johnson EF, Heard MC, Hemsell PG, Nobles BJ, Bawdon RE.** Single-dose piperacillin versus triple-dose cefoxitin prophylaxis at vaginal and abdominal hysterectomy. *South Med J* 1989;82:438–42.

74. **Hemsell DL, Bernstein SG, Bawdon RE, Hemsell PG, Heard MC, Hobles BJ.** Preventing major operative site infection after radical abdominal hysterectomy and pelvic lymphadenectomy. *Gynecol Oncol* 1989;35:55–60.

75. **Orr JW Jr, Sisson PF, Patsner B, Barrett JM, Ellington JR Jr, Jennings RH Jr, et al.** Single-dose antibiotic prophylaxis for patients undergoing extended pelvic surgery for gynecologic malignancy. *Am J Obstet Gynecol* 1990;162:718–21.

76. **Brachman PS, Dan BB, Haley RW, Hooton TM, Garner JS, Allen JR.** Nosocomial surgical infections: incidence and cost. *Surg Clin North Am* 1980;60:15–25.

77. **Garibaldi RA, Brodine S, Matsumiya S, Colemen M.** Evidence for the noninfectious etiology of early postoperative fever. *Infect Control* 1985;6:273–6.

78. **Hemsell DL.** Infections after gynecologic surgery. *Obstet Gynecol Clin North Am* 1989;16: 381–5.

79. **Bartzen PJ, Hafferty FW.** Pelvic laparotomy without an indwelling catheter. A retrospective review of 949 cases. *Am J Obstet Gynecol* 1987;156:1426–30.

80. **Kingdom JCP, Kitchener HC, MacLean AB.** Postoperative urinary tract infection in gynecology: implications for an antibiotic prophylaxis policy. *Obstet Gynecol* 1990;76:636–40.

81. **Ireland D, Tacchi D, Bint AJ.** Effect of single-dose prophylactic co-trimoxazole on the incidence of gynaecological post-operative urinary tract infection. *Br J Obstet Gynaecol* 1982; 89:578–82.

82. **Boyd ME.** Postoperative gynecologic infections. *Can J Surg* 1987;30:7–12.

83. **Kunin CM.** Urinary tract infections. *Surg Clin North Am* 1980;60:223–7.

84. **Harkness GA, Bentley DW, Roghmann KJ.** Risk factors for nosocomial pneumonia in the elderly. *Am J Med* 1990;89:457–60.

85. **Eikhoff TC.** Pulmonary infections in surgical patients. *Surg Clin North Am* 1980;60:175–80.

86. **Tomford JW, Hershey CO, McLaren CE, Porter DK, Cohen DI.** Intravenous therapy team and peripheral venous catheter-associated complications. *Arch Intern Med* 1984;144:1191–4.

87. **Hershey Co, Tomford JW, McLaren CE, Porter DK, Cohen DI.** The natural history of intravenous catheter-associated phlebitis. *Arch Intern Med* 1984;144;1373–5.

88. **Cruse PJE, Ford R.** The epidemiology of wound infection: a 10-year prospective study of 62,939 wounds. *Surg Clin North Am* 1980;60:27–32.

89. **Brown SE, Allen HH, Robins RN.** The use of delayed primary wound closure in preventing wound infections. *Am J Obstet Gynecol* 1977;127:713–7.

90. **Crombleholme WR, Schachter J, Ohm-Smith M, Luft J, Whidden R, Sweet RL.** Efficacy of single-agent therapy for the treatment of acute pelvic inflammatory disease with ciprofloxacin. *Am J Med* 1989;87:142–50.

91. **Crombleholme WR, Ohm-Smith M, Robbie MO, DeKay V, Sweet RL.** Ampicillin/sulbactam versus metronidazole/gentamicin in the treatment of soft tissue infections. *Am J Obstet Gynecol* 1987;156:507–12.

92. **Cunningham FG.** Treatment and prevention of female pelvic infection: the quest for single agent therapy. *Am J Obstet Gynecol* 1987;157:485–90.

93. **Hemsell DL, Heard MC, Hemsell PG.** Single-agent therapy for women with acute polymicrobial pelvic infections. *Am J Obstet Gynecol* 1987;157:488–92.

94. **Riseman JA, Zamboni WA, Curtis A, Graham DR, Konrad HR, Ross DS.** Hyperbaric oxygen therapy for necrotizing fasciitis reduces mortality and the need for debridements. *Surgery* 1990;108:847–51.

95. **Meleney RL.** Hemolytic streptococcus gangrene. *Arch Surg* 1925;9:317–21.

96. **Umbert IJ, Winkelmann MD, Oliver GF, Peters MS.** Necrotizing fasciitis: a clinical, microbiologic, and histopathologic study of 14 patients. *J Am Acad Dermatol* 1989;20:774–81.

97. **Wilkerson R, Paull W, Coville FV.** Necrotizing fasciitis: review of the literature and case report. *Clin Orthop* 1987;216:187–92.

98. **Marrie TJ, Costerton JW.** In vivo ultrastructural study of microbes in necrotizing fasciitis. *Eur J Clin Microbiol Infect Dis* 1988;7:51–8.

99. **Clayton MD, Fowler JE, Sharifi R, Pearl RK.** Causes, presentation and survival of fifty-seven patients with necrotizing fasciitis of the male genitalia. *Surg Gynecol Obstet* 1990; 170:49–53.

100. **Sudarsky LA, Laschinger JC, Coppa GF, Spencer FC.** Improved results from a standardized approach in treatment patients with necrotizing fasciitis. *Ann Surg* 1989;206:661–7.

101. **Fisher JR, Conway MJ, Takeshita RT, Sandoual MR.** Necrotizing fasciitis: importance of roentgenographic studies for soft tissue gas. *JAMA* 1979;241:803–9.

102. **Hirn M, Niinikoski J.** Management of perineal necrotizing fasciitis (Fournier's gangrene). *Ann Chir Gynaecol* 1989;78:277–81.

103. **Stamenkovic I, Lew PD.** Early recognition of potentially fatal necrotizing fasciitis. The use of frozen-section biopsy. *N Engl J Med* 1984;310:1689–92.

104. **Rothman PA, Wiskind AK, Dudley AG.** Amniotic membranes in the treatment of necrotizing fasciitis complicating vulvar herpes virus infection. *Obstet Gynecol* 1989;74:483–9.

105. **Hoffman MS, Turhquist DT.** Necrotizing fasciitis of the vulva during chemotherapy. *Obstet Gynecol* 1989;74:483–9.

106. **Cruikshank SH, McLauchlan L.** A de novo case of vulvar synergistic necrotizing fasciitis. *Obstet Gynecol* 1987;69:516–20.

107. **Frolich EP, Schein M.** Necrotizing fasciitis arising from Bartholin's abscess: case report and review of literature. *Isr J Med Sci* 1989;25:644–9.

108. **Cederna JP, Davies BW, Farkas SA, Sonta JA, Sworniowski T.** Necrotizing fasciitis of the total abdominal wall after sterilization by partial salpingectomy. *Am J Obstet Gynecol* 1990;163:138–9.

109. **Ahrenholz DH.** Surgical spectrum. Clinical skin and soft tissue infection. *Physicians World Communications (Monograph).* West Point, PA: Merck, Sharpe and Dohme, 1988:16–24.

110. **Eltorai IM, Hart GB, Strauss MB, Montroy R, Juler GL.** The role of hyperbaric oxygen in the management of Fournier's gangrene. *Int Surg* 1986;71:53–8.

111. **Kaiser PE, Cerra FB.** Progressive necrotizing surgical infections: a unified approach. *J Trauma* 1981;21:349–53.

112. **Robson MC, Krizek TJ, Koss N, Samburg JC.** Amniotic membranes as a temporary wound dressing. *Surg Gynecol Obstet* 1973;136:904–9.

113. **Beck DE, Harford FJ, DiPalma JA.** Comparison of cleansing methods in preparation for colonic surgery. *Dis Colon Rectum* 1985;28:491–5.

114. **Clarke JS, Condon RE, Bartlett JG, Gorbach SL, Nichols RL, Ochi S.** Preoperative oral antibiotics reduce septic complications of colon operations: results of prospective, randomized, double-blind clinical study. *Ann Surg* 1977;186:251–9.

115. **Fry DE.** Antibiotics in surgery: an overview. *Ann Surg* 1988;155(5A):11–5.

116. **Menaker GJ.** The use of antibiotics in surgical treatment of the colon. *Gynecol Obstet* 1987; 164:581–6.

117. **Wolfson PJ, Bauer JJ, Gelernt IM, Kreel I, Aufses AH Jr.** Use of the long tube in the management of patients with small intestinal obstruction due to adhesions. *Arch Surg* 1985;120: 1001–6.

118. **Ratcliff JB, Kapernick P, Brooks GG, Dunnihoo DR.** Small bowel obstruction and previous gynecologic surgery. *South Med J* 1983;76:1349–50, 1360.

119. **Jeffcoate TNA, Tindall VR.** Venous thrombosis and embolism in obstetrics and gynecology. *Aust N Z J Obstet Gynaecol* 1965;5:119–30.

120. **Kimball AM, Hallum VA, Cates W.** Deaths caused by pulmonary thromboembolism after legally induced abortion. *Am J Obstet Gynecol* 1978;132:169–74.

121. **Clarke-Pearson DL, Jelovsek FR, Creasman WT.** Thromboembolism complicating surgery for cervical and uterine malignancy: incidence, risk factors, and prophylaxis. *Obstet Gynecol* 1983;61:87–94.

122. **Creasman WT, Weed JC Jr.** Radical hysterectomy. In: **Schaefer G, Grager EA,** eds. *Complications in Obstetrics and Gynecology Surgery.* Hagerstown, MD: Harper & Row, 1981: 389–98.

123. **Clayton JK, Anderson JA, McNicol GP.** Preoperative prediction of postoperative deep vein thrombosis. *BMJ* 1976;2(6041):910–2.

124. **Clarke-Pearson DL, DeLong E, Synan IS, Coleman RE, Creasman WT.** Variables associated with postoperative deep venous thrombosis: a prospective study of 411 gynecology patients and creation of a prognostic model. *Obstet Gynecol* 1987;69(2):146–50.

125. **Kakkar VV.** Prevention of fatal postoperative pulmonary embolism by low dose heparin. An international multicenter trial. *Lancet* 1975;2:145–51.

126. **Ballard RM, Bradley-Watson PJ, Johnstone FD, Kenney A, McCarthy TG.** Low doses of subcutaneous heparin in the prevention of deep venous thrombosis after gynecologic surgery. *J Obstet Gynaecol Br Commonw* 1973;80:469–72.

127. **Taberner DA, Poller L, Burslem RW, Jones JB.** Oral anticoagulants controlled by British comparative thromboplastin versus dose heparin prophylaxis of deep venous thrombosis. *BMJ* 1978;1:272–4.

128. **Clarke-Pearson DL, Coleman RE, Synan IS, Hinshaw W, Creasman WT.** Venous thromboembolism prophylaxis in gynecologic oncology: a prospective controlled trial of low-dose heparin. *Am J Obstet Gynecol* 1983;145:606–13.

129. **Clarke-Pearson DL, DeLong E, Synan IS, Soper JT, Creasman WT, Coleman RE.** A controlled trial of two low-dose heparin regimens for the prevention of postoperative deep vein thrombosis. *Obstet Gynecol* 1990;75:684–9.

130. **Clarke-Pearson DL, DeLong E, Synan IS, Creasman WT, et al.** Complications of low-dose heparin prophylaxis in gynecologic oncology surgery. *Obstet Gynecol* 1984;64:689–94.

131. **Docherty PW, Goodman JD, Hill JG, Pickles BG, Boardman J, Taylor CG, et al.** The effect of low-dose heparin on blood loss at abdominal hysterectomy. *Br J Obstet Gynaecol* 1983;90:759–62.

132. **Catalona WJ, Kadmon D, Crane DB.** Effect of mini-dose heparin on lymphocele formation following extraperitoneal pelvic lymphadenectomy. *J Urol* 1979;123:890–5.

133. **Piver MS, Malfetano JH, Lele SB, Moore RH.** Prophylactic anticoagulation as a possible cause of inguinal lymphocyst after radical vulvectomy and inguinal lymphadenectomy. *Obstet Gynecol* 1983;62:17–21.

134. **Clarke-Pearson DL, Synan IS, Coleman RE, Hinshaw W, Creasman WT.** The natural history of postoperative venous thromboembolism in gynecologic oncology: a prospective study of 283 patients. *Am J Obstet Gynecol* 1984;148:1051–4.

135. **Conti S, Daschbach M.** Venous thromboembolism prophylaxis: a survey of its use in the United States. *Arch Surg* 1982;117:1036–40.

136. **Scurr JH, Ibrahim SZ, Faber RG, Le Quesne LP.** The efficacy of graduated compression stocking in the prevention of deep vein thrombosis. *Br J Surg* 1977;64:371–3.

137. **Allenby F, Boardman L, Pflug JJ, Calnan JS.** Effects of external pneumatic intermittent compression on fibrinolysis in man. *Lancet* 1973;2:1412–4.

138. **Salzman EW, Ploet J, Bettlemann M, Skillman J, Klein L.** Intraoperative external pneumatic calf compression to afford long-term prophylaxis against deep vein thrombosis in urological patients. *Surgery* 1980;87:239–42.

139. **Nicolaides AN, Fernandes e Fernandes J, Pollock AV.** Intermittent sequential pneumatic compression of the legs in the prevention of venous stasis and postoperative deep venous thrombosis. *Surgery* 1980;87:69–76.

140. **Clarke-Pearson DL, Synan IS, Hinshaw W, Coleman RE, Creasman WT.** Prevention of postoperative venous thromboembolism by external pneumatic calf compression in patients with gynecologic malignancy. *Obstet Gynecol* 1984;63:92–8.

141. **Clarke-Pearson DL, Creasman WT, Coleman RE, Synan IS, Hinshaw WM.** Perioperative external pneumatic calf compression as thromboembolism prophylaxis in gynecologic oncology: report of a randomized controlled trial. *Gynecol Oncol* 1984;18:226–32.

142. **Slazman EW, Davies GC.** Prophylaxis of venous thromboembolism: analysis of cost effectiveness. *Ann Surg* 1980;191:207–18.

143. **Haegger K.** Problems of acute deep vein thrombosis. *Angiology* 1969;20:219–22.

144. **Palko Pa, Namson EM, Fedonik SO.** The early detection of deep venous thrombosis using ^{135}I-tagged fibrinogen. *Can J Surg* 1964;7:215–20.

145. **Athanasoulis CA.** *Phlebography for the Diagnosis of Deep Leg Vein Thrombosis, Prophylactic Therapy of Deep Venous Thrombosis and Pulmonary Embolism.* DHEW Publication No. 76–886. Washington, DC: National Institutes of Health, 1975:62–76.

146. **Wheeler HB, O'Donnel JA, Anderson FA.** Occlusive cuff impedance phlebography: a diagnostic procedure for venous thrombosis and pulmonary embolism. *Prog Cardiovasc Dis* 1974;17:199–204.

147. **Clarke-Pearson DL, Creasman WT.** Diagnosis of deep vein thrombosis in obstetrics and gynecology in impedance phlebography. *Obstet Gynecol* 1981;58:52–9.

148. **Yao JST, Groumos C, Hobbs JT.** Detection of proximal vein thrombosis by Doppler ultrasound flow-detection method. *Lancet* 1972;1:1–6.

149. **Lensing AWA, Pradoni P, Bandjes D, Huisman PM, Vigo M, Tomasella G, et al.** Detection of deep-vein thrombosis by real-time B-mode ultrasonography. *N Engl J Med* 1989;320:342–8.

150. **Mintz MC, Levy DW, Axel L, Kressel HY, Arger PH, Coleman BG, et al.** Puerperal ovarian vein thrombosis: MR diagnosis. *AJR* 1987;149:1273–9.

151. **Clarke-Pearson DL, Synan IS, Creasman WT.** Anticoagulation therapy for venous thromboembolism in patients with gynecologic malignancy. *Am J Obstet Gynecol* 1983;147:369–72.

152. **Moser KM, Fedullo PR.** Venous thromboembolism: three simple decisions. *Chest* 1983;83:256–60.

153. **Hull RD, Raskob GE, Rosenbloom D, Panju AA, Brill-Edwards P, Ginsberg JS, et al.** Heparin for 5 days as compared with 10 days in the initial treatment of proximal venous thrombosis. *N Engl J Med* 1990;322:1260–4.

154. **Bell WR, Royal RM.** Heparin induced thrombocytopenia: a comparison of three heparin regimens. *N Engl J Med* 1980;303:902–7.

155. **Reynolds C.** Management of the diabetic surgical patient. *Postgrad Med* 1985;77:266–79.

156. **Alberti KGGM, Thomas DJB.** The management of diabetes during surgery. *Br J Anaesth* 1979;51:693–710.

157. **Walts LF.** Perioperative management of diabetes mellitus. *Anesthesiology* 1981;55:104–8.

158. **Galloway JA, Shuman CR.** Diabetes and surgery. A study of 667 cases. *Am J Med* 1963;34:177–91.

159. **Zonszein J, Santangele RP, Mackin JF, Lee TC, Coffey RJ, Canary JJ, et al.** Propanol therapy in thyrotoxicosis: a review of 84 patients undergoing surgery. *Am J Med* 1979;66:411.

160. **Goldman DR.** Surgery in patients with endocrine dysfunction. Preoperative consultation. *Med Clin North Am* 1987;71:499–6.

161. **James ML.** Endocrine disease and Anesthesia. *Anesth Analg* 1970;25:232–52.

162. **Weinberg AD, Brennan MD, Gorman CA, Marsh HM, O'Fallon WM, et al.** Outcome of anesthesia and surgery in hypothyroid patients. *Arch Intern Med* 1983;143:893.

163. **Ladenson Z, Levin AA, Ridgway EC, Daniels GH.** Complications of surgery in hypothyroid patients. *Am J Med* 1984;77:261–6.

164. **Grader AL, Neg KL, Nicholson WE, Islanel DP, Liddle GW.** Nature history of pituitary-adrenal recovery following long-term suppression with corticosteriods. *J Clin Endocrinol Metab* 1965;25:11.

165. **Kehlet H, Binder C.** Value of ACTH test in assessing HPA function in glucocorticoid-treated patients. *BMJ* 1973;1:47.

166. **Becker RC, Underwood DA.** Myocardial infarction in patients undergoing noncardiac surgery. *Cleve Clin J Med* 1987;54:25–8.

167. **Goldman L.** Cardiac risk factors and complications in non-cardiac surgery. *Medicine* 1978; 57:357–70.

168. **Steen PA, Tinder JH, Tarhan S.** Myocardial reinfarction after anesthesia and surgery. *JAMA* 1978;239:2366–70.

169. **Von Knorring J.** Postoperative myocardial infarction: a prospective study in a risk group of surgical patients. *Surgery* 1981;90:55–60.

170. **Rao TLK, Jacobs KJ, El-Etr AN.** Reinfarction following anesthesia in patients with myocardial infarction. *Anesthesiology* 1983;59:499.

171. **Tarhan S, Moffitt EA, Taylor WF, Giuliani ER.** Myocardial infarction after general anesthesia. *Anesth Analg* 1977;56:455–61.

172. **Goldman L.** Multifactorial index of cardiac risk in noncardiac surgical procedures. *N Engl J Med* 1977;297:845–50.

173. **Foster ED, Davis KB, Carpenter JA, Abele S, Fray D.** Risk of noncardiac operation in patients with defined coronary disease: the Coronary Artery Surgery Study (CASS) registry experience. *Ann Thorac Surg* 1986;41:42–9.

174. **Carliner NH, Fisher ML, Plotnick GD, Garbart H, Rapaport A, Keleman MH, et al.** Routine preoperative exercise testing in patients undergoing major noncardiac surgery. *Am J Cardiol* 1985;56:51–8.

175. **Cutler BS, Wheeler HB, Paraskos JA, Cardullo PA.** Applicability and interpretation of electrocardiographic stress testing in patients with peripheral vascular disease. *Am J Surg* 1981;141:501–6.

176. **Boucher CA, Brewster DC, Darling RC, Okada RD, Strauss HW, Pohost GM.** Determination of cardiac risk of dipyridamole-thallium imaging before peripheral vascular surgery. *N Engl J Med* 1985;312:389–94.

177. **Eagle KA, Singer DE, Brewster DC, Darling RC, Mulley AG, Boucher CA.** Dipyridamole-thallium scanning in patients undergoing vascular surgery: optimizing preoperative evaluation of cardiac risk. *JAMA* 1987;257:2185–9.

178. **Leppo J.** Noninvasive evaluation of cardiac risk before elective vascular surgery. *J Am Coll Cardiol* 1987;9:269–76.

179. **Pasternack PF.** The value of the radionuclide angiogram in the prediction of postoperative myocardial infarction in patients undergoing lower extremity revascularization procedures. *Circulation* 1985;72(Suppl II);13–7.

180. **Kaplan J.** Hemodynamic monitoring. In: **Kaplan J,** ed. *Cardiac Anesthesia.* New York: Grune & Stratton, 1987:179–226.

181. **Goldman L.** Cardiac risks and complications of non-cardiac surgery. *Ann Intern Med* 1983; 98:504–9.

182. **Driscoll AC, Hobika JH, Etsten BE, Proger S.** Clinically unrecognized myocardial infarction following surgery. *N Engl J Med* 1961;264:633–40.

183. **Pasternack PR, Imparato AM, Baumann FG, Laub G, Riles TS, Lamparello PJ, et al.** The hemodynamics of beta blockade in patients undergoing abdominal aortic aneurysm repair. *Circulation* 1987;76(Suppl III):1.

184. **Poquized SM, Sharma AD, Corr PB.** Influence of labetalol, a combined alpha and beta adrenergic blocking agent, on the dysrhythmias induced by coronary occlusion and reperfusion. *Cardiovasc Res* 1982;16:398–402.

185. **McGregor M.** The nitrates and myocardial ischemia. *Circulation* 1982;66:689–91.

186. **Coriat P, Daloz M, Bousseau D, Fusciardi J, Echter E, Viars P.** Prevention of intraoperative myocardial ischemia during noncardiac surgery with intravenous nitroglycerin. *Anesthesiology* 1984;61:193–8.

187. **Gallagher J, Moore RA, Jose AB, Botros SB, Clark DL.** Prophylactic nitroglycerin infusions during coronary artery bypass surgery. *Anesthesiology* 1986;64:785–9.

188. **Thomson I, Mutch W, Culligan J.** Failure of intravenous nitroglycerin to prevent intraoperative myocardial ischemia during fentanyl-pancuronium anesthesia. *Anesthesiology* 1984;61:385–90.

189. **Lacche A, Basaglia P.** Hypertensive emergencies: effects of therapy by nifedipine administrated sublingually. *Curr Ther Res* 1983;34:879–82.

190. **Pedersen O, Christensen N, Ramsch K.** Comparison of acute effects of nifedipine in normotensive and hypertensive man. *J Cardiovasc Pharmacol* 1980;2:357–61.

191. **O'Mailia J, Saunder G, Giles T.** Nifedipine associated myocardial ischemia or infarction in the treatment of hypertensive urgencies. *Ann Intern Med* 1989;107:185–90.

192. **Howat DDC.** Cardiac disease, anesthesia and operation for noncardiac conditions. *Br J Anaesth* 1971;43:288–98.

193. **Cooperman LH, Price HL.** Pulmonary edema in the operative and postoperative period: a review of 40 cases. *Ann Surg* 1970;172:883–91.

194. **Kuner J.** Cardiac arrythmias during anesthesia. *Dis Chest* 1967;52:580–7.

195. **Vanik PE, Davis HS.** Cardiac arrythmias during halothane anesthesia. *Anesth Analg* 1968;47:299–307.

196. **Bertrand CA, Steiner NV, Jameson AG, Lopez M.** Disturbances of cardiac rhythm during anesthesia and surgery. *JAMA* 1971;216:1615–7.

197. **Vandam LK, McLemore GA Jr.** Circulatory arrest in patients with complete heart block during anesthesia and surgery. *Am J Med* 1957;47:518.

198. **Frye RL.** Guidelines for permanent cardiac pacemaker implantation, May 1984: a report of the joint American College of Cardiology/American Heart Association task force on assessment of cardiovascular procedures (Subcommittee on pacemaker implantation). *Circulation* 1984;70:331A–9.

199. **Lerner SM.** Suppression of a demand pacemaker by transurethral electrocautery. *Anesth Analg* 1973;52:703–6.

200. **Rooney SM, Goldner PL, Muss E.** Relationship of right bundle branch block and marked left axis deviation to complete heart block during general anesthesia. *Anesthesiology* 1976;44:64–6.

201. **Bellocci F, Santarelli P, DiGennaro M, Ansalone G, Fenici R.** The risk of cardiac complications in surgical patients with bifascicular block. A clinical and electrophysiologic study in 98 patients. *Chest* 1980;77:343–8.

202. **Berg GR, Kofler MN.** The significance of bilateral bundle branch block in the preoperative patient. A retrospective electrocardiographic and clinical study in 30 patients. *Chest* 1971;59:62–7.

203. **Skinner JF, Pearce ML.** Surgical risk in the cardiac patient. *J Chron Dis* 1964;17:57–72.

204. **Maille JG, Dyrda I, Paiement B, Boulanger M.** Patients with cardiac valve prosthesis: subsequent anesthetic management for noncardiac surgical procedures. *Can Anaesth Soc J* 1973;20:207–16.

205. **Katholi RE, Nolan SP, McGuire LB.** The management of anticoagulation during noncardiac operations in patients with prosthetic heart valves. A prospective study. *Am Heart J* 1978;96:163–5.

206. **Tinker JH, Tarhan S.** Discontinuing anticoagulant therapy in surgical patients with cardiac valve prostheses: observations in 180 operations. *JAMA* 1978;239:738–9.

207. **Ryhanen P, Saarela E, Hollmen A, Horttonen L.** Blood pressure changes during and after anesthesia in treated and untreated hypertensive patients. *Ann Chir Gynaecol* 1978;67:180–4.

208. **Strandgaard S, Olesen J, Skinhoj E, Lassen NA.** Autoregulation of brain circulation in severe arterial hypertension. *BMJ* 1973;1:507–10.

209. **Samaan HA.** Risk of operation in a patient with unsuspected pheochromocytoma. *Br J Surg* 1970;57:462–5.

210. **Swan HJ, Ganz W, Forrester J, Marcus H, Diamond G, Chonette D.** Catheterization of the heart in man with the use of flow-directed balloon-tipped catheter. *N Engl J Med* 1970;283:447–52.

211. **Linman JW.** Physiologic and pathophysiologic effects of anemia. *N Engl J Med* 1968; 279:812–8.

212. **Lundsgaard-Hansen P.** Blood transfusion and capillary function. In: **Ikkala E, Nyhanen A,** eds. *Transfusion and Immunology.* Helsinki: International Society of Blood Transfusions, 1975.

213. **National Institutes of Health.** Summary of NIH consensus development conference on perioperative red cell transfusion. *Am J Hematol* 1989;31:144–50.

214. **Goodnough LT.** Autologous blood donation. *JAMA* 1988;250:65–7.

215. **Goodnough LT.** Increased preoperative collection of autologous blood with recombinant human erythropoietin therapy. *N Engl J Med* 1989;321:1163–8.

216. **Kelton JG.** Drug-induced thrombocytopenia is associated with increased binding of IgG to platelets both in vivo and in vitro. *Blood* 1981;58:524–5.

217. **Brown CH.** Defective platelet function following the administration of penicillin compounds. *Blood* 1976;47:949–53.

218. **Marengo-Rowe AJ, Leveson JE.** Evaluation of the bleeding patient. *Postgrad Med* 1977; 62:171–5.

219. **Myers ER, Clarke-Pearson DL, Olt GJ, Soper JT, Berchuck A.** Preoperative coagulation testing on a gynecologic oncology service. *Obstet Gynecol* 1994;83:438–44.

220. **Bodey GP, Buckley M, Sathe YS, Freireich EJ.** Quantitative relationships between circulating leukocytes and infection in patients with acute leukemia. *Ann Intern Med* 1966;64: 328–40.

221. **Stehling LC.** Anesthetic management of the patient with hyperthyroidism. *Anesthesiology* 1974;41:585–95.

222. **Miller RD, Robins TO, Tong MJ, Barton SL.** Coagulation defects associated with massive blood transfusions. *Ann Surg* 1971;174:794–9.

223. **Reed RL 2nd, Ciavarella D, Heimbach DM, Baron L, Paulin E, Counts RB, et al.** Prophylactic platelet administration during massive transfusion: a prospective, randomized, double-blind clinical study. *Ann Surg* 1986;203:40–6.

224. **Harke H, Rahman S.** Hemostatic disorders in massive transfusion. *Bibl Haemat* 1980;46: 179–84.

225. **Kahn RC, Jascott D, Carlon GC, Schweizer O, Howland WS, Goldiner PL.** Massive blood replacement. Correlation of ionized calcium citrate, and hydrogen ion concentration. *Anesth Analg* 1979;58:274–80.

226. **Mohr DN, Jett JR.** Clinical reviews. Preoperative evaluation of pulmonary risk factors. *J Gen Intern Med* 1988;3:277–87.

227. **Hensley MJ, Fencl V.** Lungs and respiration. In: **Vandam LD,** ed. *To Make the Patient Ready for Anesthesia: Medical Care of the Surgical Patient.* Menlo Park, CA: Addison-Wesley Publishing Co., 1981:21–46.

228. **Hotchkiss RS.** Perioperative management of patient with chronic obstructive pulmonary disease. *Int Anesthesiol Clin* 1988;26:134–41.

229. **Stein M, Cassara EL.** Preoperative pulmonary evaluation and therapy for surgery patients. *JAMA* 1970;211:787–90.

230. **Forthman HJ, Shepard A.** Postoperative pulmonary complications. *South Med J* 1969; 62:1198–1200.

231. **Lawrence VA, Page CP, Harris GD.** Preoperative spirometry before abdominal operations. A critical appraisal of its predictive value. *Arch Intern Med* 1989;149:280–5.

232. **Aibrak JD, O'Donnell CR, Marton K.** Indications for pulmonary function testing. *Ann Intern Med* 1990;112:763–71.

233. **Sagel SS, Evens RG, Forrest JV, Branson RT.** Efficacy of routine screening and lateral chest radiographs in a hospital based population. *N Engl J Med* 1974;291:1001–4.

234. **Blosser SA, Rock P.** Asthma and chronic obstructive lung disease. In: **Breslow MJ, Miller CJ, Rogers MC,** eds. *Perioperative Management.* St. Louis: CV Mosby Co., 1990:259–80.

235. **Galang SP.** Treatment of asthma. New and time-tested strategies. *Postgrad Med* 1990;87: 229–36.

236. **Barnes PJ.** A new approach to the treatment of asthma. *N Engl J Med* 1989;321:1517–27.

237. **Reave FE, Dolovich J, Newhouse MT.** The assessment and treatment of asthma: a conference report. *J Allergy Clin Immunol* 1990;85:109–11.

238. **Flenley DC.** Chronic obstructive pulmonary disease. *Dis Mon* 1988;34:543–7.

239. **Schwaber JF.** Evaluation of respiratory status in surgical patients. *Surg Clin North Am* 1970;50:637–44.

240. **Milledge JS, Nunn JF.** Criteria of fitness for anaesthesia in patients with chronic obstructive lung disease. *BMJ* 1975;3:670–3.

241. **Tarhan S, Moffitt EA, Sessler AD, Douglas WW, Taylor WF.** Risk of anesthesia and surgery in patients with chronic bronchitis and chronic obstructive pulmonary disease. *Surgery* 1973;74:720–6.

242. **Gracey DR, Divertie MB, Didier EP.** Preoperative pulmonary preparation of patients with chronic obstructive pulmonary disease. *Chest* 1979;76:123–9.

243. **Stein M, Koota GM, Simon M, Frank HA.** Pulmonary evaluation of surgical patients. *JAMA* 1962;181:765–70.

244. **Thoren L.** Post-operative pulmonary complications. Observations on their prevention by means of physiotherapy. *Acta Chir Scand* 1953;107:193–205.

245. **Castillo R, Haas A.** Chest physical therapy: comparative efficacy of preoperative and postoperative in the elderly. *Arch Phys Med Rehabil* 1985;66:376–9.

246. **Anderson ME, Belani KG.** Short-term preoperative smoking abstinence. *Am Fam Physician* 1990;41:1191–4.

247. **Warner MA, Offord KP, Warner ME, Lennon RL, Conover MA, Jansson-Schumacher U.** Role of preoperative cessation of smoking and other factors in postoperative pulmonary complications: a blinded prospective study of coronary artery bypass patients. *Mayo Clin Proc* 1989;64:609–16.

248. **Wellman JJ, Smith BA.** Respiratory complications of surgery. In Lubin MR, ed. *Medical Management of the Surgical Patient*. Boston: Butterworth, 1988:9–10.

249. **Cebul RD, Beck RJ.** Biochemical profiles: applications in ambulatory screening and preadmission testing of adults. *Ann Intern Med* 1987;106:403–13.

250. **Batchelder BM, Cooperman LH.** Effects of anesthetics on splanchnic circulation and metabolism. *Surg Clin North Am* 1975;55:787–94.

251. **Child CG, Turcotte JG.** Surgery and portal hypertension. In: **Child CG,** ed. *The Liver and Portal Hypertension*. 3rd ed. Philadelphia: WB Saunders, 1964:1–85.

252. **Garrison RN, Cryer HM, Howard DA, Polk HC Jr.** Clarification of risk factors for abdominal operations in patients with hepatic cirrhosis. *Ann Surg* 1984;199:648–55.

253. **Terblanche J.** Sclerotherapy for prophylaxis of variceal bleeding. *Lancet* 1986;1:961–3.

254. **LaMont JT.** The liver. In: **Vandam LD,** ed. *To Make the Patient Ready for Anesthesia: Medical Care of the Surgical Patient*. Menlo Park, CA: Addison-Wesley, 1984:47–66.

255. **Blamey SL, Fearon KCH, Gilmour WH, Osborne DH, Carter DC.** Prediction of risk in biliary surgery. *Br J Surg* 1983;70:535–8.

256. **Czaja Aj, Summerskill WH.** Chronic hepatitis. To treat or not to treat? *Med Clin North Am* 1978;62:71–85.

257. **Perrillo RP, Schiff ER, Davis GL, Bodenheimer HC Jr, Lindsay K, Payne J, et al.** A randomized controlled trial of interferon alpha-IIB alone and after prednisone withdrawal for the treatment of chronic hepatitis B. *N Engl J Med* 1990;323:295–301.

258. **Immunization Practices Advisory Committee.** Recommendations for protection against viral hepatitis. *Ann Intern Med* 1985;103:391–402.

259. **Greenwood SM, Leffler CT, Minkowtiz S.** The increased mortality rate of open liver biopsy in alcoholic hepatitis. *Surg Gynecol Obstet* 1972;134:600–4.

260. **Matloff DS, Kapkan MM.** Gastroenterology. In: **Molitch ME,** ed. *Management of Medical Problems in Surgical Patients*. Philadelphia: FA Davis, 1982:219–52.

261. **Block RS, Allaben RD, Walt AJ.** Cholecystectomy in patients with cirrhosis: a surgical challenge. *Arch Surg* 1985;120:669–72.

262. **Sirinek KR, Burk RR, Brown M, Levine BA.** Improving survival in patients with cirrhosis undergoing major abdominal operations. *Arch Surg* 1987;122:271–3.

263. **Broyer M, Brunner FP, Brynger H, Fasskinder W, Rizzoni G, Challad S, et al.** Demography of dialysis and transplantation in Europe, 1984. *Nephrol Dial Transplant* 1986;1:1–8.

264. **Blumberg A, Weidman P, Shaw S, Gnadinger M.** Effect of various therapeutic approaches on plasma potassium and major regulating factors in terminal renal failure. *Am J Med* 1988;85:507–12.

265. **Lewis SL, Van Epps DE.** Neutrophil and monocyte alterations in chronic dialysis patients. *Am J Kidney Dis* 1987;9:381–95.

266. **Hellem A, Borchgrevink C, Ames S.** The role of red cells in hemostasis. The relationship between hematocrit, bleeding time, and platelet adhesiveness. *Br J Haematol* 1961;7:42–50.

267. **Remuzzi G.** Bleeding disorders in uremia. *Adv Nephrol* 1989;18:171–4.

268. **Sherrard DJ.** Aluminum toxicity. In: **Ferris TF,** ed. *The Kidney.* Washington, DC: National Kidney Foundation, 1988;20(6):31–6.

269. **Hostetter TH, Olson JL, Rennke HG, Venkatachalam MA, Brenner BM.** Hyperfiltration in remnant nephrons: a potentially adverse response to renal ablation. *Am J Physiol* 1981;241:85–93.

270. **Gallop DG, Taller DE, King LA.** Primary mass closure of midline incisions with continuous running monofilament suture in gynecologic patients. *Obstet Gynecol* 1989;73:67–70.

271. **Miller RD.** Pharmacology of muscle relaxants and their antagonists. In: **Miller RD,** ed. *Anesthesia.* 2nd ed. New York: Churchill-Livingstone, 1986:920.

272. **Mazze RI.** Anesthesia for patients with abnormal renal function and genitourinary problems. In: **Miller RD,** ed. *Anesthesia.* 2nd ed. New York: Churchill-Livingstone, 1986:1648.

273. **Hunter JM, Jones RS, Utting JE.** Use of the muscle relaxant atracurium in anephric patients: preliminary communication. *J R Soc Med* 1982;72:336–40.

274. **Bevan DR, Donati F, Gyasi H, Williams A.** Vecuronium in renal failure. *Can Anaesth Soc J* 1984;31:491–6.

275. **Roth F, Wuthrich H.** The clinical importance of hyperkalemia following suxamethonium administration. *Br J Anaesth* 1969;41:311–5.

276. **Hou SH.** Hospital-acquired renal insufficiency: a prospective study. *Am J Med* 1983;74:243–8.

277. **Bullock ML, Umen AJ, Finkelstein MS.** The assessment of risk factors in 462 patients with acute renal failure. *Am J Kidney Dis* 1985;5:97–103.

278. **Meyer RD.** Risk factors and comparison of clinical nephrotoxicity of aminoglyosides. *Am J Med* 1986;80(S6B):119–25.

279. **Shusterman N, Strom BL, Murray TG, Morrison G, West SL, Maislin G.** Risk factors and outcome of hospital-acquired acute renal failure: clinical epidemiologic study. *Am J Med* 1987;83:65–71.

280. **Harkonen S, Kjellstrand CM.** Contrast nephropathy. *Am J Nephrol* 1981;1:69–72.

281. **Bush HL, Huse JB, Johnson WC, Johnson WC, O'Hara ET, Nabseth DC, et al.** Prevention of renal insufficiency after abdominal aortic aneurysm resection by optimal volume loading. *Arch Surg* 1981;116:1517–24.

20 Incontinence, Prolapse, and Disorders of the Pelvic Floor

L. Lewis Wall

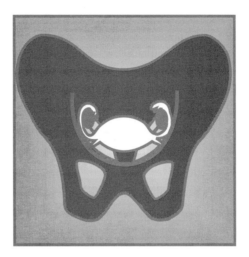

The genital and urinary tracts are intimately associated anatomically and embryologically from the earliest stages of their development. The bladder is located directly above the anterior vaginal wall and the urethra is fused to it. Both of these structures, as well as other structures of the pelvic floor, are placed at risk during pregnancy and childbirth. The term "urogynecology" has been coined to describe the area of gynecology that deals with disorders of the female lower urinary tract; however, it has become apparent that urinary tract disorders are only one facet of a wide range of pelvic floor disorders that afflict women.

Each organ system in the pelvic floor—urinary, genital, intestinal—traverses the pelvis and exits through its own orifice. Thus, these systems are intricately related in function and anatomic support (1). Disorders of each of these components should be evaluated in light of their impact on the function of the surrounding structures and the functional anatomy of the pelvic floor.

Functional Anatomy of the Pelvic Floor

The striated muscles of the pelvic floor, in combination with their fascial attachments, work together across the entire pelvis to prevent pelvic organ displacement, to maintain continence, and to control expulsive activities. An appreciation of the fact that these organ systems have complex interrelationships should help clinicians realize that patients' problems are not necessarily limited to a single organ but rather that each disturbance of pelvic support or continence exists within a complex pelvic "ecosystem" and, as a result, may be linked to problems in other organ systems.

Pelvic Support

The bony pelvis surrounds and protects its contents but, by itself, actually provides them with little support. The pelvic organs are supported primarily by the muscular activity of the pelvic floor, aided by ligamentous attachments. Rather than functioning as a rigid structure, the pelvic floor muscles provide dynamic support through constant ac-

619

tivity, functioning more like a self-regulating trampoline that continually adjusts its tension in response to changing circumstances (2, 3).

The functional anatomy of the muscles of the pelvic floor (the levator ani) has been studied for many years but remains poorly understood (4). The pelvic floor muscles contract to maintain urinary and fecal incontinence and relax to permit bowel and bladder emptying. It plays a role in normal female sexual responsiveness (5). The pelvic floor must distend tremendously to allow the delivery of a term infant, but it must contract again during the postpartum period to allow its varied functions to continue. Because the urethra, bladder, rectum, and the supporting structures of the pelvis are all part of the pelvic floor, the functions of these organs cannot really be understood without an understanding of the pelvic musculature (see Chapter 5) (6, 7).

Levator Ani Muscle

The nomenclature of the pelvic muscles has long been subject to debate. The *levator ani muscle* (the broad general term for most of the muscles of the pelvic floor) has been described as consisting of a diaphragmatic portion (*iliococcygeus*) and the more important "pubovisceral" portion (8). The iliococcygeus (or "diaphragmatic") portion of the levator ani consists of a thin muscular sheet that arises from the pelvic sidewall on either side of the arcus tendinous and ischial spine and inserts into a midline raphe behind the rectum. The *pubovisceral* (*"pubococcygeus"*) portion of the levator ani muscle consists of a thick U-shaped band of muscle arising from the pubic bone and attaching to the lateral walls of the vagina and rectum (Fig. 20.1). Therefore, the rectum is supported by a muscular sling

Figure 20.1   The levator ani muscles, as seen from below. (From **Goss CM,** ed. *Gray's Anatomy of the Human Body.* 28th ed. Philadelphia, Lea & Febiger, 1966:447.)

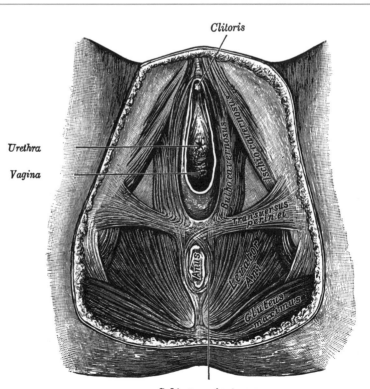

that pulls it toward the pubic bones when these muscles contract. This muscular band is often called the *puborectalis* or the *pubococcygeus* muscle, but a more accurate term is the "*pubovisceral muscle,*" because these muscles arise from the pubic bone and insert directly onto pelvic viscera or provide a supporting sling for them.

When the pubovisceral muscle contracts, it pulls the rectum, vagina, and urethra anteriorly toward the pubic bone and constricts the lumens of these pelvic organs (Fig. 20.2). **It is this contractile property that is so important in maintaining urinary and fecal continence and in providing support for the genital organs (vagina, cervix, uterus) that lie upon and are supported by the levator plate.** The medial portions of the pubovisceral muscle (levator ani) pass laterally to the arcus tendinous fasciae of the pelvis and attach to the endopelvic fascia surrounding the vaginal wall at a point opposite to the upper half of the urethra (9–11) (Fig. 20.3). The pubovisceral muscle attaches to a web of endopelvic fascia rather than directly to the urethra in this area. This portion of the muscle (puborectalis) contains large quantities of *type I* ("*slow-twitch*") muscle fibers that are tonically contracted. This base-line level of muscular activity provides constant resilient support for the urethra. At the same time, *type II* ("*fast-twitch*") fibers allow the pubovisceral muscle to respond quickly to rapid changes in intra-abdominal pressure (coughing, sneezing) and to maintain urethral closure under such conditions (12). Reflex contraction of both types of muscle fibers helps support all of the contents of the pelvis.

As with the external anal sphincter, the levator ani muscles exhibit constant base-line tone in addition to their ability to contract and offset increases in intra-abdominal pressure that would force pelvic contents downward. The phenomenon of constant base-line tone is separate from the ability of these muscles to contract forcefully. This aspect of pelvic muscle function is poorly understood, but it is critical for proper pelvic support because closure of the pelvic floor allows the pelvic viscera to rest on a muscular shelf. The constant adjustments in muscle activity maintain pelvic floor closure in response to changing circumstances and keep the pelvic ligaments from stretching.

Pelvic Ligaments

It is often erroneously believed that the various pelvic "ligaments" are the most important factors in pelvic support. Ligaments are poorly suited to maintaining support over time because fibrous tissues elongate when subjected to constant tension. The pelvic ligaments serve mainly to keep structures in positions where they can be supported by muscular activity rather than as weight-bearing structures themselves. The loss of normal muscular

Figure 20.2   *A,* **The pubovisceral muscle at rest.** *B,* **Contraction of the pubovisceral muscle constricts the lumens of the urethra, vagina, and rectum, augmenting closure of all three organs.**

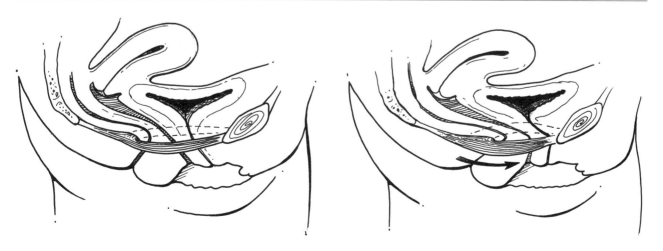

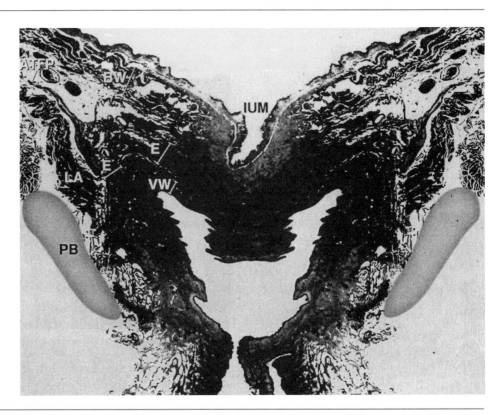

Figure 20.3   Frontal section of the cadaver of a 21-year-old woman at the vesical neck showing the supportive layer formed by the vaginal wall (VW) and the endopelvic fascia (E) attached to the pelvic wall at the arcus tendinous fasciae pelvis (ATFP) on the inner surface of the levator ani (LA) at the level of the proximal urethral and internal urinary meatus (IUM). The area where the pubic bones were removed is shaded (PB). The image is reconstructed from a specimen made from the left side of the body by reflecting it across the midline. (Reproduced with permission from **Delancey J.** Structural support of the urethra as it relates to stress urinary incontinence: the hammock hypothesis. *Am J Obstet Gynecol* 1994;170:1715.)

support leads to sagging and widening of the urogenital hiatus and predisposes patients to the development of pelvic organ prolapse (13) (Fig. 20.4).

Although fascia and ligaments are believed to be essential for support of the pelvic organs, this belief comes more from the amount of attention given to these structures in the performance of gynecologic surgery than from any empiric evidence regarding their role in pelvic support. However, the pelvic ligaments (i.e., the round, infundibulopelvic, and cardinal) are loose condensations of areolar tissue, blood vessels, and muscle fibers. By themselves, they have little supportive strength but function as "moorings" to hold the uterus and vagina in place. The pelvic ligaments and the endopelvic fascia attach the uterus and vagina to the pelvic sidewalls so these structures can be supported by the muscles of the pelvic floor. The entire complex then rests on the levator plate, where it can be closed by increases in intra-abdominal pressure by a "flap-valve" effect (14).

Connective Tissue

Connective tissue is the "glue" of the body. It is composed primarily of elastin and collagen fibers in a polysaccharide ground substance. The composition of connective tissue is not constant but varies in different sites throughout the body. Connective tissue forms capsules to help maintain the structural integrity of organs, and it forms the fascia that covers muscles and the tendons and allows them to attach to other structures in the body. If con-

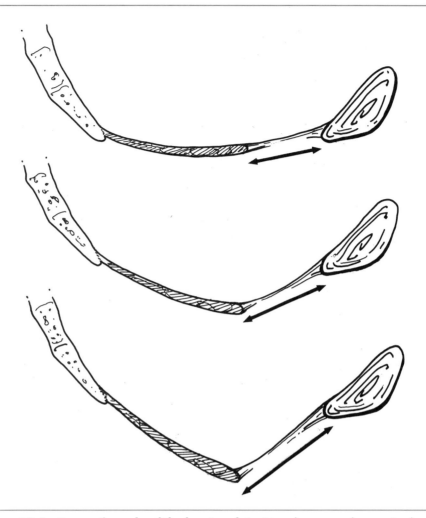

Figure 20.4   Supportive role of the levator plate. Note how muscle tone in the levator muscle complex keeps the urogenital hiatus constricted and relatively closed (*top*). As muscle tone is lost, the levator plate sags, gradually widening the levator hiatus and predisposing patients to the development of prolapse (*bottom*).

nective tissue fails, muscular support will be weak, because the attachments that permit muscles to exercise their functions will be unreliable (15). Connective tissue is not static; instead, it is a dynamic tissue which undergoes constant turnover and remodeling in response to stress. Connective tissue turnover and repair are especially important in relation to wound healing and recovery from surgery. Hormonal changes seem to have significant effects on collagen, and these effects are probably of great importance during pregnancy and parturition, as well as in aging (16–18). Exercise seems to increase collagen turnover, as measured by increased proline hydroxylase activity in 69-year-old women who exercised for 8 weeks (19). Nutrition has an important role in the maintenance of connective tissue integrity. Vitamin C deficiency (scurvy) produces defects in collagen synthesis and repair that can result in the breakdown of seemingly normal connective tissue, even including the reopening of old, previously healed wounds (20).

Studies suggest that connective tissue abnormalities are a significant factor contributing to prolapse and related conditions. For example, joint hypermobility is a common clinical marker for abnormal collagen levels. Two studies have now shown an association between joint hypermobility and genital prolapse (21, 22), and one study has shown an association between joint hypermobility and rectal prolapse (23). Fibroblasts grown in

623

tissue culture from the fascia of women with recurrent genital prolapse have an imbalance of collagen types, with excessive synthesis of weaker type III collagen (24). Both collagen content and collagen strength seem to be decreased in the fascia of women with stress incontinence (25, 26). However, pelvic support defects are affected by many different factors, and the ultimate clinical presentation (and perhaps the surgical solution) may be different for each patient (27).

Lower Urinary Tract Function

The bladder is a complex organ that has a relatively simple function: to store urine effortlessly, painlessly, and without leakage and to discharge urine voluntarily, effortlessly, completely, and painlessly. To meet these demands, the bladder must have normal anatomic support as well as normal neurophysiologic function.

Normal Urethral Closure

Normal urethral closure is maintained by a combination of intrinsic and extrinsic factors. The *extrinsic factors* include the levator ani muscles, the endopelvic fascia, and their attachments to the pelvic sidewalls and the urethra. This forms a hammock beneath the urethra that responds to increases in intra-abdominal pressure by remaining tense, allowing the urethra to be closed against the posterior supporting shelf (Fig. 20.5). When this supportive mechanism becomes faulty for some reason—the endopelvic fascia has detached from its normal points of fixation, muscular support has weakened, or a combination of these two processes—normal support is lost and anatomic hypermobility of the urethra and bladder neck develops. For many women, this loss of support is severe enough to cause

Figure 20.5 Lateral view of the pelvic floor drawn from a three-dimensional reconstruction with the urethra, vagina, and fascial tissues transected at the level of the vesical neck. Note how the urethra is compressed against the underlying supportive tissues by the downward force (*arrow*) generated by a cough or sneeze. (Reproduced with permission from **Delancey J.** Structural support of the urethra as it relates to stress urinary incontinence: the hammock hypothesis. *Am J Obstet Gynecol* 1994;170:1718.)

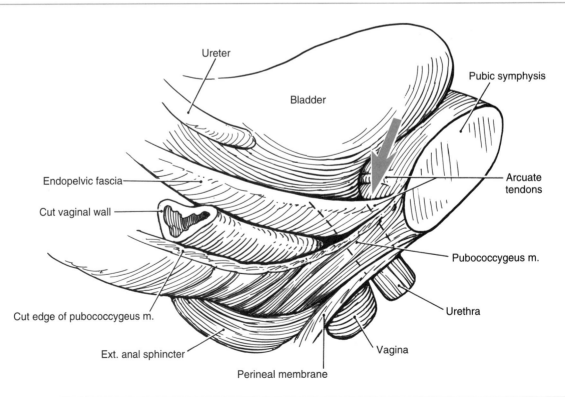

loss of closure during periods of increased intra-abdominal pressure, and stress incontinence results. However, many women remain continent when urethral support is lost (11).

The *intrinsic factors* contributing to urethral closure include the striated muscle of the urethral wall, vascular congestion of the submucosal venous plexus, the smooth muscle of the urethral wall and associated blood vessels, the epithelial coaptation of the folds of the urethral lining, urethral elasticity, and the tone of the urethra as mediated by alpha-adrenergic receptors of the sympathetic nervous system. The intrinsic competence of the urethral closure mechanism can be affected by congenital developmental defects, scarring from trauma or multiple unsuccessful surgical procedures, estrogen deficiency, and neurological injury. Stress incontinence resulting from intrinsic sphincteric deficiency is more difficult to correct than that occurring from loss of proper anatomic support. Urethral support alone, however, is not responsible for ensuring the integrity of the closure mechanism. The bladder is an autonomic organ under voluntary control and neurophysiology plays a role in its function, although understanding of these complex processes is limited (28).

The Bladder

The bladder is a bag of smooth muscle that stores urine and contracts to expel urine under voluntary control. It is a low-pressure system that expands to accommodate increasing volumes of urine without an appreciable rise in pressure. This function seems to be mediated primarily by the sympathetic nervous system. During bladder filling, there is an accompanying increase in outlet resistance. This action is manifest as increasing muscle fiber recruitment, as seen with electromyography of the pelvic floor and urethra while performing filling cystometry. The bladder muscle (the detrusor) should remain inactive during bladder filling, without involuntary contractions. When the bladder has filled to a certain volume, fullness is registered by tension-stretch receptors, which signal the brain to initiate a micturition reflex. This reflex is permitted or not permitted by cortical control mechanisms, depending on the social circumstances and the state of the patient's nervous system. Normal voiding is accomplished by voluntary relaxation of the pelvic floor and urethra, accompanied by sustained contraction of the detrusor muscle, leading to complete bladder emptying.

Innervation

The lower urinary tract receives its innervation from three sources: the sympathetic and parasympathetic divisions of the autonomic nervous system and the neurons of the somatic nervous system (external urethral sphincter). The *autonomic nervous system* consists of all efferent pathways with ganglionic synapses that lie outside the central nervous system. Although knowledge of the neurophysiology of the autonomic nervous system is incomplete, it seems that the sympathetic system primarily controls bladder storage and the parasympathetic nervous system controls bladder emptying. The *somatic nervous system* plays only a peripheral role in neurologic control of the lower urinary tract through its innervation of the pelvic floor and external urethral sphincter.

The *sympathetic nervous system* originates in the thoracolumbar spinal cord, principally T11 through L2–L3. The ganglia of the sympathetic nervous system are located close to the spinal cord and use acetylcholine as the preganglionic neurotransmitter. The postganglionic neurotransmitter in the sympathetic nervous system is norephedrine, and it acts on two types of receptors: alpha receptors, located principally in the urethra and bladder neck, and beta receptors, located principally in the bladder body. Stimulatino of alpha receptors increases urethral tone and thus promotes closure. Alpha blockers have the opposite effect. Stimulation of beta receptors decreases tone in the bladder body.

The *parasympathetic nervous system* controls bladder motor function—bladder contraction and bladder emptying. The parasympathetic nervous system originates in the sacral spinal cord, primarily in S2–S4, as does the somatic innervation of the pelvic floor, urethra, and external anal sphincter. Sensation in the perineum is also controlled by sensory fibers that connect with the spinal cord at this level. For this reason, examination of perineal sensation, pelvic muscle reflexes, and pelvic muscle or anal sphincter tone are relevant to clinical evaluation of the lower urinary tract. The parasympathetic neurons have long preganglionic neurons and short postganglionic neurons, which are located in the end organ. Both the preganglionic and postganglionic synapses use acetylcholine as their neurotransmitter, acting on muscarinic receptors. Because acetylcholine is the main neurotransmitter used in bladder muscle contraction, virtually all drugs used to control detrusor muscle overactivity have anticholinergic properties. Unfortunately, cholinergic stimulants seem to be ineffective in promoting bladder emptying, even though they will cause bladder muscle strips to contract in a laboratory setting.

Bladder storage and bladder emptying involve the interplay of the sympathetic and parasympathetic nervous systems. The modulation of these activities seems to be influenced by a variety of nonadrenergic, noncholinergic neurotransmitters and neuropeptides, which fine-tune the system at various facilitative and inhibitory levels in the spinal cord and higher areas of the central nervous system (29–31). Thus, neuropathology at almost any level of the neurourologic axis can have an adverse effect on lower urinary tract function.

Micturition

Micturition is triggered via the peripheral nervous system controlled by the central nervous system. It is useful to consider this event as occurring at a micturition threshold, a bladder volume at which reflex detrusor contractions occur. The threshold volume is not fixed but is variable, and it can be altered depending on the contributions made by sensory afferents from the perineum, bladder, colon, and rectum as well as input from the higher centers of the nervous system. The micturition threshold is, therefore, a floating threshold that can be altered or reset by various influences.

The spinal cord and higher centers of the nervous system have complex patterns of inhibition and facilitation. The most important facilitative center above the spinal cord is the pontine-mesencephalic gray matter of the brain stem, often called the pontine micturition center, which serves as the final common pathway for all bladder motor neurons. Transection of the tracts below this level leads to disturbed bladder emptying, whereas destruction of tracts above this level leads to detrusor hyperreflexia. The cerebellum serves as a major center for coordinating pelvic floor relaxation and the rate, force, and range of detrusor contractions, and there are multiple interconnections between the cerebellum and the brain-stem reflex centers. Above this level, the cerebral cortex and related structures exert inhibitory influences on the micturition reflex. Thus, the upper cortex exerts facilitative influences that release inhibition, permitting the anterior pontine micturition center to send efferent impulses down the complex pathways of the spinal cord, where a reflex contraction in the sacral micturition center generates a detrusor contraction that causes bladder emptying.

Colorectal Function

The sigmoid (S-shaped) colon begins at the pelvic brim and straightens as it enters the pelvis to become the rectum. Below the cul-de-sac, it expands into the rectal ampulla, filling the posterior pelvis from the left side. An anorectal angle of 90° is formed at this point by the action of the puborectalis portion of the levator ani muscle complex, separating the anal canal below from the rectum above. **The anorectal angle is believed to be one factor among several that are important in the maintenance of normal anal continence. The puborectalis muscle maintains this angle through its normal tone, and during normal defecation, it relaxes to depress the pelvic floor and then contracts to elevate the pelvic floor during and after bowel emptying.**

The anorectal continence mechanism consists of an *internal sphincter* composed of smooth muscle and an *external sphincter* composed of striated muscle. The internal sphincter is a visceral muscle under autonomic control and normally has a high resting tone. The external sphincter is a striated muscle under voluntary control. In addition, there are sensory nerves in the rectum and pelvic floor. Continence is maintained at the level of the internal anal sphincter by gradual increases in the level of tonic contraction of the internal anal sphincter. This seal works only if the anal lining is sufficiently bulky to permit closure, and it is maintained by a combination of vascularity and infolding of the anal lining. The contractile efficiency of the internal sphincter is aided by contraction of the external anal sphincter. Rapid rectal distention causes a reflex relaxation of the internal anal sphincter. Under these circumstances, continence is maintained by contraction of the external sphincter. The efficiency of this process is closely linked to rectal sensation. Afferent sensation from the rectum appears to travel with the parasympathetic nerves to sacral segments S2–S4. Sensation from the anal canal also travels to these sacral segments via the inferior hemorrhoidal branches of the pudendal nerve. The sensory apparatus of the rectum allows patients to distinguish between solid feces, liquid stool, and flatus. Impairment of this ability can have serious social consequences.

Innervation

The innervation of the gut is similarly complex. There are two ganglionic complexes in the bowel wall: a *myenteric plexus* between the longitudinal and circular muscle coats and a *submucosal plexus*. The innervation of the smooth muscle of the bowel involves excitatory and inhibitory nonadrenergic, noncholinergic neurotransmitters and cotransmitters, primarily acetylcholine, substance P, and vasoactive intestinal polypeptide. The sphincters seem to be under separate neuronal control from nonsphincteric smooth muscle of the bowel. Sympathetic stimulation (norepinephrine) seems to cause contraction of the internal anal sphincter, whereas parasympathetic stimulation causes relaxation of the internal anal sphincter. The internal anal sphincter receives sympathetic innervation via the hypogastric nerves from L5, and the parasympathetic innervation comes from sacral segments S1–S3. The external anal sphincter is innervated by branches of the pudendal nerve, originating in the sacral segments S2–S4, with some branches from the coccygeal nerve plexus (S4–S5).

Like the bladder, the colon and rectum undergo a filling and emptying cycle; unlike the bladder, the lower end of the gastrointestinal tract is not a closed viscus but rather a one-way conduit through which waste matter passes (32). Like the bladder, colorectal function can be categorized into storage (continence) and emptying (defecation) components.

Anal Continence

Anal continence is maintained by a combination of colonic compliance and mechanisms for retention in the rectosigmoid that keep the distal rectum collapsed and empty. The forces of retention are both mechanical and physiological. The mechanical forces promoting retention of stool involve the S-shaped anterior-posterior angulations of the sigmoid colon and the spiral folds in the lumen formed by the valves of Houston. Also, the puborectalis muscle creates a sharp angulation of the anorectum, which is accentuated by contraction of this muscle. Increases in intra-abdominal pressure accentuate these angulations. These pressure increases have been postulated to create a flap-valve effect, which helps occlude the upper anal canal during periods of increased intra-abdominal pressure (33); however, the principal mechanism of action may actually be a sphincter-like function exerted by puborectalis contraction (34). A flutter valve effect may also be created in the collapsed anorectum (32, 35). Retention of stool is further helped by a reverse pressure gradient between the rectum and the rectosigmoid colon. Waves of muscle contraction are both more frequent and of higher amplitude in the rectum than they are in the sigmoid.

The most important factors in maintaining fecal continence are sphincteric factors. The anus has both internal and external sphincters. Both of these sphincters are tonically contracted in the resting state, with the internal sphincter more so than the external sphincter. The external sphincter contains both slow-twitch and fast-twitch fibers. It remains tonically contracted even during sleep. In addition to its tonic base-line contractility, the external anal sphincter can respond with a quick, forceful contraction during periods of stress to maintain anal control, and its degree of contraction varies with posture and activity. The internal sphincter is at or near its state of maximal contraction all of the time. It relaxes only to allow the passage of stool when the rectum reaches a threshold of distention. When this occurs, relaxation of the internal sphincter allows the passage of matter into the distal anal canal. This stimulates multiple nerve endings to give warning of an impending movement of matter, which is detected as solid, liquid, or gaseous in nature. Continence is maintained by a reflex contraction of the external anal sphincter, which occurs concurrently with internal sphincter relaxation. Voluntary contraction of the anal sphincter, in conjunction with rectal compliance, allows the individual to withhold a bowel movement until it is appropriate to release it.

Defecation

Defecation is the emptying phase of the colonic cycle. This may occur involuntarily in certain pathologic states or as a response to prolonged overdistension of the rectum, but defecation usually is a voluntary process. Voluntary defecation begins with closure of the glottis, which helps increase intra-abdominal pressure, and by closure of the muscles of the pelvic floor. The diaphragm descends and the muscles of the abdominal wall are contracted, raising intra-abdominal pressure. The anal sphincter also contracts, further increasing intra-abdominal pressure. Segmental contractions in the colon are inhibited. When the bolus of feces reaches the upper rectum, the muscles of the pelvic floor relax, the pelvic floor descends, and the acute rectal angle that existed at rest is straightened. Constriction of the distal muscles allows pressure to build up in the rectum, and when the internal sphincter relaxes, the bolus of stool is expelled. As the bolus passes, there is complete inhibition of electrical activity in the external sphincter, which contracts again only after the stool has been passed. The act of defecation represents the only known condition in which the external sphincter responds to increased intra-abdominal pressure by relaxation rather than by contraction. At the end of defecation, the pelvic floor is elevated to its normal position and the sphincters return to their tonically contracted resting state ("the closing reflex").

The complex intricate mechanisms involved in maintenance of continence and defecation are poorly understood, grossly undervalued, and generally taken for granted until impairment occurs (32). The same is undoubtedly true for all aspects of pelvic floor function.

Lower Urinary Tract Dysfunction

Symptoms arising in the lower urinary tract account for a significant number of patient visits to gynecologists. Disturbances in bladder function produce a wide variety of urinary tract symptoms. To help the clinician organize an initial patient evaluation, these symptoms can be classified according to whether they are disturbances of storage, emptying, sensation, or bladder contents (Table 20.1).

Urinary Incontinence

Urinary incontinence is defined as involuntary loss of urine that is a social or hygienic problem and that is objectively demonstrable (36). Urinary incontinence is a symptom, not a diagnosis. It is not a normal part of aging, although the prevalence of the problem increases with age, and it is not a trivial complaint. The National Institutes of Health have estimated that there are over 10 million adult Americans (7 million women) with urinary incontinence, resulting in a cost of over $10.3 billion per year (37). The differential diagnosis of urinary incontinence is extensive (Table 20.2); however, urinary incontinence is almost always treatable. It can almost always be improved and frequently can be cured, often using relatively simple, nonsurgical interventions.

Table 20.1   Classification and Definition of Lower Urinary Symptoms In Women

I. Abnormal Storage

Incontinence: Involuntary urine loss that is a social or hygienic problem.
Stress incontinence: Incontinence occurring under conditions of increase intra-abdominal pressure.
Urge incontinence: Incontinence accompanied by a strong desire to void.
Mixed incontinence: Stress and urge incontinence occurring together.
Unconscious incontinence: Incontinence occurring without urgency and without conscious recognition of leakage.
Frequency: The number of voids per day, from waking in the morning until falling asleep at night.
Nocturia: The number of times the patient is awakened from sleep to void at night.
Nocturnal enuresis: Urinary incontinence during sleep.

II. Abnormal Emptying

Hesitancy: Trouble initiating voiding.
Straining to void: Voiding accompanied by abdominal straining.
Poor stream: Decreased force of flow of the urinary stream.
Intermittent stream: A "stop-and-start" pattern of urination.
Incomplete emptying: A persistent feeling of bladder fullness after voiding.
Postmicturition dribble: Urine loss occurring just after normal voiding has been completed.
Acute urinary retention: Sudden inability to void resulting in painful bladder overdistention and the need for catheterization to obtain relief.

III. Abnormal Sensation

Urgency: A strong desire to void.
Dysuria: Burning pain with urination.
Bladder pain: Conscious, hurting, suprapubic pain in the bladder.
Flank pain: Pain between the lower rib cage and the ilial crest.
Pressure: A feeling of heaviness or constant force being exerted in the bladder or lower pelvis.
Loss of bladder sensation: Decreased sensation in the bladder.

IV. Abnormal Bladder Contents

Abnormal color
Abnormal smell
Hematuria
Pneumaturia
Stones
Foreign bodies

Principles of Investigation

The initial evaluation of most patients with incontinence is not difficult, but it requires a systematic approach to consider all possible causes. The following items should be part of the basic evaluation:

1. History

2. Physical examination

3. Urinalysis, with urine culture and cytology as appropriate

4. Measurement of postvoid residual urine

5. Frequency/volume bladder chart

When these steps have been completed, some patients will benefit from urodynamic studies to create a more comprehensive bladder biophysical profile before treatment.

Table 20.2   Differential Diagnosis Of Urinary Incontinence

I. Extraurethral incontinence

   A. Congenital
      1. Ectopic ureter
      2. Bladder exstrophy
      3. Other
   B. Acquired (fistulas)
      1. Ureteric
      2. Vesical
      3. Urethral
      4. Complex combinations

II. Transurethral incontinence

   A. Genuine stress incontinence
      1. Bladder neck displacement (anatomic hypermobility)
      2. Intrinsic sphincteric dysfunction
      3. Combined
   B. Detrusor overactivity
      1. Idiopathic detrusor instability
      2. Neuropathic detrusor hyperreflexia
   C. Mixed incontinence
   D. Urinary retention with bladder distention and overflow
      1. Genuine stress incontinence
      2. Detrusor hyperactivity with impaired contractility
      3. Combinations
   E. Urethral diverticulum
   F. Congenital urethral abnormalities (e.g., epispadias)
   G. Uninhibited urethral relaxation ("urethral instability")
   H. Functional and transient incontinence

History

Every incontinent patient should undergo a thorough history, including a review of symptoms, general medical history, review of past surgery, and current medications. It is helpful to write down the patient's chief complaint in her own words and expand the history from this point. The patient's most troubling symptoms must be ascertained—how often she leaks urine, how much urine she leaks, what provokes urine loss, what helps the problem or makes it worse, and what treatment (if any) she has had in the past.

The general medical history will often reveal systemic illnesses that have a direct bearing on urinary incontinence, such as diabetes mellitus (which produces osmotic diuresis if glucose control is poor), vascular insufficiency (which can lead to incontinence at night when peripheral edema is mobilized into the vascular system, resulting in increased diuresis), chronic pulmonary disease (which can lead to stress incontinence from chronic coughing), or a wide variety of neurological conditions that can affect the neurourologic axis at any point from the cerebral cortex to the peripheral nervous system.

Many medications affect the lower urinary tract (38, 39).

  1. *Sedatives* such as the benzodiazepines may accumulate in the patient's system and cause confusion and secondary incontinence, particularly for elderly patients.

  2. *Alcohol* may have similar effects to benzodiazepines and also impairs mobility as well as produces diuresis.

  3. *Anticholinergic drugs* may impair detrusor contractility and may lead to voiding difficulty and overflow incontinence. Drugs with anticholinergic properties are widespread and include antihistamines, antidepressants, antipsychotics, opiates, antispasmodics, and drugs used to treat Parkinson's disease.

4. *Alpha-adrenergic agents* may have a profound effect on the lower urinary tract. α Agonists, which are often found in over-the-counter cold remedies, increase outlet resistance and may lead to voiding difficulty; conversely, these drugs are often useful in treating some cases of stress incontinence.

5. *Alpha blockers,* which are often used in the treatment of hypertension (e.g., *prazosin, terazosin*), may decrease urethral closure and lead to stress incontinence (40).

6. *Calcium channel blockers* may reduce bladder smooth muscle contractility and lead to voiding problems or incontinence; they may also cause peripheral edema, which may lead to nocturia or nighttime urine loss.

Physical Examination

The physical examination of the patient with incontinence should include detection of general medical conditions that may affect the lower urinary tract. Such conditions include cardiovascular insufficiency, pulmonary disease, occult neurologic processes (e.g., multiple sclerosis, stroke, Parkinson's disease, and anomalies of the spine and lower back), as well as abnormalities of genitourinary development. The pelvic examination, including an evaluation of urethral support, is of crucial importance:

1. Patients with urinary incontinence should be examined with a full bladder, particularly if stress incontinence is a complaint.

2. The patient should stand with her feet separated to shoulder width and cough several times to see if the physical sign of stress incontinence can be demonstrated. If urine loss occurs, confirm with the patient that this is the problem that has been bothering her. Many multiparous women may lose a small amount of urine during such an examination but not be bothered by it.

3. Many women with urge incontinence caused by detrusor overactivity may demonstrate urine loss during a cough stress test, but this finding may not be relevant to their real complaint. The physical findings must be set within the context of the patient's history to be relevant.

4. **The patient's complaint should be reproduced by the physician and confirmed with the patient, particularly if surgery is contemplated.**

Urinalysis

Examination of the urine by dipstick testing and microscopy is necessary to exclude infection, metabolic abnormalities, and kidney disease.

1. Urine culture will help rule out infection, which can be associated with incontinence.

2. Urine cytology is useful as a screening test for urinary tract malignancy, but the utility of the test depends greatly on the accuracy of the laboratory performing the cytology. Routine urinary cytology is not helpful, but testing should be performed in women older than 50 years of age with irritative urinary tract symptoms, particularly if those symptoms are of sudden onset.

3. Hematuria should be evaluated with cytology, intravenous urography, and cystoscopy. Bladder biopsy should be performed by the surgeon who will treat the patient in the event that a malignancy is discovered.

Measurement of Postvoid Residual Urine

Incomplete bladder emptying is a frequent cause of incontinence. Patients with a large postvoid residual urine have a diminished functional bladder capacity because of the dead

631

space occupied in the bladder by retained urine. This stagnant pool of urine is also a frequent source of urinary tract infections, because the major defense of the bladder against infection is frequent, complete emptying.

A large postvoid residual can contribute to urinary incontinence in two ways. If the bladder is overdistended, increases in intra-abdominal pressure can force urine past the urethral sphincter, causing stress incontinence. In some cases, bladder overdistention may provoke an uninhibited contraction of the detrusor muscle, leading to incontinence. Both conditions may exist together, further complicating the problem.

Patients with an elevated postvoid residual urine should begin a regimen of clean, intermittent self-catheterization to improve bladder emptying. In many cases, this technique may be the only therapy needed to correct the incontinence and eliminate recurrent urinary tract infections.

Frequency/Volume Bladder Chart

A frequency/volume bladder chart is an invaluable aid in the evaluation of patients with urinary incontinence, but use of this tool often is neglected (41, 42). A frequency/volume chart is a voiding record kept by the patient for several days. Use of a plastic measuring "hat" that fits over the patient's toilet bowl is very useful in keeping accurate records. Patients should be instructed to write down the time of every void on the chart and measure the amount of urine voided. The time of any incontinent episodes should be recorded, and it is also helpful to maintain an annotated record of symptoms or activities associated with urine loss. If desired, the patient can also be instructed to keep a record of fluid intake, although in most cases intake can be estimated with some accuracy from the amount of urine produced.

A frequency/volume bladder chart gives an accurate record of 24-hour urinary output, the total number of daily voids, the average voided volume, and the functional bladder capacity (largest volume voided in normal daily life). This information allows the clinician to confirm complaints of urinary frequency with objective data and to determine whether part of the patient's problem is an abnormally high (or low) urinary output. For example, incontinence is a common complaint for many patients with diabetes, and the first step in the management of such patients is to control their blood glucose levels and decrease their urinary output rather than using medications or surgery, which will often be ineffective. Conversely, many patients with incontinence decrease their fluid intake dramatically in an attempt to control their urine loss, not realizing that the resulting highly concentrated urine is often much more irritating to their bladders than a higher volume of a more diluted urine. **As a rule, daily urine output should be 1500–2500 ml, with an average voided volume of approximately 250 ml, a functional bladder capacity (largest voided volume) of 400–600 ml, and seven or eight voids per day.** The frequency/volume chart is the foundation for conservative management of urinary incontinence based on fluid manipulation and behavioral management of voiding habits.

Urodynamic Studies

At its most basic level, a urodynamic study is anything that provides objective evidence about lower urinary tract function (43). In this sense, measurement of a patient's voided urine volume and catheterization to determine her postvoid residual urine are urodynamic studies. A frequency/volume chart is also a valuable urodynamic study. Obtaining clinically useful information does not always require the use of expensive, complex technology.

Bladder Filling Test

If a patient with a complaint of urinary incontinence comes for her examination without a full bladder, a great deal of information can be obtained by a simple *bladder filling test*

632

(44). The patient should urinate and measure the volume she voids. The residual urine can be measured by draining it through a 10-French or 12-French red rubber catheter placed into the bladder. Once the residual urine has been drained out, a bag of sterile water or saline attached to the catheter can be used to fill the patient's bladder at a rate of 60–75 ml/min until her functional bladder capacity is reached.

If the patient experiences urgency with accompanying urine loss during bladder filling, it is highly likely that she has motor *urge incontinence* caused by detrusor overactivity. If the patient leaks an isolated spurt of urine each time she coughs, and this leakage is demonstrated repetitively and confirmed as the problem for which she is seeking help, she has *stress incontinence*. Further evaluation is required for patients who exhibit *mixed incontinence* (the presence of both stress and urge incontinence), who exhibit prolonged leakage with coughing (suggestive of a cough-induced detrusor contraction), or for whom the complaint cannot be verified.

Multichannel Urodynamic Studies

Multichannel urodynamic studies produce a biophysical profile of a patient's bladder and urethral function, but such studies are only helpful if they are interpreted with reference to the patient's history and her physical examination. Clinicians recommend that patients who undergo urodynamic studies as part of a diagnostic "fishing expedition" without a careful history and a thorough physical examination are likely to obtain useless or irrelevant information.

A wide variety of sophisticated studies of bladder and urethral function have been developed to measure various aspects of bladder storage and bladder emptying. These studies include uroflowmetry, filling cystometry, pressure-flow voiding studies (with and without simultaneous electromyography of the pelvic floor), urethral pressure profilometry, and determination of leak-point pressure.

The bladder is affected by neural impulses running along afferent and efferent sensory pathways and generates a pressure/volume relationship in the cycle of micturition (Fig. 20.6). As bladder volume increases, tension-stretch receptors in the bladder wall are activated, and the afferent sensory impulses gradually lead to a desire to void. Normally, this occurs between 150 and 250 ml. A normal patient will be able to suppress a micturition reflex until an appropriate time. She should then be able to relax the pelvic floor and generate a sustained contraction of the bladder detrusor muscle until emptying is complete, after which the detrusor relaxes and the cycle begins again.

Cystometry

Cystometry is the technique by which the pressure/volume relationship of the bladder is measured. It can be divided into two phases: filling cystometry and voiding cystometry (also called a pressure-flow study). Simple cystometry is carried out when bladder pressure only is measured during filling. Because the bladder is an intra-abdominal organ, however, the pressure recorded in the bladder is a combination of several other pressures, most notably the pressure created by the activity of the detrusor muscle itself and the pressure exerted on the bladder by the weight of the surrounding intra-abdominal contents (e.g., uterus, intestines, straining or exertion). For this reason, the technique of *subtracted cystometry* is used.

Subtracted Cystometry Subtracted cystometry is an attempt to measure the pressure exerted in the bladder by the activity of the detrusor muscle. Subtracted cystometry is carried out by measuring *total intravesical pressure* (**P**ves) with a bladder pressure catheter, approximating *intra-abdominal pressure* (**P**abd) by measuring either rectal or vaginal pressure, and using an electronic instrument to subtract the latter from the former to give the *true detrusor pressure* (**P**det) or the subtracted pressure:

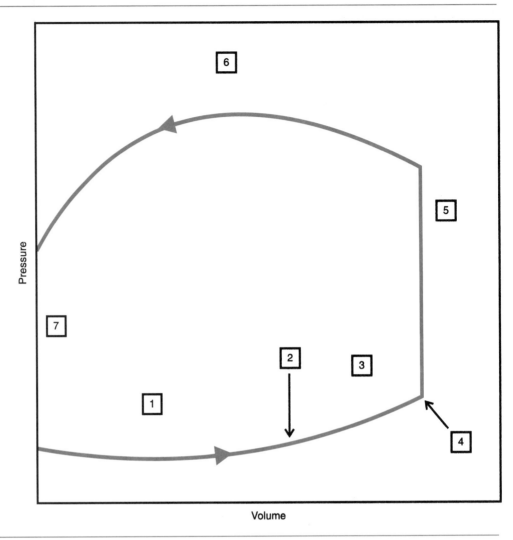

Figure 20.6   Pressure/volume relationship of the micturition cycle. 1) The normal bladder accommodates increasing urine volumes without a significant increase in pressure. 2) At around 200 ml, the first sensation of bladder fullness is appreciated. 3) The micturition reflex can be suppressed until a socially acceptable time and place for urination presents itself. 4) At this time, a voluntary detrusor contraction is initiated, in conjunction with pelvic floor relaxation. 5) There is a brief isometric pressure rise before the bladder neck is open and flow starts. 6) Normal voiding is accomplished by a sustained detrusor contraction until bladder emptying is complete. 7) The detrusor muscle then relaxes and the process of filling begins anew. (Reproduced with permission from **Wall LL, Addison WA.** Basic cystometry in gynecologic practice. *Postgrad Obstet Gynecol* 1988;26(2):2.)

$$Pdet = Pves - Pabd$$

Measurements can be made using either expensive electronic microtip transducer pressure catheters or inexpensive fluid-filled pressure lines.

The technique for such a study is shown in Figure 20.7.

1.   Fluid (usually sterile water or saline, sometimes radiographic contrast dye) is infused at a rate of 50–100 ml/min. The volume infused and the pressure mea-

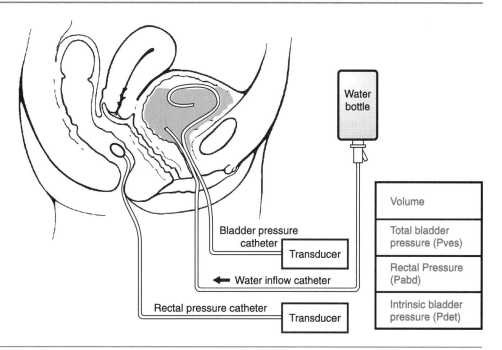

Figure 20.7   Subtracted filling cystometry. Pressure catheters are in place in the bladder and rectum. An additional filling catheter has been placed in the bladder. Volume infused, total bladder pressure, rectal (abdominal) pressure, and subtracted detrusor pressure (intrinsic bladder pressure) are recorded. (Reproduced with permission from **Wall LL, Addison WA.** Basic cystometry in gynecologic practice. *Postgrad Obstet Gynecol* 1988;26(2):3.)

surements are recorded continuously. The patient's bladder may be filled with her lying supine, in a modified lithotomy position, sitting, or standing. When possible, standing cystometry is usually preferable, because most patients with incontinence complain of this problem when they are erect.

2. The point at which any leakage occurs should be noted carefully.

3. During filling, the point at which the first desire to void is experienced should be noted, along with the point at which the patient experiences a strong desire to void, urgency, and her cystometric capacity.

4. Provocative maneuvers are performed, such as coughing, heel-bouncing, and listening to the sound of running water in an attempt to produce urinary incontinence and to provoke any uninhibited detrusor contractions, which may be the cause of the patient's symptoms.

Normal cystometric values for women are shown in Table 20.3.

At *cystometric capacity* (ideally, the same as the patient's functional bladder capacity), the filling catheter should be removed, leaving only the pressure-measurement lines in place (Fig. 20.8). If the pressures are allowed to equilibrate for 1 minute, *bladder compliance* can be calculated by dividing the bladder volume in milliliters by the pressure of water in centimeters. The patient should then void. The urine flow rate can be measured and correlated with the detrusor pressure. This technique allows a better assessment of voiding function than measurement of urine flow rate alone.

Table 20.3   Approximate normal values of female bladder function

Residual urine <50 ml

First desire to void occurs between 150 and 250 ml infused

Strong desire to void does not occur until >250 ml

Cystometric capacity between 400 and 600 ml

Bladder compliance between 20 and 100 ml/cm H_2O measured 60 seconds after reaching cystometric capacity

No uninhibited detrusor contractions during filling, despite provocation

No stress or urge incontinence demonstrated, despite provocation

Voiding occurs because of a voluntarily initiated and sustained detrusor contraction

Flow rate during voiding is >15 ml/sec with a detrusor pressure of less than 50 cm H_2O

Reproduced with permission from **Wall LL, Norton P, DeLancey J.** *Practical Urogynecology.* Baltimore: Williams & Wilkins, 1993.

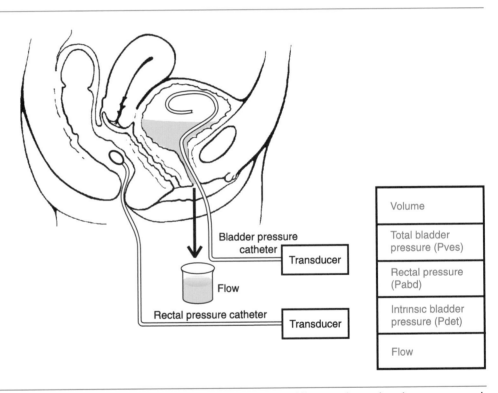

Figure 20.8   Pressure-flow voiding study. The filling catheter has been removed. Volume voided, urine flow rate, total bladder pressure, rectal (abdominal) pressure, and subtracted detrusor pressure are recorded. (Reproduced with permission from **Wall LL, Addison WA.** Basic cystometry in gynecologic practice. *Postgrad Obstet Gynecol* 1988;26(2):3.)

Urethral Pressure Profile   In addition to an assessment of filling and emptying, specific urodynamic tests allow some quantitative assessment of sphincteric integrity. The *urethral pressure profile* is a test designed to measure urethral closure. Because continence requires the pressure in the urethra to be higher than the pressure in the bladder, it was believed that measuring the pressure differential between the two would provide useful clinical information. The urethral pressure profile is generated by slowly pulling a pressure-sensitive catheter through the urethra from the bladder, which is usually filled with a consistent volume of fluid (Fig. 20.9). The *urethral closure pressure* (**P**close) is the difference between the *urethral pressure* (**P**ure) and the *bladder pressure* (**P**ves):

$$Pclose = Pure - Pves$$

Although this pressure can be used to differentiate normal women from those with stress incontinence (women with stress incontinence tend to have higher urethral pressure levels than those who do not), there is considerable overlap between the two groups. It has also been suggested that women with stress incontinence with low urethral closure pressure (<20 cm H_2O) have a poorer prognosis for surgical outcome than women who do not have this condition; however, there is considerable debate about this (45–47). Because stress incontinence, by definition, occurs during increases in intra-abdominal pressure that are generated by some kind of physical activity, it is not obvious why measurement of resting urethral pressure should be relevant to stress-related leakage, which is a dynamic event. In general, the urethral pressure profile has been a disappointing test with questionable clinical utility.

Leak-Point Pressure Test

A more promising test seems to be the *leak-point pressure* test (48). The idea behind this test is quite simple: the amount of force that it takes to produce stress incontinence should be related to the severity of the stress incontinence and to the strength of the sphincteric unit. **The leak-point pressure is the intravesical (or sometimes intra-abdominal) pres-**

Figure 20.9   Parameters normally measured during urethral pressure profile studies. (International Continence Society.)

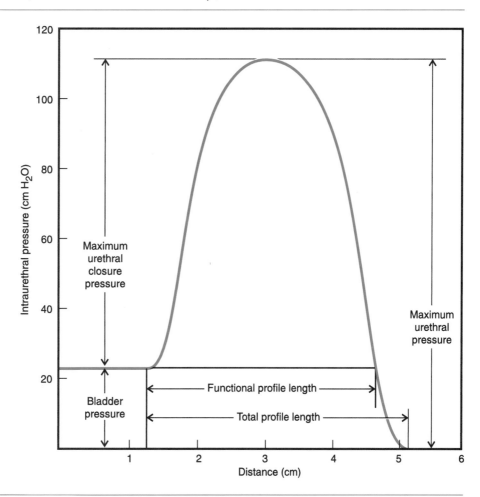

sure measured at the moment that stress incontinence occurs. It is usually determined at a bladder volume of around 200 ml, but the technique has not been completely standardized. When the appropriate bladder volume has been reached, patients are asked to strain slowly to increase intravesical pressure gradually. The lowest pressure at which leakage occurs is recorded as the Valsalva leak-point pressure. If leakage does not occur during Valsalva, the patient can be asked to cough several times, gradually increasing the intensity of each cough until leakage occurs. If leakage is not demonstrated, the highest pressure that has been obtained can be recorded with the notation "no leakage" to the specified pressure as measured in cm H_2O. This figure seems to give a reasonable estimation of sphincteric strength.

Extraurethral Causes of Incontinence

Involuntary urine loss can occur through two basic routes. Most urinary incontinence represents unwanted urine loss through the urethra (transurethral incontinence); however, urine loss can also occur through abnormal openings. These openings can be created by congenital causes or some form of trauma. The congenital causes of urinary incontinence are not common and usually are easy to diagnose. The most extreme cases are caused by *bladder exstrophy,* in which there is a congenital absence of the lower anterior abdominal wall and anterior portion of the bladder, resulting in the entire bladder opening directly to the outside (49). Such cases are always diagnosed at birth, and before the advent of modern reconstructive surgery, these infants all died very early in life from sepsis.

Ectopic Ureter

The most common, and far more subtle, congenital anomaly causing extraurethral urine loss is an ectopic ureter (50). Generally, ectopic ureters are also detected early in life, but occasionally one may escape detection until adolescence or early adulthood. In infancy, an ectopic ureter should be suspected when a mother seeks care for her baby whom she says is never dry. Normally, infants have periods of dryness interspersed with periods of wetness. If a parent notes that every time the baby is checked her diaper is wet, this is the first clue that an ectopic ureter may exist, because this ureter will most likely drain to the outside, causing continuous urinary leakage. Most commonly, the ectopic ureter drains into the vagina, but occasionally it may drain into the urethra distal to the point of continence. This condition can be diagnosed easily by excretory urography.

Urinary Fistula

A traumatic opening between the urinary tract and the outside is called a *fistula*. Worldwide, the most common cause of fistulas is obstructed labor. This was also true in the Western world 150 years ago, but advances in the provision of basic obstetric services and advanced obstetrical intervention have virtually eliminated this problem in developed countries. The rest of the world is not so fortunate.

Obstructed labor often occurs in rural areas where girls are married young (sometimes as early as 9 or 10 years of age) and where transportation is poor and access to medical services is limited. In such circumstances, pregnancy often occurs shortly after menstruation begins and before maternal skeletal growth is complete. When labor begins, cephalopelvic disproportion is common, and little can be done to correct fetal malpresentations. Women may be in labor as long as 5–6 days without intervention, and if they survive, they usually give birth to a stillborn infant. In such cases, the soft tissues of the pelvis have been crushed by constant pressure from the fetal head, leading to an ischemic vascular injury and subsequent tissue necrosis. When this tissue sloughs, a genitourinary or rectovaginal fistula develops. Many of these patients have complex or multiple fistulas, involving total destruction of the urethra and sloughing of the entire bladder base. Obstetric fistulas are frequently as large as 5–6 cm.

After such fistulas develop, the lives of these young women (most of whom are younger than 20 years of age) are disrupted unless they can gain access to curative surgical services.

638

The constant, uncontrolled dribble of urine makes them offensive to their husbands and family members. They can no longer live with their families. Most of them eventually become destitute social outcasts—and yet these are otherwise healthy functional young women. The social and economic costs of this problem are enormous, but the problem has largely been neglected by the world medical community. The morbidity associated with obstetric fistulas remains, along with the related problem of maternal mortality, one of the single most neglected issues in international women's health care (51).

In the industrialized world, the most common causes of genitourinary fistulas are surgery, malignancy, and radiation therapy or the interrelation of all three factors. Most often, a vesicovaginal fistula develops after an otherwise uncomplicated vaginal or abdominal hysterectomy in which a small portion of the bladder was inadvertently trapped in a surgical clamp or was transfixed by a suture. These fistulas most often occur at the vaginal apex and are no larger than 1–2 mm. The amount of urine that can leak through a fistula of any size, however, is enormous and constant.

A wide variety of techniques are available for fistula repair (52, 53). **Fistula repair is best performed after a waiting period of 3 months to allow the resolution of inflammation and formation of scar tissue.** This is particularly important in the case of obstetric fistulas, in which the extent of the vascular injury to the soft tissues of the pelvis may not be apparent for many weeks. The keys to closure of a vesicovaginal fistula include wide mobilization of tissue planes so that the fistula edges can be approximated without any tension, close approximation of tissue edges, closure of the fistula in several layers, and meticulous attention to postoperative bladder drainage for 10–14 days. The closure of large fistulas will be enhanced by the use of tissue grafts (e.g., Martius labial fat-pad grafts, gracilis muscle flaps) that bring an additional blood supply to nourish an area that has sustained vascular injury.

Stress Urinary Incontinence

Stress incontinence occurs during periods of increased intra-abdominal pressure (e.g., sneezing, coughing, or exercise) when the intravesical pressure rises higher than the pressure that the urethral closure mechanism can withstand, and urine loss results. Stress urinary incontinence is the most common form of transurethral urinary incontinence in women. A community survey of 1060 randomly selected women older than 18 years of age in South Wales, for example, revealed that 22% of women had this complaint (54). In a survey of 144 collegiate female varsity athletes, 27% complained of stress incontinence while participating in their sport (55). The activities most likely to produce urinary loss were jumping, high-impact landings, and running. Even in otherwise fit and vigorous women, the continence mechanism is particularly susceptible to stress incontinence.

The term "stress incontinence" refers to three distinct entities: a symptom, a sign, and a condition (38). Confusion can occur if the differences between these three entities are not appreciated.

Symptoms and Signs

The *symptom* of stress incontinence refers to the patient's complaint that she leaks urine when intra-abdominal pressure is increased. Such urine leakage may result from a variety of conditions: genuine stress incontinence, a detrusor contraction provoked by coughing or change of position, incomplete bladder emptying, or a urethral diverticulum. The patient's complaint of stress incontinence makes it likely, but not certain, that she has this problem, but the complaint must be confirmed by some objective means. A patient should never undergo surgery for stress incontinence on the basis of symptoms alone.

The *sign* of stress incontinence refers to the physical demonstration of urine loss during conditions of increased intra-abdominal pressure (e.g., coughing) while the patient is being examined. Mere demonstration of stress urinary leakage during a physical examination does not mean that the patient has a clinical problem with stress incontinence. According to the International Continence Society's definition, incontinence exists when urine loss becomes a social or hygienic problem (38). Many women experience occasional stress urinary leakage that is merely annoying or inconvenient. These women do not consider themselves incontinent nor do they need surgery; however, studies have also shown that there is little relationship between the volume of urine lost and the distress that it causes a patient with incontinence (56).

Genuine Stress Incontinence

A specific technical term, *"genuine stress incontinence,"* is used to refer to the urodynamic diagnosis of stress incontinence (38). Genuine stress incontinence is said to exist when a patient has demonstrable urinary leakage when intravesical pressure exceeds the maximum urethral closure pressure in the absence of a detrusor contraction. This term can only be used for a patient who has undergone urodynamic testing and who has met these test criteria, which prove that her urine loss is caused by ineffective urethral closure during periods of increased intra-abdominal pressure (Fig. 20.10).

Figure 20.10   Subtracted cystometrogram showing a stable bladder with genuine stress incontinence. During the filling phase (*A*), there is no rise in detrusor pressure. When the patient stands (*B*), there is a rise in intravesical and rectal pressure as the position of the intra-abdominal contents changes, but the subtracted detrusor pressure remains stable. When the patient coughs in the standing position, the detrusor remains stable. Coughs appear as sharp, isolated pressure spikes (*C*) on the intravesical and rectal pressure tracings, but there are no spikes on the subtracted detrusor tracing. The presence of leakage occurring simultaneously with each cough (*arrows*) confirms that the patient has genuine stress incontinence caused by ineffective urethral closure rather than incontinence from detrusor overactivity.

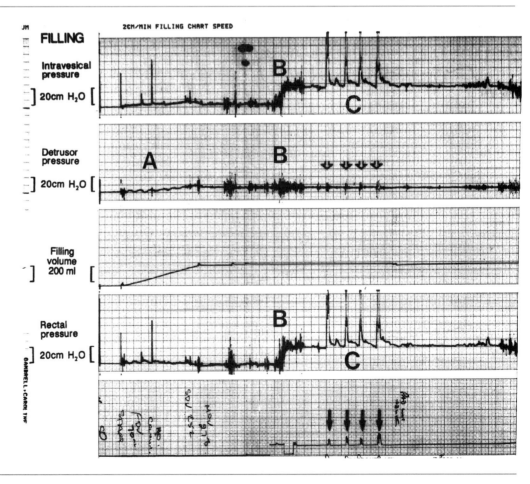

This urodynamic diagnosis must be analyzed with reference to the patient's complaint; one may have genuine stress incontinence that is nonetheless not a clinical problem or is a less severe problem than urge incontinence caused by detrusor muscle overactivity.

The clinical *condition* of stress incontinence includes a spectrum of symptoms ranging in severity. At one end of the spectrum is the female athlete who leaks only a tiny amount during vigorous physical activity; at the other end of the spectrum is the frail elderly woman who leaks large amounts of urine during minimal physical effort. The degree to which either woman is bothered by her leakage is influenced by her cultural values and expectations regarding urinary continence and incontinence.

Biobehavioral Model   **A biobehavioral model of stress incontinence can be created by examining the interaction of three variables: the biologic strength of the sphincteric mechanism, the level of physical stress placed on the closure mechanism, and the woman's expectations about urinary control** (Fig. 20.11). This model explains the enormous variation that exists among the symptoms, the degree of demonstrable leakage, and a patient's response to her stress incontinence. Modification of any one of these factors may influence the patient's clinical status. For example, many patients give up certain physical activities (e.g., running, dancing, aerobics) when they experience stress incontinence. Lim-

Figure 20.11   A biobehavioral model of stress incontinence. Clinical stress urinary incontinence results from the interaction of three distinct components: the inherent biological strength of the urinary sphincter, the level of physical stress placed on the sphincter, and the psychosocial milieu in which the patient lives (i.e., her personal and cultural expectations concerning urinary control and urinary incontinence).

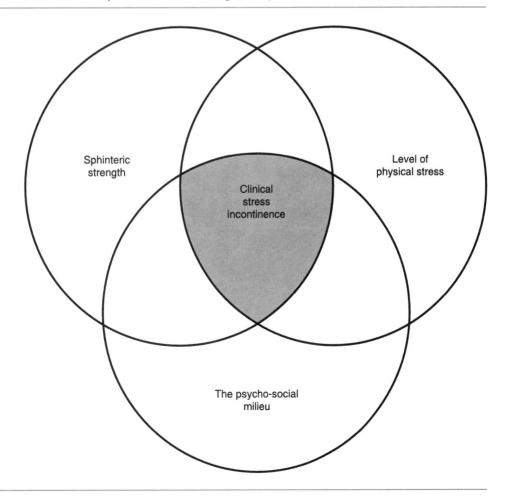

iting their activities may eliminate the incontinence problem, but it does so at a certain cost to their quality of life. Other women learn to cope with stress incontinence by adopting new body postures during physical activities that cause them to leak or by strengthening their pelvic muscles to compensate for increased exertion. Other women may be profoundly relieved to find out that the small amount of leakage they experience from time to time is not abnormal. In any case, the interaction of these three biopsychosocial factors opens up a variety of strategies for the management of stress incontinence. Surgical intervention is only one strategy, and it only addresses the biological competence of the sphincteric mechanism rather than either of the other factors that interact to produce the clinical problem.

Interaction of Extrinsic and Intrinsic Urethral Support   Effective urethral closure is maintained by the interaction of *extrinsic urethral support* and *intrinsic urethral integrity,* each of which is influenced by several factors (i.e., muscle tone and strength, innervation, fascial integrity, urethral elasticity, coaptation of urothelial folds, urethral vascularity). In the clinical setting, damaged urethral support is manifest clinically by urethral hypermobility, which often results in incompetent urethral closure during physical activity and presents as stress urinary incontinence. Intrinsic urethral functioning is more complicated and is not nearly as well understood as urethral support (57).

Clinical appreciation of the importance of extrinsic support and intrinsic urethral function have led surgeons to separate stress incontinence into two broad types:

1. That caused by anatomic hypermobility of the urethra, which produces faulty urethral closure under stress

2. That caused by intrinsic sphincteric weakness or deficiency

The former type is more prevalent, probably accounting for somewhere between 80 and 90% of stress urinary incontinence.

The latter type is less common and more challenging to treat. Although this concept is useful, in most cases, patients cannot be divided into one category or another but instead are affected by both aspects that interact to produce the clinical condition (Fig. 20.12). The challenge is deciding which factor predominates, because this decision will have a direct bearing on the type of treatment chosen.

Figure 20.12 Interaction of anatomic urethral hypermobility with intrinsic sphincteric deficiency in patients with stress incontinence. The problem is not an either/or dichotomy but rather one of degree.

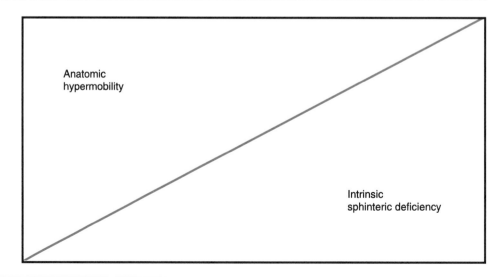

Nonsurgical Treatment

Many extrinsic, as well as intrinsic, factors influence urethral closure, and surgery is not the only option, nor is it always the best choice, for this condition. **Nonsurgical approaches to stress incontinence are based on manipulation of the factors that contribute to the condition. These approaches may involve reducing factors that worsen the problem** (e.g., obesity, smoking, or excessive fluid intake) **or by intervening actively to enhance the ability of the patient's pelvic floor to compensate for increased intraabdominal pressure** (e.g., making adaptive changes in posture, rehabilitating pelvic muscles, improving estrogen status, using alpha-adrenergic stimulants, or wearing a device to improve urethral support).

Muscle Strengthening

By its connection with the endopelvic fascia, the musculature of the levator ani complex provides substantial support for the urethra, vagina, and rectum as they descend through the pelvic floor (58). The periurethral levator ani muscles contain both type I (slow-twitch) and type II (fast-twitch) muscle fibers, which allows them to maintain tone over a long period and to increase tone suddenly to compensate for the increased abdominal pressure that occurs with coughing, sneezing, and straining. These muscle groups can be rehabilitated through exercise and physical therapy (59). There are two possible ways in which this therapy improves stress urinary incontinence. First, strengthening the striated urogenital sphincter could enhance its ability to constrict the urethral lumen, yielding a stronger closure force in the urethra at rest or increasing the forces of urethral closure generated during a cough or other stressful situations. Second, because the levator ani muscles play an important role in pelvic and urethral support, exercise could improve the support of the proximal urethra, generating improved continence during a cough, when the muscles are active, without producing a noticeable rise in resting urethral pressure measurements.

Kegel Exercises   Kegel was the first person to investigate pelvic floor muscle strengthening. He developed the patient's awareness of the pubococcygeus muscle and instructed her in exercises to strengthen this muscle with a crude pneumatic biofeedback device called a perineometer. He stressed the importance of supervised instruction and encouragement in the performance of these exercises and reported good success rates in relieving symptomatic stress incontinence by his program. Although nearly all gynecologists are familiar with these exercises, they rarely are taught and used as Kegel did originally, and this form of therapy has often degenerated into a few brief words of oral instruction in which the patient is told to stop and start her urine stream a few times each day while voiding. Programs based on this approach are not only disappointing in their results but also can train women to become dysfunctional voiders.

For muscular rehabilitation of the pelvic floor to be effective, exercises must be supervised, performed regularly, and aided by some form of feedback so the patient can judge her progress. Careful supervision makes a dramatic difference in the degree of success that can be obtained (59, 60). Using an intensive program of physical therapy over 3 months with pretherapy and posttherapy urodynamic and radiographic evaluations, Benvenuti and colleagues cured 32% of their patients with genuine stress incontinence and brought about marked improvement in symptoms in the remaining 68%. Both tonic and phasic contractility of the pubococcygeus muscle were improved, and there was clear-cut improvement of bladder neck support, as seen on radiographic evaluation in 13 of 15 patients who underwent repeat studies. After 12–36 months of follow-up, 77% reported that they had maintained the functional level they had attained at the end of treatment (61).

Similarly, Peattie and co-workers trained 30 premenopausal women with genuine stress incontinence in pelvic muscle rehabilitation with an ingenious form of resistive therapy using a set of weighted vaginal cones (62). These cones are of the same size but of increasing weight (from 20–100 g). After inserting a cone into the vagina, it can only be retained in place by contracting the pelvic floor. As one cone is successfully retained for 15 minutes, the next heaviest cone is used, thus progressively increasing the retained weight. The feeling that the cone is slipping out of the vagina results in a form of sensory biofeedback that causes an increased contraction in the pelvic floor in an attempt to retain it. At the end of 1 month of therapy, 19 patients (70%) reported cure or significant improvement of symptoms and only 11 (37%) opted for subsequent surgical intervention.

Physical therapy will not cure or improve all cases of stress incontinence; however, properly supervised and rigorously performed techniques for pelvic muscular rehabilitation can play a significant role in the treatment of genuine stress incontinence (59). Patients can expect improvement in their symptoms by tensing the musculature of the pelvic floor and holding these contractions for 5 seconds each, 15–20 times per session, three sessions per day. This will strengthen slow-twitch muscle fibers. Patients should also practice a similar number of rapid contractions to strengthen the fast-twitch muscle fibers. Pelvic muscle exercises should be taught to patients one-on-one during a pelvic examination, because many patients contract the wrong muscles; teaching Kegel exercises to large groups in classrooms is not worthwhile. Because pelvic muscle rehabilitation is virtually without side effects, involves the patient in her own care, and may prevent the development of subsequent pelvic organ prolapse if used regularly, physicians should be encouraged to incorporate pelvic muscle exercises into routine health maintenance programs for women.

Drug Therapy

Alpha-Adrenergic Drugs   The tone of the urethra and bladder neck is maintained in large part by alpha-adrenergic activity from the sympathetic nervous system. For this reason, many pharmacologic agents have been used with varying degrees of success to treat stress incontinence (Table 20.4). These drugs include *imipramine* (which has a concomitant relaxing effect on the detrusor), *ephedrine, pseudoephedrine, phenylpropanolamine,* and *norepinephrine*. Unfortunately, many of these compounds also increase vascular tone and may, therefore, lead to problems with hypertension, a condition that afflicts many postmenopausal women with stress incontinence. These effects may preclude the use of alpha agonists in such patients. Of equal importance, however, is the role of alpha blockers such as *prazosin* in the development of stress incontinence. These drugs are commonly used in treating hypertension because of their relaxing effects on vascular smooth muscle. They may also relax the bladder neck and urethra to the point at which incontinence develops. For patients who have symptoms of stress incontinence while taking this or a related drug, their antihypertensive medication should be changed before surgery is considered because their incontinence may resolve spontaneously with a change of medication (40).

Estrogen Therapy   **Postmenopausal women with urogenital atrophy resulting from estrogen deprivation and concurrent urinary incontinence should receive hormone replacement therapy as part of their therapeutic regimen unless such therapy is con-**

Table 20.4   Pharmacologic Agents Useful in the Treatment of Stress Incontinence

Drug	*Dose**
Imipramine	10–25 mg p.o. b.i.d./t.i.d.
Phenylpropanolamine	50–75 mg p.o. b.i.d.
Pseudoephedrine	30–60 mg p.o. t.i.d./q.i.d.
Ephedrine	15–30 mg p.o. b.i.d./t.i.d.
Norephedrine	100 mg p.o. b.i.d.

*p.o., by mouth; b.i.d., two times per day; t.i.d., three times per day; q.i.d., four times per day.

traindicated. Not only will many complaints of urgency, frequency, and irritation often disappear, but evidence suggests that estrogen replacement enhances the effectiveness of alpha-adrenergic receptors in the urethra (63, 64).

Electrical Stimulation

In addition to physical therapy and selected pharmacologic agents, electrical stimulation therapy has been used to treat stress incontinence. Passage of an electrical current through the muscles of the pelvic floor causes them to contract and simultaneously causes a reflex inhibition of detrusor activity. The stimulus can be applied transvaginally or transrectally in either continuous or intermittent fashion. Although many authors have reported good success rates using these devices, patient acceptance of the technique is often poor and the device may fail because of mechanical problems. Although this mode of therapy remains an option for patients with stress incontinence, it is unlikely to be used extensively at present outside a research setting (65).

Surgical Management

Operations for stress incontinence can be classified into four broad categories (66–68):

1. Traditional anterior vaginal colporrhaphy

2. Operations to correct stress incontinence resulting from anatomic hypermobility (retropubic bladder neck suspension operations and needle suspension procedures)

3. Operations for stress incontinence resulting from intrinsic sphincteric weakness or dysfunction (sling operations and periurethral injections)

4. Salvage operations (intentionally obstructive sling operations, implantation of an artificial urinary sphincter, urinary diversion)

Anterior Colporrhaphy

Anterior vaginal repair is the oldest operation for stress incontinence in gynecology. It was described by Howard Kelly in 1914 (69). He believed that stress incontinence was caused by an open vesical neck, rather than from loss of urethral support, and designed an operation to cure this condition by pulling the bladder neck closed using periurethral Kelly plication sutures. This operation remained the standard first approach to stress incontinence until the middle of this century and still is popular among many practitioners.

Many different operations have been lumped together under the term anterior colporrhaphy, including simple plication of the bladder neck, elevation of the bladder neck by plicating the fascia under the urethra, and elevation and fixation of the bladder neck by passing sutures lateral to the urethra and driving the needles anteriorly into the back of the pubic symphysis for fixation.

The mechanism of action of this operation, when it works, is preventing excessive displacement of endopelvic fascia beneath the urethra so the urethra can be closed during coughing or sneezing. The main advantage of this operation is that it avoids an abdominal incision, which may not be well tolerated by older women. It also allows the operation to be performed in conjunction with other vaginal surgery, such as vaginal hysterectomy for uterine prolapse.

The problem with most techniques of anterior colporrhaphy is that they do not hold up well over time (70–73). In essence, this operation attempts to take weak support from below and to push it back up from below, in hopes that these structures will maintain their strength and position over time. Although there have been excellent long-term results shown with anterior colporrhaphy, most of these reports use specific techniques requiring skillful dissection of the endopelvic fascia, deep bold bites of suture, and fixation of permanent sutures to the pubic bone from below: in essence, a transvaginal retropubic bladder neck suspension (74, 75). Most surgical series that have evaluated techniques of anterior colporrhaphy for stress incontinence show long-term success rates of only 35–65%, a figure that most would regard as unacceptably low. **Anterior colporrhaphy should be reserved primarily for patients requiring cystocele repair who do not have significant stress incontinence.**

Retropubic Bladder Neck Surgery, Needle Suspensions

Retropubic Urethropexy   The modern era of retropubic surgery for stress incontinence began in 1949, when *Marshall, Marchetti, and Krantz* described their technique for urethral suspension in a male with postprostatectomy incontinence (76). Since that time, **a variety of modifications of this operation have been described, all of which share at least two characteristics: they are performed through a low abdominal incision into the Retzius' space, and they all involve attachment of the periurethral/perivesical endopelvic fascia to some other supporting structure in the anterior pelvis** (Fig. 20.13). In the Marshall, Marchetti, and Krantz operation, the periurethral fascia is attached to the back of the pubic symphysis. Another approach, the *Burch colposuspension,* involves the attachment of the fascia at the level of the bladder neck to the iliopectineal ligament (Cooper's ligament) (77, 78). With the paravaginal repair, the lateral endopelvic fascia along the urethra and bladder is reattached to the arcus tendinous fascia pelvis (79, 80). In the *Turner-Warwick vagino-obturator shelf procedure,* the endopelvic fascia or vagina or both are attached to the fascia of the obturator internus muscle (81, 82). All of these operations cure stress incontinence by correcting anatomic hypermobility of the urethra and bladder neck. The long-term success rate for patients undergoing these operations as primary procedures for stress incontinence is in the range of 80–90% (83–88).

No operation is perfect, however (89, 90). Depending on how high and tight the suspending sutures are tied, these operations may also introduce an element of urethral kinking or

Figure 20.13   Points of reattachment of the endopelvic fascia during retropubic bladder neck suspension operations. *A,* Arcus tendinous fascia pelvis. *B,* Periosteum of the pubic symphysis. *C,* Iliopectineal ligament (Cooper's ligament). *D,* Obturator internus fascia. (Reproduced with permission from **Wall LL.** Stress urinary incontinence. In: **Rock JA, Thompson JD,** eds. *TeLinde's Operative Gynecology.* 8th ed. Philadelphia: JB Lippincott, 1996.)

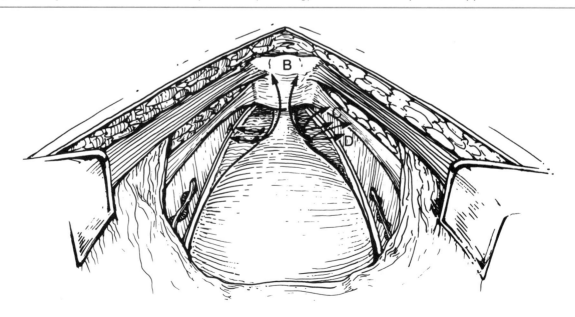

obstruction, with subsequent voiding difficulty (91–93). This can be a significant long-term complication for patients undergoing this type of surgery. Operations that put sutures directly into the pubic symphysis may cause debilitating osteitis pubis, which can disable an otherwise healthy woman for several months. The normal vaginal axis is almost horizontal, with the vagina resting on top of the levator plate (Fig. 20.14). Because the vagina is a tubular structure, pulling up on the anterior vagina also elevates the posterior vagina. This can pull the posterior vagina up out of its normal position, opening the rectouterine pouch of Douglas and thereby predisposing patients to enterocele formation, uterine prolapse, and vaginal vault eversion. For this reason, many authors recommend performance of a careful culdoplasty at the time of bladder neck suspension to reduce the incidence of future prolapse (94).

Transvaginal Urethropexy   Needle suspension procedures are so named because they suspend the urethra and bladder neck through a technique that involves passage of sutures between the vagina and anterior abdominal wall using a specially designed long needle carrier. To perform these operations, a vaginal incision is typically made at the level of the bladder neck, the endopelvic fascia is perforated, the Retzius' space is entered from below, and a permanent suture is passed down through a low abdominal incision through the Retzius' space, where it is fixed to the endopelvic fascia at the level of the bladder neck. The long needle is then passed back up through the retropubic space to the abdominal incision, where it is tied in place (Figure 20.15). The first needle suspensions were performed by a gynecologist, Dr. Armand Pereyra, in the 1950s, but many urologic surgeons have since made modifications to the technique (95–100).

These operations are designed to correct stress incontinence resulting primarily from anatomic hypermobility of the bladder neck and urethra. If the suspending sutures are pulled too tight, an element of obstruction can be created. They are relatively

Figure 20.14   Normal location of structures over the pelvic floor. Note that the normal vagina is almost horizontal, lying over the levator plate. Any operation that pulls the vagina forward, away from its normal location, increases the risk of enterocele formation and the development of rapidly progressive prolapse.

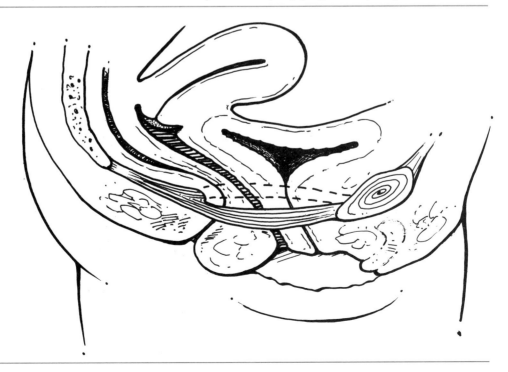

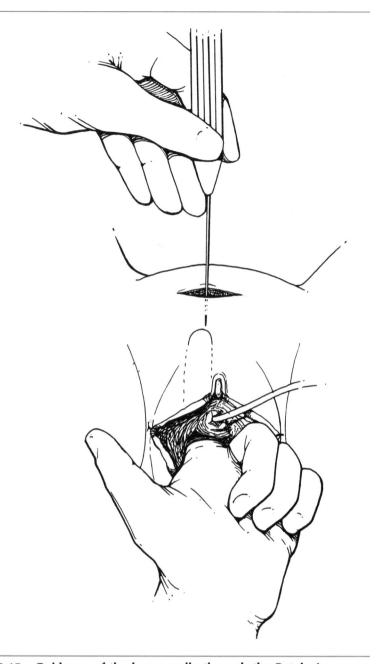

Figure 20.15   Guidance of the long needle through the Retzius' space using the surgeon's index finger. (Reproduced with permission from **Wall LL.** Stress urinary incontinence. In: **Rock JA, Thompson JD,** eds. *TeLinde's Operative Gynecology.* 8th ed. Philadelphia: JB Lippincott, 1996.)

simple and take less time to perform than open procedures, but this advantage is often offset by the fact that they are not as effective in curing stress incontinence. Initial cure rates are between 70 and 90%, but these rates seem to decrease significantly over time in many series, with 5-year success rates of 50% or less (83, 101–104). In addition to a lower success rate, other complications include perforation of the bladder or urethra by the long needles, infections, formation of granulation tissue around sutures and the synthetic bolsters often used in fixing the sutures to the fascia at the bladder neck or abdominal wall, development of prolapse as a result of changes created in the vaginal axis, chronic pulling pelvic pain created by the suspension sutures, and nerve entrapment syndromes (105–109).

Sling Procedures and Periurethral Injections

Sling Operations **Sling operations are used principally for patients with complicated stress incontinence, usually resulting from intrinsic sphincteric damage or weakness. Probably no more than 15–20% of women with stress incontinence need a sling procedure to be cured.** Patients requiring a sling typically have demonstrable stress incontinence with normal urethral support or stress incontinence with a low leak-point pressure. Other candidates might be women with stress incontinence who engage in very heavy occupational lifting, who have severe chronic obstructive lung disease, and who have posthysterectomy vaginal vault eversion. Such patients seem to have an increased risk of surgical failure if their stress incontinence is treated with an anterior colporrhaphy, retropubic operation, or needle suspension. Although sling operations do provide urethral support, they work primarily by compressing the urethral lumen at the level of the bladder neck to compensate for a faulty urethral closure mechanism; that is, they work by creating some degree of outlet obstruction (Fig. 20.16).

Sling operations are performed using a combined vaginal and abdominal approach. The anterior vagina is opened, the Retzius' space is dissected on each side of the bladder neck, and a sling is passed around the bladder neck and urethra and is then attached to the anterior rectus fascia or some other structure to cradle the urethra in a supporting hammock. This both supports the urethra and allows it to be compressed during periods of increased intra-abdominal pressure (110–118). The sling can be made of organic or inorganic materials. Organic materials can be autologous tissues harvested from the patient herself (e.g., fascia lata, rectus fascia, tendon, round ligament, rectus muscle, vagina) or heterologous tissues harvested from another species and processed for surgical use (e.g., ox dura mater, porcine dermis). Synthetic materials (e.g., Silastic, Gore-Tex, Marlex) are popular because

Figure 20.16   Mechanism of action of sling procedures for stress incontinence. *A,* Normal urethra. *B,* Incompetent urethra with intrinsic sphincteric deficiency. The lumen is gaping, scarred, and has lost its normal coaptation and pliability. *C,* Correction of intrinsic sphincteric deficiency using a sling operation. The urethra is supported and the urethral lumen is partially compressed by the sling. (Reproduced with permission from **Wall LL.** Stress urinary incontinence. In: **Rock JA, Thompson JD,** eds. *TeLinde's Operative Gynecology.* 8th ed. Philadelphia: JB Lippincott, 1996.)

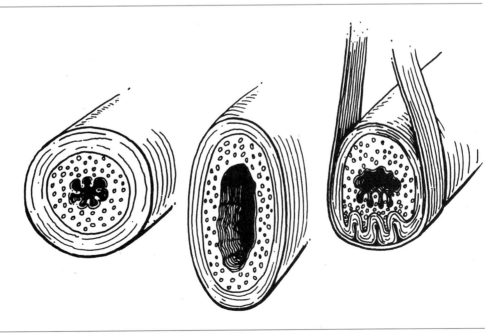

of their consistent strength and easy availability, but these substances are often plagued by problems with erosion and infection when they are used around the urethra.

The most common problem encountered by patients for whom a sling procedure has been performed is obstructed voiding after surgery. The sling does not have to be pulled tight to work, but the common temptation of less experienced surgeons is to make the sling too tight in hopes of ensuring that the patient is cured. Not infrequently, patients with a sling require long-term bladder drainage using either a suprapubic catheter or clean intermittent self-catheterization. The symptoms of obstructed voiding—urgency, frequency, urge incontinence, incomplete emptying, low flow, intermittent stream, hesitancy, and increased residual urine—typically improve over time and often resolve. Some patients, however, will require long-term self-catheterization. This possibility should be discussed with patients before surgery.

Periurethral Injections   A less invasive treatment of intrinsic urethral failure is attempting to restore urethral closure by injecting a material around the periurethral tissues to facilitate their coaptation under conditions of increased intra-abdominal pressure (119–124). This approach has been tried for years with only limited success, but recent advances in chemistry have allowed the development of materials better suited to the injection procedure, namely polytetrafluoroethylene past (*Polytef*) and glutaraldehyde cross-linked bovine collagen (*Contigen*). A small-gauge needle is inserted into the periurethral tissues and the material is injected along the urethra at the level of the bladder neck. This seems to work by bulking up the bladder neck, allowing enhanced urethral closure under stress, rather than by changing the resting urethral pressure. Teflon is harder to work with and requires the use of a power-injector. It also has been shown to migrate to other areas of the body under some circumstances. *Contigen* can be passed easily through small-bore needles under local anesthesia, but requires preoperative skin testing to check for possible allergic reactions (<3%). Both techniques may require several injections to achieve continence, and the long-term success of these operations remains poorly studied.

Salvage Operations

The best opportunity to cure stress incontinence occurs at the time of the initial operation. Subsequent surgeries have a lower success rate, and the chances of success seem to diminish with each subsequent operation (57). In some cases, the surgeon is faced with a scarred, fibrotic nonfunctional urethra in a hopelessly incontinent patient. This type of patient requires what can best be called "salvage" operations—a last ditch effort for cure. Such patients may benefit from periurethral collagen injections. Others may benefit from the placement of a deliberately obstructive sling, with the plan that the patient will drain her bladder by self-catheterization for the rest of her life. Still others may benefit from the implantation of an artificial urinary sphincter, a high-technology approach to incontinence that seems to works better for males than females (125, 126). Finally, others may require urinary diversion. Only a small percentage of women with stress incontinence will require such measures.

| Urinary Incontinence Caused by Detrusor Overactivity | **Although stress incontinence is the most common type of urinary continence in women, urge incontinence caused by detrusor overactivity is the most common form of incontinence in older women, and the second most common form of urinary incontinence overall (127).** In this condition, urine loss is caused not by failure of urethral support or closure but rather by uninhibited contractions of the detrusor muscle. Patients with this condition typically experience sudden, unexpected loss of large volumes of urine or leakage associated with a sudden urge to urinate that cannot be controlled. In both cases, urine loss occurs from an unsuppressed contraction of the bladder muscle, a failure to inhibit the micturition reflex. **When this occurs as the result of a known neuropathologic process relevant to bladder disorders (e.g., stroke, Parkinson's disease, multiple sclerosis), it is referred to as *detrusor hyperreflexia*. For cases in which there is no evi-** |

650

dence of neuropathology (in most cases), the condition is referred to as *detrusor instability.* **Both conditions can be called** *detrusor overactivity* (56). Detrusor overactivity should be suspected for all cases in which the patient has symptoms of urgency, frequency, and urge incontinence. For patients who have frequency and urgency without incontinence, detrusor overactivity rarely is the cause of their problem. For most such cases, the cause of the symptoms is a disorder of bladder sensation (128, 129).

Diagnosis

The diagnosis of incontinence caused by detrusor overactivity can be confirmed by cystometry. A rule for all incontinence evaluations is to demonstrate incontinence and confirm with the patient that what has been demonstrated reproduces her complaint. Subtracted filling cystometrography for patients with an overactive detrusors should show phasic pressure waves that produce urgency and urge incontinence (Fig. 20.17). False-negative and

Figure 20.17   Subtracted cystometrogram showing detrusor overactivity. Notice that the rectal pressure stays relatively constant throughout bladder filling in the supine position, whereas there are phasic changes in intravesical pressure and subtracted detrusor pressure. These changes are diagnostic of uninhibited contractions of the detrusor muscle. In this patient, these contractions produced a large amount of urine loss. Note that the rise in rectal pressure that occurs when the patient stands (S) provokes an additional detrusor contraction.

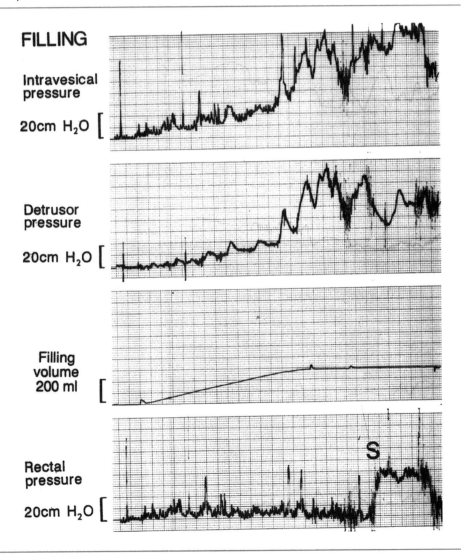

false-positive results can occur. False-positive results occur for patients with asymptomatic detrusor activity, detrusor activity that is irrelevant to their complaint, or detrusor activity that is situational (e.g., caused by test anxiety). The false-negative results occur because 20-minute cystometrography is not always an accurate measure of daily bladder activity. Looking for detrusor instability with such a test is like looking for an episodic cardiac arrhythmia by doing 12-lead electrocardiography, as opposed to looking for the arrhythmia using a 24-hour Holter monitor. The sensitivity of the latter test is far greater than the former. The same principles apply to stationary subtracted cystometry when compared with long-term ambulatory urodynamic studies (130–133). For most patients with a strong history of urge incontinence, a detrusor problem is the cause of leakage.

Treatment

Detrusor overactivity can be treated using drugs or behavioral modification (127). **The best initial choice is probably a combination of the two therapies.** If possible, long-term management of this condition should be based on behavioral therapy for two main reasons. The first is that the drugs used in treating detrusor instability have unpleasant anticholinergic side effects. Most patients will tire of tolerating these problems over time and will discontinue medications. Secondly, the cure rates with behavorial treatment are comparable to drug therapy, and any drug therapy for this condition will be enhanced by modifying the behavior that contributes to detrusor overactivity.

Drug Therapy   The drugs used in treating detrusor muscle overactivity can be grouped into different categories according to their pharmacologic characteristics; however, for all practical purposes, these drugs are *anticholinergic agents* that exert their effects on the bladder by blocking the activity of acetylcholine at muscarinic receptor sites. Most of these drugs have a short half-life, which means that they must be taken frequently. All of these drugs have side effects, the most common of which are dry mouth resulting from decreased saliva production, increased heart rate because of vagal blockade, feelings of constipation resulting from decreased gastrointestinal motility, and occasionally, blurred vision caused by blockade of the sphincter of the iris and the ciliary muscle of the lens of the eye. Other drugs, such as *imipramine,* may produce orthostatic hypotension and cardiac arrhythmias. Patients should be encouraged to titrate their medication to their symptoms and to vary the dosage (within acceptable limits) according to their needs.

A list of medications and the usual dosage ranges are given in Table 20.5. In general, it is best to start with a lower dose (particularly for elderly patients) and to increase it as needed to a higher, more frequent dosage. Patients with *neuropathic detrusor hyperreflexia* generally need more medication than patients with idiopathic detrusor instability. Patients should be warned of the anticholinergic side effects, but if patients do not notice them, they may not be taking their medications. Patients should be particularly advised about the symptom of a dry mouth and told that this is not due to thirst. Some patients will increase their fluid intake to combat this problem, with a subsequent worsening of their inconti-

Table 20.5   Drugs Useful In Treating Detrusor Overactivity

Drug	Dose*
Propantheline bromide	15–30 mg p.o. q.i.d.
Hyoscyamine sulfate	0.125–0.25 mg p.o. q. 4–6 hours
Hyoscyamine sulfate, extended release	0.375 mg p.o. b.i.d.
Oxybutynin chloride	5–10 mg p.o. t.i.d./q.i.d.
Dicyclomine hydrochloride	20 mg p.o. q.i.d.

*p.o., by mouth; b.i.d., two times per day; t.i.d., three times per day; q.i.d., four times per day.

nence. If dry mouth is a problem, patients should relieve it by chewing gum, sucking on a piece of hard candy, or eating a piece of moist fruit.

Behavioral Therapy   **Behavioral therapy for detrusor instability is based on the assumption that the underlying pathophysiology is the escape of the detrusor from the cortical control over micturition that had previously been established during childhood toilet-training.** The object of bladder retraining (or bladder drill, as it is sometimes called) is to reestablish the authority of the cerebral cortex over bladder function. This is performed through a regimen of timed voiding, gradually increasing the intervals between voids until the cycle of urgency, frequency, and urge incontinence is broken.

Behavioral therapy is carried out as follows:

1. The patient is instructed to void on a timed schedule, starting with a relatively frequent interval of every hour while she is awake.

2. When she wakes up in the morning, she voids at 6:00 AM, 7:00 AM, 8:00 AM, throughout the day. If it is 7:00 AM, and she does not feel the need to void, she must do so anyway. The object is to make her bladder do what she wants it to do, instead of responding to the whims of her bladder. If it is 7:55 AM and she is desperate to urinate, she cannot do so. She must wait until 8:00 AM, even if this means that she leaks some urine onto a pad. When the appropriate time arrives, she can empty her bladder.

3. At night, the patient is allowed to void only when she is awakened from sleep by the need to do so.

4. When she can maintain this schedule for 1 week, the voiding interval is increased by 15 minutes. It is increased gradually by 15 minutes every week until a normal voiding interval of 2.5–3 hours has been established.

This program works very well for patients with detrusor instability. The secret of success is gradual increases in the interval between voids. The best predictor of success is patient compliance; those who follow this program get excellent results. Unfortunately, **patients who have suffered a neurologic insult that has resulted in detrusor hyperreflexia do not respond very well to bladder retaining, because the problem is actually one of neural pathway destruction rather than the need to reestablish cortical control mechanisms.** Frequently, these patients have a trigger volume of urine that sets off a contraction that they cannot control voluntarily. Such patients may benefit from a timed voiding schedule in which they void at regular intervals (such as every 2 hours) to keep their bladder volume below the trigger point, but attempting to lengthen the interval between voids often does not work well.

Mixed Incontinence

Patients are said to have mixed incontinence when they have motor urge incontinence as a result of detrusor overactivity as well as stress incontinence. Because most patients have mixed symptoms, every effort should be made to confirm the diagnosis and to demonstrate objectively stress and urge incontinence before establishing such a diagnosis. Patients with mixed incontinence often pose complicated management problems, and controversy exists regarding the best method of treating them. In the confirmed presence of both types of urinary incontinence, one reasonable approach is to try to determine which symptom is more bothersome to the patient — stress incontinence or urge incontinence — and to proceed from that point (134). Others advocate using conservative therapy to treat urge incontinence first and proceeding with surgery only if stress incontinence persists. Because patients with mixed incontinence have a lower continence rate after surgery than patients with genuine stress incontinence alone, this approach is reasonable. However, it must be realized that some patients experience the *de novo* onset of detrusor overactivity after stress incontinence surgery, and that detrusor instability resolves in some patients with mixed incontinence after surgery for stress incontinence. **Bladder neck suspension surgery is contraindicated for patients with detrusor instability alone as the cause of their incontinence. Patients with mixed incontinence, a small functional bladder capacity, and high-pressure detrusor contractions on filling cystometry should undergo operations for stress incontinence only after careful consideration of their individual circumstances and a comprehensive clinical and urodynamic evaluation.**

Functional or Transient Incontinence

In addition to stress incontinence and incontinence caused by detrusor overactivity, a variety of other conditions may cause involuntary urine loss that is a social or hygienic problem (Table 20.2). Among the most important of these causes are those that are loosely categorized as functional or transient. The factors leading to urinary incontinence of this type are medically reversible conditions. This gives them heightened importance (particularly for older women), because appropriate medical intervention can cure or improve the continence problem without resorting to other forms of treatment.

Resnick has invented the useful mnemonic "DIAPPERS" to help remember these factors (Table 20.6) (135, 136). *Delirium* is an acute confusional state that may result in incontinence caused by disorientation. It is often associated with serious underlying pathology. *Infection* may lead to detrusor overactivity, which can be reversed by appropriate antimicrobial therapy. *Atrophic* urethritis and vaginitis can be a significant cause of urgency and frequency in older women. *Pharmacologic* agents of many types can have an adverse impact on urinary tract function. *Psychiatric* diagnoses may also be accompanied by incontinence. *Excessive* urine production, such as that found in diabetes, hypercalcemia, or excessive fluid intake, often leads to incontinence by overwhelming a bladder's capabilities to deal with large volumes of fluid. *Restricted* mobility is often associated with incontinence, particularly for elderly patients who, because of arthritis or unsteady gait, cannot reach toilet facilities or undress themselves quickly enough when the urge to urinate arises. Bowel disorders are often found in association with urinary tract problems, partly because of the shared innervation of these organ systems. *Stool* impaction is often found in elderly patients with urinary incontinence; relief of the impaction by prescribing a good bowel regimen to prevent the problem from recurring is often associated with improvement in the function of both organ systems. All of these factors argue strongly for the inclusion of a good medical evaluation as part of the workup of any patient with urinary incontinence.

Disorders of Bladder Emptying, Storage, and Contents

Voiding Difficulty

For women, disorders of urine storage (incontinence) are more common than disorders of bladder emptying (voiding difficulty), which tend to be the predominant problems in men

---

Table 20.6   Reversible Causes of Incontinence

D elirium
I nfection
A trophic urethritis and vaginitis
P harmacologic causes
P sychological causes
E xcessive urine production
R estricted mobility
S tool impaction

Modified with permission from **Resnick N, Yalla S.** Management of urinary incontinence in the elderly. *N Engl J Med* 1985;313:800–5.

because of the longer urethra and the presence of a potentially enlarged and obstructing prostate gland. Nonetheless, **women do suffer from voiding difficulties, which may be defined as emptying dysfunction resulting from a failure of pelvic floor relaxation or failure of the detrusor muscle to contract appropriately.** True outflow obstruction (defined as a detrusor pressure >50 cm H_2O in association with a urine flow rate <15 ml/sec) is rare in women, and when seen, is usually found in patients who have undergone obstructive bladder neck surgery for stress incontinence (92, 137).

For normal voiding to occur, the pelvic floor and urethral sphincter must relax, which should occur in conjunction with a coordinated contraction of the detrusor muscle that leads to complete bladder emptying. Of course, the bladder may be emptied by other mechanisms, such as by abdominal straining in the absence of a detrusor contraction, or simply by relaxation of the pelvic floor if the closure mechanism is exceptionally weak; however, complete bladder emptying is not the same as normal voiding. Some women may empty their bladders completely, but only by expending great effort over several minutes. In such cases, voiding is clearly abnormal, even though the bladder is empty when voiding ceases. In the worst cases, voiding is both difficult and incomplete.

An example of voiding difficulty is the *detrusor-sphincter dyssynergia* that occurs in some patients with multiple sclerosis (138, 139). With this condition, there is a lack of coordination between detrusor contraction and urethral relaxation, and the urethral sphincter contracts at the same time as the detrusor. This means that outlet resistance to voiding increases at the same time that intravesical pressure is increasing, so voiding becomes difficult if not impossible. Great effort is required to overcome urethral resistance; the patient voids with an interrupted stop-and-start stream and usually leaves a significant amount of residual urine.

Treatment

Voiding difficulty can be managed in several different ways, depending on the cause of the condition. Patients with pelvic floor spasticity (in the absence of a neurologic insult) can often be trained to relax the pelvic floor through biofeedback therapy and to void normally.

Drug Therapy   Mild sedatives are sometimes helpful in this process, as are alpha blockers, which reduce urethral tone (e.g., *prazosin, phenoxybenzamine*). For patients who are unable to generate a detrusor contraction, attempts have been made to enhance detrusor contractility using a cholinergic agonist such as *bethanechol chloride*. Although cholinergic medications are successful in making strips of bladder muscle contract in a laboratory, there is little evidence that such drugs are helpful clinically (140).

Self-Catheterization   **The mainstay in the treatment of voiding difficulty, therefore, is clean intermittent self-catheterization** (141). The implementation of self-catheterization programs revolutionized the treatment of voiding difficulties and urinary retention by eliminating the use of chronic indwelling catheters for many patients. **The most important protection against urinary tract infection is frequent and complete bladder emptying rather than avoidance of the introduction of a foreign body into the bladder.** Self-catheterization allows the patient to accomplish this task using a small (14 French) plastic catheter that she inserts through the urethra into the bladder, draining its contents. The catheter is then removed, washed with soap and water, dried, and stored in a clean, dry place. Elaborate sterile procedures are not necessary. Although bacteria are introduced into the bladder in this process, frequent emptying through self-catheterization greatly reduces the risk of urinary tract infection for these patients. The urine of women after self-catheterization regimens will always be colonized with bacteria; however, this condition should not be treated unless symptomatic infection occurs.

Suppressive Antibiotics   Voiding difficulty and stress incontinence pose special surgical problems, and many women with these conditions do not void normally after surgery, particularly if an obstructive operation is performed. After surgery, voiding difficulty can be managed with self-catheterization and reassurance. If outflow obstruction is diagnosed on a pressure-flow voiding study (low flow in the presence of high pressure), however, it may be beneficial to take down the obstructive operative procedure and resuspend the bladder neck at a lower, less obstructed, level (92).

Chronic suppressive antibiotic therapy should not be used; instead, acute infections should be treated with an appropriate antibiotic for 3 days. This treatment prevents the selection of potentially dangerous drug-resistant bacteria, which pose a risk for these patients.

Acute Urinary Retention

Acute urinary retention exists when there is a sudden inability to void (142). The condition is painful, and upon catheterization, a large volume of urine is released. Sometimes, the explanation is found readily, as in the case of a woman who develops urinary retention after having an epidural anesthetic during childbirth or a painful posterior colporrhaphy that results in pelvic floor spasm. A careful search should always be made to determine the cause of the retention, particularly if any neurologic signs are present. The patient should be catheterized to decompress her bladder and prevent overdistension. Most patients should be taught self-catheterization. This procedure not only gives patients a better method of long-term bladder emptying than an indwelling catheter but also provides them with a safety valve in the event that the problem recurs unexpectedly in the future.

Disorders of Bladder Sensation

Most patients with disorders of bladder sensation experience pain rather than lack of bladder sensation. The cause of most painful bladder conditions is unknown, and the therapies currently used in treatment are only partially successful, similar to the treatment of most chronic pain syndromes. As a result, disorders of bladder sensation are among the most frustrating urogynecologic conditions.

Diagnosis

A careful history should be obtained, along with a sterile urine specimen for analysis and culture. Many women treated repetitively for chronic cystitis will have taken multiple courses of antibiotics on the basis of symptoms without ever having had a culture-proven infection. Detrusor instability may be the cause of frequency, urgency, and urge incontinence but is not usually a factor for dysuria or painful urination. **Women older than 50 years of age (particularly smokers or workers exposed to chemicals) are at risk for bladder cancer, and this possibility must be considered, especially if hematuria is present. Urinary cytology is sometimes helpful in detecting early tumors of the urinary tract, and cystoscopy and intravenous urography are mandatory in the evaluation of patients with hematuria.**

Interstitial cystitis is a syndrome that presents as urgency, frequency, and bladder pain in the presence of a small bladder capacity, with bladder pain experienced on filling and relieved by voiding. Many different pathophysiologic processes factor into this condition, which compounds treatment (143). A number of possible causes must be considered in the differential diagnosis of painful voiding, including urethral diverticulae; vulvar disease; endometriosis; chemical irritation from soaps, bubble bath, or feminine hygiene products; urinary stones; urogenital atrophy from estrogen deprivation; and sexually transmitted diseases (144).

Treatment

Typically, the clinician has no definitive diagnosis at the end of the evaluation and must rely on symptomatic treatment.

1. Frequency-urgency syndromes should be managed with a careful voiding regimen (similar to that used in the treatment of detrusor instability) and local care.

2. The use of urinary tract analgesics such as *Urised* is often helpful in reducing urethral irritation. *Urised* is a polypharmaceutical agent containing a mixture of *methenamine, methylene blue, phenyl salicylate, benzoic acid, atropine sulfate,* and *hyoscyamine,* which has a soothing effect on many irritative urethral symptoms.

3. Restricting the patient's intake of alcohol, caffeine, fruit juice, spices, artificial sweeteners, and food colorings is often helpful.

4. Instruction in the basics of vulvar and perineal hygiene is also important (thorough drying; avoidance of most body powders, perfumes, or colored irritating soaps; avoidance of tight-fitting undergarments).

5. Some patients will benefit from the instillation of 50 ml of a 50% solution of *dimethylsulfoxide (DMSO)* for 20–30 minutes every other week for four or five sessions.

6. Because it has been theorized that bladder pain may result from increased histamine release, some patients benefit from medications that block these inflammatory mediators, such as *diphenhydramine hydrochloride* 25–50 mg orally three times per day in combination with 300 mg of *cimetidine* three times per day.

Pelvic Organ Prolapse

Pelvic support problems account for thousands of gynecologic surgical procedures each year, and yet our understanding of these conditions has advanced remarkably slowly in the past century. An increased appreciation of the various contributions of muscle, nerve, and connective tissue to support pelvic organs will probably change this within the next decade. Many basic questions have not yet been asked, and many basic clinical issues (such as a standard definition and classification of prolapse) remain unresolved.

Definition and Classification of Prolapse

A prolapse is a downward or forward displacement of one of the pelvic organs from its normal location. Traditionally, prolapse has referred to displacement of the bladder, the uterus, or the rectum. These displacements have usually been graded on a scale of 0–3 (or 0–4); the grade increases with increasing severity of the prolapse, with 0 referring to no prolapse and 3 (or 4) referring to total prolapse ("procidentia"). All forms of female genital prolapse are described with reference to the vagina. True rectal prolapse (as contrasted to a rectocele) will be discussed separately.

A variety of terms are used to describe female genital prolapse. Although these terms are generally unsatisfactory and somewhat inaccurate, they are so fixed in the literature that it is impossible to avoid using them.

- A *cystocele* is a downward displacement of the bladder.
- A *cystourethrocele* is a cystocele that includes the urethra as part of the prolapsing organ complex.
- A *uterine prolapse* is descent of the uterus and cervix down the vaginal canal toward the vaginal introitus.
- A *rectocele* is a protrusion of the rectum into the posterior vaginal lumen.
- An *enterocele* is a herniation of the small bowel into the vaginal lumen.

Unfortunately, these descriptive terms are inaccurate and misleading. They prejudge the true nature of any prolapse by focusing attention on the bladder, rectum, or uterus rather than focusing on the specific defects that are responsible for alterations in vaginal support. Furthermore, these terms are used in combination with an imprecise (and usually unspecified) system of grading, and they do not convey useful comparative information. The lack of an accurate system of classification of pelvic support defects has hampered progress in the clinical evaluation and treatment of patients with prolapse.

What is observed during a pelvic examination of patients with these conditions is an alteration in vaginal anatomy: anterior vaginal wall descent, posterior vaginal wall descent, a lateral vaginal support defect, cervical descent, or descent of the vaginal apex (in patients who have had a hysterectomy). To name these areas of vaginal descent after the organs that are presumed to be responsible for them prejudges many clinical issues and can lead the surgeon into problems for which he or she may not be prepared, such as, for example, when an "occult" enterocele is discovered during a rectocele repair or when vaginal eversion occurs after surgery because its apex was not believed to be involved in the support defect. Similarly, lumping defects of vaginal support into organ compartments or broad categories such as "cystocele" or "rectocele" draws attention from the precise nature and location of the defects of pelvic support that are present.

The way in which pelvic support defects are classified and described should be improved. A committee of the International Continence Society has been charged with developing a uniform international system for the description and classification of pelvic support defects. Until such a generally accepted system has been developed, reports on prolapse should specify the technique of examination used. The prolapse should be described as it exists at its maximal protrusion, as noted by the patient during her daily activities. The physical examination of the patient should not stop until this degree of prolapse has been observed by the examiner. Of prime importance is the concept of describing and evaluating site-specific defects of pelvic support: anterior vaginal support, lateral vaginal support (particularly the vaginal attachments along the arcus tendinous), posterior vaginal support, support of the vaginal apex, and total vaginal length (145–150). When possible, prolapse should be described with respect to fixed anatomic points, such as the plane of the hymen or the ischial spines. **Clinicians should be encouraged to describe the defects clearly and specifically and to avoid the use of general grades or classes of poorly defined entities. For example, a uterine prolapse could be described by saying that the cervix protrudes 2 cm below the hymenal ring during straining. A cystocele could be described by saying that the anterior vaginal wall descends through the hymenal plane and distends the hymenal ring to a diameter of 5 cm.**

Symptoms of Prolapse

Asymptomatic pelvic prolapse generally does not require treatment, but the patient should be informed that she is losing some aspects of pelvic support, which may require treatment in the future. Symptomatic prolapse may be manifest in several different ways. The most common symptom is a feeling of pressure or that something is protruding from the vagina. Patients often say they feel like they are sitting on an egg or they may complain of a dragging discomfort, which is described as a low backache or feeling of heaviness. Generally, this feeling is relieved by lying down, is less noticeable in the morning, and worsens as the day progresses, particularly if patients are on their feet for long periods of time. Specific types of prolapse may be associated with specific symptoms. Loss of anterior vaginal support often leads to urethral hypermobility, which in turn often (but not necessarily) results in stress urinary incontinence. A large anterior vaginal prolapse (or vaginal vault eversion) can produce symptoms of voiding difficulty. In such cases, the large prolapse comes out below the urethra, either compressing it from below or kinking it so that bladder emptying is incomplete or intermittent. An anterior protrusion of the rectum into the vaginal canal ("rectocele") can cause symptoms of inefficient rectal emptying, often described by the patient as constipation. In severe cases, the patient may have to splint the posterior vagina, thereby reducing the pocket that is trapping stool back into its normal position. It should be noted, however, that in most cases, constipation in women has causes other than a rectocele. The symptoms that result from a massive prolapse in which the entire uterus or vagina protrudes below the pelvic floor are self explanatory.

Examination of the Patient with Prolapse

In examining a patient with pelvic organ prolapse, all aspects of vaginal support should be carefully surveyed. Each area of vaginal anatomy should be described separately, and **because prolapse is almost invariably worse when the patient is upright, the clinician should become accustomed to examining patients in the standing position as well as in the standard dorsal lithotomy position.** The patient should stand on the floor with one foot elevated on a well-supported footstool. The examining gown can be lifted slightly to expose the genital region (Fig. 20.18). A standing pelvic examination allows the prolapse to be assessed when it is at its worst. A *rectovaginal examination* performed in this position is the best way of detecting an occult enterocele, because the small bowel can be palpated easily in the cul-de-sac between the thumb and forefinger. A standing pelvic examination can be conducted quickly and efficiently.

For a patient with prolapse, the traditional speculum examination of the vagina should be supplemented with a site-specific examination of the vagina using either a single-bladed speculum (such as a Sims speculum) or by taking a traditional Graves speculum apart and using the posterior blade and a single-sided retractor. This allows the clinician to obtain a better view of the anterior, posterior, and lateral vagina, looking for specific defects of vaginal support. When the nature of a prolapse is unclear, an examination of this kind will usually allow the problem to be identified (Fig. 20.19A–C).

After the prolapse has been identified to its maximal extent, the clinician should examine each aspect of vaginal support separately by retracting the anterior, posterior, and lateral

Figure 20.18   Standing examination of the patient to detect the extent of pelvic organ prolapse. An enterocele is detected during a standing rectovaginal examination by palpating the small bowel between the thumb and index finger.

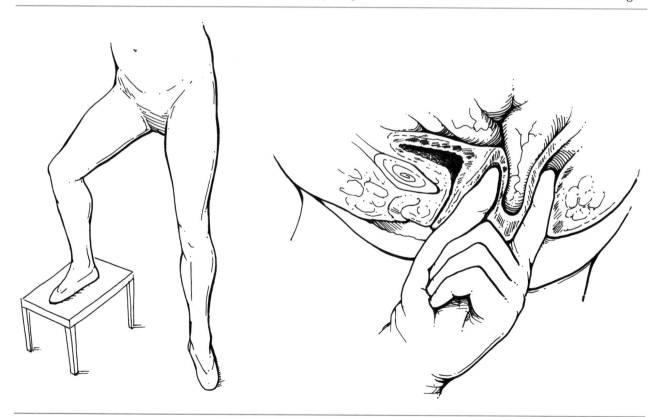

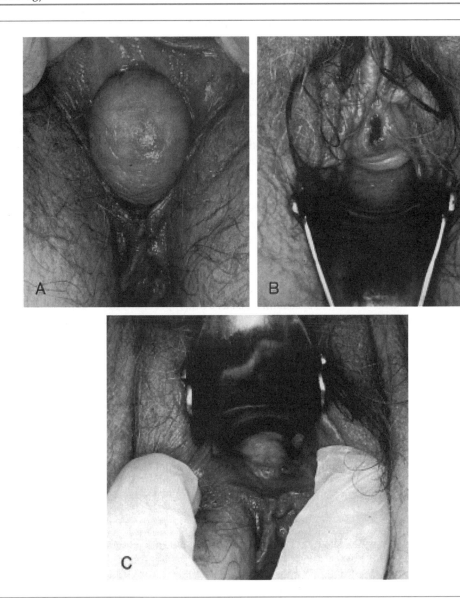

Figure 20.19   Examination of a prolapse in which the nature is unclear. *A,* Without more careful examination, the components of this prolapse are uncertain. When a speculum is place posteriorly (*B*) and anteriorly (*C*) to inspect each vaginal wall separately, the prolapse goes away. This indicates that the patient has a prolapse of the vaginal apex, which has been elevated by the speculum in each instance. (Reproduced with permission from **Wall LL, Norton P, DeLancey J.** *Practical Urogynecology.* Baltimore: Williams & Wilkins, 1993:307.)

vaginal walls with the single-bladed speculum and examining what remains. This is important because a large prolapse of one side of the vagina may hold a smaller prolapse from the other side in place, resulting in misdiagnosis, such as when a large cystocele obscures the presence of a large rectocele or when eversion of the vaginal apex is mistaken for a large cystocele. As a general rule, any prolapse that lies within the vaginal lumen above the plane of the hymenal ring is of limited significance, particularly if the patient is asymptomatic.

Treatment of Pelvic Organ Prolapse

Asymptomatic prolapse does not need treatment. An exception is a woman with stress incontinence and prolapse who is about to undergo surgical bladder neck suspension. Most operations for stress incontinence elevate the anterior vagina and, in doing so, pull the posterior vagina forward. This opens the cul-de-sac, pulling it off the levator plate and thereby creating an opening for enterocele formation, the development of uterine prolapse, vaginal vault eversion, or worsening of an asymptomatic rectocele (94). Under these conditions, additional surgery in the form of a culdoplasty, rectocele or enterocele repair, or in some cases, hysterectomy, may be advisable.

Symptomatic prolapse can be treated conservatively or surgically, depending on the individual. Although pelvic muscle exercises may be of benefit to women with stress incontinence by strengthening urethral support, they have not proven beneficial for patients with significant prolapse. The pelvic muscles provide most of the support for the pelvic organs; after this support has become inefficient, increasing stress is placed on the connective tissue involved in pelvic support. When fascial attachments have been disrupted in the presence of poor muscular tone and clinically significant prolapse has developed, attempts to correct the problem by restoring muscular tone are not efficient. Pelvic muscle exercises are virtually never harmful, but under these circumstances, they are not likely to correct the problem.

Pessary

Conservative management of prolapse usually involves fitting the patient with a pessary. A wide variety of shapes and sizes of pessaries are available. The use of pessaries is an important part of gynecologic practice that has been neglected in contemporary gynecologic residency training programs (151–152). Each patient should be fitted individually with her pessary, much as each individual is fitted for a contraceptive diaphragm. The patient who is using a pessary should have a well-estrogenized vagina. Postmenopausal women should be given hormone replacement therapy, or alternatively, they should use intravaginal estrogen cream on a regular basis. **For women who are past menopause, it is preferable to use intravaginal estrogen cream 4–6 weeks before the pessary is inserted, because this makes the pessary more comfortable to wear and dramatically increases compliance and promotes long-term use.**

Complications of pessary use include chronic irritation and erosion of a pessary into the bladder, creating a vesicovaginal fistula (153, 154). All such cases are caused by neglect rather than the pessary itself. Patients who are using pessaries, particularly older women, should be examined on a regular basis. Some pessaries, such as the silicone doughnut pessary, can be left in place for months at a time without removal or inspection. Other pessaries, such as the cube pessary, which provides vaginal support through a gentle suction effect, ideally should be removed by the patient at bedtime each night and replaced in the morning to avoid erosions. The exact schedule of care should be based on individual circumstances. At the initial fitting, the patient should be encouraged to insert and remove the pessary herself. If the pessary fits and the patient is comfortable, it is helpful to reexamine her within 1 week and every 4–6 months thereafter.

Surgery

Traditionally, prolapse has been treated by surgery, the nature of which depends on the type of prolapse. The goal of surgery should be to relieve the patient of her symptoms by repairing each aspect of abnormal pelvic support in a durable and long-lasting manner. A detailed description of the various operations for managing pelvic support defects is beyond the scope of this chapter and can be obtained elsewhere (155, 156); however, a few general remarks are in order.

Most patients with prolapse have defects in more than one location, so attention should be paid to correcting all defects during the same operation. Operations for prolapse are generally, but not always, carried out through the vaginal rather than through the abdominal surgical route. Some conditions, such as stress urinary incontinence, are more reliably handled by an abdominal operation.

Operations for Vaginal Prolapse

Vaginal Hysterectomy   **Uterine prolapse is generally treated with vaginal hysterectomy, which may be accomplished by several different techniques.** The advantage of vaginal hysterectomy is that it allows other vaginal surgery (e.g., anterior and posterior colporrhaphy or enterocele repair) to be performed at the same time, without the need for a separate incision or for repositioning the patient. At the time of hysterectomy for prolapse, special attention should be paid to closing the cul-de-sac using a *McCall culdoplasty* and to reattaching the endopelvic fascia and the uterosacral ligaments to the vaginal cuff to provide additional support (157). These same steps should be performed with abdominal hysterectomy (158).

Manchester/Fothergill Operation   An alternative to hysterectomy for patients with uterine prolapse is the *Manchester operation,* originally described in 1888 by Donald and subsequently modified by *Fothergill.* In this operation, the bladder is dissected off the cervix, which is then amputated. The cardinal ligaments are sewn to the anterior cervical stump, and the posterior vagina is closed over the rest of the opening. This operation is usually performed in conjunction with an anterior-posterior colporrhaphy, and it is usually done for the sake of expediency in patients who are poor surgical risks and who do not desire future fertility.

Uteropexy   Occasionally, marked uterine prolapse may develop in a young nulliparous patient who desires to retain her fertility. If prolapse cannot be managed successfully with a pessary, such patients present a surgical challenge. The older abdominal uterine suspension operations (Baldy-Webster, Gilliam, ventrofixation or hysteropexy) frankly do not work for patients with significant uterine prolapse. There is anecdotal evidence of success in such patients using *sacrospinous ligament fixation* or *retroperitoneal abdominal uterosacropexy,* suturing mesh or fascia to the uterosacral ligaments and then to the anterior longitudinal ligament of the sacrum. There is little information available regarding long-term follow-up of such patients.

Paravaginal Defect Repair Operation   Anterior vaginal prolapse has been treated with anterior colporrhaphy, plicating the endopelvic fascia in the midline under the bladder neck. If the anterior vaginal prolapse results from a lateral detachment of the endopelvic fascia from the lateral pelvic sidewall, however, better results will be obtained by performing a lateral repair. In this technique, the endopelvic fascia is reattached to the arcus tendinous fasciae pelvis through what is referred to as a *paravaginal defect repair operation* (79, 146, 147). Generally, this procedure is performed through an abdominal incision, operating in the Retzius' space, although some surgeons are now performing it through a vaginal incision.

Posterior Colporrhaphy   Repair of posterior vaginal prolapse for rectocele and enterocele is also performed vaginally using *posterior colporrhaphy.* In a rectocele repair, the posterior vagina is opened, the rectum is dissected away from the pararectal fascia, and the levator ani muscles are plicated over the rectum in the midline, after which the vaginal epithelium is closed. An enterocele is a peritoneal hernia over the rectum, often seen as a second bump higher up in the vaginal canal on examination. The peritoneal sac should be carefully identified, opened, and closed with several purse-string sutures of permanent material; the sac should be excised, and the vagina should be closed once more over the defect. If the perineal body is noted to be deficient and the patient has a gaping introitus, this deficit may be repaired by a *perineorrhaphy* or *perineoplasty,* in which the vaginal fourchette is opened and the base of the levator ani muscle is pulled together in the midline, providing renewed support for the lateral vagina at its outlet.

Operations for Complete Eversion of the Vagina

Among the most challenging cases are those involving *complete eversion of the vagina* in patients who have had a previous hysterectomy. This condition virtually always requires surgical correction because of the large size of the prolapse, its propensity to increase over time because of increases in intra-abdominal pressure, and the rare danger of vaginal evisceration if it is not treated.

Colpectomy and Colpocleisis   For some patients, particularly elderly women who are not sexually active and who lead a sedentary lifestyle, the condition can be managed by surgically removing the vagina and closing off the space (*colpectomy* and *colpocleisis*).

Colpopexy   Another procedure is required for younger women and women who wish to retain sexual function. For these women, the condition can be managed transvaginally or transabdominally. With the transvaginal approach, vaginal eversion is corrected by suturing one side of the vaginal apex (usually the right side) to the sacrospinous ligament with one or two sutures—a *transvaginal sacrospinous colpopexy*. In the transabdominal approach, the vaginal apex is suspended from the anterior longitudinal ligament along the sacrum using a graft of fascia or artificial mesh that is sutured to the vagina and to the sacrum in a retroperitoneal position—a *transabdominal sacral colpopexy*. Both operations are highly successful in resuspending the vaginal apex (159, 160). Because the lines of force produced by increases in intra-abdominal pressure are directed across the vagina differently after the two operations, patients who have recurrent prolapse postoperatively tend to have different problems. As a rule, recurrent anterior vaginal prolapse is more common for patients with vaginal eversion if they have had a sacrospinous ligament fixation, whereas recurrent posterior vaginal prolapse is more common if they have undergone an abdominal sacral colpopexy.

Colorectal Dysfunction

Disorders of colon and rectal function are disproportionately prevalent among women and often are neglected (1). To develop a more complete understanding of pelvic floor disorders, the diagnosis and treatment of common disorders of colorectal functioning must be understood. Among the more common conditions are anal incontinence, rectal prolapse, constipation, fecal impaction, and irritable bowel syndrome (see Chapter 14).

Anal Incontinence

Anal incontinence is the involuntary loss of feces or flatus (161). Most patients with anal incontinence are women. Although it is becoming socially more acceptable to discuss urinary incontinence, anal incontinence remains a virtual taboo and is often neglected even by patients who have severe anorectal symptoms. The physician will often have to elicit this complaint by sensitive direct questioning of the patient.

Normal continence depends on the interaction of many factors, including anal sphincter function, anorectal sensation and reflexes, colonic transit, rectal distensibility, stool consistency, stool volume, and the patient's mental functioning. As in the case of urinary incontinence, there are multiple potential causes of anal incontinence. These have been summarized by Madoof and colleagues (161) (Table 20.7), among others (162–164).

Diagnosis

History   A thorough history regarding bowel function should give an understanding of the nature and frequency of anal loss. In general, loss of flatus alone represents minimal incontinence, whereas frequent loss of formed stool is a much more severe problem. If the history is uncertain, administration of an enema of normal saline will often be beneficial in determining whether anal incontinence is a problem. The patient who can retain 1000–1500 ml of normal saline without leakage is unlikely to have a significant problem with anal incontinence (165). Changes in stool frequency or consistency, history of blood in the stool, associated medical conditions (especially diabetes and related neurologic

Table 20.7   Causes Of Fecal Incontinence

Normal Pelvic Floor

Diarrheal states
  Infectious diarrhea
  Inflammatory bowel disease
  Short-gut syndrome
  Laxative abuse
  Radiation enteritis

Overflow
  Impaction
  Encopresis
  Rectal neoplasms

Neurologic conditions
  Congenital anomalies (e.g., myelomeningocele)
  Multiple sclerosis
  Dementia, strokes, tabes dorsalis
  Neuropathy (e.g., diabetes)
  Neoplasms of brain, spinal cord, cauda equina
  Injuries to brain, spinal cord, cauda equina

Abnormal Pelvic Floor

Congenital anorectal malformation
Trauma
  Accidental injury (e.g., impalement, pelvic fracture)
  Anorectal surgery
  Obstetrical injury

Aging

Pelvic-floor denervation (idiopathic neurogenic incontinence)
  Vaginal delivery
  Chronic straining at stool
  Rectal prolapse
  Descending perineum syndrome

Reproduced with permission from **Madoof RD, Williams JG, Caushaj PF.** Fecal incontinence. *N Engl J Med* 1992;326:1002–7.

problems), medication use, obstetric history, and any history of pelvic surgery are all important pieces of information. It is also important to determine whether the patient ever notices anything protruding from the anus, because rectal prolapse is associated with anal incontinence in a high percentage of cases.

Physical Examination   The perineum should be carefully inspected, to determine the state of hygiene, the presence of fissures, and the anal sphincter. In all patients with anal incontinence, pelvic muscle reflexes should be checked, and a vaginal and bimanual examination should be performed. The possibility of a disrupted sphincter or a rectovaginal fistula cannot be ignored. All patients must undergo a digital rectal examination with testing of the stool for occult blood. At least 50% of rectal carcinomas lie within reach of the examiner's finger. Many patients with fecal incontinence will have a fecal impaction, which should be removed (166, 167). The puborectalis muscle should be palpated through the posterior rectum. When the patient contracts this muscle, the examiner's finger should move anteriorly. Poor sphincter tone is indicated by the rectum gaping when the puborectalis muscle is depressed.

Anal Function Tests   Patients should undergo anoscopy or proctosigmoidoscopy. A barium enema and upper gastrointestinal radiographic series using swallowed contrast material with small-bowel follow-through are indicated if defects are suspected higher in the gastrointestinal tract than originally thought. Other useful tests include *anorectal manometry* to check the resting and squeeze pressures generated by the internal and external anal sphincters, a *balloon distention test* to check the rectal sensory threshold (168), and *pelvic floor electromyographic studies,* including concentric needle or single-fiber *electromyography* of the anal sphincter and pudendal nerve terminal motor latency studies. Electrophysiologic testing is helpful in diagnosing idiopathic denervation of the pelvic floor and anal sphincter, which can occur with childbirth injury, descending perineum syndrome, or chronic constipation (58). Impaired rectal sensation, as indicated by a delayed sensation of fullness when a balloon catheter is inflated, is often associated with anal incontinence (168).

Treatment

Treatment of anal incontinence depends on its etiology. Patients with sphincteric rupture from obstetric trauma or those with a rectovaginal fistula will benefit from surgical repair of the appropriate defect. Patients with pelvic floor denervation often do not respond well to sphincter repair operations; for this reason, screening for this problem with pudendal nerve terminal motor latency studies and related neurophysiologic techniques is helpful in planning an appropriate surgical strategy. Rectal cancers should be resected and inflammatory bowel conditions can be treated medically (sometimes surgically). Antiflatulence preparations such as *Beano* (AKPharma, Pleasantville, NJ) are often very helpful. High-fiber diets and stool bulking agents will help the patient develop a more consistent stool that can be controlled more easily by the sphincters. Antidiarrheal agents, such as *loperamide* or *diphenoxylate* with *atropine,* also help. Daily tap water enemas can be used to help keep the rectum empty and to plan daily bowel movements.

Biofeedback training is useful in helping patients regain control of sphincteric activity, especially when they have impaired rectal sensation. This technique allows patients to strengthen the muscles of the pelvic floor, to sense smaller volumes of stool in the rectum, and to improve their control over the anal sphincter mechanism, often with surprisingly good results (169).

For some patients, construction of an anal neo-sphincter using transplanted gracilis muscle driven by an implanted pacemaker may be of benefit (170). Patients who have severe persistent incontinence after biofeedback therapy, medical management, and surgical treatment may be candidates for colostomy.

Rectal Prolapse

Rectal prolapse is relatively uncommon but nonetheless is a significant clinical problem for those unfortunate enough to experience it. Approximately 90% of patients with rectal prolapse are women (171). Normally, the rectum is attached firmly to the levator ani muscle complex through an extensive interweaving of longitudinal muscle fibers. This attachment is important because the rectum undergoes multiple changes in position and location during the act of normal defecation. Without this attachment, the rectum would slip down through the levator muscle hiatus during defecation. In rectal prolapse, this actually occurs. An intussusception of the rectum develops (for reasons not totally clear), and gradually over time, the intussusception pulls the rectum away from its sacral attachments until it appears at or through the anal verge. Predisposing factors associated with rectal prolapse as outlined by Corman are summarized in Table 20.8 (171).

Most patients with rectal prolapse complain of the presence of the prolapse itself as the major problem. Many patients complain of constipation; however, fecal incontinence is also commonly associated with rectal prolapse. Stretch injury of the pudendal and pelvic nerves may cause denervation injury to the rectum and resultant incontinence, but this finding is not always present. As the prolapse worsens, patients must replace the rectum manually to defecate. Occasionally, a rectal prolapse may become incarcerated; rarely, there is a transanal evisceration of small bowel from a ruptured rectal prolapse.

Table 20.8   Factors Associated With Or Predisposing To Rectal Prolapse

Poor bowel habits (especially constipation)
Neurologic disease (e.g. congenital anomaly, cauda equina lesion, spinal cord injury, senility)
Female sex
Nulliparity
Redundant rectosigmoid
Deep Douglas' pouch
Patulous anus (weak internal sphincter)
Diastasis of levator ani muscle (defect in pelvic floor)
Lack of fixation of rectum to sacrum
Intussusception (also secondary to colonic lesions)
Operative procedure (e.g., hemorrhoidectomy, fistulectomy, abdominoanal pull-through)

Reproduced with permission from **Corman ML.** Rectal prolapse. In: *Colon and Rectal Surgery.* 2nd ed. Philadelphia: JB Lippincott, 1989:209–47.

Diagnosis

Patients with rectal prolapse should be examined while straining. If their sphincter tone is poor and the anus is patulous, subsequent surgical repair may not be satisfactory. If the tone of the pelvic muscles is good, however, the prognosis is more favorable. An important point is whether the prolapse is a full-thickness prolapse of the rectum or whether it is only a prolapse of the rectal mucosa. Examination of patients with rectal prolapse should include both digital examination as well as a thorough proctosigmoidoscopic examination because a colonic cancer or sigmoidal polyp may be the point at which an intussusception develops. All patients with a rectal prolapse should undergo a barium enema or colonoscopic examination, or both. Changes associated with the solitary rectal ulcer syndrome are frequently seen in patients with early rectal prolapse. Radiographic studies performed during defecation (*defecography*) with the patient in a sitting position help to further characterize this problem, although unfortunately, many radiologists are uncomfortable or unwilling to perform such studies (172–174).

Treatment

Partial or incomplete rectal mucosal prolapse generally can be treated with anal surgery, often involving only excision of the affected area. Complete rectal prolapse is a more complicated; more than 200 operations are described for the treatment of this condition (171). These operations include or combine several modes of therapy such as narrowing the anal orifice, obliteration of the cul-de-sac, restoration of the pelvic floor, resection of bowel, and suspension or fixation of the rectum. Surgical treatment of this condition has been summarized by a number of authors (175, 176). In general, some form of rectopexy seems to have the highest success rate, the lowest recurrence rate, and an acceptable level of complications. A full preoperative evaluation of patients in a colorectal laboratory, including manometry, cinedefecography, and neurophysiologic studies, will lead to improved surgical outcome in the treatment of this condition.

Constipation and Fecal Impaction

Constipation is a subjective disorder for which there is no standard definition. Commonly used definitions include frequent straining at stool (more than 25% of the time) or fewer than three bowel movements per week. Nearly 95% of normal individuals have between three bowel movements per day and three bowel movements per week. In surveys of patients not seeking medical care for gastrointestinal disorders, between 10 and 20% seem to have symptoms of constipation; most of these individuals are female (177, 178). Constipation is less frequent among the young and increases to its highest prevalence in old age.

As might be expected with a condition that is so widespread, the causes of constipation are many and varied (Table 20.9) (179). It appears that some degree of constipation is prevalent in the population at large and may be a normal variaion in bowel habits for many people. In other cases of severe constipation, the etiology is unknown (chronic idiopathic constipation).

Treatment

Because of its high prevalence among women, physicians should be well versed in the treatment of constipation. The goal of treatment for patients with chronic constipation is restoration of normal frequency and consistency of stools without the need to strain during defecation (180). Restoration should be accomplished with as little artificial intervention as possible, and it should result in the diminution of any associated symptoms such as crampy abdominal pain or bloating. Because stool of normal consistency is about 70% water, the mainstays in the treatment of constipation are water and fiber. The fiber serves as a bulking agent that can trap water and promote an increased mass of stool. The normal dietary fiber intake should be 14 g/day. Unprocessed bran is the most readily available fiber supplement. If it is not available, psyllium can also be used. The type of fiber is not nearly as important as adequate fiber intake.

Table 20.9   Causes of Constipation

Disorders	
Anorectal	Anal fissure, anal stenosis, anterior mucosal prolapse, descending perineum syndrome, hemorrhoids, perineal abscess, rectocele, tumors.
Colonic	Irritable bowel syndrome, diverticular disease, tumors, strictures, carcinoma, Crohn's disease, diverticulitis, ulcerative colitis, ischemic colitis, tuberculosis, amebiasis, syphilis, lymphogranuloma venereum, hernias, volvulus, intussusception, ulcerative colitis with right-sided fecal stasis, pneumatosis cystoides intestinalis, idiopathic slow transit constipation.
Pelvic causes	Pregnancy and the puerperium, ovarian and uterine tumors, endometriosis.
Neuromuscular causes	Peripheral causes: Hirschsprung's disease, autonomic neuropathy, Chaga's disease, intestinal pseudo-obstruction. Central causes: cerebrovascular accident, cerebral tumors, Parkinson's disease, meningocele disseminated sclerosis, tabes dorsalis, paraplegia, cauda equina tumor, trauma to the lumbosacral cord or cauda equina, Shy-Drager syndrome. Muscular causes: dermatomyositis, dystrophia myotonica, progressive systemic sclerosis.
Psychiatric	Depression, anorexia nervosa, denied bowel action.
Endocrine causes	Diabetes mellitus, hypercalcemia, hypothyroidism, hypopituitarism, pheochromocytoma.
Metabolic causes	Hypokalemia, lead poisoning, porphyria, uremia.
Environmental causes	Debility; dehydration; immobilization; use of a bed pan
Drug-induced	Anesthetics, analgesics, antacids containing aluminum and calcium, anticholinergics, anticonvulsants, antidepressants, antihypertensives, anti-Parkinsonian drugs, diuretics, ganglion-blocking drugs, iron, habitual abuse of laxatives, monoamine oxidase inhibitors, oral contraceptives, psychotherapeutic agents.

Reproduced with permission from **Moriarty KJ, Irving MH.** Constipation. *BMJ* 1992;304:1237–40.

Laxatives are an important adjunct to fiber and water in the treatment of constipation. Literally hundreds of laxative preparations are available. They can be divided into two main groups: stimulant laxatives and mechanical laxatives. Stimulant laxatives (e.g., *cascara, senna, castor oil, bisacodyl,* and *diphenylmethane*) cause increased peristaltic activity in the colon. These irritant laxatives are useful in the treatment of acute constipation or constipation associated with prolonged bedrest, but prolonged use of such cathartics may result in dependency, which can be difficult to manage. Stimulant laxatives, such as *bisacodyl, docusate sodium,* or *senna,* may be used occasionally but long-term use should be avoided as much as possible because the bowel may become dependent on them. Side effects of stimulant laxatives can include cramps and urgent, explosive defecation. The mechanical laxatives include salts such as sodium phosphate or magnesium sulfate, mineral oil, and surfactants such as *docusate sodium.* These agents increase peristalsis by changing stool consistency or increasing stool bulk. Agents such as *lactulose* produce an osmotic catharsis. Oral agents such as mineral oil work by decreasing water absorption from the stool, thereby keeping it soft. If taken orally, mineral oil should be used with caution, because inhalation can lead to aspiration pneumonia, particularly in elderly or debilitated patients.

Enemas and suppositories are also useful. An enema is particularly helpful in removing an acute fecal impaction. The best enemas are usually the simplest: warm tap water or equal parts of water, glycerin, and mineral oil. The use of these agents is preferable to soap enemas or hypertonic phosphate enemas, which are particularly irritating. Injudicious use of enemas can cause electrolyte imbalances or colonic perforation. Suppositories are helpful in the periodic evacuation of the lower bowel. Insertion of a *simple glycerin* suppository will usually initiate defecation within 1 hour without chemical stimulation of the colon.

Attention should always be paid to other factors influencing the normal action of the gut. Patients should be taught not to suppress defecation but to make use of the normal gastrocolic reflex that promotes a call to stool approximately 30 minutes after a meal (usually breakfast). Regular meals help promote regular bowel movements. Regular exercise, even exercise as simple as a brisk walk, has an important influence on regular defecation, as well as on general fitness and well-being.

Attention to good bowel habits, adequate fiber intake, and occasional laxative use should help prevent fecal impaction. This condition can occur at any age, but elderly and institutionalized patients are at particular risk for developing it (166). Continued passage of stool does not rule out an impaction, and many patients develop diarrhea and anal incontinence, as well as nausea, anorexia, vomiting, and abdominal pain. The diagnosis can usually be established by rectal examination, although fecal impaction can also occur high in the colon. The stool may be hard or soft, a single mass or multiple pellets. If the patient's presentation suggests an impaction but its presence is not confirmed by rectal examination, flat-plate radiography of the abdomen may be useful to detect masses of stool or unusual air-fluid levels. Once diagnosed, the impaction should be removed by fragmenting the fecal mass manually and then removing it in pieces. This usually can be done with local anesthesia using *lidocaine* jelly and liberal amounts of lubricant, aided by posterior pressure exerted through the vagina. After the mass has been broken up, expulsion may be aided by tap water enemas and *bisacodyl* suppositories. The patient should then be placed on a good bowel regimen to prevent the occurrence of future impactions.

Conservative measures, including adequate fluid intake, a high fiber diet, and occasional laxative use, should allow most women with constipation to regain normal bowel habits of at least three movements per week. If a trial of 3–6 months of conservative therapy in a compliant patient is unsuccessful in relieving the constipation, further evaluation should be undertaken. Constipation is not a diagnosis but is a symptom that may be associated with many different pathologic states. The further examination of patients with constipation should include endoscopic examination of the colon and rectum, an air-contrast barium enema, and referral to a colorectal function laboratory for more sophisticated studies, including segmental colonic transit studies, pelvic floor electromyography, and defecography (181). If blood is present in the stool, if the constipation is painful, if constipation is the result of a sudden change in bowel habits, or if the clinician is otherwise suspicious of a more serious disease process, these studies should be performed earlier in the course of treatment.

When the usual sets of studies reveal no etiology, constipation is considered functional or nonorganic (182). Most patients with severe functional constipation are young women (183–185). Many of these women seem to have disordered colonic motility of unknown etiology, and many of them exhibit paradoxical contraction (rather than relaxation) of the external anal sphincter during defecation, resulting in fecal outflow obstruction. This condition has been termed the *spastic pelvic floor syndrome*. Although they are refractory to treatment by fiber supplementation and laxatives, some of these patients seem to benefit from biofeedback therapy that enables them to learn normal patterns of defecation and to relax the pelvic floor during a bowel movement (186).

References

1. **Wall LL, DeLancey JOL.** The politics of prolapse: a revisionist approach to disorders of the pelvic floor in women. *Perspect Biol Med* 1991;34:486–96.

2. **Parks AG, Porter NH, Melzack J.** Experimental study of the reflex mechanism controlling the muscles of the pelvic floor. *Dis Colon Rectum* 1962;5:407–14.

3. **Zacharin RF.** Pulsion enterocele: review of functional anatomy of the pelvic floor. *Obstet Gynecol* 1980;55:135–40.

4. **Dickinson RL.** Studies of the levator ani muscle. *Am J Obstet Dis Women* 1889;22:897–917.

5. **Kegel AJ.** Sexual functions of the pubococcygeus muscle. *West J Obstet Gynecol* 1952;60:521–4.

6. **Gillan P, Brindley GS.** Vaginal and pelvic floor responses to sexual stimulation. *Psychophysiology* 1979;16:471–81.

7. **Wall LL.** The muscles of the pelvic floor. *Clin Obstet Gynecol* 1993;36:910–25.

8. **Lawson JO.** Pelvic anatomy I: pelvic floor muscles. *Ann R Coll Surg Engl* 1974;54:244–52.

9. **DeLancey JOL.** Structural aspects of the extrinsic continence mechanism. *Obstet Gynecol* 1988;72:296–301.

10. **DeLancey JOL.** Correlative study of paraurethral anatomy. *Obstet Gynecol* 1986;68:91–7.

11. **DeLancey JOL.** Structural support of the urethra as it relates to stress urinary incontinence: the hammock hypothesis. *Am J Obstet Gynecol* 1994;170:1713–23.

12. **Gosling JA, Dixson JS, Critchley HOD, Thompson SA.** A comparative study of the human external sphincter and periurethral levator ani muscles. *Br J Urol* 1981;53:35–41.

13. **Berglas B, Rubin IC.** Study of the supportive structures of the uterus by levator myography. *Surg Gynecol Obstet* 1953;97:677–92.

14. **DeLancey JOL.** Anatomy and biomechanics of genital prolapse. *Clin Obstet Gynecol* 1993;36:897–909.

15. **Norton PA.** Pelvic floor disorders: the role of fascia and ligaments. *Clin Obstet Gynecol* 1993;36:926–38.

16. **Bird J.** The effects of pregnancy on joint mobility. *J Orthop Res* 1984;41:345–9.

17. **Brincat M, Versi E, Moniz C, Magos A, de Trafford J, Studd J.** Skin collagen changes in postmenopausal women receiving different regimens of estrogen. *Obstet Gynecol* 1987;70:123–7.

18. **Castelo-Branco C, Duran M, Gonzalez-Merlo J.** Skin collagen changes related to age and hormone replacement therapy. *Maturitas* 1992;15:113–9.

19. **Suominen H, Heikken E, Parkatti T.** Effects of eight weeks physical training on muscle and connective tissue of the m. vastus lateralis in 69-year-old-men and women. *J Gerontol* 1977;32:33–7.

20. **Lind J.** *A Treatise on the Scurvy.* 3rd ed. London, 1772:113.

21. **Al-Rawi R, Al-Rawi L.** Joint hypermobility in multiparous Iraqi women with genital prolapse. *Lancet* 1982;1:439–41.

22. **Norton P, Baker J, Sharp H, Warenski J.** Genitourinary prolapse: its relationship with joint mobility. *Neurourol Urodyn* 1990;9:321–2.

23. **Marshman D, Percy J, Fielding I, Delbridge L.** Rectal prolapse: relationship with joint mobility. *Aust N Z J Surg* 1987;57:827–9.

24. **Norton P, Boyd C, Deak S.** Abnormal collagen ratios in women with genitourinary prolapse. *Neurourol Urodynam* 1992;11:2–4.

25. **Ulmsten U, Ekman G, Giertz G, Malmstrom A.** Different biochemical composition of connective tissue in continent and stress incontinent women. *Acta Obstet Gynecol Scand* 1987;66:455–7.

26. **Kondo A, Narushima M, Yoshikawa Y, Hayashi H.** Pelvic fascia strength in women with stress urinary incontinence in comparison with those who are continent. *Neurourol Urodyn* 1994;13:507–13.

27. **Ball T.** Anterior and posterior cystocele: cystocele revisited—an account of the twilight hours of some antifascialists and fascialists as I knew them. *Clin Obstet Gynecol* 1964;9:1062–4.

28. **Torrens M, Morrison JFB.** *The Physiology of the Lower Urinary Tract.* New York: Springer-Verlag, 1987.

29. **Burnstock G.** Nervous control of smooth muscle by transmitters, co-transmitters, and modulators. *Experientia* 1985;41;869–74.

30. **Burnstock G.** The changing face of autonomic neurotransmission. *Acta Physiol Scand* 1986;126:67–91.

31. **Daniel EE, Cowan W, Daniel VP.** Structural bases of neural and myogenic control of human detrusor muscle. *Can J Physiol Pharmacol* 1983;61:1247–73.

32. **Schuster MM.** The riddle of the sphincters. *Gastroenterology* 1975;69:249–62.

33. **Parks AG.** Anorectal incontinence. *Proc R Soc Med* 1975;68:681–90.

34. **Bartolo DCC, Roe AM, Locke-Edmunds JC, Virjee J, Mortensen NJM.** Flap-valve theory of anorectal continence. *Br J Surg* 1986;73:1012–4.

35. **Phillips SF, Edwards DAW.** Some aspects of anal continence and defecation. *Gut* 1965;6:396–406.

36. **Abrams P, Blaivas JG, Stanton SL, Anderson JT.** The standardisation of terminology of lower urinary tract function. *Scand J Urol Nephrol* 1988;114:5–18.

37. **Rowe JW, Besdine RW, Ford AB, Gartley CB, Gleason DM, Greiss FC, et al.** Urinary incontinence in adults: NIH Consensus Development Conference. *JAMA* 1989;261:26885–90.

38. **Bissada NK, Finkbeiner AE.** Urologic manifestations of drug therapy. *Urol Clin North Am* 1988;15:725–36.

39. **Ostergard DR.** The effect of drugs on the lower urinary tract. *Obstet Gynecol Surv* 1979;34:424–32.

40. **Wall LL, Addison WA.** Prazosin-induced stress incontinence. *Obstet Gynecol* 1990;75:558–60.

41. **Larrson G, Victor A.** Micturition patterns in a healthy female populations, studied with a frequency/volume chart. *Scand J Urol Nephrol* 1988;114:53–7.

42. **Wyman JF, Choi SC, Harkins SW, Wilson MS, Fantl JA.** The urinary diary in the evaluation of incontinent women: a test-retest analysis. *Obstet Gynecol* 1998;71:812–7.

43. **Wall LL, Norton PA, DeLancey JOL.** Practical urodynamics. In: *Practical Urogynecology.* Baltimore: Williams & Wilkins, 1993:83–124.

44. **Wall LL, Wiskind AK, Taylor PA.** Simple bladder filling with a cough stress test compared to subtracted cystometry in the diagnosis of urinary incontinence. *Am J Obstet Gynecol* 1994;171:1472–9.

45. **Hilton P, Stanton SL.** Urethral pressure measurement by microtransducer: the results in symptom-free women and in those with genuine stress incontinence. *Br J Obstet Gynecol* 1983;90:919–33.

46. **Sand PK, Bowen LD, Panganiban R, Ostergard DR.** The low pressure urethra as a factor in failed retropubic urethropexy. *Obstet Gynecol* 1987;69:399–402.

47. **Richardson DA, Ramahi A, Chalas E.** Surgical management of stress incontinence in patients with low urethral pressure. *Obstet Gynecol Invest* 1991;31:106–9.

48. **McGuire EJ, Fitzpatrick CC, Wan J, Bloom D, Sanvordenker J, Ritchey M, et al.** Clinical assessment of urethral sphincter function. *J Urol* 1993;150:1452–4.

49. **Stanton SL.** Gynecologic complications of epispadias and bladder exstrophy. *Am J Obstet Gynecol* 1974;119:749–54.

50. **Mitchell RJ.** An ectopic vaginal ureter. *J Obstet Gynaecol Br Commw* 1961;68:299–302.

51. **Tahzib F.** Epidemiological determinants of vesicovaginal fistulas. *Br J Obstet Gynaecol* 1983; 90:387–91.

52. **Fitzpatrick C, Elkins TE.** Plastic surgical techniques in the repair of vesicovaginal fistulas: a review. *Int Urogynecol J* 1993;4:287–95.

53. **Arrowsmith SD.** Genitourinary reconstruction in obstetric fistulas. *J Urol* 1994;152:403–6.

54. **Yarnell JW, Voyle GJ, Richards CJ, Stephenson TP.** The prevalence and severity of urinary incontinence in women. *J Epidemiol Comm Health* 1981;35:71–4.

55. **Nygaard I, DeLancey JO, Arnsdorf L, Murphy E.** Exercise and incontinence. *Obstet Gynecol* 1990;75:848–51.

56. **Frazer MI, Haylen BT, Sutherst JR.** The severity of urinary incontinence in women: comparison of subjective and objective tests. *Br J Urol* 1989;63:14–5.

57. **Wall LL, Helms M, Peattie AB, Pearce M, Stanton SL.** Bladder neck mobility and the outcome of surgery for genuine stress incontinence: a logistic regression analysis of lateral bead-chain cystourethrograms. *J Reprod Med* 1994;39:429–35.

58. **Wall LL.** The muscles of the pelvic floor. *Clin Obstet Gynecol* 1993;36:910–25.

59. **Wall LL, Davidson TG.** The role of muscular re-education by physical therapy in the treatment of genuine stress incontinence. *Obstet Gynecol Surv* 1992;47:322–31.

60. **Bo K, Larsen S.** Pelvic floor muscle exercise for the treatment of stress urinary incontinence: classification and characterization of responders. *Neurourol Urodyn* 1992;11:497–508.

61. **Benvenuti F, Caputo GM, Bandinelli S, Mayer F, Biagini C, Sommavilla A.** Reeducative treatment of female genuine stress incontinence. *Am J Phys Med* 1987;66:155–68.

62. **Peattie AB, Plevnik S, Stanton SL.** Vaginal cones: a conservative method of treating genuine stress incontinence. *Br J Obstet Gynaecol* 1988;95:1049–53.

63. **Fantl JA, Wyman JF, Anderson RL, Matt DW, Bump RC.** Postmenopausal urinary incontinence: comparison between non-estrogen supplemented and estrogen-supplemented women. *Obstet Gynecol* 1988;71:823–8.

64. **Schrieter F, Fuchs P, Stockamp K.** Estogenic sensitivity of alpha-receptors in the urethra musculature. *Urol Int* 1976;31:13–9.

65. **Meyer S, Dhenin T, Schmidt N, De Grandi P.** Subjective and objective effects of intravaginal electrical myostimulation and biofeedback in patients with genuine stress incontinence. *Br J Urol* 1992;69:584–8.

66. **Hurt G.** *Urogynecologic Surgery.* Gaithersburg, MD: Aspen Publishers, 1992.

67. **Stanton SL, Tanagho EA.** *Surgery of Female Incontinence.* 2nd ed. London: Springer-Verlag, 1986.

68. **Wall LL.** Stress urinary incontinence. In: **Rock JA, Thompson JD,** eds. *TeLinde's Operative Gynecology.* 8th ed. Philadelphia: JB Lippincott, 1996.

69. **Kelly HA, Dumm WM.** Urinary incontinence in women without manifest injury to the bladder. *Surg Gynecol Obstet* 1914;18:444–50.

70. **Bailey KV.** A clinical investigation into uterine prolapse with stress incontinence: treatment by modified Manchester colporrhaphy. *J Obstet Gynaecol Br Emp* 1954;61:291–301.

71. **Low JA.** Management of anatomic urinary incontinence by vaginal repair. *Am J Obstet Gynecol* 1967;97:308–15.

72. **Stanton SL, Norton C, Cardozo LD.** Clinical and urodynamic effects of anterior colporrhaphy and vaginal hysterectomy for prolapse with and without incontinence. *Br J Obstet Gynaecol* 1982;89:459–63.

73. **Stanton SL, Cardozo LD.** A comparison of vaginal and suprapubic surgery in the correction of incontinence due to urethral sphincter incompetence. *Br J Urol* 1979;51:497–9.

74. **Beck RP, McCormick S.** Treatment of urinary stress incontinence with anterior colporrhaphy. *Obstet Gynecol* 1982;59:269–74.

75. **Beck RP, McCormick S, Nordstrom L.** A 25-year experience with 519 anterior colporrhaphy procedures. *Obstet Gynecol* 1991;78:1011–8.

76. **Marshall VF, Marchetti AA, Krantz KE.** The correction of stress incontinence by simple vesicourethral suspension. *Surg Gynecol Obstet* 1949;88:509–18.

77. **Burch JC.** Urethrovaginal fixation to Cooper's ligament for correction of stress incontinence, cystocele and prolapse. *Am J Obstet Gynecol* 1961;81:281–90.

78. **Burch JC.** Cooper's ligament urethrovesical suspension for stress incontinence: nine years experience—results, complications, technique. *Am J Obstet Gynecol* 1968;100:764–74.

79. **Richardson AC, Lyon JB, Williams NL.** Treatment of stress urinary incontinence due to paravaginal fascial defect. *Obstet Gynecol* 1981;57:357–62.

80. **Shull BL, Baden WFA.** A six-year experience with paravaginal defect repair for stress urinary incontinence. *Am J Obstet Gynecol* 1989;160:1432–40.

81. **Turner-Warwick R.** Turner-Warwick vagino-obturator shelf urethral repositioning procedure. In: **Gingell C, Abrams P,** eds. *Controversies and Innovations in Urologic Surgery.* New York: Springer-Verlag, 1988:195–200.

82. **German KA, Kynaston H, Weight S, Stephenson TP.** A prospective randomized trial comparing a modified needle suspension procedure with the vagina/obturator shelf procedure for genuine stress incontinence. *Br J Urol* 1994;74:188–90.

83. **Bergman A, Ballard CA, Kooning PP.** Comparison of three different surgical procedures for genuine stress incontinence: prospective randomized study. *Am J Obstet Gynecol* 1989;160:1102–6.

84. **Van Geelen JM, Theeuwes AG, Eskes TK, Martin CB Jr.** The clinical and urodynamics effects of anterior vaginal repair and Burch colposuspension. *Am J Obstet Gynecol* 1988;159:137–44.

85. **Hilton P, Stanton SL.** A clinical and urodynamic assessment of the Burch colposuspension for genuine stress incontinence. *Br J Obstet Gynaecol* 1983;90:934–9.

86. **Stanton SL, Cardozo LD.** Results of the colposuspension operation for incontinence and prolapse. *Br J Obstet Gynaecol* 1978;86:693–7.

87. **Herbertsson G, Iosif C.** Surgical results and urodynamic studies 10 years after retropubic colpocystourethropexy. *Acta Obstet Gynecol Scand* 1993;72:298–301.

88. **Mainprize TCF, Drutz HP.** The Marshall-Marchetti-Krantz procedure: a critical review. *Obstet Gynecol Surv* 1988;43:724–9.

89. **Persky L, Guerriere K.** Complications of Marshall-Marchetti-Krantz urethropexy. *Urology* 1976;8:469–71.

90. **Galloway NTM, Davies N, Stephenson TP.** The complications of colposuspension. *Br J Urol* 1987;60:122–4.

91. **Zimmern PE, Hadley HR, Leach GE, Raz S.** Female urethral obstruction after Marshall-Marchetti-Krantz operation. *J Urol* 1987;138:517–20.

92. **Webster GD, Kreder KJ.** Voiding dysfunction following cystourethropexy: its evaluation and management. *J Urol* 1990;144:670–3.

93. **Lose G, Jorgensen L, Mortensen SO, Molsted-Pedersen L, Kristensen JK.** Voiding difficulties after colposuspension. *Obstet Gynecol* 1987;69:33–8.

94. **Wiskind AK, Creighton SM, Stanton SL.** The incidence of prolapse after the Burch colposuspension. *Am J Obstet Gynecol* 1992;167:399–405.

95. **Pereyra AJ.** A simplified surgical procedure for the correction of stress incontinence in women. *West J Surg* 1959;67:223–56.

96. **Pereyra AJ, Lebherz TB.** Combined urethral vesical suspension vaginal urethroplasty for correction of urinary stress incontinence. *Obstet Gynecol* 1967;30:537–46.

97. **Pereyra AJ, Lebherz TB.** The revised Pereyra procedure. In: **Buchsbaum H, Schmidt JD,** eds. *Gynecologic and Obstetric Urology.* Philadelphia: WB Saunders, 1978:208–22.

98. **Stamey TA.** Endoscopic suspension of vesical neck for urinary incontinence in females. *Ann Surg* 1980;192:465–71.

99. **Hadley HR, Zimmern PE, Staskin DR, Raz S.** Transvaginal needle bladder neck suspension. *Urol Clin North Am* 1985;12:291–303.

100. **Gittes RF, Loughlin KR.** No-incision pubovaginal suspension for stress incontinence. *J Urol* 1987;138:568–70.

101. **O'Sullivan DC, Chilton CP, Munson KW.** Should Stamey colposuspension be our primary surgery for stress incontinence? *Br J Urol* 1995;75:457–60.

102. **Hilton P, Mayne C.** The Stamey endoscopic bladder neck suspension: a clinical and urodynamic investigation including actuarial follow-up over four years. *Br J Obstet Gynaecol* 1991; 98:1141–9.

103. **Peattie A, Stanton S.** The Stamey operation for correction of genuine stress incontinence in the elderly woman. *Br J Obstet Gynaecol* 1989;96:983–6.

104. **Handley-Ashken M.** Follow-up results with Stamey operation for stress incontinence of urine. *Br J Urol* 1990;65:168–9.

105. **Birhle W, Tarantino AF.** Complications of retropubic bladder neck suspension. *Urology* 1990;35:213–4.

106. **Miyazaki F, Shook G.** Ilioinguinal nerve entrapment during needle suspension for stress incontinence. *Obstet Gynecol* 1992;80:246–8.

107. **Varner RE.** Retropubic long-needle suspension procedures for stress urinary incontinence. *Am J Obstet Gynecol* 1990;163:551–7.

108. **Weiss RE, Cohen E.** Erosion of buttress following bladder neck suspension. *Br J Urol* 1992; 69:656–7.

109. **Zedric SA, Burros HM, Hanno PM, Dudas N, Whitmore KE.** Bladder calculi in women after urethrovesical suspension. *J Urol* 1988;139:1047–8.

110. **Parker RT, Addison WA, Wilson CJ.** Fascia lata urethrovesical suspension for recurrent stress urinary incontinence. *Am J Obstet Gynecol* 1979;135:843–52.

111. **Beck RP, Lai AR.** Results in treating 88 cases of recurrent urinary stress incontinence with the Oxford fascia lata sling procedure. *Am J Obstet Gynecol* 1982;142:649–51.

112. **Beck RP, McCormick S, Nordstrom L.** The fascia lata sling procedure for treating recurrent genuine stress incontinence. *Obstet Gynecol* 1988;72:699–703.

113. **Jarvis GJ, Fowlie A.** Clinical and urodynamic assessment of the porcine dermis bladder sling in the treatment of genuine stress incontinence. *Br J Obstet Gynaecol* 1985;92:1189–91.

114. **McGuire EJ, Lytton B.** Pubovaginal sling procedure for stress incontinence. *J Urol* 1978;119:82–4.

115. **McGuire EJ, Bennet CJ, Konnak JA, Sonda LP, Savastano JA.** Experience with pubovaginal slings for urinary incontinence at the University of Michigan. *J Urol* 1987;138:525–6.

116. **Stanton SL, Brindley GS, Holmes DM.** Silastic sling for urethral sphincter incompetence. *Br J Obstet Gynaecol* 1985;92:747–50.

117. **Horbach NS, Blanco JS, Ostergard DR, Bont AE, Cornella JL.** A suburethral sling procedure with polytetrafluoroethylene for the treatment of genuine stress incontinence with low urethral closure pressure. *Obstet Gynecol* 1988;71:648–52.

118. **Rottenberg RD, Weil A, Brioschi PA, Bischof P, Krauer F.** Urodynamic and clinical assessment of the Lyodura sling operation for urinary stress incontinence. *Br J Obstet Gynaecol* 1985;92:829–34.

119. **Murless BC.** The injection treatment of stress incontinence. *J Obstet Gynaecol Brit Emp* 1938;45:67–73.

120. **Beckingham IJ, Wemyss-Holden G, Lawrence WT.** Long-term follow-up of women treated with periurethral Teflon injections for stress incontinence. *Br J Urol* 1992;69:580–3.

121. **Appell RA.** Injectables for urethral incompetence. *World J Urol* 1990;8:208–11.

122. **Malizia AA, Reiman HM, Meyers RP, Sande JR, Barham SS, Benson RC Jr, et al.** Migration and granulomatous reaction after periurethral injection of Polytef (Teflon). *JAMA* 1984;251:3277–81.

123. **Appell RA.** Periurethral collagen injection for female incontinence. *Prob Urol* 1991;5:134–40.

124. **Kieswetter H, Fischer M, Wober L, Flamm J.** Endoscopic implantation of collagen (GAX) for the treatment of urinary incontinence. *Br J Urol* 1992;69:22–5.

125. **Webster GD, Perez LM, Khoury JM, Timmons SL.** Management of type III stress incontinence using artificial urinary sphincter. *Urology* 1992;39:499–503.

126. **Diokno AC, Hollander JB, Alderson TP.** Artificial urinary sphincter for recurrent female urinary incontinence: indications and results. *J Urol* 1987;138:778–80.

127. **Wall LL.** Diagnosis and management of urinary incontinence due to detrusor instability. *Obstet Gynecol Surv* 1990;45:1S–47S.

128. **Koefoot RB, Webster GD.** Urodynamic evaluation in women with frequency, urgency symptoms. *Urology* 1983;6:648–51.

129. **Coolsaet BLRA, Blok C, van Venrouji GEFM, Tan B.** Subthreshold detrusor instability. *Neurourol Urodyn* 1985;4:309–11.

130. **Van Waalwijk Van Doorn ESC, Remmers A, Janknegt RA.** Conventional and extramural ambulatory urodynamic testing of the lower urinary tract in female volunteers. *J Urol* 1992;147:1319–26.

131. **Griffiths CJ, Assi MS, Styles RA, Ramsden PD, Neal DE.** Ambulatory monitoring of bladder and detrusor pressure during natural filling. *J Urol* 1989;142:780–4.

132. **Bhatia NN, Bradley WE, Haldeman S.** Urodynamics: continuous monitoring. *J Urol* 1982;128:963–8.

133. **James D.** Continuous monitoring. *Urol Clin North Am* 1979;6:125–35.

134. **Wall LL, Norton PA, DeLancey JOL.** Mixed incontinence. In: *Practical Urogynecology.* Baltimore: Williams & Wilkins, 1993:215–20.

135. **Resnick N, Yalla S.** Management of urinary incontinence in the elderly. *N Engl J Med* 1985;313:800–5.

136. **Resnick N, Yalla S, Laurino E.** An algorithmic approach to urinary incontinence in the elderly. *Clin Res* 1986;34:832–7.

137. **Massey J, Abrams P.** Obstructed voiding in the female. *Br J Urol* 1988;61:36–9.

138. **McGuire EJ, Savastano JA.** Urodynamic findings and long term outcome management of patients with multiple sclerosis induced lower urinary tract dysfunction. *J Urol* 1984;132:713–5.

139. **Philp T, Read DJ, Higson RH.** The urodynamic characteristics of multiple sclerosis. *Br J Urol* 1981;53:672–5.

140. **Finkbeiner A.** Is bethanechol chloride clinically effective in promoting bladder emptying. *J Urol* 1985;134:443–9.

141. **Lapides J, Diokno A, Silber S, Lowe B.** Clean intermittent self-catheterization in the treatment of urinary tract disease. *J Urol* 1972;107:458–61.

142. **Preminger GM.** Acute urinary retention in female patients: diagnosis and treatment. *J Urol* 1983;130:112–3.

143. **Hanno PM, Staskin DR, Krane RJ, Wein AJ.** *Interstitial Cystitis.* New York: Springer-Verlag, 1990.

144. **Wall LL, Norton PA, DeLancey JOL.** Sensory disorders of the bladder and urethra: frequency/urgency/dysuria/bladder pain. In: *Practical Urogynecology.* Baltimore: Williams & Wilkins, 1993:255–73.

145. **Baden WF, Walker T.** Genesis of the vaginal profile. *Clin Obstet Gynecol* 1972;15:1048–54.

146. **Richardson AC, Lyon JB, Williams NL.** A new look at pelvic relaxation. *Am J Obstet Gynecol* 1976;126:568–73.

147. **Shull BL, Capen CV, Riggs MW, Huehl TJ.** Preoperative and postoperative analysis of site-specific pelvic support defects in 81 women treated with sacrospinous ligament suspension and pelvic reconstruction. *Am J Obstet Gynecol* 1992;166:1764–71.

148. **Baden WF, Walker T.** *Surgical Repair of Vaginal Defects.* Philadelphia: JB Lippincott, 1992.

149. **Shull BL.** Clinical evaluation of women with pelvic support defects. *Clin Obstet Gynecol* 1993;36:939–51.

150. **Wall LL, Hewitt JK.** Urodynamic characteristics of women with complete post-hysterectomy vaginal vault prolapse. *Urology* 1994;44:336–42.

151. **Zeitlin MP, Lebherz TB.** Pessaries in the geriatric patient. *J Am Geriatr Soc* 1992;40:635–9.

152. **Shulak PT.** Vaginal pessaries and their use in pelvic relaxation. *J Reprod Med* 1993;38: 919–23.

153. **Russell JK.** The dangerous vaginal pessary. *BMJ* 1961;1:1595–7.

154. **Goldstein I, Wise GJ, Tancer ML.** A vesicovaginal fistula and intravesical foreign body: a rare case of the neglected pessary. *Am J Obstet Gynecol* 1990;163:589–91.

155. **Nichols DH, Randall CL.** *Vaginal Surgery.* 3rd ed. Baltimore: Williams & Wilkins, 1989.

156. **Thompson JD, Rock JA.** *TeLinde's Operative Gynecology.* 7th ed. Philadelphia: JB Lippincott, 1992.

157. **McCall M.** Posterior culdoplasty: surgical correction of enterocele during vaginal hysterectomy; a preliminary report. *Obstet Gynecol* 1957;10:595–602.

158. **Wall LL.** A technique for modified McCall culdoplasty at the time of abdominal hysterectomy. *J Am Coll Surg* 1994;178:507–9.

159. **Morley GW, DeLancey JOL.** Sacrospinous ligament fixation for eversion of the vagina. *Am J Obstet Gynecol* 1988;158:872–81.

160. **Addison WA, Livengood CH, Sutton GP, Parker RT.** Abdominal sacral colpopexy with Mersilene mesh in the retroperitoneal position in the management of posthysterectomy vaginal vault prolapse and enterocele. *Am J Obstet Gynecol* 1985;153:140–6.

161. **Madoof RD, Williams JG, Caushaj PF.** Fecal incontinence. *N Engl J Med* 1992;326: 1002–7.

162. **Toglia MR, DeLancey JOL.** Anal incontinence and the obstetrician-gynecologist. *Obstet Gynecol* 1994;84:731–40.

163. **Jorge JMN, Wexner SD.** Etiology and management of fecal incontinence. *Dis Colon Rectum* 1993;36:77–97.

164. **Kiff ES.** Faecal incontinence. *BMJ* 1992;305:702–4.

165. **Read NW, Harford WV, Schmulen AC, Read MG, Ana CS, Fordtran JS.** A clinical study of patients with fecal incontinence and diarrhea. *Gastroenterology* 1979;76:747–56.

166. **Wrenn K.** Fecal impaction. *N Engl J Med* 1989;321:658–62.

167. **Read NW, Abouzekry L.** Why do patients with faecal impaction have faecal incontinence? *Gut* 1986;27:283–7.

168. **Sun WM, Read NW, Miner PB.** Relationship between rectal sensation and anal function in normal subjects and patients with faecal incontinence. *Gut* 1990;31:1056–61.

169. **Enck P.** Biofeedback training in disordered defecation: a critical review. *Dig Dis Sci* 1993; 38:1953–60.

170. **Seccia M.** Study protocols and functional results in 86 electrostimulated gracilosphincters. *Dis Colon Rectum* 1994;37:897–904.

171. **Corman ML.** Rectal prolapse. In: *Colon and Rectal Surgery.* 2nd ed. Philadelphia: JB Lippincott, 1989:209–47.

172. **Kuijpers JHC, De Morree H.** Toward a selection of the most appropriate procedure in the treatment of complete rectal prolapse. *Dis Colon Rectum* 1988;31:355–7.

173. **Broden B, Snellman B.** Procidentia of the rectum studied with cineradiography: a contribution to the discussion of causative mechanism. *Dis Colon Rectum* 1968;11:330–47.

174. **Kelvin FM, Maglinte DDT, Benson JT.** Evacuation proctography (defecography): an aid to the investigation of pelvic floor disorders. *Obstet Gynecol* 1994;83:307–14.

175. **Kuijpers HC.** Treatment of complete rectal prolapse: to narrow, to wrap, to suspend, to fix, to encircle, to plicate or to resect? *World J Surg* 1992;16:826–30.

176. **Duthie GS, Bartolo DCC.** Abdominal rectopexy for rectal prolapse: a comparison of techniques. *Br J Surg* 1992;79:107–113.

177. **Thompson WG, Heaton KW.** Functional bowel disorders in apparently healthy people. *Gastroenterology* 1980;79:283–8.

178. **Drossman DA, Sandler RS, McKee DC, Lovitz AJ.** Bowel patterns among subjects not seeking health care: use of a questionnaire to identify a population with bowel dysfunction. *Gastroenterology* 1982;83:529–34.

179. **Moriarty KJ, Irving MH.** ABC or colorectal disease. Constipation. *BMJ* 1992;304:1237–40.

180. **Shafik A.** Constipation: pathogenesis and management. *Drugs* 1993;45:528–40.

181. **Kuijpers HC.** Application of the colorectal laboratory in diagnosis and treatment of functional constipation. *Dis Colon Rectum* 1990;33:35–9.

182. **Kamm MA.** Idiopathic constipation: any movement? *Scand J Gastroenterol Suppl* 1992;192: 106–9.

183. **Read NW, Timms JM, Barfield LJ, Donnelly TC, Bannister JJ.** Impairment of defecation in young women with severe constipation. *Gastroenterology* 1986;90:53–60.

184. **Preston DM, Lennard-Jones JE.** Severe chronic constipation of young women: idiopathic slow transit constipation. *Gut* 1986;27:41–8.

185. **Preston DM, Lennard-Jones JE.** Anismus in chronic constipation. *Dig Dis Sci* 1985;30: 413–8.

186. **Bleijenberg G, Juijpers HC.** Treatment of spastic pelvic floor syndrome with biofeedback. *Dis Colon Rectum* 1987;30:108–11.

21 Gynecologic Endoscopy

Malcolm G. Munro

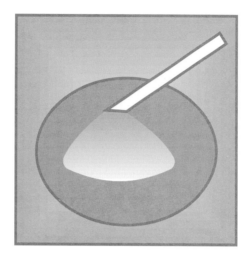

Endoscopy is a procedure that uses a narrow telescope to view the interior of a viscus space. Although the first medical endoscopic procedures were performed more than 100 years ago, the potential of this method was only recently realized. Endoscopes are currently used to perform a variety of operations. In gynecology, endoscopes are used most often to diagnose conditions by direct visualization of the peritoneal cavity (laparoscopy) or the inside of the uterus (hysteroscopy).

When used appropriately, endoscopic surgery offers the benefits of reduced pain, improved cosmesis, less cost, and faster recovery. The indications for endoscopic surgery are outlined here and detailed in the appropriate chapters. The technology, potential uses, and complications of laparoscopy and hysteroscopy are summarized.

Laparoscopy

The past two decades have witnessed rapid progress and technological advances in laparoscopy (1–12). Operative laparoscopy was developed by the 1970s, and by the early 1980s, laparoscopy was first used to direct the application of electrical or laser energy for the treatment of advanced stages of endometriosis (6–10). The use of high-resolution, lightweight video cameras in operative laparoscopy has facilitated visibility of the pelvis during the performance of complex procedures. Subsequently, many other procedures that were previously performed using traditional techniques, e.g., hysterectomy, became feasible with the laparoscope (11). However, the endoscopic approach may have drawbacks in some patients. Although some laparoscopic procedures seem to reduce the cost and morbidity associated with surgery, others have not been shown to be effective replacements for more traditional operations. The techniques and indications for operative endoscopy are evolving.

Diagnosis

The objective lens of a laparoscope can be positioned to allow wide-angle or magnified views of the peritoneal cavity. Laparoscopy is the standard method for the diagnosis of endometriosis and adhesions, because no other imaging technique provides the same degree of sensitivity and specificity.

677

However, there are limitations to laparoscopy. The view is restricted, and if tissue or fluid becomes attached to the lens, vision may be obscured. Also, soft tissues or the inside of a hollow viscus cannot be palpated. For assessment of soft tissue, imaging modalities such as ultrasonography, computed tomography (CT), or magnetic resonance imaging (MRI) scans are superior. Because of its ability to view soft tissue, ultrasonography is more accurate than laparoscopy for the evaluation of the inside of adnexal masses. The intraluminal contour of the uterus can be demonstrated only by hysteroscopy or contrast imaging. Ultrasonography, in combination with serum assays of β-human chorionic gonadotropin (β-hCG) and progesterone, can be used to diagnose ectopic pregnancy, usually allowing medical therapy to be given without laparoscopic confirmation (12). As a result of the advances in blood tests and imaging technology, laparoscopy is more often used to confirm a clinical impression than for initial diagnosis.

Laparoscopy may disclose abnormalities that are not necessarily related to the patient's problem. Although endometriosis, adhesions, leiomyomas, and small cysts in the ovaries are common, they are frequently asymptomatic. Thus, diagnostic laparoscopy must be performed prudently, interpreting findings in the context of the clinical problem and other diagnoses.

Therapy

The role of laparoscopy in the operative management of gynecologic conditions is still being defined. Many procedures previously in the domain of traditional abdominal and vaginal operations are feasible with laparoscopy. In addition to the benefits of endoscopic procedures in general, laparoscopic surgery is less likely than laparotomy to form adhesions. Because sponges are not used, the amount of direct peritoneal trauma is reduced substantially and contamination of the peritoneal cavity is minimized. The lack of exposure to air allows the peritoneal surface to remain more moist and, therefore, less susceptible to injury and adhesion formation.

Despite these advantages, there are potential limitations. For example, exposure of the operative field can be reduced, manipulation of the pelvic viscera is limited, and the caliber of the suture required may be larger than otherwise desired. In many cases, the cost of hospitalization increases, despite a shortened stay, because of prolonged operating room time and the use of more expensive surgical equipment and supplies. Efficacy may be reduced because surgeons may not adequately replicate the abdominal operation. In some patients, there is an increased risk of complications, which can be attributed to the innate limitations of laparoscopy, the level of surgical expertise, or both. With an adequate combination of ability, training, and experience, however, operative time and complications are comparable to traditional abdominal surgery.

Tubal Surgery

Sterilization   Laparoscopic sterilization has been extensively used since the late 1960s and can be performed under local or general anesthesia. The tubes may be occluded by suture, clips, or silastic rings, but electrosurgical desiccation with bipolar energy is the technique used most often (see Chapter 10). If an operative laparoscope is used, only one incision is required. Otherwise, a second port is needed for the introduction of the occluding instrument. Patients remain in the hospital for several hours, even when general anesthesia is used. Postoperative pain is usually minor and related to the effects of the anesthesia, gas that remains in the peritoneal cavity (shoulder pain, dyspnea), and in the case of occlusive devices, pain at the surgical site. These effects normally disappear within a few days. The failure rate is about 5.4 per 1000 women years (13, 14).

Ectopic Gestation   Ectopic gestation can be managed using laparoscopy to perform the same procedures done with laparotomy, including salpingostomy, salpingectomy, and segmental resection of a portion of the oviduct (see Chapter 17) (15). Salpingostomy is performed with scissors, a laser, or an electrosurgical electrode after carefully injecting the mesosalpinx with a dilute *vasopressin*-containing solution (20 units/100 ml normal saline). For salpingectomy, the vascular pedicles are usually secured with electrosurgical desiccation, ligatures, clips, or a combination thereof. Tissue is removed from the peritoneal cavity via one of the laparoscopic ports.

When salpingostomy is performed by any route, there is about a 5% chance that trophoblastic tissue remains. In such instances, medical treatment with *methotrexate* is considered appropriate (see Chapter 17). Consequently, β-hCG levels should be measured weekly until there is confidence that complete excision has occurred (16, 17).

Ovarian Surgery

Ovarian Masses   Laparoscopic removal of selected ovarian masses is a well-established procedure (18, 19). However, controversy exists regarding the selection of tumors that can be removed via laparoscopy, because of concerns about an adverse effect on prognosis with malignant tumors (20). Preoperative ultrasonography is mandatory. Sonolucent lesions with thin walls and no solid components are at very low risk for malignancy and, therefore, are suitable for laparoscopic removal. For postmenopausal women, the measurement of CA125 may be useful in identifying candidates for laparoscopic management (21, 22). Lesions with sonographic findings suggestive of mature teratoma (dermoid) may also be suitable for endoscopic management (23). The ovarian tumors should be assessed by frozen histologic section, and any malignancy should be managed expeditiously by laparotomy (22, 24).

Oophorectomy and cystectomy are performed similar to those for laparotomy (16). For cystectomy, scissors are used to separate the cyst from the ovary; if oophorectomy is performed, the vascular pedicles are ligated with sutures, clips, linear cutting staplers, electrosurgical desiccation, or a combination thereof. Most cysts are drained before extraction, via either a laparoscopic cannula or a posterior colpotomy. If there is concern about the impact of spilled cyst contents, the specimen can be removed in a retrieval bag inserted into the peritoneal cavity.

Although in the past the ovary has routinely been closed after cystectomy, this practice may be unnecessary and could contribute to the formation of adhesions (25). However, complete disruption of the ovarian cortex may make closure necessary. If so, the edges of the ovarian incision can be sutured.

Other Ovarian Surgery   Many cases of ovarian torsion previously treated by laparotomy and oophorectomy can be managed laparoscopically (26, 27). If there is no apparent necrosis, the adnexa should be untwisted. Otherwise, adnexectomy is indicated.

Polycystic ovarian syndrome can be treated laparoscopically using electrosurgery and laser vaporization (28–30). Although such procedures have been shown to be successful, the occurrence of postoperative adhesions in 15–20% of patients underscores the need to first exhaust medical treatment (31, 32).

Uterine Surgery

Myomectomy   Laparoscopic myomectomy, although feasible, is rarely performed, in part because its efficacy is yet to be established, especially as it relates to the treatment of infertility and menorrhagia (33, 34). Also, laparoscopic myomectomy requires more technical skills than many other endoscopic procedures.

Unless the myoma involves the endometrial cavity, it is unlikely to contribute to heavy menstrual bleeding. Leiomyomas that cause pressure are often large and located in or near vital vascular structures. Myomectomy should be performed only when indicated (as opposed to expectant or medical management), and laparotomy should be used if there are technical limitations (35). **The only leiomyomas that are clearly appropriate candi-**

dates for laparoscopic excision are those pedunculated subserosal lesions that cause pain in association with torsion (16, 36).

Hysterectomy   In many patients, hysterectomy can be performed under laparoscopic direction. *Laparoscopic hysterectomy* encompasses a variety of procedures ranging from the facilitation of vaginal hysterectomy by variable amounts of endoscopic dissection to entire uterine removal with the assistance of the laparoscope (37). The procedure is performed with scissors, sutures, electricity, clips, and, in some instances, linear cutting and stapling devices to dissect or ligate pedicles.

Laparoscopic hysterectomy offers no advantage for women in whom vaginal hysterectomy is possible, because the endoscopic approach is more expensive and does not have a lower risk of postoperative morbidity (38, 39).

Fertility Operations

Laparoscopic treatment of infertility includes operations used to reconstruct the normal anatomic relationships altered by an inflammatory process: fimbrioplasty, adhesiolysis, and salpingostomy for distal obstruction. Fimbrioplasty is distinguished from salpingostomy because it is performed in the absence of preexisting complete distal obstruction. Endometriosis associated with adnexal distortion can be treated by laparoscopic adhesiolysis. There is no known additional benefit of laparoscopic (or medical) treatment to coexistent active endometriosis. Laparoscopy has been superseded by ultrasound for the retrieval of oocytes for *in vitro* fertilization but is still used for procedures in which gametes (gamete intrafallopian transfer—GIFT) or zygotes (zygote intrafallopian transfer—ZIFT) are placed into the fallopian tube.

Adhesiolysis may be accomplished by blunt or sharp dissection with scissors, laser, or an electrosurgical electrode. These instruments are usually passed through an ancillary port; those who use laser energy frequently use the channel of the operating laparoscope. Although there has been controversy regarding the most appropriate modality, both methods are probably equally effective in appropriately trained hands.

Laparoscopic operations for the treatment of mechanical infertility are probably equally effective to similar procedures performed via laparotomy. In patients with extensive adhesions, however, the effectiveness of all procedures is limited. Assisted reproductive technologies such as *in vitro* fertilization and embryo transfer are necessary in these situations (16, 40).

Endometriosis

The laparoscopic management of endometriomas parallels that of adnexal masses, although the sonographic complexity of endometriomas may make it difficult to preoperatively distinguish them from a neoplasm. The relationship of the endometrioma to the ovarian cortex and stroma makes it difficult to find surgical dissection planes. There is a tendency to either compromise the function of the remaining ovary by attempting complete removal or to leave part of the endometrioma in place. Therefore, for women who want to retain their fertility, electrosurgical or laser ablative techniques may be used to treat endometriotic tissue that is adherent to the remaining ovary.

Multifocal endometriosis may be treated by mechanical excision or ablation, the latter using coagulation or vaporization with either electrical or laser energy. With proper use, each energy source creates approximately the same amount of thermal injury (41–43). Endometriosis is frequently deeper than appreciated, making excisional techniques valuable in many instances (16, 40).

Pelvic Floor Disorders

Laparoscopy can be used to guide procedures to treat pelvic floor prolapse, including enterocele repair, vaginal vault suspension, and retropubic cystourethropexy for urinary stress incontinence. Although these conditions can be treated vaginally, the abdominal approach may offer benefits, particularly with retropubic urethropexy. There is some evidence that this procedure is effective when compared with the traditional approaches (44). The laparoscopic treatment of enterocele and vault prolapse may be useful in patients who require abdominal approaches after failure of a previous vaginal procedure.

Gynecologic Malignancy

The role of laparoscopy in the management of gynecologic malignancy has not been clearly established (24, 45, 46). However, a number of ongoing research protocols relating cervical, endometrial, and ovarian cancer should document this role. Lymph node biopsies performed by laparoscopy can be coupled with vaginal hysterectomy for the management of early-stage endometrial cancer. The potential for laparoscopic lymphadenectomy has fostered a resurgence of interest in vaginal radical hysterectomy for stage I carcinoma of the cervix. Laparoscopy is also being investigated for the staging of early ovarian malignancy and for second-look surgery.

Patient Preparation and Communication

The prospective patient must understand the rationale, alternatives, risks, and potential benefits of the selected approach. She should know what would probably happen if the procedure is not done and expectant management is used.

The expectations and risks of diagnostic laparoscopy, as well as those of any other procedures that may be needed, must be explained. The risks of laparoscopy include those associated with anesthesia, infection, bleeding, and injury to the abdominal and pelvic viscera. Infection is uncommon with laparoscopic surgery. For procedures involving extensive dissection, there is a higher risk of visceral injury. The potential for these risks should be clearly presented. The patient should be given realistic expectations regarding postoperative disability. After diagnostic or brief operative procedures, patients can be discharged on the day of surgery and will usually require 24–72 hours away from work or school. If extensive dissection is performed or the surgery lasts longer than 2 hours, hospital admission may be necessary and the period of disability may be longer.

If the colon may be involved, mechanical bowel preparation should be performed to help improve visualization and minimize the need for a colostomy if the colon is entered. The patient should arrange for a friend or family member to discuss the results of the procedure and to drive her home if she is discharged the same day. Mild analgesia is often necessary.

Laparoscopic Technique

Laser and electrical sources of energy manifest their effect via conversion to thermal energy. Highly focused energy produces vaporization or cutting, while less focused energy causes desiccation and tissue coagulation. Animal studies fail to demonstrate differences in injury characteristics (41–43). Randomized controlled studies have shown no differences in fertility outcomes in women undergoing CO_2 laser surgery and electrosurgery (47, 48). Therefore, differences in results are more likely to be caused by other factors such as patient selection, extent of disease, and degree of surgical expertise. With proper education, modern equipment, and adherence to safety protocols, these techniques can be safely used. To facilitate the discussion of laparoscopic equipment, supplies, and techniques, it is useful to divide procedures into "core competencies," which are as follows:

1. Patient positioning

2. Operating room organization

3. Peritoneal access

4. Visualization

5. Manipulation of tissue and fluid

6. Cutting, hemostasis, and tissue fastening

7. Tissue extraction

8. Incision management

Patient Positioning

Proper positioning of the patient is essential for safety, comfort of the operator, and optimal visualization of the pelvic organs. Laparoscopy is performed on an operating table that can be rotated around the patient's long axis and tipped to create a steep, head-down (Trendelenburg) position. The footrest can be dropped to allow access to the perineum. The patient is placed in the *low lithotomy position,* with the legs supported in stirrups and the buttocks protruding slightly from the lower edge of the table (Fig. 21.1). The thighs are usually kept in the neutral position to preserve the sacroiliac angle, reducing the tendency of bowel to slide into the peritoneal cavity. The lateral aspect of the knee should be protected with padding or a special stirrup to avoid peroneal nerve injury. The knees should be kept in at least slight flexion to minimize stretching of the sciatic nerve and to provide more stability in the Trendelenburg position. The arms are positioned at the patient's side to allow freedom of movement for the surgeon and to lower the risk of brachial plexus injury (Fig. 21.2). Care must be exercised to protect the fingers and hand from injury when

Figure 21.1   Patient positioning: the low lithotomy position. The patient's buttocks are positioned so that the perineum is at the edge of the table. The legs are well supported with stirrups with the thighs in slight flexion. Too much flexion may impede the manipulation of laparoscopic instruments while in the Trendelenburg (head down) position.

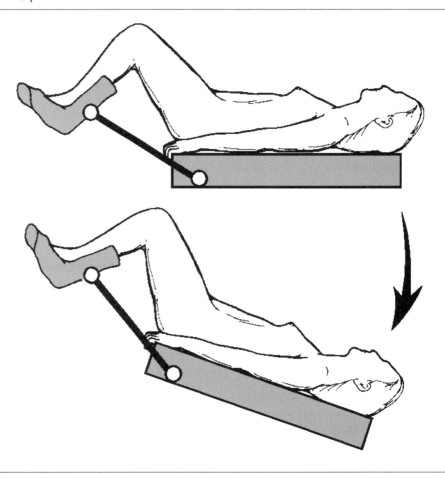

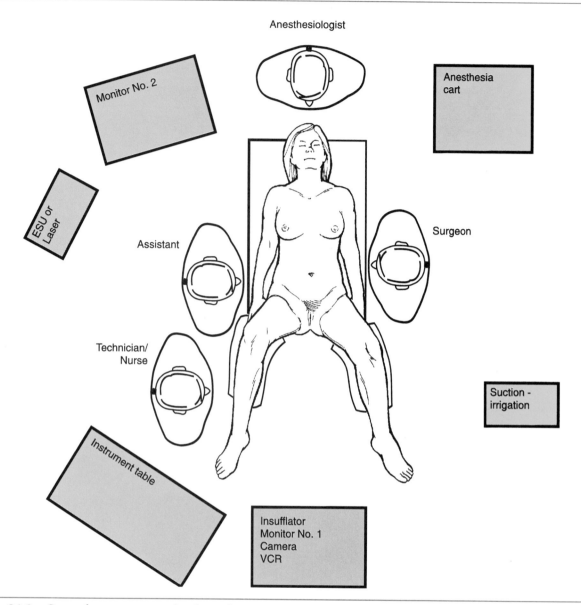

Figure 21.2   Operating room organization. The patient's arms are at the sides. The right-handed surgeon stands on the patient's left. Instruments and equipment are distributed around the patient within view of the surgeon. For pelvic surgery, the monitor should be located between the patient's legs. For upper abdominal surgery, or when operating from below, a monitor should be placed near the patient's head.

the foot of the table is raised or lowered. After the patient is properly positioned, the bladder should be emptied with a catheter and a uterine manipulator attached to the cervix.

Operating Room Organization

The arrangement of instruments and equipment is important for safety and efficiency. The orientation depends on the operation, the instruments used, and whether the surgeon is right- or left-handed. An orientation for a right-handed operator is shown in Figure 21.2.

For pelvic surgery, the monitor should be placed at the foot of the table within the angle formed by the patient's legs. If a second monitor is used, one should be positioned at each foot of the patient. If upper abdominal surgery is also to be performed, the additional monitor should be moved to the head of the operating table.

The surgeon stands by the patient's left side, at an angle facing the patient's contralateral foot. The nurse or technician and instrument table are positioned near the foot of the operating table to avoid obscuring the video monitor. The insufflator is placed on the patient's right side, in front of the surgeon, to allow continuous monitoring of the inflation rate and intra-abdominal pressure. The electrosurgical generator is also positioned on the patient's right side to permit visualization of the power output. When a laser is used through a second puncture site, it is also placed to the patient's right. When the laser is passed though the channel of an operating laparoscope, however, it is situated on the patient's left side, beside the surgeon.

Peritoneal Access

Before inserting the laparoscope, a cannula or port must be positioned in the abdominal wall to establish access to the peritoneal cavity. The *closed technique* is a blind approach in which the cannula is introduced with a sharp trocar used to penetrate the abdominal layers. In *open laparoscopy,* entry into the peritoneal cavity is achieved by a minilaparotomy, with the cannula fixed into position with sutures or other suitable techniques. Gynecologists have generally favored a closed technique, preinflating the peritoneal cavity with CO_2 via a hollow needle. In either case, additional cannulas are inserted via sharp trocars under direct vision to allow the use of laparoscopic hand instruments such as scissors, probes, and other manipulating devices.

Cannula insertion is aided by an understanding of the normal anatomy, especially the location of vessels (Fig. 21.3). A "safety zone" exists inferior to the sacral promontory in the area bounded cephalad by the bifurcation of the aorta, posteriorly by the sacrum, and laterally by the iliac vessels. In women placed in the Trendelenburg position, the great vessels are situated more cephalad and anterior, making them more vulnerable to injury un-

Figure 21.3   Vascular anatomy of the anterior abdominal wall. Location of the vessels that can be traumatized when inserting trocars into the anterior abdominal wall.

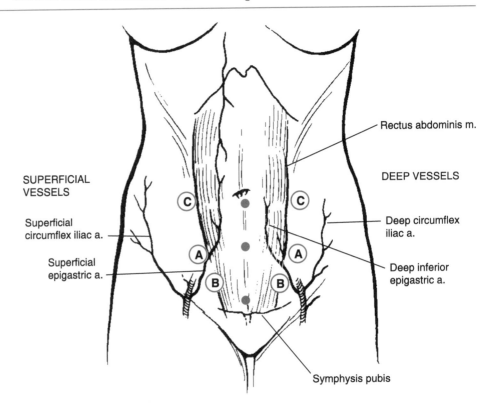

SUPERFICIAL VESSELS

Superficial circumflex iliac a.

Superficial epigastric a.

Rectus abdominis m.

DEEP VESSELS

Deep circumflex iliac a.

Deep inferior epigastric a.

Symphysis pubis

less appropriate adjustments are made in the angle of insertion (Fig. 21.4). Therefore, positioning of the insufflation needle, the initial trocar, and the cannula are best accomplished with the patient in a horizontal position. This approach also facilitates the evaluation of the upper abdomen, which is limited if the intraperitoneal contents are shifted cephalad by the head-down position.

Insufflation Needles

Virtually all insufflation needles are modifications of the hollow needle designed by Verres (Fig. 21.5). In cases uncomplicated by previous pelvic surgery, the preferred site for insertion is as close as possible to (or within) the umbilicus, where the abdominal wall is the thinnest.

Figure 21.4   Vascular anatomy. Location of the great vessels and their changing relationship to the umbilicus with increasing patient weight (from left to right).

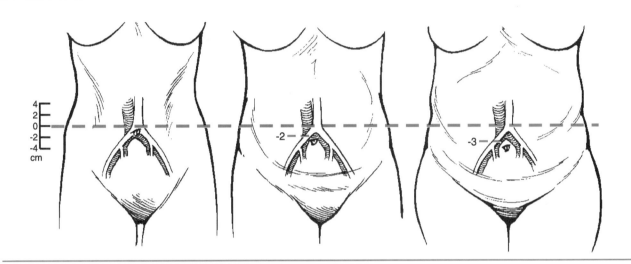

Figure 21.5   Insufflation needle (Ethicon Endosurgery, Inc., Cincinnati, OH). When pressed against tissue such as fascia or peritoneum, the spring-loaded blunt obturator is pushed back into the hollow needle, revealing its sharpened end. When the needle enters the peritoneal cavity, the obturator springs back into position, protecting the intra-abdominal contents from injury. The handle of the hollow needle allows the attachment of a syringe or tubing for insufflation of the distension gas.

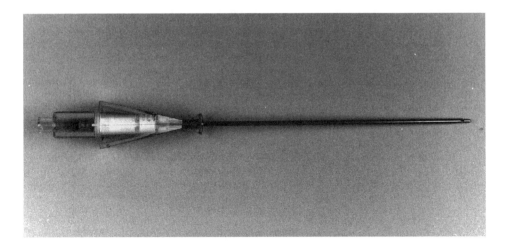

1. *A 3-mm incision adequate for the needle is made with a small scalpel and the abdominal wall is elevated by gripping it in the midline below the umbilicus.* Safe insertion of the insufflation needle mandates that the instrument be maintained in a midline, sagittal plane while the operator directs the tip between the iliac vessels, anterior to the sacrum but inferior to the bifurcation of the aorta and the proximal aspect of the vena cava. Therefore, in women of average weight, the insufflation needle is directed at a 45° angle to the patient's spine. In heavy to obese individuals, this angle may be increased incrementally to nearly 90°, accounting for the increasing thickness of the abdominal wall and the tendency of the umbilicus to gravitate caudad with increasing abdominal girth (49). The needle's shaft is held by the tips of the fingers and steadily but purposefully guided into position only far enough to allow the tip's entry into the peritoneal cavity. The tactile and visual feedback created when the needle passes through the facial and peritoneal layers of the abdominal wall may provide guidance and help prevent overaggressive insertion attempts. This proprioceptive feedback is less apparent with disposable needles than with the classic Verres needle. With the former, the surgeon must listen to the "clicks" as the needle obturator retracts when it passes through the rectus fascia and the peritoneum. The needle should never be forced.

2. *In instances in which the umbilicus has known or suspected intra-abdominal adhesions, alternative sites for insufflation needle insertion should be used.* These include the pouch of Douglas, the fundus of the uterus, and the left upper quadrant, most often at the left costal margin (Fig. 21.6). The left upper quadrant is preferred if there has been no previous surgery in this area. In such patients, the stomach must be decompressed with a nasogastric or orogastric tube prior to the puncture.

3. *Before insufflation, the operator should try to detect whether the insufflation needle has been malpositioned in the omentum, mesentery, blood vessels, or hollow organs such as the stomach or bowel.* Using a syringe attached to the insufflation needle, blood or gastrointestinal contents may be aspirated. This examination may be facilitated by injecting a small amount of saline into the syringe. If the needle is appropriately positioned, negative intra-abdominal pressure is created by lifting the abdominal wall. This negative pressure may be demonstrated by aspiration of a drop of saline placed over the open, proximal end of the needle or, preferably, by using the digital pressure gauge on the insufflator.

4. *Additional signs of proper placement may be sought after starting insufflation.* The intra-abdominal pressure reading should be low, reflecting only systemic resistance to the flow of CO_2. Consequently, there should be little deviation from a base-line measurement, generally less than 10 mm Hg. The pressure varies with respiration and is slightly higher in obese patients. The earliest reassuring sign is the loss of liver "dullness" over the lateral aspect of the right costal margin. However, this sign may be absent if there are dense adhesions in the area, usually the result of previous surgery. Symmetrical distension is unlikely to occur when the needle is positioned extraperitoneally. Proper positioning can also be shown by lightly compressing the xiphoid process, which increases the pressure measured by the insufflator.

5. *The amount of gas transmitted into the peritoneal cavity should depend on the measured intraperitoneal pressure, not the volume of gas inflated.* Intraperitoneal volume capacity varies significantly between individuals. Many surgeons prefer to insufflate to 20 mm Hg for positioning of the cannulas. This level usually provides enough counterpressure against the peritoneum, facilitating trocar introduction and potentially reducing the chance of bowel or posterior abdominal wall and vessel trauma. After placement of the cannulas, the pressure should be dropped to 10–12 mm Hg, which essentially eliminates hypercarbia or decreased venous return of blood to the heart.

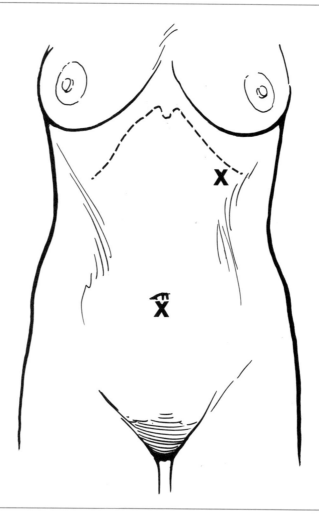

Figure 21.6   Insufflation needle and cannula insertion sites. In most instances, both the insufflation needle, if used, and the primary cannula are inserted through the umbilicus. When subumbilical adhesions are known or suspected, the insufflation needle may be placed through the pouch of Douglas or in the left upper quadrant following evacuation of the gastric contents with an orogastric tube.

Primary Cannulas

Laparoscopic cannulas are necessary to allow the insertion of laparoscopic instruments into the peritoneal cavity while maintaining the pressure created by the distending gas (Figs. 21.7 and 21.8). Cannulas are hollow tubes with a valve or sealing mechanism at or near the proximal end. The cannula may be fitted with a Luer-type port that allows attachment to tubing connected with the CO_2 insufflator. Larger-diameter cannulas (8–12 mm) may be fitted with adapters or specialized valves that allow the insertion of smaller diameter instruments without loss of intraperitoneal pressure.

The trocar is a longer instrument of slightly smaller diameter that is passed through the cannula, exposing its tip. Most trocars have sharp tips, allowing penetration of the abdominal wall after a small skin incision. Many disposable trocar-cannula systems are designed with a "safety-mechanism"—usually a pressure-sensitive spring that either retracts the trocar or deploys a protective sheath around its tip after passage through the abdominal wall. None of these protective devices has been shown to make the procedure safer; however, they do increase the cost.

Cannulas can be inserted following minilaparotomy (*open laparoscopy*), after the successful creation of a pneumoperitoneum (*secondary puncture*), or without previously in-

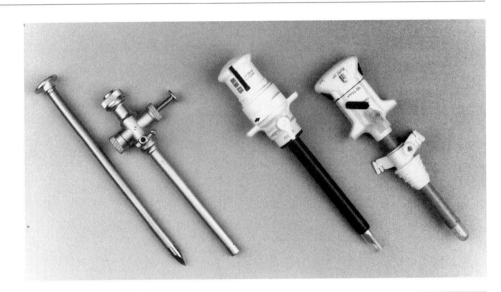

Figure 21.7   Primary laparoscopic cannulas. *Left to right:* a nondisposable 10-mm cannula with the obturator removed (Olympus America, Inc., Woodbury, NY), a disposable 5- to 12-mm cannula with a "safety" sheath (Autosuture, Inc, Norwalk, CT), and a Hasson cannula used in open laparoscopy (Ethicon Endosurgery, Inc., Cincinnati, OH).

Figure 21.8   Ancillary laparoscopic cannulas: 5-mm laparoscopic cannulas for ancillary instruments. *Top:* Apple Medical, Boston, MA (disposable). *Middle:* Wolf, Laguna Niguel, CA (nondisposable). These cannulas neither have or require ports or "safety" sheaths and are therefore less expensive than other cannulas. *Bottom:* Core Surgical Inc. (Jacksonville, FL).

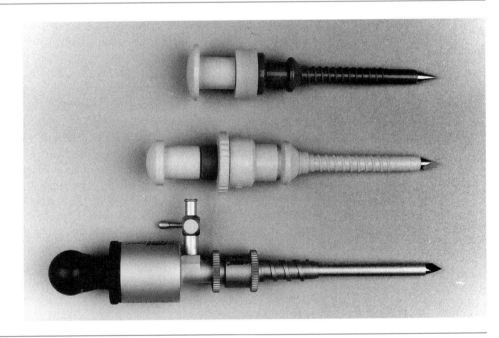

stilling intraperitoneal gas (*primary puncture*). With open laparoscopy, there is less risk of injury to blood vessels and abdominal viscera. However, open laparoscopy cannot prevent all insertion accidents because intestine can be entered inadvertently no matter how small the laparotomy. There is little evidence that secondary puncture is necessary, at least when there are no preexisting abdominal wall adhesions. Therefore, in women with no previous surgery, the primary puncture can be performed with a sharp-tipped, trocar-cannula system, which lowers the cost by eliminating the need for the insufflation needle and by reducing operating time. The first, or primary, cannula must be of sufficient caliber to permit passage of the laparoscope and is usually inserted in or at the lower border of the umbilicus. The incision should be extended only enough to allow insertion of the cannula; otherwise, leakage of gas may occur around the sheath. For the primary puncture, an assistant should elevate the abdominal wall. For the secondary puncture, it is unnecessary to lift the abdominal wall during insertion. Both hands can be positioned on the device, using one to provide counter-pressure and control to prevent "overshoot" and resultant injury to bowel or vessels. The angle of insertion is the same as for the insufflation needle; adjustments are made according to the patient's weight and body habitus. The laparoscope should be inserted to confirm proper intraperitoneal placement before the insufflation gas is allowed to flow. Laparoscope cannulas can become dislodged and slip out of the incision during a procedure. There are a variety of cannula attachments designed to prevent slippage.

Previous abdominal surgery increases the incidence of adhesions of the bowel to the anterior abdominal wall, frequently near the umbilicus and in the path of the primary trocar. In such patients, another primary insertion site should be selected, even if it is used solely for conveying a narrow "scout" laparoscope, some types of which can be inserted through an insufflation needle (Fig. 21.9). Using such a laparoscope, the presence of adhesions under the incision can be confirmed or excluded and the umbilical cannula can be inserted under direct vision. Alternate insertion sites for primary cannulas are shown in Figure 21.6. Of these locations, the left upper quadrant is the most useful because adhesions are rarely present. Nasogastric or orogastric suction must be applied preceding insertion to improve vision and reduce the risk of gastric injury.

Figure 21.9   Scout laparoscopes. *Top,* the 2.7-mm-diameter Olympus/Ethicon Endosurgery system. The Imagyn outer sheath is introduced with a standard diameter 15-cm insufflation needle, and the Olympus/Ethicon system is inserted with a 3-mm needle. *Bottom,* the 2-mm-diameter Imagyn laparoscope (Imagyn, Inc., Laguna Niguel, CA).

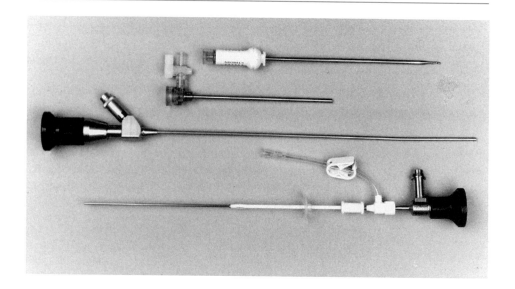

Ancillary Cannulas

Ancillary cannulas are necessary to perform most diagnostic and operative laparoscopic procedures. Most of the currently available disposable ancillary cannulas are identical to those designed for insertion of the primary cannula. However, many of the integrated design features for the primary cannula are unnecessary for ancillary cannulas. Consequently, simple cannulas without safety sheaths and insufflation ports are sufficient (Fig. 21.8).

Proper positioning of these cannulas depends on a sound knowledge of the abdominal wall vascular anatomy. They should always be inserted under direct vision because injury to bowel or major vessels can occur. Prior to insertion, the bladder should be drained with a urethral catheter. The insertion sites depend on the procedure, the disease, the patient's body habitus, and the surgeon's preference. The most useful and cosmetically acceptable site for an ancillary cannula is usually in the midline of the lower abdomen, about 2–4 cm above the symphysis. The ancillary cannula should not be inserted too close to the symphysis, because it limits the mobility of the ancillary instruments and access to the cul-de-sac.

Lower-quadrant cannulas are useful for operative laparoscopy, but the inferior epigastric vessels must be located in order to avoid injury (Fig. 21.3). Transillumination of the abdominal wall from within will permit the identification of the *superficial inferior epigastric* vessels in most thin women. However, the *deep inferior epigastric* vessels cannot be identified by this mechanism because of their location deep to the rectus sheath. The most consistent landmarks are the median umbilical ligaments (obliterated umbilical arteries) and the entry point of the round ligament into the inguinal canal. At the pubic crest, the deep inferior epigastric vessels begin their cephalad course between the medially located umbilical ligament and the laterally positioned exit point of the round ligament. The trocar should be inserted medial or lateral to the vessels if they are visualized. If the vessels cannot be seen and it is necessary to position the cannula laterally, it should be placed 3–4 cm lateral to the median umbilical ligament or lateral to the lateral margin of the rectus abdominis muscle. However, if the insertion is placed too far laterally, it will endanger the deep circumflex epigastric artery. The risk of injury can be minimized by placing a 22-gauge spinal needle through the skin at the desired location, directly observing the entry via the laparoscope. This provides reassurance that a safe location has been identified and allows visualization of the peritoneal needle hole, which provides a precise target for inserting the trocar.

Even after a proper incision, the abdominal wall vessels can be injured if the trocar is directed medially. Large-diameter trocars are more likely to cause injury; therefore, the smallest cannulas necessary to perform the procedure should be used. Ancillary cannulas should not be placed too close together, because this results in "knitting" of the hand instruments, which compromises access and maneuverability.

Visualization

During endoscopy, the image must be transferred through an optical system. Although direct optical viewing is feasible and often used for diagnostic purposes, virtually all operative laparoscopy is performed using video guidance.

Operative Versus Diagnostic Equipment   Laparoscopes used for operative purposes have a straight channel, parallel to the optical axis, for the introduction of operating instruments. The advantages of such an endoscope are that it provides an additional port for the insertion of instruments and the tangential application of laser energy. However, they are of relatively larger caliber than diagnostic laparoscopes and have smaller fields of view and increased electrosurgical risks. Diagnostic laparoscopes permit better visualization at a given diameter and are associated with fewer electrosurgical risks.

Diameter   Narrow-diameter laparoscopes allow limited transfer of light both into and out of the peritoneal cavity; therefore, they require a more sensitive camera or a more powerful light source for adequate illumination. Ideal illumination is provided by 10-mm diagnostic laparoscopes, but improvements in optics are making more procedures feasible with smaller-caliber devices (Fig. 21.10).

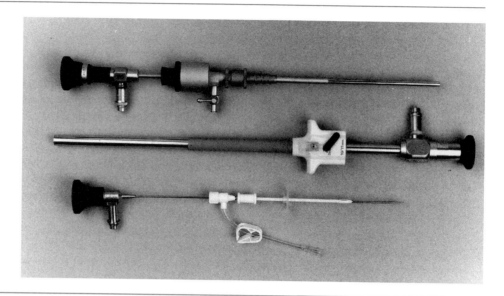

Figure 21.10 Laparoscopes. *Top to bottom:* 5-mm-diameter (Olympus, Inc., Woodbury, NY), 10-mm-diameter (Karl Storz, Agoura Hills, CA), and 2-mm-diameter (Imagyn, Inc., Laguna Niguel, CA) laparoscopes. The 2-mm laparoscope can be inserted via a very narrow cannula passed through an insufflation needle.

Lenses Most laparoscope lenses are made of optical quality glass. The use of fibers is necessary for very small-caliber laparoscopes (<3-mm diameter) because lens integrity is not well protected by the flexible sheath. Relatively large-caliber fibers tend to "pixellate" the image, although the use of densely packed, fine-caliber fibers reduces this tendency, and with an adequate number and quality of fibers, it is eliminated altogether.

Viewing Angle The viewing angle depicts the relationship of the visual field to the axis of the endoscope and is usually either 0° or 30° to the horizontal. The 0° scope is the standard for gynecologic surgery. However, the 30° angle provides some advantage in difficult situations such as the performance of retropubic urethropexy.

Imaging Systems

Video Cameras The video camera captures the image transmitted by the endoscope with one or three light-sensitive, charged-coupled-device (CCD) chips located in the camera head and coupled with the endoscope. Generally, the camera is attached to the eyepiece of the laparoscope, but with newer instruments, the chip will be affixed to the end of the device ("chip-on-a-stick"), obviating the need for an optical channel. In either case, the image is transmitted to the body of the camera located outside the operative field, where it is processed and sent to a recording device or monitor.

The key functional features of a camera are its light sensitivity and its horizontal resolution. Light sensitivity is measured in *lux* (1 lux = 1 lumen/M^2); lower minimum lux ratings reflect increased sensitivity of the chips in the camera. The most sensitive cameras are rated at 1 lux, but for adequate imaging, the rating should be no higher than 5 lux when used with a 10-mm laparoscope and a 250- to 300-watt light source. Horizontal resolution is measured in lines; the best single-chip and triple-chip resolutions are about 500 and 700 lines, respectively. The images with the highest resolution are provided by cameras that separate chrominance from luminance (sometimes referred to as Y/C or S-Video) or by those that separate the three components of color (RGB-red, green, blue). These cameras are to be distinguished from the lower-resolution composite signals that are provided with standard coaxial cable television. However, the additional cost of triple-chip technology at this time is justified only for the creation of teaching videos or still images for publication.

Monitors The resolution capability of the monitor should be at least equal to that provided by the camera. The best available monitors have the potential to display about 800 horizontal lines of resolution. This degree of resolution is not produced by S-Video or RGB systems; therefore, expensive Y/C- or RGB-capable cameras are unnecessary.

Light Sources The more light transmitted via the endoscope, the better the visualization. The best currently available output is achieved from 250–300 watts, usually using xenon or metal halide bulbs. Most camera systems are integrated with the light source to automatically vary light output depending on the amount of exposure required.

Light Cables Light guides or cables transmit light from the source to the endoscope. They may be constructed of densely packed fibers (fiberoptic) or can be fluid-filled. Fiberoptic cables lose function over time, particularly if they are bent at sharp angles, which breaks the fibers. Fluid-filled guides may initially supply more light but are less convenient than fiberoptic cables because they are heavier and less flexible.

Camera-Endoscope Couplers These instruments connect the video camera to the laparoscope. Couplers with a beam splitter allow direct visualization by the surgeon with simultaneous video monitoring for the assistants. By sending the image through two optical channels, however, the brightness of each is reduced. Couplers also vary in focal length, which affects both the amount of screen occupied by the circular image and the depth of field in focus. For example, a coupler with a wide-angled 28° lens will fill all of the screen but will have less depth of field in focus than the smaller image of a 32° lens.

Some laparoscopes attach directly to the camera, making a coupler unnecessary. This feature further enhances light transmission and reduces problems with fogging of the lens.

Intraperitoneal Distension

Insufflation Machines The insufflator delivers CO_2 from a gas cylinder to the patient via tubing connected to one of the ports on the laparoscope. Most insufflators can be set to maintain a predetermined intra-abdominal pressure. High flow rates (9–20 l/min) are especially useful for maintaining exposure when suction of smoke or fluid depletes the volume of intraperitoneal gas.

Laparoscopic Lifting Systems Intraperitoneal retractors attached to a pneumatic or mechanical lifting system can be used to create an intraperitoneal space much like a tent. This "gasless" or "apneumic" technique may have some advantages over pneumoperitoneum, particularly in patients with cardiopulmonary disease. Also, airtight cannulas are not necessary and instruments do not need to have a uniform, narrow, cylindrical shape. Consequently, some conventional instruments may be used directly through the incisions.

Manipulation of Fluid and Tissue

Fluid Management

Fluid may be instilled into the peritoneal cavity via wide-caliber arthroscopy or cystoscopy tubing using pressure provided by gravity, an infusion cuff, or a high-pressure mechanical pump. The pumps deliver fluid faster than the other techniques, and the highly pressurized stream of fluid may facilitate blunt dissection (*hydro-* or *aqua-dissection*). Removal of small volumes of fluid can be performed with a syringe attached to a cannula, but for large volumes, it is necessary to use suction generated by a machine or a wall source.

The cannulas used for suction and irrigation depend on the irrigation fluid used and the fluid being removed. For ruptured ectopic gestations or other procedures in which there is a large amount of blood and clots, large-diameter cannulas (7–10 mm) are preferred. Cannulas with narrow tips are more effective in generating the high pressure needed for hydrodissection.

If large volumes of fluid are required, isotonic fluids should be used to avoid fluid overload and electrolyte imbalance. If electrosurgery is to be performed, however, small volumes of nonelectrolyte-containing solutions such as glycine or sorbitol can be used for hemostasis and irrigation. Heparin can be added to irrigating solution to prevent blood from clotting, thus allowing it to be removed more easily (1000–5000 U/l).

Tissue Manipulation

Uterine Manipulators   A properly designed uterine manipulator should have an intrauterine component, or obturator, and a method for fixation of the device to the uterus. A hollow obturator attached to a port allows intraoperative instillation of liquid dye to demonstrate tubal patency. Articulation of the probe will permit acute anteversion or retroversion, which are extremely useful maneuvers. If the uterus is large, longer and wider obturators are used so that the manipulations can be performed more effectively. An articulated uterine manipulator is shown in Figure 21.11.

Grasping Forceps   The forceps used during laparoscopy should replicate those used in open surgery. Disposable instruments generally do not have the quality, strength, and precision of nondisposable forceps. Instruments with teeth (toothed forceps) are necessary to securely grasp the peritoneum or the edge of ovary to remove an ovarian cyst. Minimally traumatic instruments designed like Babcock clamps are needed to safely retract the fallopian tube. Tenaculum-like instruments are desirable to retract leiomyomas or the uterus. A ratchet is useful to hold tissue in the absence of hand pressure. The instrument should be insulated and capable of transmitting unipolar or bipolar electrical energy for hemostasis.

Cutting, Hemostasis, and Tissue Fixation

Cutting can be achieved by mechanical means, electricity, laser energy, and ultrasonic energy (Fig. 21.12). The methods for maintaining or securing hemostasis include sutures,

Figure 21.11   Uterine manipulators. The disposable "Clearview" (Ethicon Endosurgery, Cincinnati, OH) manipulator is demonstrated. Inset is a demonstration of the ability of the obturator to articulate, allowing the uterus to be anteverted or retroverted more easily and completely.

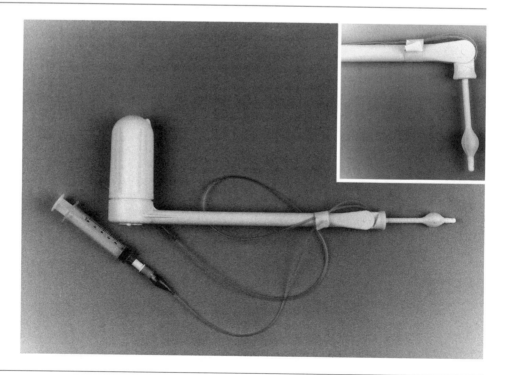

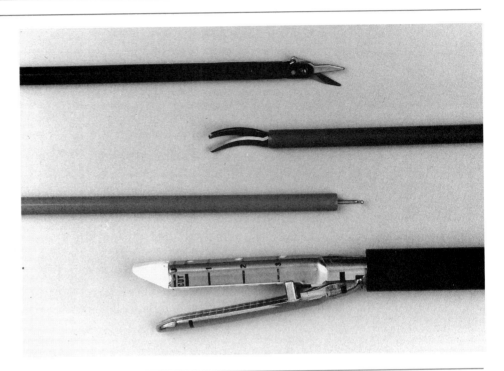

Figure 21.12 Laparoscopic cutting devices. *Top to bottom:* pointed "micro" scissors (Ethicon Endosurgery, Cincinnati, OH), curved dissecting scissors (Microsurge, Needham, MA), a narrow-angled electrode (Ethicon, Cincinnati, OH), a GIA-30 linear cutter stapler (Autosuture, U.S. Surgical, Norwalk, CT).

clips, linear staplers, energy sources, and topical or injectable substances (Fig. 21.13). Secure apposition or tissue fixation may be accomplished with sutures, clips, or staples. Because of the visual, tactile, and mechanical limitations of laparoscopy, prevention of bleeding is important.

Cutting The most useful cutting instruments are scissors. Because it is difficult to sharpen laparoscopic scissors, most surgeons prefer disposable instruments that may be used until dull and then discarded. Another mechanical cutting tool is the *linear stapler-cutter* that can simultaneously cut and hemostatically staple the edges of the incision. The cost and large dimensions of the instruments limit their practical use to only a few highly selected situations such as separation of the uterus from the ovary and fallopian tube during laparoscopic hysterectomy.

Electrosurgical electrodes that are narrow or pointed are capable of generating the high-power densities necessary to vaporize or cut tissue. Continuous or modulated, usually unipolar sine-wave outputs are used. For optimal results, they should be used in a noncontact fashion, following (not leading) the energy. Specially designed bipolar cutting probes are available that have one integrated electrode shaped as a needle and the other band-shaped electrode designed to be dispersive. Laparoscopic scissors with unipolar or bipolar electrosurgical attachments are designed to cut mechanically with energy used simultaneously for desiccation and hemostasis when cutting tissue that has small blood vessels.

Laser energy can be focused to vaporize and cut tissue. The most efficient cutting instrument is the CO_2 laser, which has the drawback of requiring linear transmission because light cannot be effectively conducted along bendable fibers. The potassium-titanyl-phosphate (KTP) and neodymium:yttrium, aluminum, garnet (Nd:YAG) lasers are also effective cutting tools. They are capable of propagating energy along bendable quartz fibers but

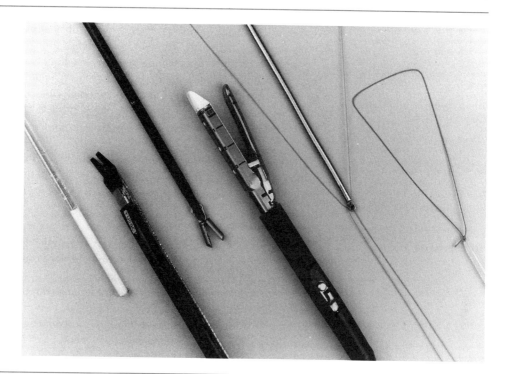

Figure 21.13   Hemostatic devices. *Left to right:* preloaded microfibrillar collagen (MedChem Products Inc., Woburn, MA), 1-cm clip applier (U.S. Surgical, Norwalk, CT), monopolar grasping forceps (Ethicon Endosurgery, Cincinnati, OH), GIA-30 linear with stapler (Autosuture, U.S. Surgical, Norwalk, CT), Clarke knot manipulator (Marlow, Inc., Willoughby, OH), Endoloop pretied ligature (Autosuture, U.S. Surgical, Norwalk, CT).

result in slightly greater thermal injury than electrical or CO_2 laser energy. Because of such limitations and the additional expense, these lasers are of limited value.

A laparoscopic instrument has been developed that uses ultrasonic energy for cutting. The device consists of a vibrating pizo electrode located in a handle that causes linear oscillation of a probe tipped with a blade, hook, or clamp. The rapid oscillation (55 kHz) of the probe allows the tip to cut mechanically or create hemostasis via tissue coagulation. In low-density tissue, cutting is augmented by the process of *cavitation,* in which reduction of local atmospheric pressure allows vaporization of intracellular water at body temperature.

Hemostasis and Tissue Fixation   Electricity is the least expensive and most versatile method for achieving hemostasis during laparoscopy. The process of *electrical desiccation* (coagulation) is achieved by contacting the tissue, activating the electrode using continuous "cutting" current of adequate power to heat and coagulate the tissue. For large-caliber vessels, the tissue should be compressed before the electrode is activated, allowing the edges of the vessel to seal or coapt. Either unipolar or bipolar grasping devices may be used. *Fulguration* is near-contact spraying of tissue with unipolar, high-voltage energy from the "coagulation" side of the electrosurgical generator. This technique is useful for control of superficial bleeding.

Clips may be placed with specially designed laparoscopic instruments. Nonabsorbable clips made of titanium are useful for relatively narrow vessels, and longer, self-retaining clips are generally preferred for larger vessels. Clips may be of particular value when securing relatively large vessels near an important structure such as the ureter.

Laparoscopic suturing has only recently become accepted as a method of maintaining hemostasis (50). The co st of materials is far less than clips or linear staplers, although operating time may be longer. The two basic methods for securing a ligature around a blood vessel are with intracorporeal and extracorporeal knots, depending on where the suture is tied. Intracorporeal knots are derived from the standard instrument knot and are formed within the peritoneal cavity. Extracorporeal knots are created outside the abdomen under direct vision and then transferred into the peritoneal cavity by knot manipulators (Fig. 21.13) (51).

Topical agents such as microfibrillar collagen are available in 5- and 10-mm-diameter laparoscopic applicators (Fig. 21.13). Local injection of diluted vasopressin may be used to maintain hemostasis for myomectomy or removal of ectopic pregnancy.

Removal of Tissue

After excising tissue, it is usually necessary to remove it from the peritoneal cavity. Small samples can be pulled through an appropriately sized cannula with grasping forceps; however, larger specimens may not fit. If the specimen is cystic, it may be drained via a needle or incised, shrinking it to a size suitable for removal through the cannula or one of the small laparoscopic incisions. An alternative is to place the specimen in an endoscopic retrieval bag prior to drainage, because of the concern for malignancy. More solid tissue may be morcellated with scissors, ultrasonic equipment, or electrosurgery. Electrosurgical morcellation requires special bipolar needles or, if the monopolar technique is used, that the specimen remain attached to the patient to preserve the integrity of the electrical circuit.

Larger specimens may be removed by inserting a larger cannula through an incision in the cul-de-sac (posterior culdotomy) or by extending one of the laparoscopy incisions. With the exception of colpotomy, extension of the umbilical incision may be the most cosmetic approach because removal of the tissue can be directed from an endoscope positioned in one of the ancillary ports.

Incision Management

Dehiscence and hernia risk increase when the fascial incision is made by a trocar that is larger than 10 mm in diameter (52). Closure of the fascia should take place under direct laparoscopic vision to prevent the accidental incorporation of bowel into the incisions. A small-caliber laparoscope passed through one of the narrow cannulas can be used to direct the fascial closure using curved needles or a ligature carrier especially designed for this purpose.

Complications

Laparoscopic procedures can be complicated by infections, trauma, or hemorrhage, as well as by problems associated with anesthetic use. The incidence of infection is lower than with procedures performed via laparotomy. Conversely, problems associated with visualization in conjunction with the change in anatomical perspective may increase the risk of damage to blood vessels or vital structures such as the bowel, ureter, or bladder.

Some complications are more common with laparoscopy than with procedures performed via laparotomy or vaginally. The instillation of large amounts of fluid into the peritoneal cavity may contribute to electrolyte disturbances or fluid overload. The prolonged use of intraperitoneal gas under pressure may cause metabolic abnormalities or may adversely affect cardiorespiratory function. The intraperitoneal use of electrical or laser energy creates the potential for a variety of complications that can be minimized by knowledge of the energy source, meticulous technique, and maintenance of the instruments.

Anesthetic and Cardiopulmonary Complications

One-third of the deaths associated with minor laparoscopic procedures such as sterilization are secondary to complications of anesthesia (52). The potential complications of general anesthesia include hypoventilation, esophageal intubation, gastroesophageal reflux, bronchospasm, hypotension, narcotic overdose, cardiac arrhythmias, and cardiac arrest. These risks can be enhanced by some of the inherent features of gynecologic laparoscopy. For example, the Trendelenburg position, in combination with the increased intraperitoneal pressure provided by pneumoperitoneum, places greater pressure on the diaphragm, increasing the risk of hypoventilation, hypercarbia, and metabolic acidosis. This position, combined with anesthetic agents that relax the esophageal sphincter, promotes regurgitation of gastric content, which in turn can lead to aspiration, bronchospasm, pneumonitis, and pneumonia.

Parameters of cardiopulmonary function associated with both CO_2 and N_2O insufflation include reduced PO_2, O_2 saturation, tidal volume, and minute ventilation and an increased respiratory rate. The use of intraperitoneal CO_2 as a distension medium is associated with an increase in PCO_2 and a decrease in pH. Elevation of the diaphragm may be associated with basilar atelectasis, resulting in right-to-left shunt and a ventilation perfusion mismatch (53).

Carbon Dioxide Embolus   Carbon dioxide is the most widely used peritoneal distension medium, largely because of the rapid absorption of CO_2 in blood. However, if large amounts of CO_2 gain access to the central venous circulation, if there is peripheral vasoconstriction, or if the splanchnic blood flow is decreased by excessively high intraperitoneal pressure, severe cardiorespiratory compromise may result.

The signs of CO_2 embolus include sudden and otherwise unexplained hypotension, cardiac arrhythmia, cyanosis, and heart murmurs. The end-tidal CO_2 may increase, and findings consistent with pulmonary edema may occur. Accelerating pulmonary hypertension may occur, resulting in right-sided heart failure.

Because gas embolism may result from direct intravascular injection via an insufflation needle, the proper placement of the needle must be ensured. The intraperitoneal pressure should be maintained at less than 20 mm Hg and, except for the initial placement of trocars, at 8–12 mm Hg. The risk of CO_2 embolus is also reduced by careful hemostasis, because open venous channels are the portal of entry for gas into the systemic circulation. The anesthesiologist should continuously monitor the patient's color, blood pressure, heart sounds, heart beat, and end-tidal CO_2 to allow early recognition of the signs of CO_2 embolus.

If CO_2 embolus is suspected or diagnosed, the surgeon must evacuate the CO_2 from the peritoneal cavity and place the patient in the left lateral decubitus position, with the head below the level of the right atrium. A large-bore central venous line should be inserted immediately to allow aspiration of gas from the heart. Because the findings are nonspecific, other causes of cardiovascular collapse should be excluded.

Cardiovascular Complications   Cardiac arrhythmias occur relatively frequently during laparoscopic surgery and are related to a number of factors, the most significant of which are hypercarbia and acidemia. Early reports of laparoscopy-associated arrhythmia were associated with spontaneous respiration; therefore, most anesthesiologists have adopted the practice of mechanical ventilation during laparoscopic surgery. The incidence of hypercarbia is reduced by operating with intraperitoneal pressures less than 12 mm Hg (54).

The risk of cardiac arrhythmia may also be reduced by using NO_2 as a distending medium. However, although NO_2 is associated with a decreased incidence of arrhythmia, it is insoluble in blood. External lifting systems avoid the complication of hypercarbia and can also provide protection against cardiac arrhythmia.

Hypotension can occur because of decreased venous return secondary to very high intraperitoneal pressure, and this condition may be potentiated by volume depletion. Vagal discharge may occur in response to increased intraperitoneal pressure, which can cause hypotension secondary to cardiac arrhythmias (55). All of these side effects are more dangerous for patients with preexisting cardiovascular disease.

697

Gastric Reflux   Gastric regurgitation and aspiration can occur during laparoscopic surgery, especially in patients with obesity, gastroparesis, hiatal hernia, or gastric outlet obstruction. In these patients, the airway must be maintained with a cuffed endotracheal tube, and the stomach must be decompressed, e.g., with a nasogastric tube. The lowest necessary intraperitoneal pressure should be used to minimize the risk of aspiration. Patients should be moved out of the Trendelenburg position prior to being extubated. Routine preoperative administration of *metoclopramide*, H_2 blocking agents, and nonparticulate antacids will also reduce the risk.

Extraperitoneal Insufflation

The most common causes of extraperitoneal insufflation are preperitoneal placement of the insufflating needle or leakage of CO_2 around the cannula sites. Although this condition is usually mild and limited to the abdominal wall, subcutaneous emphysema can become extensive, involving the extremities, the neck, and the mediastinum. Another relatively common site for emphysema is the omentum or mesentery, a circumstance that may be mistaken for preperitoneal insufflation.

Subcutaneous emphysema may be identified by the palpation of crepitus, usually in the abdominal wall. Emphysema can extend along contiguous fascial plains to the neck, where it can be visualized directly. Such a finding may reflect mediastinal emphysema, which may indicate impending cardiovascular collapse (56–58).

The risk of subcutaneous emphysema is reduced by the proper positioning of the insufflation needle and by maintaining a low intraperitoneal pressure after placement of the desired cannulas. Other approaches that reduce the chance of subcutaneous emphysema include open laparoscopy and the use of abdominal wall lifting systems that make gas unnecessary.

If the insufflation has occurred extraperitoneally, the laparoscope can be removed and the procedure can be repeated. However, difficulty may ensue because of the altered anterior peritoneum. Open laparoscopy or the use of an alternate site, such as the left upper quadrant, should be considered. One approach is to leave the laparoscope in the expanded preperitoneal space while the insufflation needle is reinserted under direct vision through the peritoneal membrane caudad to the tip of the laparoscope (59).

In mild cases of subcutaneous emphysema, the findings quickly resolve after evacuation of the pneumoperitoneum, and no specific intraoperative or postoperative therapy is required. When the extravasation extends to the neck, it is usually preferable to terminate the procedure, because pneumomediastinum, pneumothorax, hypercarbia, and cardiovascular collapse may result.

At the end of the procedure, it is prudent to obtain a chest x-ray. The patient's condition should be managed expectantly unless a tension pneumothorax results, when immediate evacuation must be performed using a chest tube or a wide-bore needle (14–16 gauge) inserted in the second intercostal space in the midclavicular line.

Electrosurgical Complications

Complications of electrosurgery occur secondary to thermal injury from unintended or inappropriate use of the active electrode(s), current diversion to an undesirable path, and injury at the site of the dispersive electrode. Active electrode injury can occur with either unipolar or bipolar instruments, whereas trauma secondary to current diversion or dispersive electrode accidents occurs only with unipolar technique. Complications of electrosurgery are reduced by adherence to safety protocols coupled with a sound understanding of the principles of electrosurgery and the circumstances that can lead to injury (16).

Active Electrode Trauma   If the foot pedal is accidentally depressed, tissue adjacent to the electrode will be traumatized. Commonly, the bowel or ureter is involved, or, if the electrode lies on the abdomen, the skin is burned. Direct extension injuries occur when the zone of vaporization or coagulation extends to large blood vessels or vital structures such as the bladder, ureter, or bowel. Bipolar technique may reduce but does not eliminate the risk of thermal injury to adjacent tissue (60). Therefore, blood vessels should be isolated prior to desiccation, especially when they are near vital structures, and appropriate amounts of energy must be applied to allow an adequate margin of noninjured tissue.

The diagnosis of direct thermal visceral injury may be difficult. If unintended activation of the electrode occurs, nearby intraperitoneal structures should be evaluated carefully. The appearance can be affected by several factors, including the output of the generator, the type of electrode, its proximity to tissue, and the duration of its activation. The diagnosis of visceral thermal injury is often delayed until signs and symptoms of fistula or peritonitis appear. Because these complications may not manifest until 2–10 days after surgery, patients should be advised to report any postoperative fever or increasing abdominal pain.

Unintended activation injuries are prevented if the surgeon is always in direct control of electrode activation and if all electrosurgical hand instruments are removed from the peritoneal cavity when not in use. When removed from the peritoneal cavity, the instruments should be detached from the electrosurgical generator or they should be stored in an insulated pouch near the operative field. These measures prevent damage to the patient's skin if the electrode is accidentally activated.

Thermal injury to the bowel, bladder, or ureter that is recognized at the time of laparoscopy should be managed immediately with laparotomy, taking into consideration the potential extent of the zone of coagulative necrosis. Incisions made with the focused energy from a pointed electrode will be associated with a minimal amount of surrounding thermal injury. Prolonged or even transient contact with a relatively large-caliber electrode may produce thermal necrosis that extends several centimeters. In such cases, wide excision or resection will be necessary.

Current Diversion   Current diversion can occur when electrons find a direct path out of the patient's body via grounded sites other than the dispersive electrode. Alternatively, the current can be diverted directly to other tissues before it reaches the tip of the active electrode. In either case, if the power density becomes high enough, unintended and severe thermal injury can result.

Alternate Ground Site Burns   These injuries can occur only with "ground-referenced" electrosurgical generators (ESUs) because they lack an isolated circuit. In such generators, when the dispersive electrode becomes detached, unplugged, or otherwise ineffective, the current will seek any grounded conductor. If the conductor has a small surface area, the current or power density may become high enough to cause thermal injury (Fig. 21.14A). Examples include electrocardiograph patch electrodes or the conductive metal components of the operating table.

Modern ESUs are designed with isolated circuits and impedance monitoring systems that shut down the machine if dispersive electrode detachment occurs. Because ground-referenced machines without such safeguards are still in use, it is important to know the type of ESU used in the operating room.

Insulation Defects   If the insulation coating the shaft of an electrosurgical electrode becomes defective, it can allow current diversion to adjacent tissue, often bowel, potentially resulting in significant injury (Fig 21.15A). Therefore, the instruments should be examined before each procedure to detect worn or obviously defective insulation. When applying unipolar electrical energy, the shaft of the instrument should be kept away from vital structures and, if possible, totally visible in the operative field.

699

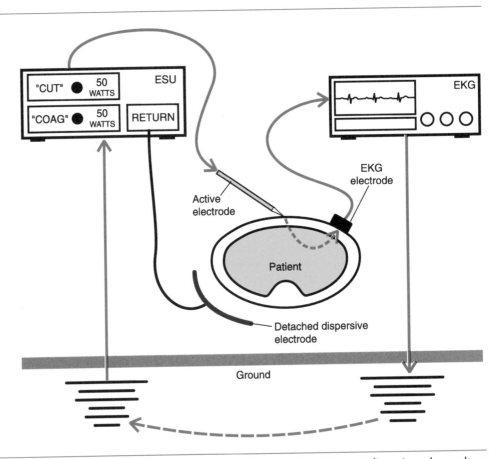

Figure 21.14   Risk of ground-referenced generators. Current diversion along alternate pathways is a risk associated with ground referenced electrosurgical generators, particularly if the dispersive electrode is detached. In the example depicted, the relatively high current density at the EKG electrode site may result in a skin burn.

Direct Coupling   Direct coupling occurs when an activated electrode touches and energizes another metal conductor such as a laparoscope, cannula, or other instrument, especially one that is not insulated. If the conductor is near or in contact with other tissue, a thermal injury can result (Fig 21.15*B*). Direct coupling can be prevented by removal of the electrode when it is not in use and by visually confirming that there is no contact with other conductive instruments prior to activation.

Capacitive Coupling   Capacitance is the ability of a conductor to establish an electrical current in an unconnected but nearby circuit. An electrical field is established around the shaft of any activated laparoscopic unipolar electrode, a circumstance that makes the electrode a capacitor. This field is harmless if the circuit is completed via a dispersive, low-power density pathway (Fig. 21.16). For example, if capacitative coupling occurs between the laparoscopic electrode and a metal cannula positioned in the abdominal wall, the current harmlessly "returns" to the abdominal wall, where it traverses to the dispersive electrode (Fig. 21.16*A*). However, if the metal cannula is anchored to the skin by a nonconductive plastic retaining sleeve or anchor (a hybrid system), the current will not return to the abdominal wall because the sleeve acts as an insulator (Fig. 21.16*B*). Instead, the capacitor will have to "look" elsewhere to complete the circuit. Therefore, bowel or any other nearby conductor can become the target of a relatively high-power density discharge (Fig. 21.16*C*). This mechanism can also occur when a unipolar electrode is inserted through an operating laparoscope that, in turn, is passed through a nonconductive plastic laparoscopic cannula. In this configuration, the plastic port acts as the insulator. If the electrode capac-

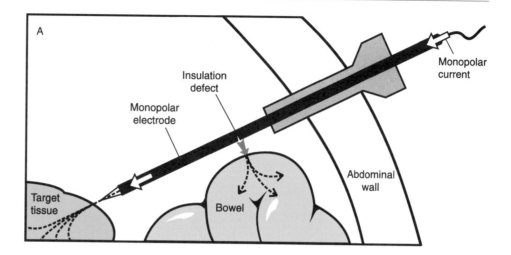

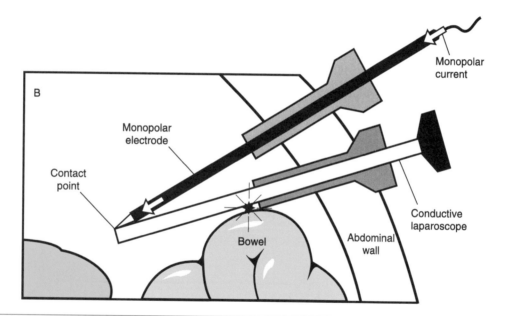

Figure 21.15   Direct coupling. Direct coupling is a potential complication of monopolar electrosurgery and may occur secondary to defects in the insulation (*A*) or, classically, to contract with a conductive instrument that in turn touches other intraperitoneal structures. In the example depicted (*B*), the active electrode is touching the laparoscope, and current is transferred to bowel via a small enough contact point that thermal injury results. Another common target of such coupling is to noninsulated hand instruments.

itively couples with the metal laparoscope, nearby bowel will be at risk for significant thermal injury (61, 62).

Capacitative coupling can be prevented by avoiding the use of hybrid laparoscope-cannula systems that contain a mixture of conductive and nonconductive elements. Instead, it is preferred that all-plastic or all-metal cannula systems be used. When operating laparoscopes are used, all-metal cannula systems should be the rule unless there is no intent to perform unipolar electrosurgical procedures through the operating channel.

Dispersive Electrode Burns   The use of isolated-circuit electrosurgical generators with return electrode monitors has virtually eliminated dispersive-electrode-related thermal in-

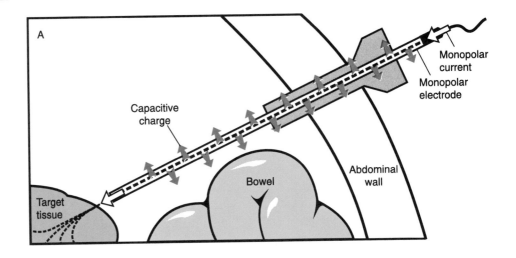

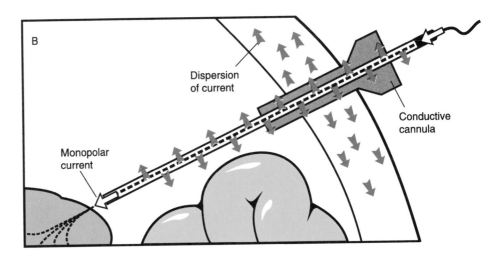

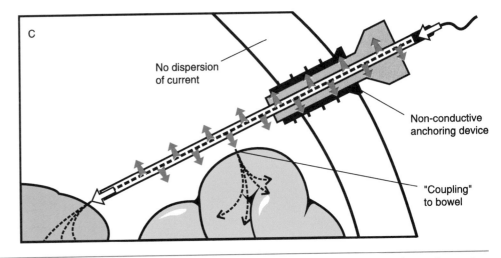

Figure 21.16 Capacitive coupling. *A,* All activated monopolar electrodes emit a surrounding charge, proportional to the voltage of the current. This makes the electrode a potential capacitor. *B,* Generally, as long as the charge is allowed to disperse through the abdominal wall, no sequelae result. However, if the "return" to the dispersive electrode is blocked by insulation, such as a plastic anchor (*C*), the current can couple to a conductive cannula or directly to bowel.

jury. Return electrode monitoring (REM) is actually accomplished by measuring the impedance in the dispersive electrode (patient pad), which should always be low because of the large surface area. Without such devices, partial detachment of the "patient pad" could result in a thermal injury, because reducing the surface area of the electrode raises the current density (Fig. 21.17).

Hemorrhagic Complications

Great Vessel Injury   The most dangerous hemorrhagic complications are injuries to the great vessels, including the aorta and the vena cava, the common iliac vessels and their branches, and the internal and external iliac arteries and veins. The injuries most often occur secondary to insertion of an insufflation needle but may be created by the tip of the primary or ancillary trocars. The vessels most frequently damaged are the aorta and the right common iliac artery as it branches from the aorta in the midline. The anatomically more posterior location of the vena cava and the iliac veins provides relative protection, but not immunity, from injury (63). Although most of these injuries are small and amenable to repair with suture, some are larger and require ligation with or without the insertion of a vascular graft. Deaths have been reported.

After vascular injury, patients usually develop profound hypotension with or without hemoperitoneum. In some instances, blood is aspirated via the insufflation needle prior to the introduction of the distending gas. Frequently, the bleeding may be contained in the retroperitoneal space, which usually delays the diagnosis and, consequently, hypovolemic shock may develop. To avoid late recognition, the course of each great vessel must be identified prior to completing the procedure.

If blood is withdrawn from the insufflation needle, it should be left in place while immediate preparations are made to obtain blood products and perform laparotomy. If hemoperitoneum is diagnosed upon initial visualization of the peritoneal cavity, a grasping instrument may be used, if possible, to temporarily occlude the vessel. Upon entry into the peritoneal cavity, the aorta and vena cava should immediately be compressed just below the level of the renal vessels to gain at least temporary control of blood loss. The most appropriate course of action will depend on the site and extent of injury.

Figure 21.17   Dispersive electrode burns. If the dispersive electrode becomes partially detached, the current density may increase to the point that a skin burn results.

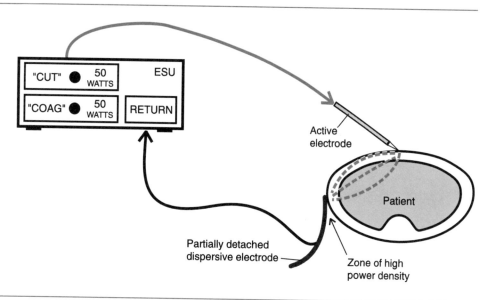

Abdominal Wall Vessel Injury   The abdominal wall vessels most commonly injured during laparoscopy are the *superficial inferior epigastric* vessels as they branch from the femoral artery and vein and course cephalad in each lower quadrant. They are invariably damaged by the initial passage of an ancillary trocar or by the introduction of a wider device later in the procedure. The problem may be recognized immediately by the observation of blood dripping along the cannula or out through the incision. However, the bleeding may be obstructed by the cannula until it is withdrawn at the end of the operation.

The more serious injuries are those to the deep inferior epigastric vessels, which are branches of the external iliac artery and vein that course cephalad but are deep to the rectus fascia and often deep to the muscles (Fig. 21.3). More laterally located are the deep circumflex iliac vessels which are not often encountered in laparoscopic surgery. Laceration of these vessels may cause profound blood loss, particularly when the trauma is unrecognized and causes extraperitoneal bleeding.

Signs of injury include blood dripping down the cannula or the postoperative appearance of shock, abdominal wall discolorization or hematoma located near the incision. In some instances, the blood may track to a more distant site, presenting as a pararectal or vulvar mass. Delayed diagnosis may be prevented by laparoscopic evaluation of each peritoneal incision after removal of the cannula.

Superficial inferior epigastric vessel trauma usually stops spontaneously; therefore, expectant management is appropriate. A straight ligature carrier can be used to repair lacerated deep inferior epigastric vessels. If a postoperative hematoma develops, local compression should be used initially. Open removal or aspiration of the hematoma should not be undertaken, because it may inhibit the tamponade effect and increase the risk of abscess. However, if the mass continues to enlarge or if signs of hypovolemia develop, the wound must be explored.

Intraperitoneal Vessel Injury   Hemorrhage may result from inadvertent entry into a vessel or failure of a specific occlusive technique. In addition to delayed hemorrhage, there may be a further delay in diagnosis at laparoscopy as a result of the restricted visual field and the temporary occlusive pressure exerted by CO_2 in the peritoneal cavity.

Inadvertent division of an artery or vein is usually evident immediately. Transected arteries may go into spasm and bleed minutes to hours later, going unnoticed temporarily because of the limited visual field of the laparoscope. Therefore, at the end of the procedure, all areas of dissection must be carefully examined. CO_2 should be vented, which decreases the intraperitoneal pressure so that blood vessels temporarily occluded by higher pressure can be recognized.

Gastrointestinal Complications

The stomach, the small bowel, and the colon can be injured during laparoscopy. Mechanical entry into the large or small bowel can occur 10 times more often when laparoscopy is performed in patients who have had prior intraperitoneal inflammation or abdominal surgery. Loops of intestine can adhere to the abdominal wall under the insertion site and be injured (64–66).

Insufflation Needle Injuries   Needle entry into the gastrointestinal tract may be more common than reported, often occurring unnoticed and without further complication. Gastric entry may be identified by the increased filling pressure, asymmetric distension of the peritoneal cavity, or the aspiration of gastric particulate matter through the lumen of the needle. Initially, the hollow, capacious stomach may allow the insufflation pressure to remain normal. Signs of bowel entry are the same as those for gastric injury, with the addition of feculent odor.

If particulate debris are identified, the needle should be left in place and an alternate insertion site should be identified, such as the left upper quadrant. Immediately after successful entry into the peritoneal cavity, the site of injury is identified. Defects must be repaired immediately.

Trocar Injuries   Damage caused by a sharp trocar is usually more serious than needle injury. Inadvertent gastric entry usually results from stomach distension because of aerophagia, difficult or improper intubation, or mask induction with inhalation anesthetic. Most often, the injury is created by the primary trocar, although ancillary cannulas may also result in visceral injury.

The risk of gastric perforation can be minimized with the selective use of preoperative nasogastric suction when left upper quadrant entries are used or if the intubation was difficult. Open laparoscopy can reduce but not eliminate the risk of gastrointestinal complications. For high-risk patients, left upper quadrant needle insertion with a properly decompressed stomach may be preferable (67–69).

If the trocar of a primary cannula penetrates the bowel, the condition is usually diagnosed when the mucosal lining of the gastrointestinal tract is visualized. If the large bowel is entered, a feculent odor may be noted. However, the injury may not be immediately recognized because the cannula may not stay within the bowel or it may pass through the lumen. Such injuries usually occur when a single loop of bowel is adherent to the anterior abdominal wall. The injury may not be recognized until peritonitis, abscess, enterocutaneous fistula, or death occurs (70, 71). Therefore, at the end of the procedure, the removal of the primary cannula must be viewed either through the cannula or an ancillary port, a process facilitated by routine direct visualization of closure of the incision of the primary port.

Trocar injuries to the stomach and bowel require repair as soon as they are recognized. If the injury is small, a trained operator can repair the defect via laparoscopy using a double layer of running 2-0 or 3-0 absorbable suture. Extensive lesions may require resection and reanastomosis, which in most instances requires laparotomy. The preoperative use of mechanical bowel preparation in selected high-risk cases will minimize the need for laparotomy or colostomy.

Dissection and Thermal Injury   It is often easier to recognize intestinal injury that occurs during dissection than thermal injury to the bowel, particularly if the latter was created with electrical or laser energy. Even if thermal injury is recognized, it is difficult to estimate by visual inspection the extent of the damage, because the zone of desiccation may exceed the area of visual damage. In some patients, the diagnosis is delayed until the development of peritonitis and fever develop, usually a few days later but occasionally not for several weeks (72). When mechanical bowel trauma is recognized during the dissection, treatment is the same as described for trocar injury. If the diagnosis is delayed until the postoperative recognition of peritonitis, a laparotomy must be performed immediately.

Thermal injury may be handled expectantly if the lesion seems superficial and confined. In a study of 33 women with such injuries who were managed expectantly in the hospital, only two required laparotomy for perforation (72).

Urologic Injury

Laparoscopy-associated damage to the bladder or ureter may occur secondary to mechanical or thermal trauma. Ideally, such injury should be prevented; otherwise, it is essential that the lesion be identified intraoperatively.

Bladder Injury   Bladder injury can occur from a trocar perforation of the undrained bladder but may also occur while dissecting the bladder from adherent structures or from the anterior uterus (73, 74). The injury may be readily apparent by direct visualization. If an indwelling catheter is in place, hematuria or pneumaturia (CO_2 in the catheter drainage system) may be noticed. A bladder laceration can be confirmed by injecting sterile milk or a diluted methylene blue solution via a transurethral catheter. Thermal injury to the bladder, however, may not be initially apparent and, if missed, can present as peritonitis or a fistula.

Routine preoperative bladder drainage usually prevents trocar-related cystotomies. Separation of the bladder from the uterus or other adherent structures requires good visualization, appropriate retraction, and excellent surgical technique. Sharp mechanical dissection is preferred, particularly when relatively dense adhesions are present.

Very-small-caliber injuries to the bladder (1–2 mm) may be treated with bladder catheterization for 5–7 days. If repair is undertaken immediately, catheterization is unnecessary. When a larger injury is identified, it can be repaired laparoscopically (73–75). However, if the laceration is near the trigone or involves the trigone, an open procedure should be used. The mechanism of injury should be taken into consideration in making this evaluation, because electrical injuries often extend beyond the visible limits of the apparent defect.

For small lesions, closure may be performed with layers of absorbable 2-0 to 3-0 sutures. If there is thermal injury, the coagulated portion should be excised. Postoperative catheterization with either a transurethral or suprapubic catheter should be maintained for 2–5 days for small fundal lacerations and for 10–14 days for injuries to the trigone.

Ureteral Injury   The most common cause of ureteral injury during laparoscopy is electrosurgical trauma (76, 77). However, ureteral injury can occur after mechanical dissection and the use of linear cutting and stapling devices (78–80). Although intraoperative recognition of ureteral injury is possible, the diagnosis is usually delayed (76). Ureteral lacerations may be confirmed intraoperatively visually or with the intravenous injection of indigo carmine. Thermal injury will present up to 14 days after surgery with fever, abdominal or flank pain, and peritonitis. Leukocytosis may be present and intravenous pyelography will show extravasation of urine or a urinoma. Mechanical obstruction from staples or a suture can be recognized intraoperatively only by direct visualization. Ureteral obstruction presents a few days to 1 week after surgery with flank pain and often fever (80). Abdominal ultrasound may be helpful, but intravenous pyelography can more precisely identify the site and degree of the obstruction.

Discharge or continuous incontinence are delayed signs of ureterovaginal or vesicovaginal fistulae. A bladder fistula can be confirmed by detecting dye on a tampon previously placed in the vagina after filling the bladder with methylene blue. With a ureterovaginal fistula, the methylene blue will not pass into the vagina, but it can be detected with the intravenous injection of indigo carmine.

Knowledge of the course of the ureter through the pelvis is a prerequisite to reducing the risk of injury. The ureter can usually be seen through the peritoneum of the pelvic sidewall between the pelvic brim and the attachment of the broad ligament. However, because of variation from one patient to another or the presence of disease, the location of the ureter can become obscured, making it necessary to enter the retroperitoneal space. The techniques used for retroperitoneal dissection are also important factors in reducing the risk of ureteric injury. Blunt and sharp dissection with scissors is preferred, although hydrodissection can be used (81). The selective placement of ureteral stents may also be helpful.

Ureteral injury can be treated immediately if it is diagnosed intraoperatively. Although very limited damage may heal over a ureteral stent left in place for 10–21 days, repair is indicated in most patients. Although laparoscopic repair of ureteric lacerations and transsections has been performed, most injuries require laparotomy (76, 82).

When the diagnosis of ureteral injury is delayed, the bladder should be drained with a catheter. Incomplete or small obstructions or lacerations may be treated successfully with either a retrograde or anterograde ureteral stent. Urinomas may be drained percutaneously. If a stent cannot be placed successfully, a percutaneous nephrostomy should be performed before operative repair is undertaken.

Neurologic Injury

Peripheral nerve injury is usually related either to poor positioning of the patient or to excessive pressure exerted by the surgeons. Nerve injury may also occur as a result of the surgical dissection.

In the extremities, the trauma may be direct, such as when the common peroneal nerve is compressed against the stirrups. The femoral nerve or the sciatic nerve or its branches may be overstretched and damaged by inappropriate positioning of the hip or the knee joint (83, 84). Brachial plexus injuries may occur secondary to the surgeon or assistants leaning against the abducted arm during the procedure. If the patient is placed in a steep Trendelenburg position, the brachial plexus may be damaged because of the pressure exerted on the shoulder joint (85). In most cases, sensory or motor deficits are found as the patient emerges from anesthesia. The likelihood of brachial plexus injury can be reduced with adequate padding and support of the arms and shoulders or by placing the patient's arms in an adducted position.

Most injuries to peripheral nerves recover spontaneously. The time to recovery depends on the site and severity of the lesion. For most peripheral injuries, full sensory nerve recovery occurs in 3–6 months. Recovery may be facilitated by physical therapy, appropriate braces, and electrical stimulation of the affected muscles. Open microsurgery should be performed for transection of major intrapelvic nerves.

Incisional Hernia and Wound Dehiscence

Incisional hernia after laparoscopy has been reported in more than 900 cases (51). Although no incision is immune to the risk, defects that are larger than 10 mm in diameter are particularly vulnerable (86, 87). In most cases, these defects can be prevented by proper technique and closure of large defects. All ancillary cannulas should be removed under direct vision to ensure that bowel is not drawn into the incision. Incisions larger than 10 mm in diameter should have the fascia closed while viewing the defect with the laparoscope to minimize the risk of intestinal injury. A small-diameter laparoscope should be used through a narrow cannula to facilitate incisional closure.

The most common defect is when intestinal hernia develops in the immediate postoperative period. The patient may be asymptomatic or, within the first postoperative week, may experience pain, fever, periumbilical mass, obvious evisceration, and the symptoms and signs of mechanical bowel obstruction.

Because Richter's hernias contain only a portion of the intestine in the defect, the diagnosis is often delayed. Hernias most often occur in incisions lateral to the midline. The initial symptom is usually pain, because the incomplete obstruction still allows the passage of intestinal contents. Fever can be present if incarceration occurs, and peritonitis may result from subsequent perforation. The condition is difficult to diagnose, requires a high index of suspicion, and may be confirmed with an ultrasound or a CT scan (88).

The management of laparoscopic incisional defects depends on the time of presentation and the presence of entrapped bowel and its condition. Evisceration always requires surgical intervention. If the condition is diagnosed immediately, the intestine is replaced into the peritoneal cavity (if there is no evidence of necrosis or intestinal defect) and the incision is repaired, usually with laparoscopic guidance. If the diagnosis is delayed or the

707

bowel is incarcerated or at risk of perforation, laparotomy is necessary to repair or resect the intestine.

Infection

Wound infections after laparoscopy are uncommon; most are minor skin infections that can be treated successfully with expectant management, drainage, or antibiotics (89). Severe necrotizing fasciitis can occur rarely (90). Bladder infection, pelvic cellulitis, and pelvic abscess have been reported (91).

The risk of infection associated with laparoscopy is much lower than that associated with open abdominal or vaginal surgery. Prophylactic antibiotics should be offered to selected patients, e.g., those with enhanced risk for bacterial endocarditis and those for whom hysterectomy is planned. Patients should be instructed to monitor temperature after discharge and to immediately report fever higher than 38°C.

Hysteroscopy

The hysteroscopic lysis of intrauterine adhesions was first described in 1973 (92). The technique of endoscopically guided electrosurgical resection was adapted from urology to gynecology for the removal of uterine leiomyomas (93). Hysteroscopic division of uterine septa was developed using a technique in which scissors are passed along the outside of the endoscope (94). Hysteroscopic destruction of the endometrium has been reported using Nd:YAG laser vaporization, electrosurgical resection, and electrosurgical coagulation (95–97).

The use of diagnostic and operative hysteroscopy has been limited by the difficulties in obtaining a consistently acceptable image (i.e., inadequate distension, bleeding) and the perception that its therapeutic potential is low. Although hysteroscopic technology and techniques are still being developed, the current quality of the images is excellent because smaller-diameter endoscopes have been made possible by improvements in fiber technology. The concomitant use of ultrasound imaging can provide a view of the myometrial wall during resectoscopic procedures.

Because diagnostic hysteroscopy can be performed in an office or clinic setting without anesthetic, its widespread use has been advocated to investigate abnormal uterine bleeding. Hysteroscopic surgical procedures include removal of polyps, excision of leiomyomas, endometrial ablation, and division of adhesions and uterine septa. Some of these procedures are well established and others, although promising, require more clinical investigation. Hysteroscopy has been suggested as a method to replace blind sampling of the uterine cavity because it may provide better results at a lower cost (98, 99).

Diagnostic Hysteroscopy

Diagnostic hysteroscopy can provide information that cannot be obtained by blind endometrial sampling (98–104). In most cases, the additional findings visible with hysteroscopy are endometrial polyps or submucous leiomyomas (101, 102, 104, 105). Malignant or hyperplastic processes can be identified with hysteroscopy and directed biopsy (103). Hysteroscopic examination is probably superior to hysterography in the evaluation of the endometrial cavity (106, 107). However, in some situations (e.g., endometritis, hyperplasia), curettage provides information not otherwise available by hysteroscopic evaluation, even when it is combined with directed biopsy (101, 102, 104, 108). The principal advantage of diagnostic hysteroscopy is that structural anomalies (congenital or acquired) are more easily detected and defined. Potential indications for diagnostic hysteroscopy are as follows.

1. Unexplained abnormal uterine bleeding
   • Premenopausal
   • Postmenopausal

708

2. Selected infertility cases
- Abnormal hysterogram
- Unexplained infertility

3. Recurrent spontaneous abortion

In most patients, diagnostic hysteroscopy can be performed in an office or clinic with minimal discomfort and at a much lower cost than in an operating room. For some patients, concerns about patient comfort or a preexisting medical condition may preclude office hysteroscopy.

Although hysteroscopy can, in many patients, provide more information than blind curettage, it should still be used prudently. For most patients, other investigative or therapeutic measures can be undertaken prior to, or instead of, diagnostic hysteroscopy. For women with perimenopausal and postmenopausal bleeding, office endometrial biopsy or curettage should be performed before diagnostic hysteroscopy. If a satisfactory diagnosis cannot be established, or if bleeding continues without explanation, office hysteroscopy and directed biopsy or repeat curettage is appropriate. For women in their reproductive years, medical or expectant management may be used initially, depending on the severity and inconvenience of the bleeding. For those who do not respond to medical regimens such as oral contraceptives, office hysteroscopy with biopsy or curettage can be performed for diagnosis (109).

For women with infertility, hysterosalpingography is the best initial imaging step because it provides information about the patency of the oviducts. In the presence of a suspicious or identified abnormality in the endometrial cavity, hysteroscopy can be performed to confirm the diagnoses, to define the abnormality, and perhaps to direct the removal of the lesion. Some consider hysteroscopy to be mandatory for these patients because of the high occurrence of false-negative radiologic images in those with intrauterine anomalies. However, there has been no evidence that identification and treatment of these "missed" anomalies improves pregnancy rates. Confirmation of patency of the oviduct is unnecessary in women who have recurrent abortions; therefore, they can be evaluated primarily with hysteroscopy.

Operative Hysteroscopy

Adhesiolysis, division of a uterine septum, resection of myomas, and endometrial destruction via resection, electrosurgical desiccation, or vaporization with the Nd:YAG laser can be performed hysteroscopically. Hysteroscopy may also be used to remove foreign bodies or to position instruments in the fallopian tube.

Foreign Body   If the string of an intrauterine device is absent, the device usually can be removed with a specially designed hook or a toothed curette (e.g., Novak). When removal is difficult or impossible, the location of the device may be confirmed by hysteroscopy, allowing removal with a grasping forceps.

Septum   When a single uterus with a divided cavity is present, hysteroscopic division of uterine septa improves reproductive outcome at a rate comparable to abdominal metroplasty with reduced morbidity and cost (110–113). The procedure may be performed mechanically with scissors or with energy-based techniques such as the Nd:YAG laser or an electrosurgical knife or loop. Because most septa have few vessels, scissors can be used easily, and the minimal risk of thermal damage is avoided.

Endometrial Polyps   **Although endometrial polyps can be removed with blind curettage, many are missed** (101, 102, 104, 105). Therefore, known or suspected endometrial polyps are more successfully treated with hysteroscopic guidance, which can often be performed in a clinic or office using local anesthesia. Hysteroscopy may be used either to evaluate the result of blind curettage, or preferably, to guide a grasping forceps. Alternatively, for larger polyps, a uterine resectoscope may be used to sever the stalk or morcellate the lesion.

Leiomyomas Hysteroscopy may be used to remove intracavitary leiomyomas in women with menorrhagia or infertility (114–121). However, this approach is limited by the location and size of the leiomyomas. In some patients, excision is relatively easy, whereas in others, laparotomy is necessary.

Pedunculated leiomyomas may be removed by transecting the stalk with scissors or a resectoscope. For larger lesions, electrosurgical morcellation with a resectoscope may be necessary prior to removal. In some patients, hysteroscopy can be used to direct the attachment of a tenaculum so that the lesion can be twisted off. Although preferable, it is not absolutely necessary to remove the leiomyoma because it will be expelled spontaneously.

Selected submucous leiomyomas that extend into the uterine wall may be resected using a loop electrode. The extent of intramural involvement may be evaluated by performing abdominal ultrasound with saline instilled into the endometrial cavity (i.e., sonohysterography) (121). If the leiomyoma is too deeply imbedded in the myometrium, it may not be resectable or the uterus might be perforated if overzealous attempts are made to remove the tumor. Selected intramural leiomyomas may be removed completely during a second procedure performed after a suitable interval (119). Instead of a second procedure, the Nd:YAG laser or bipolar electrosurgery can be used to desiccate the remaining portion of the leiomyomas, although the efficacy of this approach is unclear (115). Preoperative gonadotropin-releasing hormone (GnRH) agonists may help shrink submucous myomas, facilitating their complete removal (122–124).

Menorrhagia Menorrhagia that does not respond to medications may be managed by endometrial ablation or resection (95–97, 117, 124–132). Ablation may be performed with the laser (95, 125, 126) or by electrosurgical desiccation using a uterine resectoscope equipped with a blunt ball- or barrel-shaped electrode (97, 131, 132). Resection is performed with an electrosurgical loop electrode that can shave the endometrium (96, 127, 128). Complications of the procedure include fluid overload, electrolyte imbalances, bleeding, perforation, and intestinal injury (133). The risk of uterine perforation can be reduced by using a combination of resection and electrosurgical ablation; the latter is most suitable for the thinner areas of the myometrium in the cornu and on the lateral walls of the endometrial cavity (117). The preoperative use of GnRH analogues or danazol may reduce operating time, bleeding, and the amount of fluid required (134, 135).

For many women, these procedures are successful in reducing or eliminating menses without hysterectomy or long-term medical therapy. Success rates vary and depend on the duration of follow-up and the definition of success. For many patients, amenorrhea is the goal, whereas for others, normalization of menses is the objective. Approximately 75–95% of patients are satisfied with the surgical procedure after 1 year, and 30–90% of patients have amenorrhea. In comparative studies, there is no advantage of laser over electrosurgical techniques (125, 130).

The long-term efficacy and impact of ablation or resection on women with adenomyosis is unknown. Because some endometrium inevitably cannot be ablated, there is the potential for endometrial cancer; therefore, postmenopausal hormonal replacement therapy should include a progestin (136).

Sterilization Hysteroscopic sterilization can be performed without entering the peritoneal cavity. Because the tubal ostia are usually visible during hysteroscopy, there are several potential options for sterilization: insertion of a plug, injection of a sclerosing agent, or destruction of the intramural portion of the oviduct. These procedures are being developed and should be performed only as part of an approved clinical trial (36).

Synechiae Asherman's syndrome is the presence of adhesions in the endometrial cavity resulting in infertility or recurrent spontaneous abortion with or without amenorrhea.

These synechiae may be detected on a hysterogram but are best demonstrated at the time of diagnostic hysteroscopy. Relatively thin, fragile synechiae may be divided with the tip of a rigid diagnostic hysteroscope (137). Thicker lesions may require division by semirigid or rigid scissors or energy-based instruments such as a resectoscope or an operative hysteroscope with a Nd:YAG laser. Reproductive outcome depends on the extent of the preoperative endometrial damage (138–140).

Patient Preparation

Most diagnostic hysteroscopy procedures are performed in the office or clinic, whereas operative hysteroscopy is performed in an operating room or hospital surgicenter. The patient should understand the rationale for either procedure as well as the anticipated discomfort, the potential risks, and the expectant medical and surgical alternatives. The patient must understand the nature of the procedure and the chance of therapeutic success. A realistic estimate of success based on the operator's experience must be presented to the patient.

Diagnostic Hysteroscopy   Diagnostic hysteroscopy is designed to identify or exclude the presence of anatomic or structural abnormalities in the endometrial cavity that may contribute to bleeding, infertility, or recurrent pregnancy loss. The risks of diagnostic hysteroscopy are few, and they rarely have severe consequences. However, those related to anesthesia, perforation, bleeding, and the distension media should be discussed. After diagnostic hysteroscopy, most patients have slight vaginal bleeding and lower abdominal cramps. Severe cramps, dyspnea, and upper abdominal and right shoulder pain can develop if CO_2 passes into the peritoneal cavity. Consequently, the patient should be accompanied by a friend or relative to escort her home.

Operative Hysteroscopy   Counseling before operative hysteroscopy varies depending on the planned procedure and the type of anesthesia used. The risks of operative hysteroscopy are higher and are potentially more dangerous than with diagnostic hysteroscopy. The use of large volumes of hypotonic distension media may not be tolerated in some patients if there is significant intravascular absorption, especially in patients with underlying cardiovascular disease. The patient must be aware of the risk of damage to the intestines or to the urinary tract. If damage occurs during the procedure, it may not be possible to complete the surgery and laparotomy may be necessary to repair the problem.

Equipment and Technique

The equipment required depends on the goals of the procedure. The surgeon must be knowledgeable about the equipment, its mechanisms, and the technical specifications to facilitate efficiency, optimal clinical outcome, and a decreased probability of complications (Fig. 21.18). A typical hysteroscopy setup for diagnostic and minor operative procedures is shown in Figure 21.19. Core competencies required for hysteroscopy are as follows:

1. Patient positioning and cervical exposure

2. Anesthesia

3. Cervical dilation

4. Uterine distension

5. Imaging

6. Intrauterine manipulation

Patient Positioning and Exposure

Hysteroscopy is performed in a modified dorsal lithotomy position; the patient is supine and the legs are held in stirrups. For hysteroscopic procedures performed while the patient

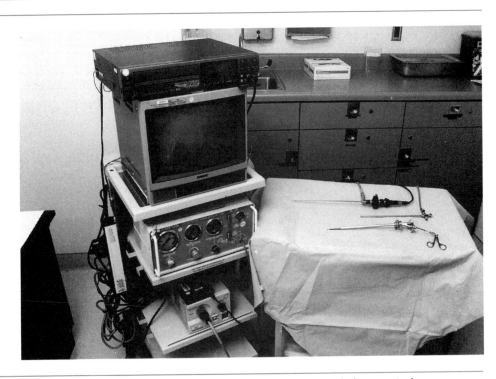

Figure 21.18   Office hysteroscopy equipment. A typical diagnostic hysteroscopy setup. On the table are a hysteroscope, a video camera mount, and diagnostic instruments. On the cart is (*from top*) a super VHS 1/2-inch videotape recorder, a Sony high-resolution monitor, an Olympus hysteroscopic insufflator, and the Olympus video camera base and light source.

Figure 21.19   Diagnostic and minor operative hysteroscopic instruments. *Top to bottom:* a 4-mm-diameter hysteroscope in a 5-mm diagnostic sheath with attached CCD video camera, light cable and insufflation tubing; two semirigid hysteroscopic instruments—scissors and a biopsy forceps; the obturator for the operative sheath; the 7-mm operative sheath with two ports on the right side, allowing the introduction of the semirigid instruments.

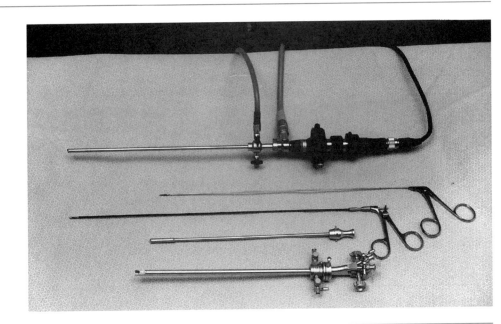

is conscious, comfort must be considered in conjunction with the need to gain good exposure of the perineum. Stirrups that hold and support the knees, calves, and ankles will permit prolonged procedures. "Candy cane" stirrups should be avoided for hysteroscopic surgery on conscious patients.

The smallest speculum possible should be used to expose the cervix. A bivalve speculum hinged on only one side allows its removal without disturbing the other instruments needed. The use of weighted specula should be avoided in conscious patients.

Anesthesia

The anesthetic requirements for hysteroscopy vary greatly, depending on the patient's level of anxiety, the status of her cervical canal, the procedure, and the outside diameter of the hysteroscope or sheath. In some patients, diagnostic hysteroscopy is possible without anesthesia, especially if the patient is parous or if narrow-caliber (<3 mm outside diameter) hysteroscopes are used. The pain of cervical dilation will also be avoided or minimized by inserting a laminaria tent in the cervix 3–8 hours prior to the procedure. However, if left in place too long (e.g., longer than 24 hours) the cervix may overdilate, which is counterproductive for CO_2 insufflation.

For most diagnostic procedures, effective cervical anesthesia is obtained with an intracervical block. A spinal needle can be used to instill approximately 3 ml of 0.5–1% *lidocaine* into the anterior lip of the cervix. A tenaculum is used to grasp the cervix. An intracervical block is administered evenly around the circumference of the internal os. A paracervical block may also be injected into the uterosacral ligaments at the 4- and 8-o'clock positions, if necessary (141, 142). Care must be taken to avoid intravascular injection. Additional topical anesthesia may be given by injecting 5 ml of 2% *mepivacaine* into the endometrial cavity with a syringe (141). Many operative procedures can be performed with this technique combined with intravenous anxiolytics or analgesics, as necessary. Alternatively, regional or general anesthesia may be used.

Cervical Dilation

Dilation of the cervix, although apparently simple, can be incorrectly performed in a way that compromises the whole procedure. If the objective lens of the hysteroscope cannot be placed in the endometrial cavity, the hysteroscopy cannot be done. The cervix should be dilated as atraumatically as possible. A uterine sound should not be used, because it can traumatize the canal or the endometrium, causing unnecessary bleeding and uterine perforation.

Uterine Distension

Distension of the endometrial cavity is necessary to create a viewing space. The choices include CO_2 gas, high-viscosity 32% *Dextran 70,* and a number of low-viscosity fluids including glycine, sorbitol, saline, and dextrose in water. A pressure of 45 mm Hg or higher is required for adequate distension of the uterine cavity, To minimize extravasation, this pressure should not exceed the mean arterial pressure. For each of the fluids, there are several methods used to create this pressure by infusion into the endometrial cavity.

Sheaths   A rigid hysteroscope is passed into the endometrial cavity via an external sheath. The design and diameter of the sheath reflects both the dimensions of the endoscope and the purpose of the instrument. Diagnostic hysteroscopes have a sheath slightly wider than the telescope, allowing infusion of the distension media. Sheaths for operative hysteroscopes have one or two additional channels that permit the passage or efflux of distension media or the insertion of semirigid instruments or laser fibers. These sheaths are usually 7–8 mm in diameter, and some allow continuous flow of distension media in and out of the endometrial cavity (Fig. 21.16).

Media   Carbon dioxide provides an excellent view for diagnostic purposes, but it is unsuitable for operative hysteroscopy or for diagnostic procedures when the patient is bleeding, because there is no effective way to remove blood and other debris from the endometrial cavity. To prevent CO_2 embolus, the gas must be instilled by an insufflator that is specially designed for the procedure—the intrauterine pressure is kept below 100 mm Hg and the flow rate is maintained at less than 100 ml/minute.

Normal saline is a useful and safe medium for procedures that do not require electricity. Even if there is absorption of a significant volume of solution, saline does not cause electrolyte imbalance. Therefore, saline is a good fluid for minor procedures performed in the office.

Dextran 70 is useful for patients who are bleeding, because it does not mix with blood. However, it is expensive and tends to "caramelize" on instruments, which must be disassembled and thoroughly cleaned in warm water immediately after each use. Anaphylactic reactions, fluid overload, and electrolyte disturbances can occur.

For operative hysteroscopy, low-viscosity, nonconductive fluids such as 1.5% glycine and 3% sorbitol are used most often. These solutions can be used with electricity, because there are no electrolytes to disperse the current and impede the electrosurgical effect. Both 1.5% glycine and 3% sorbitol are inexpensive and are readily available in 3-l bags suitable for continuous-flow hysteroscopy. Because each fluid is hypotonic, extravasation into the systemic circulation can be associated with fluid and electrolyte disturbances. Therefore, uterine "absorption" must be monitored continuously by collecting outflow from the sheath and subtracting it from the total infused volume. Absorbed volumes greater than 1 liter mandate the measurement of electrolyte levels. If there is more than 2 liters of extravasated fluid, the procedure should be stopped. Excessive circulating sorbitol may cause hyperglycemia, and large volumes of glycine may elevate levels of ammonia in the blood (143).

Delivery Systems   Syringes can be used for office diagnostic procedures and are especially good for infusing *Dextran* solution. The syringe can be operated by the surgeon and is either connected directly to the sheath or attached via connecting tubing. Because this technique is so tedious, it is suited only for simple operations.

Continuous hydrostatic pressure is effectively achieved by elevating the vehicle containing the distension media above the level of the patient's uterus. The achieved pressure is the product of the width of the connecting tubing and the elevation—for operative hysteroscopy with 10-mm tubing, intrauterine pressure ranges from 70 to 100 mm Hg when the bag is between 1 and 1.5 meters above the uterine cavity.

A pressure cuff may be placed around the infusion bag to elevate the pressure in the system. Caution must be exercised, however, because this technique will cause extravasation if intrauterine pressure rises above the mean arterial pressure.

A variety of infusion pumps are available, ranging from simple devices to instruments that maintain a preset intrauterine pressure. Simple pump devices continue to press fluid into the uterine cavity regardless of resistance, whereas the pressure-sensitive pumps reduce the flow rate when the preset level is reached, thereby impeding the efflux of blood and debris and compromising the view.

Imaging

Endoscopes   Hysteroscopes are available in two basic types—flexible and rigid. Flexible hysteroscopes have lower resolution than rigid instruments of a similar diameter and are most useful for cannulation of the fallopian tube. For other uses, rigid hysteroscopes are more durable and provide a superior image. The most commonly used hysteroscopes are 4 mm in diameter, although those smaller than 3 mm in diameter are available. Small-diameter endoscopes have a somewhat lower resolution but are easier to pass through the cervix.

Oblique endoscopes are more useful for hysteroscopy than laparoscopy and are available in 0°, 12–15°, and 25–30° models (Fig. 21.20). The 0° telescope provides a panoramic view and is best for diagnostic procedures. Hysteroscopes with 25–30° angles are most often used for both diagnosis and therapy, although the 12–15° types are a suitable compromise useful for diagnosis, ablation, and resection.

Light Sources and Cables   Adequate illumination of the endometrial cavity is essential. Because it runs from a standard 110- or 220-volt wall outlet, the light source requires no special electrical connections. For most cameras and endoscopes, the element must have at least 150 watts of power for direct viewing and preferably 250 watts or more for video and operative procedures.

Video Imaging   Although diagnostic hysteroscopy may be performed with direct visualization, it is best to use video guidance for prolonged operations. Video imaging is important for teaching and to record pathology and procedures. The cameras used for operative hysteroscopy often have greater technical requirements than those used for laparoscopy. The camera must be more sensitive because of the narrow diameter of the endoscope and the frequently dark background of the endometrial cavity, particularly when it is enlarged (Fig. 21.18).

Intrauterine Manipulation   The instruments available for use via operative hysteroscopes include grasping, cutting, and punch biopsy devices. These tools are narrow and flexible enough to navigate the 1- to 2-mm-diameter operating channel (Fig. 21.21). Their value is limited by their small size and flimsy construction. However, the scissors can be used to divide adhesions, the biopsy forceps can be used to sample targeted lesions, and the grasping forceps can be used to remove small polyps or intrauterine devices. Some operative hysteroscopes are designed to allow passage of fibers for the conduction of Nd:YAG laser.

The uterine resectoscope is similar to the one used in urology and is designed to apply electrical energy in the endometrial cavity (Fig. 21.22). An understanding of the principles of

Figure 21.20   Hysteroscope optics. Panoramic (0°) and oblique (15° and 30°) viewing angles.

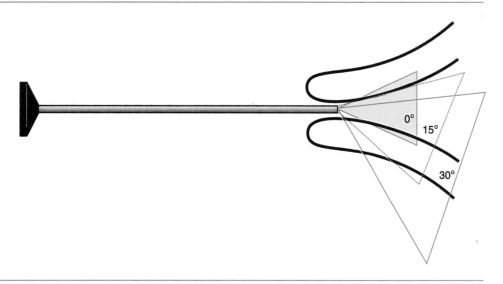

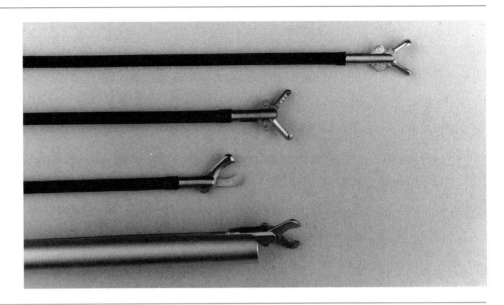

Figure 21.21   Hysteroscopy hand instruments. *From top:* biopsy forceps, grasping forceps, and scissors, each of which pass through the instrument channel of an operating hysteroscope. *Bottom,* a rigid sheath with integrated scissors.

electrosurgery is mandatory for safe and effective use of this instrument. By sliding the "working element," one of a variety of electrode tips can be manipulated back and forth within the cavity. Tissue can be divided with a pointed electrode, excised with a loop, or desiccated with a rolling ball or bar. A clear operative field is maintained by the continuous flow of nonconductive distending media in and out of the cavity. Although basic design modifications have made the resectoscope more useful in gynecology, extraction of resected fragments is time consuming. The most effective approach is the periodic use of a uterine curette or polyp forceps inserted after removal of the hysteroscope.

Other Instruments   For any hysteroscopic procedure, it is necessary to have a cervical tenaculum, dilators, uterine curette, and suitably sized vaginal specula. When using the resectoscope, it is helpful to have a modern, solid-state, isolated circuit electrosurgical generator capable of delivering both modulated and nonmodulated radiofrequency current. Laparoscopy or laparotomy may be necessary for emergencies secondary to uterine perforation.

Complications

The potential risks of diagnostic hysteroscopy include uterine perforation, infection, excessive bleeding, and complications related to the distention media (144). The latter include CO_2 embolus and pulmonary edema secondary to overinfusion of 32% *Dextran 70* (*Hyskon*) or low-viscosity fluids. Diagnostic hysteroscopy performed in the office has a low rate of complications (0–1%) (98–100). The risks of operative hysteroscopy are related to one of five aspects of the procedure performed: anesthesia, perforation, bleeding, the use of energy, and the distension media.

Anesthesia

Local anesthesia is provided by the intracervical or paracervical injection of 0.5–2% *lidocaine* or *mepivacaine* solution, with or without a local vasoconstrictor such as *adrenaline*. Overdosage is prevented by ensuring that intravascular injection is avoided and by not exceeding the maximum recommended doses (*lidocaine*, 4 mg/kg; *mepivacaine*, 3 mg/kg). The use of a vasoconstrictor reduces the amount of systemic absorption of the agent, doubling the maximum dose that can be used.

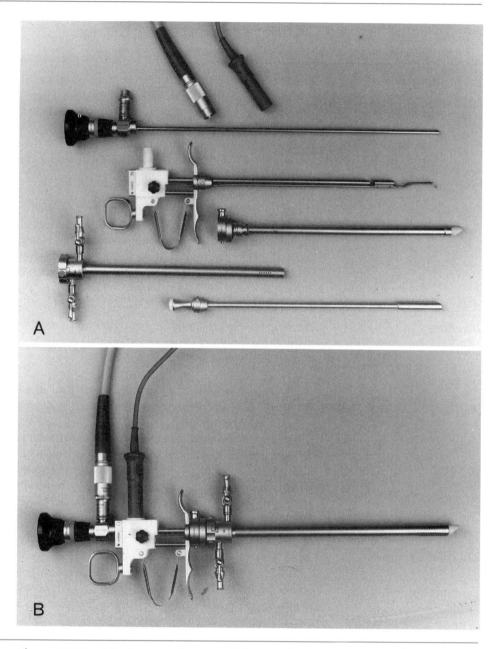

Figure 21.22   Uterine resectoscope (Olympus America, Inc., Woodbury, NY). *A, From top:* light guide (*left*) and monopolar electrosurgical cord (*right*); a 4-mm 12° endoscope; the Iglesas working element; an inner sheath; an outer sheath; the obturator. *B,* Fully assembled resectoscope.

Complications of intravascular injection or anesthetic overdose include allergy, neurologic effects, and impaired myocardial conduction. Allergy is characterized by the typical symptoms of agitation, palpitations, pruritus, coughing, shortness of breath, urticaria, bronchospasm, shock, and convulsions. Treatment measures include administration of oxygen, isotonic intravenous fluids, intramuscular or subcutaneous adrenaline, and intravenous prednisolone and aminophylline. Cardiac effects related to impaired myocardial conduction include bradycardia, cardiac arrest, shock, and convulsions. Emergency treatment measures include the administration of oxygen, intravenous *atropine* (0.5 mg), and intravenous *adrenaline* and the initiation of appropriate cardiac resuscitation. The most common central nervous system manifestations are paresthesia of the tongue, drowsiness, tremor, and convulsions. Options for therapy include intravenous *diazepam* and respiratory support.

Perforation

Perforation may occur during dilation of the cervix or during the hysteroscopic procedure. With perforation, the endometrial cavity does not distend and the visual field is lost. When perforation occurs during dilation of the cervix, the procedure must be terminated, but usually there are no other injuries. If the uterus is perforated by a hysteroscopic instrument, the tip of a laser, or an activated electrode, there is a risk of bleeding or injury to the adjacent viscera. Therefore, the operation must be stopped and the instruments must be withdrawn under hysteroscopic guidance.

If there is evidence of bleeding or presumed visceral injury, laparoscopy or laparotomy should be performed. Injury to the uterus is relatively easy to detect with a laparoscope. However, mechanical or thermal injury to the bowel, ureter, or bladder are more difficult and may require laparotomy. If the patient's condition is managed expectantly, she should be advised of the situation and asked to report any symptoms of bleeding or visceral trauma.

Bleeding

Bleeding that occurs during or after hysteroscopy results from trauma to the vessels in the myometrium or injury to other vessels in the pelvis. Myometrial vessels can be lacerated during the resectoscopic procedures.

In planning operations that involve deep resection, autologous blood can be obtained prior to surgery. The risk of bleeding may be reduced by the preoperative injection of diluted vasopressin into the cervical stroma (145). The risk of injury to branches of the uterine artery can be lowered by minimizing the depth of resection in the lateral endometrial cavity near the uterine isthmus, where ablative techniques should be used. When bleeding is encountered during resectoscopic procedures, the ball electrode can be used to desiccate the vessel electrosurgically. Intractable bleeding may respond to the injection of diluted vasopressin or to the inflation of a 30-ml Foley catheter balloon in the endometrial cavity (117).

Thermal Trauma

The temperature of the uterine serosa does not rise significantly during electrosurgical coagulation of the endometrium, even at the cornu, which is the thinnest area of the myometrium (146). However, if an activated electrode or laser fiber penetrates the uterus, surrounding structures such as bowel, urinary tract, and blood vessels are at risk. An activated electrode or fiber should never be advanced, but if an activated electrode has penetrated the uterine wall, direct examination of the pelvic viscera is mandatory. Laparoscopy is the appropriate first step. The site of the perforation should be examined to exclude the presence of significant bleeding. Most perforations do not need to be repaired. However, the pelvic sidewalls, the bladder, and the small and large bowel should be carefully inspected. If the intestines are damaged, laparotomy is indicated to repair the damage (147).

Thermal injury to the intestine or ureter may be difficult to diagnose, and symptoms may not occur for several days to 2 weeks. Therefore, the patient should be advised of the symptoms that could indicate peritonitis.

Distension Media

Carbon Dioxide   Carbon dioxide can cause emboli and result in serious intraoperative morbidity and death (148–150). These risks can be eliminated by not using CO_2 with operative procedures and by ensuring that the insufflation pressure is always lower than 100 mm Hg and the flow rate is lower than 100 ml/min. The insufflator used must be especially designed for hysteroscopy; it is difficult to set laparoscopic insufflator flow rates below 1000 ml/min.

Dextran 70 *Dextran 70* is a hyperosmolar medium that can induce an allergic response, coagulopathy, and, if sufficient volumes are infused, vascular overload and heart failure (151, 152). Because *Dextran* is hydrophilic, it can draw six times its own volume into the systemic circulation. Consequently, the volume of this agent used should be limited to less than 300 ml, particularly for office use.

Low-Viscosity Fluids The low-viscosity fluids 1.5% glycine and 3% sorbitol are most often used, largely because of their low cost, compatibility with electrosurgery, and availability in large-volume bags. However, the use of a continuous-flow system with hypotonic media can create fluid and electrolyte disturbances.

1. Before undertaking a procedure using the resectoscope, base-line serum electrolyte levels should be measured. Women with cardiopulmonary disease should be evaluated carefully. The selective preoperative use of agents such as GnRH agonists may reduce operating time and media absorption.

2. In the operating room, media infusion and collection should take place in a closed system to allow accurate measurement of the "absorbed" volume. The volume should be calculated every 5 minutes or at least every 15 minutes.

3. The lowest intrauterine pressure necessary for adequate distension should be used to complete the operation, usually at a level that is below the mean arterial pressure. A good range is 70–80 mm Hg, which can be achieved with a specially designed pump or by maintaining the meniscus of the infusion bag 1 m above the level of the patient's uterus.

4. Deficits of more than 1 l equire measurement of electrolyte levels. The procedure should be completed expeditiously. If the deficit is more than 2 l, the procedure should be terminated and diuretics such as *mannitol* or *furosemide* should be used as needed. In patients with cardiovascular compromise, deficits must be avoided (36).

Image Documentation

A small video camera can be used to teach and to better coordinate the procedure with the operating room team. It also allows the operation to be recorded for future reference. A video recorder may be attached to a video camera system. For optimal recording, the camera should be attached directly to the recorder so the image is transmitted to the monitor for viewing during the operation. A number of video recording formats are available, each with inherent advantages and disadvantages. The best quality still images are obtained with a 35-mm single-lens reflex still camera and coupler. The use of a camera is often cumbersome, but the images taken from a standard still camera are of higher resolution than those obtained from videotape. Some video printers provide images suitable for a medical record. Newer digital cameras provide video still images, slides, or prints that are suitable for publication or teaching.

References

1. **Shapiro HI, Adler DH.** Excision of an ectopic pregnancy through the laparoscope. *Am J Obstet Gynecol* 1973;117:290–1.

2. **Gomel V.** Laparoscopic tubal surgery in infertility. *Obstet Gynecol* 1975;46:47–8.

3. **Gomel V.** Salpingostomy by laparoscopy. *J Reprod Med* 1977;18:265–7.

4. **Mettler L, Giesel H, Semm K.** Treatment of female infertility due to tubal obstruction by operative laparoscopy. *Fertil Steril* 1979;32:384–8.

5. **Steptoe PC, Edwards RG.** Birth after the reimplantation of a human embryo. *Lancet* 1978;2:366.

6. **Daniell JF.** Operative laparoscopy for endometriosis. *Semin Reprod Endocrinol* 1985;3:353.

7. **Feste JR.** Laser laparoscopy, a new modality. *J Reprod Med* 1985;40:413–7.

8. **Nezhat C, Crowgey SR, Garrison CP.** Surgical treatment of endometriosis via laser laparoscopy. *Fertil Steril* 1986;45:778–83.

9. **Martin DC.** CO$_2$ laser laparoscopy for endometriosis associated with infertility. *J Reprod Med* 1986;31:1089–94.

10. **Davis GD.** Management of endometriosis and its associated adhesions with the CO$_2$ laser laparoscope. *Obstet Gynecol* 1986;68:422–5.

11. **Reich H, DeCaprio J, McGlynn F.** Laparoscopic hysterectomy. *J Gynecol Surg* 1989;5:213–6.

12. **Stovall G, Ling FW, Gray LA.** Single dose methotrexate for treatment of ectopic pregnancy. *Obstet Gynecol* 1991;77:754–7.

13. **Bhiwandiwala PP, Mumbord SD, Feldblum PJ.** A comparison of different laparoscopic sterilization occlusion techniques in 24,939 procedures. *Am J Obstet Gynecol* 1982;144:319–31.

14. **Cittadini E, La Sala G, Perino A.** Endoscopy for contraception. *Acta Eur Fertil* 1988;19:309–14.

15. **Maruri F, Azziz R.** Laparoscopic surgery for ectopic pregnancies: technology assessment and public health implications. *Fertil Steril* 1993;59:487–98.

16. **Gomel V, Taylor PJ.** *Diagnostic and Operative Laparoscopy.* St. Louis: CV Mosby, 1995.

17. **Gomel V.** Management of ectopic gestation; surgical treatment is usually best. *Clin Obstet Gynecol* 1995;38:353–61.

18. **Mecke H, Lehmann-Willenbrock E, Ibrahim M, Semm K.** Pelviscopic treatment of ovarian cysts in premenopausal women. *Gynecol Obstet Invest* 1992;34:36–42.

19. **Canis M, Mage G, Pouly J, Wattiez H, Bruhat M.** Laparoscopic diagnosis of adnexal cystic masses: a twelve year experience with long-term followup. *Obstet Gynecol* 1994;83:707–12.

20. **Maiman M, Seltzer V, Boyce J.** Laparoscopic excision of ovarian neoplasms subsequently found to be malignant. *Obstet Gynecol* 1991;77:563–5.

21. **Parker WH, Berek JS.** Management of selected cystic adnexal masses in postmenopausal women by operative laparoscopy. A pilot study. *Am J Obstet Gynecol* 1990;163:1574–7.

22. **Parker WH, Levine R, Howard F, Sansone B, Berek JS.** A multicenter study of laparoscopic management of selected cystic adnexal masses in postmenopausal women. *J Am Coll Surg* 1994;179:733–7.

23. **Albini S, Benadiva C, Haverly K, Luciano A.** Management of benign cystic teratomas: laparoscopy compared with laparotomy. *J Am Assoc Gynecol Laparosc* 1994;1:219–22.

24. **Parker WH.** Laparoscopic management of the adnexal mass in postmenopausal women. *J Gynecol Tech* 1995;1:3–6.

25. **Operative Laparoscopy Study Group.** Postoperative adhesion development after operative laparoscopy: evaluation at early second-look laparoscopy. *Fertil Steril* 1991;55:700–4.

26. **Mage G, Canis M, Manhes H, Pouly JL, Bruhat MA.** Laparoscopic management of adnexal torsion. *J Reprod Med* 1989;34:520–4.

27. **Vancaillie T, Schmidt EH.** Recovery of ovarian function after laparoscopic treatment of adnexal torsion. *J Reprod Med* 1987;32:561–2.

28. **Gjönnaess H.** Polycystic ovarian syndrome treated by ovarian electrocautery through the laparoscope. *Fertil Steril* 1984;41:20–5.

29. **Kovacs G, Buckler H, Bangah M, Outch R, Burger H, Healy D, et al.** Treatment of anovulation due to polycystic ovarian syndrome by laparoscopic ovarian cautery. *Br J Obstet Gynaecol* 1991;98:30–5.

30. **Huber J, Hosmann J, Spona J.** Polycystic ovarian syndrome treated by laser through the laparoscope. *Lancet* 1988;2(8604):215.

31. **Gürgan T, Kisnisci H, Yarali H, Develioglu O, Zeyneloglu H, Asku T.** Evaluation of adhesion formation after laparoscopic treatment of polycystic ovarian disease. *Fertil Steril* 1991;56:1176–8.

32. **Naether OGJ, Fischer R.** Adhesion formation after laparoscopic electrocoagulation of the ovarian surface in polycystic ovary patients. *Fertil Steril* 1993;60:95–8.

720

33. **Hasson H, Rotman C, Rana N, Sistos F, Dmowski W.** Laparoscopic myomectomy. *Obstet Gynecol* 1993;82:897–900.

34. **Daniell J, Gurley L.** Laparoscopic treatment of clinically significant symptomatic uterine fibroids. *J Gynecol Surg* 1991;7:37.

35. **Parker WH, Rodi I.** Patient selection for laparoscopic myomectomy. *J Am Assoc Gynecol Laparosc* 1994;2:23–6.

36. **Sutton C, Diamond MP.** *Endoscopic Surgery for Gynecologists.* St. Louis: CV Mosby, 1993:169–71.

37. **Munro MG, Parker WH.** A classification system for laparoscopic hysterectomy. *Obstet Gynecol* 1993;82:624–9.

38. **Summitt RL, Stovall TG, Lipscomb GH, Ling FW.** Randomized comparison of laparoscopy-assisted vaginal hysterectomy with standard vaginal hysterectomy with standard vaginal hysterectomy in and outpatient setting. *Obstet Gynecol* 1992;80:895–901.

39. **Munro MG, Deprest JA.** Laparoscopic hysterectomy, does it work? Bicontinental review of the literature and clinical commentary. *Clin Obstet Gynecol* 1995;38(2):401–24.

40. **Munro MG, Gomel V.** Fertility-promoting laparoscopically-directed procedures. *Reprod Med Rev* 1994;3:29–42.

41. **Luciano AA, Whitman G, Maier D, Randolf J, Maenza R.** Comparison of thermal injury, healing patterns and postoperative adhesion formation following CO_2 laser and electromicrosurgery. *Fertil Steril* 1987;48:1025–9.

42. **Filmar S, Jetha N, McComb P, Gomel V.** A comparative histologic study on the healing process after tissue transection. I. Carbon dioxide laser and electromicrosurgery. *Am J Obstet Gynecol* 1991;77:563–5.

43. **Munro MG, Fu YS.** A randomized comparison of thermal injury characteristics of an electrosurgical laparoscopic loop electrode and the CO_2 laser in the rat uterine horn. *Am J Obstet Gynecol* 1995;172(4):1257–62.

44. **Lyons TL.** Minimally invasive treatment of urinary stress incontinence and laparoscopically directed repair of pelvic floor defects. *Clin Obstet Gynecol* 1995;38:380–91.

45. **Montz FJ, Schlaerth JB.** Laparoscopic surgery: does it have a role in the management of gynecologic malignancies? *Clin Obstet Gynecol* 1995;38(2):426–35.

46. **Fowler JM, Carter JR.** Laparoscopic management of the adnexal mass in postmenopausal women. *J Gynecol Tech* 1995;1:7–10.

47. **Tulandi T, Vilos GA.** A comparison between laser surgery and electrosurgery for bilateral hydrosalpinx: a 2-year followup. *Fertil Steril* 1985;44:846–8.

48. **Tulandi T.** Salpingo-ovariolysis: a comparison between laser surgery and electrosurgery. *Fertil Steril* 1986;45:489–91.

49. **Hurd WW, Bude RO, DeLancey JO, Pearl ML.** The relationship of the umbilicus to the aortic bifurcation: implications for laparoscopic technique. *Obstet Gynecol* 1992;80:48–51.

50. **Munro MG.** Laparoscopic suturing techniques. In: **Stovall T, Sammarco M, Steege J,** eds. *Gynecologic Endoscopy: Principles in Practice.* Baltimore: Williams & Wilkins, 1996:193–246.

51. **Montz FR, Holschneider CH, Munro MG.** Incisional hernia following laparoscopy: a survey of the American Association of Gynecologic Laparoscopists. *Obstet Gynecol* 1994;84:881–4.

52. **Peterson HB, DeStefano F, Rubin GL, Greenspan JR, Lee NC, Ory HW.** Deaths attributable to tubal sterilization in the United States, 1977 to 1981. *Am J Obstet Gynecol* 1982;146:131–6.

53. **Brady CE III, Harklerood LE, Pierson WP.** Alterations in oxygen saturation and ventilation after intravenous sedation of peritoneoscopy. *Arch Intern Med* 1989;149:1029–32.

54. **Ishizaki Y, Bandai Y, Shimomura K, Abe H, Ohtomo Y, Idezuki Y.** Safe intra-abdominal pressure of carbon dioxide pneumoperitoneum during laparoscopic surgery. *Surgery* 1993;114:549–54.

55. **Myles PS.** Brady arrhythmias and laparoscopy: a prospective study of heart rate changes with laparoscopy. *Aust N Z J Obstet Gynecol* 1991;31:171–3.

56. **Kent RB.** Subcutaneous emphysema and hypercarbia associated with laparoscopy. *Arch Surg* 1991;126:1154–6.

57. **Bard PA, Chen L.** Subcutaneous emphysema associated with laparoscopy. *Anesth Analg* 1990;71:101–2.

58. **Kalhan SB, Reaney JA, Collins RL.** Pneumomediastinum and subcutaneous emphysema during laparoscopy. *Cleve Clin J Med* 1990;57:639–42.

59. **Kabukoba JJ, Skillern LH.** Coping with extraperitoneal insufflation during laparoscopy: a new technique. *Obstet Gynecol* 1992;80:144–5.

60. **Grainger DA, Soderstrom RM, Schiff SF, Glickman MG, DeChernay AH, Diamond MP.** Ureteral injuries at laparoscopy: insights into diagnosis, management, and prevention. *Obstet Gynecol* 1990;75:839–43.

61. **Corson SL.** Electrosurgical hazards in laparoscopy. *JAMA* 1974;227:1261.

62. **Engel T.** The electrical dynamics of laparoscopic sterilization. *J Reprod Med* 1975;15:33–42.

63. **Baadsgarrd SE, Bille S, Egeblad K.** Major vascular injury during gynecologic laparoscopy. *Acta Obstet Gynecol Scand* 1989;68:283–5.

64. **Chi IC, Feldblum PJ.** Laparoscopic sterilization requiring laparotomy. *Am J Obstet Gynecol* 1982;142:712–3.

65. **Chi IC, Feldblum PJ, Baloh SA.** Previous abdominal surgery as a risk factor in interval laparoscopic sterilization. *Am J Obstet Gynecol* 1983;145:841–6.

66. **Franks AL, Kendrick JS, Peterson HB.** Unintended laparotomy associated with laparoscopic tubal sterilization. *Am J Obstet Gynecol* 1987;157:1102–5.

67. **Penfield AJ.** How to prevent complications of open laparoscopy. *J Reprod Med* 1985;30:660–3.

68. **Reich H.** Laparoscopic bowel injury. *Surg Laparosc Endosc* 1992;2:74–8.

69. **Childers JM, Brzechfta PR, Surwit EA.** Laparoscopy using the left upper quadrant as the primary trocar site. *Gynecol Oncol* 1993;50:221–5.

70. **Deziel DJ, Millikan KW, Economou SG, Doolas A, Sung-Tao K, Airan MC.** Complications of laparoscopic cholecystectomy: a national survey of 4292 hospitals and an analysis of 77,614 cases. *Am J Surg* 1993;165:9–14.

71. **Wolfe BM, Gardiner BN, Leary BF, Frey CF.** Endoscopic cholecystectomy; an analysis of complications. *Arch Surg* 1991;126:1192–8.

72. **Wheeless CR.** Thermal gastrointestinal injuries. In: **Phillips JM,** ed. *Laparoscopy.* Baltimore: Williams & Wilkins, 1977:231–5.

73. **Reich H, McGlynn F.** Laparoscopic repair of bladder injury. *Obstet Gynecol* 1990;75:909–10.

74. **Font GE, Brill AI, Stuhldreher PV, Rosenweig BA.** Endoscopic Management of incidental cystotomy during operative laparoscopy. *J Urol* 1993;149:1130–1.

75. **Reich H, McGlynn F.** Laparoscopic repair of bladder injury. *Obstet Gynecol* 1990;75:909–10.

76. **Gomel V, James C.** Intraoperative management of ureteral injury during operative laparoscopy. *Fertil Steril* 1991;55:416–9.

77. **Grainger DA, Soderstrom RM, Schiff SF, Glickman MG, DeCherney AH, Diamond MP.** Ureteral injuries at laparoscopy: insights into diagnosis, management, and prevention. *Obstet Gynecol* 1990;75:839–43.

78. **Steckel J, Badillo F, Waldbaum RS.** Uretero-fallopian tube fistula secondary to laparoscopic fulguration of pelvic endometriosis. *J Urol* 1993;149:1128–9.

79. **Kadar N, Lemmerling L.** Urinary fistulas during laparoscopic hysterectomy: causes and prevention. *Am J Obstet Gynecol* 1994;170:47–8.

80. **Woodland MB.** Ureter injury during laparoscopy-assisted hysterectomy with the endoscopic linear stapler. *Am J Obstet Gynecol* 1992;167:756–7.

81. **Nezhat C, Nezhat FR.** Safe laser endoscopic excision or vaporization of peritoneal endometriosis. *Fertil Steril* 1989;52:149–51.

82. **Nezhat C, Nezhat F.** Laparoscopic repair of ureter resected during operative laparoscopy. *Obstet Gynecol* 1992;80:543–4.

83. **Loffler FD, Dent D, Goodkin R.** Sciatic nerve injury in a patient undergoing laparoscopy. *J Reprod Med* 1978;21:371–2.

84. **al Hakin M, Katirjic B.** Femoral neuropathy induced by the lithotomy position: a report of 5 cases with a review of the literature. *Muscle Nerve* 1993;16:891–5.

85. **Reich H.** Laparoscopic treatment of extensive pelvic adhesions, including hydrosalpinx. *J Reprod Med* 1987;32:736–42.

86. **Bloom DA, Ehrlich RM.** Omental evisceration through small laparoscopy port sites. *J Endourol* 1993;7:31–3.

87. **Plaus WJ.** Laparoscopic trocar site hernias. *J Laparoendosc Surg* 1993:3:567–70.

88. **Maco A, Ruchman RB.** CT diagnosis of post laparoscopic hernia. *J Comput Assist Tomogr* 1991;15:1054–5.

89. **Chamberlain GVP, Carron-Brown J.** *Gynaecological Laparoscopy.* London: Royal College of Obstetricians & Gynecologists, 1978.

90. **Sotrel G, Hirsch E, Edelin KC.** Necrotizing fascitis following diagnostic laparoscopy. *Obstet Gynecol* 1982;62(Suppl 3):675–95.

91. **Glew RH, Pokoly TB.** Tubovarian abscess following laparoscopic sterilization with silicone rubber bands. *Obstet Gynecol* 1980;50:760–2.

92. **Levine RU, Neuwirth RS.** Simultaneous laparoscopy and hysteroscopy for intrauterine adhesions. *Obstet Gynecol* 1973;42:441–5.

93. **Neuwirth RS, Amin JH.** Excision of submucous fibroids with hysteroscopic control. *Am J Obstet Gynecol* 1976;126:95–9.

94. **Chervenak FA, Neuwirth RS.** Hysteroscopic resection of uterine septa. *Am J Obstet Gynecol* 1981;141:351–3.

95. **Goldrath MH, Fuller TA, Segal S.** Laser photovaporization of endometrium for the treatment of menorrhagia. *Am J Obstet Gynecol* 1983;147:869–72.

96. **DeCherney AH, Polan ML.** Hysteroscopic management if intrauterine adhesions and intractable uterine bleeding. *Obstet Gynecol* 1983;61:392–7.

97. **Townsend DE, Richart RM, Paskowitz RA, Woolfork RE.** "Rollerball" coagulation of the endometrium. *Obstet Gynecol* 1987;679:679–82.

98. **Goldrath MH, Sherman AI.** Office hysteroscopy and suction curettage: can we eliminate the hospital diagnostic dilatation and curettage? *Am J Obstet Gynecol* 1985;152:220–9.

99. **Gimpelson RJ.** Office hysteroscopy. *Clin Obstet Gynecol* 1992;35:270–81.

100. **Itzkowic DJ, Laverty CR.** Office hysteroscopy and curettage: a safe diagnostic procedure. *Aust N Z J Obstet Gynecol* 1990;30:150–3.

101. **Gimpelson R, Rappold H.** A comparative study between panoramic hysteroscopy with directed biopsies and curettage. A review of 276 cases. *Am J Obstet Gynecol* 1988;158:489–92.

102. **Loffer FD.** Hysteroscopy with selective endometrial sampling compared with D&D for abnormal uterine bleeding: the value of a negative hysteroscopic view. *Obstet Gynecol* 1989;73:16–20.

103. **Iossa A, Cianferoni L, Ciatto S, Cecchini S, Campatelli C, Lo Stumbo F.** Hysteroscopy and endometrial cancer diagnosis: a review of 2007 consecutive examinations in self-referred patients. *Tumori* 1991;77:479–83.

104. **Crescini C, Artuso A, Repetti F, Reale D, Pezzica E.** Hysteroscopic diagnosis in patients with abnormal uterine hemorrhage and previous endometrial curettage. *Minerva Ginecol* 1992;44:233–5.

105. **Brooks PG, Serden SP.** Hysteroscopic findings after unsuccessful dilatation and curettage for abnormal uterine bleeding. *Am J Obstet Gynecol* 1988;158:1354–7.

106. **Valle RF.** Hysteroscopy in the evaluation of female infertility. *Am J Obstet Gynecol* 1980;317:425–31.

107. **Golan A, Ron-El R, Herman A, Soffer Y, Bukobsky I, Caspi E.** Diagnostic hysteroscopy: its value in an *in vitro* fertilization transfer unit. *Hum Reprod* 1992;7:1433–4.

108. **Marty R, Amouroux J, Haouet S, De Brux J.** The reliability of endometrial biopsy performed during hysteroscopy. *Int J Gynaecol Obstet* 1991;34:151–5.

109. **Chambers JT, Chambers SK.** Endometrial sampling: When? Where? Why? With what? *Clin Obstet Gynecol* 1992;35:28–39.

110. **DeCherney AH, Russell JB, Graebe RA, Polan ML.** Resectoscopic management of müllerian fusion defects. *Fertil Steril* 1986;45:726–8.

111. **Valle RF, Sciarra JJ.** Hysteroscopic treatment of the septate uterus. *Obstet Gynecol* 1986; 67:253–7.

112. **March CM, Israel R.** Hysteroscopic management of recurrent abortion caused by the septate uterus. *Am J Obstet Gynecol* 1987;156:834–42.

113. **Daly DC, Maier D, Soto-Albers C.** Hysteroscopic metroplasty: six years' experience. *Obstet Gynecol* 1989;61:392–7.

114. **Loffer FD.** Removal of large symptomatic growths by the hysteroscopic resectoscope. *Obstet Gynecol* 1990;76:836–40.

115. **Donnez J, Gillerot S, Bourgonjon D, Clerckx F, Nisolle M.** Neodymiuim:YAG laser hysteroscopy in large submuous fibroids. *Fertil Steril* 1990;54:999–1003.

116. **Derman SG, Rehnstrom J, Neuwirth RS.** The long-term effectiveness of hysteroscopic treatment of menorrhagia and leiomyomas. *Obstet Gynecol* 1991;77:591–4.

117. **Serden SP, Brooks PG.** Treatment of abnormal uterine bleeding with the gynecologic resectoscope. *J Reprod Med* 1991;36:697–9.

118. **Itzkowic D.** Submucous fibroids: clinical profile and hysteroscopic management. *Aust N Z J Obstet Gynecol* 1993;33:63–7.

119. **Wamsteker K, Emanuel MH, de Kruif JH.** Transcervical hysteroscopic resection of submucous fibroids for abnormal uterine bleeding: results regarding the degree of intramural extension. *Obstet Gynecol* 1993;82:736–40.

120. **Indman PD.** Hysteroscopic treatment of menorrhagia associated with uterine leiomyomas. *Obstet Gynecol* 1993;81:716–20.

121. **Cicinelli E, Romano F, Anastasio PS, Blasi N, Parisi C, Galantino P.** Transabdominal sonohysterography, transvaginal sonography and hysteroscopy in the evaluation of submucous myomas. *Obstet Gynecol* 1995;85:42–7.

122. **Brooks PG.** Hysteroscopic surgery using the resectoscope: myomas, ablation, septa, synechiae. Does pre-operative medication help? *Clin Obstet Gynecol* 1992;35:249–55.

123. **Mencaglia L, Tantini C.** GnRH agonist analogues and hysteroscopic resection of myomas. *Int J Gynaecol Obstet* 1993;43:285–8.

124. **Ke RW, Taylor PJ.** Endometrial ablation to control excessive uterine bleeding. *Hum Reprod* 1991;6:574–80.

125. **Petrucco OM, Gillespie A.** The neodymium:YAG laser and the resectoscope for the treatment of menorrhagia. *Med J Aust* 1991;154:518–20.

126. **Lomano J.** Endometrial ablation for the treatment of menorrhagia: a comparison of patients with normal, enlarged and fibroid uteri. *Lasers Surg Med* 1991;11:8–12.

127. **Magos AL, Baumann R, Lockwood GM, Turnbull AC.** Experience with the first 250 endometrial resections for menorrhagia. *Lancet* 1991;337:1074–8.

128. **Wortman M, Daggett A.** Hysteroscopic endomyometrial resection: a new technique for the treatment of menorrhagia. *Obstet Gynecol* 1994;83:295–8.

129. **Gillespie A.** Endometrial ablation: a conservative alternative to hysterectomy for menorrhagia? *Med J Aust* 1991;154:791–2.

130. **Pinion SB, Parkin DE, Abramovich DR, Naji A, Alexander DA, Russell IT, et al.** Randomised trial of hysterectomy, endometrial laser ablation and transcervical endometrial resection for dysfunctional uterine bleeding. *BMJ* 1994;309:979–83.

131. **Vancaillie TG.** Electrocoagulation of the endometrium with the ball-end resectoscope. *Obstet Gynecol* 1989;74:425–7.

132. **Daniell JF, Kurtz BR, Ke RW.** Hysteroscopic endometrial ablation using the rollerball electrode. *Obstet Gynecol* 1992;80:329–32.

133. **Itzkowic D, Beale M.** Uterine perforation associated with endometrial ablation. *Aust N Z J Obstet Gynaecol* 1992;32:359–61.

724

134. **Perino A, Chianchiano N, Petronio M, Cittadini E.** Role of leuprolide acetate depot in hysteroscopic surgery: a controlled study. *Fertil Steril* 1993;59:507–10.

135. **Goldrath MH.** Use of danazol in hysteroscopic surgery for menorrhagia. *J Reprod Med* 1990;35:91–6.

136. **Wood C, Rogers P.** A pregnancy after planned partial endometrial resection. *Aust N Z J Obstet Gynaecol* 1993;33:316–8.

137. **Sugimoto O.** Diagnostic and therapeutic hysteroscopy for traumatic intrauterine adhesions. *Am J Obstet Gynecol* 1978;131:539–47.

138. **March CM, Israel R.** Gestational outcome following hysteroscopic lysis of adhesions. *Fertil Steril* 1981;36:455–9.

139. **Valle RF, Schiarra JJ.** Intrauterine adhesions: classification, treatment and reproductive outcome. *Am J Obstet Gynecol* 1988;158:1459–70.

140. **Schlaff WD, Hurst BS.** Preoperative sonographic measurement of endometrial pattern predicts outcome of surgical repair in patients with severe Asherman's syndrome. *Fertil Steril* 1995;63:410–3.

141. **Zupi E, Luciano AA, Valli E, Marconi D, Maneschi F, Romanini C.** The use of topical anesthesia in diagnostic hysteroscopy and endometrial biopsy. *Fertil Steril* 1995;63:414–6.

142. **Vercellini P, Colombo A, Mauro F, Oldani S, Bramante T, Crosignani PG.** Paracervical anesthesia for outpatient hysteroscopy. *Fertil Steril* 1994;62:1083–5.

143. **Hoekstra PT, Kahnoski R, McCamish MA, Bergen W, Heetderks DR.** Transurethral resection syndrome—a new perspective: encephalopathy with associated hyperammonemia. *J Urol* 1983;130:704–7.

144. **Finikiotis G.** Side effects and complications of outpatient hysteroscopy. *Aust N Z J Obstet Gynecol* 1993;33:61–2.

145. **Corson SL, Brooks PG, Serden SP, Batzer FR, Gocial B.** Effects of vasopressin administration during hysteroscopic surgery. *J Reprod Med* 1994;39:419–23.

146. **Indman PD, Brown WW 3rd.** Uterine surface temperature changes caused by electrosurgical endometrial coagulation. *J Reprod Med* 1992;37:667–70.

147. **Sullivan B, Kenney P, Seibel M.** Hysteroscopic resection of fibroid with thermal injury to sigmoid. *Obstet Gynecol* 1992;80;546–7.

148. **Obenhaus T, Maurer W.** CO_2 embolism during hysteroscopy. *Anaesthetist* 1990;39:243–6.

149. **Vo Van JM, Nguyen NQ, Le Bervet JY.** A fatal gas embolism during a hysteroscopy-curettage. *Cah Anesthesiol* 1992;40:617–8.

150. **Brundin J, Thomasson K.** Cardiac gas embolism during carbon dioxide hysteroscopy: risk and management. *Eur J Obstet Gynecol* 1989;33:241–5.

151. **Cholban MJ, Kalhan SB, Anderson RJ, Collins R.** Pulmonary edema and coagulopathy following intrauterine instillation of 32% dextran-70 (Hyskon). *J Clin Anesth* 1991;3:317–9.

152. **Golan A, Siedner M, Bahar M, Ron-El R, Herman A, Caspi E.** High-output left ventricular failure after dextran use in an operative hysteroscopy. *Fertil Steril* 1990;54:939–41.

22 Hysterectomy

Thomas G. Stovall

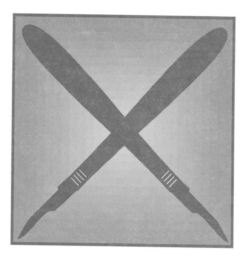

Hysterectomy is one of the most common surgical procedures performed; after cesarean delivery, it is the second most frequently performed major surgical procedure in the U.S. (1). In 1965, there were 426,000 hysterectomies performed in the U.S. with an average length of hospital stay of 12.2 days. This number peaked in 1985, when 724,000 procedures were reported with the length of stay decreasing to 9.4 days. Since that time, the number of hysterectomies has declined, and in 1991 there were only 544,000 hysterectomies performed in the U.S., with an average length of stay of 4.5 days. Of these 544,000 hysterectomies, 408,000 (75%) were performed abdominally and 136,000 (25%) were performed vaginally (2, 3). Using 1987 age-specific hysterectomy rates and the population projections supplied by the U.S. Census Bureau, it has been projected that there will be 824,000 hysterectomies in the year 2005 (4, 5).

The rate of hysterectomy has varied between 6.1 and 8.6 per 1000 women of all ages; women between the ages of 20 and 49 years constituted the largest segment of women undergoing the procedure. The average age of a woman undergoing hysterectomy is 42.7 years and the median age is 40.9 years, which has remained constant during the past 2 decades. Approximately 75% of all hysterectomies are performed in women between the ages of 20 and 49 years. The rates of hysterectomy vary by region of the country. The highest overall rate is in the southern states, where the rate tends to be higher for women aged 15–44 years. The lowest rates have consistently been in the northeastern portion of the U.S. Hysterectomy is more often performed in African-Americans than in Caucasians and is performed more frequently by male gynecologists than female gynecologists (6–9).

Indications

The indications for hysterectomy are listed in Table 22.1. Uterine leiomyomas are the leading indication for hysterectomy. As expected, the indications differ with the patient's age (10). For instance, whereas pelvic relaxation accounts for 16% of hysterectomies, this diagnosis is responsible for over 33% of hysterectomies in women older than 55 years of age. More complete discussions of these indications are presented in the specific chapters indicated below.

727

Table 22.1   Hysterectomy Indication Profile

Indication	Number of Patients	Percentage	Percentage Confirmed*
Acute condition (emergencies)			
A-1 Pregnancy catastrophe[1]	27	1.5	93
A-2 Severe infection[2]	2	<1	100
A-3 Operative complication[1]	1	<1	100
Benign disease			
B-1 Leiomyomas[2]	522	29	86
B-2 Endometriosis[2]	95	5.3	92
B-3 Adenomyosis[2]	27	1.5	44
B-4 Chronic infection[2]	29	1.6	100
B-5 Adnexal mass[2]	146	8.1	100
B-6 Other[2]	1	<1	100
Cancer or premalignant disease (known)			
C-1 Invasive cancer[2]	164	9.1	100
C-2 Preinvasive disease[2]	137	7.6	100
C-3 Adjacent or distant cancer[2]	6	<1	100
Discomfort (chronic or recurrent)			
D-1 Chronic pelvic pain[1]	144	8	80
D-2 Pelvic relaxation[1]	189	10.5	100
D-3 Stress urinary incontinence[1]	86	4.8	100
D-4 Abnormal uterine bleeding[1]	225	12.5	94
Extenuating circumstances (peer reviewed)			
E-1 Sterilization[3]	3	<1	100
E-2 Cancer prophylaxis[3]	5	<1	100
E-3 Other[3]	2	<1	100
Total:	1811	100	92

*Validated by the American College of Obstetricians and Gynecologists criteria sets[1] or verified by tissue pathology[2] or preoperative peer review.[3]
Information based on single designated (first-listed) preoperative diagnosis for 1811 operations performed at Naval Hospitals in San Diego and Camp Pendleton, CA and UCLA Medical Center.
Adapted from **Gambone JC, Reiter RC.** Nonsurgical management of chronic pelvic pain: a multidisciplinary approach. *Clin Obstet Gynecol* 1990;33(1):205–11.

Leiomyomas

Uterine leiomyomas are the most common pelvic tumors in women; therefore, this condition is responsible for a large number of hysterectomies (10). Hysterectomy for uterine leiomyomas should be considered only in patients who do not desire future fertility. Otherwise, fertility-preserving surgical management (myomectomy) is possible in most patients with leiomyomas. The decision to perform a hysterectomy for leiomyomas is usually based on the need to treat symptoms—abnormal uterine bleeding, pelvic pain, or pelvic pressure. Other indications for intervention have included "rapid" uterine enlargement (although this finding is poorly defined), ureteral compression, or growth following menopause. The concept of "rapid growth" has recently been challenged (11), because such patients have not been shown clearly to have malignant conditions. Furthermore, there is no clearly reproducible definition of "rapid growth."

The removal of the uterus because it reaches a certain size is widely debated. Some investigators suggest that if the uterus is the size of 12 weeks of gestation or greater, it should be removed even if it is asymptomatic. The reasons given for such an intervention include the inability to palpate the ovaries on bimanual examination and the assumption that, as the uterus enlarges, the morbidity for hysterectomy increases. Malignancy is uncommon in premenopausal patients, however, and adnexal palpation is not possible in many patients whose ovaries are of normal size.

No difference in surgical morbidity exists between patients with a 12-week-sized uterus and those with a 20-week-sized uterus if the procedures are performed abdominally (12). **Available data strongly suggest that hysterectomy for leiomyomas should be considered only in symptomatic patients who do not desire future fertility (12).**

To reduce uterine size, patients with large leiomyomas may be pretreated with a gonadotropin-releasing hormone (GnRH) agonist (13–15). In many cases, the reduction of uterine size will be sufficient to permit vaginal hysterectomy when, otherwise, an abdominal hysterectomy would have been necessary. In one prospective trial, premenopausal patients with leiomyomas the size of 14–18 weeks of gestation were randomized to receive either 2 months preoperative depot GnRH agonist or no GnRH agonist (15). Treatment with a short course (8 weeks) of *leuprolide acetate* prior to surgery enabled patients to be converted safely from an abdominal hysterectomy to a vaginal hysterectomy. This preoperative regimen was associated with a rise in hematocrit prior to surgery and, because patients were more likely to have vaginal rather than abdominal hysterectomy, shortening of the hospital stay and convalescent period.

Dysfunctional Uterine Bleeding

Dysfunctional uterine bleeding is the indication for approximately 20% of hysterectomies. Because dysfunctional uterine bleeding usually is the result of anovulation, the bleeding can be controlled by medical interventions with progestin, estrogen, a combination of progestin and estrogen, oral contraceptives, or nonsteroidal anti-inflammatory agents (see Chapter 13). In most patients, the bleeding requires no therapy unless anemia is present or bleeding is excessive. In patients older than 35 years of age, endometrial sampling should always be performed prior to hysterectomy. Dilation and curettage is not an effective means of controlling bleeding and is not necessary before hysterectomy (16). Therefore, hysterectomy should be reserved for patients who do not respond to or who cannot tolerate medical therapy. Alternatives to hysterectomy (e.g., endometrial ablation or resection) should be considered in selected patients because these operations may be cost-effective and have a lower morbidity rate (see Chapter 21).

Intractable Dysmenorrhea

Approximately 10% of adult women are incapacitated for up to 3 days per month as a result of dysmenorrhea (see Chapter 14) (17). Dysmenorrhea can be treated with nonsteroidal anti-inflammatory agents used alone or in combination with oral contraceptives (18, 19). Hysterectomy is only rarely required for the treatment of primary dysmenorrhea. In patients with secondary dysmenorrhea, the underlying condition (e.g., leiomyomas, endometriosis) should be treated primarily. Nonsteroidal anti-inflammatory agents may be effective. **Hysterectomy should be considered only if medical therapy fails or if the patient does not want to preserve fertility (20–22).**

Pelvic Pain

In a review of 418 women in whom hysterectomy was performed for a variety of nonmalignant conditions, 18% had chronic pelvic pain and only preoperative laparoscopy was performed in only 66% of these patients. After hysterectomy, there was a significant reduction in symptoms associated with an improvement in the patient's quality of life (23). Stovall and colleagues reviewed 104 patients who underwent hysterectomy for chronic pelvic pain that was believed to be of uterine origin. Patients were followed for a mean of 21.6 months after hysterectomy and 78% experienced improvement in their pain (24). However, 22% of patients had no improvement or exacerbation of their pain. **Hysterectomy should be performed only in those patients whose pain is of uterine origin and does not respond to nonsurgical treatments** (18) (see Chapter 14).

Cervical Intraepithelial Neoplasia

In the past, hysterectomy was performed as primary treatment of cervical intraepithelial neoplasia. However, the maximum depth of dysplasia at the squamocolumnar junction is 5.2 mm; 99.7% of dysplasias (including carcinoma *in situ*) are located within 3.8 mm from the epithelial surface (25). Therefore, more conservative treatments such as cryotherapy,

729

laser, or loop electrosurgical excision procedure can be effective in treating the disease, making hysterectomy unnecessary in most women with these conditions (see Chapter 16). For patients with recurrent high-grade dysplasia who do not desire to preserve fertility, hysterectomy is an appropriate treatment option. Even after hysterectomy, however, patients are at increased risk of vaginal intraepithelial neoplasia.

Genital Prolapse

Hysterectomy for symptomatic genital prolapse accounts for approximately 15% of hysterectomies performed in the U.S. (7). **Unless there is an associated condition requiring an abdominal incision, vaginal hysterectomy is the preferred approach for genital prolapse.** Uterine prolapse typically is not an isolated event and is most often associated with a variety of pelvic support defects (see Chapter 20). Each defect must be corrected to optimize the surgical outcome and decrease the chance for future development of pelvic support defects.

Obstetric Emergency

Most emergency hysterectomies are performed because of postpartum hemorrhage resulting from uterine atony. Other indications include uterine rupture that cannot be repaired or a pelvic abscess that does not respond to medical therapy. Hysterectomy may be required for patients with placenta accreta or placenta increta.

Pelvic Inflammatory Disease

The uterus, tubes, and ovaries should not be removed in a patient with pelvic inflammatory disease unless the patient has not responded to intravenous antibiotic therapy (see Chapter 15). Whether one proceeds with conservative surgical management, abscess drainage, or organ removal is a subjective decision that must be based on the individual. If accessible, some pelvic abscesses may be drained successfully by percutaneous catheter drainage guided by ultrasonography or computerized tomography (CT) scanning. Surgical intervention also is necessary if the patient has acute abdominal findings associated with peritonitis and signs of sepsis in the presence of a ruptured tubo-ovarian abscess. **For the patient who desires future fertility, consideration should be given to unilateral adnexectomy or partial bilateral adnexectomy without hysterectomy.** For the patient in whom bilateral adnexectomy is required, the uterus can be left in place for possible ovum donation and *in vitro* fertilization (see Chapter 27).

Endometriosis

Medical and conservative surgical procedures generally are successful for treatment of endometriosis (see Chapter 26). Therefore, adnexectomy with or without hysterectomy should be performed only in patients who do not respond to conservative surgical (resection or ablation of endometriotic implants) or medical therapy. Most patients with endometriosis who require hysterectomy have unrelenting pelvic pain or dysmenorrhea. Other less common situations include patients who do not desire future fertility who have endometriosis involving other pelvic organs such as the ureter or colon.

Cancer

Metastases from nongynecologic sites may cause symptoms requiring hysterectomy. As a primary procedure, hysterectomy with bilateral salpingo-oophorectomy should be considered for patients with colorectal carcinoma because these patients are at risk for either synchronous pelvic cancers or occult metastases (26, 27).

Benign Ovarian Tumor

Benign ovarian tumors that are persistent or symptomatic require surgical treatment. Obviously, if the patient desires fertility, the uterus should be conserved. If fertility is not an issue, however, or if the patient is peri- or postmenopausal, a decision must be made regarding whether the uterus should be removed. Gambone and colleagues reviewed 100 patients who underwent adnexectomy plus hysterectomy for benign adnexal disease and compared these patients to a group of risk-matched women who underwent adnexectomy without hysterectomy for the same indication (28). There was a significant increase in operative morbidity, estimated blood loss, and the length of hospital stay for patients in whom hysterectomy was performed.

Vaginal Versus Abdominal Hysterectomy

The proportion of abdominal versus vaginal hysterectomies has not changed significantly over the last 20 years—about 75% of hysterectomies are abdominal (2, 3, 7, 29–32). There are no specific criteria that can be used to determine the route of hysterectomy. The route chosen should be individualized. Absolute and relative contraindications have been proposed (27–29).

In a large, multicenter retrospective study conducted by the U.S. Centers for Disease Control between 1978 and 1981, the risks and outcome of abdominal and vaginal hysterectomy were compared (32). The study included 1851 patients aged 15–44 years in whom hysterectomy was performed for benign gynecologic disorders (568 vaginal, 1283 abdominal). Surgical complications were classified into six categories. The overall complication rate was 24.5 per 100 for vaginal hysterectomy compared with 42.8 per 100 women for abdominal hysterectomy. **The risk of one or more complications after abdominal hysterectomy was 1.7 times the risk after vaginal hysterectomy.** The two major categories of complications were febrile morbidity and hemorrhage requiring transfusion. **The risk of febrile morbidity was 2.1 times higher for abdominal hysterectomy than for vaginal hysterectomy, and the risk of transfusion was 1.9 times higher for abdominal surgery.** Since the collection of these data, transfusion practices within the U.S. have changed as a result of increased awareness of the human immunodeficiency virus. Although only one-fourth of hysterectomies are performed vaginally, this proportion could probably be increased substantially. In a recent study of 617 hysterectomies, 548 were performed vaginally; laparoscopic assistance was used in 63 patients, and an abdominal approach was required in only six patients (33). If feasible, vaginal hysterectomy is the preferred approach.

Supracervical/Subtotal Hysterectomy	The indications for supracervical hysterectomy are somewhat vague. Among potential indications are endometriosis with obliteration of the anterior and posterior cul-de-sac, cesarean hysterectomy when the cervix is fully dilated and difficult to identify, and concern for sexual function. During a technically difficult surgical procedure (e.g., obliteration of the cul-de-sac), there may be concern about the potential morbidity associated with the removal of the cervix. However, **the cervix can almost always be removed.** Some women desire to conserve the cervix because they believe that it is important for sexual satisfaction, although there are no sound scientific data to prove this perception. Some authors (which currently represent the minority view) believe that the cervix should not be removed unless there is a specific reason. They suggest that removal of the cervix leads to a decrease in sexual pleasure, increased operative and postoperative morbidity, vaginal shortening, vault prolapse, abnormal cuff granulations, and the potential for oviductal prolapse (34, 35).

There is a debate about the effects of leaving the cervix *in situ.* Kilkku et al. reported on a group of 210 patients who underwent hysterectomy, half of whom had total abdominal hysterectomies and half who had supracervical hysterectomies (36). Studies of the same population disclosed an increase in psychiatric symptoms in both groups (34–36). Sexual desire and functioning was unchanged, although there was a decrease in dyspareunia in both groups. Patients undergoing supracervical hysterectomy were reported to have increased orgasmic frequency when compared with patients in which the cervix was left intact (36–39). Regardless of the reason for leaving the cervix at the time of hysterectomy, preoperative Papanicolaou (Pap) test results must be normal and appropriate consent must be obtained from the patient.

The Role of Laparoscopy	Laparoscopy has been used diagnostically prior to hysterectomy (see Chapter 21). Kovac et al. (33) performed laparoscopy in 46 patients who had been advised to have abdominal hysterectomies, and the findings suggested that uterine size had been overestimated and uterine

mobility had been underestimated by the referring physicians. All 14 patients who were referred for adnexal pathology had none. In 91% (42 of 46) of the patients, a vaginal hysterectomy was completed. In another study of seven patients who were candidates for vaginal hysterectomy, except that they had a history suggestive of adhesions, six of the patients underwent laparoscopy, which did not reveal any adhesive disease (40), and were able to undergo vaginal hysterectomy. These findings are consistent with the other data demonstrating that **the presence of pelvic adhesions cannot be predicted based on either history or physical examination** (41). However, if laparoscopy is performed on patients with risk factors for adhesions or endometriosis, many patients will undergo the procedure needlessly and approximately one-half of those with adhesions or endometriosis will be overlooked. Thus, the role of diagnostic laparoscopy immediately prior to hysterectomy seems limited.

The use of operative laparoscopy to complete some or all of the hysterectomy has been widely reported (42–52) (see Chapter 21). However, in most of these studies, the patient population has been neither randomized nor defined. Furthermore, the reasons why the patient would require an abdominal approach are unclear. **The criteria for patient selection for laparoscopy-assisted vaginal hysterectomy (LAVH) versus abdominal hysterectomy have not been clearly established.**

Summitt et al. (46) published a randomized, prospective, controlled trial in which patients who were candidates for vaginal hysterectomy were randomized to either LAVH or a standard vaginal approach. All procedures were performed on an outpatient basis; included were patients who had uterine leiomyomas up to the size of 16 weeks of gestation. There was no difference between the groups in terms of uterine weight, febrile morbidity, or the need for transfusion. Patients undergoing LAVH had a lower hematocrit value on the first and second postoperative days and required more pain mediation on the second postoperative day. Although these findings are not significant clinically, they suggest that LAVH does not reduce perioperative morbidity when compared with a vaginal approach. The cost of LAVH is significantly higher ($7905 vs. $4891) than for vaginal hysterectomy; the largest component of this difference resulted from the use of disposable equipment. **This study demonstrates that there is no advantage of LAVH over traditional vaginal hysterectomy.**

It has been suggested that LAVH may be helpful in treating patients with documented endometriosis, known pelvic adhesive disease, an adnexal mass that requires hysterectomy, and lack of uterine mobility (Chapter 21). Depending on the circumstances, LAVH may be appropriate in some patients with stage I endometrial cancer or previous episodes of multiple major pelvic surgery. For example, if the patient has had endometriosis that has been treated previously or adhesions that have been lysed previously and now require hysterectomy, a vaginal approach can most likely be taken. Davis et al. reported a group of patients with stage III and stage IV endometriosis in whom the procedure was successful in 40 of 46 patients (53). Even in the hands of expert laparoscopic surgeons, however, the rate of complications was high.

Mild pelvic adhesions do not preclude vaginal hysterectomy. If the patient has intensive adhesions that involve the adnexa, bowel, and uterus, however, an abdominal approach is usually needed (54). In such patients, laparoscopy may be a better alternative than hysterectomy.

It is uncertain whether LAVH is preferable in patients with limited uterine mobility. The major supporting structures of the uterus are the uterosacral ligaments and lower cardinal complex (55), which are not generally transected laparoscopically. Transection of the utero-ovarian ligament, round ligament, and the broad ligament does not improve mobility.

Both LAVH and pelvic lymphadenectomy may be useful in selected patients with endometrial carcinoma (56). The data suggest that a lymphadenectomy can be performed successfully, and that hospital stay and morbidity are decreased when compared with the standard transabdominal approach. Long-term prospective studies are needed to address these questions.

A laparoscopic approach should not be used for hysterectomy solely for the purpose of removal of the ovaries. Although not every ovary can be removed through the vagina, it has been shown clearly that most can be removed in this manner (57).

Concurrent Surgical Procedures

Prophylactic Oophorectomy

Prophylactic oophorectomy is the most common surgical procedure performed concurrently with hysterectomy. Oophorectomy prophylactically is performed to prevent ovarian cancer and to eliminate the potential need for further surgery for either benign or malignant disease. **Arguments against prophylactic oophorectomy center around the need for earlier and more prolonged hormone replacement.** Although hormone replacement therapy is generally well tolerated and provides good symptomatic relief, it may not be as effective as normal ovarian function, and the implications of long-term replacement therapy are not fully known. Therefore, the decision to proceed with oophorectomy should be considered carefully after the patient has been informed of the risks and benefits.

The risk of developing ovarian cancer after hysterectomy for benign disease is lower than would be expected based on its prevalence. Of those women who have no history of ovarian tumors and normal-appearing ovaries at the time of abdominal hysterectomy, 0.14% subsequently develop ovarian cancer in their conserved ovaries (58). Considering that as many as 1.4% of women are expected to get ovarian cancer, this is about one-tenth the expected rate. Presumably, this lower rate occurs because the cohort of women with normal-appearing ovaries in whom hysterectomy is performed for benign disease is a "selected" population. In women who do not have ovarian disease at the time of hysterectomy, the risk of developing benign ovarian tumors is <5% (59). The risk of ovarian cancer in women with a strong family history is 3–50%, depending on the pedigree (60, 61) (see Chapter 33).

Long-term compliance with post-hysterectomy estrogen replacement therapy is low (62). Only 20–40% of women who initiate treatment after hysterectomy and bilateral oophorectomy continue to take estrogen for more than 5 years. Therefore, it should not be assumed that patients will receive adequate replacement estrogen after oophorectomy. Women who subsequently develop breast cancer may be advised not to take estrogen.

Appendectomy

Appendectomy may be performed concurrently with hysterectomy to prevent appendicitis and to remove disease that may be present. The former use is of limited value, however, because the peak incidence of appendicitis is between 20 and 40 years of age, whereas the peak age for hysterectomy is 10–20 years later (63). Appendectomy is effective in removing previously undetected disease, but the likelihood that these abnormalities would cause any clinical problems is uncertain. In one study, histologic abnormalities were found in 71% (32 of 45) of appendices removed at the time of hysterectomy, and two had asymptomatic carcinoid tumors (64). In another study, 22% of appendices removed at the time of hysterectomy showed evidence of pathologic alterations, and five carcinoid tumors were identified (65).

There is no increase in morbidity associated with appendectomy performed at the time of hysterectomy (65–67), although it does require an average of 10 minutes additional operating time (59). Appendectomy has also been performed with vaginal hysterectomy without additional intraoperative or postoperative morbidity (68–71).

Cholecystectomy

Gallbladder disease is approximately four times more common in women than men, and its highest incidence occurs between 50 and 70 years of age, when hysterectomy is most often performed. Thus, women may require both procedures. A combined procedure does not appear to result in increased febrile morbidity or length of hospital stay (72, 73).

Abdominoplasty	Abdominoplasty performed at the time of hysterectomy is associated with a shorter hospital stay, a shorter operating time, and a lower intraoperative blood loss than when the two operations are performed separately (74, 75). Liposuction also can be performed safely at the time of vaginal hysterectomy (76).

Hysterectomy Technique

Negative results of a Pap test performed within the year should be obtained before performing a hysterectomy for benign disease. If the patient is 40 years of age or older and has not recently had a recent mammography, this examination should be performed. Endometrial sampling is recommended if the patient has reported abnormal uterine bleeding. In patients older than 40 years of age, a stool guaiac test should be performed.

The technique of radical hysterectomy and its modifications are presented in Chapter 32.

Abdominal Hysterectomy

Preoperative Preparation   A cleansing enema of tap water or soap is given on the evening prior to or the morning of the scheduled hysterectomy. To reduce the amount of skin bacteria, the patient is asked to shower. Hair surrounding the incision area may be removed at the time of surgery. Hair clipping is preferable to shaving because it decreases the incidence of incisional infection (77).

Patient Positioning   The patient is placed in the dorsal supine position for the procedure. After the patient is anesthetized adequately, her legs are placed in the stirrups and a pelvic examination is performed to validate the pelvic findings. A Foley catheter is placed in the bladder, and the vagina is cleansed with an iodine solution. The patient's legs are then straightened.

Skin Preparation   Several methods for skin cleaning can be recommended, including a 5-minute iodine solution scrub followed by application of iodine solution, iodine solution scrub followed by alcohol with application of an iodine-impregnated occlusive drape, or an iodine/alcohol combination with or without application of an iodine-impregnated occlusive drape.

Surgical Technique   *Incision*   The choice of incision should be determined by the following considerations:

1. Simplicity of the incision

2. The need for exposure

3. The potential need for enlarging the incision

4. The strength of the healed wound

5. Cosmesis of the healed incision

6. The location of previous surgical scars

The skin is opened with a scalpel and the incision is carried down through the subcutaneous tissue and fascia. With traction applied to the lateral edges of the incision, the fascia is divided. The peritoneum is opened similarly. This technique minimizes the possibility of inadvertent enterotomy entering the abdominal cavity.

734

Abdominal Exploration   After entering the peritoneal cavity, the upper abdomen and the pelvis are explored systematically. The liver, gallbladder, stomach, kidneys, para-aortic lymph nodes, and large and small bowel should be examined and palpated. Cytologic sampling of the peritoneal cavity, if needed, should be performed before abdominal exploration.

Retractor Choice and Placement   A variety of retractors have been designed for pelvic surgery. The Balfour and the O'Connor-O'Sullivan retractors are used most often. The Bookwalter retractor has a variety of adjustable blades that can be helpful, particularly in obese patients.

Elevation of the Uterus   The uterus is elevated by placing broad ligament clamps at each cornu so it crosses the round ligament. The clamp tip may be placed close to the internal os. This placement provides uterine traction and prevents back bleeding (Fig. 22.1).

Round Ligament Ligation   The uterus is deviated to the patient's left side, stretching the right round ligament. With the proximal portion held by the broad ligament clamp, the distal portion of the round ligament is ligated with a suture ligature or simply transected with Bovie cautery (Fig. 22.2). The distal portion can be grasped with forceps, and the round ligament is cut to separate the anterior and posterior leaves of the broad ligament. The anterior leaf of the broad ligament is incised with Metzenbaum scissors or electrocautery

Figure 22.1   The uterus is elevated by placement of clamps across the broad ligament. (From **Mann WA, Stovall TG.** *Gynecologic Surgery.* New York: Churchill Livingstone, 1996.)

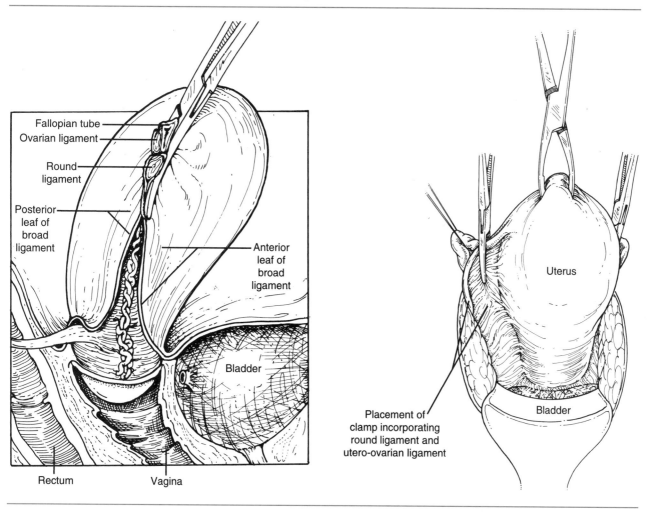

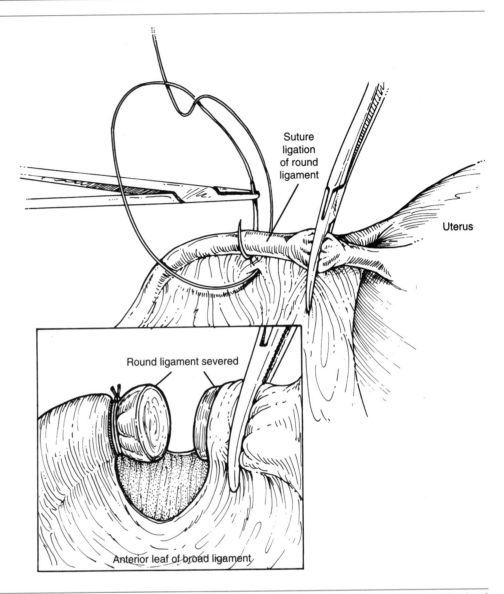

Figure 22.2   The round ligament is transected and the broad ligament is incised and opened. (From **Mann WA, Stovall TG.** *Gynecologic Surgery.* New York: Churchill Livingstone, 1996.)

along the vesicouterine fold, separating the peritoneal reflection of the bladder from the lower uterine segment (Fig. 22.3).

Ureter Identification **The retroperitoneum is entered by extending the incision cephalad on the posterior leaf of the broad ligament.** Care must be taken to remain lateral to both the infundibulopelvic ligament and iliac vessels. The external iliac artery courses along the medial aspect of the psoas muscle and is identified by bluntly dissecting the loose alveolar tissue overlying it. **By following the artery cephalad to the bifurcation of the common iliac artery, the ureter is identified crossing the common iliac artery. The ureter should be left attached to the medial leaf of the broad ligament to protect its blood supply** (Fig. 22.4).

Utero-Ovarian or Infundibulopelvic Ligament Ligation If the ovaries are to be preserved, the uterus is retracted toward the pubic symphysis and deviated to one side, plac-

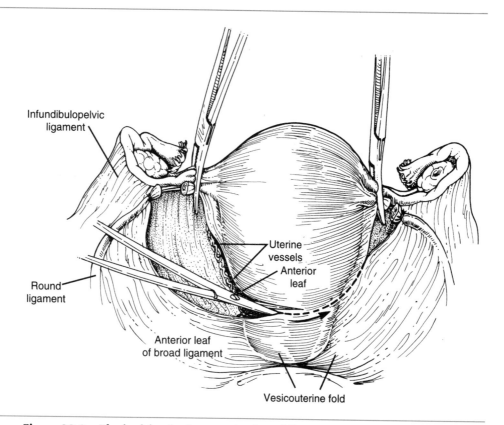

Figure 22.3   The incision in the anterior broad ligament is extended along the vesicouterine fold. (From **Mann WA, Stovall TG.** *Gynecologic Surgery.* New York: Churchill Livingstone, 1996.)

ing tension on the contralateral infundibulopelvic ligament, the tube, and the ovary. **With the ureter under direct visualization, a window is created in the peritoneum of the posterior leaf of the broad ligament under the utero-ovarian ligament and fallopian tube.** The tube and utero-ovarian ligament are clamped on each side with a curved Heaney or Ballentine clamp, cut and ligated with both a free-tie and a suture ligature. The medial clamp at the uterine cornu should control back bleeding; if it does not, the clamp should be repositioned to do so (Fig. 22.5).

If the ovaries are to be removed, the peritoneal opening is enlarged and extended cephalad to the infundibulopelvic ligament and caudad to the uterine artery. This opening allows proper exposure of the uterine artery, the infundibulopelvic ligament, and the ureter. In this manner, the ureter is released from its proximity to the uterine vessels and the infundibulopelvic ligament.

A curved Heaney or Ballentine clamp is placed lateral to the ovary (Fig. 22.6); care is taken to ensure that the entire ovary is included in the surgical specimen. The infundibulopelvic ligament on each side is cut and doubly ligated (Fig. 22.7). Alternatively, free ties can be passed around the infundibulopelvic ligament, two cephalad and one caudad, before the ligament is cut.

Bladder Mobilization   Using Metzenbaum scissors, with the tips pointed toward the uterus, the bladder is sharply dissected from the lower uterine segment and cervix. Alternatively, Bovie electrocautery can be used. An avascular plane, which exists between the lower uterine segment and the bladder, allows for this mobilization. Tonsil clamps

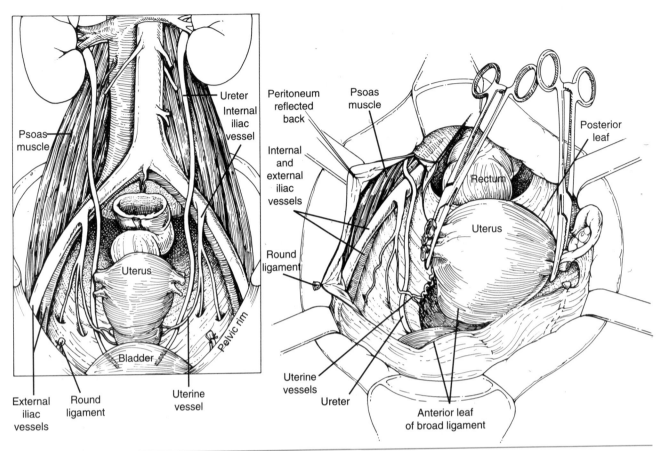

Figure 22.4   Identification of the ureter in the retroperitoneal space on the medial leaf of the broad ligament.
(From **Mann WA, Stovall TG.** *Gynecologic Surgery.* New York: Churchill Livingstone, 1996.)

may be placed on the bladder edge to provide countertraction and easier dissection (Fig. 22.8).

Uterine Vessel Ligation   The uterus is retracted cephalad and deviated to one side of the pelvis, stretching the lower ligaments. The uterine vasculature is dissected or "skeletonized" from any remaining areolar tissue, and a curved Heaney clamp is placed perpendicular to the uterine artery at the junction of the cervix and body of the uterus. Care is taken to place the tip of the clamp adjacent to the uterus at this anatomic narrowing. The vessels are cut and the suture is ligated. The same procedure is repeated on the opposite side (Fig. 22.9).

Incision of Posterior Peritoneum   If the rectum is to be mobilized from the posterior cervix, the posterior peritoneum between the uterosacral ligaments just beneath the cervix and rectum may be incised (Fig. 22.10). A relatively avascular tissue plane exists in this area, allowing mobilization of the rectum inferiorly out of the operative field. A sponge may be placed to control the venous oozing that often occurs.

Cardinal Ligament Ligation   The cardinal ligament is divided by placing a straight Heaney clamp medial to the uterine vessel pedicle for a distance of 2–3 cm parallel to the uterus. The ligament is then cut and the pedicle suture is ligated. This step is repeated on each side until the junction of the cervix and vagina is reached (Fig. 22.11).

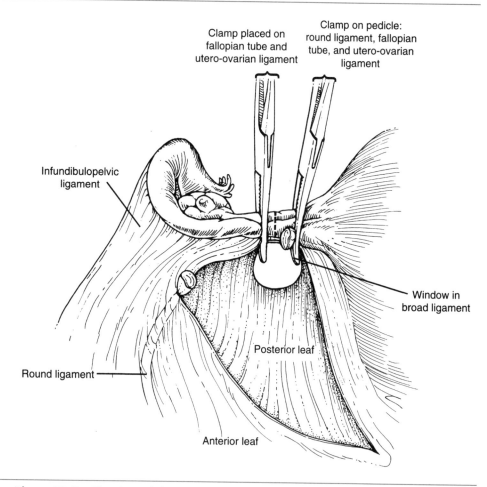

Figure 22.5 **Ligation of the utero-ovarian ligament.** (From **Mann WA, Stovall TG.** *Gynecologic Surgery.* New York: Churchill Livingstone, 1996.)

Figure 22.6 **Ligation of the infundibulopelvic ligament.** (From **Mann WA, Stovall TG.** *Gynecologic Surgery.* New York: Churchill Livingstone, 1996.)

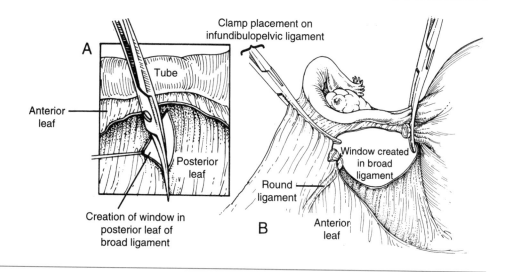

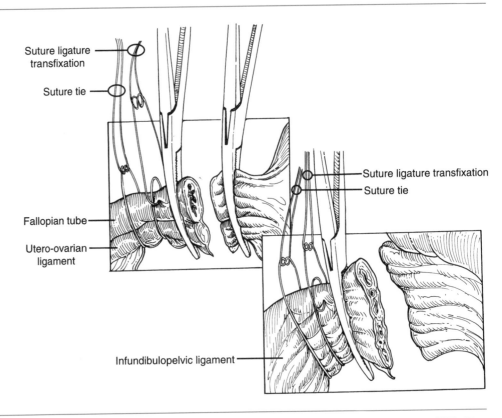

Labels in figure: Suture ligature transfixation; Suture tie; Fallopian tube; Utero-ovarian ligament; Suture ligature transfixation; Suture tie; Infundibulopelvic ligament

Figure 22.7   Transection of the infundibulopelvic ligament. (From **Mann WA, Stovall TG.** *Gynecologic Surgery.* New York: Churchill Livingstone, 1996.)

Removal of the Uterus   The uterus is placed on traction cephalad and the tip of the cervix is palpated. Curved Heaney clamps are placed bilaterally, incorporating the uterosacral ligament and upper vagina just below the cervix. **Care should be taken to avoid foreshortening the vagina.** The uterus is then removed with heavy curved scissors (Fig. 22.12).

Vaginal Cuff Closure   Several techniques of vaginal cuff closure have been described. A figure-of-eight suture of 0 braided absorbable material is placed between the tips of the two clamps. The suture is used for both traction and hemostasis. Sutures are also placed at the tip of each clamp, and the pedicles are sutured with a Heaney stitch, thereby incorporating the uterosacral and cardinal ligament at the angle of the vagina (Fig. 22.13). Alternatively, the vaginal cuff can be left open to heal secondarily. If this method is utilized, a running-locking suture is used for hemostasis along the cuff edge (Fig. 22.14).

Irrigation and Hemostasis   The pelvis is thoroughly irrigated with saline or lactated Ringer's solution. Meticulous care is taken to ensure hemostasis throughout the pelvis, particularly of the vascular pedicles. Ureteral position and integrity are checked again to ensure that they are intact and do not appear dilated.

Peritoneal Closure   The pelvic peritoneum is not reapproximated. Research using animal models suggests that reapproximation may increase tissue trauma and promote adhesion formation (77).

If the ovaries have been retained, they may be suspended to the pelvic sidewall to minimize the risk of their becoming retroperitoneal or adherent to the vaginal cuff.

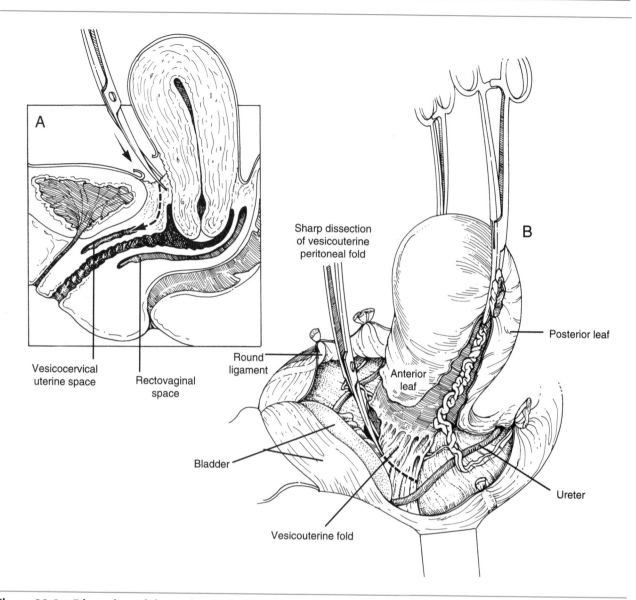

Figure 22.8   Dissection of the vesicouterine plane to mobilize the bladder. (From **Mann WA, Stovall TG.** *Gynecologic Surgery.* New York: Churchill Livingstone, 1996.)

Incision Closure   The parietal peritoneum is not reapproximated as a separate layer. Fascia can be closed with an interrupted or a suture of 0 or 1 monofilament absorbable suture. A continuous suture may reduce the risk of necrosis, which may occur when interrupted sutures are tied too tightly (77). As with interrupted sutures, bites should be taken approximately 1 cm from the cut edge of the fascia and approximately 1 cm apart to prevent wound dehiscence.

Skin Closure   The subcutaneous tissue should be irrigated with careful attention given to maintaining hemostasis. Subcutaneous sutures are not used because they may increase the incidence of wound infection (77). Skin staples or subcuticular sutures are used to reapproximate the skin edges. A bandage is applied and left in place for approximately 24 hours.

Intraoperative Complications

Most intraoperative injuries during abdominal hysterectomy can be traced to poor lighting, unsatisfactory assistance, undue haste, anatomic variants, or involvement of the injured or-

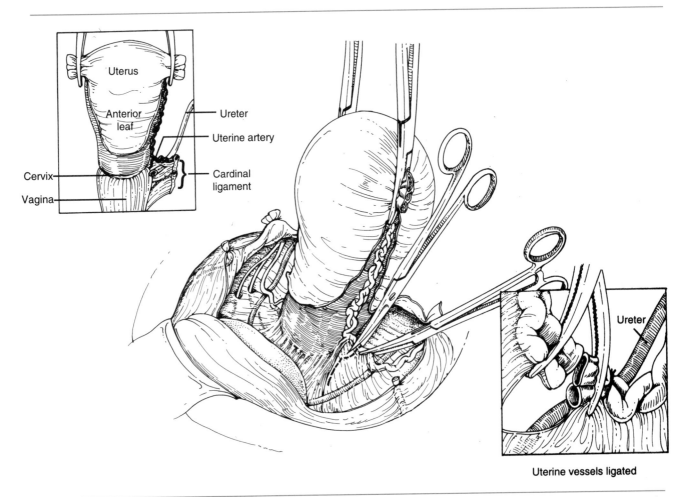

Figure 22.9   Ligation of the uterine blood vessels. (From **Mann WA, Stovall TG.** *Gynecologic Surgery.* New York: Churchill Livingstone, 1996.)

gan in the disease process (78). Some of these factors can be eliminated with careful attention to detail and use of proper surgical technique. However, some operative injuries cannot be avoided by even the most skilled surgeons. The surgeon, therefore, must be prepared to recognize and repair these injuries.

Ureteral Injuries

Injury to the pelvic ureter is one of the most formidable complications of hysterectomy (79–81). Because of the risk of subsequent renal impairment, injury to the ureter is far more serious than injury to the bladder or bowel (82, 83).

It is essential to be aware of the proximity of the ureter to the other pelvic structures at all times. **Most ureteral injuries can be avoided by opening the retroperitoneum and directly identifying the ureter.** The use of ureteral catheters as a substitute for direct visualization is often of little help in patients with extensive fibrosis or scarring resulting from endometriosis, pelvic inflammatory disease, or ovarian cancer. In these instances, a false sense of security may actually increase an already high risk of ureteral injury (84).

Direct visualization is accomplished by opening the retroperitoneum lateral to the external iliac artery. Blunt dissection of the loose areolar tissue is performed to directly visualize the artery. The artery may then be traced cephalad to the bifurcation of the

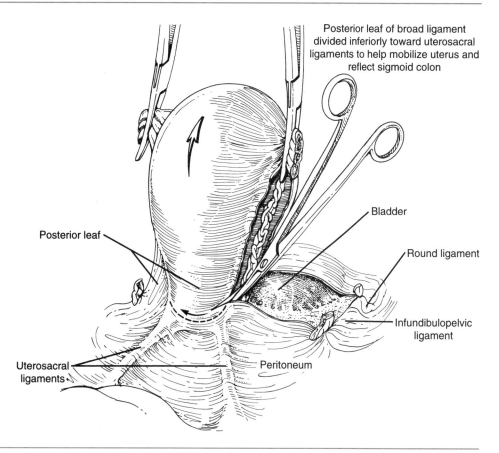

Posterior leaf of broad ligament divided inferiorly toward uterosacral ligaments to help mobilize uterus and reflect sigmoid colon

Bladder

Round ligament

Infundibulopelvic ligament

Posterior leaf

Peritoneum

Uterosacral ligaments

Figure 22.10   Incision of the rectouterine peritoneum and mobilization of the rectum from the posterior cervix. (From **Mann WA, Stovall TG.** *Gynecologic Surgery.* New York: Churchill Livingstone, 1996.)

internal and external iliac arteries. The ureter crosses the common iliac artery at its bifurcation and may be followed throughout its course in the pelvis.

Despite these precautions, ureteral injuries may occur. Prompt consultation is necessary if the surgeon has not been trained in ureteral repair. If a ureteral obstruction is suspected, confirmation may be obtained by intravenous injection of one ampule of indigo carmine dye, opening the dome of the bladder, and observing the presence or absence of bilateral spill of tinted urine. Alternatively, ureteral patency may be established by opening the dome of the bladder and positioning retrograde ureteral stents. Cystoscopic evaluation may replace opening the bladder to evaluate the spill of tinted urine (79–84).

Bladder Injury

Because of the close anatomic relationship of the bladder, uterus, and upper vagina, the bladder is the segment of the lower urinary tract that is most vulnerable to injury (82, 84). Bladder injury may occur on opening the peritoneum or, more frequently, during the dissection of the bladder off the cervix and upper vagina (85). Unless there is involvement of the bladder trigone, a bladder laceration is easily repaired. In the nonirradiated bladder, a one- or two-layer closure with a small-caliber braided absorbable suture such as a 3-0 polyglycolic acid is adequate. The bladder should be drained postoperatively. The length of time that drainage is required is controversial. In the noncompromised bladder, drainage should be continued at least until gross hematuria clears, which may occur as soon as 48

743

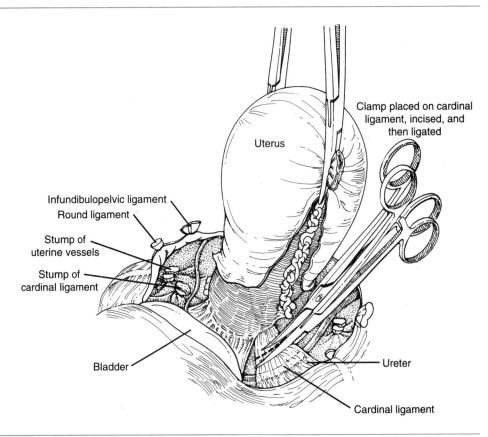

Figure 22.11   Ligation of the cardinal ligament. (From **Mann WA, Stovall TG.** *Gynecologic Surgery.* New York: Churchill Livingstone, 1996.)

hours postoperatively. A more conservative practice is to continue drainage until the patient is ready for discharge, usually a total of 3–4 days. Elective incision into the dome of the bladder is performed similarly (85). If the trigone is involved, a surgeon trained in complicated urologic repair should be consulted.

Bowel Injury

Small bowel injuries are the most common intestinal injuries in gynecologic surgery (86). Small defects of the serosa or muscularis may be repaired utilizing a single layer of continuous or interrupted 3–0 braided absorbable suture. Although single-layer closure of the small bowel has proven adequate, it is safer to close defects involving the lumen in two layers using a 3–0 braided absorbable suture. **The defect should be closed in a direction perpendicular to the intestinal lumen.** If a large area has been injured, resection with reanastomosis may be necessary (85, 87).

Because the bacterial flora of the ascending colon is similar to that of the small bowel, injuries can be repaired in a similar manner. The transverse colon rarely is injured in normal gynecologic procedures because it is well outside the operative field. However, the descending colon and the rectosigmoid colon are intimately involved with the pelvic structures and are at significant risk of injury during gynecologic surgery. Injuries not involving the mucosa may be repaired with a single running layer of 2-0 or 3-0 braided absorbable suture. If the laceration involves the mucosa, it may be closed as with small bowel injuries if the colon has been prepared adequately. Otherwise, diverting colostomy may be necessary in some patients to protect the repair site from fecal conta-

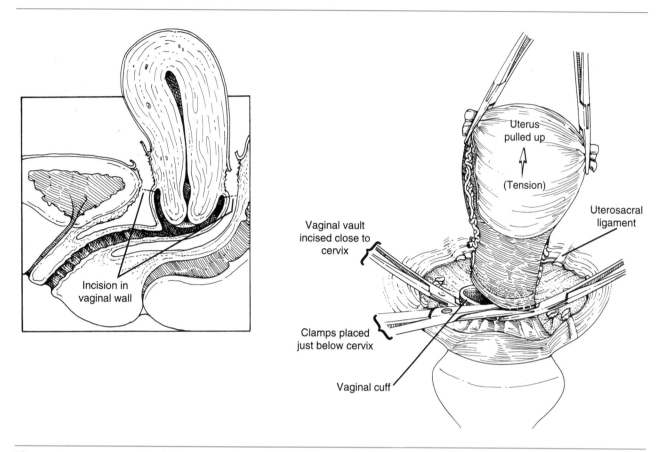

Uterus
pulled up

(Tension)

Uterosacral
ligament

Vaginal vault
incised close to
cervix

Clamps placed
just below cervix

Vaginal cuff

Incision in
vaginal wall

Figure 22.12   Removal of the uterus by transection of the vagina. (From **Mann WA, Stovall TG.** *Gynecologic Surgery.* New York: Churchill Livingstone, 1996.)

mination, especially if the defect is larger than 5 cm or if there is spillage of the bowel contents (85, 87).

Hemorrhage

Significant arterial bleeding usually arises from the uterine arteries or the ovarian vessels near the insertion of the infundibulopelvic ligaments (88). Blind clamping of these vessels presents a risk of ureteral injury; therefore, the ureters should be identified in the retroperitoneal space and traced to the area of bleeding to avoid inadvertent ligation. It is best to apply a pressure pack to tamponade the bleeding and then slowly remove the pack in an effort to visualize, isolate, and individually clamp the bleeding vessels. Mass ligatures should be avoided. The use of surgical clips may be helpful. Venous bleeding, while less dramatic, is often more difficult to manage, particularly in the presence of extensive adhesions and fibroids. This type of bleeding can be controlled with pressure alone or with suture ligation. Bleeding from peritoneal edges or denuded surfaces may be controlled with pressure, application of topical agents such as thrombin or collagen, or cautery with the Bovie or the argon beam laser.

Postoperative Care   ***Bladder Drainage***   Overdistension of the female bladder resulting from bladder trauma or the patient's reluctance to initiate the voluntary phase of voiding is one of the most common complications following abdominal hysterectomy (89). For this reason, an indwelling bladder catheter should be used for the first 18–24 postoperative hours.

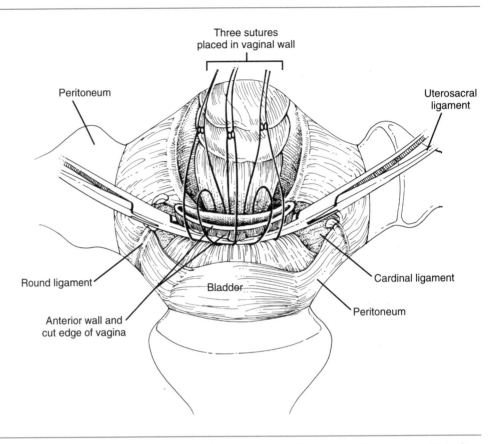

Figure 22.13   Vaginal cuff closure incorporating the uterosacral and cardinal ligaments. (From **Mann WA, Stovall TG.** *Gynecologic Surgery.* New York: Churchill Livingstone, 1996.)

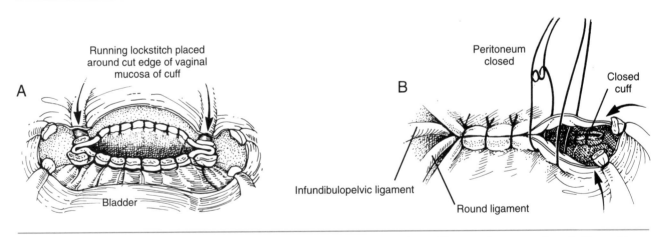

Figure 22.14   *A,* Vaginal cuff left open with a running suture along the cuff. *B,* Peritoneum closed. (From **Mann WA, Stovall TG.** *Gynecologic Surgery.* New York: Churchill Livingstone, 1996.)

If retropubic urethropexy has been performed, consideration should be given to using a suprapubic catheter, which allows postvoid residual levels to be checked without repetitive catheterizations. This catheter may be removed when satisfactory postvoid residual levels of <100 ml have been obtained.

Diet   In anticipation of the rare case in which the patient must be returned to the operating room, the patient is allowed only ice chips on the day of surgery. On the first postoperative day, assuming bowel sounds are present, diet is resumed, beginning with clear liquids and advancing to solid foods as tolerated. This dietary regimen assumes minimal intraoperative bowel manipulation and dissection. In patients who have undergone pelvic and para-aortic lymph node dissection, bowel surgery, or other extensive dissections, clear liquids should not be given until flatus has been passed. The diet should be advanced only as tolerated.

Activity   Early ambulation decreases the incidence of thrombophlebitis and pneumonia. Patients are encouraged to begin ambulation on their first postoperative day and to progressively increase their time out of bed as their strength improves. On discharge, the patient is instructed to avoid lifting more than 20 pounds for 6 weeks, thereby minimizing stress on fascia to allow full healing. Sexual intercourse is not recommended until 6 weeks postoperative. Patients are instructed to avoid driving until full mobility returns because postoperative pain and tenderness may hinder sudden braking or steering maneuvers in emergency situations. With these exceptions, the patient is encouraged to return to normal activities as soon as she feels comfortable doing so.

Wound Care   The abdominal incision normally requires little attention, except for ordinary hygienic measures. The wound is kept covered with a sterile bandage for the first 24 hours following surgery, by which time the incision has sealed itself. After the bandage has been removed, the incision should be cleaned daily with mild soap and water and kept dry.

Vaginal Hysterectomy

Preoperative Evaluation   ***Evaluation of Pelvic Support***   The most important observation in determining the feasibility of a vaginal hysterectomy is the demonstration of uterine mobility (89, 90). A vaginal approach should not be chosen if the uterus is not freely mobile. Pelvic support structures are elevated at the initial pelvic examination. In patients with no apparent prolapse, poor pelvic support can often be demonstrated by observing descent of the uterus with a series of Valsalva maneuvers. Although vaginal hysterectomy is easier to perform when the uterine supporting ligaments are lax, it is not an absolute requirement. Some gynecologists advocate the application of a tenaculum to the anterior cervical lip with subsequent traction applied as the patient bears down. Although this exercise may give some indication of uterine mobility, it is uncomfortable and not necessarily predictive of the success of vaginal hysterectomy. Therefore, the practice of applying traction to the cervix with a tenaculum to demonstrate descent of an apparently well-supported uterus is not recommended.

Evaluation of Pelvis   After assessment of pelvic support, the bony pelvis should be evaluated. Ideally, the angle of the pubic arch should be 90° or greater, the vaginal canal should be ample, and the posterior vaginal fornix should be wide and deep. The surgeon may use a closed fist to approximate the bituberous diameter, which should exceed 10 cm. The size and shape of the female pelvis contributes to increased exposure.

Surgical Considerations   ***Patient Positioning***   Once the patient is in the dorsal lithotomy position, the buttocks should be positioned just over the table's edge. Several stirrup types are available, including those that support the entire leg and those that suspend the legs in straps. To avoid nerve injury, adequate padding should be used; marked flexion of the thigh and pressure points should be avoided. Trendelenberg (10–15°) positioning aids with intravaginal visualization are needed during surgery.

Preparation   A povidone-iodine solution is applied to the vagina, the bladder is drained, and the catheter is removed. Several methods for draping have been proposed, including individual or single-piece drapes; the method chosen is at the surgeon's discretion. There is usually no need to shave or clip the pubic hair. Individual drapes with an adhesive barrier should be used to hold the drapes in place and prevent the pubic hair from compromising the field.

Instruments   Instruments that are useful in performing a vaginal hysterectomy include right-angled retractors, narrow Deaver retractors, weighted specula, Heaney needle holders, and an assortment of Briesky-Navratil vaginal retractors. Heaney and Heaney-Ballentine hysterectomy clamps are preferable. Several other clamps also are commonly used, including the Masterson clamp.

Lighting   Overhead high-intensity lamps should be used and positioned to direct light over the operator's shoulder. In addition, the surgeon may prefer a headlight, which can be worn to provide direct horizontal lighting. Although not routinely used, a fiberoptic-lighted irrigating suction system can provide additional light and transilluminate tissue planes.

Suture Material   Various suture materials have been advocated for gynecologic surgery. The type of suture material chosen should be based on the surgeon's preference. A synthetic delayed absorbable polyglactin or polyglycolic acid suture and atraumatic needles are generally preferable.

The Surgical Procedure

Examination Under Anesthesia   The patient is examined while anesthetized to confirm prior findings and to assess uterine mobility and descent. The decision is then made whether to proceed vaginally or abdominally.

Grasping and Circumscribing the Cervix   The anterior and posterior lips of the cervix are grasped with a single- or double-toothed tenaculum. With downward traction applied on the cervix, a circumferential incision is made in the vaginal epithelium at the junction of the cervix (Fig. 22.15).

Dissection of Vaginal Mucosa   After the initial incision is made, the vaginal epithelium may be dissected sharply from the underlying tissue or pushed bluntly with an open sponge (Fig. 22.16). If the initial incision is made too close to the external cervical os, there is a greater amount of dissection required and associated bleeding. Therefore, this circumscribing incision should be made just below the bladder reflection. It is important to continue the dissection in the correct cleavage plane, because dissection in the wrong plane will increase blood loss.

Posterior Cul-De-Sac Entry   The peritoneal reflection of the posterior cul-de-sac (cul-de-sac of Douglas) can be identified by stretching the vaginal mucosa and underlying connective tissue with forceps (Fig. 22.17). If difficulty is encountered (for example, if the cervix is elongated and the peritoneum is not evidence), the vaginal mucosa may be incised vertically to the point at which the cul-de-sac becomes more apparent.

If vaginal mucosal has been dissected in the wrong plane, the hysterectomy may be begun extraperitoneally by clamping and cutting the uterosacral and cardinal ligaments close to the cervix. The posterior cul-de-sac will then become readily identifiable.

If the peritoneal reflection of the posterior cul-de-sac still cannot be identified, entry into the anterior peritoneum is attempted and a finger is hooked into the posterior cul-de-sac to place tension on the peritoneum. The peritoneum is opened with Mayo scissors. An interrupted suture is placed to approximate the peritoneum and vaginal cuff and thus provide hemostasis (Fig. 22.18).

The posterior pelvic cavity is examined for pathologic alterations of the uterus or adhesive disease of the cul-de-sac. The weighted speculum is placed into the posterior cul-de-sac.

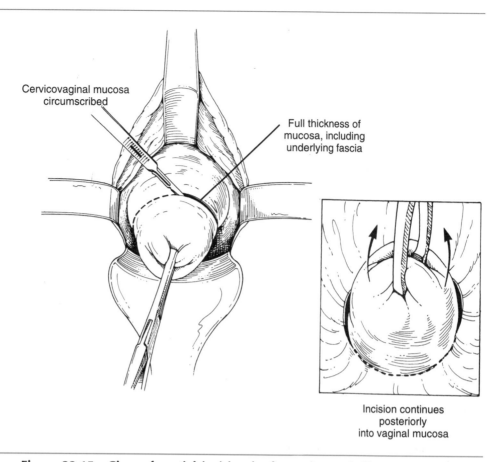

Figure 22.15   Circumferential incision in the vagina to infiltrate a vaginal hysterectomy. (From **Mann WA, Stovall TG.** *Gynecologic Surgery.* New York: Churchill Livingstone, 1996.)

Uterosacral Ligament Ligation   With retraction of the lateral vaginal wall and countertraction on the cervix, the uterosacral ligaments are clamped, with the tip of the clamp incorporating the lower portion of the cardinal ligaments (Fig. 22.19). The clamp is placed perpendicular to the uterine axis, and the pedicle is cut close to the clamp and sutured. A small pedicle (0.5 cm) distal to the clamp is optimal because a larger pedicle becomes necrotic and the tissue sloughs, which may present culture medium for microorganisms. The pedicle should be incised no more than one-half to three-fourths of the way around the tip of the clamp. Limiting the incision prevents the next pedicle, which may be vascular, from being cut.

When suturing any pedicle, the needle point is placed at the tip of the clamp, and the needle is passed through the tissue by a rolling motion of the operator's wrist. Once ligated, the uterosacral ligaments may be transfixed to the posterolateral vaginal mucosa (Fig. 22.20). This suture may lend additional support to the vagina and provides hemostasis at this point on the vaginal mucosa. This suture is held with a hemostat to facilitate location of any bleeding at the completion of the procedure and to aid in the closure of vaginal mucosa.

Entry Versus Nonentry into the Vesicovaginal Space (Cul-De-Sac)   Downward traction is placed on the cervix. Using either Mayo scissors, with the points directed toward the uterus, or an open moistened 4×8 gauze sponge, the bladder is advanced. If the vesicovaginal peritoneal reflection is easily identified at this point, the vesicovaginal space may be entered. Otherwise, it may be preferable to delay entry. There is no danger in delaying entry as long as the operator has ascertained that the bladder has been advanced.

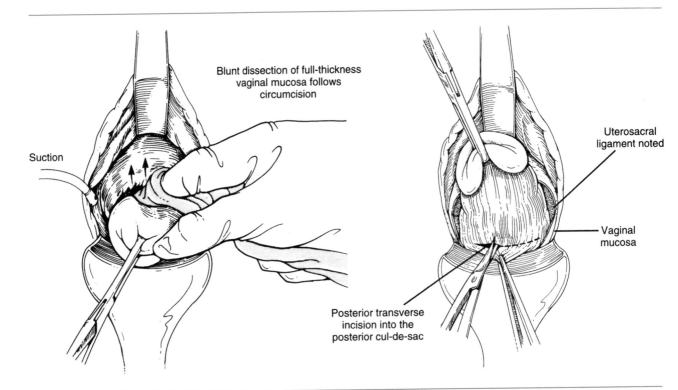

Figure 22.16   Dissection of the vaginal mucosa. (From **Mann WA, Stovall TG.** *Gynecologic Surgery.* New York: Churchill Livingstone, 1996.)

Figure 22.17   Entry into the posterior cul-de-sac. (From **Mann WA, Stovall TG.** *Gynecologic Surgery.* New York: Churchill Livingstone, 1996.)

Figure 22.18   Interrupted suture is placed on posterior vaginal cuff and peritoneum for hemostasis. (From **Mann WA, Stovall TG.** *Gynecologic Surgery.* New York: Churchill Livingstone, 1996.)

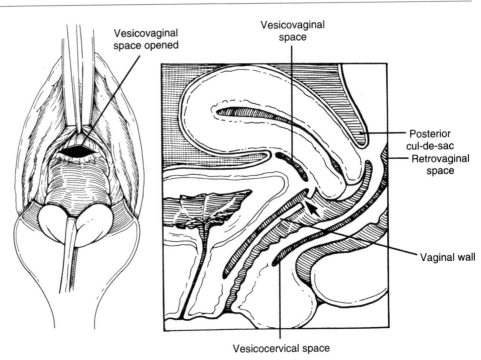

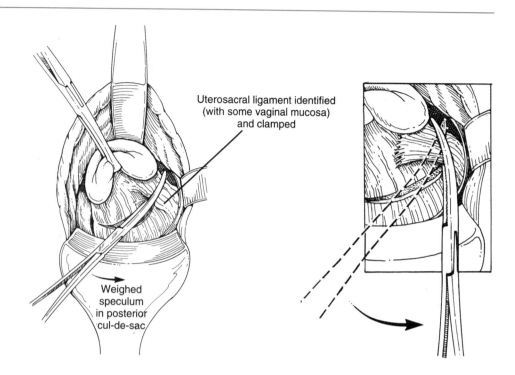

Figure 22.19   Ligation of the uterosacral ligaments. (From **Mann WA, Stovall TG.** *Gynecologic Surgery.* New York: Churchill Livingstone, 1996.)

After the bladder has been advanced, a curved Deaver or Heaney retractor is placed in the midline, holding the bladder out of the operative field. This process precedes each step of the vaginal hysterectomy until the vesicovaginal space is entered.

Cardinal Ligament Ligation   With traction on the cervix continued, the cardinal ligaments are identified, clamped, and cut and the suture is ligated (Fig. 22.21).

Advancement of Bladder   The bladder again is advanced out of the operative field. A blunt dissection technique may be used; however, sharp dissection may be helpful if the patient has had previous surgery such as cesarean delivery, which may have scarred the bladder reflection.

Uterine Artery Ligation   Contralateral and downward traction is placed on the cervix. With an effort to incorporate the anterior and posterior leaves of the visceral peritoneum, the uterine vessels are identified, clamped, and cut and the suture is ligated (Fig. 22.22). A single suture and single clamp technique is adequate and decreases the potential risk of ureteral injury. When the uterus is large or when a fibroid distorts the anatomical relationships, a second suture may be required to ligate any remaining branches of the uterine artery.

Entry into the Vesicovaginal Space   The anterior peritoneal fold usually can be identified readily just before or after clamping and suture ligation of the uterine arteries. The anterior peritoneal cavity should not be opened blindly because of the increased risk of bladder injury (Fig. 22.23). The peritoneum is grasped with forceps, tented, and opened with scissors with the tips pointed toward the uterus. A Heaney or Deaver retractor is then placed and the peritoneal contents are identified. This retractor serves to keep the bladder out of the operative field.

Delivery of the Uterus   A tenaculum is placed onto the uterine fundus in a successive fashion to deliver the fundus posteriorly (Fig. 22.24). The operator's index finger is used to identify the utero-ovarian ligament and aid in clamp placement.

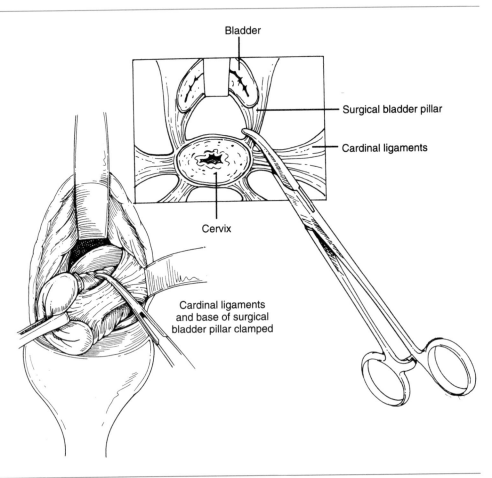

Figure 22.20   Transfixion of the uterosacral ligament to the posterolateral vaginal mucosa. (From **Mann WA, Stovall TG.** *Gynecologic Surgery.* New York: Churchill Livingstone, 1996.)

Utero-Ovarian and Round Ligament Ligation   With the posterior and anterior peritoneum opened, the remainder of the broad ligament and utero-ovarian ligaments are clamped, cut, and ligated (Fig. 22.25). The utero-ovarian and round ligament complexes are double-ligated with a suture tie followed by a ligature medial to the first suture. A hemostat is placed on the second suture to aid in the identification of any bleeding and to assist with peritoneal closure. A hemostat should not be placed on the first suture or any other vascular pedicle in order to avoid the risk of loosening the tie.

Removal of the Ovaries   When the adnexa are removed, the round ligaments should be removed separately from the adnexal pedicles. Traction is placed on the utero-ovarian pedicle. The ovary is drawn into the operative field by grasping it with a Babcock clamp. A Heaney clamp is placed across the infundibulopelvic ligament and the ovary and tube are excised (Fig. 22.26). A transfixion tie and suture ligature are placed on the infundibulopelvic ligament. The surgeon should not be reluctant to remove the fallopian tube separately from the ovary if taking them together risks loss of the tissue pedicle or injury to the ureter or nearby blood vessels.

Hemostasis   A retractor or tagged sponge is placed into the peritoneal cavity, and each of the pedicles is visualized and inspected for hemostasis. If additional sutures are required, they should be placed precisely with care to avoid the ureter or bladder.

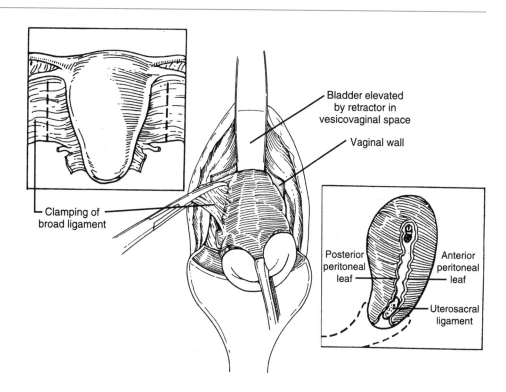

Figure 22.21   Ligation of the cardinal ligament. (From **Mann WA, Stovall TG.** *Gynecologic Surgery.* New York: Churchill Livingstone, 1996.)

Figure 22.22   Ligation of the uterine artery. (From **Mann WA, Stovall TG.** *Gynecologic Surgery.* New York: Churchill Livingstone, 1996.)

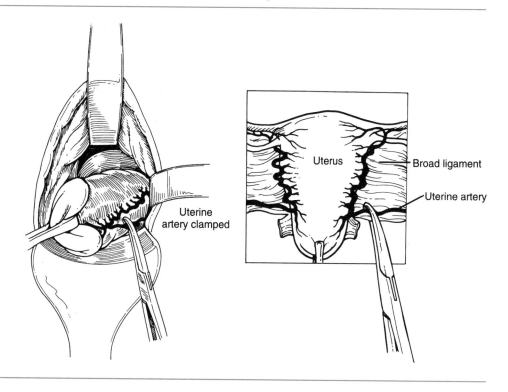

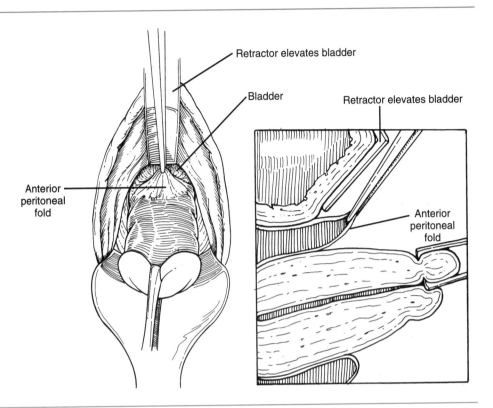

Labels in figure: Retractor elevates bladder; Bladder; Retractor elevates bladder; Anterior peritoneal fold; Anterior peritoneal fold

Figure 22.23   Entry into the vesicovaginal space. (From **Mann WA, Stovall TG.** *Gynecologic Surgery.* New York: Churchill Livingstone, 1996.)

Peritoneal Closure   Because the pelvic peritoneum does not provide support and reforms in 24 hours after surgery, the peritoneum need not be reapproximated routinely. If it is believed to be important, the anterior peritoneal edge is identified and grasped with forceps. A continuous absorbable 0 suture is begun at the 12-o'clock position. The suture is continued in a purse-string fashion and incorporates the distal portion of the left upper pedicle and the left uterosacral ligament (Fig. 22.27). Tension is applied to the suture placed at the beginning of the procedure that incorporates the posterior peritoneum and vaginal mucosa. This allows for high posterior reperitonealization, which shortens the cul-de-sac and thus helps to prevent future enterocele formation. The right uterosacral ligament and the distal portion of the right upper pedicle are incorporated, and this continuous suture ends at the point on the anterior peritoneum where it was begun.

The intra-abdominal tagged sponge is removed and inspected for the presence of blood at its distal end. The slack of the purse-string peritoneal suture is taken up by pulling the suture tight. Before tying the peritoneal suture, the surgeon should make certain that no prolapse of viscera has occurred.

Vaginal Mucosa Closure   The vaginal mucosa can be reapproximated in a vertical or horizontal manner, using either interrupted or continuous sutures (Fig. 22.28). The vaginal mucosa is, in this case, reapproximated horizontally with interrupted absorbable sutures. The sutures are placed through the entire thickness of the vaginal epithelium, with care to avoid entering the bladder anteriorly. These sutures will obliterate the underlying dead space and produce an anatomic approximation of the vaginal epithelium, thereby decreasing the postoperative formation of granulation tissue.

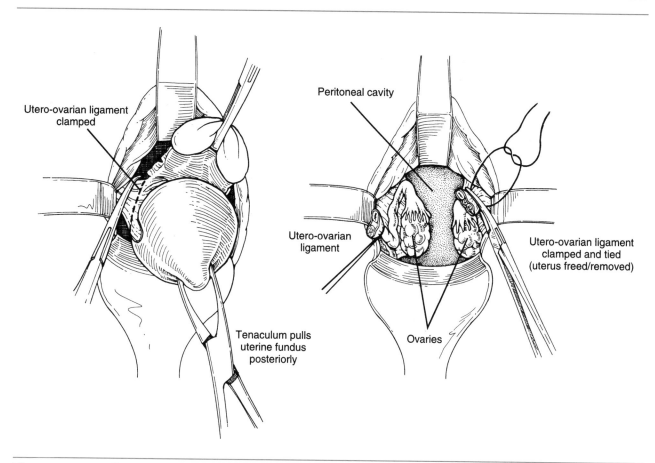

Figure 22.24   Delivery of the uterine fundus posteriorly. (From **Mann WA, Stovall TG.** *Gynecologic Surgery.* New York: Churchill Livingstone, 1996.)

Figure 22.25   Ligation of the utero-ovarian and round ligaments. (From **Mann WA, Stovall TG.** *Gynecologic Surgery.* New York: Churchill Livingstone, 1996.)

Bladder Drainage   After completion of the procedure, the bladder is drained. Unless an anterior or posterior colporrhaphy or other reconstructive procedure is performed, a bladder catheter or vaginal packing is not mandatory.

Surgical Techniques for Selected Patients

Injection of Vaginal Mucosa   The use of paracervical and submucosal injection of 20–30 ml of 0.5% *lidocaine* with 1:200,000 *epinephrine* prior to incision of the vaginal mucosa is believed by some to decrease postoperative pain and facilitate identification of surgical planes. There is no need to inject the cervix.

Areas to be injected include the bladder pillars, lower portion of the cardinal ligament, uterosacral ligaments, and paracervical tissue.

Morcellation of the Large Uterus   Uterine morcellation is a well known but often underutilized surgical procedure whereby the uterus is removed piecemeal. Several methods of uterine morcellation have been described (91), including hemisection or bivalving, wedge or "V" incisions, or intramyometrial coring. Prior to beginning any morcellation procedure, the uterine vessels must be ligated and the peritoneal cavity must be entered.

755

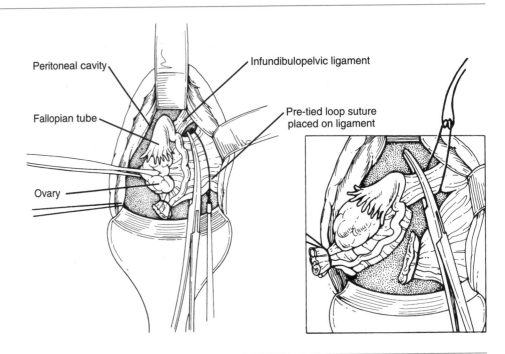

Figure 22.26   Removal of the ovaries and fallopian tubes by clamping across the infundibulopelvic ligament. (From **Mann WA, Stovall TG.** *Gynecologic Surgery.* New York: Churchill Livingstone, 1996.)

Figure 22.27   Closure of the peritoneum. (From **Mann WA, Stovall TG.** *Gynecologic Surgery.* New York: Churchill Livingstone, 1996.)

Figure 22.28   Closure of the vaginal mucosa. (From **Mann WA, Stovall TG.** *Gynecologic Surgery.* New York: Churchill Livingstone, 1996.)

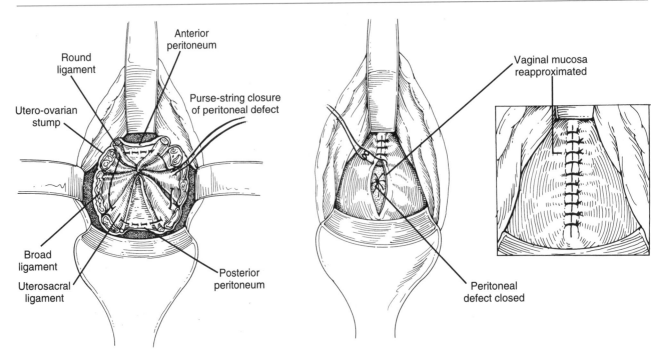

When uterine hemisection or bivalving is performed, the cervix is split at the midline and the uterus is cut into halves, which are removed separately (92, 93). This method seems best suited for fundal, midline leiomyomas.

Wedge morcellation is best suited for anterior or posterior fibroids or for fibroids in the other broad ligaments (i.e., when the fibroids are away from the midline) (93–97). The cervix is amputated, and the myometrium is grasped with clamps. Wedge-shaped portions of myometrium are removed from the anterior or posterior uterine wall. The apex of the wedge is kept in the midline, thereby reducing the bulk of the myometrium. This process is repeated until the uterus can be removed or until a pseudocapsule of a fibroid can be grasped with a Leahy clamp or towel clip. Traction is then applied, and a "myomectomy" is performed.

When the intramyometrial coring technique is utilized, the myometrium above the site of the ligated vessels is incised parallel to the axis of the uterine cavity and serosa of the uterus. This incision is continued around the full circumference of the myometrium in a symmetrical fashion beneath the uterine serosa. Traction is maintained on the cervix, and the avascular myometrium is cut to allow the undisturbed endometrial cavity, with a thick layer of myometrium, to be delivered with the cervix. As a result, the inside of the uterus with its unopened endometrial cavity is brought closer to the operator. Incision of the lateral portions of the myometrium medial to the remaining attachment of the broad ligament results in considerable additional descent of the uterus and greatly increases the mobility of the uterine fundus. The uterus is converted from a globular to an elongated tissue mass. The cored uterus is removed by clamping the utero-ovarian pedicle and fallopian tubes.

McCall Culdoplasty

McCall culdoplasty may help decrease future enterocele formation (96). An absorbable suture is placed through the full thickness of the posterior vaginal wall at the point of the highest portion of the vaginal vault. The patient's left uterosacral ligament pedicle is grasped and sutured. The suture then incorporates the posterior peritoneum, between the uterosacral ligaments, and the right uterosacral ligament. The suture is completed by passing the needle from the inside to the outside at the same point at which it was begun. The suture is tied, thereby approximating the uterosacral ligaments and the posterior peritoneum.

Schuchardt's Incision

When vaginal exposure is difficult, the Schuchardt's incision may be utilized (96). If the surgeon is right-handed, the incision is made on the patient's left side. To decrease blood loss, the area can be infiltrated with *lidocaine*-containing *epinephrine*. The incision follows a curved line from the 4 o'clock position at the hymenal margin to a point halfway between the anus and the ischial tuberosity. The incision may be continued as high as necessary in the vaginal vault to gain exposure. The depth of the incision is the medial portion of the pubococcygeus muscle, which may be divided in extreme cases. The incision must be closed in layers at the completion of the procedure.

Intraoperative Complications

Bladder Injury

Injury to the urinary bladder is one of the most common intraoperative complications associated with hysterectomy. **If the bladder is inadvertently entered, repair generally should be performed when the injury is discovered and not delayed until completion of surgery** (84). When bladder injury is recognized, the edges of the wound should be mobilized to assess the full extent of the injury and to allow repair without tension. This assessment should include visualization of the trigone to exclude injury to that area. The bladder may then be repaired with a single- or double-layered closure with a small-caliber absorbable suture. Methylene blue or a dye sterile milk formula can be instilled into the bladder to ensure that the repair is adequate..

Bowel Injury

Because patients with suspected pelvic adhesions or obvious pelvic disease are excluded as candidates for vaginal hysterectomy, bowel injuries do not often occur. Bowel injuries more often are associated with the performance of a posterior colporrhaphy and are usually confined to the rectum (84, 96).

If the rectum is entered, the injury is repaired with a single- or double-layer closure using a small-caliber absorbable suture, followed by copious irrigation. Postoperatively, the patient should be given a stool softener and a low-residue diet.

Hemorrhage

Intraoperative hemorrhage invariably is the result of failure to securely ligate a significant blood vessel, bleeding from the vaginal cuff, slippage of a previously placed ligature or avulsion of tissue prior to clamping (96). Most intraoperative bleeding can be avoided with adequate exposure and good surgical technique. Using square knots with attention to proper knot-tying mechanisms will prevent bleeding in most cases. Likewise, the use of Heaney-type sutures minimizes ligature slippage and subsequent bleeding. When bleeding does occur, blind clamping, which may endanger the ureter, should be avoided. The bleeding vessel should be identified and precisely ligated with visualization of the ureter if necessary. If the location of the ureter is in question, it should be visualized prior to suturing a bleeding vessel. Although excessive blood loss occasionally will occur despite these precautions, it should be infrequent.

Perioperative Care

Bladder Drainage   Postoperative bladder drainage should be employed after any procedure in which spontaneous, complete voiding is not anticipated. Reasons to consider closed bladder drainage include significant local pain, additional vaginal reparative procedures, surgery for stress incontinence, the use of a vaginal pack, and patient anxiety.

Following vaginal hysterectomy without additional repair, most patients can void spontaneously and, therefore, catheter drainage is not required. The relative amount of pain after a vaginal hysterectomy is less than with abdominal hysterectomy and, in the absence of additional repairs or a pack, no obstructive effect should be present.

If the patient does not tolerate pain well postoperatively or is extremely anxious, the transurethral insertion of a 16-Fr catheter after completing surgery is warranted. This catheter may also be inserted postoperatively if the patient is unable to void spontaneously on two attempts. Closed-catheter drainage after vaginal hysterectomy usually is not necessary for longer than 24 hours. The catheter is removed without clamping and there is no need to obtain a urine specimen for culture and sensitivity.

Diet   Although little manipulation of the bowel occurs during vaginal hysterectomy, there is some slowing of gastrointestinal motility. This slowing rarely occurs to a degree that limits some form of oral intake soon after surgery. Most patients experience some degree of nausea after surgery, which, combined with drowsiness from analgesics, usually makes them disinterested in food on the evening after surgery. A clear liquid diet is suitable during the first 24 hours postoperatively. On the first full postoperative day, a regular diet can usually be consumed. The patient is often the best judge of what she can tolerate.

Perioperative Complications of Hysterectomy

A comprehensive discussion of postoperative complications after gynecologic surgery is presented in Chapter 19.

Wound Infections

Wound infections occur after 4–6% of abdominal hysterectomies (29). Measures believed to reduce the incidence of wound infections include a preoperative shower, no removal of hair, removal of hair with clippers in the operating room if hair removal is necessary, use of adhesive drapes and prophylactic antibiotics, and delayed primary closure (see Chapter 19).

Hemorrhage

Hemorrhage immediately after hysterectomy may present in one of two ways (88). First, bleeding from the vagina may be noted by the nursing staff or physician within the first few hours after surgery. Second, and less commonly, the patient may be noted to have little bleeding from the vagina but deteriorating vital signs manifest by low blood pressure and rapid pulse, falling hematocrit level, and flank or abdominal pain. The first presentation usually represents bleeding from the vaginal cuff or one of the pedicles. The second presentation may represent a retroperitoneal hemorrhage. Each situation is approached differently in its evaluation and treatment, but both involve the same general principles of rapid diagnosis, stabilization of vital signs, appropriate fluid and blood replacement, and constant surveillance of the patient's overall condition (98).

After vital signs are assessed, attention should be directed to the amount of bleeding. A small amount of bleeding is expected after any vaginal hysterectomy. However, steady bleeding 2–3 hours after surgery suggests lack of hemostasis. The patient should be taken promptly to the examining room, where the operative site is viewed using a large speculum and good lighting. If bleeding is not excessive, the vaginal cuff can be inspected and, in many instances, bleeding from the cuff edge will be found. Hemostasis can easily be achieved with one or two sutures placed through the mucosa.

If bleeding is excessive or appears to be coming from above the cuff, or if the patient is too uncomfortable to tolerate adequate examination, she should be taken to the operating room. General anesthesia should be administered and the vaginal operative site should be thoroughly explored. Any bleeding point may be sutured or ligated. However, bleeding that is coming from above the cuff or is extremely brisk usually cannot be controlled through the vaginal route. An exploratory laparotomy is necessary to examine the pelvic floor, identify and isolate the bleeding vessel, and achieve hemostasis. The ovarian vessels and uterine arteries should be thoroughly inspected because they often are the source of excessive vaginal bleeding. If it is difficult to localize bleeding to a specific pelvic vessel, ligation of the hypogastric artery may be necessary.

In the patient with little vaginal bleeding in whom vital signs have deteriorated, retroperitoneal hemorrhage should be suspected. Input and output should be monitored. Hematocrit assessment along with cross-matching should be be performed immediately. Examination may reveal tenderness and dullness in the flank. In cases of intraperitoneal bleeding, abdominal distension may occur. Diagnostic radiologic studies can be used to confirm the presence of retroperitoneal or intra-abdominal bleeding. Ultrasonography is one option for viewing low pelvic hematomas. Computerized tomography provides better visualization of retroperitoneal spaces, however, and can delineate a hematoma.

If the patient's condition stabilizes rapidly with intravenous fluids, one of two approaches may be used for continued care. The first is to give the patient a transfusion and follow serial hematocrit assessments and vital signs. In many instances, retroperitoneal bleeding will tamponade and stop, forming a hematoma that may eventually be resorbed. The risk with this approach is that the hematoma will later become infected, necessitating surgical drainage. In some instances when the patient's condition is stable, radiologic embolization may be considered.

Another option is to perform abdominal exploratory surgery while the patient's condition is stable. This approach adds the morbidity of a second procedure but avoids the possibility of the patient's condition deteriorating with continued delay or the formation of a pelvic abscess. Once adequate exposure is obtained, the peritoneum over the hematoma should be opened and the blood should be evacuated. All bleeding vessels should be identified and ligated. Again, if control of bleeding is difficult, consideration should be given to unilateral or bilateral ligation of the anterior division of the internal iliac artery. Once hemostasis is achieved, the pelvis should be drained using a closed system.

Urinary Tract Complications of Hysterectomy

Urinary Retention

Urinary retention after hysterectomy is an uncommon occurrence (32). If the urethra is unobstructed and retention occurs, it is usually the result of either pain or bladder atony resulting from anesthesia. Both are temporary effects.

If a catheter was not placed after surgery, retention can be initially relieved with the insertion of a Foley catheter for 12–24 hours. Most patients are able to void after the catheter is removed 1 day later. If the patient still has trouble voiding and urethral spasm is suspected, success often can be achieved with a skeletal muscle relaxant such as *diazepam* (2 mg twice a day). In most cases, waiting is the best course and voiding usually occurs spontaneously.

Ureteral Injury

In patients with flank pain developing soon after vaginal hysterectomy, ureteral obstruction should be suspected. The incidence of ureteral injury is lower with vaginal hysterectomy than with abdominal hysterectomy (83). One risk factor for its occurrence is total uterine prolapse, in which the ureters are drawn outside the bony pelvis.

In a patient with flank pain in whom ureteral obstruction is suspected, intravenous pyelography and urinalysis should be performed (80). If obstruction is noted on intravenous pyelography, it is usually present near the ureterovesical junction. The first immediate step should be attempted passage of a catheter through the ureter under cystoscopic guidance. If a catheter can be passed through the ureter, it should be left in place for at least 4–6 weeks, allowing sutures to absorb and the obstruction or kinking to release. If the catheter cannot be passed through the ureter, the best course is to perform abdominal exploratory surgery and repair the ureter at the site of obstruction (79–84).

Vesicovaginal Fistula

Vesicovaginal fistulas occur most often after total abdominal hysterectomy for benign gynecologic disease (83). Intraoperative steps to avoid the formation of a vesicovaginal fistula include correct identification of the proper plane between the bladder and cervix, sharp rather than blunt dissection of the bladder, and care in clamping and suturing the vaginal cuff. The development of a postoperative vesicovaginal fistula following hysterectomy is rare; the incidence is as low as 0.2% (82, 83).

The patient with a postoperative vesicovaginal fistula presents 10–14 days after surgery with a watery vaginal discharge. Some fistulas resulting from surgery are noted as early as the first 48–72 hours postoperatively (84). After vaginal examination with a speculum, the diagnosis can usually be confirmed with the insertion of a cotton tampon into the vagina followed by the instillation of *methylene blue* or *indigo carmine* dye via a transurethral catheter. If the tampon stains blue, a vesicovaginal fistula is present. If no staining occurs, however, the presence of a ureterovaginal fistula must be ruled out by the intravenous injection of 5 ml *indigo carmine* dye. Within 20 minutes, the tampon should stain blue if a ureterovaginal fistula is present. Intravenous pyelography should also be performed to rule out ureteral obstruction.

If a vesicovaginal fistula is diagnosed, a Foley catheter should be inserted for prolonged drainage. As many as 15% of fistulas will spontaneously close with 4–6 weeks of continuous bladder drainage. If closure has not occurred by 6 weeks, operative correction is necessary. Waiting 3–4 months from the time of diagnosis before operative repair is recommended to allow reduction of inflammation and to improve vascular supply. After vaginal hysterectomy, the fistula site is above the bladder trigone and away from the ureters. Vaginal repair can be anticipated in most patients. The surgical correction is generally undertaken in a four-layered closure: the bladder mucosa, the seromuscular layer, the endopelvic fascia, and the vaginal epithelium.

Incidental cystotomy at the time of hysterectomy is more common than vesicovaginal fistula. When repaired correctly, cystotomy rarely results in the development of a fistula (82).

Prolapse of the Fallopian Tube

Posthysterectomy prolapse of the fallopian tube is a rare event and is often confused with granulation tissue at the vaginal apex (32). Predisposing factors for the development of fallopian tube prolapse include development of a hematoma and an abscess developing at the vaginal apex. As many as 50% of patients undergoing vaginal hysterectomy will form some granulation tissue at the vaginal vault. In patients in whom granulation tissue persists after attempts to cauterize it or pain is experienced with attempts to remove it, fallopian tube prolapse should be suspected. A biopsy of the area is warranted and will usually reveal tubal epithelium if a fallopian tube is present.

If fallopian tube prolapse is diagnosed, it should be repaired with surgery. In general, the surrounding vaginal mucosa should be opened and undermined widely. The tube is then ligated high and removed followed by closure of the vaginal mucosa.

Discharge Instructions

Before discharging the patient, instructions should be reviewed. Printed postoperative instructions are helpful to the patient and should include the following information:

1. Avoid strenuous activity for the first 2 weeks and increase activity level gradually.

2. Avoid heavy lifting, douching, or sexual intercourse until the instructed by the doctor.

3. Bathing may consist of showering or tub baths.

4. Follow a regular diet.

5. Avoid straining for a bowel movement or urination. For constipation, use Milk of Magnesia or Metamucil (1 tsp in juice).

6. Call the physician if excessive vaginal bleeding or fever occurs.

7. Schedule a return appointment at the time specified by the doctor.

The physician should provide phone numbers for emergencies both during and after office hours. Typically, the first postoperative visit is scheduled approximately 4 weeks after discharge from the hospital. At the time of that visit, the patient should be ambulating well and vaginal discharge or bleeding should be minimal. Speculum examination of the cuff should be gentle and cursory, but the patient should be assured that the healing process is proceeding normally. Finally, the patient's questions should be answered and advice should be given on increasing her activity level, including sexual activity, work, and normal household activity.

Psychosomatic Aspects of Hysterectomy

The decision to proceed with hysterectomy should be made jointly by the patient and her physician. Factors leading a patient or her physician to choose hysterectomy and reasons that patients with similar conditions choose different treatments are uncertain. For many patients, the decision to undergo hysterectomy may be sudden. They face the potential risks of anesthesia and surgery, and, if premenopausal, they must also cope with the loss of menstruation and the ability to procreate. Many women are concerned that the procedure will result in a loss of femininity, a decrease in sexual satisfaction, or an increase in interpersonal problems with their spouses. The concern over the loss of the reproductive tract is greater than that related to the loss of other intra-abdominal organs (99). To minimize the possibility that the patient has a poor outcome, preoperative counseling and preparation are essential.

Drellich and Bieber studied 23 women after hysterectomy. Most of these women regretted the loss of menstruation, which was true even for women who had experienced dysmenorrhea (100). Several of these women viewed the menstrual cycle as a way for the body to "rid itself of waste," and they felt better after the menstrual phase of their cycle.

Depression

There is wide variation in women's responses to hysterectomy. Most studies suggest that there is little evidence that hysterectomy increases the risk of depression. Some investigators have reported depression and an increased incidence of psychiatric symptoms after hysterectomy (101, 102). Hollender reported that almost twice as many women were admitted to a psychiatric hospital after pelvic operations compared with other types of surgery (103). However, other authors have not found such an association (104), and some report a decrease in symptoms after hysterectomy (105–109). The impact of hysterectomy on the development of depression is unknown because most studies are retrospective and not well controlled for preoperative depression (Chapter 12).

Patients who had a moderate amount of preoperative anxiety do much better postoperatively than patients with little or no anxiety or patients who had an exaggerated response (110). Both long delays prior to surgery and a very short time before surgery increase patients' anxiety. Thus, women should be scheduled for surgery several weeks in advance to avoid this problem (110). Women who planned to have children in the future had more problems during the immediate postoperative period. The patient's response to previous loss (e.g., death of family members) predicted her response after hysterectomy (111).

Sexuality

The incidence of sexual dysfunction after hysterectomy ranges from 10 to 40%. Estimates vary based on study variations, cultural variations, and the definitions used to make the diagnosis. Some report a decrease in libido after hysterectomy, whereas others suggest that libido is increased because of the reduced fear of unwanted pregnancy (102, 112). Humphries found that most patients do not have a change in their sexual practices after hysterectomy (113), whereas others report a deterioration of sexual relations (114). Preoperative anxiety about sexual functioning is often associated with an overall deterioration of sexual relations (115).

The literature supports that hysterectomy does not cause psychiatric sequelae or diminished sexual functioning in most patients. The best predictor of satisfaction after hysterectomy is the patient's preoperative understanding of the procedure. **The best predictor of postoperative sexual functioning is the patient's preoperative sexual satisfaction.** Preoperatively, these issues should be discussed with the patient, and her questions and concerns should be addressed to decrease the fear and anxiety.

References

1. **Benrubi GI.** History of hysterectomy. *J Fla Med Assoc* 1988;75:533–8.

2. **U.S. Department of Health and Human Services, Public Health Services, Center for Disease Control.** *National Hospital Discharge Survey, Annual Summary.* (Vital and Health Statistics. Series 13, Data from the National Health Survey). Hyattsville, MD: U.S. Department of Health and Human Services, 1991.

3. **Pokras R.** Hysterectomy: past, present and future. *Stat Bull Metrop Insur Co* 1989;70:12.

4. **Spencer G.** *Projections of the Population of the United States, by Age, Sex, and Race, 1983 to 2080.* (Current Population Reports. Population estimates and projections. Series P-25; no. 952). Washington, DC: U.S. Dept. of Commerce, Bureau of the Census, 1984.

5. **Pokras R, Hufnagel VG.** Hysterectomy in the United States, 1965-84. *Am J Public Health* 1988;78:852–3.

6. **Roos NP.** Hysterectomy: variations in rates across small areas and across physicians' practices. *Am J Public Health* 1984;74:327–35.

7. **Dicker RC, Scally MJ, Greenspan JR, Layde PM, Ory HW, Maze JM, et al.** Hysterectomy among women of reproductive age: trends in the United States, 1970–1978. *JAMA* 1982;248: 323–7.

8. **Domenighetti G, Luraschi P, Marazzi A.** Hysterectomy and sex of the gynecologist. *N Engl J Med* 1985;313:1482.

9. **Kjerulff KH, Guzinski GM, Langenberg PW, Stolley PD, Moyee NEA, Kazandjian VA.** Hysterectomy and race. *Obstet Gynecol* 1993;82:757–64.

10. **Gambone JC, Reifer RC.** Hysterectomy. *Clin Obstet Gynecol* 1990;33:205–11.

11. **Parker WH, Fu YS, Berek JS.** Uterine sarcoma in patients operated for presumed leiomyomata and presumed rapidly growing leiomyoma. *Obstet Gynecol* 1994;83:814–78.

12. **Friedman AJ, Haas ST.** Should uterine size be an indication for surgical intervention in women with myomas? *Am J Obstet Gynecol* 1993;168:751–5.

13. **Coddington CC, Collins RL, Shawker THE.** Long-acting gonadotropin hormone-releasing analog used to treat uteri. *Fertil Steril* 1986;45:624–9.

14. **West CP, Lumsden MA, Lawson S.** Shrinkage of uterine fibroids during therapy with Goserelin (Zoladex): a leutinizing hormone-releasing hormone agonist administered as a monthly subcutaneous depot. *Fertil Steril* 1987;48:45–51.

15. **Stovall TG, Ling FW, Henry LC.** A randomized trial evaluating leuprolide acetate prior to hysterectomy for leiomyomata. *Am J Obstet Gynecol* 1991;164:1420–5.

16. **Nilsson L, Rybo G.** Treatment of menorrhagia. *Am J Obstet Gynecol* 1971;110:713–20.

17. **Dawood MY.** Current concepts in the etiology and treatment of primary dysmenorrhea. *Acta Obstet Gynecol Scan Suppl* 1986;138:7–10.

18. **Halbert DR, Demers LM, Fontana J, Jones DE.** Prostaglandin levels in endometrial jet wash specimens in patients with dysmenorrhea before and after indomethacin therapy. *Prostaglandins* 1975;10:1047–56.

19. **Chan WY, Dawood MY, Fuchs F.** Prostaglandins in primary dysmenorrhea: comparison of prophylactic and nonprophylactic treatment with ibuprofen and use of oral contraceptives. *Am J Med* 1981;70:535–41.

20. **Gambone JC, Reiter RC.** Nonsurgical management of chronic pelvic pain: a multidisciplinary approach. *Clin Obstet Gynecol* 1990;33:205–11.

21. **Reiter RC, Gambone JC.** Demographic and historic variables in women with idiopathic chronic pelvic pain. *Obstet Gynecol* 1990;75:428–32.

22. **Rapkin AJ, Kames LD.** The pain management approach to chronic pelvic pain. *J Reprod Med* 1987;32:323–7.

23. **Carlson KJ, Miller BA, Fowler FJ.** The Maine women's health study: I. Outcomes of hysterectomy. *Obstet Gynecol* 1994;83:556–65.

24. **Stovall TG, Ling FW, Crawford DA.** Hysterectomy for chronic pelvic pain of presumed uterine etiology. *Obstet Gynecol* 1990;75:676–9.

25. **Anderson MC, Hartley RB.** Cervical crypt involvement by intraepithelial neoplasia. *Obstet Gynecol* 1980;55:546–50.

26. **Enblad P, Adami HO, Glimelius B, Krusemou U, Pahlman L.** The risk of subsequent primary malignant diseases after cancers of the colon and rectum: a nationwide cohort study. *Cancer* 1990;65:2091–100.

27. **Stearns MW Jr.** Benign and malignant neoplasms of colon and rectum: diagnosis and management. *Surg Clin North Am* 1978;58:605–18.

28. **Gambone JC, Reiter RC, Lench JB.** Short-term outcome of incidental hysterectomy at the time of adnexectomy for benign disease. *J Womens Health* 1992;1:197–200.

29. **Easterday CL, Grimes DA, Riggs JA.** Hysterectomy in the United States. *Obstet Gynecol* 1983;62:203–12.

30. **Copenhaver EH.** Hysterectomy: vaginal versus abdominal. *Surg Clin North Am* 1965;45:751–63.

31. **White SC, Wartel LJ, Wade ME.** Comparison of abdominal and vaginal hysterectomies: a review of 600 operations. *Obstet Gynecol* 1971;37:530–7.

32. **Dicker RC, Greenspan JR, Strauss LT, Cowart MR, Scally MJ, Peterson HB, et al.** Complications of abdominal and vaginal hysterectomy among women of reproductive age in the United States: the collaborative review of sterilization. *Am J Obstet Gynecol* 1982;144:841–8.

33. **Kovac SR.** Guidelines to determine the route of hysterectomy. *Obstet Gynecol* 1995;85:18–23.

34. **Hasson HM.** Cervical removal at hysterectomy for benign disease: risks and benefits. *J Reprod Med* 1993;38:781–90.

35. **Drife J.** Conserving the cervix at hysterectomy. *Br J Obstet Gynaecol* 1994;101:563–4.

36. **Kilkku P, Lehtinen V, Hirvonen T, Gronroos M.** Abdominal hysterectomy versus supravaginal uterine amputation: psychic factors. *Ann Chir Gynaecol Suppl* 1987;76:62–7.

37. **Kilkku P, Hirvonen T, Gronroos M.** Supra-vaginal uterine amputation vs. abdominal hysterectomy: the effects on urinary symptoms with special reference to pollakisuria, nocturia and dysuria. *Maturitas* 1981;3:197–204.

38. **Kilkku P, Gronroos M, Hirvonen T, Rauramo L.** Supravaginal uterine amputation vs. hysterectomy. *Acta Obstet Gynecol Scand* 1983;62:147–52.

39. **Kilkku P.** Supravaginal uterine amputation vs. hysterectomy: effects on coital frequency and dyspareunia. *Acta Obstet Gynecol Scand* 1983;62:141–5.

40. **Cartwright DS.** Diagnostic laparoscopy immediately preceding elective hysterectomy. *Proc Am Assoc Gynecol Laparosc* 1992;18:88–9.

41. **Stovall TG, Elder RE, Ling FW.** Predictors of pelvic adhesions. *J Reprod Med* 1989;34:345–8.

42. **Howard FM, Sanchez R.** A comparison of laparoscopically assisted vaginal hysterectomy and abdominal hysterectomy. *J Gynecol Surg* 1993;9:83–90.

43. **Jones RA.** Laparoscopic hysterectomy: a series of 100 cases. *Med J Aust* 1993;159:447–9.

44. **Kovac SR, Cruikshank SH, Retto HF.** Laparoscopic-assisted vaginal hysterectomy. *J Gynecol Surg* 1990;6:185–93.

45. **Saye WB, Espy GB III, Bishop MR, Slinkard P, Miller W, Hertzmann P.** Laparoscopic Doderlein hysterectomy: a rational alternative to traditional abdominal hysterectomy. *Surg Laparosc Endosc* 1993;3:88–94.

46. **Summitt RL Jr, Stovall TG, Lipscomb GH, Ling FW.** Randomized comparison of laparoscopic-assisted vaginal hysterectomy with standard vaginal hysterectomy in an outpatient setting. *Obstet Gynecol* 1992;80:895–901.

47. **Johns DA, Diamond MP.** Laparoscopically assisted vaginal hysterectomy. *J Reprod Med* 1994;39:424–8.

48. **Liu CY.** Laparoscopic hysterectomy. Report of 215 cases. *Gynaecol Endos* 1992;1:73–7.

49. **Nezhat F, Nezhat CH, Admon D, Gordon S, Nezhat C.** Complications and results of 361 hysterectomies performed at laparoscopy. *J Am Coll Surg* 1995;180:307–16.

50. **Raju KS, Auld BJ.** A randomized prospective study of laparoscopic vaginal hysterectomy versus abdominal hysterectomy each with bilateral salpingo-oophorectomy. *Br J Obstet Gynaecol* 1994;101:1068–71.

51. **Nezhat F, Nezhat C, Gordon S, Wilkins E.** Laparoscopic versus abdominal hysterectomy. *J Reprod Med* 1992;37:247–50.

52. **Daniell JF, Kurtz BR, McTavish G, Gurley LD, Shearer RA, Chambers JF, et al.** Laparoscopically assisted vaginal hysterectomy: the initial Nashville, Tennessee, experience. *J Reprod Med* 1993;38:537–42.

764

53. **Davis GD, Wolgamott G, Moon J.** Laparoscopically assisted vaginal hysterectomy as definitive therapy for stage III and IV endometriosis. *J Reprod Med* 1993;38:577–81.

54. **Coulam CB, Pratt JH.** Vaginal hysterectomy: is previous pelvic operation a contraindication? *Am J Obstet Gynecol* 1973;116:252–60.

55. **Mengert WF.** Mechanisms of uterine support and position. I. Factors influencing uterine support (an experimental study). *Am J Obstet Gynecol* 1936;31:775–82.

56. **Photopulos GJ, Stovall TG, Summitt RL Jr.** Laparoscopic-assisted vaginal hysterectomy, bilateral salpingo-oophorectomy, and pelvic lymph node sampling for endometrial cancer. *J Gynecol Surg* 1992;8:91–4.

57. **Sheth SS.** The place of oophorectomy at vaginal hysterectomy. *Br J Obstet Gynaecol* 1991;98: 662–6.

58. **Schweppe KW, Beller FK.** Prophylactic oophorectomy. *Geburtshilfe Frauenheilkd* 1979; 39(12):1024–32.

59. **Randall CL, Hall DW, Armenia CS.** Pathology in the preserved ovary after unilateral oophorectomy. *Am J Obstet Gynecol* 1962;84(9):1233–41.

60. **Lynch HT, Guirgis HA, Albert S, Brennan M, Lynch J, Kraft C, et al.** Familial association of carcinoma of the breast and ovary. *Surg Gynecol Obstet* 1974;138(5):717–24.

61. **American College of Obstetricians and Gynecologists.** Familiar ovarian cancer. *ACOG Technical Bulletin.* Washington DC, American College of Obstetricians and Gynecologists, 1993.

62. **Ryan PJ, Harrison R, Blake GM, Fogelman I.** Compliance with hormone replacement therapy (HRT) after screening for postmenopausal osteoporosis. *Br J Obstet Gynaecol* 1992;99:1325–8.

63. **Storer EH.** Appendix. In: **Schwartz SI,** ed. *Principles of Surgery.* 3rd ed. New York: McGraw-Hill, 1979:1257–67.

64. **Melcher DH.** Appendectomy with abdominal hysterectomy. *Lancet* 1971;1:810–11.

65. **Waters EG.** Elective appendectomy with abdominal and pelvic surgery. *Obstet Gynecol* 1977; 50:511–7.

66. **Loeffler F, Stearn R.** Abdominal hysterectomy with appendicectomy. *Acta Obstet Gynecol Scand* 1967;46:435–43.

67. **Voitk AJ, Lowry JB.** Is incidental appendectomy a safe practice? *Can J Surg* 1988;31:448–51.

68. **Massoudnia N.** Incidental appendectomy in vaginal surgery. *Int Surg* 1975;60:89–90.

69. **Reiner IJ.** Incidental appendectomy at the time of vaginal surgery. *Tex Med* 1980;76:46–50.

70. **McGowan L.** Incidental appendectomy during vaginal surgery. *Am J Obstet Gynecol* 1966;95: 588.

71. **Kovac SR, Cruikshank SH.** Incidental appendectomy during vaginal hysterectomy. *Int J Gynecol Obstet* 1993;43:62–3.

72. **Pratt JH, O'Leary JA, Symmonds RE.** Combined cholecystectomy and hysterectomy: a study of 95 cases. *Mayo Clin Proc* 1967;42:529–35.

73. **Murray JM, Gilstrap LC, Massey FM.** Cholecystectomy and abdominal hysterectomy. *JAMA* 1980;244:2305–6.

74. **Hester TR, Baird W, Bostwick J, Nahai F, Cukic J.** Abdominoplasty combined with other major surgical procedures: safe or sorry? *Plast Reconstr Surg* 1989;83:997–1004.

75. **Voss SC, Sharp HC, Scott JR.** Abdominoplasty combined with gynecologic surgical procedures. *Obstet Gynecol* 1986;67:181–6.

76. **Kovac SR.** Vaginal hysterectomy combined with liposuction. *Mo Med* 1989;86:165–8.

77. **Sanz L, Smith S.** Mechanisms of wound healing, suture material, and wound closure. In: **Buchsbaum HJ, Walton LA,** eds. *Strategies in Gynecologic Surgery.* New York: Springer-Verlag, 1986:53–76.

78. **Richardson AC, Lyon JB, Geraham EE.** Abdominal hysterectomy: relationship between morbidity and surgical technique. *Am J Obstet Gynecol* 1973;115:953–61.

79. **Masterson BJ.** Total abdominal hysterectomy. In: *Manual of Gynecologic Surgery.* 2nd ed. New York: Springer-Verlag, 1986:187–218.

80. **Masterson BJ.** Ureteral injuries. In: *Manual of Gynecologic Survey.* 2nd ed. New York: Springer-Verlag, 1986:339–49.

81. **Mattingly RF, Thompson JD.** Operative injuries of the ureter. In: *TeLinde's Operative Gynecology.* 6th ed. Philadelphia: JB Lippincott, 1985:325–44.

82. **Symmonds RE.** Ureteral injuries associated with gynecologic surgery: prevention and management. *Clin Obstet Gynecol* 1976;19:623–44.

83. **Symonds RE.** Incontinence: vesical and ureteral fistulas. *Clin Obstet Gynecol* 1984; 27:499–514.

84. **Buchsbaum HJ, Walton LA.** *Strategies in Gynecological Surgery.* New York: Springer-Verlag, 1986:77–104.

85. **Berek JS.** Surgical techniques. In: **Berek JS, Hacker NF,** eds. *Practical Gynecologic Oncology.* 2nd ed. Baltimore: Williams & Wilkins, 1994:519–60.

86. **Walker FW.** Small intestine operative procedures. In: **Shackerford RT, Zuideema GE.** *Surgery for the Alimentary Tract.* 2nd ed. Philadelphia: WB Saunders, 1986:46–56.

87. **Shakerford RT, Zuideema GE.** *Surgery in the Alimentary Tract.* 2nd ed. Philadelphia: WB Saunders, 1986:312–35.

88. **Mitchell GW, Massey FM.** Bleeding 3 hours following vaginal hysterectomy. In: **Nichols DH,** ed. *Clinical Problems, Injuries and Complications of Gynecologic Surgery.* Baltimore: Williams & Wilkins, 1988:151–3.

89. **Buchsbaum HJ.** Avoiding urinary tract injuries. In: **Buchsbaum HJ, Walton LA,** eds. *Strategies in Gynecological Surgery.* New York: Springer-Verlag, 1986:77–85.

90. **Copenhaver EH.** Vaginal hysterectomy: an analysis of indications and complications among 1,000 operations. *Am J Obstet Gynecol* 1962;84:123–8.

91. **Grody MHT.** Vaginal hysterectomy: the large uterus. *J Gynecol Surg* 1989;5:301–12.

92. **Kaser SR, Ikle FA, Hirsch HA.** *Atlas of Gynecologic Surgery.* 2nd ed. Philadelphia: WB Saunders, 1985.

93. **Kovac SR.** Intramyometrial coring as an adjunct to vaginal hysterectomy. *Obstet Gynecol* 1986;67:131–6.

94. **Lash AF.** A method for reducing the size of the uterus in vaginal hysterectomy. *Am J Obstet Gynecol* 1941;42:452–9.

95. **Lash AF.** Technique for removal of abnormally large uteri without entering the cavities. *Clin Obstet Gynecol* 1961;4:210–9.

96. **Nichols DH, Randall CL.** *Vaginal Surgery.* 3rd ed. Baltimore: Williams & Wilkins, 1989:206–9.

97. **Pratt JH, Gunnar H.** Vaginal hysterectomy by morcellation. *Mayo Clin Proc* 1970;45: 374–87.

98. **Shires GT, Canzaro PC, Lowry SF.** Fluid, electrolyte, and nutritional management of the surgical patient. In: **Schartz SL,** ed. *Principles of Surgery.* 4th ed. New York: McGraw-Hill, 1984:45–80.

99. **Massler DJ, Devanesan MM.** Sexual consequences of gynecologic operations. In: **Comfort A,** ed. *Sexual Consequences of Disability.* Philadelphia: George F. Stickley, 1978:153–81.

100. **Drellich MG, Bieber I.** The psychological importance of the uterus and its function. *J Nerv Ment Dis* 1958;126:322–36.

101. **Lindemann E.** Observations on psychiatric sequelae to surgical operations in women. *Am J Psychiatry* 1941;98:132–7.

102. **Richards DH.** Depression after hysterectomy. *Lancet* 1973;2:430–32.

103. **Hollender MH.** A study of patients admitted to a psychiatric hospital after pelvic operations. *Am J Obstet Gynecol* 1960;79:498–503.

104. **Bragg RL.** Risk of admission to mental hospital following hysterectomy or cholecystectomy. *Am J Public Health* 1965;55:1403–10.

105. **Martin RL, Roberts WV, Clayton PJ.** Psychiatric status after hysterectomy: a one year prospective follow-up. *JAMA* 1980;244:350–3.

106. **Moore JT, Tolley DH.** Depression following hysterectomy. *Psychosomatics* 1976;17:86–9.

107. **Hamptom PT, Tarnasky WG.** Hysterectomy and tubal ligation: a comparison of the psychological aftermath. *Am J Obstet Gynecol* 1974;119:949–52.

108. **Gath D, Cooper P, Day A.** Hysterectomy and psychiatric disorder: I. Levels of psychiatric morbidity before and after hysterectomy. *Br J Psychiatry* 1982;140:335–42.

109. **Lalinec-Michaud M, Engelsmann F, Marino J.** Depression after hysterectomy: a comparative study. *Psychosomatics* 1988;29:307–13.

110. **Janis IL.** *Psychological Stress; Psychoanalytical Behavioral Studies of Surgical Patients.* New York: John Wiley and Sons, 1958.

111. **Menzer D, Morris T, Gates P, Sabbath J, Robey H, Plaut T, et al.** Patterns of emotional recovery from hysterectomy. *Psychosom Med* 1957;19:379–88.

112. **Huffman JW.** The effect of gynecologic surgery on sexual relations. *Am J Obstet Gynecol* 1950;59:915–7.

113. **Humphries PT.** Sexual adjustment after a hysterectomy. *Issues Health Care Women* 1980; 2:1–14.

114. **Dennerstein L, Wood C, Burrows GD.** Sexual response following hysterectomy and oophorectomy. *Obstet Gynecol* 1977;49:92–6.

115. **Lindgren HC.** *Personality as a Social Phenomenon.* 2nd ed. New York: John Wiley and Sons, 1973:225–99.

REPRODUCTIVE
ENDOCRINOLOGY

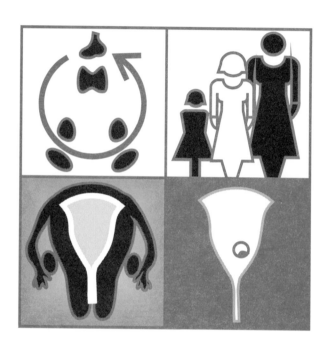

23 Puberty

Robert W. Rebar

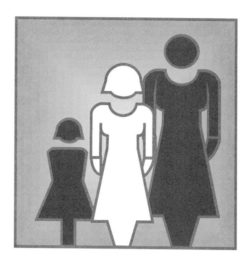

Puberty is defined as the period during which secondary sexual characteristics begin to develop and the capability of sexual reproduction is attained. The physical changes accompanying pubertal development result directly or indirectly from maturation of the hypothalamus, stimulation of the sex organs, and the secretion of sex steroids. Hormonally, puberty in humans is characterized by the resetting of the classic negative gonadal steroid feedback loop, alterations in circadian and ultradian (frequent) gonadotropin rhythms, and the acquisition in the woman of a positive estrogen feedback loop, controlling the monthly rhythm as an interdependent expression of gonadotropins and ovarian steroids.

The ability to evaluate and treat aberrations of pubertal development requires an understanding of the normal hormonal and physical changes that occur at puberty. An understanding of these changes is also important in evaluating young women with amenorrhea.

Normal Pubertal Development

Factors Affecting Time of Onset

The major determinant of the timing of the onset of puberty is no doubt genetic, but a number of other factors appear to influence both the age at onset and the progression of pubertal development. Among these influences are nutritional state, general health, geographic location, exposure to light, and psychologic state (1). The concordance of the age of menarche in mother-daughter pairs and between sisters and in ethnic populations illustrates the importance of genetic factors (1). Typically, the age of menarche is earlier than average in children with moderate obesity (up to 30% above normal weight for age), whereas delayed menarche is common in those with severe malnutrition. Children who live in urban settings, closer to the equator, and at lower altitudes typically begin puberty earlier than those who live in rural areas, farther from the equator, and at higher elevations. Blind girls apparently undergo menarche earlier than sighted girls, suggesting some influence of light (2).

771

In western Europe, the age of menarche declined 4 months each decade between 1850 and 1960 (1). It appears that this trend has now halted (3). It has been presumed that these changes represent improved nutritional status and healthier living conditions.

One of the more controversial hypotheses has centered around the role of total body weight and body composition on the age of menarche. Frisch has argued that a girl must reach a critical body weight (47.8 kg) prior to menarche (4). More importantly, body fat must increase to 23.5% from the typical 16% of the prepubertal state, which presumably is influenced by nutritional status (5). This hypothesis is supported by observations that menarche occurs earliest in obese girls, followed by normal weight girls, then underweight girls, and lastly anorectic girls (Fig. 23.1). The importance of other factors is indicated by observations that menarche is often delayed in morbidly obese girls, those with diabetes, and those who exercise intensely but are of normal body weight and percent body fat. Moreover, girls with precocious puberty may undergo menarche even if they have a low percent body fat, and other girls show no pubertal development with a percent body fat of 27% (6). The hypothesis linking menarche to body weight and composition does not always seem valid because menarche is a late event in pubertal development.

Physical Changes During Puberty

The changes associated with puberty occur in an orderly sequence over a definite time frame. Any deviation from this sequence or time frame should be regarded as abnormal. Moreover, the pubertal changes, their relationships to each other, and the ages at which they occur are distinctly different in girls and in boys. Although this chapter focuses on girls, changes in boys will be considered briefly as well.

Tanner Stage

In girls, pubertal development typically requires 4.5 years (Fig. 23.2). Although generally the first sign of puberty is accelerated growth, breast budding is usually the first recognized pubertal change, followed by the appearance of pubic hair, peak growth velocity, and menarche. The stages initially described by Marshall and Tanner are often used to describe breast and pubic hair development (7).

With regard to breast development (Fig. 23.3), Tanner *stage 1* refers to the prepubertal state and includes no palpable breast tissue, with the areolae generally less than 2 cm in diameter. The nipples may be inverted, flat, or raised. In *stage 2*, breast budding occurs, with a visible and palpable mound of breast tissue. The areolae begin to enlarge, the skin of the areolae thins, and the nipple develops to varying degrees. *Stage 3* is reflected by further growth and elevation of the entire breast. When the individual is seated and viewed from the side, the nipple is generally at or above the midplane of breast tissue. In most individuals, *stage 4* is defined by projection of the areola and papilla above the general breast contour in a secondary mound. Breast development is incomplete until Tanner *stage 5*, in which the breast is mature in contour and proportion. In most women, the nipple is more pigmented than earlier in development and Montgomery's glands are visible around the circumference of the areola. The nipple is generally below the midplane of breast tissue when the woman is seated and viewed from the side. Full breast development usually occurs over 3–3.5 years but may occur in as little as 2 years or not progress beyond stage 4 until the first pregnancy. Breast size is no indication of breast maturity.

Pubic hair staging is related both to quantity and distribution (Fig. 23.4). In Tanner *stage 1*, there is no sexually stimulated pubic hair present, but some nonsexual hair may be present in the genital area. *Stage 2* is characterized by the first appearance of coarse, long, crinkly pubic hair along the labia majora. In *stage 3*, coarse, curly hair extends onto the mons pubis. *Stage 4* is characterized by adult hair in thickness and texture, but the hair is not distributed as widely as in adults and typically does not extend onto the inner aspects of the thighs. Except in certain ethnic groups, including Asians and American Indians, pubic hair extends onto the thighs in Tanner *stage 5*.

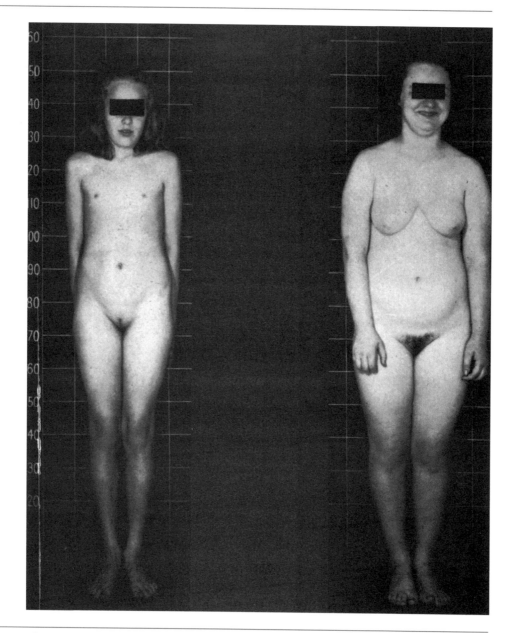

Figure 23.1   Normal twins at 12 years of age. The heavier twin (weighing 143 lb) is clearly more advanced in puberty than the lighter twin (weighing 87 lb). Anecdotal photographs and data such as these served to provide the basis for the theory that body fat, body mass, and menarche are linked. (Reproduced with permission from **Wilkins L.** *The Diagnosis and Treatment of Endocrine Disorders in Childhood and Adolescence.* 3rd ed. Springfield, IL: Charles C. Thomas, 1965:218.)

The staging of male pubertal sexual maturation is based on genital size and pubic hair development. *Stage 1* is prepubertal. *Stage 2* of genital growth begins when testicular enlargement is first evident. Testis length along the longitudinal axis ranges from 2.5–3.2 cm. The size of the penis increases as well. Pigmented, curly, pubic hair is first visible around the base of the penis. In Tanner *stage 3*, there is further growth of the penis in both length and diameter, the scrotum develops further, and testis length increases to 3.3–4.0 cm. Thicker, curly hair extends above the penis. *Stage 4* involves further growth of the genitalia, with testis length ranging from 4.0–4.5 cm. Extension of pubic hair over the geni-

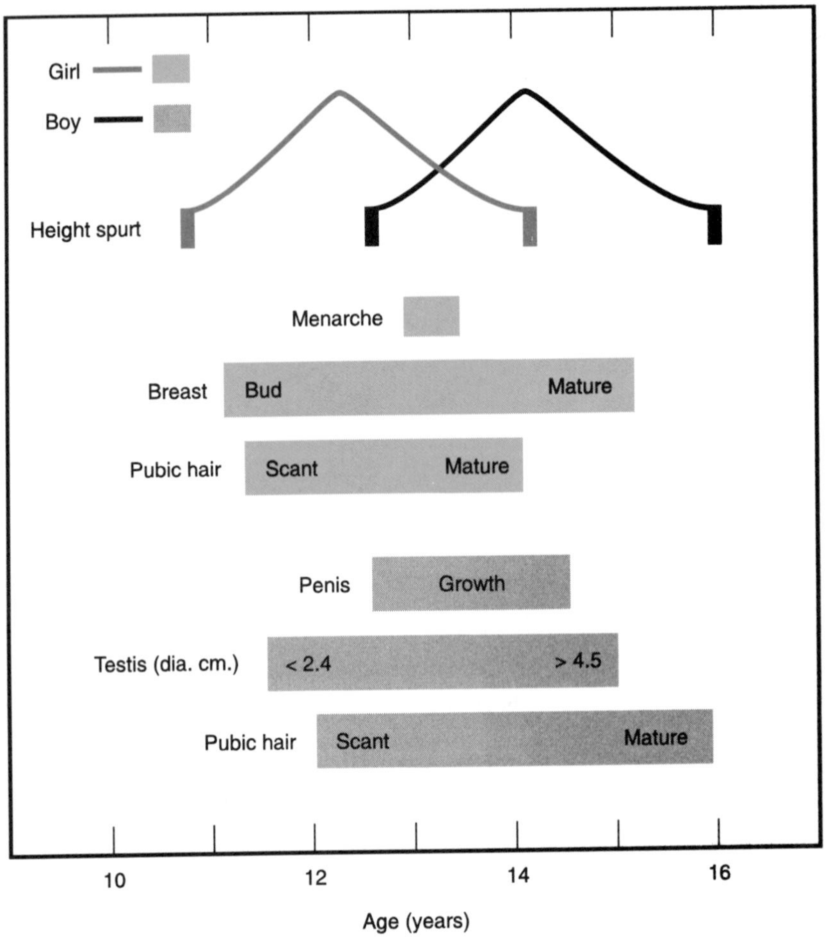

Figure 23.2   Schematic sequence of events at puberty. An idealized average girl (upper panel) and an idealized average boy (lower panel) are represented. (Reproduced with permission from **Rebar RW.** Practical evaluation of hormonal status. In: **Yen SSC, Jaffe RB,** eds. *Reproductive Endocrinology: Physiology, Pathophysiology and Clinical Management.* 3rd ed. Philadelphia: WB Saunders, 1991:830. Based on data from **Marshall WA, Tanner JM.** Variations in patterns of pubertal changes in girls. *Arch Dis Child* 1969;44:291–303; and **Marshall WA, Tanner JM.** Variation in the pattern of pubertal changes in boys. *Arch Dis Child* 1970;45:13–23.)

area continues, but the volume is less than in the adult. At this stage, the prostate gland is palpable by rectal examination. In Tanner *stage 5,* the genitalia are within the adult range in size. Stretched penile length measured along the dorsum averages 15.7 cm in adult men. Pubic hair spreads laterally onto the medial thighs. Hair may or may not extend from the pubic area toward the umbilicus and anus.

Pigmented pubic hair is often the first recognized sign of male puberty even though it typically occurs 6 months after genital growth begins. Tanner stage 3 puberty is often accompanied by symmetric or asymmetric gynecomastia, and mature sperm first can be identified with microscopic urinalysis.

Height and Growth Rate   **Plotting height increments (i.e., growth velocity) against the phases of puberty allows one to see relationships during puberty** (Fig. 23.2). Girls reach peak height velocity early in puberty prior to menarche. As a consequence, they have limited growth potential

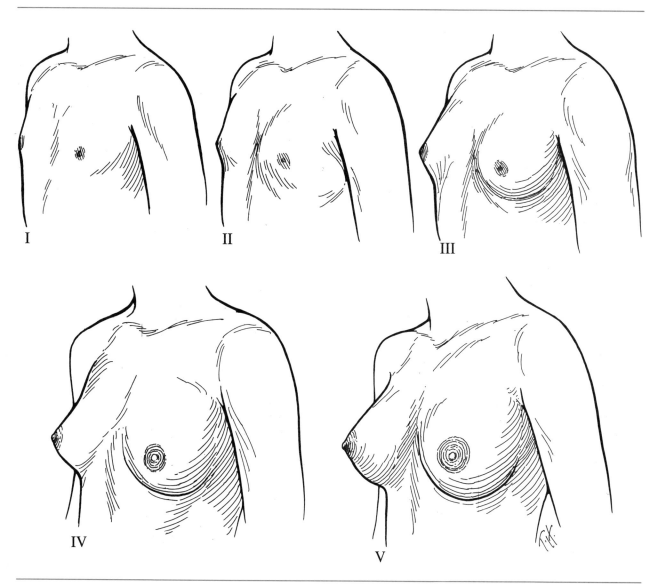

Figure 23.3   Diagrammatic depiction of Tanner breast stages in adolescent women. (Reproduced with permission from **Ross GT, VandeWiele RL, Frantz AG.** The ovaries and the breasts. In: **Williams RH,** ed. *Textbook of Endocrinology.* 6th ed. Philadelphia, WB Saunders, 1981:355; as adapted from **Marshall WA, Tanner JM.** Variations in patterns of pubertal changes in girls. *Arch Dis Child* 1969;44:291–303.)

following menarche. In contrast, boys reach peak height velocity approximately 2 years later than girls. Boys grow an average of 28 cm during the growth spurt in comparison to a mean of 25 cm for girls. Adult men eventually are an average of 10 cm taller than adult women largely because they are taller at the onset of the growth spurt. Hormonal control of the pubertal growth spurt is complex. Growth hormone, insulin-like growth factor 1 (IGF-1), and gonadal steroids play major roles. Adrenal androgens appear to be less important.

During the growth spurt associated with puberty, the long bones in the body lengthen and the epiphyses ultimately close. The bone or skeletal age of any individual can be estimated closely by comparing x-rays documenting the development of bones in the nondominant hand (most commonly), knee, or elbow to standards of maturation for the normal population. The Greulich and Pyle atlas (8) is used most often for this purpose. Skeletal age is more closely correlated with pubertal stage than with chronologic age during puberty.

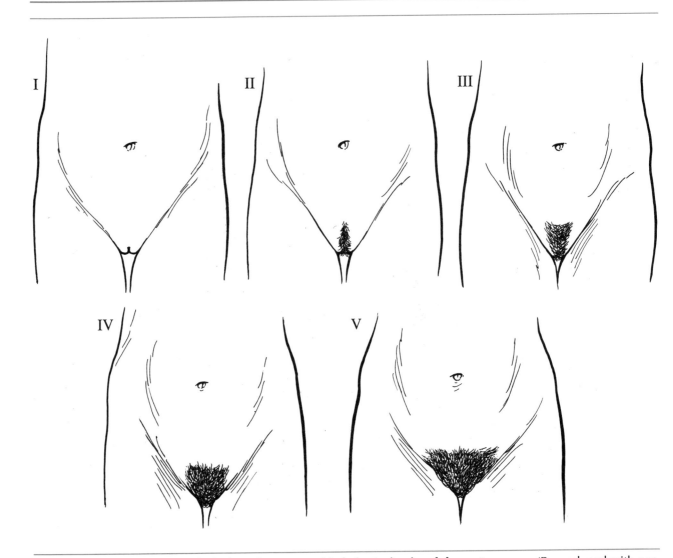

Figure 23.4   Diagrammatic depiction of Tanner pubic hair staging in adolescent women. (Reproduced with permission from **Ross GT, VandeWiele RL, Frantz AG.** The ovaries and the breasts. In: **Williams RH,** ed. *Textbook of Endocrinology.* 6th ed. Philadelphia: WB Saunders, 1981:355; as adapted from **Marshall WA, Tanner JM.** Variations in patterns of pubertal changes in girls. *Arch Dis Child* 1969;44:291–303.)

With height and chronologic age, an individual's bone age can be used to predict final adult height using the Bayley-Pinneau tables (9).

Another practical clinical approach to predicting adult height involves utilizing midparental height. **The adjusted midparental height is calculated by adding 13 cm to the mother's height (for boys) or subtracting 13 cm from the father's height (for girls) and then determining the mean of the heights of the parents, including the adjusted height of the opposite-sex parent. Adding and subtracting 8.5 cm to the calculated predicted height will approximate the target range of the 3rd to the 97th percentile for the anticipated adult height of the child.** This quick calculation can be of assistance in evaluating individuals with delayed or precocious pubertal development and those with short stature.

Several changes in body composition also occur during pubertal development. Although lean body mass, skeletal mass, and body fat are equal in prepubertal boys and girls, by maturity men have 1.5 times the lean body mass and almost 1.5 times the skeletal mass of women, whereas women have twice as much body fat as men (1). The changes in body contour in girls, with accumulation of fat at the thighs, hips, and buttocks, occur during the pubertal growth spurt. Voice and other changes also are associated with the changes in body composition.

Hormonal Changes During Puberty

It is now clear that by 10 weeks of gestation, gonadotropin-releasing hormone (GnRH) is present in the hypothalamus and luteinizing hormone (LH) and follicle-stimulating hormone (FSH) are present in the pituitary gland (10). Gonadotropin levels are elevated in both female and male fetuses before birth; the levels of FSH are higher in females. At birth, gonadotropin and sex steroid concentrations are still high, but the levels decline during the first several weeks of life and remain low during the prepubertal years. The hypothalamic-pituitary unit appears to be suppressed by the extremely low levels of gonadal steroids present in childhood. Gonadal suppression of gonadotropin secretion is demonstrated by higher gonadotropin levels in children with gonadal dysgenesis and those who undergo gonadectomy before puberty (11).

Several of the hormonal changes associated with pubertal development begin before any of the physical changes are obvious. Early in puberty, there is increased sensitivity of LH to GnRH. Sleep-entrained increases in both LH and FSH can be documented early in puberty (12). In boys, the nocturnal increases in gonadotropin levels are accompanied by simultaneous increases in circulating testosterone levels (13). In contrast, in girls, the nighttime increases in circulating gonadotropin levels are followed by increased secretion of estradiol the next day (14) (Fig. 23.5). This delay in estradiol secretion is believed due to

Figure 23.5   Patterns of circulating luteinizing hormone (LH), follicle-stimulating hormone (FSH), and estradiol in a stage 3 pubertal girl over a 24-hour period with the encephalographic stage of sleep indicated. (Reproduced with permission from **Boyar RM, Wu RHK, Roffwarg H, Kapen S, Hellman L, Weitzman ED, et al.** Human puberty: 24-hour estradiol patterns in pubertal girls. *J Clin Endocrinol Metab* 1976;43:1418–21.)

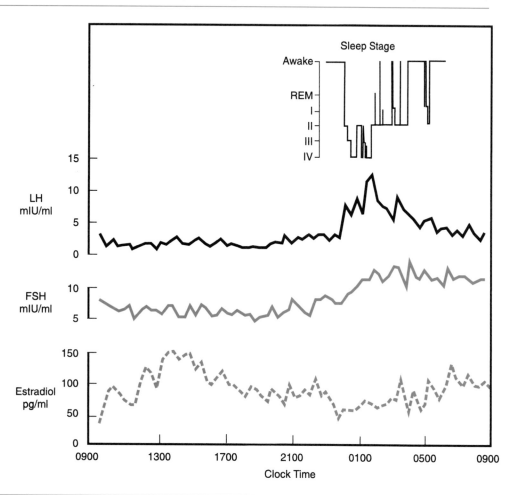

the additional synthetic steps required in the aromatization of estrogens from androgens. Basal levels of both FSH and LH increase through puberty. The patterns differ in boys and girls, with LH levels (measured in mIU/ml) eventually becoming greater than FSH (15) (Fig. 23.6). Although it now appears that gonadotropins are always secreted in an episodic or pulsatile fashion, even before puberty, the pulsatile secretion of gonadotropins is more easily documented as puberty progresses and basal levels increase (16).

Increased adrenal androgen secretion is important in stimulating adrenarche, the appearance of pubic and axillary hair, in both boys and girls. Pubarche specifically refers to the appearance of pubic hair. Progressive increases in circulating levels of the major adrenal androgens, dehydroepiandrosterone (DHEA) and its sulfate (DHEAS), begin as early as 2 years of age, accelerate at 7–8 years of age, and continue until 13–15 years of age (17–19). The accelerated increases in adrenal androgens begin about 2 years before the increases in gonadotropin and gonadal sex steroid secretion when the hypothalamic-pituitary-gonadal unit is still functioning at a low prepubertal level.

In girls, estradiol, secreted predominantly by the ovaries, increases steadily during puberty (15). Although, as noted, increases in estradiol first appear during the daytime hours, basal

Figure 23.6   Increases (± standard error) in circulating levels of gonadotropins and adrenal and gonadal steroids through puberty in girls. DHEA, dehydroepiandrosterone; DHEAS, dehydroepiandrosterone sulfate. (Reproduced with permission from **Emans SJH, Goldstein DP.** The physiology of puberty. In: **Emans SJH, Goldstein DP,** eds. *Pediatric and Adolescent Gynecology.* 3rd ed. Boston: Little, Brown & Co., 1990:95.)

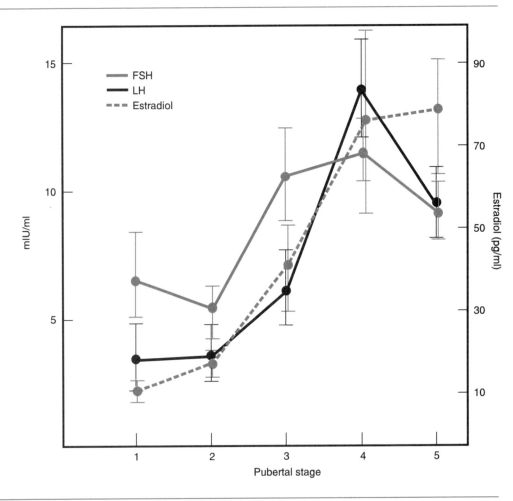

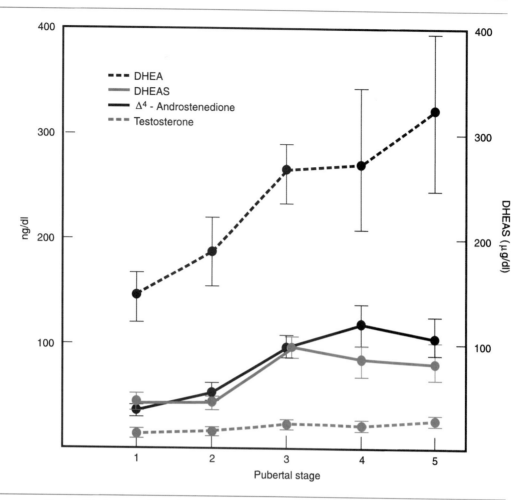

Figure 23.6—*continued*

levels increase during both the day and night. Estrone, which is secreted in part by the ovaries and arises in part from extraglandular conversion of estradiol and androstenedione, also increases early in puberty but plateaus by midpuberty. Thus, **the ratio of estrone to estradiol decreases throughout puberty, indicating that ovarian production of estradiol becomes increasingly important and peripheral conversion of androgens to estrone becomes less important during maturation.**

In boys, most of the testosterone in the circulation arises from direct secretion by the Leydig cells of the testis. Testosterone induces development of a male body habitus and voice change, whereas dihydrotestosterone (DHT), produced following 5α reduction within target cells, induces enlargement of the penis and prostate gland, beard growth, and temporal hair recession during puberty. Mean plasma testosterone levels rise progressively during puberty, with the greatest increase occurring during Tanner stage 2 (20).

Mechanisms Underlying Puberty

The mechanisms responsible for the numerous hormonal changes occurring during puberty are poorly understood, although it is recognized that a "CNS program" must be responsible for initiating puberty. It appears that the hypothalamic-pituitary-gonadal axis in girls develops in two distinct stages during puberty. First, sensitivity to the negative or inhibitory effects of the low levels of circulating sex steroids present in childhood decreases early in puberty. Second, late in puberty, there is maturation of the positive or stimulatory feedback response to estrogen, which is responsible for the ovulatory midcycle surge of LH.

Current evidence suggests that the central nervous system inhibits the onset of puberty until the appropriate time (21). Based on this theory, the neuroendocrine control of puberty is mediated by GnRH-secreting neurons in the medial basal hypothalamus, which act together as an endogenous pulse generator. At puberty, the GnRH pulse generator is reactivated (i.e., disinhibited), leading to increased amplitude and frequency of GnRH pulses. In turn, the increased GnRH secretion results in increased gonadotropin and then gonadal steroid secretion. What causes this "disinhibition" of GnRH release is unknown.

Aberrations of Pubertal Development

Classification

Several aberrations of pubertal development, as detailed in Table 23.1, can occur in girls. Pubertal aberrations can be classified in four broad categories:

1. *Delayed or interrupted puberty* **exists in girls who fail to develop any secondary sex characteristics by age 13, have not had menarche by age 16, or in whom 5 or more years have passed since the onset of pubertal development without attainment of menarche.**

2. *Asynchronous pubertal development* **is characterized by pubertal development that deviates from the normal pattern of puberty.**

3. *Precocious puberty* **is pubertal development beginning before the age of 8 years.** Precocious pubertal development is characterized in several ways. In isosexual precocious puberty, the early changes are common to the phenotypic sex of the individual. In heterosexual precocious puberty, the development is characteristic of the opposite sex. Precocious puberty is sometimes termed "true" when it is of central origin with activation of the hypothalamic-pituitary unit. In precocious pseudopuberty, also known as precocious puberty of peripheral origin, secretion of hormones in the periphery (commonly by neoplasms) stimulates pubertal development.

4. *Heterosexual puberty* **is characterized by development that is characteristic of the opposite sex occurring at the expected age of normal puberty.**

Disorders of sexual development and amenorrhea may be considered in relation to this classification of the aberrations of puberty. It is very helpful to document the growth of the individual and to plot the individual's height and weight on one of several commonly available growth charts (Fig. 23.7).

Delayed or Interrupted Puberty

The history and physical examination, with particular attention to growth, are most important in the evaluation of individuals with delayed puberty. One possible approach to evaluation is depicted in Figure 23.8.

Anatomic Abnormalities of the Genital Outflow Tract

Those girls who have mature secondary sex characteristics and any of a number of disorders of the outflow tract and uterus, often termed müllerian agenesis and dysgenesis, are most often identified on examination (Fig. 23.9). One of the most logical classification schemes that has been proposed is shown in Table 23.2 (22). The incidence of these anomalies was estimated to be 0.02% of the female population several years ago (23), but the incidence may have increased as a result of the maternal ingestion of *diethylstilbestrol (DES)* and the resultant increase in anomalies of the lumen of the uterus (class VI) (24). Of the disorders unrelated to drugs, the septate uterus (class V) is most common.

Table 23.1   Aberrations of Pubertal Development

I. Delayed or interrupted puberty
- **A.** *Anatomic abnormalties of the genital outflow tract*
  1. Müllerian dysgenesis (*Rokitansky-Küster-Hauser syndrome*)
  2. Distal genital tract obstruction
     a. Imperforate hymen
     b. Transverse vaginal septum
- **B.** *Hypergonadotropic (follicle-stimulating hormone >30 mIU/ml) hypogonadism (gonadal "failure")*
  1. Gonadal dysgenesis with stigmata of *Turner's syndrome*
  2. Pure gonadal dysgenesis
     a. 46XX
     b. 46XY
  3. Early gonadal "failure" with apparent normal ovarian development
- **C.** *Hypogonadotropic (LH and FSH <10 mIU/ml) hypogonadism*
  1. Constitutional delay
  2. Isolated gonadotropin deficiency
     a. Associated with midline defects (*Kallmann's syndrome*)
     b. Independent of associated disorders
     c. Prader-Labhardt-Willi syndrome
     d. Laurence-Moon-Bardet-Biedl syndrome
     e. Many other rare syndromes
  3. Associated with multiple hormone deficiencies
  4. Neoplasms of the hypothalamic-pituitary area
     a. Craniopharyngiomas
     b. Pituitary adenomas
     c. Other
  5. Infiltrative processes (Langerhans-cell type histiocytosis)
  6. After irradiation of the central nervous system
  7. Severe chronic illnesses with malnutrition
  8. Anorexia nervosa and related disorders
  9. Severe hypothalamic amenorrhea (rare)
  10. Antidopaminergic and gonadotropin-releasing hormone inhibiting drugs (especially psychotropic agents, opiates)
  11. Primary hypothyroidism
  12. *Cushing's syndrome*

II. Asynchronous pubertal development
- **A.** Complete androgen insensitivity syndrome (testicular feminization)
- **B.** Incomplete androgen insensitivity syndrome

III. Precocious puberty
- **A.** *Central (true) precocious puberty*
  1. Constitutional (idiopathic) precocious puberty
  2. Hypothalamic neoplasms (most commonly hamartomas)
  3. Congenital malformations
  4. Infiltrative processes (Langerhans-cell-type histiocytosis)
  5. After irradiation
  6. Trauma
  7. Infection
- **B.** *Precocious puberty of peripheral origin (precocious pseudopuberty)*
  1. Gonadotropin-secreting neoplasms
     a. Human chorionic gonadotropin-secreting
        i. Ectopic germinomas (pinealomas)
        ii. Choriocarcinomas
        iii. Teratomas
        iv. Hepatoblastomas
     b. Luteinizing hormone-secreting (pituitary adenomas)
  2. Gonadal neoplasms
     a. Estrogen-secreting
        i. Granulosa-theca cell tumors
        ii. Gonadal sex-cord tumors
     b. Androgen-secreting
        i. Arrhenoblastomas
        ii. Teratomas
  3. Congenital adrenal hyperplasia
     a. 21-Hydroxylase (P450c21) deficiency

Table 23.1—continued

III. Precocious puberty
> b. 11 β-Hydroxylase (P450c11) deficiency
> c. 3 β-Hydroxysteroid dehydrogenase deficiency
> **4.** Adrenal neoplasms
>> a. Adenomas
>> b. Carcinomas
> **5.** Autonomous gonadal hypersecretion
>> a. Cysts
>> b. *McCune-Albright syndrome*
> **6.** Iatrogenic ingestion/absorption of estrogens or androgens

IV. Heterosexual puberty
> **A.** Polycystic ovarian syndrome
> **B.** Nonclassic forms of congenital adrenal hyperplasia
> **C.** Idiopathic hirsutism
> **D.** Mixed gonadal dysgenesis
> **E.** Rare forms of male pseudohermaphroditism (*Reifenstein syndrome,* 5α-reductase deficiency)
> **F.** *Cushing's syndrome* (rare)
> **G.** Androgen-secreting neoplasms (rare)

Disorders of the outflow tract and uterus often occur as a part of a syndrome of malformations that include abnormalities of the skeletal and renal systems (*Rokitansky-Küster-Hauser syndrome*). The most simple single disorder is the imperforate hymen, which prevents the passage of endometrial tissue and blood. These products can accumulate in the vagina (*hydrocolpos*) or uterus (*hydrometrocolpos*) and result in a bulging hymen that is often bluish in color. The affected individual often will have a history of vague abdominal pain with approximately monthly exacerbations. It is sometimes difficult to distinguish an imperforate hymen from a transverse vaginal septum, and in most situations, examination under anesthesia would be required.

Regardless of the cause, uterine anomalies not involving segmental müllerian agenesis or hypoplasia (class I) are compatible with normal pregnancy. However, increased fetal wastage has been reported (25). Uterine malformations have been associated with spontaneous abortion, premature labor, abnormal presentations, and complications of labor (i.e., retained placenta). Many of these uterine anomalies can be identified with hysterosalpingography (HSG) (Fig. 23.9), but a septate uterus (class V) can be distinguished from a bicornuate uterus (class IV) only by diagnostic laparoscopy in addition to HSG or by magnetic resonance imaging (MRI).

Obstruction or malformation of the distal genital tract must be distinguished from androgen insensitivity. Individuals with androgen insensitivity have breast development in the absence of significant pubic and axillary hair development; the vagina may be absent or foreshortened in these women.

Hypergonadotropic and Hypogonadotropic Hypogonadism

Basal levels of FSH and prolactin should be determined in individuals in whom secondary sex characteristics have not developed to maturity (Fig. 23.8). Bone age should be estimated from x-rays of the nondominant hand. If prolactin levels are elevated, thyroid function should be assessed to determine whether the individual has primary hypothyroidism. Paradoxically, primary hypothyroidism can result in precocious puberty as well. If thyroid function is normal, a hypothalamic or pituitary neoplasm is possible, and careful evaluation of the hypothalamic and pituitary area by MRI or computed tomography (CT) is indicated.

The karyotype should be determined in any individual with delayed puberty and increased basal FSH concentrations. Regardless of the karyotype, the individual with hypergonadotropic hypogonadism has some form of ovarian "failure."

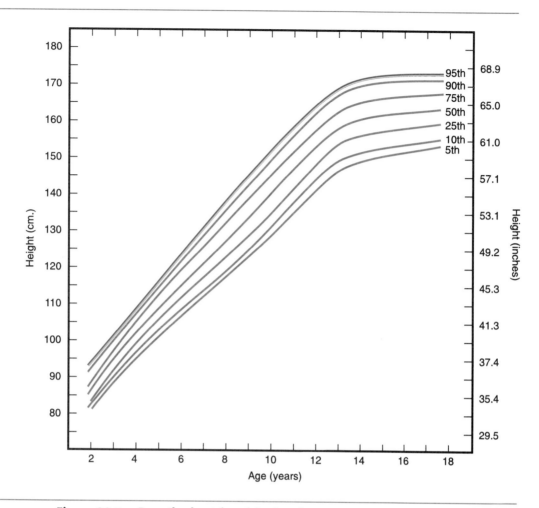

Figure 23.7   Growth chart for girls showing stature by age percentiles for girls aged 2 to 18 years. Weight can be plotted in a similar fashion. Several excellent growth charts are available to clinicians, including those from Ross Laboratories (Columbus, OH), Serono Laboratories (Randolph, MA), and Genentech, Inc. (South San Francisco, CA). (Reproduced with permission **Hamill PVV, Drizd TA, Johnson CL, Reed RB, Roche AF, Moore WM.** Physical growth: National Center for Health Statistics percentiles. *Am J Clin Nutr* 1979;32:607–29. Based on data from the National Center for Health Statistics.)

Forms of Gonadal Failure

Turner's Syndrome   **Most affected individuals have a 45X karyotype and Turner's syndrome; still others have mosaic karyotypes (i.e., 45X/46XX; 45X/46XY) and may present with the Turner's phenotype as well.** These patients generally grow slowly, beginning in the second or third year of life. They typically have many of the associated stigmata, including lymphedema at birth; a webbed neck; multiple pigmented nevi; disorders of the heart, kidneys (most commonly horseshoe), and great vessels (most commonly coarctation of the aorta); and small hyperconvex fingernails (26) (Fig. 23.10). Diabetes mellitus, thyroid disorders, essential hypertension, and other autoimmune disorders are often present in individuals with 45X karyotypes. Most 45X patients have normal intelligence, but many affected individuals have an unusual cognitive defect characterized by an inability to appreciate the shapes and relations of objects with respect to one another (i.e., space-form blindness). As they grow older, affected children typically are shorter than normal. Although they do not develop breasts at puberty, some pubic or axillary hair may develop because appropriate adrenarche can occur with failure of thelarche (i.e., breast de-

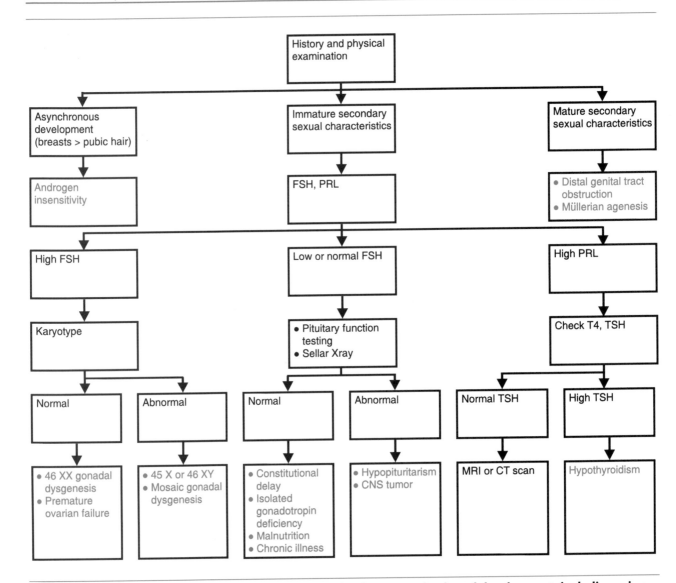

Figure 23.8   Flow diagram for the evaluation of delayed or interrupted pubertal development, including primary amenorrhea, in phenotypic females. Individuals with asynchronous development often present because of failure to menstruate. (Reproduced with permission from **Rebar RW.** Normal and abnormal sexual differentiation and pubertal development. In: **Moore TR, Reiter RC, Rebar RW, Baker VV,** eds. *Gynecology and Obstetrics. A Longitudinal Approach.* New York: Churchill Livingstone, 1993:97–133.)

velopment). **Although less severe short stature and some adolescent development may occur with chromosomal mosaicism, it is reasonable to assume that any short, slowly growing, sexually infantile girl has Turner's syndrome until proved otherwise because this disorder is so prevalent (approximately one in 2500 newborn phenotypic females). In fact, the 45X karyotype is the single most frequent chromosomal disorder in humans, but most affected fetuses are aborted spontaneously early in pregnancy. However, trisomy is the most common chromosomal type or category of abnormality in first-trimester losses.**

Even in the presence of typical Turner stigmata, a karyotype is indicated to eliminate any possibility of any portion of a Y chromosome. If a Y chromosome is identified, surgical extirpation of the gonads is warranted to eliminate any possibility of a germ cell neoplasm (estimated 20–30% prevalence) (27, 28). In individuals in whom there is no evidence of neoplastic dissemination, the uterus may be left *in situ* for donor *in vitro* fertilization and embryo transfer. The evaluation of other commonly involved organ systems should in-

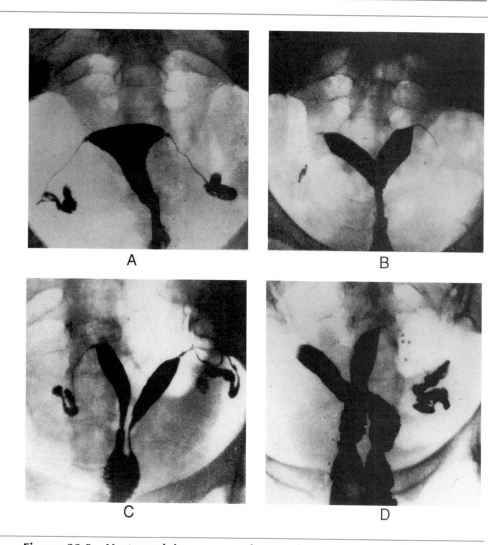

Figure 23.9 Hysterosalpingograms of normal and abnormal female genital tracts. The radiographic photographs have been reversed to accentuate the uterine cavities. *A,* Normal study with bilateral spill. *B,* Bicornuate uterus. *C,* Uterus didelphis. *D,* Uterus didelphis with double vagina. (Courtesy of Dr. A. Gerbie. Reproduced with permission from **Spitzer IB, Rebar RW.** Counselling for women with medical problems. Ovary and reproductive organs. In: **Hollingsworth D, Resnik R,** eds. *Medical Counselling Before Pregnancy.* New York: Churchill Livingstone, 1988:213–48.)

clude a careful physical examination, with special attention to the cardiovascular system, and thyroid function tests (including antibody assessment), fasting blood glucose, renal function tests, and intravenous pyelogram or a renal ultrasound scan.

Treatment of Turner's Syndrome In order to increase final adult height, treatment strategies utilizing exogenous growth hormone (GH) are commonly accepted (29). It is not yet known what dose of GH is optimal or if an anabolic steroid such as oxandrolone will provide additional growth. However, GH in doses 25% greater than those recommended for GH deficiency are proving safe and effective, with a net increase in height of 8.1 cm over the average height of approximately 146 cm in untreated individuals.

The treatment of patients with Turner's syndrome is as follows:

Table 23.2   Classification of Müllerian Anomalies*

Class I. Segmented Müllerian agenesis or hypoplasia
  A. Vaginal
  B. Cervical
  C. Fundal
  D. Tubal
  E. Combined

Class II. Unicornuate uterus
  A. With a rudimentary horn
    1. With a communicating endometrial cavity
    2. With a noncommunicating cavity
    3. With no cavity
  B. Without any rudimentary horn

Class III. Uterus didelphis

Class IV. Bicornuate uterus
  A. Complete to the internal os
  B. Partial
  C. Arcuate

Class V. Septate uterus
  A. With a complete septum
  B. With an incomplete septum

Class VI. Uterus with internal luminal changes

Adapted from **Buttrarm VC Jr, Gibbons WE.** Müllerian anomalies: a proposed classification (an analysis of 144 cases). *Fertil Steril* 1979;32:40.

1. **To promote sexual maturation, therapy with exogenous estrogen should be initiated when the patient is psychologically ready, at approximately 12–13 years of age, and after GH therapy is completed.**

2. Because the intent is to mimic normal pubertal development, low-dose estrogen alone (such as 0.3–0.625 mg *conjugated estrogens* orally each day) should be initiated.

3. Progestins (5–10 mg *medroxyprogesterone acetate* given orally for 12–14 days every 1–2 months) can be added to prevent endometrial hyperplasia after the patient first experiences vaginal bleeding or after 6 months of unopposed estrogen use if the patient has not yet had any bleeding.

4. The dose of estrogen is increased slowly over 1–2 years until the patient is taking about twice as much estrogen as is administered to postmenopausal women.

5. Girls with gonadal dysgenesis must be monitored carefully for the development of hypertension with estrogen therapy.

6. The patients and their parents should be counseled regarding the emotional and physical changes that will occur with therapy.

Mosaic Forms of Gonadal Dysgenesis   Individuals with rare mosaic forms of gonadal dysgenesis may develop normally at puberty. The decision to initiate therapy with exogenous estrogen should be based mainly on circulating FSH levels, because FSH levels in the normal range for the patient's age imply the presence of functional gonads. Pregnancies can be achieved in these individuals, with success rates of over 50%, by using donor oocytes (30).

Pure Gonadal Dysgenesis   The term *pure gonadal dysgenesis* refers to 46XX or 46XY phenotypic females who have streak gonads. This condition may occur spo-

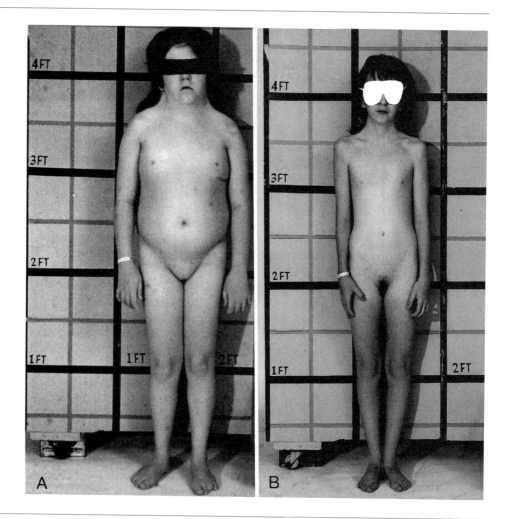

Figure 23.10   Typical appearance of two individuals with 45X gonadal dysgenesis.
A, This 16-year-old individual has obvious short stature, a webbed neck, shortened fourth metatarsals, and a thoracotomy scar from the repair of the coarctation of the aorta that was performed at 13 years of age. *B,* This 13-year-old individual had evidence of adrenarche with some pubic and axillary hair development. She is quite short, but the stigmata of Turner's syndrome are less obvious than in the patient in *A.*

radically or may be inherited as an autosomal recessive trait or as an X-linked trait in XY gonadal dysgenesis (Fig. 23.11). Affected girls are typically of average height and have none of the stigmata of Turner's syndrome, but they have elevated levels of FSH because the streak gonads produce neither steroid hormones nor inhibin. When gonadal dysgenesis occurs in 46XY individuals, it is sometimes termed *Swyer's syndrome.* Surgical extirpation is warranted in individuals with a 46XY karyotype to prevent development of germ cell neoplasms. Both 46XX and 46XY forms of gonadal dysgenesis benefit from exogenous estrogen and are potential candidates for donor oocytes.

In early gonadal failure, the ovaries apparently develop normally but contain no oocytes by the expected age of puberty. These disorders are considered further in the discussion delineating the evaluation of amenorrhea (Chapter 24).

Hypogonadotropic Hypogonadism

Hypothalamic-pituitary disturbances are usually associated with low levels of circulating gonadotropins (with both LH and FSH <10 mIU/ml) (31). There are both sporadic and fa-

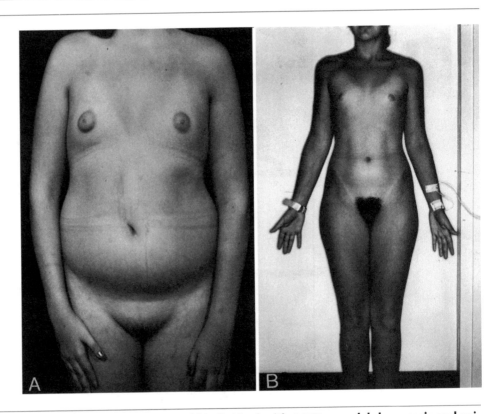

Figure 23.11 *A,* **A 16-year-old individual with 46XX gonadal dysgenesis and primary amenorrhea.** Circulating FSH levels were markedly elevated. The small amount of breast development (Tanner stage 2) is unusual, but some pubertal development may occur in such patients. *B,* **A 16-year-old individual with 46XY gonadal dysgenesis who presented with primary amenorrhea and markedly elevated FSH levels.** Most affected individuals do not present with as much pubic and axillary hair development. The right gonad contained a dysgerminoma, but there was no evidence of metastases. (Reproduced with permission from **Rebar RW.** Normal and abnormal sexual differentiation and pubertal development. In: **Moore TR, Reiter RC, Rebar RW, Baker VV,** eds. *Gynecology and Obstetrics. A Longitudinal Approach.* New York: Churchill Livingstone, 1993:97–133.)

milial causes of hypogonadotropic hypogonadism, and the differential diagnosis is extensive. It is important to remember, however, that low levels of LH and FSH are normally present in the prepubertal years; thus, girls with constitutionally delayed puberty may be mistakenly presumed to have hypogonadotropic hypogonadism. In fact, **constitutional delay is the most common cause of delayed puberty.** Constitutional delayed growth and adolescence can be diagnosed only after careful evaluation excludes other causes of delayed puberty and longitudinal follow-up documents normal sexual development. The farther below the third percentile for height that the young girl is, the less likely it is that constitutional explanations are correct.

Isolated Gonadotropin Deficiency   Isolated gonadotropin deficiency occurs as part of a number of syndromes in which there is a disorder of the GnRH pulse generator rather than a failure of the pituitary gland to produce gonadotropin. As originally described in 1944 (32), *Kallmann syndrome* consisted of the triad of anosmia, hypogonadism, and color blindness in men. Women may be affected as well, and other associated defects may include cleft lip and palate, cerebellar ataxia, nerve deafness, and abnormalities of thirst and vasopressin release. Because autopsy studies have shown partial or complete agenesis of the olfactory bulb, the term *olfactogenital dysplasia* has also been used to describe the disorder. These anatomic findings coincide with embryologic studies documenting that GnRH neurons originally develop in the epithelium of the olfactory placode and normally migrate into the hypothalamus (33). Gene defects have been found in the proteins that facilitate this neuronal migration, thus leading to an absence of GnRH neurons in the hypothalamus and olfactory bulbs and consequent hypogonadotropic hypogonadism and anosmia (*Kallmann syndrome*) (34). The gene defect resulting in loss of this facilatory adhesion protein has been localized to the X chromosome in the X-linked form of the syndrome, and this locus has been designated KALIG-1 (*Kallmann syndrome interval gene-1*). Isolated gonadotropin deficiency is so heterogeneous, however, that it appears likely that this disorder forms a structural continuum with other midline defects; septo-optic dysplasia represents the most severe disorder.

Clinically, affected individuals typically present with sexual infantilism and an eunuchoid habitus, but some degree of breast development may occur (Fig. 23.12). Primary amenorrhea is the rule. The ovaries are usually small, with follicles seldom developed beyond the primordial stage. Circulating gonadotropin levels are usually very low but almost invariably measurable. Affected individuals respond readily to pulsatile administration of exogenous GnRH, and clearly this is the most physiologic approach to ovulation induction (34). For women not seeking pregnancy, replacement therapy with exogenous estrogen and progestin is indicated.

Isolated gonadotropin deficiency can also occur in association with the *Prader-Labhardt-Willi syndrome,* which is characterized by obesity, short stature, hypogonadism, small hands and feet (acromicria), mental retardation, infantile hypotonia, and the *Laurence-Moon-Bardet-Biedl syndrome,* which is characterized by retinitis pigmentosa, postaxial polydactyly, obesity, and hypogonadism.

Multiple pituitary hormone deficiencies, which are usually hypothalamic in origin, may be congenital and either part of an inherited constellation of findings or sporadic. If growth hormone (GH) or thyroid-stimulating hormone (TSH) concentrations are subnormal, growth in addition to pubertal development will be affected. Thus, the condition should be diagnosed before the age of puberty.

Tumors of the Hypothalamus and Pituitary   Several different tumors of the hypothalamic and pituitary regions may also lead to hypogonadotropic hypogonadism (Fig. 23.13A) (35). Except for craniopharyngiomas, these tumors are relatively uncommon in children. Craniopharyngiomas are usually suprasellar in location and may be asymptomatic well into the second decade of life. Such tumors may present as headache, visual disturbances, short stature or growth failure, delayed puberty, or diabetes insipidus. Visual field defects (including bilateral temporal hemianopsia), optic atrophy, or papilledema may be seen on physical examination. Laboratory evaluation should document hypogonadotropinism and may also reveal hyperprolactinemia as a result of interruption of hypothalamic dopamine inhibition of prolactin release. Radiographically, the tumor may be either cystic or solid and may show areas of calcification. Appropriate therapy for hypothalamic-pituitary tumors may involve surgical excision or radiotherapy (with adequate pituitary hormone replacement therapy) and is best decided by an involved team of physicians including an endocrinologist, a neurosurgeon, and a radiotherapist.

Other Central Nervous System Disorders   Other central nervous system disorders that may lead to delayed puberty include infiltrative diseases, such as Langerhans-type histiocytosis, particularly the form known previously as Hand-Schüller-Christian disease (Fig. 23.13B). Diabetes insipidus is the most common endocrinopathy (because of infiltration of the supraoptic nucleus in the hypothalamus), but short stature resulting from GH deficiency, and delayed puberty caused by gonadotropin deficiency are not uncommon in this disorder (36).

Irradiation of the central nervous system for treatment of any neoplasm or leukemia may result in hypothalamic dysfunction. Although GH deficiency occurs most often, partial or complete gonadotropin deficiency may develop in some patients.

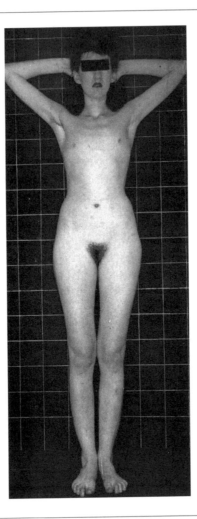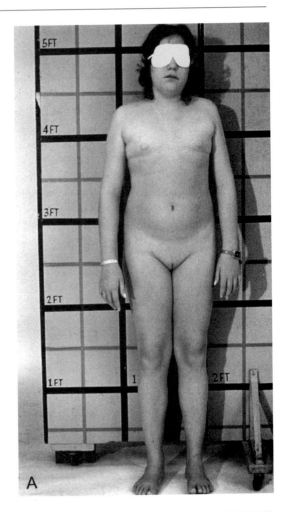

Figure 23.12   A 21-1/2-year-old woman with Kallmann's syndrome. Note that the patient has some pubic and axillary hair. Bone age was 16 years. It is rare to see affected individuals today who were not given oral contraceptive agents to induce menses (with some consequent breast developments. (Reproduced with permission from **Wilkins L.** *The Diagnosis and Treatment of Endocrine Disorders in Childhood and Adolescence.* 3rd ed. Springfield, IL: Charles C. Thomas, 1965.)

Figure 23.13   *A,* **A 16-year-old girl with delayed puberty.** Breast budding began at age 11, but there was no further development. During the year before presentation, her scholastic performance in school deteriorated, she gained 25 lb, she became increasingly lethargic, and nocturia and polydypsia were noted. Initial evaluation documented low follicle-stimulating hormone, elevated prolactin, and a bone age of 10.5 years. Computed tomography scanning documented a large hypothalamic neoplasm that proved to be an ectopic germinoma. The patient was also documented to be hypothyroid and hypoadrenal and to have diabetes insipidus. Despite the elevated prolactin, she had no galactorrhea because of the minimal breast development. (Reproduced with permission from **Rebar RW.** Normal and abnormal sexual differentiation and pubertal development. In: **Moore TR, Reiter RC, Rebar RW, Baker VV,** eds. *Gynecology and Obstetrics. A Longitudinal Approach.* New York: Churchill Livingstone, 1993:97–133.)

Severe chronic illnesses, often accompanied by malnutrition, may also lead to slowed growth in childhood and delayed adolescence. **Regardless of the cause, weight loss to less than 80–85% of ideal body weight often will result in hypothalamic GnRH deficiency.** If adequate body weight and nutrition are maintained in chronic illnesses such as Crohn's disease or chronic pulmonary or renal disease, sufficient gonadotropin secretion usually is present to initiate and maintain pubertal development.

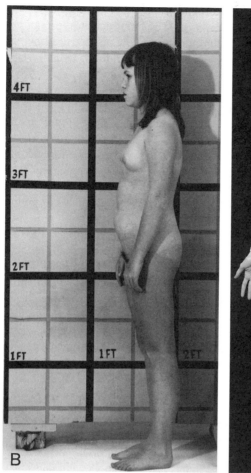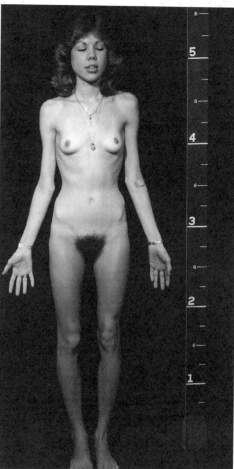

Figure 23.13 *B,* **A 16-year-old girl with primary amenorrhea who progressed in puberty until approximately 12 years of age.** Breast budding occurred at about 10 years of age. Her short stature is obvious. She proved to have hypopituitarism. Classical radiographic findings established the diagnosis of Langerhans-cell-type histiocytosis (Hand-Schüller-Christian disease).

Figure 23.14   An 18-year-old female with anorexia nervosa. As is true of most such patients, pubertal development had been completed and menses initiated before anorexia led to marked weight loss.

Anorexia Nervosa and Bulimia   Significant weight loss and psychologic dysfunction occur simultaneously with anorexia nervosa (37, 38). **Although many anorectic girls experience amenorrhea after pubertal development has begun, if the disorder begins sufficiently early, pubertal development may be delayed or interrupted** (Fig. 23.14). The following constellation of associated findings confirms anorexia nervosa in most individuals:

1. Relentless pursuit of thinness

2. Amenorrhea, sometimes preceding the weight loss

3. Extreme inanition

4. Obsessive-compulsive personality often characterized by overachievement

5. Distorted and bizarre attitude toward eating, food, or weight

6. Distorted body image

Because normal body weight is commonly maintained in bulimia, it is unusual for bulimic patients to experience either delayed development or amenorrhea. Girls with anorexia nervosa may have partial diabetes insipidus, abnormal temperature regulation, chemical hypothyroidism with low serum triiodothyronine (T3) and high reverse T3 levels, and elevated circulating cortisol levels in the absence of evidence of hypercortisolism in addition to hypogonadotropic hypogonadism (39).

Fear of obesity, a syndrome of self-induced malnutrition common among teenage gymnasts and ballet dancers, also may slow growth and delay pubertal development (40). These children voluntarily reduce their caloric intake as much as 40%, leading to nutritional growth retardation. Any additive role for endurance training in the delayed development is possible, but the mechanisms are unclear at this point. These conditions are essentially severe forms of hypothalamic amenorrhea. It is clear, however, that delayed puberty will occur inevitably unless adequate caloric intake is provided.

Hyperprolactinemia   Low levels of LH and FSH may be associated with hyperprolactinemia. As noted, galactorrhea cannot occur in the absence of complete breast development. Pituitary prolactinomas are rare during adolescence but must be considered when certain signs and symptoms are present. Many individuals with prolactinomas have a history of delayed menarche. The association between the ingestion of certain drugs (most often psychotropic agents and opiates in this age group) is well established. Primary hypothyroidism also is associated with hyperprolactinemia because increased levels of thyrotropin-releasing hormone (TRH) stimulate secretion of prolactin. The *empty sella syndrome,* in which the sella turcica is enlarged but has been replaced by cerebrospinal fluid, may also be associated with hyperprolactinemia.

Asynchronous Puberty

Asynchronous pubertal development is characteristic of androgen insensitivity (i.e., *testicular feminization*). Affected individuals typically present with breast development (usually only to Tanner stage 3) out of proportion with the amount of pubic and axillary hair (Fig. 23.15). In this disorder, 46XY individuals have bilateral testes, female external genitalia, a blindly ending vagina (often foreshortened and sometimes absent), and no müllerian derivatives (i.e., uterus and fallopian tubes) (41). Infrequently, patients may have clitoral enlargement and labioscrotal fusion at puberty, which is referred to as *incomplete androgen insensitivity.*

Asynchronous puberty is heterogeneous but is always related to some abnormality of the androgen receptor or of androgen action (42). In perhaps 60–70% of cases, androgen receptors cannot be detected (i.e., the patient is receptor negative). In the remaining cases, androgen receptors are present (i.e., receptor positive), but mutations in the androgen receptor have been detected or there is a defect at a more distal step in androgen action (i.e., a postreceptor defect). Receptor-positive individuals are indistinguishable clinically from receptor-negative individuals. Several different mutations in the androgen receptor gene, most of which occur within the androgen-binding domain of the receptor, have been identified in affected individuals who are receptor positive.

Because the Sertoli cells of the testis make antimüllerian hormone (AMH), müllerian derivatives are absent in this disorder; thus, müllerian regression occurs normally. The testes are often normal in size and may be located anywhere along the path of embryonic testicular descent, in the abdomen, inguinal canal, or labia. One-half of all individuals with androgen insensitivity develop inguinal hernias. Recognizing that most such girls will be 46XX, it is important to determine the karyotype in prepubertal girls with inguinal hernias, especially if a uterus cannot be detected with certainty by ultrasound.

The frequency of gonadal neoplasia is increased with this condition, but the extent is uncertain (27). Most clinicians believe the risk of neoplasia is low before the 25 years of age; thus, the testes should be left in place until after pubertal feminization, especially because

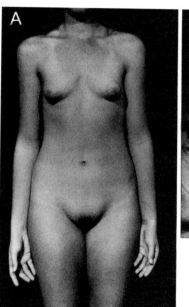
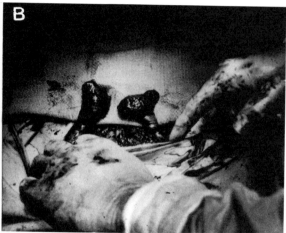

Figure 23.15   *A,* **This 17-year-old individual presented with primary amenorrhea and was found to have a blind-ending vagina and bilateral inguinal masses.** Circulating levels of testosterone were at the upper limits of the normal range for men and the karyotype was 46XY, confirming androgen insensitivity. *B,* **Two inguinal testes (arrows) were found at surgery.** (Reproduced with permission from **Simpson JL, Rebar RW.** Normal and abnormal sexual differentiation and development. In: **Becker KL,** ed. *Principles and Practice of Endocrinology and Metabolism.* 2nd ed. Philadelphia: JB Lippincott, 1995:788–822.)

the risk of neoplasia appears to increase with age. Exogenous estrogen should be provided after gonadectomy.

The diagnosis is often suspected by the typical physical findings and strongly suggested by normal (or even somewhat elevated) male levels of testosterone, normal or somewhat elevated levels of LH, and normal levels of FSH. The diagnosis is confirmed by a 46XY karyotype.

Interacting with the patient and family requires sensitivity and care. It may be inadvisable to begin by informing the patient of the karyotype; the psychological implications may be devastating because the patient has been reared as a female. Family members should be informed that müllerian aplasia occurred and that the risk of neoplasia mandates gonadectomy after puberty. Because the disorder can be inherited in X-linked recessive fashion, families should undergo appropriate genetic counseling and screening to identify the possible existence of other affected family members.

Precocious Puberty

Although precocious pubertal development may be classified in several ways, it is perhaps simplest to think of the development as *gonadotropin-dependent* (in which case it is almost invariably of central origin) or *gonadotropin-independent* (of peripheral origin). The evaluation of precocious puberty is as follows:

1. **Measurement of basal gonadotropin levels is the first step in the evaluation of a child with sexual precocity** (Fig. 23.16).

2. Thyroid function should also be evaluated to rule out primary hypothyroidism as the cause of precocious development.

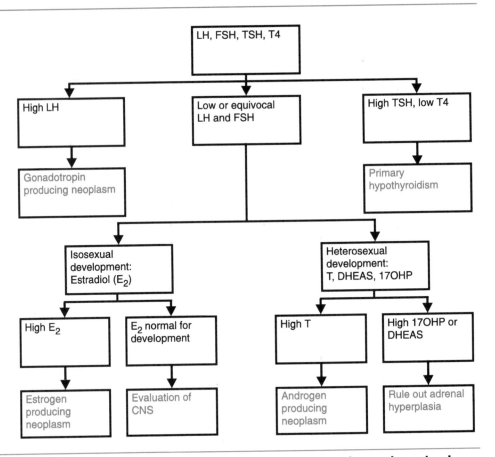

Figure 23.16   Flow diagram for the evaluation of precocious puberty in phenotypic females. (Reproduced with permission from **Rebar RW.** Normal and abnormal sexual differentiation and pubertal development. In: **Moore TR, Reiter RC, Rebar RW, Baker VV,** eds. *Gynecology and Obstetrics. A Longitudinal Approach.* New York: Churchill Livingstone, 1993:97–133.)

3. High levels of LH (which really may be human chorionic gonadotropin detected because of cross-reactivity with LH in immunoassays) suggest a gonadotropin-producing neoplasm, most often a pinealoma (ectopic germinoma) or choriocarcinoma and less often a hepatoblastoma. (Gonadotropin-producing neoplasms are the only causes of precocious puberty in which the gonadotropin dependence does not equate with central precocious puberty.)

4. Low or pubertal levels of gonadotropins indicate the need to determine circulating estradiol concentrations in girls with isosexual development and in girls with heterosexual development to assess androgen levels, specifically testosterone, dehydroepiandrosterone sulfate, and 17α-hydroxyprogesterone.

5. Increased estradiol levels suggest an estrogen-secreting neoplasm, probably of ovarian origin.

6. Increased testosterone levels suggest an androgen-producing neoplasm of the ovary or the adrenal gland. Such neoplasms may be palpable on abdominal or rectal examination. Increased 17α-hydroxyprogesterone levels are diagnostic of 21-hydroxylase deficiency (i.e., congenital adrenal hyperplasia [CAH]).

7. Dehydroepiandrosterone sulfate levels are elevated in various forms of CAH as well.

8. If the estradiol levels are compatible with the degree of pubertal development observed, evaluation of the central nervous system by magnetic resonance imaging or computed tomography scanning is warranted.

9. Bone age should always be assessed in evaluating an individual with sexual precocity.

Perhaps the most difficult decision for the gynecologist is to decide just how much evaluation is warranted for the young girl brought in by her mother for precocious breast budding only (*precocious thelarche*) or the appearance of pubic or axillary hair alone (*precocious pubarche* or *adrenarche*). In such cases, it is acceptable to many clinicians to merely follow the patient at frequent intervals and to proceed with evaluation if there is evidence of pubertal progression. The feasibility of this approach may depend on the concerns of the parents. Premature thelarche may be caused by increased sensitivity of the breasts to low levels of estrogen or to increased estradiol secretion by follicular cysts. Premature adrenarche or pubarche may be due to increased sensitivity to low levels of androgens and must be distinguished from late-onset (nonclassical) CAH. If there is no evidence of both breast development and the appearance of sexually stimulated hair (i.e., precocious puberty) or of progression, these conditions are virtually always benign.

Constitutional sexual precocity is the most common cause of precocious puberty. It is often familial and represents the so-called "tail" of the Gaussian curve (i.e., the early 2.5% for the age distribution for the onset of puberty).

Central (True) Precocious Puberty

In central precocious puberty, GnRH prematurely stimulates increased gonadotropin secretion. Central precocious puberty may occur in children in whom there is no structural abnormality, in which case it is termed *constitutional* or *idiopathic*. Alternatively, central precocious puberty may result from a tumor, infection, congenital abnormality, or traumatic injury affecting the hypothalamus. Tumors of the hypothalamus include hamartomas and, less frequently, neurogliomas and pinealomas. It appears that hamartomas produce GnRH in a pulsatile manner and thus stimulate gonadotropin secretion (Fig. 23.17) (43). A number of congenital malformations, including hydrocephalus, craniostenosis, arachnoid cysts, and septo-optic dysplasia, can also be associated with precocious puberty (as well as with sexual infantilism).

Precocious Puberty of Peripheral Origin

In gonadotropin-independent precocious puberty, production of estrogens or androgens from the ovaries, adrenals, or rare steroid-secreting neoplasms leads to early pubertal development. Small functional ovarian cysts, typically asymptomatic, are common in children and may cause transient sexual precocity (44). Simple cysts (with a benign ultrasonographic appearance) can be observed and usually resolve over time. Of the various ovarian neoplasms that can secrete estrogens, granulosa-theca cell tumors occur most frequently but are still rare (45). Although such tumors may grow rapidly, more than two-thirds are benign.

The *McCune-Albright syndrome* is characterized by polyostotic fibrous dysplasia of bone, irregular *café au lait* spots on the skin, and hyperfunctioning endocrinopathies. Girls develop sexual precocity as a result of functioning ovarian cysts. Other endocrinopathies may include hyperthyroidism, hypercortisolism, hyperprolactinemia, and acromegaly. It is now known that mutations of the $G_{S\alpha}$ subunit of the G protein, which couples extracellular hormonal signals to the activation of adenylate cyclase, are responsible for the autonomous hyperfunction of the endocrine glands and, presumably, for the other defects present in this disorder (46). Exposure to exogenous estrogens can mimic gonadotropin-independent precocious puberty. Ingestion of oral contraceptives, other estrogen-containing pharmaceutical agents, and estrogen-contaminated foods and the topical

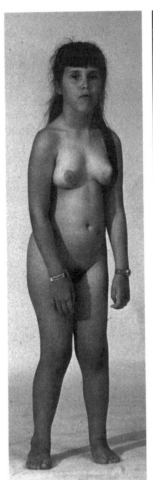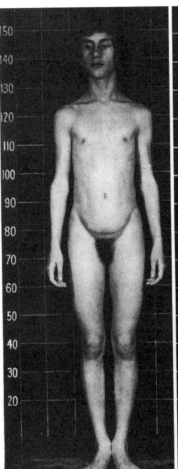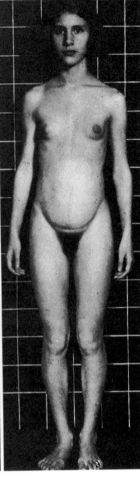

Figure 23.17   A 7-1/2-year-old girl with Tanner stage 4 pubertal development who began menstruating 1 month earlier. She was 57 inches tall (above the 95 percentile). Luteinizing hormone and follicle-stimulating hormone levels were consistent with her development. A large neoplasm that proved to be a hypothalamic hamartoma was present on computed tomography scan. Pubertal development began at about 5 years of age.

Figure 23.18   *Left,* **A 10-1/2-year-old girl with 21-hydroxylase deficiency before treatment.** 17-Ketosteroid (KS) excretion was 34 mg/day. *Right,* **The same patient after 9 months of therapy with cortisone** (17-KS excretion: 4.6 mg/day). (Reproduced with permission from **Wilkins L.** *The Diagnosis and Treatment of Endocrine Disorders in Childhood and Adolescence.* 3rd ed. Springfield, IL: Charles C. Thomas, 1965:439.)

use of estrogens have been implicated in cases of precocious development in infants and children. Severe primary hypothyroidism has also been associated with sexual precocity; associated hyperprolactinemia may result in galactorrhea in affected individuals.

Congenital Adrenal Hyperplasia

Heterosexual precocious puberty is always of peripheral origin and is most often caused by CAH. Three adrenal enzyme defects—21-hydroxylase deficiency, 11β-hydroxylase deficiency, and 3β-hydroxysteroid dehydrogenase deficiency–can lead not only to heterosexual precocity but also to virilization of the external genitalia because of increased androgen production beginning *in utero* (47).

21-Hydroxylase Deficiency   **Most patients with classic CAH have 21-hydroxylase deficiency** (Fig. 23.18). Neonatal screening suggests an incidence of approximately one in 15,000 births. This disorder is inherited as an autosomal recessive trait closely linked to the human leukocyte antigen (HLA) major histocompatibility complex on the short arm of chromosome 6. Thus, siblings with 21-hydroxylase deficiency usually have identical HLA types. There are various forms of 21-hydroxylase deficiency, including *simple virilizing* or classic (typically identified at birth because of genital ambiguity), *salt-wasting* (in which there is impairment of mineralocorticoid as well as glucocorticoid secretion), and *late-onset* or nonclassical (in which heterosexual development occurs at the expected age of puberty). All types involve alleles at the same locus. The nonclassical form is discussed in the following section on heterosexual pubertal development.

21-Hydroxylase deficiency results in the impairment of the conversion of 17α-hydroxyprogesterone to 11-deoxycortisol and of progesterone to deoxycorticosterone (Fig. 23.19). As a consequence, precursors accumulate and there is increased conversion to adrenal androgens. Because the development of the external genitalia is controlled by androgens, in the classic form, girls are born with ambiguous genitalia, including an enlarged clitoris, fusion of the labioscrotal folds, and the urogenital sinus. The internal female organs (including the uterus, fallopian tubes, and ovaries) develop normally because they are not affected by the increased androgen levels. Almost two-thirds of affected newborns rapidly develop salt-wasting 21-hydroxylase deficiency, hyponatremia, hyperkalemia, and hypotension. During childhood, untreated girls with either the classic or salt-wasting form grow rapidly but have advanced bone ages, enter puberty early, experience early closure of their epiphyses, and ultimately are short in stature as adults. CAH, with appropriate therapy, is the only inherited disorder of sexual differentiation in which normal pregnancy and childbearing are possible. The classic and salt-wasting forms of 21-hydroxylase deficiency are easily diagnosed based on the presence of genital ambiguity and markedly elevated levels of 17α-hydroxyprogesterone. Some states have initiated neonatal screening programs to detect 21-hydroxylase deficiency at birth.

3β-Hydroxysteroid Dehydrogenase   Deficiency of 3β-hydroxysteroid dehydrogenase (3β-HSD) affects the synthesis of glucocorticoids, mineralocorticoids, and sex steroids. Typically, levels of 17-hydroxypregnenolone and DHEA are elevated (Fig. 23.19). The classic form of the disorder, detectable at birth, is quite rare, and affected girls may be masculinized only slightly. In severe cases, salt-wasting may also be present.

A nonclassic form of this disorder may be associated with heterosexual precocious pubertal development (as is the classic form if untreated), but postpubertal hyperandrogenism occurs more often. The androgen excess in individuals with nonclassic 3β-HSD deficiency appears to result from androgens derived from the peripheral conversion of increased serum concentrations of DHEA. This disorder is inherited in autosomal recessive fashion, with allelism at the 3β-HSD gene on chromosome 1 believed to be responsible for the varying degrees of enzyme deficiency.

11-Hydroxylase Deficiency   The classic form of 11-hydroxylase deficiency is believed to constitute 5–8% of all cases of CAH. Deficiency in 11-hydroxylase results in the ability to convert 11-deoxycortisol to cortisol, with accumulation of androgen precursors (Fig. 23.19). Markedly elevated levels of 11-deoxycortisol and deoxycorticosterone are present in the disorder. Because deoxycorticosterone acts as a mineralocorticoid, many individuals with this disorder become hypertensive. A mild nonclassic form of 11-hydroxylase deficiency has been reported but is apparently very uncommon.

Treatment of Congenital Adrenal Hyperplasia   **The treatment of CAH involves providing replacement doses of the deficient steroid hormones.** *Hydrocortisone* (10–20 mg/m^2 body surface area) or its equivalent is given daily in divided doses to suppress the elevated levels of pituitary corticotropin present and thus suppress the elevated androgen

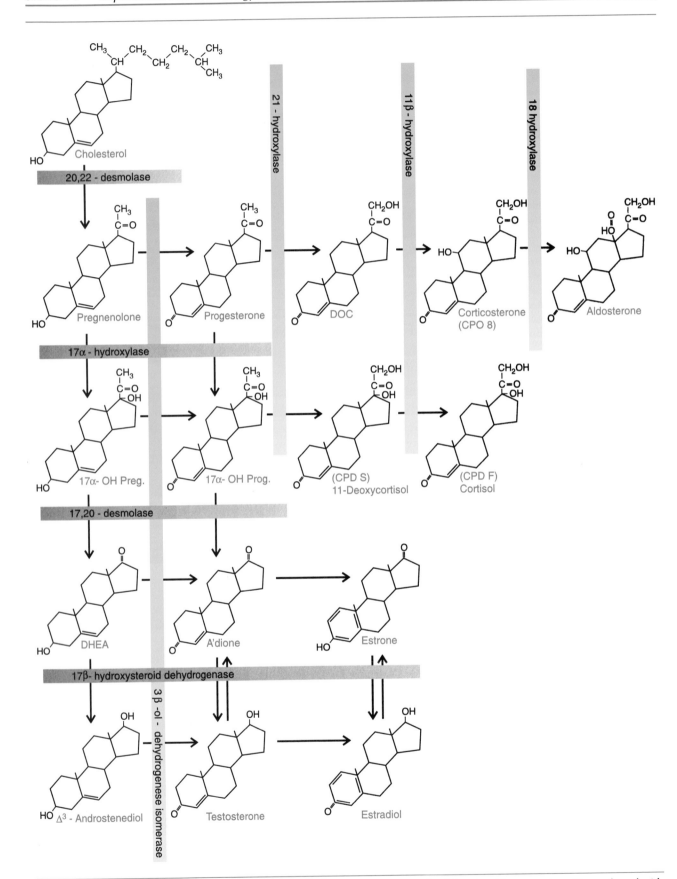

Figure 23.19   Gonadal and adrenal steroid pathways and the enzymes required for steroid conversion. (Reproduced with permission from **Rebar RW, Kenigsberg D, Hodgen GD.** The normal menstrual cycle and the control of ovulation. In: **Becker KL,** ed. *Principles and Practice of Endocrinology and Metabolism.* 2nd ed. Philadelphia: JB Lippincott, 1995:868–80.)

levels. With such treatment, signs of androgen excess should regress. In children, growth velocity and bone age should be monitored carefully because both over- and underreplacement can result in premature closure of the epiphyses and short stature.

Mineralocorticoid replacement is generally required in individuals with 21-hydroxylase deficiency whether or not they are salt-losing. The intent of glucocorticoid therapy should be to suppress morning 17α-hydroxyprogesterone levels to between 300 and 900 ng/dl. Sufficient *fluorocortisone* should be given daily to suppress plasma renin activity to <5 mg/ml/hour. Girls with ambiguous genitalia may require reconstructive surgery, including clitoral recession and vaginoplasty. Timing of such surgery is debated, but the girl must be of appropriate size to permit the surgery to be as simple as possible.

Heterosexual Pubertal Development

The most common cause of heterosexual development at the expected age of puberty is polycystic ovarian syndrome (PCO) (Fig. 23.20). Because the syndrome is heterogeneous and poorly defined, clinical difficulties result in diagnosis and management (48). For the sake of simplicity, **PCO may be defined as LH-dependent hyperandrogenism** (49). Most clinical manifestations arise as a consequence of the hyperandrogenism and often include hirsutism beginning at or near puberty and irregular menses from the age of menarche because of oligo-ovulation or anovulation and are as follows:

1. Affected girls may be but are not necessarily somewhat overweight.

2. In rare instances, menarche may be delayed, and primary amenorrhea also may occur.

3. Basal levels of LH tend to be elevated in most affected individuals, and androgen production is invariably increased, even though circulating levels of androgens may be near the upper limits of the normal range in many affected women.

4. In anovulatory women, estrone levels are typically greater than estradiol levels.

5. Because circulating levels of estrogens are not diminished in PCO and androgen levels are only mildly elevated, affected girls become both feminized and masculinized at puberty. This is an important feature because girls with classic forms of CAH who do not experience precocious puberty (and even those who do) only become masculinized at puberty (i.e., they do not develop breasts).

Differential Diagnosis and Evaluation

Distinguishing PCO from the nonclassic forms of CAH is problematic and controversial (50, 51). The evaluation is as follows:

1. Some clinicians advocate measurement of 17α-hydroxyprogesterone in all women who develop hirsutism. Although values of 17α-hydroxyprogesterone are commonly elevated more than 100-fold in individuals with classic 21-hydroxylase deficiency, they may or may not be elevated in nonclassic late-onset forms of the disorder.

2. Measurement of 17α-hydroxyprogesterone also can identify women with various forms of 11-hydroxylase deficiency.

3. Basal levels of DHEAS as well as 17α-hydroxyprogesterone may be moderately elevated in PCO patients, making the diagnosis even more difficult.

4. To screen for CAH, 17α-hydroxyprogesterone should be measured in early morning.

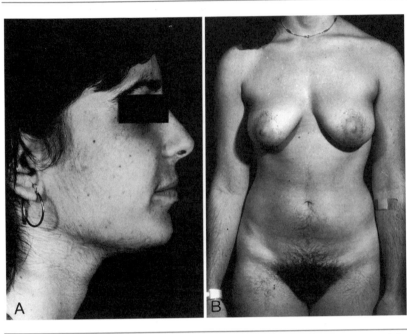
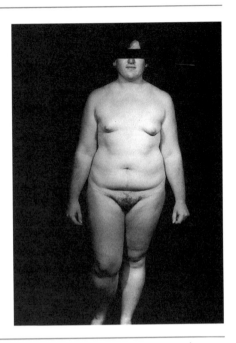

Figure 23.20   Typical appearance of a young 21-year-old woman with polycystic ovarian syndrome. *A,* The patient is well feminized but has apparent hirsutism on her face, and *B,* on her torso..

Figure 23.21   A 19-year-old girl with secondary amenorrhea and severe acne and hirsutism beginning at the normal age of puberty. Stimulatory testing with corticotropin documented nonclassic 21-hydroxylase deficiency. Flattening of the breasts is apparent. She was shorter than her one sister and her mother.

5. In women with regular cyclic menses, it is important to measure 17α-hydroxyprogesterone only in the follicular phase, because basal levels increase at midcycle and in the luteal phase.

Such measurements appear to be of value in populations at high risk of nonclassic late-onset 21-hydroxylase deficiency. In the white population, the gene frequency is only about one in 1000, but it is one in 27 in Ashkenazic Jews, one in 40 in Hispanics, one in 50 in Yugoslavs, and one in 300 in Italians (47). The incidence is also increased among Eskimos and French Canadians. Alternatively, screening might be restricted to hirsute teenagers presenting with the more "typical" features of nonclassic 21-hydroxylase deficiency, including severe hirsutism beginning at puberty, "flattening" of the breasts (i.e., defeminization), shorter stature than other family members, and increased DHEAS levels (between 5000 and 7000 ng/ml). Women with a strong family history of hirsutism or hypertension might be screened as well (Fig. 23.21) (31).

Basal Levels of 17α-Hydroxyprogesterone   Basal levels of 17α-hydroxyprogesterone higher than 800 ng/dl are virtually diagnostic of CAH. Levels between 300 and 800 ng/dl require stimulatory testing with corticotropin to distinguish between PCO and CAH. To complicate the situation even further, nonclassic 21-hydroxylase deficiency may occur even when basal levels of 17α-hydroxyprogesterone are below 300 ng/dl, thus requiring stimulatory testing in those cases as well.

Cosyntropin Stimulation Test   The most commonly used stimulatory test involves measurement of 17α-hydroxyprogesterone 30 minutes after administration of a bolus of 250 μg of synthetic *Cortrosyn* (*cosyntropin*) (52). In normal women, this value seldom exceeds 400 ng/dl. Patients with classic 21-hydroxylase deficiency achieve peak levels of 3000 ng/dl or higher. Patients with nonclassic 21-hydroxylase deficiency commonly achieve levels of 1500 ng/dl or more. Heterozygous carriers achieve peak levels up to approximately 1000 ng/dl. In hirsute women with hypertension, 11-deoxycortisol levels can be determined during the test. If both 11-deoxycortisol and 17α-hydroxyprogesterone levels are increased, the rare 11-hydroxylase deficiency is present. Only measurements of several steroid precursors after corticotropin stimulation can identify individuals with nonclassic forms of 3β-HSD deficiency.

The elevated levels of 17α-hydroxyprogesterone present in all forms of 21-hydroxylase deficiency are rapidly suppressed by administration of exogenous corticoids. Even a single dose of a glucocorticoid such as *dexamethasone* will suppress 17α-hydroxyprogesterone in CAH but not in virilizing ovarian and adrenal neoplasms.

Hirsutism   It has been suggested that androgen-receptor blockade may be preferable to glucocorticoids as primary treatment of nonclassic 21-hydroxylase deficiency (53). Although menses usually (but not always) become regular shortly after beginning therapy with glucocorticoids, the hirsutism in this disorder has proved to be remarkably refractory to glucocorticoids.

Distinguishing nonclassic forms of CAH from idiopathic hirsutism also may be problematic. Individuals with idiopathic hirsutism have regular ovulatory menses, thus effectively eliminating PCO from consideration. Confusion can be created by the fact that some women with nonclassic CAH may continue to ovulate. Basal levels of 17α-hydroxyprogesterone are normal in idiopathic hirsutism, as is the response to ACTH stimulation. Recent studies document that idiopathic hirsutism represents enhanced androgen action at the hair follicle (54).

Mixed Gonadal Dysgenesis	**The term *mixed gonadal dysgenesis* is used to designate individuals with asymmetrical gonadal development with a germ cell tumor or a testis on one side and an undifferentiated streak, rudimentary gonad, or no gonad on the other side.** Most individuals with this rare disorder have a mosaic karyotype of 45X/46XY and are raised as females who then virilize at puberty. Gonadectomy is indicated to remove the source of androgens and eliminate any risk of neoplasia.
Reifenstein Syndrome	Rare forms of male pseudohermaphroditism, especially 5α-reductase deficiency (the so-called "penis at 12" syndrome) and the *Reifenstein syndrome,* generally have ambiguous female genitalia with variable virilization at puberty. Cushing syndrome, too, may occur rarely during the pubertal years, as may adrenal or ovarian androgen-secreting neoplasms.

Genital Ambiguity at Birth

Because of the concerns of the parents and the need to prevent life-threatening complications, the infant with genital ambiguity should be evaluated promptly. Evaluation and treatment is best conducted by a team of physicians. The initial evaluation is as follows:

1. Cytogenetic and endocrine studies should be initiated promptly. Use of specific probes for the Y chromosome and fluorescent *in situ* hybridization can assist in obtaining a karyotype within 48 hours. Probes for many of the specific inherited disorders are now available as well.

2. To exclude CAH, the most common cause of genital ambiguity, serum levels of sodium, potassium, and 17α-hydroxyprogesterone and urinary excretion of 17-ketosteroids, pregnanetriol, and tetrahydrodeoxycortisol should be measured. Infants should be monitored closely to prevent development of dehydration, hyponatremia, and hyperkalemia.

3. It has been suggested that antimüllerian hormone be measured in infants with genital ambiguity because it is elevated in males and undetectable in females in the first several years of life (55).

During the 3–4 days required for evaluation, it is important to be supportive of the parents. Many clinicians believe that it is important not to attach any unusual significance to the genital ambiguity and to treat the abnormality as just another "birth defect." Physicians should emphasize that the child should undergo normal psychosexual development regardless of the sex-of-rearing selected. Either a name compatible with either sex should be chosen or the naming of the infant should be delayed until the studies have been completed.

Physical Signs

Although the diagnosis is not usually obvious on examination, there are some helpful distinguishing features (Fig. 23.22). In normal males, there is only a single midline frenulum on the ventral side of the phallus; in normal females, there are two frenula lateral to the midline. A female with clitoral enlargement still has two frenula, and a male with hypospadias has a single midline frenulum or several irregular fibrous bands (chordee).

It is important to determine if any müllerian derivatives are present. Recent studies suggest that MRI may be the most effective way of evaluating the infant for the presence of müllerian tissue (56).

Figure 23.22   Two newborn girls with 46XX karyotypes and genital ambiguity. Both had clitoral hypertrophy, paired frenula, so-called scrotalization of the labia, and a common urogenital sinus (shown by the probe in *B*). Both were shown to have 21-hydroxylase deficiency. (Reproduced with permission from **Rebar RW.** Normal and abnormal sexual differentiation and pubertal development. In: **Moore TR, Reiter RC, Rebar RW, Baker VV,** eds. *Gynecology and Obstetrics. A Longitudinal Approach.* New Yorkk: Churchill Livingstone, 1993:97–133.)

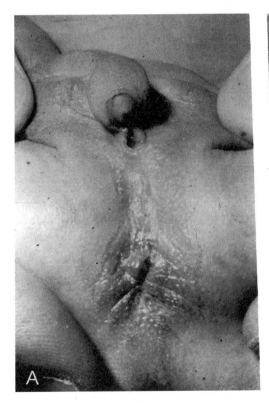
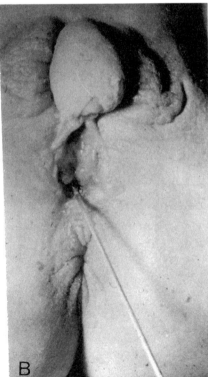

The location or consistency of the gonad may be helpful in deducing its composition. A gonad located in the labial or inguinal regions almost always contains testicular tissue. A testis is generally softer than an ovary or a streak gonad and is more apt to be surrounded by blood vessels imparting a reddish cast. An ovary is more often white, fibrous, and convoluted. A gonad that varies in consistency may be an ovotestis or a testis or a streak gonad that has undergone neoplastic transformation. If a well-differentiated fallopian tube is absent on only one side, the side without the tube probably contains a testis or ovotestis.

Diagnosis and Management

Although genital ambiguity is usually identified at birth, it may not be recognized for several years. Questions about changing the sex-of-rearing may arise. It has been believed that sex-of-rearing may be changed before 2 years of age without psychologically damaging the child, but experience with individuals with 5α-reductase deficiency suggest that gender changes may be made after 2 years of age in certain instances (57). In any case, surgery for genital ambiguity to make the external genitalia (and development) as compatible with the sex-of-rearing of the child is warranted but has not always been proven to be successful. Clitoral recession and clitorectomy are the most frequently performed surgical procedures.

It is possible to diagnose prenatally 21-hydroxylase deficiency in patients known to be at risk (47). The diagnosis is established by documenting elevated levels of 17α-hydroxyprogesterone or 21-deoxycortisol in amniotic fluid. Genetic diagnosis utilizing specific probes and cells obtained by chorionic villus sampling or amniocentesis is also possible. Unfortunately, prenatal treatment of the fetus by administering *dexamethasone* to the mother is usually but not always successful in preventing genital ambiguity (58). Moreover, maternal complications including hypertension, massive weight gain, and overt Cushing syndrome have been noted in about 1% of pregnancies in which the mothers are given low doses of *dexamethasone*. Despite the risks and the nonuniformity of beneficial outcome to affected female fetuses, many parents may choose prenatal medical treatment because of the psychological impact of ambiguous genitalia.

Teratogens

It is important to recognize that ambiguous genitalia can result from the maternal ingestion of various teratogens, most of which are synthetic steroids (Table 23.3). Exposure to the teratogen must occur early in pregnancy during genital organogenesis. Moreover, not all exposed fetuses manifest the same anomalies or even the presence of any anomalies.

In principle, most synthetic steroids with androgenic properties, including weakly androgenic progestins, can affect female genital differentiation. However, the doses required to

Table 23.3   Androgens and Progestogens Potentially Capable of Producing Genital Ambiguity*

Proved	*No Effect*	*Insufficient Data*
Testosterone enanthate	Progesterone	Ethynodiol diacetate
Testosterone propionate	17α-hydroxyprogesterone	Dimethisterone
Methylandrostenediol	Medroxyprogesterone	Norgestrel
6α-methyltestosterone	Norethynodrel	Desogestrel
Ethisterone		Gestodene
Norethindrone		Norgestimate
Danazol		

*Those agents proved to cause genital ambiguity do so only when administered in relatively high doses. Insufficient data exist regarding effects of *dimethisterone* and *norgestrel*. In low doses (e.g., as in oral contraceptives), progestins, even including *norethindrone,* seem unlikely to virilize a female fetus.

produce genital ambiguity are generally so great that the concern is only theoretical. The one agent that clearly can lead to genital ambiguity when ingested in clinically used quantities is *danazol*. There is no evidence that inadvertent ingestion of oral contraceptives, which contain relatively low doses of either *mestranol* or *ethinyl estradiol* and a 19-norsteroid, results in virilization (59, 60).

References

1. **Tanner JM.** *Growth at Adolescence.* 2nd ed. Oxford: Blackwell Scientific Publications, 1962.

2. **Zacharias L, Wurtman RJ.** Blindness: its relation to age of menarche. *Science* 1964;144: 1154–5.

3. **Zacharias L, Rand WM, Wurtman JR.** A prospective study of sexual development and growth in American girls: the statistics of menarche. *Obstet Gynecol Surv* 1976;31:325–37.

4. **Frisch RE.** Body fat, menarche, and reproductive ability. *Semin Reprod Endocrinol* 1985;3: 45–9.

5. **Maclure M, Travis LB, Willett W, MacMahon B.** A prospective cohort study of nutrient intake and age at menarche. *Am J Clin Nutr* 1991;54:649–56.

6. **deRidder CM, Thijssen JHH, Bruning PF, Van den Brande JL, Zonderland ML, Erich WBM.** Body fat mass, body fat distribution, and pubertal development: a longitudinal study of physical and hormonal sexual maturation of girls. *J Clin Endocrinol Metab* 1992;75:442–6.

7. **Marshall WA, Tanner JM.** Variations in patterns of pubertal changes in girls. *Arch Dis Child* 1969;44:291–303.

8. **Greulich WW, Pyle SI.** *Radiographic Atlas of Skeletal Development of the Hand and Wrist.* 2nd ed. London: Oxford University Press, 1959.

9. **Bayley N, Pinneau SR.** Tables for predicting adult height from skeletal age: revised for use with the Greulich-Pyle hand standards. *J Pediatr* 1952;40:423–41.

10. **Kaplan SL, Grumbach MM, Aubert ML.** The ontogeny of pituitary hormones and hypothalamic factors in the human fetus: maturation of central nervous system regulation of anterior pituitary function. *Recent Prog Horm Res* 1976;32:161–243.

11. **Conte FA, Grumbach MM, Kaplan SL.** A diphasic pattern of gonadotropin secretion in patients with the syndrome of gonadal dysgenesis. *J Clin Endocrinol Metab* 1975;40:670–4.

12. **Boyar RM, Finkelstein JW, Roffwarg HP, Kapen S, Weitzman ED, Hellman L.** Synchronization of augmented luteinizing hormone secretion with sleep during puberty. *N Engl J Med* 1972;287:582–6.

13. **Boyar RM, Rosenfeld RS, Kapen S, Finklestein JW, Roffwarg HP, Weitzman ED, et al.** Simultaneous augmented secretion of luteinizing hormone and testosterone during sleep. *J Clin Invest* 1974;54:609–18.

14. **Boyar RM, Wu RHK, Roffwarg H, Kapen S, Hellman L, Weitzman ED, et al.** Human puberty: 24-hour estradiol patterns in pubertal girls. *J Clin Endocrinol Metab* 1976;43:1418–21.

15. **Grumbach MM.** The neuroendocrinology of puberty. In: **Krieger DT, Hughes JC,** eds. *Neuroendocrinology.* Sunderland, MA: Sinauer Associates, Inc., 1980:249–58.

16. **Penny R, Olambiwonnu NO, Frasier SD.** Episodic fluctuations of serum gonadotropins in pre- and post-pubertal girls and boys. *J Clin Endocrinol Metab* 1977;45:307–11.

17. **Korth-Schutz S, Levine LS, New MI.** Serum androgens in normal prepubertal and pubertal children and in children with precocious adrenarche. *J Clin Endocrinol Metab* 1976;42:117–24.

18. **Ducharme J-R, Forest MG, DePeretti E, Sempé M, Collu R, Bertrand J.** Plasma adrenal and gonadal sex steroids in human pubertal development. *J Clin Endocrinol Metab* 1976;42: 468–76.

19. **Lee PA, Xenakis T, Winer J, Matsenbaugh S.** Puberty in girls: correlation of serum levels of gonadotropins, prolactin, androgens, estrogens and progestin with physical changes. *J Clin Endocrinol Metab* 1976;43:775–84.

20. **Judd HL, Parker DC, Siler TM, Yen SSC.** The nocturnal rise of plasma testosterone in pubertal boys. *J Clin Endocrinol Metab* 1974;38:710–13.

21. **Grumbach MM, Kaplan SL.** The neuroendocrinology of human puberty: an ontogenetic perspective. In: **Grumbach MM, Sizonenko PC, Aubert ML,** eds. *Control of the Onset of Puberty.* Baltimore: Williams & Wilkins, 1990:1–62.

22. **Buttram VC Jr, Gibbons WE.** Müllerian anomalies: a proposed classification (an analysis of 144 cases). *Fertil Steril* 1979;32:40–6.

23. **Smith FR.** The significance of incomplete fusion of the Müllerian ducts in pregnancy and parturition with a report on 35 cases. *Am J Obstet Gynecol* 1931;22:714–28.

24. **Herbst AL, Hubby MM, Azizi F, Makii MM.** Reproductive and gynecological surgical experience in diethylstilbestrol-exposed daughters. *Am J Obstet Gynecol* 1981;141:1019–28.

25. **Buttram VC Jr, Reiter RC.** *Surgical Treatment of the Infertile Female.* Baltimore: Williams & Wilkins, 1985:89.

26. **Simpson JL.** Localizing ovarian determinants through phenotypic-karyotypic deductions: progress and pitfalls. In: **Rosenfield R, Grumbach M,** eds. *Turner Syndrome.* New York: Marcel Dekker, Inc., 1990:65–77.

27. **Simpson JL, Photopulos G.** The relationship of neoplasia to disorders of abnormal sexual differentiation. *Birth Defects* 1976;12:15–60.

28. **Manuel M, Katayama KP, Jones HW Jr.** The age of occurrence of gonadal tumors in intersex patients with a Y chromosome. *Am J Obstet Gynecol* 1976;124:293–300.

29. **Rosenfeld RG, Frane J, Attie KM, Brazel JA, Burstein S, Cara JF, et al.** Six-year results of a randomized prospective trial of human growth hormone and oxandrolone in Turner syndrome. *J Pediatr* 1992;121:49–55.

30. **Rebar RW, Cedars MI.** Hypergonadotropic amenorrhea. In: **Filicori M, Flamigni C,** eds. *Ovulation Induction: Basic Science and Clinical Advances.* Amsterdam: Elsevier Science B.V., 1994:115–21.

31. **Kustin J, Rebar RW.** Hirsutism in young adolescent girls. *Pediatr Ann* 1986;15:522.

32. **Kallmann FJ, Schoenfeld WA, Barrera SE.** The genetic aspects of primary eunuchoidism. *Am J Ment Defic* 1944;48:203–36.

33. **Schwanzel-Fukuda M, Jorgenson KL, Bergen HT, Weesner GD, Pfaff DW.** Biology of normal luteinizing hormone-releasing hormone neurons during and after their migration from olfactory placode. *Endocr Rev* 1992;13:623–34.

34. **Crowley WF Jr, Jameson JL.** Clinical counterpoint: gonadotropin-releasing hormone deficiency: perspectives from clinical investigation. *Endocr Rev* 1992;13:635–40.

35. **Vance ML.** Hypopituitarism. *N Engl J Med* 1994;330:1651–62.

36. **Braunstein GD, Whitaker JN, Kohler PO.** Cerebellar dysfunction in Hand-Schüller-Christian disease. *Arch Intern Med* 1973;132:387–90.

37. **Spitzer R.** *Diagnostic and Statistical Manual of Mental Disorders.* 4th ed. Washington, DC: American Psychiatric Association, 1994:53.

38. **Vigersky RA, Loriaux DL, Andersen AE, Lipsett MB.** Anorexia nervosa: behavioral and hypothalamic aspects. *Clin Endocrinol Metab* 1976;5:517–35.

39. **Gold PW, Gwirtsman H, Avgerinos PC, Nieman LK, Gallucci WT, Kaye W, et al.** Abnormal hypothalamic-pituitary-adrenal function in anorexia nervosa: pathophysiologic mechanisms in underweight and weight-corrected patients. *N Engl J Med* 1986;314:1335–42.

40. **Vigersky RA, Andersen AE, Thompson RH, Loriaux DL.** Hypothalamic dysfunction in secondary amenorrhea associated with simple weight loss. *N Engl J Med* 1977;297:1141–5.

41. **Morris JM.** The syndrome of testicular feminization in male pseudohermaphrodites. *Am J Obstet Gynecol* 1953;65:1192.

42. **Griffin JE.** Androgen resistance the clinical and molecular spectrum. *N Engl J Med* 1992;326:611–18.

43. **Mahachoklertwattana P, Kaplan SL, Grumbach MM.** The luteinizing hormone-releasing hormone-secreting hypothalamic hamartoma is a congenital malformation: natural history. *J Clin Endocrinol Metab* 1993;77:118–24.

44. **Lyon AJ, DeBruyn R, Grant DB.** Transient sexual precocity and ovarian cysts. *Arch Dis Child* 1985;60:819–22.

45. **Ein SH, Darte JM, Stephens CA.** Cystic and solid ovarian tumors in children: a 44-year review. *J Pediatr Surg* 1970;5:148–56.

46. **Weinstein LS, Shenker A, Gejman PV, Merino MJ, Friedman E, Spiegal AM.** Activating mutations of the stimulatory G protein in the McCune-Albright syndrome. *N Engl J Med* 1991; 325:1688–95.

47. **Speiser PW.** Congenital adrenal hyperplasia. In: **Becker KL,** ed. *Principles and Practice of Endocrinology and Metabolism.* 2nd ed. Philadelphia: JB Lippincott, 1995:686–95.

48. **Futterweit W.** Pathophysiology of polycystic ovarian syndrome. In: **Redmond GP,** ed. *Androgenic Disorders.* New York: Raven Press, 1995:77–166.

49. **Rebar RW.** Disorders of menstruation, ovulation, and sexual response. In: **Becker KL,** ed. *Principles and Practice of Endocrinology and Metabolism.* 2nd ed. Philadelphia: JB Lippincott, 1995:880–99.

50. **Lobo RA, Goebelsmann U.** Adult manifestation of congenital hyperplasia due to incomplete 21-hydroxylase deficiency mimicking polycystic ovarian disease. *Am J Obstet Gynecol* 1980;138:720–6.

51. **Chrousos GP, Loriaux DL, Mann DL, Cutler GB.** Late-onset 21-hydroxylase deficiency mimicking idiopathic hirsutism or polycystic ovarian disease. *Ann Intern Med* 1982;96:143–8.

52. **New MI, Lorenzen F, Lerner AJ, Kohn B, Oberfield SE, Pollack MS, et al.** Genotyping steroid 21-hydroxylase deficiency: hormonal reference data. *J Clin Endocrinol Metab* 1983; 57:320–6.

53. **Spritzer P, Billaud L, Thalabard J-C, Birman P, Mowszowicz I, Raux-Demay MC, et al.** Cyproterone acetate versus hydrocortisone treatment in late-onset adrenal hyperplasia. *J Clin Endocrinol Metab* 1990;70:642–6.

54. **Horton R, Hawks D, Lobo R.** $3\alpha < 17\beta$-Androstanediol glucuronide in plasma: a marker of androgen action in idiopathic hirsutism. *J Clin Invest* 1982;69:1203–6.

55. **Gustafson ML, Lee MM, Asmundson L, MacLaughlin DT, Donahoe PK.** Müllerian inhibiting substance in the diagnosis and management of intersex and gonadal abnormalities. *J Pediatr Surg* 1993;28:439–44.

56. **Hricak H, Chang YCF, Thurner S.** Vagina: evaluation with MR imaging, Part I: Normal anatomy and congenital anomalies. *Radiology* 1991;179:593.

57. **Imperato-McGinley J, Guerrero L, Gautier T, Peterson PE.** Steroid 5α-reductase deficiency: an inherited form of male pseudohermaphroditism. *Science* 1974;186:1213–5.

58. **Pang SY, Pollack MS, Marshall RN, Immken L.** Prenatal treatment of congenital adrenal hyperplasia due to 21-hydroxylase deficiency. *N Engl J Med* 1990;322:111–5.

59. **Schardein JL.** Congenital abnormalities and hormones during pregnancy: a clinical review. *Teratology* 1980;22:251–70.

60. **Bracken MB.** Oral contraception and congenital malformations in offspring: a review and meta-analysis of the prospective studies. *Obstet Gynecol* 1990;76:552–7.

61. **Wilkins L.** *The Diagnosis and Treatment of Endocrine Disorders in Childhood and Adolescence.* 3rd ed. Springfield, IL: Charles C. Thomas, 1965.

62. **Rebar RW.** Practical evaluation of hormonal status. In: **Yen SSC, Jaffe RB,** eds. *Reproductive Endocrinology: Physiology, Pathophysiology and Clinical Management.* 3rd ed. Philadelphia: WB Saunders, 1991:830.

63. **Marshall WA, Tanner JM.** Variation in the pattern of pubertal changes in boys. *Arch Dis Child* 1970;45:13–23.

64. **Ross GT, VandeWiele RL, Frantz AG.** The ovaries and the breasts. In: **Williams RH,** ed. *Textbook of Endocrinology.* 6th ed. Philadelphia: WB Saunders, 1981:355.

65. **Emans SJH, Goldstein DP.** The physiology of puberty. In: **Emans SJH, Goldstein DP,** eds. *Pediatric and Adolescent Gynecology.* 3rd ed. Boston: Little, Brown & Co., 1990:95.

66. **Hamill PVV, Drizd TA, Johnson CL, Reed RB, Roche AF, Moore WM.** Physical growth: National Center for Health Statistics percentiles. *Am J Clin Nutr* 1979;32:607–29.

67. **Rebar RW.** Normal and abnormal sexual differentiation and pubertal development. In: **Moore TR, Reiter RC, Rebar RW, Baker VV,** eds. *Gynecology and Obstetrics. A Longitudinal Approach.* New York: Churchill Livingstone, 1993:97–133.

68. **Spitzer IB, Rebar RW.** Counselling for women with medical problems. Ovary and reproductive organs. In: **Hollingsworth D, Resnik R,** eds. *Medical Counselling Before Pregnancy.* New York: Churchill Livingstone, 1988:213–48.

69. **Simpson JL, Rebar RW.** Normal and abnormal sexual differentiation and development. In: **Becker KL,** ed. *Principles and Practice of Endocrinology and Metabolism.* 2nd ed. Philadelphia: JB Lippincott, 1995:788–822.

70. **Rebar RW, Kenigsberg D, Hodgen GD.** The normal menstrual cycle and the control of ovulation. In: **Becker KL,** ed. *Principles and Practice of Endocrinology and Metabolism.* 2nd ed. Philadelphia: JB Lippincott, 1995:868–80.

71. **Buttram VC Jr, Gibbons WE.** Müllerian anomalies: a proposed classification (an analysis of 144 cases). *Fertil Steril* 1979;32:40–6.

24 Amenorrhea

Wendy J. Scherzer
Howard McClamrock

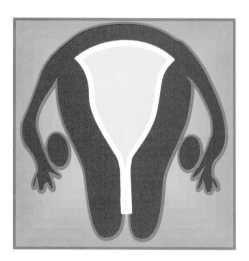

A complex hormonal interaction must take place in order for normal menstruation to occur. The hypothalamus must secrete gonadotropin-releasing hormone (GnRH) in a pulsatile fashion, which is modulated by neurotransmitters and hormones. The GnRH stimulates secretion of follicle-stimulating hormone (FSH) and luteinizing hormone (LH) from the pituitary, which promotes ovarian follicular development and ovulation. A normally functioning ovarian follicle secretes estrogen; after ovulation, the follicle is converted to a corpus luteum and progesterone is secreted in addition to estrogen. These hormones stimulate endometrial development. If pregnancy does not occur, estrogen and progesterone secretion decrease, and withdrawal bleeding begins. If any of the components (hypothalamus, pituitary, ovary, outflow tract and feedback mechanism) are nonfunctional, bleeding cannot occur.

Primary amenorrhea is defined as the absence of menses by 16 years of age in the presence of normal secondary sexual characteristics or by 14 years of age when there is no visible secondary sexual characteristic development. The definition represents approximately two standard deviations from the mean age when secondary sexual characteristic development and menstruation should occur. **A woman who has previously menstruated can develop secondary amenorrhea, which is defined as absence of menstruation for three normal menstrual cycles or 6 months.**

Patients may develop slight alterations in the hypothalamic-pituitary-ovarian axis that are not severe enough to cause amenorrhea but instead cause anovulation. Anovulatory patients usually have irregular menses and may bleed excessively during menstruation because estrogen is unopposed. This often occurs at the beginning and end of the reproductive years. Luteal phase defect is caused by minimal alterations in the hypothalamic-pituitary-ovarian axis, and patients have regular menses along with infertility or recurrent pregnancy loss. Except for anatomic and chromosomal etiologies, luteal phase defects and anovulation have causes similar to those of amenorrhea, but the hypothalamic, pituitary, or ovarian hormonal dysfunction is less severe or of shorter duration than with amenorrhea.

In order to detect the cause of amenorrhea, it is useful to determine whether secondary sexual characteristics are present (Fig. 24.1). The absence of secondary sexual characteristics indicates that a women has never been exposed to estrogen stimulation.

809

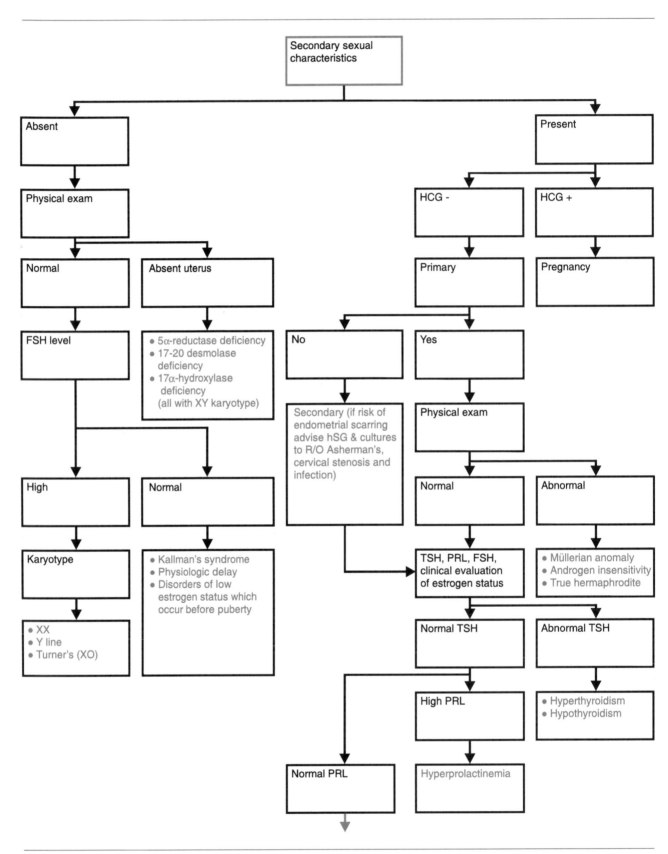

Figure 24.1   Decision tree for evaluation of amenorrhea.

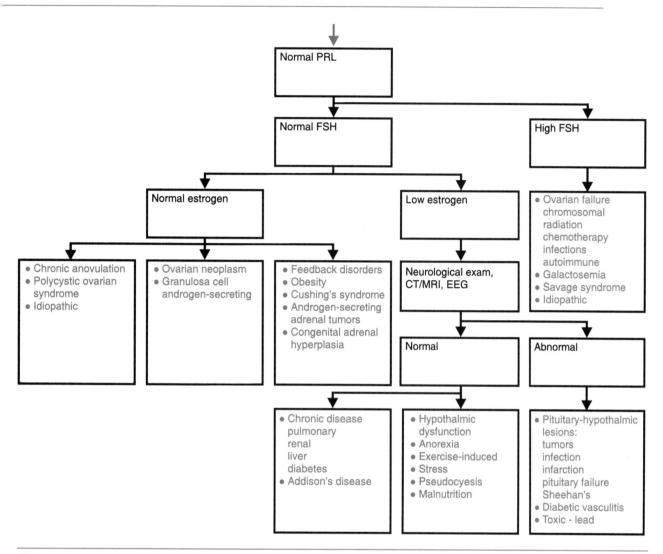

Figure 24.1—*continued*

Amenorrhea Without Secondary Sexual Characteristics

Although the diagnosis and treatment of disorders associated with hypogonadism have been discussed in Chapter 23, they will also be mentioned here because these conditions may present as primary amenorrhea. Abnormal findings on physical examination may suggest certain enzyme deficiencies (Fig. 24.1). Because these conditions are very rare, however, it seems easier to discuss the causes on the basis of the gonadotropin status.

Causes of Primary Amenorrhea

Hypergonadotropic Hypogonadism

Primary gonadal failure and the resulting impaired secretion of gonadal steroids is manifest by elevated levels of LH and FSH that result from decreased negative feedback. Gonadal failure as well as primary amenorrhea are most often associated with genetic abnormalities (Table 24.1). **Approximately 30% of patients with primary amenorrhea have**

Table 24.1   Amenorrhea Associated with a Lack of Secondary Sexual Characteristics

Abnormal Physical Examination

5α-reductase deficiency in XY individual
17–20 desmolase deficiency in XY individual
17α-hydroxylase deficiency in XY individual

Hypergonadotropic Hypogonadism

Gonadal dysgenesis
Pure gonadal dysgenesis
Partial deletion of X chromosome
Sex chromosome mosaicism
Environmental and therapeutic ovarian toxins
17α-hydroxylase deficiency in XX individual
Galactosemia
Other

Hypogonadotropic Hypogonadism

Physiological delay
Kallman's syndrome
Central nervous system tumors
Hypothalamic/pituitary dysfunction

an associated genetic abnormality (1). **The syndrome of gonadal dysgenesis, or Turner's syndrome, and its variants represent the most common form of hypogonadism in women** (see Chapter 23). Other disorders associated with primary amenorrhea include structurally abnormal X chromosomes, mosaicism, pure gonadal dysgenesis (46XX and 46XY with gonadal streaks), and 17α-hydroxylase deficiency. Individuals with these conditions have gonadal failure and cannot synthesize ovarian steroids. Therefore, gonadotropin levels are elevated because of the lack of negative estrogen feedback on the hypothalamic-pituitary axis. Patients with 17α-hydroxylase deficiency have primordial follicles, but gonadotropin levels are elevated because the enzyme deficiency prevents synthesis of sex steroids. Most patients with these conditions have primary amenorrhea and lack secondary sexual characteristics. However, occasionally patients with a partial deletion of the X chromosome, mosaicism, or pure gonadal dysgenesis (46XX) may synthesize enough estrogen in early puberty to induce breast development and a few episodes of uterine bleeding. Ovulation and, occasionally, pregnancy are possible.

Genetic Disorders

Gonadal Dysgenesis   **Turner's syndrome (45X) is the most common chromosomal abnormality causing gonadal failure and primary amenorrhea** (1, 2). Turner's syndrome is discussed in Chapter 23.

Partial Deletions of the X Chromosome   Individuals with partial deletions of the X chromosome have the karyotype 46XX with part of one of the X chromosomes missing. The phenotype is variable depending on the amount and location of the missing genetic material. Patients with a deletion of part of the long arm of the X chromosome (Xq-) often have sexual infantilism, normal stature, no somatic abnormalities, and streak gonads (3,4). Some patients may be eunuchoid in appearance and have delayed epiphyseal closure. Patients with a deletion of the short arm of the X chromosome (Xp-) and patients with isochrome of the long arm of the X chromosome, with or without mosaicism, usually are phenotypically similar to individuals with Turner's syndrome (5).

Mosaicism   **Primary amenorrhea is associated with various mosaic states, the most common of which is 45X/46XX** (6). As discussed in Chapter 23, the clinical findings in 45X/47XXX and 45X/46XX/47XXX are similar to those in 45X/46XX and vary in estrogen and gonadotropin production depending on the number of follicles in the gonads. When compared to the pure 45X cell line, individuals with 45X/46XX are taller and have fewer abnormalities, although 80% of those with 45X/46XX mosaics are shorter than their peers and 66% have some somatic abnormalities. **Spontaneous menstruation occurs in approximately 20% of these patients** (6).

Pure Gonadal Dysgenesis   **Pure gonadal dysgenesis refers to individuals who are phenotypically female with sexual infantilism, have primary amenorrhea with normal stature, and have no chromosomal abnormalities (46XX or 46XY). The gonads are usually streaks, but there may be some development of secondary sexual characteristics as well as a few episodes of uterine bleeding.**

Enzyme Deficiencies

17α-Hydroxylase Deficiency   **17α-hydroxylase deficiency may be associated with either 46XX or 46XY karyotypes. The uterus is absent in individuals with 46XY karyotype, a feature distinguishing them from individuals with 46XX karyotype. Individuals with 17α-hydroxylase deficiency have primary amenorrhea, no secondary sexual characteristics, female phenotypes, hypertension, and hypokalemia** (7). The diminished levels of 17α-hydroxylase that characterize this disorder lead to a reduction in cortisol production, which in turn causes an increase in adrenocorticotropic hormone (ACTH). 17α-hydroxylase is not required for production of mineralocorticoids; thus, excessive amounts of mineralocorticoid are produced, resulting in sodium retention, loss of potassium, and hypertension.

17-20 Desmolase Deficiency   **Complete block in the δ-4 pathway of 17-20 desmolase leads to a female phenotype in individuals with an XY karotype. The uterus is absent, and sexual development does not occur at puberty.** Although cortisol levels respond normally to ACTH stimulation, testosterone levels are low and do not respond to human chorionic gonadotropin (hCG) stimulation (8).

Other Causes of Primary Ovarian Failure	Amenorrhea and premature ovarian failure can occur in association with irradiation of the ovaries (9), chemotherapy with alkylating agents, e.g., *cyclophosphamide* (10), or combinations of radiation and other chemotherapeutic agents. Galactosemia in girls is often associated with premature ovarian failure, but it usually is detected by newborn screening programs. Gonadotropin resistance, autoimmune ovarian failure, and ovarian failure due to infectious and infiltrative processes have also been described.
Hypogonadotropic Hypogonadism	Primary amenorrhea resulting from hypogonadotropic hypogonadism occurs when the hypothalamus fails to secrete adequate amounts of GnRH or when a pituitary disorder associated with inadequate production or release of pituitary gonadotropins is present.

Physiologic Delay   **Physiologic or constitutional delay of puberty is the most common manifestation of hypogonadotropic hypogonadism. Amenorrhea may result from the delay of physical development caused by delayed reactivation of the GnRH pulse generator.** Levels of GnRH are functionally deficient in relation to chronologic age but normal in terms of physiologic development.

Kallmann's Syndrome   **The second most common hypothalamic cause of primary amenorrhea associated with hypogonadotropic hypogonadism is insufficient pulsatile secretion of GnRH (Kallmann's syndrome), which has varied modes of genetic transmission,** as discussed in Chapter 23. Insufficient pulsatile secretion of GnRH leads to deficiencies in FSH and LH. Deficiencies in GnRH may also be caused by developmental or genetic defects, inflammatory processes, tumors, vascular lesions, or trauma. Patients with isolated deficiencies of LH and FSH usually are a normal height for their age, whereas patients with physiologic delay of puberty are usually short for their chronologic age but normal for their bone age (11).

Central Nervous System Tumors   Central nervous system tumors that lead to primary amenorrhea, the most common of which is craniopharyngioma, are usually extracellular masses that interfere with synthesis and secretion of GnRH or stimulation of pituitary gonadotropins. Virtually all of these patients have disorders in the production of other pituitary hormones as well as LH and FSH (12, 13). Prolactin-secreting pituitary adenomas are rare in childhood and more commonly occur after development of secondary sexual characteristics.

Enzyme Deficiencies

5α-Reductase Deficiency   5α-Reductase deficiency should also be considered as a cause of amenorrhea (14). Patients with this disorder are genotypically XY, frequently experience virilization at puberty, have testes (because of functioning Y chromosomes), and have no müllerian structures due to functioning müllerian-inhibiting factor (MIF). 5α-Reductase converts testosterone to its more potent form, dihydrotestoterone. **Patients with 5α-reductase deficiency differ from patients with androgen insensitivity because they do not develop breasts at puberty and have low gonadotropin levels as a result of testosterone levels sufficient to suppress breast development and allow normal feedback mechanisms to remain intact.** Normal male differentiation of the urogenital sinus and external genitalia do not occur, because dihydrotestosterone is required for this development. However, normal internal male genitalia derived from the Wolffian ducts are present because this development requires testosterone only.

Other Hypothalamic/Pituitary Dysfunctions

Functional gonadotropin deficiency results from malnutrition, malabsorption, weight loss or anorexia nervosa, stress, excessive exercise, chronic disease, neoplasias, and marijuana use (15–19). Hypothyroidism, Cushing's syndrome, hyperprolactinemia, and infiltrative disorders of the central nervous system are rare causes of primary amenorrhea (20,21).

Diagnosis

A careful history and physical examination are necessary to appropriately diagnose and manage patients with primary amenorrhea associated with hypogonadism. The physical examination may be particularly helpful in patients with Turner's syndrome. A history of short stature but consistent growth rate, a family history of delayed puberty, and normal physical findings (including assessment of smell, optic disks, and visual fields) may suggest physiologic delay. Headaches, visual disturbances, short stature, symptoms of diabetes insipidus, and weakness of one or more limbs suggest central nervous system lesions (13). Galactorrhea may be seen with prolactinomas, and the history of galactorrhea is also helpful when diagnosing postinfectious, inflammatory, or vascular lesions of the central nervous system; trauma; anorexia nervosa; stress-related amenorrhea; or other systemic disease processes.

The diagnostic workup is summarized as follows:

1. Assessment of the serum FSH level should be performed as the initial laboratory test unless the history and physical examination suggest otherwise. The FSH level differentiates hypergonadotropic and hypogonadotropic forms of hypogonadism. If the FSH level is elevated, a karyotype is obtained. An elevated FSH level in combination with a 45X karyotype confirms the diagnosis of Turner's syndrome. Partial deletion of the X chromosome, mosaicism, pure gonadal dysgenesis, and mixed gonadal dysgenesis are diagnosed by obtaining a karyotype.

2. Because of the association with coarctation of the aorta and thyroid dysfunction, patients with Turner's syndrome should undergo echocardiography and thyroid function studies.

3. If the karyotype is normal and the FSH is elevated, it is important to consider the diagnosis of 17α-hydroxylase deficiency because it may be a life-threatening disease if untreated. This diagnosis should be considered when testing indicates elevated serum progesterone (>3 ng/ml) levels, a low 17α-hydroxyprogesterone (<0.2 ng/ml) level, and an elevated serum deoxycorticosterone level (DOS) (22). The diagnosis is confirmed with an ACTH stimulation test. After ACTH bolus administration, affected individuals have markedly increased levels of serum progesterone compared with base line levels and no change in serum 17α-hydroxyprogesterone levels.

4. If the screening FSH level is low, the diagnosis hypogonadotropic hypogonadism is established.

5. If the history suggests the presence of a central nervous system lesion or galactorrhea, imaging of the head using computed tomography (CT) or magnetic resonance imaging (MRI) is helpful in the diagnosis. Suprasellar or intrasellar calcification in an abnormal sella is found in approximately 70% of patients with craniopharyngioma (13).

6. Physiologic delay is a diagnosis of exclusion that is difficult to distinguish from insufficient GnRH secretion. The diagnosis can be supported by a history suggesting physiologic delay, an x-ray showing delayed bone age, and the absence of a central nervous system lesion on CT or MRI scanning.

7. Gonadotropin-deficient patients can usually be distinguished from patients with physiologic delay by their response to GnRH stimulation. Patients with physiologic delay have a normal LH response to GnRH stimulation for their bone age, in contrast to gonadotropin-deficient patients, in whom the LH and FSH responses are low (23).

Treatment of Primary Amenorrhea

Individuals with primary amenorrhea asociated with all forms of gonadal failure and hypergonadotropic hypogonadism need cyclic estrogen and progestin therapy to initiate, mature, and maintain secondary sexual characteristics. Prevention of osteoporosis and cardiac disease are additional benefits of estrogen therapy as follows:

1. Therapy is usually initiated with 0.625 mg/day of *conjugated estrogens* or 1 mg of *estradiol*.

2. If the patient is short in stature, higher doses should not be used in an attempt to prevent premature closure of the epiphyses. However, most of these patients are of normal height, and higher estrogen doses may be used initially and then reduced to the maintenance doses after several months.

3. Estrogens can be given daily or 25 days per month and progestin (*medroxyprogesterone acetate* 5–10 mg) should be added 12–14 days every 1–2 months to prevent unopposed estrogen stimulation of the endometrium and breast.

4. In patients with estrogen-free intervals, the progestin should be added during the last 12–14 days of each estrogen cycle.

5. Alternatively, estrogen and progestin may be given daily.

6. Occasionally, individuals with mosaicism and gonadal streaks may ovulate and conceive either spontaneously or after the institution of estrogen replacement therapy (5).

7. If 17α-hydroxylase deficiency is confirmed, treatment is instituted with corticosteroid replacement as well as estrogen and progestin.

815

If possible, therapeutic measures are aimed at correcting the primary cause as follows:

1. Craniopharyngiomas may be resected with a transphenoidal approach or at craniotomy, depending on the size of the tumor. Some studies have showed improved prognosis with radiation therapy used in combination with limited tumor removal (13, 24).

2. Germinomas are highly radiosensitive, and surgery is rarely indicated (25).

3. Prolactinomas and hyperprolactinemia often may respond to *bromocriptine* therapy (26).

4. Specific therapies are directed to malnutrition, malabsorption, weight loss, anorexia nervosa, exercise amenorrhea, neoplasia, and chronic diseases.

5. Logically, it would appear that patients with hypogonadotropic hypogonadism of hypothalamic origin should be treated with long-term administration of pulsatile GnRH. This form of therapy is impractical, however, because of the necessity for the use of an indwelling catheter and a portable pump for prolonged periods. Therefore, these patients should be treated with cyclic estrogen and progestin therapy.

6. Patients with Kallman's syndrome, as well as patients with exercise and stress amenorrhea and anorexia and weight loss, are treated with estrogen replacement.

7. If the patient has physiologic delay of puberty, the only management required is reassurance that the anticipated development will occur eventually (27).

Individuals whose karyotypes contain a Y cell line (45X/46XY mosaicism, or pure gonadal dysgenesis 46XY) are predisposed to gonadal ridge tumors such as gonadoblastomas, dysgerminomas, and yolk sac tumors. The gonads of these individuals should be removed when the condition is diagnosed to prevent malignant transformation (11, 22). There is some evidence that hirsute individuals without Y chromosomes should also undergo gonad removal. A patient with hirsutism and the karyotype 45X was noted to have a streak gonad with the contralateral gonad being dysgenic and containing both follicular development and well-differentiated seminiferous tubules and Leydig cells. This patient was found to be H-Y antigen positive (28).

Clomiphene citrate is ineffective in inducing ovulation in patients with hypogonadism who desire pregnancy because such patients are hypoestrogenic. Ovulation induction in patients with hypogonadism with human menopausal gonadotropins (hMG) is generally successful and pulsatile treatment with GnRH may be used in patients who have normal pituitary function. In patients without ovarian function, oocyte donation may be appropriate. Because most patients with hypogonadism and lack of sexual development are young, usually pregnancy is not desired.

Amenorrhea with Secondary Sexual Characteristics and Anatomic Abnormalities

Causes

Anatomic Abnormalities   Amenorrhea will occur if there is blockage of the outflow tract or if the outflow tract is missing (Table 24.2). An intact outflow tract includes a patent vagina as well a function-

Table 24.2   Anatomic Causes of Amenorrhea

Absent Secondary Sexual Characteristics

Müllerian anomalies
  Imperforate hymen
  Transverse vaginal septum
  Mayer-Rokitansky-Küster-Hauser syndrome
Androgen insensitivity
True hermaphrodites
Absent endometrium
Asherman's syndrome
  Secondary to prior uterine or cervical surgery
    Currettage, especially postpartum
    Cone biopsy
    Loop electroexcision procedure
  Secondary to infections
    Pelvic inflammatory disease
    IUD-related
    Tuberculosis
    Schistosomiasis

ing cervix and uterus. Any transverse blockage of the müllerian system (Buttram and Gibbons Classification I) will cause amenorrhea (29). Such outflow obstructions include imperforate hymen, transverse vaginal septum, and hypoplasia or absence of the uterus, cervix, and or vagina (*Mayer-Rokitansky-Küster-Hauser syndrome*). Of the patients with Mayer-Rokitansky-Küster-Hauser syndrome, 15% have an absent kidney, 40% have a double urinary collecting system (30), and 5–12% have skeletal abnormalities (31). Transverse blockage of the outflow tract with an intact endometrium frequently cause cyclic pain without menstrual bleeding in adolescents. The blockage of blood flow can cause hematocolpos, hematometria, or hemoperitoneum. Endometriosis may develop.

When the findings of the physical examination are normal, anatomic abnormalities may still be considered. A congenitally absent endometrium is a rare finding in patients with primary amenorrhea. Asherman's syndrome, which is more common with secondary amenorrhea or hypomenorrhea, may occur in patients with risk factors for endometrial or cervical scarring, such as a history of uterine or cervical surgery, infections related to use of an intrauterine device, and severe pelvic inflammatory disease. It is found in 39% of patients undergoing hysterosalpingography who have previously undergone postpartum curettage (32). Infections such as tuberculosis and schistosomiasis may cause Asherman's syndrome but are rare in the United States. Cervical stenosis resulting from surgical removal of dysplasia (cone biopsy, loop electroexcision procedure) may also lead to amenorrhea.

Androgen Insensitivity

Phenotypic females with complete congenital androgen insensitivity (previously called testicular feminization) develop secondary sexual characteristics but do not have menses. These patients are male pseudohermaphrodites. Genotypically, they are male (XY) but have a defect that prevents normal androgen receptor function, leading to the development of the female phenotype. Defects in the androgen receptor gene located on the X chromosome include absence of the gene that encodes for the androgen receptor and abnormalities in the androgen binding domain of the receptor. Postreceptor defects also exist (33). Total serum testosterone concentration is in the range of normal males. Because antimüllerian hormone is present and functions normally in these patients, internal female (müllerian) structures such as a uterus, vagina, and fallopian tubes are absent. Testes rather than ovaries are present in the abdomen or in inguinal hernias because of the presence of normally functioning genes on the Y chromosome. Patients have a blind vaginal pouch, and scant or absent axillary and pubic hair. These patients experience abundant breast development at puberty; however, the nipples are immature and the areolae are pale. Testosterone is not present during development to suppress the formation of breast tissues, and at puberty, the conversion of testosterone to estrogen stimulates breast growth. Patients are unusually tall with eunuchnoidal tendency (long arms with big hands and feet) (Fig. 24.2).

True Hermaphrodites

True hermaphroditism is a rare condition that should be considered as a possible cause of amenorrhea. Both male and female gonadal tissue is present in these patients, in whom XX, XY, and mosaic genotypes have been found. Two-thirds of the patients menstruate, but menstruation has never been reported in XY genotypes. The external genitalia is usually ambiguous, and breast development frequently occurs in these individuals.

Diagnosis

Most congenital abnormalities can be diagnosed by physical examination:

1. An imperforate hymen is diagnosed by the presence of a bulging membrane that distends during valsalva maneuver. Ultrasound or MRI is useful to identify the

Figure 24.2 *A,* **A well-developed patient with complete androgen insensitivity.** Note the characteristic paucity of pubic hair and well-developed breasts. (From **Yen SSC, Jaffe RB.** *Reproductive Endocrinology.* 3rd ed. Philadelphia: WB Saunders, 1991:497.) *B,* **Another patient with androgen insensitivity syndrome with a contrasting thin body habitus.** This is a 17-year-old twin 46XY. (Reproduced with permission from **Jones HW Jr, Scott WW.** *Hermaphrodism, Genital Anomalies, and Related Endocrine Disorders.* 2nd ed. Baltimore: Williams & Wilkins, 1971.)

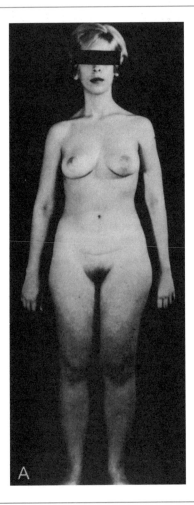 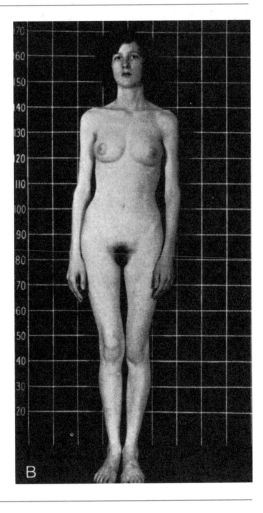

müllerian anomaly when the abnormality cannot be identified by physical examination. The patient should also be examined for skeletal malformations and assessed with intravenous pyelography to detect concomitant renal abnormalities.

2. It is difficult to differentiate a transverse septum or complete absence of the cervix and uterus in a female from a blind vaginal pouch in a male pseudohermaphrodite. Androgen insensitivity is diagnosed when pubic and axillary hair is absent. To confirm the diagnosis, a karyotype should be performed to determine whether a Y chromosome is present. In some patients, the defect in the androgen receptor is not complete and virilization occurs.

3. An absent endometrium is an outflow tract abnormality that cannot be diagnosed by physical examination in a patient with primary amenorrhea. This abnormality is so rare that in a patient with a normal physical findings, it may be advisable to proceed with evaluation of endocrine abnormalities. The absence of the endometrium should be suspected in patients with primary amenorrhea and normal secondary sexual characteristics when the results of hormonal studies are normal and they do not bleed after withdrawal of combined estrogen and progesterone replacement.

4. *Asherman's syndrome* also cannot be diagnosed by physical examination. It is diagnosed by performing hysterosalpingography or hysteroscopy. These tests will show either complete obliteration or multiple filling defects caused by synechiae (Fig. 24.3). If tuberculosis or schistosomiasis is suspected, endometrial cultures should be performed.

Treatment

The treatment of congenital anomalies can be summarized as follows:

1. **Treatment of an imperforate hymen involves making a cruciate incision to open the vaginal orifice.** Most imperforate hymens are not diagnosed until after a hematocolpos forms. It is unwise to place a needle into the hematocolpos without completely removing the obstruction because it may convert a hematocolpos into a pyocolpos.

Figure 24.3   *A,* **Intrauterine adhesion seen on hysterosalpingogram in a patient with Asherman's syndrome.** *B,* **Hysteroscopic view of intrauterine adhesion in a patient with Asherman's syndrome.** (From **Donnez J, Nisolle M.** *The Encyclopedia of Visual Medicine Series—An Atlas of Laser Operative Laparoscopy and Hysteroscopy.* New York: The Parthenon Publishing Group, 1994:306.)

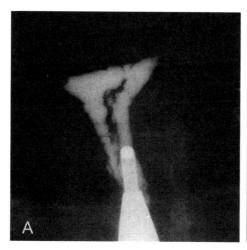 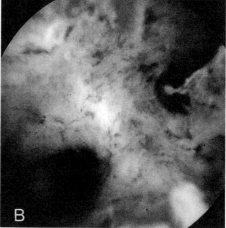

2. **If a transverse septum is present, surgical removal is required.** Forty-six percent of transverse septa occur in the upper one-third of the vagina, and 40% occur in the middle one-third of the vagina (34). Frank dilators should be used to distend the vagina until it is healed to prevent vaginal adhesions (35). Patients have a fully functional reproductive system after surgery; however, patients with repaired high transverse septa have lower pregnancy rates (36).

3. **Hypoplasia or absence of the cervix in the presence of a functioning uterus is more difficult to treat than other outflow obstructions.** Surgery to repair the cervix has not been successful, and hysterectomy is required (37). Endometriosis is a common finding, and it is questionable whether this condition should be treated with initial surgery or if it will resolve spontaneously after surgical repair of the obstruction. The ovaries should be retained to provide the benefits of estrogen and to allow for the possibility of reproducing by removing mature oocytes for *in vitro* fertilization and using a surrogate uterus for implantation.

4. **If the vagina is absent or short, progressive dilation is usually successful in making it functional** (35,38). If dilation fails or the patient is unable to perform dilation, the *McIndoe split thickness graft* technique may be performed (39,40). The initial use of vaginal dilators is required to maintain a functional vagina.

5. **In patients with complete androgen insensitivity, the testes should be removed after pubertal development is complete to prevent malignant degeneration** (41). In patients with testes, 52% develop a neoplasia, most often a gonadoblastoma. Almost one-half of the testicular neoplasms are malignant (dysgerminomas), but transformation usually does not occur until after puberty (42). In patients who develop virilization and have an XY karyotype, the testes should be removed immediately to preserve the female phenotype and to promote female gender identity. Bilateral laparoscopic gonadectomy is the preferred procedure for removal of intra-abdominal testes.

6. **Adhesions in the cervix and uterus (Asherman's syndrome) can be removed using hysteroscopic resection with scissors or electrocautery.** A pediatric Foley catheter should be placed in the uterine cavity for 7–10 days postoperatively (along with administration of systemic broad-spectrum antibiotic therapy) and a 2-month course of high-dose estrogen therapy with monthly progesterone withdrawal is used to prevent reformation of adhesions. Eighty percent of patients thus treated achieve pregnancy, but complications including miscarriage, premature labor, placenta previa, and placenta accreta are common (43). Cervical stenosis can be treated by cervical dilation.

Amenorrhea with Secondary Sexual Characteristics and Nonanatomic Causes

Pregnancy must be considered in all women of reproductive age with amenorrhea. Thyroid dysfunction and hyperprolactinemia are also frequent causes of amenorrhea and are discussed further in Chapter 25. The three major causes of amenorrhea with secondary sexual characteristics are ovarian failure, pituitary/hypothalamic lesions, and abnormal hypothalamic GnRH secretion.

Causes

Ovarian Failure

Ovarian failure is a normal occurrence during menopause. Once a patient is exposed to estrogen, estrogen withdrawal causes hot flashes and vaginal dryness. This occurs in approximately 50% of patients, whether ovarian failure is premature or occurs at the normal age (44). Physical examination reveals vaginal mucosal atrophy and no cervical mucus. When ovarian failure occurs before 40 years of age, it is pathologic. Earlier failure may be caused by decreased follicular endowment or accelerated follicular atresia. If ovarian failure occurs before puberty, the patient's breasts will not develop (i.e., Turner's syndrome), and gonadal agenesis results (Tables 24.1 and 24.3).

Despite the array of causes of ovarian failure, in most cases the etiology cannot be determined. In some patients, ovarian failure resolves spontaneously. Pregnancies have been reported to occur after the diagnosis of ovarian failure in <0.09–8.2% (44,45). Cigarette smoking has been shown to shorten the reproductive years (46).

Genetic Disorders   Mosaicism of an XO or XY cell line may cause ovarian failure in patients younger than 30 years of age. A deletion of a portion of the X chromosome may be present in patients with premature ovarian failure. The Xq26-28 region is critical (47). Individuals with a 47XXX karyotope also may develop ovarian failure. Familial ovarian failure is inherited by dominant Mendelian inheritance in some cases (48).

Iatrogenic Causes   Radiation, chemotherapy (especially alkylating agents such as *cyclophosphamide*) (49), surgical interference with ovarian blood supply, and infections can cause ovarian failure from early loss of follicles. At a radiation dose of 800 cGy, all patients become sterile. Ovarian failure can be caused by as little as 150 cGy in some patients, especially if they are older than 40 years of age with limited follicle reserves.

Autoimmune Disorders   Premature ovarian failure may be part of a polyglandular autoimmune syndrome. Antibodies are present in a variable number of patients with premature ovarian failure, depending on the autoimmune studies performed. One study showed that 92% of patients with premature ovarian failure had autoantibodies (50). However, only 20% of these patients exhibited signs of immunologic dysfunction, most frequently a thyroid disorder (45). Rarely, premature ovarian failure is associated with myasthenia gravis, idiopathic thrombocytopenic purpura, rheumatoid arthritis, vitiligo, autoimmune hemolytic anemia, diabetes mellitus, and other autoimmune disorders (51–53).

Galactosemia   Galactosemia is caused by a lack of functional galactose-1-phosphate uridyl transferase. Galactose metabolites appear to have toxic effects on ovarian follicles, causing their premature destruction (54). There is also evidence that heterozygote carriers of this disorder may have suboptimal ovarian function (55).

Table 24.3   Causes of Ovarian Failure After Development of Secondary Sexual Characteristics

Chromosomal etiology
Iatrogenic causes
   Radiation
   Chemotherapy
   Surgical alteration of ovarian blood supply

Infections

Autoimmune disorders

Galactosemia (mild form or heterozygote)

Savage syndrome

Cigarette smoking

Idiopathic

Savage Syndrome In some patients, follicles are present but they do not mature in response to FSH because FSH receptors are absent or a postreceptor defect exists (52, 56). These patients experience ovarian resistance (*Savage syndrome*) as opposed to ovarian failure, in which no follicles are present. Ovarian biopsy is the only way to distinguish these disorders. Biopsy is not advised, however, because diagnosing resistant ovarian failure will not affect management. Although the use of GnRH agonists, estrogen therapy, and ovarian stimulation have been attempted in patients desiring pregnancy, studies have shown little success.

Pituitary/Hypothalamic Lesions

Hypothalamic Tumors In order for normal menstruation to occur, the hypothalamus must be able to secrete GnRH, and the pituitary must be able to respond with production and release of FSH and LH. Tumors of the hypothalamus or pituitary such as craniopharyngiomas, germinomas, tubercular or sarcoid granulomas, or dermoid cysts may prevent appropriate hormonal secretion. Patients with these disorders may exhibit neurologic abnormalities and abnormal secretion of other hypothalamic and pituitary hormones. Craniopharyngiomas are the most common tumors. They are located in the suprasellar region and frequently cause headaches and visual changes. The surgical and radiologic treatment of tumors may in itself cause further abnormalities in hormone secretion (Table 24.4).

Pituitary Lesions Hypopituitarism is rare because a large portion of the gland must be destroyed before decreased hormonal secretion affects the patient clinically. The pituitary gland may be destroyed by tumors (nonfunctioning or hormone secreting), infarction, infiltrating lesions such as lymphocytic hypophysitis, granulomatous lesions, and surgical or radiologic ablations. *Sheehan's syndrome* is associated with postpartum necrosis of the pituitary resulting from a hypotensive episode that, in its severe form (pituitary apoplexy), presents with the patient in shock. The patient may develop a localized severe retro-orbital headache or abnormalities in visual fields and visual acuity. Patients with a mild form of postpartum pituitary necrosis experience failure to lactate, loss of pubic and axillary hair, and failure to resume menses after delivery. Diabetic vasculitis and sickle cell anemia rarely manifest as pituitary failure. Hypopituitarism is associated with hyposecretion of ACTH and TSH as well as gonadotropins; therefore, thyroid and adrenal function also must be evaluated. If hypopituitarism occurs prior to puberty, menses and secondary sexual characteristics will not develop.

Table 24.4   Pituitary/Hypothalamic Lesions

Pituitary/Hypothalamic

Craniopharyngioma
Germinoma
Tubercular granuloma
Sarcoid granuloma
Dermoid cyst

Pituitary

Nonfunctioning adenomas
Hormone-secreting ademonas
  Prolactinoma
  Cushing's disease
  Acromegaly
  Primary hyperthyroidism
Infarction
Lymphocytic hypophysitis
Surgical or radiological ablations
Sheehan's syndrome
Diabetic vasculitis

Growth hormone (GH), TSH, ACTH, and prolactin also are secreted by the pituitary, and the excess production of each by pituitary tumors causes menstrual abnormalities. The menstrual abnormalities are caused by adverse effects of these hormones on the GnRH pulse generator and not by directly effecting the ovary.

Altered Hypothalamic GnRH Secretion	The pulsatile secretion of GnRH is modulated by interactions with neurotransmitters and peripheral gonadal steroids. Endogenous opioids, corticotropin-releasing hormones (CRH), melatonin, and α-aminobutyric acid (GABA) inhibit the release of GnRH, whereas catecholamines, acetylcholine, and vasoactive intestinal peptide (VIP) stimulate GnRH pulses. Dopamine and serotonin have variable affects (57). Chronic disease, malnutrition, stress, psychiatric disorders, and exercise inhibit GnRH pulses, thus altering the menstrual cycle (Table 24.5). Other hormonal systems that produce excess or insufficient hormones can cause abnormal feedback and adversely affect GnRH secretion. In hyperprolactinemia, Cushing's disease (excess ACTH), and acromegaly (excess GH), excess pituitary hormones are secreted that inhibit GnRH secretion. When the decrease in GnRH pulsatility is severe, amenorrhea results. With less severe alterations in GnRH pulsatility, anovulation can occur. Even slight defects in the pulsatility may result in luteal phase defect.
Anorexia Nervosa	**Anorexia nervosa is an eating disorder that affects 5–10% of adolescent women in the U.S. The criteria for anorexia nervosa as stated in the psychiatric diagnostic manual (DSM-IV) are refusal to maintain body weight above 15% below normal, an intense fear of becoming fat, altered perception of one's body image (i.e., patients see themselves as fat despite being underweight), and amenorrhea.** Patients attempt to maintain their low body weight by food restriction, induced vomiting, laxative abuse, and intense exercise. **This is a life-threatening disorder with a mortality rate as high as 9%.** Amenorrhea may pre-

Table 24.5   Abnormalities Affecting Release of Gonadotropin-Releasing Hormone

Variable Estrogen Status*

Anorexia nervosa
Exercise-induced
Stress-induced
Pseudocyesis
Malnutrition
Chronic diseases
   Diabetes mellitus
   Renal disorders
   Pulmonary disorders
   Liver disease
   Chronic infections
   Addison's disease
Hyperprolactinemia
Thyroid dysfunction

Euestrogenic States

Obesity
Hyperandrogenism
   Polycystic ovarian syndrome
   Cushing's syndrome
   Congenital adrenal hyperplasia
   Androgen-secreting adrenal tumors
   Androgen-secreting ovarian tumors
Granulosa cell tumor
Idiopathic

*Severity of the condition determines estrogen status—the more severe, the more likely to manifest as hypoestrogenism.

cede, coincide, or follow the weight loss. Multiple hormonal patterns are altered. The 24-hour patterns of FSH and LH may show constantly low levels as seen in childhood or increased LH pulsatility during sleep consistent with the pattern seen in early puberty. Hypercortisolism is present despite normal ACTH levels, and the ACTH response to CRH administration is blunted. Circulating triiodothyronine (T_3) is low, yet circulating inactive reverse T_3 concentrations are high (58). Patients may develop cold and heat intolerance, lanugo hair, hypotension, bradycardia, and diabetes insipidus. They may have yellowish discoloration of the skin resulting from elevated levels of serum carotene caused by altered vitamin A metabolism.

Exercise and Stress-Induced Disorders

In patients with exercise-induced amenorrhea, there is a decrease in the frequency of GnRH pulses, which is assessed by measuring a decreased frequency of LH pulses. These patients are usually hypoestrogenic, but less severe alterations may cause minimal menstrual dysfunction (anovulation or luteal phase defect). The decrease in LH pulsatility can be caused by hormonal alterations such as elevations in endogenous opioids, ACTH, prolactin, adrenal androgens, cortisol, and melatonin (59). Differences in body fat content have been used to explain the different rates of amenorrhea by sport. Runners and ballet dancers are at higher risk for amenorrhea than swimmers (60). Frisch and McArthur suggest that a minimum of 17% body fat is required for the initiation of menses and 22% body fat for the maintenance of menses (61). However, newer studies suggest that inappropriately low caloric intake during strenuous exercise is more important than body fat. Higher intensity training, poor nutrition, stress of competition, and associated eating disorders increase an athlete's risk for menstrual dysfunction (62).

Stress-related amenorrhea can be caused by abnormalities in neuromodulation in hypothalamic GnRH secretion, similar to those that occur with exercise and anorexia nervosa. Excess endogenous opioids and elevations in CRH secretion inhibit the secretion of GnRH (57). These mechanisms are not fully understood but appear to be the common link between amenorrhea and chronic diseases, pseudocyesis, and malnutrition.

Obesity

Most obese patients have normal menstrual cycles, but the percentage of women with menstrual disorders increases from 2.6% in normal weight patients to more than 8.4% in women above 75% ideal body weight. The menstrual disorder is more often irregular uterine bleeding with anovulation rather than amenorrhea. **Obese women have an excess number of fat cells in which extraglandular aromatization of androgens to estrogen occurs. They also have lower circulating levels of sex hormone-binding globulin, which allows a larger proportion of free androgens to be converted to estrone. Excess estrogen creates a higher risk for endometrial cancer for these women.** The decrease in sex hormone-binding globulin also allows an increase in free androgen levels, which initially are removed by an increased rate of metabolic clearance. This compensatory mechanism diminishes over time, and hirsutism can develop. Frequently, these patients are classified as having polycystic ovarian syndrome. Alterations in the secretion of endorphins, cortisol, insulin, growth hormone, and insulin-like growth factor-1 (IGF-1) may interact with the abnormal estrogen and androgen feedback to the GnRH pulse generator to cause menstrual abnormalities.

Other Hormonal Imbalances

The secretion of hypothalamic neuromodulators can be altered by feedback from abnormal levels of peripheral hormones. Excesses or deficiencies of thyroid hormone, glucocorticoids, androgens, and estrogens can cause menstrual dysfunction. Polycystic ovarian syndrome (PCO) usually causes irregular bleeding but may cause amenorrhea. It is likely that PCO is the result of peripheral alteration in IGF-1, androgen, and estrogen levels, which leads to hypothalamic dysfunction. Elevations in androgens (e.g., Sertoli-Leydig, hilus, and lipoid cell tumors) and estrogens (e.g., granulosa cell tumors) by ovarian tumors may lead to abnormal menstrual patterns, including amenorrhea. In patients who are hirsute and amenorrheic, androgen-secreting adrenal tumors and congenital adrenal hyperplasia should be considered.

Excess secretion of GH, TSH, ACTH, and prolactin from the pituitary gland can cause abnormal feedback inhibition of GnRH secretion, leading to amenorrhea. Growth hormone excess causes acromegaly, which may be associated with anovulation, hirsutism, and polycystic ovaries as a result of stimulation of the ovary by IGF-1. More commonly, GH excess is accompanied by amenorrhea, low gonadotropin levels, and elevated prolactin levels. Acromegaly is recognized by enlargement of facial features, hands, and feet; hyperhidrosis; visceral organ enlargement; and multiple skin tags. Cushing's disease is caused by an ACTH-secreting pituitary tumor manifest by truncal obesity, moon facies, hirsutism, proximal weakness, depression, and menstrual dysfunction.

Diagnosis

A pregnancy test (urine or serum human chorionic gonadotropin) should be performed in a reproductive age woman with normal secondary sexual characteristics and a normal pelvic examination who has amenorrhea. If the results of the pregnancy test are negative, the evaluation of amenorrhea is as follows:

1. Serum TSH

2. Serum prolactin

3. FSH levels

4. The estrogen status

5. Pituitary and hypothalamic assessment as necessary

TSH and Prolactin Levels

1. Sensitive TSH assays can now be used to evaluate hypothyroidism and hyperthyroidism. Further evaluation of a thyroid disorder is required if abnormalities in TSH are found.

2. Hyperprolactinemia is a common cause of anovulation in women. If elevated TSH and prolactin levels are found, the hypothyroidism should be treated before hyperprolactinemia is treated. Often, the prolactin level will normalize with treatment of hypothyroidism because thyroid-releasing hormone, which is elevated in hypothyroidism, stimulates prolactin secretion.

FSH Levels   Serum FSH levels are required to determine whether the patient has hypergonadotropic, hypogonadotropic, or eugonadotropic amenorrhea. **A circulating FSH level of >40 mIU/ml indicated on at least two blood samples is indicative of hypergonadotropic amenorrhea.** Hypergonadotropism signifies that the cause of amenorrhea is at the level of the ovary. The history should determine whether chemotherapy or radiation therapy are the cause for ovarian failure. A galactose-1 phosphate uridyl transferase level should be obtained to assess the patient for galactosemia disease or carrier status.

In patients less than 30 years of age with hypergonadotropic amenorrhea, a karyotype is required to rule out the presence of a Y cell line. *In situ* hybridization studies may prove the existence of Y chromosomal material with a Y specific probe when the karyotype is normal (63). It is important to identify Y chromosomal material so it may be removed to prevent malignant degeneration.

There is much debate regarding the extent of an autoimmune workup required for a patient with ovarian failure:

1. It is reasonable to screen patients with nonspecific tests such as those for antinuclear antibodies (ANA), rheumatoid factor (RF), and erythrocytic sedimentation rate (ESR).

2. A normal partial thromboplastin time (PTT) is sufficient to exclude lupus anticoagulant.

3. Assessments of serum electrolytes, calcium, and phosphorus concentrations can be used to evaluate the possibility that parathyroid autoantibodies are active.

4. Other assessments that should be performed include TSH, antithyroglobulin antibodies, and antimicrosomal antibodies to evaluate thyroid status and 24-hour urinary free cortisol to evaluate the presence of antiadrenal antibodies.

5. A more extensive workup may include parietal cell antibodies, eyelets of Langerhans antibodies, and antiadrenal antibodies; it is unclear, however, if these tests will alter clinical management.

Tests should be repeated yearly because of the transient nature of autoimmune disorders.

In a patient with hypergonadotropic amenorrhea, ovarian biopsy to determine whether follicles are present is not advised. Even if oocytes are found, there is not a good method of stimulating those oocytes to ovulate. Some patients with negative biopsy results later ovulated spontaneously. This can be explained by considering that the biopsies sample only a small portion of the ovary (45).

Assessment of Estrogen Status   **Traditionally, estrogen status has been determined by giving *medroxyprogesterone acetate*, either 5 mg or 10 mg for 10 days, to determine whether the patient bleeds after withdrawal of the medication (usually 2–10 days after the last dose).** There is a debate as to how much bleeding constitutes withdrawal bleeding. If vaginal bleeding does not occur after oral administration of *progesterone*, frequently 100–200 mg *progesterone* in oil is given intramuscularly. Other ways of testing for estrogen status may be quicker and easier. The development of vaginal dryness and hot flashes increase the likelihood of a diagnosis of hypoestrogenism. A sample of vaginal secretions can be obtained during the physical examination, and mucosal estrogen response can be demonstrated by the presence of superficial cells. A serum estradiol level higher than 40 pg/ml is considered adequate, but interassay discrepancies often exist.

The finding of vaginal bleeding after progesterone challenge is important when Asherman's syndrome is suspected. In a patient with primary amenorrhea and an apparently normal estrogen status, a progesterone challenge will diagnose the rare finding of congenitally absent endometrium. If estrogen status is questioned, 2.5 mg *conjugated estrogen* or 2 mg *micronized estradiol* can be given for 25 days with 5–10 mg of *medroxyprogesterone acetate* added for the last 10 days. Congenital absence of the endometrium is confirmed if no bleeding occurs with this regimen in a patient with primary amenorrhea and no physical abnormalities. If similar findings occur in patients with secondary amenorrhea, Asherman's syndrome is diagnosed. **Asherman's syndrome must be confirmed by showing filling defects on hysterosalpingography or by visualizing adhesions with hysteroscopy.**

Assessment of the Pituitary and Hypothalamus

If the patient is hypoestrogenic and the FSH level is not high, pituitary and hypothalamic lesions should be excluded.

1. A complete neurologic examination, including electroencephalography (EEG), may help localize a lesion.

2. Either CT or MRI scanning should be performed to confirm the presence of a tumor. MRI will identify smaller lesions than CT; if a lesion is too small for identification by CT, it may be clinically insignificant.

3. After anatomic lesions have been excluded, the patient's history of weight changes, exercise, eating habits, body image, and career or school achievements are important factors in differentiating anorexia nervosa, malnutrition, obesity, or exercise-induced or stress-induced menstrual disorders.

Amenorrheic patients who have hypothalamic dysfunction and are hypoestrogenic may have disorders similar to those who are well estrogenized. The hypothalamic dysfunction caused by chronic disease, anorexia nervosa, stress, and malnutrition may be more severe or may exist for a more prolonged time in hypoestrogenic patients than in euestrogenic patients.

Patients with appropriate clinical findings should undergo screening for other hormonal alterations as follows:

1. Androgen levels should be assessed in any hirsute patient to ensure that adrenal and ovarian tumors are not present as well as to diagnose PCO syndrome (Chapter 25).

2. Acromegaly is suggested by coarse facial features, large doughy hands, and hyperhidrosis and may be confirmed by measuring IGF-1 levels.

3. Cushing's syndrome should be ruled out by assessing 24-hour urinary cortisol levels or a 1-mg overnight *dexamethasone* suppression test in patients with truncal obesity, hirsutism, hypertension, and erythematous striae.

Treatment

The treatment of nonanatomic causes of amenorrhea associated with secondary sexual characteristics varies widely according to the cause. The underlying disorder should be treated whenever possible. Patients with unsuspected pregnancy may be counseled regarding the options for continued care. When thyroid abnormalities are discovered, thyroid hormone, radioactive iodine, or antithyroid drugs may be administered as appropriate. When hyperprolactinemia is discovered, treatment may include discontinuation of contributing medications, treatment with *bromocriptine,* and, rarely, surgery for particularly large pituitary tumors.

When ovarian failure causes amenorrhea, estrogen replacement is prescribed for protection against cardiac disease as well as prevention of osteoporosis. Gonadectomy is required when a Y cell line is present.

Surgical removal, radiation therapy, or a combination of both is generally advocated for treatment of central nervous system tumors other than prolactinomas. It may be necessary to treat individuals with panhypopituitarism with various replacement regimens once all the deficits have been elucidated. These regimens include estrogen replacement for lack of gonadotropins, corticosteroid replacement for lack of ACTH, thyroid hormone for lack of TSH, and *DDAVP (1-deamino-8-D-AVP)* to replace vasopressin.

The treatment of amenorrhea associated with hypothalamic dysfunction also depends on the underlying cause:

1. Hormonally active ovarian tumors are surgically removed.

2. Obesity, malnutrition/chronic disease, Cushing's syndrome, and acromegaly should be specifically treated.

3. Pseudocyesis and stress-induced amenorrhea may respond to psychotherapy.

4. Exercise-induced amenorrhea may improve with moderation of activity and weight gain where appropriate.

5. Anorexia nervosa generally demands a multidisciplinary approach, with severe cases requiring hospitalization.

6. Chronic anovulation or PCO syndrome may be treated after identifying the desires of the patient. Patients often are concerned about their lack of menstruation but do not have accompanying hirsutism or infertility. The endometrium of these individuals should be protected from the environment of unopposed estrogen that accompanies the anovulatory state. This is most often done with cyclic administration of *medroxyprogesterone acetate* to induce withdrawal bleeding. A 10-mg daily dose for 10 days per month (or even every other month) should induce withdrawal bleeding and protect the endometrium from hyperplastic transformation. This treatment option presumes an adequate estrogenic environment to induce proliferation of the endometrium and is not sufficient to cause withdrawal bleeding in patients who are hypoestrogenic (i.e., anorexia nervosa). In these individuals, estrogen replacement must be added to the progestin regimen for successful menstrual regulation. Occasionally, ovulation may be associated with cyclic progestin administration. Therefore, patients should be made aware that pregnancy is possible with these therapies and appropriate contraceptive measures should be taken where needed.

7. When chronic anovulation is caused by attenuated congenital adrenal hyperplasia, corticosteroid administration (i.e., *dexamethasone* 0.5 mg at bedtime) is sometimes successful in restoring the normal feedback mechanisms, thereby permitting regular menstruation and ovulation.

Hirsutism

Patients who have oligomenorrhea or amenorrhea resulting from chronic anovulation may have hirsutism (Chapter 25). After ruling out androgen secreting tumors and congenital adrenal hyperplasia, treatment may be aimed at decreasing course hair growth:

1. *Oral contraceptives* may be effective by decreasing ovarian androgen production as well as increasing circulating levels of sex hormone-binding globulin, leading to decreased free androgen circulation.

2. *Spironolactone* has also been used because of its ability to decrease androgen production as well as compete with androgens at the androgen-receptor level. Side effects include limited diuresis and dysfunctional uterine bleeding.

3. *Cyproterone acetate* (an antiandrogen) has been used mainly in Europe, and GnRH agonist administration with addback therapy is being used more frequently in the U.S. Administration of GnRH agonist virtually eliminates ovarian steroid production, and estrogen-progestin addback therapy allows long-term administration and protection against osteoporosis.

Ovulation Induction

A large subset of patients with amenorrhea/oligomenorrhea and chronic anovulation seek care because they are unable to conceive (Chapter 27). Ovulation induction therapy is generally the treatment of choice for such patients, but pretreatment counseling should be in sufficient detail to ensure realistic expectations. The patient should be provided with information regarding the chances of a successful pregnancy (considering age of the patient and treatment modality), potential complications (hyperstimulation and multiple gestation), expense, time, and psychological impact involved in completing the course of therapy (64). **Patients may be advised that there is no increase in congenital anomalies in children born after ovulation induction** (65). Recent studies have raised the possibility of a relationship between ovulation induction and the risk of ovarian cancer (66,67). Ongoing studies are attempting to address this issue conclusively. No change in ovulation induction practices seems warranted at present. A cause-and-effect relationship between ovulation-inducing agents and invasive ovarian carcinoma has not been firmly established, and successful pregnancy may be protective against ovarian cancer.

Clomiphene citrate **is the usual first choice for ovulation induction in suitable patients because of its relative safety, efficacy, route of administration (oral), and relatively low cost** (68). *Clomiphene citrate* is primarily indicated in patients with adequate levels of estrogen and normal levels of FSH and prolactin. It is generally ineffective in hypogonadotropic patients who already have a poor estrogen supply (69). Patients with inappropriate gonadotropin release (an increased LH to FSH ratio), such as that occurring in PCO syndrome, are also candidates for therapy with *clomiphene citrate*. Up to 80% of well-selected patients can be expected to ovulate after *clomiphene citrate* therapy, and pregnancy rates approach 40% (64). Contraindications to the use of *clomiphene citrate* include pregnancy, liver disease, and preexisting ovarian cysts. Side effects include hot flashes ($\geq$11% of patients) and poorly understood visual symptoms, which generally have been viewed as an indication to discontinue subsequent *clomiphene citrate* use. The incidence of multiple gestation ranges from 6.25% to 12.3% (64). The most commonly recommended treatment regimen is 50 mg daily for 5 days, usually beginning on the fifth day of menstrual or withdrawal bleeding. Cycles are easily monitored by measuring midcycle estradiol levels and midluteal progesterone levels to assess folliculogenesis and ovulation. With these data, it is possible to adjust immediately the dose for the subsequent cycle if a given regimen is ineffective. Dosage increases of 50 mg/day are usually used, and more than 70% of conceptions occur at doses no higher than 100 mg/day for 5 days (70). Dosages higher than 150 mg/day for five days are usually ineffective, and patients who remain anovulatory with this dosage should undergo further evaluation accompanied by changes in the therapeutic plan. Longer courses of *clomiphene citrate* therapy as well as adjunctive therapy, with glucocorticoids and hCG, have been recommended (69).

Women who fail to ovulate or to become pregnant with *clomiphene citrate*, **as well as women with hypogonadotropic hypoestrogenic anovulation, may be candidates for therapy with** *hMG*. Much higher pregnancy rates (up to 90%) occur in the latter category. Existing preparations contain FSH or equal combinations of LH and FSH purified from the urine of menopausal women. More highly purified and genetically engineered products may soon be available. Administration protocols and dosages vary widely and should be adjusted to individual needs. Safe administration requires careful monitoring of ovarian response with ultrasonography and serial estradiol measurements. In general, *hMG* is administered at a dose of 75–150 IU/day by intramuscular injection for 2–4 days, after which estradiol and follicular monitoring commence. In most cycles, gonadotropin administration lasts from 7–12 days. Ovulation is triggered by intramuscular injection of 5000–10,000 IU hCG once the lead follicle reaches 16–20 mm in diameter based on ultrasound assessments. Ovulation generally occurs approximately 36 hours after hCG administration. Luteal phase support is sometimes given with additional injections of hCG or with progesterone supplementation. The two major complications associated with induction of ovulation with hMG are multiple pregnancy (10–30%) and ovarian hyperstimulation syndrome. The incidence of both of these complications can be lowered by careful monitoring. Cycles complicated by the recruitment of numerous follicles or by estradiol levels approaching or exceeding 2000 pg/ml may be canceled by withholding the ovulatory dose of hCG. Because severe ovarian hyperstimulation syndrome may lead to prolonged hospitalization and is life-threatening, ovulation induction with hMG generally is performed by experienced practitioners who devote a significant amount of their practice to the treatment of infertility.

Ovulation induction with GnRH may be effective in patients with chronic anovulation associated with low levels of estrogen and gonadotropins. In order for therapy to be successful, a functional ovary and pituitary gland must be present. Therefore, patients with ovarian or pituitary failure do not respond to GnRH therapy. To be effective, GnRH must be administered in a pulsatile fashion either intravenously or subcutaneously by a programmable pump. Ovulation induction with GnRH, as compared with hMG, is associated with a relatively low incidence of ovarian hyperstimulation and multiple births. In addition, the need for appropriate timing of the ovulatory dose of hCG is avoided because patients treated with pulsatile GnRH have an appropriately timed endogenous LH surge. Disadvantages are mainly related to maintaining the programmable pump and injection site. After ovulation, luteal phase support is necessary and may be provided with hCG, progesterone, or continuation of the GnRH therapy.

Patients who lack oocytes (ovarian failure) and desire pregnancy may be candidates for oocyte donation. Oocytes may be harvested after ovulation induction from appropriate donors, fertilized with sperm from the recipient's husband, and transferred into the recipient's uterus after the endometrium has been appropriately prepared with hormonal regimens. Estrogen and progestins are used to prepare the endometrium for implantation of the transferred embryo(s).

References

1. **Rosen GF, Kaplan B, Lobo RA.** Menstrual function and hirsutism in patients with gonadal dysgenesis. *Obstet Gynecol* 1988;17:677–80.

2. **Turner HH.** A syndrome of infantilism, congenital webbed neck, and cubitus-valgus. *Endocrinology* 1938;23:566–74.

3. **Baughman FA, Kolk KJ, Mann JD, Valdmanis A.** Two cases of primary amenorrhea with deletion of the long arm of X chromosome (46,XXq-) *Am J Obstet Gynecol* 1968;102:1065–9.

4. **Hsu LYF, Hirschhorn K.** Genetic and clinical consideration of long arm deletion of the X chromosome. *Pediatrics* 1970;45:656–64.

5. **Rimoin DL, Schimke NR.** *Genetic Disorders of the Endocrine Glands.* St. Louis: CV Mosby, 1971:285–92.

6. **Ferguson-Smith MA.** Karyotype-phenotype correlations in gonadal dysgenesis and their bearing on the pathogenesis of malformations. *J Med Genet* 1965;2:142–55.

7. **Goldsmith O, Soloman DH, Horton R.** Hypogonadism and mineralocorticoid excess: the 17-hydroxylase deficiency syndrome. *N Engl J Med* 1967;277:673–7.

8. **Zachman M, Werder EA, Prader A.** Two types of male pseudohermaphroditism due to 17,20-desmolase deficiency. *J Clin Endocrinol Metab* 1982;55:487–90.

9. **Barrett A, Nicholls J, Gibson B.** Late effects of total body irradiation. *Radiother Oncol* 1987;9:131–5.

10. **Ahmed SR, Shalet SM, Campbell RH, Deakin DP.** Primary gonadal damage following treatment of brain tumors in childhood. *J Pediatr* 1983;103:562–5.

11. **Styne DM, Grumbach MM.** Disorders of puberty in the male and female. In: **Yen SSC, Jaffe RB,** eds. *Reproductive Endocrinology.* 3rd ed. Philadelphia: WB Saunders, 1991:511–54.

12. **Banna M.** Craniopharyngioma: based on 160 cases. *Br J Radiol* 1976;49:206–23.

13. **Thomsett JJ, Conte FA, Kaplan SL, Grumbach MM.** Endocrine and neurologic outcome in childhood craniopharyngioma: review of effective treatment in 42 patients. *J Pediatr* 1980;97:728–35.

14. **Peterson RE, Imperato-McGinley J, Gautier T, Sturla E.** Male pseudohermaphroditism due to steroid 5α reductase deficiency. *Am J Med* 1977;62:170–91.

15. **Kulin HE, Bwibo N, Mutie D, Santner SJ.** Gonadotropin excretion during puberty in malnourished children. *J Pediatr* 1984;105:325–8.

16. **Cumming DC, Rebar RW.** Exercise in reproductive function in women. *Am J Intern Med* 1983;4:113–25.

17. **Ferraris J, Saenger P, Levine L, New M, Pang S, Saxena BB, et al.** Delayed puberty in males with chronic renal failure. *Kidney Int* 1980;18:344–50.

18. **Siris ES, Leventhal BG, Vaitukaitis JL.** Effects of childhood leukemia and chemotherapy on puberty and reproductive function in girls. *N Engl J Med* 1976;294:1143–6.

19. **Copeland KC, Underwood LE, Van Wyk JJ.** Marijuana smoking and pubertal arrest. *Pediatrics* 1980;96:1079–80.

20. **Patton ML, Woolf PD.** Hyperprolactinemia and delayed puberty: a report of three cases and their response to therapy. *Pediatrics* 1983;71:572–5.

21. **Asherson RA, Jackson WPU, Lewis B.** Abnormalities of development associated with hypothalamic calcification after tuberculous meningitis. *BMJ* 1965;2:839–43.

22. **Davajan V, Kletzky OA.** Primary amenorrhea: phenotypic female external genitalia. In: **Mishell DR, Davajan V, Lobo RA,** eds. *Infertility Contraception and Reproductive Endocrinology.* 3rd ed. Cambridge, MA: Blackwell Scientific Publications, 1991:356–71.

23. **Grumbach MM, Styne DM.** Puberty: ontogeny, neuroendocrinology, physiology and disorders. In: **Wilson JB, Foster DW,** eds. *Williams Textbook of Endocrinology.* 8th ed. Philadelphia: WB Saunders, 1992.

24. **Lichter AS, Wara WM, Sheline GE, Townsend JJ, Wilson CB.** The treatment of craniopharyngiomas. *Int J Radiat Oncol* 1977;2:675–83.

25. **Wara WM, Fellows FC, Sheline GE, Wilson CB, Townsend JJ.** Radiation therapy for pineal tumors and suprasellar germinomas. *Radiology* 1977;124:221–3.

26. **Koenig MP, Suppinger K, Leichti B.** Hypoprolactinemia as a cause of delayed puberty: successful treatment with bromocriptine. *J Clin Endocrinol Metab* 1977;45:825–8.

27. **Speroff L, Glass RH, Kase NG.** *Clinical Gynecologic Endocrinology and Infertility.* 5th ed. Baltimore: Williams & Wilkins, 1994.

28. **Rosen GF, Vermesh M, d'Ablain GG, Washtel S, Lobo RA.** The endocrinologic evaluation of a 45X true hermaphrodite. *Am J Obstet Gynecol* 1987;157:1272–3.

29. **Buttram VC Jr, Gibbons WE.** Müllerian anomalies: a proposed classification. *Fertil Steril* 1979;32:40–6.

30. **Fore SR, Hammond CB, Parker RT, Anderson EE.** Urology and genital anomalies in patients with congenital absence of the vagina. *Obstet Gynecol* 1975;46:410–6.

31. **Griffin JE, Edwards C, Madden JD, Harrod MJ, Wilson JD.** Congenital absence of the vagina. *Ann Intern Med* 1976;85:224–36.

32. **Klein SM, Garcia CR.** Asherman's syndrome: a critique and current review. *Fertil Steril* 1973; 24:722–35.

33. **Amrhein JA, Meyer WJ III, Jones HW Jr, Nigeon CJ.** Androgen insensitivity in man: evidence of genetic heterogeneity. *Proc Natl Acad Sci U S A* 1976;73:891–4.

34. **Rock JA.** Anomalous development of the vagina. *Semin Reprod Endocrinol* 1986;4:1–28.

35. **Frank RT.** The formation of an artificial vagina. *Am J Obstet Gynecol* 1938;35:1053–5.

36. **Rock JA, Zacur HA, Diugi AM, Jones HW Jr, TeLinde RW.** Pregnancy success following surgical correction of imperforate hymen and complete transverse vaginal septum. *Obstet Gynecol* 1982;59:448–51.

37. **Williams EA.** Uterovaginal agenesis. *Ann R Coll Surg Engl* 1976;58:266–77.

38. **Ingram JN.** The bicycle seat stool in the treatment of vaginal agenesis and stenosis: a preliminary report. *Am J Obstet Gynecol* 1982;140:867–73.

39. **McIndoe A.** The treatment of congenital absence and obliterative condition of the vagina. *Br J Plast Surg* 1950;2:254–67.

40. **Rock JA.** Surgery for anomalies of the Müllerian ducts. In: **Thompson JD, Rock JA,** eds. *TeLinde's Operative Gynecology.* 7th ed. Philadelphia: JB Lippincott, 1992:603–46.

41. **Conte FA, Grumbach MM.** Pathogenesis, classification, diagnosis, and treatment of anomalies of sex. In: **De Groot LJ,** ed. *Endocrinology.* Philadelphia: WB Saunders, 1989:1810–47.

42. **Manuel M, Katayama KP, Jones HW Jr.** The age of occurrence of gonadal tumors in intersex patients with a Y chromosome. *Am J Obstet Gynecol* 1976;124:293–300.

43. **Doody KM, Carr BR.** Amenorrhea. *Obstet Gynecol Clin North Am* 1990;17:361–87.

44. **Aiman J, Smentek C.** Premature ovarian failure. *Obstet Gynecol* 1984;66:9–14.

45. **Rebar RW, Cedars MI.** Hypergonadotropic forms of amenorrhea in young women. *Reprod Endocrinol* 1992;21:173–91.

46. **Jick H, Porter J, Morrison AS.** Relation between smoking and age of natural menopause. *Lancet* 1977;1:1354–5.

47. **Krauss CM, Tarskoy RN, Atkins L, McLaughlin C, Brown LG, Page DC.** Familial premature ovarian failure due to interstitial deletion of the long arm of the X chromosome. *N Engl J Med* 1987;317:125–31.

48. **Mattison DR, Evan MI, Schwimmer WB.** Familial premature ovarian failure *Am J Hum Genet* 1984;36:1341–8.

49. **Stillman RJ, Schinfeld JS, Schiff I, Gelber RR, Greenberger J, Larson M, et al.** Ovarian failure in long term survivors of childhood malignancy. *Am J Obstet Gynecol* 1981;139:62–6.

50. **Mignot MH, Shoemaker J, Kleingel M, Rao BR, Drexhage HA.** Premature ovarian failure. I: the association with autoimmunity. *Eur J Obstet Gynecol Reprod Biol* 1989;30:59–66.

51. **Jones GS, de Moraes-Ruehsen M.** A new syndrome of amenorrhea in association with hypergonadotropism and apparently normal ovarian follicular apparatus. *Am J Obstet Gynecol* 1969;104:597–600.

52. **Kim MH.** "Gonadotropin-resistant ovaries" syndrome in association with secondary amenorrhea. *Am J Obstet Gynecol* 1974;120:257–63.

53. **de Moraes-Ruehsen M, Blizzard RM, Garcia-Bunuel R, Jones GS.** Autoimmunity and ovarian failure. *Am J Obstet Gynecol* 1972;112:693–703.

54. **Kaufman FR, Kogut MD, Donnell GN, Goebelsmann U, March C, Koch R.** Hypergonadotropic hypogonadism in female patients with galactosemia, N Engl J Med 1981;304: 994–8.

55. **Cramer DW, Harlow BL, Barbieri RL, Ng WG.** Galactose-1-phosphate uridyl transferase activity associated with age at menopause and reproductive history. *Fertil Steril* 1989;51: 609–15.

56. **Coulam CB.** Premature gonadal failure. *Fertil Steril* 1982;38:645–55.

57. **Genazzani AR, Petragtia F, DeRamundo BM, Genazzani AD, Amato F, Algeri L, et al.** Neuroendocrine correlates of stress-related amenorrhea. *Ann NY Acad Sci* 1991;626:125–9.

58. **Herzog DB, Copeland PM.** Eating disorders. *N Engl J Med* 1985;313:295–303.

59. **Olson BR.** Exercise induced amenorrhea. *Am Fam Physician* 1989;39:213–21.

60. **Desouza MJ, Metzger DA.** Reproductive dysfunction in amenorrheic athletic and anorexic patients: a review. *Med Sci Sports Exerc* 1991;23:995–1007.

61. **Frisch RE, McArthur JW.** Menstrual cycles: fatness as a determinant of minimum weight for height necessary for their maintenance or onset. *Science* 1974;185:949–95.

62. **Highet R.** Athletic amenorrhea: an update on a etiology, complications and management. *Sports Med* 1989;7;82–108.

63. **Medlej R, Laboaccaro JM, Berta P, Belon C, Lehep B, Toublanc JE, et al.** Screening for Y-derived sex determining gene SRY in 40 patients with Turner syndrome. *J Clin Endocrinol Metab* 1992;75:1289–92.

64. **Adashi EY, McClamrock HD.** *ACOG Technical Bulletin.* Number 197. Washington, DC: ACOG, 1994.

65. **Scialli AR.** The reproductive toxicity of ovulation induction. *Fertil Steril* 1986;45:315–23.

66. **Whittemore AS, Harris R, Itnyre J, the Collaborative Ovarian Cancer Group.** Characteristics relating to ovarian cancer risk: collaborative analysis of 12 US case-control studies. *Am J Epidemiol* 1992;136:1184–203.

67. **Rossing MA, Daling JR, Weiss NL, More DE, Self SG.** Ovarian tumors in a cohort of infertile women. *N Engl J Med* 1994;331:771–6.

68. **Adashi EY.** Clomiphene citrate-initiated ovulation: a clinical update. *Semin Reprod Endocrinol* 1986;4:255–76.

69. **McClamrock HD, Adashi EY.** Ovulation induction. I. appropriate use of clomiphene citrate. *The Female Patient* 1988;13:92–106.

70. **Rust LA, Israel R, Mishell DR Jr.** An individualized graduated therapeutic regimen for clomiphene citrate. *Am J Obstet Gynecol* 1974;120:785–90.

25 Endocrine Disorders

Avner Hershlag
C. Matthew Peterson

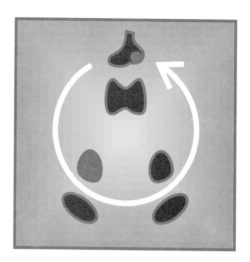

The endocrine disorders that occur most often in gynecology are those related to androgen excess, including hyperandrogenism associated with conditions of the hypothalamus and disorders of the pituitary, ovary, adrenal, and thyroid glands. Polycystic ovarian syndrome (PCOS), Cushing's syndrome, as well as functional tumors of the ovary and pituitary and their management are reviewed.

Hyperandrogenism

Diseases that reflect a state of hyperandrogenism result from either excess production of androgen such as an adrenal or ovarian tumor, from metabolic derangements such as PCOS, or from increased end-organ sensitivity.

Hirsutism

Hirsutism, which is the most frequent manifestation of androgen excess in women, is preceded by acne, chronic anovulation, and virilization. **Hirsutism is defined as the presence of hair in androgen-dependent sites in which hair does not normally appear in women.** This refers particularly to "midline hair," side burns, moustache, beard, chest or intermammary hair, and inner thigh and midline lower back hair entering the intergluteal area.

Androgens affect various types of hair differently. Hair that shows no androgen dependence includes lanugo, eyebrows, and eyelashes. Hair that is more dependent on adrenal androgens includes axillary and pubic hair. Hair that depends significantly on gonadal androgens includes midline, facial, and intermammary hair. Scalp hair is inhibited by gonadal androgens, resulting in the common temporal balding seen in males and in virilized females.

Hair demonstrates cyclic activity between growth (*anagen*), involution (*catagen*), and resting (*telogen*) phases. Both the growth and resting phases are variable in length for different areas of hair growth. Much of the influence of androgens or pharmaceutical agents depends on the phase of hair growth. Synchronization in the hair growth phase may lead to dramatic consequences, such as the hair loss occasionally encountered during pregnancy.

833

The social and clinical reaction to hirsutism may vary significantly. Androgen-dependent hair (excluding pubic and ancillary hair) occurs in only 5% of premenopausal Caucasian women and is considered abnormal in Caucasian women of North America. The presence of sexual hair in other locations is viewed as normal, however, and is socially acceptable in some ethnic groups, such as Eskimos and people of Mediterranean origin.

Two features should be distinguished from hirsutism. *Hypertrichosis* **is the term reserved for androgen-independent growth of hair that is prominent in nonsexual areas such as the trunk and extremities.** This may be an autosomal-dominant congenital disorder or may be caused by metabolic disorders (anorexia nervosa, hyperthyroidism, porphyria cutanea tarda) or medications (*phenytoin, minoxidil, cyclosporine, diazoxide*). *Virilization* **is characterized by male-pattern baldness (vertex most of the time and temples occasionally), coarsening of the voice, decrease in breast size, increase in muscle mass, loss of female body contour (obesity, particularly of the upper segment, and waist-to-hip ratio) and enlargement of the clitoris** (the mean transverse diameter of the glans is 3.4 + 1 mm and the longitudinal diameter is 5.1 + 1.4 mm) (1).

The history should focus on the age of onset and rate of progression of hirsutism or virilization. The latter is associated with a more severe degree of hyperandrogenism and should raise suspicion of ovarian and adrenal neoplasm or Cushing's syndrome. The same is true of rapid progression or onset of symptoms before or after adolescence. Anovulation, presenting as amenorrhea or oligomenorrhea, increases the probability of hyperandrogenism. Hirsutism in women with regular cycles may be associated with normal androgen levels or "idiopathic hirsutism." A tactful and sensitive approach by the physician is mandatory and should include questioning of the patient regarding whether she shaves or removes hair chemically or mechanically and, if so, how frequently. A family history should be obtained to disclose evidence of idiopathic hirsutism, PCOS, congenital adrenal hyperplasia (CAH), diabetes mellitus, and cardiovascular disease. A drug history should also be obtained. Aside from drugs that commonly cause hypertrichosis, anabolic steroids and testosterone derivatives may cause virilization. During physical examination, attention should be directed to obesity, hypertension, galactorrhea, male pattern baldness, acne (face and back), and hyperpigmentation. The presence of an androgen-producing ovarian neoplasm or Cushing's syndrome should be considered. In many cases of Cushing's syndrome, the patient's initial symptom is hirsutism. The physician should keep the possibility of Cushing's syndrome in mind and search for the physical signs of the syndrome such as "moon face," plethora, purple striae, and dorsocervical and supraclavicular fat pads. The type, pattern, and extent of hair growth are evaluated next.

Typically, clinical evaluation of the degree of hirsutism is subjective; most physicians arbitrarily classify the degree of hirsutism as mild, moderate, or severe. Objective assessment is helpful, however, especially in establishing a baseline from which therapy can be evaluated. Ferrimann and Gallway (2) suggest a hirsutism scoring scale of androgen-sensitive hair in nine body areas rated on a scale of 0–4. A score higher than 8 is defined as hirsutism.

Role of Androgens

Androgens and their precursors are produced by both the adrenal glands and the ovaries in response to their respective trophic hormones, luteinizing hormone (LH) and adrenocorticotropic hormone (ACTH) (Fig. 25.1). Biosynthesis begins with the rate-limiting conversion of cholesterol to pregnenolone by side-chain cleavage enzyme. Thereafter, pregnenolone undergoes a two-step conversion to the 17-ketosteroid dehydroepiandrosterone (DHEA) along the δ-5 steroid pathway. This conversion is accomplished via cytochrome P450 c17, an enzyme with both 17-α-hydroxylase and 17,20-lyase activities. In a parallel fashion, progesterone undergoes transformation to androstenedione in the δ-4 steroid pathway. The metabolism of δ-5 to δ-4 intermediate is accomplished via a δ-5-isomerase 3-β-hydroxysteroid dehydrogenase (3-β-HSD).

834

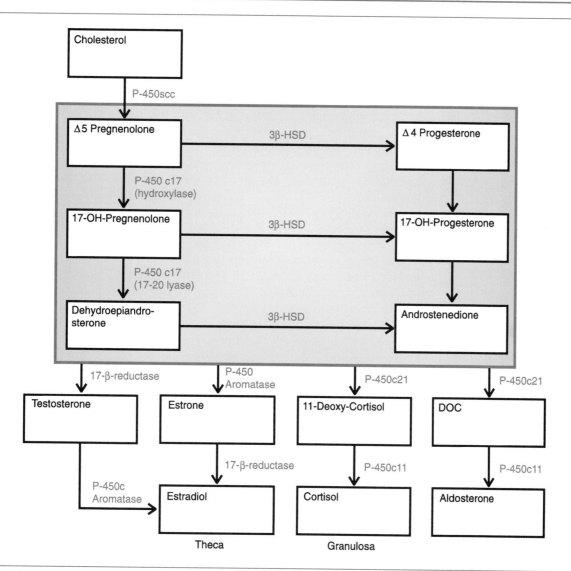

Figure 25.1   Major steroid biosynthesis pathway.

Adrenal 17-Ketosteroids   Secretion of adrenal 17-ketosteroids begins prepubertally (adrenarche) with a dramatic change in the response of the adrenal cortex to ACTH and with preferential secretion of δ-5 steroids, including 17-hydroxypronenolone, DHEA, and dehydroepiandrosterone sulfate (DHEAS). The basis for this action is related to the increase in the zona reticularis and in the increased activity of the 17-hydroxylase and the 17–20 lyase enzymes.

Testosterone   **Testosterone is the most important circulating androgen. Approximately one-half of a woman's serum testosterone is derived from peripheral conversion of secreted androstenedione, and the other one-half is derived from direct glandular secretion. The ovaries and adrenal glands contribute about equally to testosterone production in women.**

Testosterone that is circulating (85%) is bound to sex hormone-binding globulin (SHBG) and is considered biologically inactive. Thus, an increased concentration of total serum testosterone is not the only cause of androgen excess. An increase in the proportion of unbound testosterone is also a causal factor. Most of the proportion of serum testosterone that is not bound to SHBG is associated with albumin (10–15%). A small percentage (1–2%) of testosterone is entirely unbound or free.

835

The fraction of free testosterone may change in relationship to the SHBG concentration, which is increased in association with high estrogen levels such as those that occur during pregnancy and the luteal phase, when estrogen therapy (including oral contraceptives) is being taken, when thyroid hormone levels are increased, and in the presence of cirrhosis of the liver. Levels of SHBG decrease in response to androgens, androgenic medications (progestational agents, *danazol*), androgenic disorders (PCOS, Cushing's syndrome), glucocorticoids, growth hormone, prolactin, insulin, and obesity.

For testosterone to exert its biologic effects on many target tissues, it must be converted into its active metabolite, dihydrotestosterone, by 5-α-reductase, which is a cytosolic enzyme-reducing testosterone, and androstenedione. Dihydrotestosterone is more potent than testosterone, primarily because of its higher affinity and slower dissociation from the androgen receptor. The relative androgenicity of androgens is as follows: dihydrotestosterone, 300; testosterone, 100; androstenedione, 10; and DHEAS, 5.

Until adrenarche, androgens levels remain low. Around 8 years of age, adrenarche is heralded by a marked increase in DHEA and DHEAS. The half-life of free DHEA is extremely short (about 30 minutes) but extends to several hours if DHEA is sulfated. Although no clear role is identified for DHEAS, it is associated with stress and inversely related to aging.

With age, the adrenal glands produce less DHEA and DHEAS. Once the ovaries cease production of estrogen during menopause, the production of testosterone and androstenedione increases. The diurnal variation is maintained by adrenal contribution. Postmenopausally, the ovaries' contribution to elevations in circulating testosterone and androstenedione increases. These androgens are converted to estrone (E1) and estradiol (E2) via extragonadal aromatization.

Laboratory Evaluation

Initial laboratory testing for the assessment of hirsutism should include total testosterone, DHEAS, and 17-hydroxyprogesterone (17-HP) measurements (Table 25.1). If a patient is oligomenorrheic, LH, FSH, prolactin, and thyroid-stimulating hormone (TSH) values may be useful in the initial evaluation. In cases in which Cushing's syndrome is suspected, patients should undergo screening with a 24-hour urinary cortisol (most sensitive) assessment or an overnight *dexamethasone* suppression test. For this test, the patient takes 1 mg of *dexamethasone* at 11:00 PM, and a blood cortisol assessment is performed at 8:00 AM the next day. Cortisol levels of 2 μg/ml or higher require a further workup for Cushing's syndrome.

Many hirsute women manifest testosterone levels above normal [(20–80 ng/dl) (0.723 nmol/l)]. There is no direct correlation between the level of hirsutism and the total testosterone concentration, because hirsutism is caused by the action of the testosterone metabolite, dihydrotestosterone, which in turn is related to the concentration of SHBG. Low SHBG levels, which frequently occur in the presence of elevated androgen and insulin levels, increase free testosterone levels. The result is hirsutism in the absence of an increase

Table 25.1   Normal Values for Serum Androgens*

Serum Androgens	Value
Testosterone	20–80 ng/dl
Free testosterone	0.3–1.9 ng/dl
Androstenedione	20–250 ng/dl
Dehydroepiandrosterone sulfate	100–350 μg/dl
17-hydroxprogesterone (follicular phase)	30–200 ng/dl

*May vary among different laboratories.

in total testosterone. A testosterone level in the male range (>200 ng/dl) is a marker of neoplasms, which are mostly ovarian but occasionally adrenal.

In the past, testing for androgen conjugates (e.g., 3-α-androstenediol G [3-α-diol G] and androsterone G [AOG] as markers for 5-α-reductase activity in the skin) was advocated. However, routine determination of conjugates to assess hirsute patients is not recommended, because hirsutism itself is an excellent bioassay of free testosterone action on the hair follicle and because documentation identifies that these androgen conjugates arise from adrenal precursors and are likely markers of adrenal steroid production (3).

In most laboratories, the upper limit of a DHEAS level is 350 μg/dl (9.5 nmol/liter) in most laboratories. A random sample is sufficient because the level variation is minimized as a result of the long half-life of the sulfated form. The presence of normal levels essentially rules out adrenal disease, and moderate elevations are a common finding in the presence of PCOS. As a rule, a DHEAS level >700 μg/dl (20 nmol/l) is indicative of an adrenal tumor. Occasionally, ovarian tumors are associated with high DHEAS levels.

Because the 17-HP level varies significantly in the cycle, standardized testing requires evaluation in the morning during the follicular phase. A baseline follicular phase 17-HP level should be less than 200 ng/dl (6 nmol/liter). When levels >200 ng/dl but <800 ng/dl (24 nmol), ACTH testing should be performed. Levels >800 ng/dl (24 nmol) also warrant ACTH testing but are virtually diagnostic of 21 hydroxylase deficiency.

Polycystic Ovarian Syndrome

The association of amenorrhea with bilateral polycystic ovaries was first described in 1935 by Stein and Leventhal (4) and was known for decades as Stein-Leventhal syndrome. **The clinical definition of PCOS is characterized by four symptoms: 1) oligomenorrhea to amenorrhea, 2) infertility, 3) hirsutism, and 4) obesity.** Although more recent findings demonstrate the absence of one or more of these symptoms, this definition is still consistent with a diagnosis of PCOS. **In a newly accepted definition of PCOS, the diagnostic criteria include** *hyperandrogenism* **and** *chronic anovulation* **and exclude secondary causes such as neoplasm, hyperprolactinemia, and adult-onset congenital adrenal hyperplasia** (5). An elevated LH:FSH ratio is often but not always present, and cystic ovarian changes are usually present but not essential for diagnosis.

Hirsutism occurs in approximately 70% of patients in the U.S. with PCOS (6) and in only 10–20% of Japanese patients with PCOS (7). The most likely explanation for this discrepancy is genetically determined differences in skin 5-α-reductase activity (8, 9).

Patients with PCOS usually exhibit the following symptoms:

1. *Infertility*

2. *Menstrual disturbances*—patients are not necessarily aware of an increased risk of estrogen-dependent carcinomas but often are upset about irregular menstrual periods or an absence of menses. Women of the reproductive age consider regular menses as evidence of "normalcy."

3. *Hirsutism*—cosmetic concerns are typical in women in their late teens and early twenties, which is when the problem worsens or when social awareness makes patients more self-conscious.

Pathology

Macroscopically, PCOS ovaries are two to five times normal size. The sectional ovarian surface exhibits a white, thickened cortex with multiple cysts that are typically less than 1 cm in diameter (10). Microscopically, the superficial cortex is fibrotic and hypocellular and may contain prominent blood vessels. In addition to smaller atretic follicles, there is an increased number of follicles with luteinized theca interna. The stroma may contain luteinized stromal cells (10).

Pathophysiology and Laboratory Findings

The hyperandrogenism and anovulation encountered in PCOS may be caused by abnormalities in four endocrinologically active compartments: 1) the ovaries, 2) the adrenal glands, 3) the periphery (fat), and 4) the hypothalamus-pituitary compartment.

In patients with PCOS, the ovarian compartment is the most consistent contributor of androgens. Dysregulation of the cytochrome p-450c17, the androgen-forming enzyme in both the adrenals and the ovaries, may be the central pathogenetic mechanism underlying hyperandrogenism in PCOS (11). The ovarian stroma, theca, and granulosa contribute to ovarian hyperandrogenism and are stimulated by LH (12). Testosterone relates to hormone activity relative to PCOS in a number of ways:

1. Total and free testosterone levels correlate directly with LH levels (13).

2. In PCOS, the ovaries are more sensitive to gonadotropic stimulation, possibly as a result of cytochrome p-450c17 dysregulation (11).

3. Treatment with a gonadotropin-releasing hormone (GnRH) agonist effectively suppresses serum testosterone and androstenedione levels (14).

4. Androgen suppression by GnRH agonist requires larger doses of GnRH agonist than estrogen suppression (15).

The increased testosterone levels in patients with PCOS are considered ovarian in origin. The serum testosterone levels are usually no more than twice the upper normal range (20–80 ng/dl). In ovarian hyperthecosis, values may reach 200 ng/dl or more (16).

High intraovarian androgen concentrations inhibit follicular maturation. Although ovarian theca cells are hyperactive, the retarded follicular maturation results in inactive granulosa cells with minimal aromatase activity.

The adrenal compartment also plays a role in the development of PCOS. Although the hyperfunctioning, P-450c17, androgen-forming enzyme coexists in both the ovaries and the adrenal glands (11), DHEAS is increased in only about 50% of PCOS patients (17, 18). The hyperresponsiveness of DHEAS to stimulation with ACTH (17), the onset of symptoms around puberty, and the observation that 17,20-lyase activation (one of the two P-450c17 enzymes) is a key event in adrenarche have led to the concept of PCOS as an exaggerated adrenarche.

The peripheral compartment, defined as the skin and the adipose tissue, manifests its contribution to the development of PCOS in several ways:

1. The presence of 5-α-reductase in the skin largely determines the presence or absence of hirsutism (8, 9).

2. Aromatase and 17-β-hydroxysteroid dehydrogenase activities are increased in fat cells (19), and peripheral aromatization is increased with body weight (20).

3. The metabolism of estrogens, by way of reduced 2-hydroxylation and 17-α-oxidation, is decreased (21).

838

4. Whereas E2 is at a follicular phase level in PCOS patients, E1 levels are increased as a result of peripheral aromatization of androstenedione (22).

5. A chronic hyperestrogenic state results with reversal of the E1:E2 ratio.

The hypothalamic-pituitary compartment participates in aspects critical to the development of PCOS:

1. An increase in LH pulse frequency is the result of increased GnRH pulse frequency (23).

2. This increase in LH pulse frequency typically results in elevated LH and an increased LH:FSH ratio.

3. FSH is not increased with LH, probably because of the synergistic negative feedback of chronically elevated estrogen levels and normal follicular inhibin.

4. About 25% of patients with PCOS exhibit elevated prolactin levels. It is postulated that the hyperprolactinemia may result from abnormal estrogen feedback to the pituitary gland. In some patients with PCOS, *bromocriptine* has reduced LH levels and restored ovulatory function (24).

Insulin Resistance

Patients with PCOS are at risk for hyperinsulinemia and insulin resistance. The most common cause of insulin resistance and compensatory hyperinsulinemia is obesity. The insulin resistance seen in PCOS seems to be independent of the expected insulin resistance that occurs with obesity alone (25). The following observations provide evidence that the insulin resistance associated with PCOS is not the result of hyperandrogenism:

1. Hyperinsulinemia is not a characteristic of hyperandrogenism in general but is uniquely associated with PCOS (25).

2. In obese women with PCOS, 20% have glucose intolerance or frank diabetes mellitus, whereas ovulatory hyperandrogenic women have normal insulin levels and glucose tolerance (25). It seems that the negative effects of PCOS and obesity on the action of insulin are synergistic.

3. Treatment with long-acting GnRH analogs does not change insulin levels or insulin resistance (26).

4. Oophorectomy in patients with hyperthecosis accompanied by hyperinsulinemia and hyperandrogenemia does not change insulin resistance, despite a decrease in androgen levels (27).

Acanthosis nigricans **is considered a marker for insulin resistance in hirsute women. This thickened, pigmented, velvety skin lesion is most often found in the vulva and may be present on the axilla, on the nape of the neck, below the breast, and on the inner thigh** (28).

Women with severe insulin resistance sometimes develop *hair-AN syndrome* (29), **consisting of hyperandrogenism, insulin resistance, and acanthosis nigricans.** These patients usually have high testosterone levels (>1.5 ng/ml), fasting insulin levels of more than 25 μg/ml (normal <20 μg/ml), and maximal serum insulin responses to glucose load exceeding 300 μg/ml (normal is <150 μg/ml).

Insulin alters ovarian steroidogenesis independent of gonadotropin secretion in PCOS. Insulin and insulin-like growth factor 1 receptors are present in the ovarian stromal cells. A specific defect in the early steps of insulin receptor-mediated signaling (diminished autophosphorylation) has been identified in 50% of women with PCOS (30).

Clinically, it is important to realize that patients with PCOS are at increased risk for glucose intolerance or frank diabetes mellitus early in life. Therefore, it is appropriate to screen obese women with PCOS for glucose intolerance on a regular basis once or twice a year. Abnormal glucose metabolism may be improved with weight reduction, which may also reduce hyperandrogenism and restore ovulatory function (31). In obese, insulin-resistant women, caloric restriction that results in weight reduction will reduce the severity of insulin resistance (a 40% decrease in insulin level with a 10-kg weight loss) (32). This decrease in insulin levels should result in a marked decrease in androgen production (a 35% decrease in testosterone levels with a 10-kg weight loss) (32).

Radiologic Studies

Ultrasound examination may be a useful method for early detection and subsequent follow-up of PCOS (33). Generally, ovarian size is increased (34, 35). The most important ultrasonographic finding is a bilaterally increased number of microcysts measuring 0.5–0.8 cm with generally more than five microcysts in each ovary. As the number of microcysts increases and the ovarian volume enlarges, clinical and endocrine abnormalities become more obvious and the condition becomes more severe.

Long-Term Risks

Women with PCOS reportedly manifest abnormal lipid profiles (high triglycerides and low high-density lipoproteins) (36, 37). This manifestation, coupled with insulin resistance and obesity, places patients with PCOS at risk for coronary artery disease. There is a paucity of information in the literature regarding such a risk. One long-term study of patients with PCOS showed an increased prevalence of hypertension and diabetes mellitus (38).

In chronic anovulatory patients with PCOS, persistently elevated estrogen levels, uninterrupted by progesterone, increase the risk of endometrial carcinoma (39). These neoplasms are usually well-differentiated, stage I lesions with a cure rate of more than 90% (see Chapter 31). Likewise, the hyperestrogenic state is associated with an increased risk of breast cancer (40).

Treatment of Hyperandrogenism and PCOS

Treatment depends on a patient's goals. Some patients require hormonal contraception, whereas others benefit from ovulation induction. Interruption of the steady state and control of hirsutism can be accomplished simultaneously; however, for patients desiring pregnancy, effective control of hirsutism may not be possible. Treatment regimens for hirsutism are listed in Table 25.2. The induction of ovulation and treatment of infertility are discussed in Chapter 27.

Weight reduction of obese patients with PCOS may positively affect both menstrual abnormalities and hirsutism (41). Because all medications have potential side effects, weight loss should be the first line of treatment. The addition of antiandrogenic therapy to a weight loss program may further enhance its effect (32, 42).

Oral Contraceptives

Combination oral contraceptives decrease adrenal and ovarian steroid production (43–46) and reduce hair growth in nearly two-thirds of hirsute patients. Oral contraceptive treatment offers the following benefits:

1. The progestin component suppresses LH, resulting in diminished ovarian androgen production.

Table 25.2   Treatment of Hirsutism

Treatment Category	Specific Regimens
Weight loss	
Hormonal suppression	Oral contraceptives Medroxyprogesterone Gonadotropin-releasing hormone analogs Glucocorticoids
Steroidogenic enzyme inhibitors	Ketoconazole
5-α-reductase inhibitors	Finasteride
Antiandrogens	Spironolactone Cyproterone acetate Flutamide
Mechanical	Temporary Permanent (electrolysis)

2. The estrogen increases SHBG production, resulting in decreased free testosterone concentration (47, 48).

3. Circulating androgen levels are reduced, which, to some extent, is independent of the effects of both LH and SHBG (37).

4. Estrogens decrease conversion of testosterone to dihydrotestosterone in the skin by inhibition of 5-α-reductase.

5. Adrenal androgen secretion is reduced (49, 50).

When an oral contraceptive is used to treat hirsutism, a balance must be maintained between the decrease in free testosterone levels and the intrinsic androgenicity of the progestin. Three progestin compounds that are present in oral contraceptives (*norethindrone, norethindrone acetate,* and *norgestrel*), are believed to be androgen dominant. The androgenic bioactivity of these steroids may be a factor of their shared structural similarity with 19-nortesterone steroids (51). Oral contraceptives containing the "new progestins" with little or no androgenic activity (e.g., *desogestrel, gestodine,* and *norgestimate*) are now available in North America.

Low-dose oral contraceptives are as effective as high-dose formulations in improving hirsutism and acne, decreasing testosterone levels, and increasing SHBG levels (51, 52). Other benefits of oral contraceptives include contraception; control of dysfunctional uterine bleeding, iron deficiency, and dysmenorrhea; and reduced risk of pelvic inflammatory disease and ovarian and endometrial cancer.

Medroxyprogesterone Acetate

Oral or intramuscular administration of *medroxyprogesterone acetate* has been used successfully for treatment of hirsutism (53). It directly affects the hypothalamic pituitary axis by decreasing GnRH production and the release of gonadotropins, thereby reducing testosterone and estrogen levels. Despite a decrease in SHBG, total and free androgen levels are decreased significantly (54). The recommended oral dosage is 20–40 mg daily in a divided dosage or 150 mg given intramuscularly every 6 weeks to 3 months in the depot form. Up to 95% of patients note hair growth reduction (55). Other side effects of the drug include amenorrhea, headaches, fluid retention, weight gain, hepatic dysfunction, and depression.

GnRH Agonists

Administration of GnRH agonists may allow the differentiation of androgen produced by adrenal sources from that of ovarian sources (15). It has been shown to suppress ovarian steroids to castrate levels in patients with PCOS (56). Treatment with *leuprolide acetate* given intramuscularly every 28 days decreases hirsutism and hair diameter in both idiopathic hirsutism and hirsutism secondary to PCOS (57). Ovarian androgen levels are significantly and selectively suppressed. The addition of oral contraceptives or estrogen replacement therapy to treatment prevents bone loss and other side effects of menopause such as hot flushes, genital atrophy, and possible risk of heart disease. The hirsutism-reducing effect is retained (57, 58). Suppression of hirsutism is not potentiated by the addition of estrogen replacement therapy to a GnRH agonist (59).

Glucocorticoids

Dexamethasone may be used to treat patients with PCOS who have either adrenal or mixed adrenal and ovarian hyperandrogenism. Doses of *dexamethasone* as low as 0.25 mg nightly or every other night are initially used to suppress DHEAS concentrations to <400 ng/ml. Because *dexamethasone* has 40 times the glucocorticoid effect of cortisol, daily doses >0.5 mg every evening should be avoided to prevent the risk of adrenal suppression and severe cushingoid side effects. To avoid oversuppression of the pituitary adrenal access, serum cortisol levels should be monitored intermittently. Reduction in hair growth rate has been reported (60), as well as significant improvement in acne associated with adrenal hyperandrogenism.

Ketoconazole

Ketoconazole inhibits the key steroidogenic cytochromes. Administered at a low dose (200 mg/day), it has significantly reduced the levels of androstenedione, testosterone, and free testosterone (61).

Spironolactone

Spironolactone is a specific antagonist of aldosterone, which competitively binds to the aldosterone receptors in the distal tubular region of the kidney. Therefore, it is an effective potassium-sparing diuretic, which was originally marketed for treatment of hypertension. *Spironolactone* works in the treatment of hirsutism according to the following mechanisms:

1. Competitive inhibition at the intracellular receptor level for dihydrotestosterone (DHT) (62)

2. Suppression of testosterone biosynthesis by a decrease in the P-450 system (63)

3. Increase in androgen catabolism (with increased peripheral conversion of testosterone to E2)

4. Inhibition of skin 5-α-reductase activity (62)

Although total and free testosterone levels are significantly reduced in patients with both PCOS and idiopathic hirsutism (hyperandrogenism with regular menses), testosterone and free testosterone levels in patients with PCOS remain significantly elevated above those with idiopathic hirsutism following *spironolactone* treatment (64). In both groups, SHBG levels are unaltered. The reduction in circulating androgen levels observed within a few days of *spironolactone* treatment partially accounts for the progressive regression of hirsutism.

At least a modest improvement in hirsutism can be anticipated in 70–80% of women using at least 100 mg of *spironolactone* per day for 6 months (65). Most authors agree that *spironolactone* reduces the daily linear growth rate of sexual hair, hair shaft diameters, and daily hair volume production (66). The most common doses are 25–100 mg twice daily.

Women treated with 200 mg/day show a greater reduction in hair shaft diameter than women receiving 100 mg/day (67).

Maximal effect on hair growth is between 3 and 6 months but continues for 12 months. Electrolysis can be recommended thereafter for permanent hair removal.

The most common side effect of *spironolactone* is menstrual irregularity (usually metrorrhagia), which may occur in up to in 68% of patients with a dose of 200 mg/day (68). Normal menses may resume with reduction of the dosage. Infrequently, other side effects such as urticaria, mastodynia, or scalp hair loss occur (68). Nausea and fatigue can occur with high doses (65). Because *spironolactone* can raise serum potassium levels, its use is not recommended in patients with renal insufficiency or hyperkalemia. Periodic monitoring of potassium and creatinine levels is required.

Return of normal menses in amenorrheic patients is reported in up to 60% of cases (64). Patients must be counseled to use contraception with *spironolactone*, because it theoretically can feminize a male fetus.

Cyproterone Acetate

Cyproterone acetate is a synthetic progestin derived from 17-HP with potent antiandrogenic properties. The primary mechanism of *cyproterone acetate* is competitive inhibition of testosterone and dihydrotestosterone at the level of androgen receptors (69). This agent also induces hepatic enzymes and may increase the metabolic clearance rate of plasma androgens (70).

The combination of ethinyl estradiol with *cyproterone acetate,* which was commonly used in Europe for many years, significantly reduces plasma testosterone and androstenedione levels, suppresses gonadotropins, and increases SHBG (71). *Cyproterone acetate* also shows mild glucocorticoid activity (72) and may reduce DHEAS levels (73). Administered in a reverse sequential regimen (*cyproterone acetate,* 100 mg/day on days 5–15, and *ethinyl estradiol,* 30–50 μg/day on cycle days 5–26), this cyclic schedule allows regular menstrual bleeding, provides excellent contraception, and is effective in the treatment of even severe hirsutism (74) and acne. When a desired clinical response is achieved, the dose of *cyproterone acetate* may be tapered gradually at 3- to 6-month intervals.

Side effects of *cyproterone acetate* include fatigue, weight gain, decreased libido, irregular bleeding, nausea, and headaches. These symptoms occur less often when ethinyl estradiol is added. *Cyproterone acetate* administration has been associated with liver tumors in beagles and is not approved by the Food and Drug Administration for use in the U.S.

Flutamide

Flutamide, a pure nonsteroidal antiandrogen, is approved for treatment of prostate cancer. Although it has a weaker affinity to the androgen receptor than *spironolactone* or cyproterone acetate, larger doses (250 mg two or three times daily) may compensate for the reduced potency. *Flutamide* is also a weak inhibitor of testosterone biosynthesis.

In a single, 3-month study of *flutamide* alone, most patients demonstrated significant improvement in hirsutism with no change in androgen levels (75). Significant improvement in hirsutism with a significant drop in androstenedione, dihydrotestosterone, LH, and FSH levels was observed in an 8-month follow-up of *flutamide* and low-dose oral contraceptives in women who did not respond to oral contraceptives alone (76). The side effects of *flutamide* treatment combined with low-dose oral contraceptives included dry skin, hot flashes, increased appetite, headaches, fatigue, nausea, dizziness, decreased libido, and breast tenderness (77).

843

Cimetidine

Cimetidine is a histamine H2 receptor antagonist that has demonstrated a weak antiandrogenic effect as a result of its ability to occupy androgen receptors and inhibit dihydrotestosterone binding at the level of the hair follicles. Although *cimetidine* has been reported to reduce hair growth in women with hirsutsim (78), two more recent studies show no beneficial effect (79, 80).

Finasteride

Finasteride is a specific inhibitor of 5-α-reductase enzyme activity (5-α-RA) that has been approved in the U.S. for the treatment of benign prostatic hyperplasia. In a study in which *finasteride* (5 mg daily) was compared with *spironolactone* (100 mg daily) (81), both drugs resulted in similar significant improvement in hirsutism despite differing effects on androgen levels. Further studies are needed to clarify the role of this family of drugs in the treatment of hirsutism.

Ovarian Wedge Resection

Bilateral ovarian wedge resection is associated with only transient reduction in androstenedione levels and a prolonged minimal decrease in plasma testosterone (82, 83). In patients with hirsutism with PCOS after wedge resection, hair growth was reduced by approximately 16% (84, 85). Although Stein's original report cited a pregnancy rate of 85% following wedge resection and maintenance of ovulatory cycles, subsequent reports show lower pregnancy rates and a higher incidence of periovarian adhesions (86).

Laparoscopic Electrocautery

Laparoscopic ovarian electrocautery is used as an alternative to wedge resection in patients with severe PCOS whose condition is resistant to ovulation induction. In the first reported series (87), five to eight points in each ovary were cauterized for 5–6 seconds with 300–400 W. This treatment resulted in a 90% ovulation rate and a 70% conception rate. To reduce adhesion formation, a technique that cauterized the ovary only in four points led to a similar pregnancy rate (88) with a miscarriage rate of 14% (much lower than the usual miscarriage rate of 30–40% for patients with PCOS).

Most series report a decrease in both androgen and LH concentrations and an increase in FSH concentrations (89, 90). Unilateral diathermy leads to bilateral ovarian activity (91).

Further studies are anticipated to define candidates who may benefit most from such a procedure. The risk of adhesion formation should be discussed with the patient.

Physical Methods of Hair Removal

Depilatory creams remove hair only temporarily. They break down and dissolve hair by hydrolyzing disulfide bonds (92). Although depilatories can have a dramatic effect, many women cannot tolerate these irritative chemicals. The topical use of corticosteroid cream may prevent contact dermatitis.

Shaving is effective. Contrary to common belief, it does not change the quality, quantity, or texture of hair (93). However, plucking, if done unevenly and repeatedly, may cause inflammation and damage to hair follicles and render them less amenable to electrolysis. Waxing is a grouped method of plucking in which hairs are plucked out from under the skin surface. The results of waxing last longer (up to 6 weeks) than shaving or depilatory creams (92).

Bleaching removes the hair pigment through the use of hydrogen peroxide (usually 6% strength), which is sometimes combined with ammonia. Although hair lightens and softens during oxidation, this method is frequently associated with hair discoloration, skin irritation, or lack of effect (92).

Electrolysis is the only permanent means recommended for hair removal. Under magnification, a trained technician destroys each hair follicle individually. When a needle is inserted into a hair follicle, galvanic current and electrocautery alone or in combination ("the blend") destroy the hair follicle. After the needle is removed, forceps are used to remove the hair. Hair regrowth ranges from 15–50%. Problems with electrolysis include pain, scarring, pigmentation, and cost (94).

Cushing's Syndrome

The adrenal cortex produces three classes of steroid hormones—glucocorticoids, mineralocorticoids, and sex steroids (androgen and estrogen precursors). Hyperfunction of the adrenal gland can produce clinical signs of increased activity of any or all of these hormones.

Increased glucocorticoid action results in nitrogen wasting and a catabolic state. This causes muscle weakness, osteoporosis, atrophy of the skin with striae, possible nonhealing ulcerations and ecchymoses, reduced immune resistance that increases the risk of bacterial and fungal infections, and glucose intolerance resulting from enhanced gluconeogenesis and antagonism to insulin action.

Although most patients with Cushing's syndrome gain weight, some lose it. Obesity is typically central, with characteristic redistribution of fat over the clavicles around the neck and on the trunk, abdomen, and cheeks. Cortisol excess may lead to insomnia, mood disturbances, depression, and even overt psychosis. With overproduction of sex steroid precursors, women may develop some degree of masculinization (hirsutism, acne, oligomenorrhea or amenorrhea, thinning of scalp hair), and men may manifest some degree of feminization (gynecomastia and impotence). With overproduction of mineralocorticoids, patients may manifest arterial hypertension and hypokalemic alkalosis. The associated fluid retention may cause pedal edema.

The characteristic laboratory findings associated with hypercortisolism are confined mainly to a complete blood count showing evidence of granulocytosis and reduced lymphocytes and eosinophils. Increased calcium secretion may be present in the urine.

Causes

The six recognized causes of Cushing's syndrome (Table 25.3) **can be either *ACTH dependent* and *ACTH independent*.**

The ACTH-dependent causes can result from ACTH secreted by pituitary adenomas or from an ectopic source. Pituitary ACTH-secreting adenomas, or Cushing's disease, are the most common cause of Cushing's syndrome. These growths are usually microadenomas (<10 mm in diameter) that may be as small as 1 mm. They behave as if they are resistant, to a variable degree, to the "feedback" effect of cortisol. Like the normal gland, these tumors secrete ACTH in a pulsatile fashion; unlike the normal gland, the diurnal pattern of cortisol secretion is lost. ***Ectopic ACTH syndrome* is most often caused by malignant tumors.** About one-half of

Table 25.3   Causes of Cushing's Syndrome

Category	Cause	Relative Incidence
ACTH-dependent	Cushing's syndrome	75%
	Ectopic ACTH-secreting tumors	60%
	Ectopic CRH-secreting tumors	Rare
ACTH-independent	Adrenal cancer	15%
	Adrenal adenoma	10%
	Micronodular adrenal hyperplasia	Rare
	Iatrogenic	Very common

ACTH, adenocorticotropic hormone; CRH, cortical-releasing hormone.

845

these tumors are small-cell carcinomas of the lung (95). Other tumors include bronchial and thymic carcinomas, carcinoid tumor of the pancreas, and medullary carcinoma of the thyroid.

Ectopic cortical-releasing hormone (CRH) tumors are rare (95) and include such tumors as bronchial carcinoids, medullary thyroid carcinoma, and metastatic prostatic carcinoma. The presence of an ectopic CRH-secreting tumor should be suspected in patients who react biochemically like those with pituitary ACTH-dependent disease but who have rapid disease progression and very high plasma ACTH levels.

The hallmark of ACTH-dependent forms of Cushing's syndrome is the presence of normal or high plasma ACTH concentrations with increased cortisol levels. The adrenal glands are hyperplastic bilaterally.

The most common cause of ACTH-independent Cushing's syndrome is *exogenous or iatrogenic* (superphysiologic therapy with cortical steroids) or *factitious* (self-induced). Cortical steroids in pharmacologic quantities are used to treat a variety of diseases with an inflammatory component. Over time, this practice will result in Cushing's syndrome. When glucocorticoids are taken by the patient but not prescribed by a physician, the diagnosis may be especially challenging.

The diagnostic workup for Cushing's syndrome is summarized in Figure 25.2 and Table 25.4 (96, 97).

Excluding cases that are of iatrogenic or factitious etiology, ACTH-independent forms of Cushing's syndrome are adrenal in origin. Adrenal cancers are usually very large by the time Cushing's syndrome is manifest. This is because the tumors are relatively inefficient in the synthesis of steroid hormones. In general, tumors are larger than 6 cm and are easily detectable by computed tomography (CT) scanning or magnetic resonance imaging (MRI). Adrenal cancers often produce steroids other than cortisol. **Thus, when Cushing's syndrome is accompanied by hirsutism or virilization in the female or feminization in the male, adrenal cancer should be suspected.**

Adrenal adenomas are smaller than carcinomas and average 3 cm in diameter. These tumors are usually unilateral and infrequently are associated with other steroid-mediated syndromes.

Micronodular adrenal disease is a disorder of children, adolescents, and young adults. The adrenal glands contain numerous small (<3 mm) nodules, which are often pigmented and secrete sufficient cortisol to suppress pituitary ACTH. This condition can be sporadic or familial.

Treatment of Cushing's Syndrome

Surgical removal of a neoplasm is the treatment of choice (98–104). If a unilateral, well-circumscribed adenoma is identified by MRI or CT scanning, the flank approach may be the most convenient. The cure rate following surgical removal of adrenal adenomas approaches 100% (97). Several months of glucocorticoid replacement therapy are usually required.

A tumor that appears large and irregular on x-ray is suggestive of carcinoma. In these cases, a unilateral adrenalectomy through an abdominal exploratory approach is preferable. In most malignant tumors, complete resection is virtually impossible. When administered immediately after surgery, *mitotane* (O,P-DDD, adrenocorticolytic drug) may be of benefit in preventing or delaying recurrent disease (97, 105). Manifestations of Cushing's syndrome in these patients are controlled by adrenal enzyme inhibitors.

Figure 25.2   The workup of Cushing's syndrome.

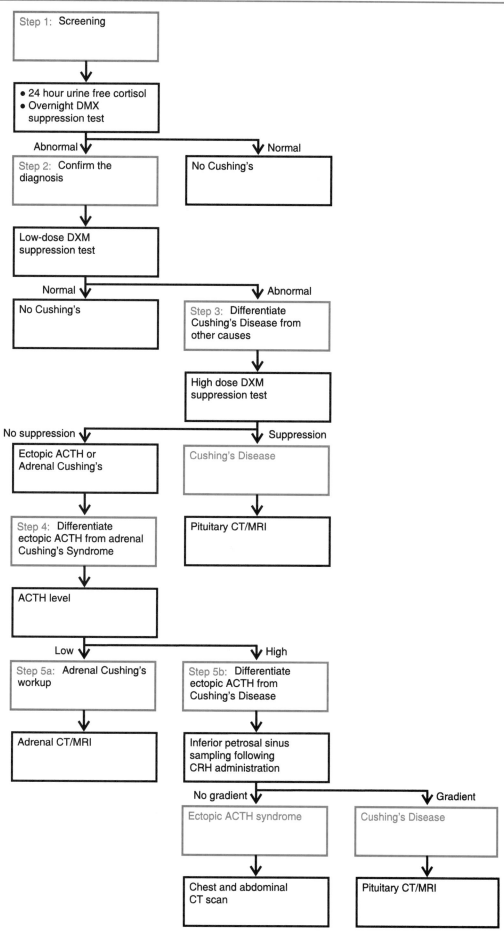

Table 25.4   Diagnostic Workup for Cushing's Syndrome

Screening	Women with hirsutism who are suspected of having Cushing's syndrome should be tested for urinary-free cortisol in a 24-hour collection and should undergo an overnight *dexamethasone* suppression test. Two consecutive collections are recommended with creatinine determination. Normal urinary free cortisol should range from 30 to 80 μg/day. The overnight *dexamethasone* suppression test is an 8:00 AM cortisol determination after the patient is given 1 mg of *dexamethasone* at 11:00 PM the previous night.
Confirmation of diagnosis	Confirmation of diagnosis at this stage can be performed by the 2-day, low-dose, *dexamethasone* suppression test of Liddle (96). The patient is given 0.5 mg of *dexamethasone* every 6 hours for 2 days. A 24-hour urine specimen is collected during the second day. Cushing's syndrome is ruled out if there is suppression of urinary 17-hydroxycorticosteroids to <3 mg/24 hr (or to 0% of baseline), suppression of plasma cortisol to <4 μg/day, or suppression of urinary free cortisol to <25 μg/24 hr.
Differentiation of Cushing's syndrome	The high-dose *dexamethasone* suppression test is used to differentiate Cushing's syndrome from other causes (2 mg every six hours). Normally, urinary 17-hydroxy corticoids should be 40% of baseline after two days. This test partially suppresses adrenocorticotropic hormone (ACTH) section with a resulting decrease in cortisol production in most patients with Cushing's syndrome; however, it has no effect on the majority of patients with ectopic or adrenal Cushing's syndrome.
Differentiation of ectopic ACTH syndrome	High-plasma ACTH (>4.5 pmol/l or >20 pg/ml) is consistent with ectopic ACTH production from adrenal. A low ACTH level (<1.1 pmol/l or <5 pg/ml) identifies a patient who most likely has adrenal Cushing's syndrome.
ACTH-independent and -dependent	A patient with ACTH-independent Cushing's syndrome should undergo an adrenal scan by MRI and should be prepared for adrenal surgery. A patient with ACTH-dependent Cushing's syndrome should initially receive an administration of cortical-releasing hormone (1 ug/kg IV over 1 minute), which is followed 3–5 minutes later by simultaneous sampling of both the inferior petrosal sinuses and of the peripheral vein. The ratio of ACTH levels from the inferior petrosal sinuses to peripheral plasma is then calculated. An inferior petrosal sinus is virtually diagnostic of a pituitary tumor. Moreover, 95% of patients with Cushing's syndrome are found to have ratios over 2. If the test indicates a patient with Cushing's syndrome, a pituitary MRI with gadolinium enhancement should be obtained in preparation for transsphenoidal surgery. If the results indicate ectopic ACTH secretion, a computed tomography scan of the chest and possibly the abdomen should be performed (97).

Treatment of Ectopic ACTH/CRH-Producing Neoplasms

Surgical excision is the treatment of choice. Unfortunately, in most cases, the tumor is nonresectable by the time the condition is diagnosed. Partial response to chemotherapy or radiation may be achieved. Adrenal enzyme inhibitors, either alone or in combination, should be used to treat Cushing's syndrome. Most patients with malignancy die within 1 year.

Surgical Treatment   The treatment of choice for Cushing's disease is transsphenoidal resection (98). The cure rate is approximately 80% in patients with microadenomas who undergo surgery by an experienced surgeon (99, 100) and is less than 50% in patients with macroadenomas (101). Transient diabetes insipidus is common (102).

Radiation Therapy   High-voltage external pituitary radiation (4200–4500 cGy) is given at a rate not exceeding 200 cGy/day. Although only 15–25% of adults show total improvement (102), approximately 80% of children respond (106).

Medical Therapy   *Mitotane* can be used to induce medical adrenalectomy during or after pituitary radiation (105). The role of medical therapy is to prepare the severely ill patient for surgery and to maintain normal cortisol levels while a patient awaits the full effect of radiation. Occasionally, medical therapy is used for patients who respond to therapy with only partial remission. Adrenal enzyme inhibitors include *aminoglutethimide, metyrapone, trilostane,* and *etomidate.*

A combination of *aminoglutethimide* and *metyrapone* may cause a total adrenal enzyme block requiring glucocorticoid replacement therapy. *Ketoconazole,* an antifungal agent, inhibits adrenal steroid biosynthesis at the side arm cleavage and 11-β hydroxylation steps. The dose of *ketoconazole* is 600–800 mg/day for 3 months to 1 year (107). *Ketoconazole* is effective for long-term control of hypercortisolism of either pituitary or adrenal origin.

Nelson's syndrome is an ACTH-secreting pituitary adenoma that develops after bilateral adrenalectomy for Cushing's disease (108). This syndrome reportedly complicates 10–50% of cases. Presently, bilateral adrenalectomy is performed rarely because medical therapy can produce an effective block to steroid overproduction, even after surgical and radiation therapy fail. This syndrome is usually caused by a macroadenoma that produces sellar pressure symptoms of headaches, visual-field disturbances, and ophthalmoplegia. Extremely high ACTH levels are associated with severe hyperpigmentation (melanocyte-stimulating hormone activity). The treatment is surgical removal or radiation.

Congenital Adrenal Hyperplasia

Congenital adrenal hyperplasia (CAH) is transmitted as an autosomal recessive disorder. Several adrenocortical enzymes necessary for cortisol biosynthesis may be affected. Failure to synthesize the fully functional enzyme has the following effects:

1. A relative decrease in cortisol production

2. A compensatory increase in ACTH levels

3. Hyperplasia of the zona reticularis of the adrenal cortex

4. An accumulation of the precursors of the affected enzyme in the bloodstream

Deficiency of 21-hydroxylase is responsible for 90–95% of all cases of CAH. The disorder produces a spectrum of conditions. Salt-wasting CAH, which is the most severe form, affects 75% of patients in whom, during the first 2 weeks of life, a hypovolemic salt-wasting crisis is manifest, accompanied by hyponatremia, hyperkalemia, and acidosis. The salt-wasting crisis results from ineffective aldosterone synthesis. The condition is usually diagnosed earlier in affected females than in males because of genital virilization (e.g., clitoromegaly, labioscrotal fusion, and abnormal urethral course).

In simple virilizing CAH, affected patients are diagnosed as virilized newborn females or as rapidly growing masculinized boys at 3 to 7 years of age.

The nonclassical type now includes the formerly termed "late onset and cryptic." Adult-onset adrenal hyperplasia typically presents as hirsutism, menstrual irregularity, or infertility. Some women with a mild gene defect demonstrate elevated circulating 17-HP concentration but no clinical symptoms or signs (cryptic).

Laboratory Testing

1. Basal follicular 17-hydroxyprogesterone (17-HP) <200 ng/dl virtually excludes the disorder; no further testing is required.

2. Basal 17-HP >500 ng/dl establishes the diagnosis; there is no need for further testing (109).

3. Basal 17-HP >200 ng/dl and <500 ng/dl requires ACTH stimulation testing.

4. In the ACTH stimulation test, plasma levels of 17-HP are checked 1 hour following intravenous administration of a bolus of 0.25 mg ACTH 1-24 (*Cotrosyn*).

5. 17-HP levels after ACTH stimulation in adult-onset adrenal hyperplasia are generally >1000 ng/dl (108, 109).

6. Individuals who are heterozygous (carriers) for both adult-onset adrenal hyperplasia and CAH reveal stimulated 17-HP values <1000 ng/dl. In many cases, an overlap with the normal population is observed (110).

Clinical Presentation

The hyperandrogenic symptoms of adult-onset CAH are mild and typically present at or after puberty. There are three phenotypic varieties (109):

1. PCOS (39%)

2. Hirsutism alone without amenorrhea (39%)

3. Cryptic (22%) (hyperandrogenism but no hyperandrogenic symptoms)

The need for screening of patients with hirsutism for adult-onset adrenal hyperplasia depends on the patient population. In the Caucasian population of North America, the frequency of nonclassical disease is 1:1000 (111). A much higher frequency is manifest in some ethnic groups: Ashkenazi Jews (1:27), Hispanics (1:53), Yugoslavs (1:63), Italians (1:50), and Yupik Eskimos (1:40) (111).

Genetics

1. The 21-hydroxylase gene is located on the short arm of chromosome 6, in the midst of the HLA region.

2. The 21-hydroxylase gene is now termed CYP 21. Its homologue is the pseudogene CYP21P (112).

3. Because CYP21P is a pseudogene, the lack of transcription renders it nonfunctional. The CYP21 is the active gene.

4. The CYP21 gene and the CYP21P pseudogene alternate with two genes called C4B and C4A, both of which code for the fourth component (C4) of serum complement (112).

5. The close linkage between the 21-hydroxylase genes and HLA alleles has allowed the study through blood HLA-typing of 21-hydroxylase inheritance patterns in families (e.g., linkage of HLA B14 was found in Ashkenazi Jews, Hispanics, and Italians) (113).

Prenatal Diagnosis and Treatment

In families at risk for CAH, first-trimester prenatal screening is advocated (112). The previously used hormonal and HLA determinations have been replaced by polymerase chain reaction (PCR) amplification of the CYP 21 gene (114). An aggressive and still controversial approach involves the use of *dexamethasone* treatment for all pregnant women at risk of having a child with CAH. The dosage is 20 μg/kg in three divided doses administered as soon as pregnancy is recognized and prior to performing chorionic villus sampling or amniocentesis. *Dexamethasone* crosses the placenta and suppresses ACTH in the fetus. If the fetus is a male, *dexamethasone* administration is stopped; if it is a female, DNA analysis is performed to detect the 21-hydroxylase gene. *Dexamethasone* therapy is discontinued if the fetus is unaffected and continued if the fetus is affected. When *dexamethasone* is administered before 9 weeks of gestation and is continued to term, it effectively reduces genital ambiguity in genetic females (112). However, at least two-thirds of treated females still require surgical repair of the genitalia. Although prenatal treatment does reduce virilization in females, the efficacy and safety to both mother and baby have not been verified. The unnecessary treatment of seven out of every eight pregnancies poses a serious ethical dilemmas (115).

11-β-Hydroxylase Deficiency

Deficiency of 11β-hydroxylase occurs less often than other defects, but it probably occurs more frequently than previously recognized. 11-β-Hydroxylase is the enzyme responsible for conversion of 11-deoxycortisol (compound S) to cortisol and deoxycorticosterone to corticosterone. Inability to synthesize a fully functional 11-β-hydroxylase enzyme causes a decrease in cortisol production, a compensatory increase in ACTH secretion, and increased production of 11-deoxycortisol, 11-deoxycorticosterone, DHEA, and androstenedione. The diagnosis of 11-β-hydroxylase-deficient late-onset adrenal hyperplasia is made when 11-deoxycortisol levels are higher than 25 ng/ml 60 minutes after ACTH 1-24 stimulation (116).

Patients with 11-β-hydroxylase deficiency may present with either a classic pattern of the disorder or symptoms of a mild deficiency (117, 118). The classic pattern is diagnosed at a younger age and is associated with more severe symptoms of virilization and frequently presence of hypertension with related cardiomyopathy and retinopathy (117, 119). In mild deficiency, patients exhibit postpubertal onset of hirsutism, acne, and amenorrhea (117, 118). When present, hypertension lends support to the diagnosis of 11-β-hydroxylase deficiency, but its absence does not rule out the diagnosis (117, 119). The 11-β-hydroxylase gene has been localized to the middle of the long arm of chromosome 8. To date, no HLA linkage has been identified.

3-β-Hydroxysteroid Dehydrogenase Deficiency

Deficiency of 3-β-hydroxysteroid dehydrogenase occurs with varying frequency in hirsute patients (121, 122). The enzyme is found in both the adrenal glands and ovaries (unlike 21- and 11-hydroxylase) and is responsible for transforming δ-5 steroids into the corresponding δ-4 compounds. The diagnosis of this disorder relies on the relationship of δ-5 and δ-4 steroids. A marked elevation of DHEA and DHEAS in the presence of normal or mildly elevated testosterone or androstenedione may be a signal to initiate a screening protocol for 3-β-hydroxysteroid dehydrogenase deficiency using exogenous ACTH stimulation (120). Following intravenous administration of 0.25 mg ACTH 1-24 bolus, 17-hydroxypregnenolone rises significantly within 60 minutes in women with 3-β-hydroxysteroid dehydrogenase deficiency compared with normal women (2276 ng/dl with normal of 1050 ng/dl). The mean poststimulation ratio between 17-hydroxypregnenolone and 17-HP was markedly elevated (mean ratio of 11 compared to 3.4 in normal controls and 0.4 in 21-hydroxylase deficiency) (121). Because of the rarity of this disorder, routine screening of hyperandrogenic patients is not justified (121, 123).

Treatment of Adult-Onset Adrenal Hyperplasia

In adults with CAH, dexamethasone has been shown to suppress the hypothalamic-pituitary axis better than cortisone acetate or hydrocortisone administered in equivalent doses and possibly to induce less fluid retention than other glucocorticoids. Evening administration is more effective (124) with a dosage of 0.25–0.5 mg. In some patients, alternative day therapy using the same dosage is sufficient. Periodic evaluation of serum cortisol is recommended. If morning serum cortisol concentrations are maintained at ≥ 2 µg/dl, oversuppression is unlikely (125).

Androgen-Secreting Ovarian and Adrenal Tumors

Patients with severe hirsutism, virilization, or recent and rapidly progressing signs of androgen excess require careful investigation for the presence of an androgen-secreting neoplasm. In prepubertal girls, virilizing tumors may cause signs of heterosexual precocious puberty in addition to hirsutism, acne, and virilization. A markedly elevated testosterone level (2.5 times the upper normal range or over 200 µg/dl) is typical of an ovarian tumor, and a DHEAS level >8 µg/ml is typical of an adrenal tumor. An adrenal tumor is unlikely when serum DHEAS and urinary 17-ketosteroid excretion measurements are in the normal basal range and the serum cortisol concentration is <3.3 µg/dl after *dexamethasone* administration (126). The results of other dynamic tests, especially testosterone suppression and stimulation, are unreliable (127).

A vaginal and abdominal ultrasound is the first step in the evaluation of an ovarian neoplasm. Duplex Doppler scanning may increase the accuracy of tumor localization (128).

CT scanning is capable of demonstrating tumors ≥ 10 mm (1 cm) in the adrenal gland but may not distinguish between different types of solid tumors (129). In the ovaries, CT scanning cannot differentiate hormonally active from functional tumors (130, 131).

MRI is comparable, if not superior, to CT scanning. When CT and selective venous catheterization fail, nuclear medicine scanning of the abdomen and pelvis after injection with *NP-59* (I-iodomethyl-norcholesterol) and after adrenal and thyroid suppression may facilitate tumor localization (131).

Selective venous catheterization allows direct localization of the tumor, if all four vessels are catheterized transfemorally. Samples are obtained for hormonal analysis, with positive localization defined as a 5-to-1 testosterone gradient, compared with lower vena cava values (131). Specificity under such circumstances approaches 80% (132), but this should be weighed against the 5% rate of significant complications such as adrenal hemorrhage and infarction, venous thrombosis, hematoma, and radiation exposure (133).

Androgen-Producing Ovarian Neoplasms

Ovarian neoplasms are the most frequent androgen-producing tumor. *Granulosa cell tumors* constitute 1–2% of all ovarian tumors and occur mostly in postmenopausal women (see Chapter 33). Usually associated with estrogen production, they are the most common functioning tumors in children and lead to isosexual precocious puberty (134). A total abdominal hysterectomy and a bilateral salpingo-oophorectomy are the treatment of choice. If fertility is desired in the absence of contralateral or pelvic involvement, unilateral salpingo-oophorectomy is justifiable. The 10-year survival rates vary from 60–90%, depending on the stage, tumor size, and histologic atypia (134).

Thecomas are rare and occur in older patients (134). In a study by Zhang et al., only 11% were found to be androgenic, even in the presence of steroid-type cells (luteinized thecomas) (135). The tumor is rarely malignant and rarely bilateral, and a simple oophorectomy is sufficient treatment.

Sclerosing stromal tumors are benign neoplasms that usually occur in patients younger than 30 years of age (134). A few cases with estrogenic or androgenic manifestations have been reported.

Sertoli-Leydig cell tumors, previously classified as androblastoma or arrhenoblastoma, account for 11% of solid ovarian tumors. They contain various proportions of Sertoli cells, Leydig cells, and fibroblasts (134).

Sertoli-Leydig cell tumors are the most common virilizing tumors in women of reproductive age. However, only one-third of patients develop masculinization. The tumor is bilateral in 1.5%. In 80% of cases, it is diagnosed at stage Ia (134). Treatment with unilateral salpingo-oophorectomy is justified in patients with stage Ia disease who desire fertility. Total abdominal hysterectomy, bilateral salpingo-oophorectomy, and adjuvant therapy are recommended for postmenopausal women who have advanced stage disease.

Pure Sertoli cell tumors are usually unilateral. For a premenopausal woman with stage I disease, a unilateral salpingo-oophorectomy is the choice of treatment. Malignant tumors are rapidly fatal (136).

Gynandroblastomas are benign tumors with well-differentiated ovarian and testicular elements. A unilateral oophorectomy or salpingo-oophorectomy is sufficient treatment.

Sex cord tumors with annular tubules (SCTAT) are frequently associated with Peutz-Jeghers syndrome (gastrointestinal polyposis and mucocutaneous melanin pigmentation) (137). Their morphologic features range between those of the granulosa cell and Sertoli cell tumors. Whereas SCTAT with Peutz-Jeghers syndrome tend to be bilateral and benign, SCTAT without Peutz-Jeghers syndrome are almost always unilateral and are malignant in one-fifth of cases (134).

Steroid Cell Tumors

According to Young and Scully (134), this group includes tumors composed entirely of steroid-secreting cells subclassified into stromal luteoma, Leydig cell tumors (hilar and nonhilar), and steroid cell tumors that are not otherwise specific. Virilization or hirsutism is encountered in three-fourths of tumors, in one-half of steroid cell tumors that are not otherwise specific, and in 12% of stromal luteomas.

Nonfunctioning Ovarian Tumors

Ovarian neoplasms, which are usually nonsteroid producing, are occasionally associated with androgen excess and include serous and mucinous cystadenomas, Brenner tumors, Krukenberg tumors, benign cystic teratomas, and dysgerminomas (138). Gonadoblastomas arising in the dysgenetic gonads of patients with a Y chromosome are associated with androgen and estrogen secretion (139, 140).

Stromal Hyperplasia and Stromal Hyperthecosis

Stromal hyperplasia is a nonneoplastic proliferation of ovarian stromal cells. *Stromal hyperthecosis* is defined as the presence of luteinized stromal cells at a distance from the follicles (10). *Stromal hyperplasia,* which is typically seen in patients between 60 and 80 years of age, may be associated with hyperandrogenism, endometrial carcinoma, obesity, hypertension, and glucose intolerance (141). *Hyperthecosis* is also seen in a mild form in older patients. In patients of reproductive age, hyperthecosis may demonstrate severe clinical manifestations of virilization, obesity, and hypertension. Hyperinsulinemia and glucose intolerance may occur in up to 90% of patients with hyperthecosis and probably play a role in the etiology of stromal luteinization and hyperandrogenism (142). Hyperthecosis is found in many cases of hair-AN syndrome.

In patients with hyperthecosis, levels of ovarian androgens, including testosterone, DHT, and androstenedione, are increased usually in the male range. The predominant estrogen, as in PCOS, is estrone, which is derived from peripheral aromatization. E1:E2 ratio is increased. Unlike PCOS, gonadotropin levels are normal (143).

Wedge resection used for the treatment of mild hyperthecosis has been successful and resulted in resumption of ovulation and even in a pregnancy (144). However, in cases of more severe hyperthecosis and high free testosterone levels (1–3 ng/dl), the ovulatory response to wedge resection was only transient (143). In a study in which bilateral oophorectomy was used to control severe virilization, hypertension and glucose intolerance sometimes disappeared (145). Moreover, when a GnRH agonist was used to treat patients with severe hyperthecosis, ovarian androgen production was dramatically suppressed (146).

Virilization During Pregnancy

Luteomas of pregnancy are frequently associated with maternal and fetal masculinization. This is not a true neoplasm but rather a reversible hyperplasia, which usually regresses postpartum. A review of the literature (147) reveals a 30% incidence of maternal virilization and a 65% incidence of virilized females in the presence of a pregnancy luteoma and maternal masculinization.

Other tumors causing virilization in pregnancy include (in descending order of frequency), Krukenberg tumors, mucinous cystic tumors, Brenner tumors, serous cystadenomas, endodermal sinus tumors, and dermoid cysts. Five cases of virilization of a female child have been reported (134).

Virilizing Adrenal Neoplasms

High testosterone levels in the tumor range, accompanied by normal or only moderately elevated DHEAS levels, should not divert attention from the adrenal gland to the ovary. In fact, patients with these adenomas manifest an increased testosterone production following stimulation with human chorionic gonadotropin (hCG) or LH and decreased testosterone secretion following LH suppression.

Of the fewer than 100 reported cases of pure virilizing adrenal neoplasms, 90% were benign. Although the peak age for the diagnosis of adenomas is 20–40 years, most of the pure testosterone-producing tumors have occurred in menopausal women. With one exception, all cases of adenomas and carcinomas were unilateral. Fifty percent were abdominally palpable in children; in adults, none was solely detected by physical examination (148).

Prolactin Disorders

Prolactin was first identified as a product of the anterior pituitary in 1933 (149). Since that time, it has been found in nearly every vertebrate species. The specific activities of human prolactin (hPRL) have been further defined by the separation of its activity from growth hormone (150) and subsequently by the development of radioimmunoassays (151–153). Although the initiation and maintenance of lactation is the primary function of prolactin, many studies have documented a significant role for prolactin activity both within and beyond the reproductive system.

Prolactin Secretion

There are 199 amino acids within hPRL with a molecular weight of 23,000 daltons (Fig. 25.3). Although human growth hormone and placental lactogen have significant lactogenic activity, they have only a 16% and 13% amino acid sequence homology with prolactin, respectively.

In the basal state, three forms are released: a monomer, a dimer, and multimeric species called "little", "big," and "big-big" PRL, respectively (154–156). The two larger species can be degraded to the monomeric form by reducing disulfide bonds (157). The proportions of each of these prolactin species vary with physiologic, pathologic, and hormonal stimulation (157–160). The heterogeneity of secreted forms remains an active area of research. Overall, these studies indicate that "little" prolactin (molecular weight [MW] 23,000) constitutes more than 50% of all combined prolactin production (156, 159, 160) and is most responsive to extrapituitary stimulation or suppression. The bioactivity and immunoreactivity of "little" prolactin is influenced by glycosylation (161–164). It appears that the glycosylated form is the predominant species secreted, but the most potent biological form appears to be the 23,000 MW nonglycosylated form of prolactin (163). To some degree, the heterogeneity of prolactin forms may explain the biologic heterogeneity

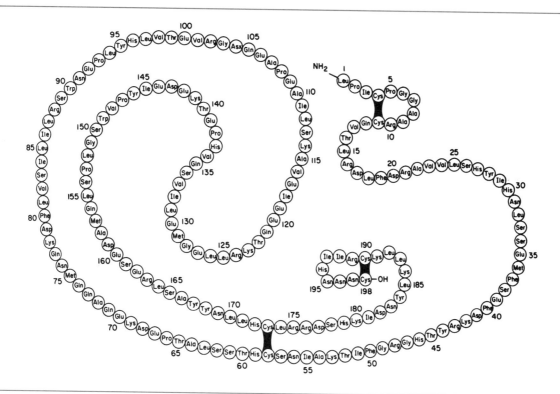

Figure 25.3   Amino acid sequence of prolactin. Three cysteine disulfide bands are located within the molecule. (Reproduced with permission from **Bondy PK.** *Rosenberg Leukocyte Esterase: Metabolic Control and Disease,* 8th ed. Philadelphia: WB Saunders, 1980.)

of this hormone, but it further complicates the physiologic evaluation of prolactin's myriad effects.

In contrast to other anterior pituitary hormones, which are controlled by hypothalamic-releasing factors, prolactin secretion is primarily under inhibitory control mediated by dopamine. Multiple lines of evidence suggest that dopamine, which is secreted by the tuberoinfundibular dopaminergic neurons into the portal hypophyseal vessels, is the primary prolactin-inhibiting factor. Dopamine receptors have been found on pituitary lactotrophs (165), and treatment with dopamine or dopamine agonists suppresses prolactin secretion (166–171). The dopamine antagonist *metaclopramide* abolishes the pulsatility of prolactin release and increases serum prolactin levels (167, 168, 172). Interference with dopamine release from the hypothalamus to the pituitary routinely raises serum prolactin levels. γ-Aminobutyric acid (GABA) and other neuropeptides may also function as prolactin-inhibiting factors (Table 25.5) (173–176). Several hypothalamic polypeptides that increase prolactin-releasing activity are also listed (Table 25.5).

Hyperprolactinemia

When evaluating prolactin levels, "physiologic" alterations or conditions may result in transient as well as persistent elevations in prolactin levels. Disorders categorized as physiologic conditions and drug-related do not always require intervention.

Evaluation

Plasma levels of immunoreactive prolactin are 5–27 ng/ml during the menstrual cycle. Samples should not be drawn soon after the patient awakes or after procedures. Prolactin is secreted in a pulsatile fashion with a pulse frequency ranging from about 14 pulses per 24 hours in the late follicular phase to about nine pulses per 24 hours in the

**Table 25.5   Chemical Factors Modulating Prolactin Release
and Conditions That Result in Hyperprolactinemia**

Inhibitory factors

Dopamine
γ-aminobutyric acid
Histidyl-proline diketopiperazine
Pyroglutamic acid
Somatostatin

Stimulatory factors

β-endorphin
17-β-estradiol
Enkephalins
Gonadotropin-releasing hormone
Histamine
Serotonin
Substance P
Thyrotropin-releasing hormone
Vasoactive intestinal peptide

Physiologic conditions

Anesthesia
Empty sella syndrome
Idiopathic
Intercourse
Major surgery and disorders of chest wall (burns, herpes, chest percussion)
Newborns
Nipple stimulation
Pregnancy
Postpartum (non-nursing: days 1–7; nursing: with suckling)
Sleep
Stress
Postpartum

Hypothalamic conditions

Arachnoid cyst
Craniopharyngioma
Cystic glioma
Cystocerosis
Dermoid cyst
Epidermoid cyst
Histiocytosis
Neurotuberculosis
Pineal tumors
Pseudotumor cerebri
Sarcoidosis
Suprasellar cysts
Tuberculosis

Pituitary conditions

Acromegaly
Addison's disease
Craniopharyngioma
Cushing's syndrome
Hypothyroidism
Histiocytosis
Lymphoid hypophysitis
Metastatic tumors (especially of the lungs and breasts)
Multiple endocrine neoplasia
Nelson's syndrome
Pituitary adenoma (microadenoma or macroadenoma)
Post oral contraception
Sarcoidosis
Thyrotropin-releasing hormone administration
Trauma to stalk
Tuberculosis

Table 25.5—continued

Metabolic dysfunction

Ectopic production (hypernephroma, bronchogenic sarcoma)
Hepatic cirrhosis
Renal failure
Starvation refeeding

Drug conditions

α methyldopa
Antidepressants (amoxapine, imipramine, amitriptyline)
Cimetidine
Dopamine antagonists (phenothiazines, thioxanthenes, butyrophenone, diphenyl butylpiperidine, dibenzoxazepine, dihydroindolone, procainamide, derivatives, metaclopramide)
Estrogen therapy
Opiates
Reserpine
Sulpiride
Verapamil

late luteal phase. There is also a diurnal variation with the lowest levels occurring the mid-morning after the patient awakes. Levels rise 1 hour after the onset of sleep and continue to rise until peak values are reached between 5:00 and 7:00 AM (177, 178). The pulse amplitude of prolactin appears to increase from early to late follicular and luteal phases (179–181). Because of the variability of secretion and inherent limitations of radioimmunoassay, an elevated level should always be rechecked. This is preferably drawn midmorning and not after stress, venipuncture, breast stimulation, or physical examination, which increases prolactin levels.

Prolactin and TSH determinations are basic evaluations in infertile women. Infertile men with hypogonadism also should be tested. Likewise, prolactin levels should be measured in the evaluation of amenorrhea, galactorrhea, galactorrhea with amenorrhea, hirsutism with amenorrhea, anovulatory bleeding, and delayed puberty (Fig. 25.4).

Physical Signs

Amenorrhea without galactorrhea is associated with hyperprolactinemia in approximately 15% of women (182–184). The cessation of normal ovulatory processes attributed to elevated prolactin levels may be related to the following gonadal and hypothalamic-pituitary effects: reduction in granulosa cell number and FSH binding (185); inhibition of granulosa cell 17 β estradiol production by interfering with FSH action (185–187); inadequate luteinization and reduced progesterone (188–190); and the suppressive effects of prolactin on GnRH pulsatile release, which may mediate most of the anovulatory effects (191–203).

Although isolated galactorrhea is commonly considered indicative of hyperprolactinemia, prolactin levels are within the normal range in nearly 50% of patients (204–206) (Fig. 25.5). In such cases, an earlier transient episode of hyperprolactinemia may have existed, which triggered persistent galactorrhea despite normal prolactin levels. This situation is very similar to nursing mothers in whom milk secretion, once established, continues despite normal prolactin levels. Repeat testing is occasionally helpful in detecting hyperprolactinemia. Approximately one-third of women with galactorrhea have normal menses. Conversely, hyperprolactinemia commonly (66%) occurs in the absence of galactorrhea, which may result from inadequate estrogenic or progestational priming of the breast.

In patients with both galactorrhea and amenorrhea (including the syndromes described and named by Forbes, Henneman, Griswold, and Albright, 1951; Chiari and Frommel, 1985; and Argonz and del Castilla, 1953), **approximately two-thirds will have hy-**

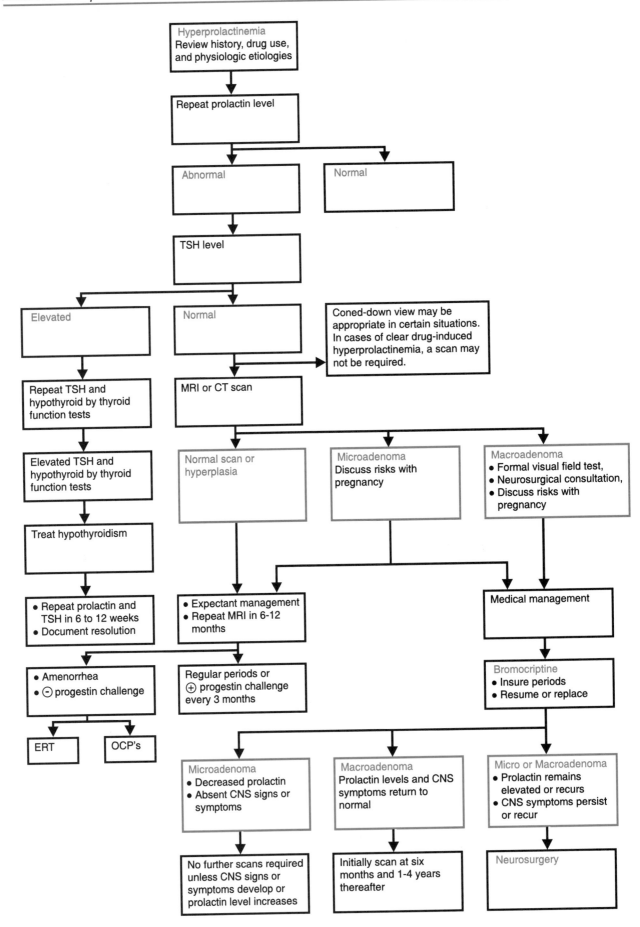

perprolactinemia. **Of that group, approximately one-third will have a pituitary adenoma** (207). Of anovulatory women, 3–10% with the diagnosis of polycystic ovarian disease are noted to be hyperprolactinemic (208, 209).

In all cases of delayed puberty, pituitary abnormalities, including craniopharyngiomas and adenomas, must be considered. Additionally, the multiple endocrine neoplasia type 1 syndrome should be considered, particularly in patients with a family history of multiple adenomas (210). Prolactin and TSH levels should be measured in all patients with delayed puberty.

Figure 25.5   Prolactin levels in 235 patients with galactorrhea. Among patients with a tumor, open triangles denote associated acromegaly, and solid circles and solid triangles denote previous radiotherapy or surgical resection, respectively. Reproduced, with permission from **Kleinberg DL, Noel GL, Frantz AG.** Galactorrhea: a study of 235 cases, including 48 with pituitary tumors. *N Engl J Med* 1977;296:589–600.

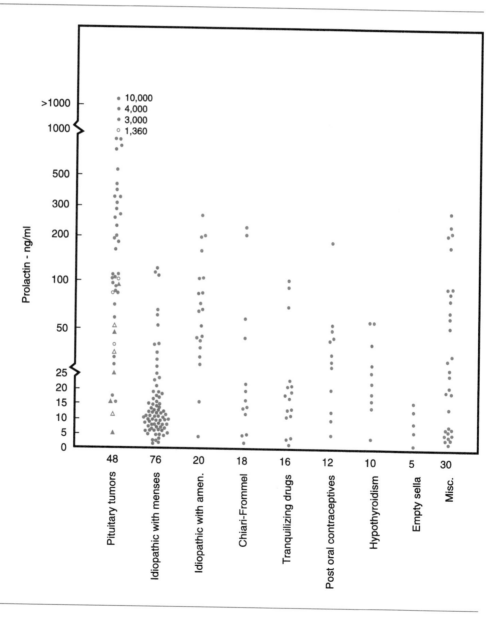

Figure 25.4   Workup for hyperprolactinemia.

859

Once an elevated prolactin level is documented, the gynecologist must be familiar with neuroanatomy as well as imaging techniques and their interpretation (see Chapter 7). Patients can be reassured that hyperprolactinemia usually is associated with a relatively benign condition (pituitary microadenoma or hyperplasia) that requires only periodic monitoring. However, it is critical for the physician to exercise vigilance and to consider the evaluation of other potential etiologies, particularly sellar/suprasellar tumors. Levels of TSH should be measured in all cases of hyperprolactinemia.

Imaging Techniques

Prolactin levels in patients with larger microadenomas and macroadenomas are usually higher than 100 ng/ml. However, levels may be lower with smaller microadenomas and other suprasellar tumors that may be missed on a "coned-down" view of the sella turcica. In patients with clearly identifiable drug-induced or physiologic etiology for hyperprolactinemia, scanning may not be necessary. Coned-down views of the pituitary are occasionally obtained as a screening technique to rule out a mass effect in the sella. The community standard of care, resources available, and expertise of the operator will influence the imaging technique: coned-down view of sella, CT scan, or MRI. An MRI is considered by neuroradiologists to be the optimal technique to evaluate the sella/suprasellar region (211) (Fig. 25.6). The cumulative radiation dose from multiple CT scans may cause cataracts, and the coned-down views or tomograms of the sella are very insensitive and likewise expose the patient to radiation. Even modest elevations of prolactin can be associated with microadenomas or macroadenomas, nonlactotroph pituitary tumors, and other central nervous system abnormalities (Table 25.6).

For patients with hyperprolactinemia who desire future fertility, MRI is indicated to differentiate a pituitary microadenoma from a macroadenoma as well as to identify other potential sellar-suprasellar masses. Although they are infrequent when pregnancy-related complications occur, sellar-suprasellar masses are associated with macroadenomas twice as often as with microadenomas, and patients should make informed decisions (Table 25.7).

Hypothalamic Disorders

Dopamine was the first of many substances demonstrated to be produced in the arcuate nucleus. Dopamine-releasing neurons innervate the external zone of the median eminence. When released into the hypophyseal portal system, dopamine inhibits prolactin release in the anterior pituitary. Lesions that disrupt dopamine release can result in hyperprolactinemia. Such lesions may arise from the suprasellar area, pituitary gland, and infundibular stalk, as well as from adjacent bone, brain, cranial nerves, dura, leptomeninges, nasopharynx, and vessels. Numerous pathologic entities and physiologic conditions in the hypothalamic-pituitary region can disrupt dopamine release and cause hyperprolactinemia (Table 25.6).

Pituitary Disorders

Microadenoma

A pituitary microadenoma or hyperplasia is the cause of hyperprolactinemia in most patients. In over one-third of women with hyperprolactinemia, a radiologic abnormality consistent with an adenoma is found. In the remainder, simple hyperplasia of the pituitary lactotrophs is assumed to be the cause. Most of these abnormalities are microadenomas (<1 cm), and patients can generally be reassured of a benign course of disease (212, 213).

Hypotheses for the formation of microadenomas and macroadenomas (>1 cm) include a reduction in dopamine concentrations in the hypophyseal portal system, vascular isolation of the tumor, or both. The tumors, which originate in the lateral aspects of the anterior pituitary, are surrounded by a pseudocapsule. They may be cystic or degenerating and are often discolored (blue, gray, or brown) as a result of hemorrhage.

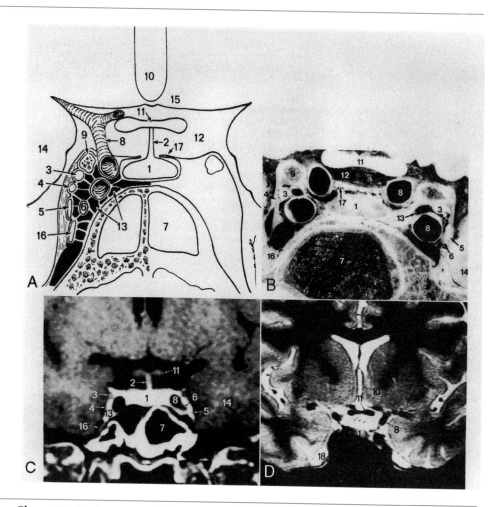

Figure 25.6   Anatomy of the intrasellar region and cavernous sinus by: *A,* anatomic diagram, *B,* coronal cytomicrotome section, *C,* coronal postcontrast T1 weighted MRI, and *D,* coronal postcontrast T2 weighted MRI. (1, Pituitary gland; 2, infundibular stalk; 3, cranial nerve (CN) III; 4, CN IV; 5, CN V$_1$; 6, CN VI; 7, sphenoid sinus; 8, internal carotid artery; 9, anterior clinoid process; 10, third ventricle; 11, optic chiasm; 12, suprasellar cistern; 13, venous spaces of cavernous sinus; 14, temporal lobe; 15, hypothalamus; 16, CN V$_2$; 17, diaphragma sellae; 18, Meckel's cave.)

Table 25.6   Sellar and Suprasellar Tumors and Conditions That May Result in Hyperprolactinemia

Abscess	Lipoma
Aneurysm	Lymphoma
Arachnoid cyst	Meningioma
Cephalocele	Meningitis (bacterial, fungal,
Chloroma (granulocytic sarcoma)	granulomatous)
Colloid cyst	Metastasis
Craniopharyngioma	Mucocele
Dermoid	Nasopharyngeal carcinoma
Ectopic neurohypophysis	Opticochiasmatic-hypothalamic
"Empty" sella	glioma
Epidermoid tumor	Osteocartilaginous tumor
Germinoma	Paracytic cyst
Hamartoma (tubercinereum/hypothalmus)	Pars intermedia cysts
Histiocytosis	Pituitary adenoma
Hyperplasia	Rathke's cleft cyst
Hypophysitis	Sarcoidosis

Table 25.7   Metabolic Parameters of T4, T3, and reverse T3 in Humans

	T4	*T3r*	*T3*
Serum concentrations (μg/dl)	8	0.14	0.025
Distribution volume (l)	10	38	90
Metabolic clearance rate (l/d)	1.1	21	110
Disposal or blood production rates			
u/d	88	30	28
nmol/d	113	46	43
Fraction from T4 (%)	—	>80	>95
Fraction of daily T4 disposal via monodeiodination (%)	—	33	38
Fraction of T4 excreted undeiodinated in feces (%)	20	—	—

T4, thyroxine; T3, triiodothyronine.
Reproduced with permission from **DeGroot LJ, Besser GM, Cahill GF Jr, et al.** *Endocrinology.* 2nd ed. Philadelphia: WB Saunders, 1989:542.

Microadenomas rarely progress to macroadenomas. Therapies include expectant, medical, or, rarely, surgical therapy. All affected women should be advised to notify their physician of chronic headaches, visual disturbances (particularly tunnel vision consistent with bitemporal hemianopsia), and extraocular muscle palsies. Formal visual field testing is rarely necessary.

Expectant Management   In women who do not desire fertility, expectant management can be utilized for both microadenomas and hyperplasia if menstrual function remains intact. Hyperprolactinemia-induced estrogen deficiency, rather than prolactin itself, is the major factor in the development of osteopenia (214). Therefore, estrogen replacement or oral contraceptives are indicated for patients with amenorrhea or irregular menses. Patients with drug-induced hyperprolactinemia can also be managed expectantly with attention to the risks of osteoporosis. Repeat imaging for microadenomas is usually performed in 6 to 12 months to ensure that there has been no further growth of the microadenoma. Less than 5% of tumors show an increase in size.

Medical Treatment   Ergot alkaloids are the mainstay of therapy. In 1985, *bromocriptine* was approved for use in the U.S. to treat hyperprolactinemia caused by a pituitary adenoma. The ergot alkaloids increase dopamine levels, thus decreasing prolactin levels. The serum half-life of bromocriptine is 3.5 hours, and twice-a-day administration is required. Ergot alkaloids are excreted via the biliary tree; therefore, caution is required in the presence of liver disease. The major adverse effects include nausea, headaches, hypotension, dizziness, fatigue and drowsiness, vomiting, headaches, nasal congestion, and constipation. Many patients tolerate the drug on the following regimen: one-half tablet every evening (1.25 mg) at bedtime for 1 week, and an increase of one-half tablet every evening in the third week and every morning in the fourth week (2.5 mg a day). The lowest dose that maintains the prolactin level in the normal range is continued.

An alternative to oral administration is the vaginal administration of *bromocriptine* tablets, which is well tolerated (215). When *bromocriptine* cannot be used, other medications such as *pergolide, cabergoline, methergoline,* and *CV205–502* may be used. In patients with a microadenoma who are receiving *bromocriptine* therapy, a repeat MRI scan may be performed at 6 to 12 months after prolactin levels are normal. Normal prolactin levels and resumption of menses should not be considered proof of tumor response to treatment. Further MRI scans should be performed only to evaluate new symptoms. Discontinuation of *bromocriptine* therapy after 2 to 3 years may be attempted because some adenomas undergo hemorrhagic necrosis and cease to function.

Macroadenomas

Macroadenomas are pituitary tumors that are larger than 1 cm in size. *Bromocriptine* is the best initial and potentially long-term treatment option, but transsphenoidal surgery may be required. Evaluation for other trophic hormone deficiencies may be indicated. Macroadenoma symptoms include severe headaches, visual field changes, and, rarely, diabetes insipidus and blindness. After prolactin has reached normal levels, a follow-up MRI is indicated within 6 months to document shrinkage or stabilization of growth. This may be performed earlier if symptoms develop or exacerbate. Normalized prolactin levels or resumption of menses should not be taken as proof of tumor response to treatment.

Medical Treatment   Macroadenomas treated with *bromocriptine* routinely show a decrease in prolactin levels and size; nearly one-half show a 50% reduction in size, and another one-fourth show a 33% reduction after 6 months of therapy. Tumor regrowth occurs in over 60% of cases after discontinuation of *bromocriptine* therapy; therefore, long-term therapy is the rule.

After stabilization of tumor size is documented, the MRI scan is repeated 6 months later and, if stable, yearly for several years. Serum prolactin levels are measured every 6 months. Because tumors may enlarge despite normalized prolactin values, reevaluation of symptoms at regular intervals (6 months) is required.

Surgical Intervention   **Tumors that are unresponsive to *bromocriptine* or that cause persistent visual field loss require surgical intervention.** Unfortunately, despite surgical resection, recurrence of hyperprolactinemia and tumor growth are not uncommon. Complications of surgery include cerebral carotid artery injury, diabetes insipidus, meningitis, nasal septal perforation, partial or panhypopituitarism, spinal fluid rhinorrhea, third nerve palsy, and recurrence. Pretreatment with *bromocriptine* may result in fibrosis, making resection more difficult. Periodic MRI scanning after surgery is indicated, particularly in patients with recurrent hyperprolactinemia.

Metabolic Dysfunction

Occasionally, patients with hypothyroid exhibit hyperprolactinemia with remarkable pituitary enlargement due to thyrotroph hyperplasia. These patients respond to thyroid replacement with reduction in pituitary enlargement and normalization of prolactin levels (216).

Hyperprolactinemia occurs in 20–75% of women with chronic renal failure. Prolactin levels are not normalized through hemodialysis but are normalized after transplantation (217–220). Occasionally, women with hyperandrogenemia also have hyperprolactinemia. Elevated prolactin levels may alter adrenal function by enhancing the release of adrenal androgens such as DHEAS (221).

Drug-Induced Hyperprolactinemia

Numerous drugs interfere with dopamine secretion (Table 25.5). The same principles utilized in the management of pituitary microadenomas or hyperplasia can be applied in these situations. If discontinuation of the drugs is feasible, resolution of hyperprolactinemia is uniformly prompt.

Use of Estrogen in Hyperprolactinemia

In rodents, rapid pituitary prolactin-secreting adenoma (prolactinoma) occurs with high-dose estrogen administration (222). However, even conditions associated with high estrogen levels, such as pregnancy, do not cause prolactinomas in humans. Indeed, pregnancy may have a favorable influence on preexisting prolactinomas (223, 224). Recent studies (225–227) and autopsy surveys (228) indicate that estrogen administration is not associated with clinical, biochemical, or radiologic evidence of growth of pituitary microadenomas or the progression of idiopathic hyperprolactinemia to an adenoma status. For these reasons, estrogen replacement or oral contraceptive use for hypoestrogenic hyperprolactinemic patients secondary to microadenoma or hyperplasia is appropriate.

Pituitary Adenomas in Pregnancy

Prolactin-secreting microadenomas rarely create complications during pregnancy. However, monitoring of patients with serial gross visual field examinations and fundoscopic examination is recommended. If persistent headaches, visual field deficits, or visual or fundoscopic changes occur, MRI scanning is advisable. Because serum prolactin levels are elevated throughout pregnancy, prolactin measurements are of no value.

Although not recommended, *bromocriptine* use during pregnancy in women with symptomatic (visual field defects, headaches) microadenoma enlargement has resulted in resolution of deficits and symptoms (229–232).

Women with previous transsphenoidal hypophysectomy and macroadenomas are monitored, as are those with microadenomas, with the addition of monthly Goldman perimetry visual field testing. Periodic MRI scanning may be necessary in women with symptoms or visual changes. *Bromocriptine* has been used on a temporary basis to resolve symptoms and visual field deficits in symptomatic macroadenoma patients to allow completion of pregnancy before initiation of definitive therapy. Breastfeeding is not contraindicated in the presence of microadenomas or macroadenomas (229–232).

Thyroid Disorders

Thyroid disorders are 10 times more common in women than men (233). Approximately 1% of the female population of the U.S. will develop overt hypothyroidism. Since the discovery of the long-acting thyroid stimulator (LATS) in women with Graves' disease in 1956, numerous investigations have demonstrated a link between these autoimmune thyroid disorders and reproductive physiology and pathology (234).

Thyroid Hormones

Iodide is actively transported into the thyroid follicular cell. The enzyme thyroid peroxidase (TPO) then oxidizes iodide near the cell-colloid surface and incorporates it into tyrosyl residues within the thyroglobulin molecule, which results in the formation of monoiodotyrosine (MIT) and diiodotyrosine (DIT). Triiodothyronine (T3) and thyroxine (T4), formed by secondary coupling of MIT and DIT, are also catalyzed by TPO. Thyroglobulin, the major protein formed in the thyroid gland, has an iodine content of 0.1–1.1% by weight. About 33% of the iodine is present in thyroglobulin in the form of T3 and T4, and the remainder is present in the iodotyrosines (MIT and DIT) and unbound iodine. Thyroglobulin provides a storage capacity capable of maintaining a euthyroid state for nearly 2 months without the formation of new thyroid hormones. TPO, the membrane-bound, heme-containing oligomer, is localized in the rough endoplasmic reticulum, Golgi vesicles, lateral and apical vesicles, and the follicular cell surface. The thyroid antimicrosomal antibodies found in patients with autoimmune thyroid disease are directed against the TPO enzyme (235, 236).

Thyroid-stimulating hormone regulates thyroidal iodine metabolism by activation of adenylate cyclase. This facilitates endocytosis, digestion of thyroglobulin-containing colloid, and the release of thyroid hormones T4, T3, and reverse T3. Thyroxine is released from the thyroid at 40–100 times the concentration of T3. The reverse T3 concentration, a histologically inactive metabolite, is 30–50% of T3 secretion and 1% of T4 concentration (Table 25.7). Of thyroid hormones released, 70% are bound. Although T4 is present in the circulating storage pool and has a slow turnover rate (about 7 days), T3 concentration is lower and has a higher turnover rate. Approximately 30% of T4 is converted to T3 in the periphery. Reverse T3 levels may help regulate the conversion of T4 to T3. Triiodothyronine is the primary physiologically functional thyroid hormone, which binds the nuclear receptor at 10 times the affinity of T4. Thyroid hormone effects on cells include increased oxygen consumption, heat production, and increased metabolism of fats, proteins, and carbohydrates. Systemically, thyroid hormone activity is responsible for the basal metabolic rate and balances fuel efficiency with performance, much as a carburetor functions in an engine. Hyperthyroid states result in excessive fuel consumption with marginal performance.

Iodide Metabolism

Normal function of the thyroid gland is dependent on iodine. The present recommended daily allowance by the U.S. National Research Council is 150–300 μg/day. Present daily consumption in the U.S. averages 200–600 μg/day. Iodine is usually ingested in the form of iodized salt (100 mg of potassium iodine/kg of salt) (237).

While the thyroid gland is dependent on iodine, sufficiency of iodine also appears to be associated with the development of autoimmune thyroid disorders (238, 239) and reduced remission rates in patients treated for Graves' disease (240). Animal studies suggest that iodine stimulates immunoglobulin production by B lymphocytes, activates macrophages, and increases the immunogenic potential of thyroglobulin because of the higher iodide content (241–244).

Factors Affecting Thyroid Function

Other potential autoimmune thyroid diseases include pollutants (plasticizers, polychlorinated biphenols, and coal processing pollutants) (245, 246) and antibodies to *Yersinia enterocolitica* (247). The female hormonal milieu and its potential effects on immune surveillance undoubtedly play a role in the increased risk of women to develop autoimmune thyroid disease. The immunoglobulins produced against the thyroid are polyclonal, and the multiple combinations of various antibodies present (stimulating versus blocking, complement fixing, and noncytotoxic) combine to create the clinical spectrum of autoimmune thyroid diseases that affect successful reproductive function.

Evaluation

Thyroid Function

Total serum T4 is measured by radioimmunoassay. Conditions that elevate the levels of thyroid-binding globulin (TBG) (pregnancy, oral contraceptives, estrogen replacement, hepatitis, and genetic abnormalities of TBG) necessitate measuring T3 resin uptake for clarification.

The T3 resin uptake determines the concentration of radiolabeled T3 bound to serum TBG and an artificial resin. The number of binding sites available in TBG is inversely proportional to the amount of labeled T3 bound to the artificial resin. Therefore, high TBG T3 receptor site availability results in a low T3 resin uptake.

The free T4 index (FTI) is obtained by multiplying the serum T4 concentration by the T3 resin uptake percentage, yielding an indirect measurement of free T4.

$$\% \text{ free T4} \times \text{T4 total} = \text{free T4}$$

Equilibrium dialysis may be used to determine the percentage of free T4. Free T4 and T3 may also be determined by radioimmunoassay.

The present TSH sandwich immunoassays are extremely sensitive and are capable of differentiating low-normal from pathological or iatrogenically subnormal values and elevations. Thus, TSH measurements provide the best single screen for thyroid dysfunction (248) and accurately predict thyroid hormone dysfunction in about 80% of cases.

Immunologic Abnormalities

Many antigen-antibody reactions affecting the thyroid gland can be detected. Antibody production to thyroglobulin obviously depends on a breech in normal immune surveillance (249, 250). Antibodies to thyroglobulin are restricted to one minor and two major epitopes. Antibodies are mainly noncomplement-fixing immunoglobulin G (IgG) polyclonal antibodies (251). Antithyroglobulin antibodies are found in patients with Hashimoto's thyroiditis, Graves' disease, acute thyroiditis, nontoxic goiter, and thyroid cancer (Table 25.8). They also appear in normal women.

Antimicrosomal antibodies directed against TPO are found in Hashimoto's thyroiditis, Graves' disease, and postpartum thyroiditis. The antibodies produced are characteristically cytotoxic, complement-fixing IgG antibodies. Antimicrosomal antibodies correlate with the histologic appearance of lymphocytic thyroiditis (Table 25.8) (235, 236).

Antibodies to T3 and T4 are present in some patients with Hashimoto's thyroiditis and Graves' disease who have antithyroglobulin antibodies (252). These antibodies can cause artifacts in the measurement of thyroid hormone levels.

The last group of antibodies important in thyroid disease is the one that binds the TSH receptor, i.e., thyroid-stimulating antibodies (TSAb) or thyroid stimulating immunoglobulin (TSI). Long-acting thyroid stimulators are monoclonol or limited polyclonal TSAb, which mimic TSH action. They are quantified by their ability to stimulate human thyroid cell cultures to produce cyclic adenosine monophosphate or to release T3.

TSH-binding inhibitor immunoglobulin (TBII) is also detectable in two varieties: those that block TSH binding and those that block both pre- and postreceptor processes. Several investigators have detected such blocking antibodies in patients with primary hypothyroidism with atrophic thyroid glands (253–255).

Thyroid growth-promoting immunoglobulins (TGI) stimulate growth but not hormone release (250–259). Their immunologic antagonists are the TGI-blocking antibodies that are capable of inhibiting TSH-mediated growth responses in patients who may have had thyroid damage by immune destruction (253–256).

Autoimmune Thyroid Disease

Autoimmune thyroid disease is the predominant class of thyroid disorders; hypothyroidism is three times more common than hyperthyroidism (260). The most common thyroid abnormalities in women, autoimmune thyroid disorders, represent the combined effects of the multiple antibodies produced. The various antigen-antibody reactions result in the varied clinical spectrum of these disorders. The transmission of these immunoglobulins transplacentally also potentially complicates thyroid function in the fetus. The presence of autoimmune thyroid disorders, particularly Graves' disease, is associated with other autoimmune conditions. Other autoimmune conditions associated with Graves' disease are Hashimoto's thyroiditis, Addison's disease, ovarian failure, rheumatoid arthritis,

Table 25.8   Autoantibodies to Thyroid Peroxidase Enzyme (Microsomal) and Thyroglobulin by Enzyme-Linked Immunosorbent Assay

Microsome	No. of Patients Studied	Antibody-Positive	*Thyroglobulin*
Normal controls	106	5 (4.7%)	13 (12.3%)
Autoimmune thyroiditis	53	29 (54.7%)	49 (92.5%)
Untreated Graves' disease	127	37 (29.1%)	118 (93%)

Reproduced with permission from **DeGroot LJ, Besser GM, Cahill GF Jr, et al.** *Endocrinology.* 2nd ed. Philadelphia: WB Saunders, 1989:542.

Sjögren's syndrome, diabetes mellitus (type I), vitiligo, pernicious anemia, myasthenia gravis, and idiopathic thrombocytopenic purpura.

Hashimoto's Thyroiditis

Hashimoto's thyroiditis or chronic lymphocytic thyroiditis, which was first described in 1912, can present as hyperthyroidism, hypothyroidism, euthyroid goiter, or diffuse goiter. High levels of antimicrosomal and antithyroglobulin antibody are usually present. Typically, glandular hypertrophy is found, but atrophic forms are also present. The composition of various antibodies (i.e., TBII, causing the atrophic form and congenital hypothyroidism in some neonates, and TGI, causing the goitrous variety) results in varied physical findings.

Three classic types of autoimmune injury are found in Hashimoto's thyroiditis: 1) complement-mediated cytotoxicity, 2) antibody-dependent cell-mediated cytotoxicity (ADCC), and 3) stimulation or blockade of hormone receptors, which results in hyper- or hypofunction or growth (Fig. 25.7).

The histologic picture of Hashimoto's thyroiditis includes cellular hyperplasia, disruption of follicular cells, and infiltration of the gland by lymphocytes, monocytes, and plasma cells. Occasionally, adjacent lymphadenopathy may be noted. Some epithelial cells are enlarged and demonstrate oxyphilic change in the cytoplasm (Askanazy cells or Hürthle

Figure 25.7   Types of autoimmune injury found in Hashimoto's thyroiditis. *A,* Complement-mediated cytotoxicity, which can be abolished by inactivating the complement system. *B,* Antibody-dependent cell-mediated cytotoxicity (ADCC) function through killer T cells, monocytes, and natural killer cells that have immunoglobulin G fragment receptors. *C,* Stimulation of blockade of hormone receptors leading to hyperfunction or hypofunction or growth, depending on the types of immunoglobulins acting on the target cell. (TBII, TSH-binding inhibitor immunoglobulin; TGI, thyroid growth promoting immunoglobulin; TSAb, thyroid-stimulating antibodies; TSH, thyroid-stimulating hormone.) (From **Coulam CB, Faulk WP, McIntyre JA.** *Immunologic Obstetrics.* New York: Norton Medical Books, 1992:658.)

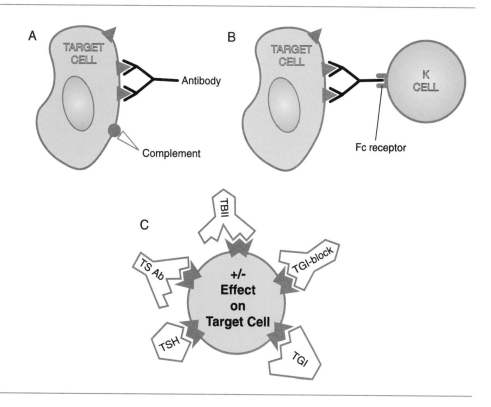

cells, which are not specific to this disorder). The interstitial cells show fibrosis and lymphocytic infiltration. Graves' disease and Hashimoto's thyroiditis may present with very similar histologic findings manifest by a similar mechanism of action. Nearly all patients with Hashimoto's thyroiditis and about two-thirds of patients with Graves' disease have sera demonstrating antibody-dependent cell-mediated cytotoxicity.

Clinical Characteristics and Diagnosis

Most patients with Hashimoto's thyroiditis are relatively asymptomatic with painless goiter and hypothyroidism. The goiter can also involve the pyramidal lobe. At later stages of the disease, hypothyroidism can be found without a goiter. Notable manifestations of hypothyroidism include cold intolerance, constipation, carotene deposition in the periorbital region, carpal tunnel syndrome, dry skin, fatigue, hair loss, lethargy, and weight gain. Hashitoxicosis (the hyperthyroid manifestation of autoimmune thyroid disease) may represent a variant of Graves' disease. This form is estimated to occur in 4–8% of patients with Hashimoto's thyroiditis. These patients often become hypothyroid in the course of treatment.

In many cases, an elevated serum level of TSH is noted during routine screening. Elevated serum antithyroglobulin and antimicrosomal antibody elevation confirm the diagnosis. The sedimentation rate may be elevated, depending on the course of the disease at the time of recognition. Other causes of hypothyroidism should be considered as listed in Table 25.9.

Treatment

Thyroxine replacement is initiated in patients with symptomatic hypothyroidism, patients who have a goiter that is cosmetically or physically bothersome and are subclinically hypothyroid, and patients who are undergoing fertility therapy and are subclinically hypothyroid. Regression of gland size usually does not occur, but treatment avoids further growth. Pregnant patients with an elevated TSH level should be treated with *l-thyroxine*. Treatment does not slow progression of the disease. Replacement therapy is monitored by TSH determinations at least 6 weeks after a change in dose. *Aluminum hydroxide* (antacids), *cholestyramine, iron*, and *sucralfate* may interfere with absorption. The half-life of *levothyroxine* is nearly 7 days; therefore, nearly 6 weeks of treatment are necessary before the effects of a dose change can be evaluated.

Reproductive Effects of Hypothyroidism	Hypothyroidism appears to be associated with decreased fertility resulting from ovulatory difficulties and not spontaneous abortion (261–264). Recent studies also suggest that early subclinical hypothyroidism is associated with menorrhagia (265).

Table 25.9   Potential Causes of Hypothyroidism

Primary

Congenital absence of thyroid gland
External thyroid gland radiation
Familial disorders and thyroxine synthesis
Hashimoto's thyroiditis
^{131}I ablation for Graves' disease
Ingestion of antithyroid drugs
Iodine deficiency
Idiopathic myxedema (autoimmune)
Surgical removal of thyroid gland

Secondary

Hypothalamic thyrotropin-releasing hormone deficiency
Pituitary or hypothalamic tumors or diseases

Severe primary hypothyroidism is associated with amenorrhea or anovulation (261, 266–268). Enhanced sensitivity of the prolactin-secreting cells to thyrotropin-releasing hormone (TRH) and defective dopamine turnover resulting in hyperprolactinemia caused by a deficiency of thyroid hormone is the apparent explanation (269–272). Hyperprolactinemia causing luteal phase defects is also associated with less severe forms of hypothyroidism (273–275). Replacement therapy appears to reverse the hyperprolactinemia and correct ovulatory defects (276–278).

Graves' Disease

A heritable specific defect in immunosurveillance by suppressor T lymphocytes is believed to result in the development of a helper T cell population that reacts to thyroid antigens and induces a B-cell-mediated response (279). TSAb are detected in the serum of 90% of patients with Graves' disease. Human leukocyte antigen (HLA) class II antigens DR, DP, DQ, and DS can present antigens to T cells and are expressed on thyroid epithelial cells. Antibodies to the TSH receptor are produced when this immunogen (TSH receptor) is presented to helper T lymphocytes with the D locus antigens (280–287). The class II antigens are upregulated by chronic stimulation of the TSH receptor (283, 284, 287), reduction in the iodinating capacity of thyroid tissue (284), viral transformation (285), and interferon α (286). The clinical use of interferon α has been associated with autoimmune thyroid disease.

Clinical Characteristics and Diagnosis

The classical triad of exophthalmos, goiter, and hyperthyroidism may be associated with frequent bowel movements, heat intolerance, irritability, nervousness, palpitations or tachycardia or both, tremor, weight loss, and lower extremity swelling. Physical findings include lid lag, nontender thyroid enlargement (two to four times normal), onycholysis, palmar erythema, proptosis, staring gaze, and thick skin. A cervical venous bruit and tachycardia are usually noted. The tachycardia does not respond to increased vagal tone produced with a Valsalva maneuver. Severe cases may demonstrate acropachy, chemosis, clubbing, dermopathy, exophthalmos with ophthalmoplegia, follicular conjunctivitis, pretibial myxedema, and vision loss.

Approximately 40% of patients with new onset of Graves' disease and many of those who have been previously treated have elevated T3 and normal T4 levels. Therefore, a T4 measurement suffices in most cases; however, a T3 measurement may also be helpful. Because normal TSH effectively rules out hyperthyroidism, such determinations should be included in laboratory tests. The TSH value may remain undetectable for some time after initiation of treatment. In most patients, antimicrosomal antibodies are present. Measurement of TSAb is useful in evaluating medical treatment, prognosis, and potential fetal complications such as neonatal thyrotoxicosis. Autonomously functioning, benign, thyroid neoplasias that present in a similar fashion include toxic adenomas and toxic multinodular goiter. Very rare conditions causing thyrotoxicosis include human chorionic gonadotropin-secreting choriocarcinoma, TSH-secreting pituitary adenomas, and struma ovarii. Factitious ingestion of thyroxine or desiccated thyroid must be considered in patients with eating disorders. Other potential causes of hyperthyroidism are listed in Table 25.10.

Treatment

Treatment of women with hyperthyroidism of an autoimmune origin presents unique challenges to the physician who must consider the patient's needs and her reproductive plans. Because the drugs used to treat this disorder have potentially harmful effects on the fetus, special attention must be given to the use of contraception and the potential for pregnancy.

131I Ablation   A single dose of radioactive ^{131}I is an effective cure in about 80% of cases and is the most commonly utilized definitive treatment in nonpregnant women. Any woman of childbearing age should be tested for pregnancy before undergoing diagnostic

Table 25.10   Potential Causes of Hyperthyroidism

Factitious hyperthyroidism
Graves' disease
Metastatic follicular cancer
Pituitary hyperthyroidism
Postpartum thyroiditis
Silent hyperthyroidism (low radioiodine uptake)
Struma ovarii
Subacute thyroiditis
Toxic multinodular goiter
Toxic nodule
Tumors secreting human chorionic gonadotropin (molar pregnancy, choriocarcinoma)

or therapeutic administration of ^{131}I. Ablation of a second-trimester fetal thyroid gland and congenital hypothyroidism from treatment in the first trimester have been reported (288, 289). Nuclear medicine professionals provide expertise in the administration of the radioactive isotope, and the endocrinologist continues to provide suppressive medical treatment for 6 to 12 weeks after administration of ^{131}I. Therefore, medical therapy is the backbone of therapy even when radioactive ^{131}I or surgery is eventually planned. Postablative hypothyroidism develops in 50% of patients within the first year after ^{131}I therapy develops and in more than 2% of patients per year thereafter.

Antithyroid Drugs   Antithyroid drugs of the thioamide class include *propylthiouracil (PTU)* and *methimazole*. Low doses of these agents block the secondary coupling reactions that form T3 and T4 from MIT and DIT. At higher doses, they also block iodination of tyrosyl residues in thyroglobulin. Only 30% of patients treated by this modality alone go into remission and become euthyroid (290).

PTU causes a reduction of hyperthyroid symptoms at a dose of 100 mg taken every 8 hours over 1 month. It blocks the intrathyroid synthesis of T3 and the peripheral conversion of T4 to T3 but does not cross the placenta as easily as *methimazole* and therefore is the drug of choice in pregnancy. Drug efficacy is monitored weekly by evaluation of appetite, emotional lability, insomnia, and tremor. A general rule is to lower the dosage by 50% when thyroid function returns to normal, which frequently correlates with the return to a normal heart rate and, subsequently, normalization of TSH levels. Thyroxine is usually the first value to become normal.

Pruritus affects 3–5% of treated patients. Serious adverse reactions include agranulocytosis (occurring 1 to 2 months after therapy in 0.02%) and a generalized drug eruption accompanied by arthralgia, fever, and sore throat. A complete blood count determination is performed if the patient develops an upper respiratory infection. If adverse reactions occur, *methimazole* (another thiomide) may be used.

Methimazole (10 mg) is given every 8 to 24 hours. Its dosage is reduced, as with *PTU*. It is not the drug of choice in pregnant women because it does not block peripheral conversion and crosses the placenta more readily than *PTU*. It does, however, have fewer adverse reactions, a longer dosing interval, and a lower cost than *PTU;* therefore, it is most often prescribed in nonpregnant women.

Other medical therapies include *iodide* and *lithium,* both of which reduce thyroid hormone release and inhibit the organification of iodine. *Iodide* also leads to the secondary coupling of T3 and T4. These medications are rarely used in women of reproductive age because of their risks to the fetal thyroid and to fetal development (*iodine* causes congenital goiter; *lithium* causes Ebstein's anomaly).

Surgery A subtotal thyroidectomy is current less commonly used as definitive therapy but is utilized if medical treatment fails or if a patient is hypersensitive to medical therapy. The risks of surgery include postoperative hypoparathyroidism, recurrent laryngeal nerve paralysis, routine anesthetic and surgical risks, hypothyroidism, and failure to release thyrotoxicosis.

β-Blockers *Propranolol* is occasionally used prior to surgery in patients who prove to be hypersensitive to other medical therapy and for symptomatic relief while awaiting a reduction in T4 caused by *PTU* or *methimazole*.

Reproductive Effects of Hyperthyroidism

High levels of TSab in women with Graves' disease have been associated with fetal neonatal hyperthyroidism (291, 292). Despite both the inhibition and elevation of gonadotropins in thyrotoxicosis (293–295), most women remain ovulatory and fertile (296). Severe thyrotoxicosis can result in weight loss, menstrual cycle irregularities, and amenorrhea (297, 298). An increased risk of spontaneous abortion is noted in women with thyrotoxicosis (299). In those who deliver, an increased incidence of congenital anomalies (6%) is noted in their offspring (287). Effective treatment appears to reduce this risk.

Postpartum Thyroid Dysfunction

This clinical entity is often difficult to diagnose, because its symptoms appear 1 to 8 months postpartum and are often attributed to postpartum depression and difficulties adjusting to the demands of the neonate and infant. Amino et al. have alerted clinicians to this condition and documented an incidence of approximately 5% in their population (300). A number of studies now describe clinical and biochemical evidence of thyroid dysfunction in 5–10% of postpartum women (301–306). These women have a 25% chance of becoming permanently hypothyroid.

Histologically, lymphocytic infiltration and inflammation are found. Antimicrosomal antibodies are also found in this disorder (307, 308). Women who are at greatest risk of developing this disorder are those with a personal or family history of the disorder, those with an autoimmune thyroid disorder, or those with an autoimmune disease.

Clinical Characteristics and Diagnosis

Patients usually present with symptoms of depression, fatigue, and palpitations at 6 to 12 weeks postpartum. Although psychotic episodes are rare, postpartum thyroid dysfunction should be considered in all women with postpartum psychosis. The thyrotoxic phase may be subclinical and overlooked, particularly in areas of low iodine intake (309). In contrast to patients with Graves' disease, the hyperthyroid form has a low radioactive isotope uptake.

The absence of thyroid tenderness, pain, fever, elevated sedimentation rate, and leukocytosis helps to rule out subacute thyroiditis (de Quervain thyroiditis). TSH, T4, T3, T3 resin uptake, and antimicrosomal antibody titer confirm the diagnosis.

Treatment

Most patients are diagnosed in the hypothyroid phase and require 6 to 12 months of T4 replacement if they are symptomatic. Because approximately 10–30% of women develop permanent hypothyroidism, TSH should be evaluated following discontinuation of replacement therapy.

Rarely, patients are diagnosed in the hyperthyroid phase (310). Antithyroid medications are not routinely utilized for these women. *Propranolol* may be used for symptomatic relief. Approximately two-thirds of these patients return to a euthyroid state and one-third return to a hypothyroid state.

Positive Antithyroid Antibody Status

Women who have thyroid autoantibodies before and after conception appear to be at an increased risk for spontaneous abortion (311–313). Nonorgan-specific antibody production and pregnancy loss are documented in cases of antiphospholipid abnormalities (314–316). The concurrent presence of organ-specific thyroid antibodies and nonorgan-specific autoantibody production is not uncommon (317, 318). In cases of recurrent pregnancy loss, thyroid autoantibodies may serve as peripheral markers of abnormal T-cell function and further implicate an immune component as the cause of reproductive failure (319).

Thyroid Nodules

Thyroid nodules are a common finding on physical examination and are demonstrated by ultrasonography in more than 50% of patients (320). Fine-needle biopsy and aspiration are required to rule out malignancy. In the case of indeterminate aspirates, 2–20% are found to be malignant; therefore, surgical biopsy is often indicated (321).

References

1. **Verkauf BS, Von Thron J, O'Brien WF.** Clitoral size in women. *Obstet Gynecol* 1992;80: 41–4.

2. **Ferrimann D, Gallway JD.** Clinical assessment of body hair growth in women. *J Clin Endocrinol Metab* 1961;21:1440.

3. **Rittmaster RS.** Clinical relevance of testosterone and dihydrotestosterone metabolism in women. *Am J Med* 1995;98(Suppl):17S–21S.

4. **Stein IF, Leventhal ML.** Amenorrhea associated with bilateral polycystic ovaries. *Am J Obstet Gynecol* 1935;29:181–91.

5. **Zawadzki JK, Dunaif A.** Diagnostic criteria for polycystic ovary syndrome towards a rational approach. In: **Dunaif A, Givens JR, Haseltine FP,** et al., eds. *Polycystic Ovary Syndrome.* Cambridge: Blackwell Scientific, 1992:377–84.

6. **Goldzieher JW, Axelrod LR.** Clinical and biochemical features of polycystic ovarian disease. *Fertil Steril* 1963;14:631.

7. **Aono T, Miyazaki M, Miyoke A, Kinugasa T, Jurachi K, Matsumoto K.** Responses of serum gonadotropins to LH-releasing hormone and estrogens in Japanese women with polycystic ovaries. *Acta Endocrinol* 1977;85:840.

8. **Serafini P, Alban F, Lobo RA.** 5 alpha reductase activity in the genital skin of hirsute women. *J Clin Endocrinol Metab* 1985;60:349–55.

9. **Lobo RA, Goebelsmann U, Horton R.** Evidence for the importance of peripheral tissue events in the development of hirsutism in polycystic ovary syndrome. *J Clin Endocrinol Metab* 1983; 57:393–7.

10. **Clement PB.** Nonneoplastic lesions of the ovary. In: **Kurman RJ,** ed. *Blaustein's Pathology of the Female Genital Tract,* 4th ed. New York: Springer Verlag, 1994:597–645.

11. **Rosenfield RL, Barnes RB, Cara JF, Lucky AW.** Dysregulation of cytochrome P450-17 alpha as the cause of polycystic ovarian syndrome. *Fertil Steril* 1990;53:785–91.

12. **McNatty KP, Makris A, De-Grazia C, Osathanondh R, Ryan KJ.** The production of progesterone, androgens, and estrogens by granulosa cells, theca tissue and stromal tissue from human ovaries in vitro. *J Clin Endocrinol Metab* 1979;49:687–99.

13. **Lobo RA, Kletzky OA, Campeau JD, Campeau JD, di Zerega GS.** Elevated bioactive luteinizing hormone in women with polycystic ovarian disease. *Fertil Steril* 1983;39:674–8.

14. **Chang RJ, Laufer LR, Meldrum DR, DeFazio J, Lu K, Vale WW,** et al. Steroid secretion in polycystic ovarian disease after ovarian suppression by a long-acting gonadotropin-releasing hormone agonist. *J Clin Endocrinol Metab* 1983;56:897–903.

15. **Biffigandi P, Massucchetti C, Molinetti GM.** Female hirsutism: pathophysiological considerations and therapeutic options. *Endocr Rev* 1984;5:498–513.

16. **Rittmaster RS.** Differential suppression of testosterone and estradiol in hirsute women with the superactive gonadotropin-releasing hormone agonist leuprolide. *J Clin Endocrinol Metab* 1988; 67:651–5.

17. **Lobo RA.** Hirsutism in polycystic ovary syndrome: current concepts. *Clin Obstet Gynecol* 1991;34:817–26.

18. **Hoffman DI, Klove K, Lobo RA.** The prevalence and significance of elevated dehydroepiandrosterone sulfate levels in anovulatory women. *Fertil Steril* 1984;42:76–81.

19. **Lobo RA.** The role of the adrenal in polycystic ovary syndrome. *Semin Reprod Endocrinol* 1984;2:251–64.

20. **Deslypere JP, Verdnock L, Vermeulen A.** Fat tissues: a steroid reservoir and site of steroid metabolism. *J Clin Endocrinol Metab* 1985;61:564–70.

21. **Edman CD, MacDonald PC.** Effect of obesity on conversion of plasma androstenedione to estrone in ovulatory and anovulatory young women. *Am J Obstet Gynecol* 1978;130:456–61.

22. **Schneider J, Bradlow HL, Strain G, Levin J, Anderson K, Fishman J.** Effect of obesity on estradiol metabolism. Decreased formation of nonuterotropic metabolites. *J Clin Endocrinol Metab* 1983;56:973–8.

23. **Judd HL.** Endocrinology of polycystic ovarian disease. *Clin Obstet Gynecol* 1978;21:99–114.

24. **Hall JE, Whitcomb RW, Rivier JE, Vale HW, Crowley WF Jr.** Differential regulation of luteinizing hormone, follicular stimulating hormone and free alpha sub-unit secretion from the gonadotrope by gonadotropin-releasing hormone (GnRH): evidence from use of two GnRH antagonists. *J Clin Endocrinol Metab* 1990;70:328–35.

25. **Seibel MM.** Toward understanding the pathophysiology and treatment of polycystic ovary disease. *Semin Reprod Endocrinol* 1984;2:297.

26. **Dunaif A, Graf M, Mandeli J, Laumas V, Dobrjansky A.** Characterization of groups of hyperandrogenic women with acanthosis nigricans, impaired glucose tolerance, and/or hyperinsulinemia. *J Clin Endocrinol Metab* 1987;65:499–507.

27. **Dunaif A, Green G, Futterweit W, Dobrjansky A.** Suppression of hyperandrogenism does not improve peripheral or hepatic insulin resistance in the polycystic ovary syndrome. *J Clin Endocrinol Metab* 1990;70:699–704.

28. **Nagamani M, Van Dinh T, Kelver ME.** Hyperinsulinemia in hyperthecosis of the ovaries. *Am J Obstet Gynecol* 1986;154:384–9.

29. **Grasinger CC, Wild RA, Parker IJ.** Vulvar acanthosis nigricans: a marker for insulin resistance in hirsute women. *Fertil Steril* 1993;59:583–6.

30. **Barbieri RL, Ryan KJ.** Hyperandrogenism, insulin resistance and acanthosis nigricans syndrome: a common endocrinopathy with unique pathophysiological features. *Am J Obstet Gynecol* 1983;147:90–101.

31. **Dunaif A.** Hyperandrogenic anovulation (PCOS): a unique disorder of insulin action associated with an increased risk of non-insulin dependent diabetes mellitus. *Am J Medication* 1995; 98:33S–39S.

32. **Kiddy DS, Hamilton-Fairley D, Bush A, Short F, Anyaoku V, Reed MJ, et al.** Improvement of endocrine and ovarian function during dietary treatment of obese women with polycystic ovary syndrome. *Clin Endocrinol* 1992;36:105–11.

33. **Pasquali R, Antenucci D, Casimirri F, Venturoli S, Paradisi R, Fabbri R, et al.** Clinical and hormonal characteristics of obese and amenorrheic hyperandrogenic women before and after weight loss. *J Clin Endocrinol Metab* 1989;68:173–9.

34. **Comparetto G, Gullo D, Venezia R, Mogauero G.** Proposal for a purely echographic classification of polycystic ovary syndrome. *Acta Ster Fertil* 1982;13:79–94.

35. **Farquhan CM, Birdsall M, Manning P.** The prevalence of polycystic ovaries on ultrasound scanning in a population of randomly selected women. *Aust N Z J Obstet Gynaecol* 1994; 34:67–72.

36. **Takahashi K, Eda Y, Okado S, Abu-musa A, Yoshino K, Kitao M.** Morphological assessment of the polycystic ovary using transvaginal ultrasound. *Hum Reprod* 1993;8:844–9.

37. **Wild RA.** Obesity, lipids, cardiovascular risk, and androgen excess. *Am J Medication* 1995; 98(Suppl):27S–32S.

38. **Burkman RT.** The role of oral contraceptives in the treatment of hyperandrogenic disorders. *Am J Med* 1995;98(Suppl):130S–136S.

39. **Dahlgren E, Johansson S, Lindstedt G, Knutsson F, Oden A, Janson PO, et al.** Women with polycystic ovary wedge resected in 1956 to 1965: a long-term follow-up focusing on natural history and circulating hormones. *Fertil Steril* 1992;57:505–13.

40. **Jafari K, Tavaheri C, Ruiz G.** Endometrial adenocarcinoma and the Stein-Leventhal syndrome. *Obstet Gynecol* 1978;51:97–100.

41. **Cowan LD, Gordis L, Tonascia JA, Jones GS.** Breast cancer incidence in women with a history of progesterone deficiency. *Am J Epidemiol* 1981;114:209–17.

42. **Bates GW, Whitworth NS.** Effect of body weight reduction on plasma androgens in obese infertile women. *Fertil Steril* 1982;38:406–9.

43. **Pasquali R, Fabbri R, Venturoli S, Paradisi R, Antenucci D, Melchionda N.** Effect of weight loss and androgenic therapy on sex hormone blood levels and insulin resistance in obese patients with polycystic ovaries. *Am J Obstet Gynecol* 1986;154:139–44.

44. **Givens JR, Andersen RN, Wiser WL, Umstot ES, Fish SA.** The effectiveness of two oral contraceptives in suppressing plasma androstenedione, testosterone, LH, and FSH and in stimulating plasma testosterone binding capacity in hirsute women. *Am J Obstet Gynecol* 1976; 124:333–9.

45. **Raj iSG, Raj MHG, Talbert LM, Sloan CS, Hicks B.** Normalization of testosterone levels using a low estrogen-containing oral contraceptive in women with polycystic ovary syndrome. *Obstet Gynecol* 1982;60:15–9.

46. **Wiebe RH, Morris CV.** Effect of an oral contraceptive on adrenal and ovarian androgenic steroids. *Obstet Gynecol* 1984;63:12–4.

47. **Wild RA, Umstot ES, Andersen RN, Givens JR.** Adrenal function in hirsutism: II. Effect of an oral contraceptive. *J Clin Endocrinol Metab* 1982;54:676–81.

48. **Marynick SP, Chakmakjian ZH, McCaffree DL, Herndon JH Jr.** Androgen excess and acne. *N Engl J Med* 1983;308:981–6.

49. **Schiavone FE, Rietschel RL, Sgoutas D, Harris R.** Elevated free testosterone levels in women with acne. *Arch Dermatol* 1983;119:799–802.

50. **Amin E, El-Sayed MM, El-Gamel BA, Nayel SA.** Comparative study of the effect of oral contraceptives containing 50 mcg of estrogen on adrenal cortical function. *Am J Obstet Gynecol* 1980;137:831–3.

51. **Goldzieher JW.** Polycystic ovarian disease. *Fertil Steril* 1981;35:371–94.

52. **Darley CS, Kirby JD, Besser GM, Munro DD, Edwards CR, Rees LH.** Circulating testosterone, sex hormone binding globulin and prolactin in women with late onset or persistent acne vulgaris. *Br J Dermatol* 1982;106:517–22.

53. **Odlind V, Carlstrom K, Michaelsson G, Vahlquist A, Victor A, Mellbin T.** Plasma androgenic activity in women with acne vulgaris and in healthy girls before, during and after puberty. *Clin Endocrinol* 1982;16:243–9.

54. **Ettinger B, Goldtich IM.** Medroxyprogesterone acetate for the evaluation of hypertestosteronism in hirsute women. *Fertil Steril* 1977;28:1285–8.

55. **Jeppson S, Gershagen S, Johannsson ED, Rannevik G.** Plasma levels of medroxyprogesterone acetate (MPA), sex-hormone binding globulin, gonadal steroids, gonadotrophins and prolactin in women during long-term use of depo MPA (Depo-Provera) as a contraceptive agent. *Acta Endocrinol* 1982;99:339–43.

56. **Gordon GG, Southern AL, Calanog A, Olivo J.** The effect of medroxyprogesterone acetate on androgen metabolism in the polycystic ovary syndrome. *J Clin Endocrinol Metab* 1972;35: 444–7.

57. **Meldrum DR, Chang RJ, Lu J, Vale W, Rivier J, Judd HL.** "Medical Oophorectomy" using a long-acting GnRH agonist—a possible new approach to the treatment of endometriosis. *J Clin Endocrinol Metab* 1982;54:1081–3.

58. **Falsetti L, Pasinetti E.** Treatment of moderate and severe hirsutism by gonadotropin-releasing hormone agonists in women with polycystic ovary syndrome and idiopathic hirsutism. *Fertil Steril* 1994;61:817–22.

59. **Morcos RN, Abdul-Malak ME, Shikora E.** Treatment of hirsutism with a gonadotropin-releasing hormone agonist and estrogen replacement therapy. *Fertil Steril* 1994;61:427–31.

60. **Tiitinen A, Simberg N, Stenman UH, Ylikurkala O.** Estrogen replacement does not potentiate gonadotropin releasing hormone agonist-induced androgen suppression in the treatment of hirsutism. *J Clin Endocrinol Metab* 1994;79:447–51.

61. **Cunningham SK, Loughlin T, Culliton M, McKenna TJ.** Plasma sex hormone-binding globulin and androgen levels in the management of hirsute patients. *Acta Endocrinol* 1973;104:365.

62. **Gal M, Orly J, Barr I, Algur N, Boldes R, Diarant Y.** Low dose ketoconazole attenuates serum androgen levels in patient with polycystic ovary syndrome and inhibits ovarian steroidogenesis in vitro. *Fertil Steril* 1994;61:823–32.

63. **Serafini PC, Catalino J, Lobo RA.** The effect of spironolactone on genital skin 5 α-reductase activity. *J Steroid Biochem Mol Biol* 1985;23:191–4.

64. **Menard RH, Guenther TM, Kon H.** Studies on the destruction of adrenal and testicular cytochrome P-450 by spironolactone. *J Biol Chem* 1979;254:1726–33.

65. **Cumming DC, Yang JC, Rebar RW, Yen SS.** Treatment of hirsutism with spironolactone. *JAMA* 1982;247:1295–8.

66. **Rittmaster R.** Evaluation and treatment of hirsutism. *Infert Reprod Med Clin North Am* 1991; 2:511–45.

67. **Barth JH, Cherry CA, Wojnarowska F, Dawber R.** Spironolactone is an effective and well tolerated systemic antiandrogen therapy for hirsute women. *J Clin Endocrinol Metab* 1989; 68:966–70.

68. **Lobo RA, Shoupe D, Serafini P, Brinton D, Horton R.** The effects of two doses of spironolactone on serum androgens and anagen hair in hirsute women. *Fertil Steril* 1985;43:200–5.

69. **Garner PR, Poznanski N.** Treatment of severe hirsutism resulting from hyperandrogenism with the reverse sequential cyproterone acetate regimen. *J Reprod Med* 1984;29:232–6.

70. **Helfer EL, Miller JL, Rose LI.** Side effects of spironolactone therapy in the hirsute woman. *J Clin Endocrinol Metab* 1988;66:208–11.

71. **Miller JA, Jacobs HS.** Treatment of hirsutism and acne with cyproterone acetate. *J Clin Endocrinol Metab* 1986;15:373–89.

72. **Mowszowicz I, Wright F, Vincens M, Rigaud C, Nahoul K, Mavier P, et al.** Androgen metabolism in hirsute patients treated with cyproterone acetate. *J Ster Biochem Mol Biol* 1984;20:757–61.

73. **Calaf-Alsina J, Rodriguez-Espinosa J, Cabero-Roura A, Lenti-Paoli O, Mora-Brugues J, Esteban-Altirriba J.** Effects of a cyproterone-containing oral contraceptive on hormonal levels in polycystic ovarian disease. *Obstet Gynecol* 1987;69:255–8.

74. **Girard J, Baumann J, Buhler U, Zappinger K, Haas HG, Staub JJ, et al.** Cyproterone acetate and ACTH adrenal function. *J Clin Endocrinol Metab* 1978;47:581–6.

75. **Rubens R.** Androgen levels during cyproterone acetate and ethinyl estradiol treatment of hirsutism. *Clin Endocrinol* 1984;20:313–25.

76. **Marcondes JA, Minnani SL, Luthold WW.** Treatment of hirsutism in women with flutamide. *Fertil Steril* 1992;57:543–7.

77. **Ciotta L, Cianci A, Marletta E, Pisana L, Agliano A, Palumbo G.** Treatment of hirsutism with flutamide and a low-dosage oral contraceptive in polycystic ovarian disease patients. *Fertil Steril* 1994;62:1129–35.

78. **Cusan L, Dupont A, Belanger A, Tremblay RR, Manhes G, Labrie F.** Treatment of hirsutism with the pure antiandrogen flutamide. *J Am Acad Dermatol* 1990;23:462–9.

79. **Vigersky RA, Mehlman I, Glass AR, Smith CE.** Treatment of hirsute women with cimetidine. *N Engl J Med* 1980;303:1042.

80. **Lissak A, Sorokin Y, Carderon I, Dirnfeld M, Lioz H, Abramovic H, et al.** Treatment of hirsutism with cimetidine: a prospective randomized controlled trial. *Fertil Steril* 1989;51:247–50.

81. **Golditch IM, Price VH.** Treatment of hirsutism with cimetidine. *Obstet Gynecol* 1990;75:911–3.

82. **Wong L, Morris RS, Chang L, Spahn MA, Lobo RA.** A prospective randomized trial comparing finasteride to spironolactone in the treatment of hirsute women. *J Clin Endocrinol Metab* 1995;80:233–8.

83. **Judd HL, Rigg LA, Anderson DC, Yen SSC.** The effects of ovarian wedge resection on circulating gonadotropin and ovarian steroid levels in patients with polycystic ovary syndrome. *J Clin Endocrinol Metab* 1976;43:347–55.

84. **Katz M, Carr PJ, Cohen BM, Millar RP.** Hormonal effects of wedge resection of polycystic ovaries. *Obstet Gynecol* 1978;51:437–44.

85. **Goldzieher JW, Green JA.** The polycystic ovary. I. Clinical and histologic features. *J Clin Endocrinol Metab* 1962;22:325–38.

86. **Stein I.** Duration of fertility following ovarian wedge resection. Stein-Leventhal syndrome. *West J Surg Obstet Gynecol* 1964;78:124–7.

87. **Adashi EY, Rock JA, Guzick D, Wentz AC, Jones GS, Jones HW Jr.** Fertility following bilateral ovarian wedge resection: a critical analysis of 90 consecutive cases of the polycystic ovary syndrome. *Fertil Steril* 1981;36:320–5.

88. **Gjonnaess H.** Polycystic ovary syndrome treated by ovarian electrocautery through the laparoscope. *Fertil Steril* 1984;41:20–5.

89. **Armar NA, Lachelin GCL.** Laparoscopic ovarian diathermy: an effective treatment for antioestrogen resistant anovulatory infertility in women with polycystic ovary syndrome. *Br J Obstet Gynecol* 1993;100:161–4.

90. **Armar NA, McGarrigle HHG, Honour JW, Jacobs HS, Lachelin GC.** Laparoscopic ovarian diathermy in the management of anovulatory infertility in women with polycystic ovaries: endocrine change and clinical outcome. *Fertil Steril* 1990;53:45–9.

91. **Rossmanith WG, Keckstein J, Spatzier K, Lauritzen C.** The impact of ovarian laser surgery on the gonadotropin secretion in women with polycystic ovarian disease. *Clin Endocrinol* 1991; 34:223–30.

92. **Balen AH, Jacobs HS.** A prospective study comparing unilateral and bilateral laparoscopic ovarian diathermy in women with the polycystic ovary syndrome. *Fertil Steril* 1994; 62:921–5.

93. **Richards RN, Uy M, Meharg G.** Temporary hair removal in patients with hirsutism: a clinical study. *Cutis* 1990;45:199–202.

94. **Lynfield YL, Mac Williams P.** Shaving and hair growth. *J Invest Dermatol* 1970;55:170–2.

95. **Wagner RF.** Physical methods for the management of hirsutism. *Cutis* 1990;45:319–21, 325–6.

96. **Orth DN.** Ectopic hormone production. In: **Felig P, Baster JD, Broadus AE, et al.,** eds. *Endocrinology and Metabolism.* New York: McGraw-Hill, 1987:1692–735.

97. **Liddle GW.** Test of pituitary-adrenal suppressibility in the diagnosis of Cushing's syndrome. *J Clin Endocrinol Metab* 1960;20:1539.

98. **Oldfield EH, Doppman JL, Nieman LK, Chrousus GP, Miller DL, Katzu DU, et al.** Petrosal sinus sampling with and without corticotropin-releasing hormone for the differential diagnosis of Cushing's syndrome. *N Engl J Med* 1991;325:897–905.

99. **Gold EM.** The Cushing's syndrome: changing views of diagnosis and treatment. *Ann Intern Med* 1979;90:829–44.

100. **Boggan JE, Tyrell JB, Wilson CB.** Transsphenoidal microsurgical management of Cushing's disease. Report of 1090 cases. *J Neurosurg* 1983;59:195–200.

101. **Bigos ST, Somma M, Rasia E, Eastman RC, Lathier A, Johnston HH, et al.** Cushing's disease: management by transsphenoidal pituitary microsurgery. *J Clin Endocrinol Metab* 1980; 50:348–54.

102. **Aron DC, Findling JW, Tyrell JB.** Cushing's disease. *J Clin Endocrinol Metab* 1987; 16:705–30.

103. **Ortho DN, Liddle GW.** Results of treatment in 108 patients with Cushing's syndrome. *N Engl J Med* 1971;285:243–7.

104. **Valimaki M, Pelkonen R, Porkka L, Sivula A, Kahri A.** Long-term results of adrenal surgery in patients with Cushing's syndrome due to adrenocortical adenoma. *Clin Endocrinol* 1984;20:229–36.

105. **Schteingart DE, Tsao HS, Taylor CI, McKenzie A, Victoria R, Therrien BA.** Sustained remission of Cushing's disease with mitotane and pituitary irradiation. *Ann Intern Med* 1980; 92:613–9.

106. **Jennings AS, Liddle GW, Orth DN.** Results of treating childhood Cushing's disease with pituitary irradiation. *N Engl J Med* 1977;297:957–62.

107. **Loli L, Berselli ME, Tagliaterri M.** Use of ketoconazole in the treatment of Cushing's syndrome. *J Clin Endocrinol Metab* 1986;63:1365–71.

108. **Nelson DH, Meakin JW, Dealy JB, Matson DO, Emerson K, Thorn GW.** ACTH-producing tumor of the pituitary gland. *N Engl J Med* 1958;85:731–4.

109. **Azziz R, Zacur HA.** 21-hydroxylase deficiency in female hyperandrogenism: screening and diagnosis. *J Clin Endocrinol Metab* 1989;69:577–83.

110. **DeWailly D, Vantyghem-Handiquet MC, Sainsard D, Buvat J, Cappoen JP, Ardaensky K, et al.** Clinical and biological phenotypes in late-onset 21-hydroxylase deficiency. *J Clin Endocrinol Metab* 1986;63:418–23.

111. **New MI, Lorenzen F, Lerner AJ, Kohn B, Oberfield SE, Pollack MS, et al.** Genotyping steroid 21-hydroxylase deficiency: hormonal reference data. *J Clin Endocrinol Metab* 1983; 57:320–6.

112. **Speiser PW, Dupont B, Rubenstein P, Piazza A, Kastelan A, New M.** High frequency of non-classical steroid 21-hyroxylase deficiency. *Am J Hum Genet* 1985;37:650.

113. **New MI.** Steroid 21-hydroxylase deficiency (congenital adrenal hyperplasia). *Am J Med* 1995;98:2S–8S.

114. **Speiser PW, New MI, White PC.** Molecular genetic analysis of nonclassic steroid 21-hydroxylase deficiency associated with HLA-B14, DRI. *N Engl J Med* 1988;319:19–23.

115. **Owerback D, Ballard AL, Draznin AB.** Salt-wasting congenital adrenal hyperplasia: detection and characterization of mutations in the steroid 21-hydroxylase gene, CYP21, using the polymerase chain reaction. *J Clin Endocrinol Metab* 1992;74:553–8.

116. **Miller WL.** Genetics, diagnosis and management of 21-hydroxylase deficiency. *J Clin Endocrinol Metab* 1994;78:241–6.

117. **Azziz R, Boots LR, Parker CR Jr, Bradley E, Zacur HA.** 11-hydroxylase deficiency in hyperandrogenism. *Fertil Steril* 1991;55:733–41.

118. **Zachmann M, Tassimari D, Prader A.** Clinical and biochemical variability of congenital adrenal hyperplasia due to 11 β-hydroxylase deficiency: a study of 25 patients. *J Clin Endocrinol Metab* 1983;56:222–9.

119. **Cathelineau G, Brerault JL, Fiet J, Julien R, Dreux C, Canivet J.** Adrenocortical 11 beta-hydroxylase defect in adult women with post menarchial onset of symptoms. *J Clin Endocrinol Metab* 1980;51:287–91.

120. **Rosler A, Leiberman E.** Enzymatic defects of steroidogenesis: 11 β-hydroxylase deficiency congenital adrenal hyperplasia. *Pediatr Adolesc Endocrinol* 1984;13:47.

121. **Brodie BL, Wentz AC.** Late onset congenital adrenal hyperplasia: a gynecologist's perspective. *Fertil Steril* 1987;48:175–88.

122. **Pang S, Lerner AJ, Stoner E, Levine LS, Oberfield SE, Engel I, New MI.** Late-onset adrenal steroid 3 β-hydroxysteroid dehydrogenase deficiency. I. A cause of hirsutism in pubertal and postpubertal women. *J Clin Endocrinol Metab* 1985;60:428–39.

123. **Azziz R, Bradley EL, Potter HD, Boots LR.** 3 β-hydroxysteroid dehydrogenase deficiency in hyperandrogenism. *Am J Obstet Gynecol* 1993;168:889–95.

124. **Nichols T, Nugent CA.** Tyler fundal height. Diurnal variation in suppression of adrenal function by glucocorticoids. *J Clin Endocrinol Metab* 1965;25:343–9.

125. **Boyers SP, Buster JE, Marshall JR.** Hypothalamic-pituitary-adrenocortical function during long-term low-dose dexamethasone therapy in hyperandrogenized women. *Am J Obstet Gynecol* 1982;142:330–9.

126. **Derksen J, Naggesser SK, Meinders AE.** Identification of virilizing adrenal tumors in hirsute women. *N Engl J Med* 1994;331:968–73.

127. **Ettinger B, Von Werder K, Thenaurs GC, Forsham PH.** Plasma testosterone stimulation-suppression dynamics in hirsute women. *Am J Med* 1971;51:170–5.

128. **Russell JB, Lambert SJ, Taylor KJW, DeCherney AH.** Androgen-producing hilus cell tumor of the ovary. *JAMA* 1987;257:962–3.

129. **Korobkin M.** Overview of adrenal imaging/adrenal CT. *Urol Radiol* 1989;11:221–6.

130. **Surrey ES, de Ziegler D, Gambone JC, Judd HL.** Preoperative localization of androgen-secreting tumors: clinical, endocrinologic and radiologic evaluation of ten patients. *Am J Obstet Gynecol* 1988;158:1313–22.

131. **Taylor L, Ayers JW, Gross MD, Peterson ED.** Diagnostic considerations in virilization: iodomethyl-norcholesterol scanning of androgen secreting tumors. *Fertil Steril* 1986;46:1005–10.

132. **Moltz L, Pickartz H, Sorensen R, Schwartz U, Hammerstein J.** Ovarian and adrenal vein steroids in seven patients with androgen-secreting ovarian neoplasms: selective catheterization findings. *Fertil Steril* 1984;42:585–93.

133. **Wentz AC, White RI, Migeon CJ, Hsu TH, Barnes H, Jones GS.** Differential ovarian and adrenal vein catheterization. *Am J Obstet Gynecol* 1976;125:1000–7.

134. **Young RH, Scully RE.** Sex-cord stromal steroid cell and other ovarian tumors with endocrine, paraendocrine, and paraneoplastic manifestations. In: **Kurman RJ,** ed. *Blaustein's Pathology of the Female Genital Tract,* 4th ed. New York: Springer-Verlag, 1994:783–847.

135. **Zhang J, Young RH, Arseneau J, Scully RE.** Ovarian stromal tumors containing lutein or Leydig cells (luteinized thecomas and stromal Leydig cell tumors): a clinopathological analysis of 50 cases. *Int J Gynecol Pathol* 1982;1:270–85.

136. **Young RH, Scully RE.** Ovarian Sertoli cell tumors: a report of 10 cases. *Int J Gynecol Pathol* 1984;2:349.

137. **Young RH, Welch WR, Dickersin GR, Scully RE.** Ovarian sex cord tumor with annular tubules: review of 74 cases including 27 with Peutz-Jeghers syndrome and four with adenoma malignum of the cervix. *Cancer* 1982;50:1384–402.

138. **Aiman J.** Virilizing ovarian tumors. *Clin Obstet Gynecol* 1991;34:835–47.

139. **Scully RE.** Gonadoblastoma. A review of 74 cases. *Cancer* 1970;25:1340–56.

140. **Ireland K, Woodruff JD.** Masculinizing ovarian tumors. *Obstet Gynecol Surv* 1976;31:83–111.

141. **Boss JH, Scully RE, Wegner KH, Cohen RB.** Structural variations in the adult ovary—clinical significance. *Obstet Gynecol* 1965;25:747–63.

142. **Nagamani M, Van Dinh T, Kelver ME.** Hyperinsulinemia in hyperthecosis of the ovaries. *Am J Obstet Gynecol* 1986;154:384–9.

143. **Judd HL, Scully RE, Herbst AL, Yen SS, Ingersol FM, Kliman B.** Familial hyperthecosis: comparison of endocrinologic and histologic findings with polycystic ovarian disease. *Am J Obstet Gynecol* 1973;117:976–82.

144. **Karam K, Hajis I.** Hyperthecosis syndrome. *Acta Obstet Gynecol Scand* 1979;58:73–9.

145. **Braithwaite SS, Erkman-Balis B, Avila TD.** Post-menopausal virilization due to ovarian stromal hyperthecosis. *J Clin Endocrinol Metab* 1978;46:295–300.

146. **Steingold KA, Judd HL, Nieberg RK, Lu JK, Chang RJ.** Treatment of severe androgen excess due to ovarian hyperthecosis with a long-acting gonadotropin-releasing hormone agonist. *Am J Obstet Gynecol* 1986;154:1241–8.

147. **Garcia-Bunuel R, Berek JS, Woodruff JD.** Luteomas of pregnancy. *Obstet Gynecol* 1975;154:407–14.

148. **Pittaway DE.** Neoplastic causes of hyperandrogenism. *Infert Reprod Med Clin North Am* 1991;2:531–45.

149. **Riddle O, Bates RW, Dykshorn S.** The preparation, identification and assay of prolactin. A hormone of the anterior pituitary. *Am J Physiol* 1933;105:191–6.

878

150. **Frantz AG, Kleinberg DL.** Prolactin: evidence that it is separate from growth hormone in human blood. *Science* 1970;170:745–7.

151. **Lewis UJ, Singh RNP, Sinha YN, VanderLaan P.** Electrophoretic evidence for human prolactin. *J Clin Endocrinol Metab* 1971;33:153–6.

152. **Hwang P, Guyda H, Friesen H.** A radioimmunoassay for human prolactin. *Proc Natl Acad Sci USA* 1971;68:1902–6.

153. **Hwang P, Guyda H, Friesen H.** Purification of human prolactin. *J Biol Chem* 1972;247:1955–8.

154. **Suh HK, Frantz AG.** Size heterogeneity of human prolactin in plasma and pituitary extracts. *J Clin Endocrinol Metab* 1974;39:928–35.

155. **Guyda HJ, Whyte S.** Heterogeneity of human growth hormone and prolactin secreted in vitro: immunoassay and radioreceptor assay correlations. *J Clin Endocrinol Metab* 1975;41:953–67.

156. **Farkough NH, Packer MG, Frantz AG.** Large molecular size prolactin with reduced receptor activity in human serum: high proportion in basal state and reduction after thyrotropin-releasing hormone. *J Clin Endocrinol Metab* 1979;48:1026–32.

157. **Benveniste R, Helman JD, Orth DN, McKenna TJ, Nicholson WE, Rabinowitz D.** Circulating big human prolactin: conversion to small human prolactin by reduction of disulfide bonds. *J Clin Endocrinol Metab* 1979;48:883–6.

158. **Jackson RD, Wortsman J, Malarkey WB.** Characterization of a large molecular weight prolactin in women with idiopathic hyperprolactinemia and normal menses. *J Clin Endocrinol Metab* 1985;61:258–64.

159. **Fraser IS, Lun ZG, Zhou JP, Herington AC, McCarron G, Caterson I, et al.** Detailed assessment of big prolactin in women with hyperprolactinemia and normal ovarian function. *J Clin Endocrinol Metab* 1989;69:585–92.

160. **Larrea F, Escorza A, Valero A, Hernandez L, Cravioto MC, Diaz-Sanchez V.** Heterogeneity of serum prolactin throughout the menstrual cycle and pregnancy in hyperprolactinemia women with normal ovarian function. *J Clin Endocrinol Metab* 1989;68:982–7.

161. **Lewis UJ, Singh RNP, Sinha YN, Vanderlaan WP.** Glycosylated human prolactin. *Endocrinology* 1985;116:359–63.

162. **Markoff E, Lee DW.** Glycosylated prolactin is a major circulating variant in human serum. *J Clin Endocrinol Metab* 1985;65:1102–6.

163. **Markoff E, Lee DW, Hollingsworth DR.** Glycosylated and nonglycosylated prolactin in serum during pregnancy. *J Clin Endocrinol Metab* 1988;67:519–23.

164. **Pellegrini I, Gunz G, Ronin C, Fenouillet E, Peyrat JP, DeLori D, et al.** Polymorphism of prolactin secreted by human prolactinoma cells: immunological, receptor binding, and biological properties of the glycosylated and nonglycosylated forms. *Endocrinology* 1988;122:2667–74.

165. **Goldsmith PC, Cronin MJ, Weiner RI.** Dopamine receptor sites in the anterior pituitary. *J Histochem Cytochem* 1979;27:1205–7.

166. **Quigley ME, Judd SJ, Gilliland GB, Yen SSC.** Effects of a dopamine antagonist on the release of gonadotropin and prolactin in normal women and women with hyperprolactinemic anovulation. *J Clin Endocrinol Metab* 1979;48:718–20.

167. **Quigley ME, Hudd SJ, Gilliland GB, Yen SSC.** Functional studies of dopamine control of prolactin secretion in normal women and women with hyperprolactinemic pituitary microadenoma. *J Clin Endocrinol Metab* 1980;50:994–8.

168. **DeLeo V, Petraglia F, Bruno MG, Lanzetta D, Inaudi P, D'Antona N.** Different dopaminergic control of plasma luteinizing hormone, follicle-stimulating hormone and prolactin in ovulatory and postmenopausal women: effect of ovariectomy. *Gynecol Obstet Invest* 1989;27:94–8.

169. **Lachelin GCL, Leblanc H, Yen SSC.** The inhibitory effect of dopamine agonists on LH release in women. *J Clin Endocrinol Metab* 1977;44:728–32.

170. **Hill MK, Macleod RM, Orcutt P.** Dibutyryl cyclic AMP, adenosine and guanosine blockade of the dopamine, ergocryptine, and apomorphine inhibition of prolactin release in vitro. *Endocrinology* 1976;99:1612–7.

171. **Lamberger L, Crabtree RE.** Pharmacologic effects in man of a potent long-acting dopamine receptor agonist. *Science* 1979;205:1151–2.

172. **Braund W, Roeger DC, Judd SJ.** Synchronous secretion of luteinizing hormone and prolactin in the human luteal phase: neuroendocrine mechanisms. *J Clin Endocrinol Metab* 1984; 58:293–7.

173. **Grossman A, Delitala G, Yeo T, Besser GM.** GABA and muscimol inhibit the release of prolactin from dispersed rat anterior pituitary cells. *Neuroendocrinology* 1981;32:145–50.

174. **Gudelsky GA, Apud JA, Masotto C, Locatelli V, Cocchi D, Racagni G, et al.** Ethanolamine-O-sulfate enhances α-aminobutyric acid secretion into hypophysial portal blood and lowers serum prolactin concentrations. *Neuroendocrinology* 1983;37:397–9.

175. **Melis GB, Paoletti AM, Mastrapasqua NM, Strigini F, Fruzzetti F, Mais V, et al.** The effects of the GABAergic drug, sodium valproate, on prolactin secretion in normal and hyperprolactinemic subjects. *J Clin Endocrinol Metab* 1982;54:485–9.

176. **Melis GB, Fruzetti F, Paoletti M, Mais V, Kemeny A, Strigini F, et al.** Pharmacological activation of α-aminobutyric acid-system blunts prolactin response to mechanical breast stimulation in puerperal women. *J Clin Endocrinol Metab* 1984;58:201–5.

177. **Sassin JF, Frantz AG, Weitzman ED, Kapen S.** Human prolactin: 24-hour pattern with increased release during sleep. *Science* 1972;177:1205–7.

178. **Sassin JE, Frantz AG, Kapen S, Weitzman ED.** The nocturnal rise of human prolactin is dependent on sleep. *J Clin Endocrinol Metab* 1973;37:436–40.

179. **Carandente F, Angeli A, Candiani GB, Crosignani PG, Dammacco F, DeCecco L.** Rhythms in the ovulatory cycle. 1st prolactin. *Chronobiologia* 1989;16:35–44.

180. **Pansini F, Bianchi A, Zito V, Mollica G, Cavallini AR, Candini GC.** Blood prolactin levels: influence of age, menstrual cycle and oral contraceptives. *Contraception* 1983;28:201–7.

181. **Pansini F, Bergamini CM, Cavallini AR, Bagni B, Burghesani F, Agnello G, et al.** Prolactinemia during the menstrual cycle. *Gynecol Obstet Invest* 1987;23:172–6.

182. **Bohnet HG, Dahlen HG, Wuhjke W, Schneider HPG.** Hyperprolactinemic anovulatory syndrome. *J Clin Endocrinol Metab* 197;42:132–43.

183. **Franks S, Murray MAF, Jequier AM, Steele SJ, Nabarro JDN, Jacobs HS.** Incidence and significance of hyperprolactinemia in women with amenorrhea. *Clin Endocrinol* 1975; 4:597–607.

184. **Jacobs HS, Hull MGR, Murray MAF, Frank S.** Therapy oriented diagnosis of secondary amenorrhea. *Horm Res* 1975;6:268–7.

185. **McNatty KP.** Relationship between plasma prolactin and the endocrine microenvironment of the developing human antral follicle. *Fertil Steril* 1979;32:433–8.

186. **Dorrington J, Gore-Lanton RE.** Prolactin inhibits oestrogen synthesis in the ovary. *Nature* 1981;290:600–2.

187. **Cutie RE, Andino NA.** Prolactin inhibits the steroidogenesis in midfollicular phase human granulosa cells cultured in a chemically defined medium. *Fertil Steril* 1988;49:632–7.

188. **Adashi EY, Resnick CE.** Prolactin as an inhibitor of granulosa cell luteinization: implications for hyperprolactinemia-associated luteal phase dysfunction. *Fertil Steril* 1987;48:131–9.

189. **Soto EA, Tureck RW, Strauss JF III.** Effects of prolactin on progestin secretion by human granulosa cells in culture. *Biol Reprod* 1985;32:541–5.

190. **Demura R, Ono M, Demura H, Shizume K, Oouchi H.** Prolactin directly inhibits basal as well as gonadotropin-stimulated secretion of progesterone and 17 β-estradiol in the human ovary. *J Clin Endocrinol Metab* 1985;54:1246–50.

191. **Boyar RM, Kapen S, Finkelstein JW, Perlow M, Sassin JF, Fukushima DK, et al.** Hypothalamic-pituitary function in diverse hyperprolactinemic states. *J Clin Invest* 1974;53: 1588–98.

192. **Bohnet HG, Dahlen HG, Wuttke W, Schneider HPG.** Hyperprolactinaemic anovulatory syndrome. *J Clin Endocrinol Metab* 1976;42:132–44.

193. **Franks S, Murray MAF, Jequier AM, Steele SJ, Nabarro JDN, Jacobs HS.** Incidence and significance of hyperprolactinemia in women with amenorrhea. *Clin Endocrinol (Oxf)* 1975; 4:597–607.

194. **Moult PJA, Rees LH, Besser GM.** Pulsatile gonadotrophin secretion in hyperprolactinaemic amenorrhoea and the response to bromocriptine therapy. *Clin Endocrinol* 1982;16:153–62.

195. **Buckman MT, Peake GT, Srivastava L.** Patterns of spontaneous LH release in normo- and hyperprolactinaemic women. *Acta Endocrinol* 1981;97:305–10.

196. **Aono T, Miyake A, Yasuda T, Kolke K, Kurachi K.** Restoration of oestrogen positive feedback on LH release by bromocriptine in hyperprolactinemic patients with galactorrhea-amenorrhea. *Acta Endocrinol* 1979;91:591–600.

197. **Travaglini P, Ambrosi B, Beck-Pecoz P, Elli R, Rodena M, Trotto G.** Hypothalamic-pituitary-ovarian function in hyperprolactinemic women. *J Clin Invest* 1978;1:39–45.

198. **Glass MR, Shaw RW, Butt WR, London DR.** An abnormality of oestrogen feedback in amenorrhea galactorrhea. *BMJ* 1975;111:274–5.

199. **Koike K, Aono T, Tsutsumi H, Miyake A, Kurachi K.** Restoration of oestrogen-positive feedback effect on LH release in women with prolactinoma by transsphenoidal surgery. *Acta Endocrinol* 1982;100:492–8.

200. **Quigley ME, Judd SJ, Gilliland GB, Yen SSC.** Effects of a dopamine antagonist on the release of gonadotropin and prolactin in normal women with hyperprolactinemic anovulation. *J Clin Endocrinol Metab* 1979;48:718–20.

201. **Boyar RM, Kapen S, Finkelstein JW, Parlow M, Sassin JF, Fukushima DK.** Hypothalamic-pituitary function in diverse hyperprolactinemic states. *J Clin Invest* 1974;53:1588.

202. **Rakoff J, VandenBerg G, Siler TM, Yen SSC.** An integrated direct functional test of the adenohypophysis. *Am J Obstet Gynecol* 1974;119:358–68.

203. **Zarate A, Jacobs S, Canales ES, Schally AV, Cruz A, Sorra J, et al.** Functional evaluation of pituitary reserve in patients with the amenorrhea-galactorrhea syndrome utilizing luteinizing hormone-releasing hormone (LH-RH), L-dopa and chlorpromazine. *J Clin Endocrinol Metab* 1973;37:855.

204. **Kleinberg DL, Noel GL, Frantz AG.** Galactorrhea: a study of 235 cases, including 48 with pituitary tumors. *N Engl J Med* 1977;296:589–600.

205. **Tolis G, Somma M, Van Campenhout J, Friesen H.** Prolactin secretion in 65 patients with galactorrhea. *Am J Obstet Gynecol* 1974;118:91–101.

206. **Boyd AE III, Reichlin S, Tuskoy RN.** Galactorrhea-amenorrhea syndrome: diagnosis and therapy. *Ann Intern Med* 1977;87:165–75.

207. **Schlechte J, Sherman B, Halmi N, Van Gilder J, Chapler FK, et al.** Prolactin-secreting pituitary tumors. *Endocr Rev* 1980;1:295–308.

208. **Minakami H, Abe N, Oka N, Kimura K, Tamura T, Tamata T.** Prolactin release in polycystic ovarian syndrome. *Endocrinol J* 1988;35:303–10.

209. **Murdoch AP, Dunlop W, Kendall-Taylor P.** Studies of prolactin secretion in polycystic ovary syndrome. *Clin Endocrinol* 1986;24:165–75.

210. **Lythgoe K, Dotson R, Peterson CM.** Multiple endocrine neoplasia I presenting as primary amenorrhea. A case report. *Obstet Gynecol* 1995;86:683–6.

211. **Bohler HCL Jr, Jones EE, Briner ML.** Marginally elevated prolactin levels require magnetic imaging and evaluation for acromegaly. *Fertil Steril* 1994;61:1168–70.

212. **Sisan DA, Sheehan JP, Sheeler LR.** The natural history of untreated microprolactinomas. *Fertil Steril* 1987;48:67–71.

213. **Schlechte J, Dolan K, Sherman B, Chapler F, Ulciano A.** The natural history of untreated hyperprolactinemia: a prospective analysis. *J Clin Endocrinol Metab* 1989;412–8.

214. **Klibanski A, Biller BMK, Rosenthal DI, Schoenfeld DA, Saxe V.** Effects of prolactin and estrogen deficiency in amenorrheic bone loss. *J Clin Endocrinol Metab* 1988;67:124–30.

215. **Katz E, Weiss BE, Hassell A, Schran H, Adashi EY.** Increased circulating levels of bromocriptine after vaginal compared to oral administration. *Fertil Steril* 1991;55:882–4.

216. **Abram M, Brue T, Marange I, Girard N, Guibout M, Jaquet P.** Pituitary tumor syndrome and hyperprolactinemia in peripheral hypothyroidism. *Ann Endocrinol (Paris)* 1992;53:215–23.

217. **Chirito E, Bonda A, Friesen HG.** Prolactin in renal failure. *Clin Res* 1972;20:423.

218. **Nagel TC, Freinkel N, Bell RH, et al.** Gynecomastia, prolactin, and other peptide hormones in patients undergoing chronic hemodialysis. *J Clin Endocrinol Metab* 1973;36:428–32.

219. **Olgaard K, Hagen C, McNeilly AS.** Pituitary hormones in women with chronic renal failure: the effect of chronic haemo- and peritoneal dialysis. *Acta Endocrinol* 1975;80:237–46.

220. **Hagen C, Olgaard K, McNeilly AS, Fisher R.** Prolactin and the pituitary-gonadal axis in male uremic patients on regular dialysis. *Acta Endocrinol* 1976;82:29–38.

221. **Thorner MO, Edwards CRW, Hanker JP.** Prolactin and gonadotropin interaction in the male. In: **Troen P, Nankin H,** eds. *The Testis in Normal and Infertile Men.* New York: Raven Press, 1977:351–66.

222. **Lloyd RV.** Estrogen-induced hyperplasia and neoplasia in the rat anterior pituitary gland; an immunohistochemical study. *Am J Pathol* 1983;113:198–206.

223. **Scheithauer BW, Sano T, Kovacs KT, Young W, Ryan N, Randall RV.** The pituitary gland in pregnancy: a clinico-pathologic and immunohistochemical study of 69 cases. *Mayo Clin Proc* 1990;65:461–74.

224. **Well C.** The safety of bromocriptine in hyperprolactinemic female infertility; a literature review. *Curr Med Res Opin* 1986;10:172–95.

225. **Shy KK, McTiernan AM, Daling JR, Weiss NS.** Oral contraceptive use and the occurrence of pituitary prolactinoma. *JAMA* 1983;249:2204–7.

226. **Corenblum B, Taylor PJ.** Idiopathic hyperprolactinemia may include a distinct entity with a natural history different from that of prolactin adenomas. *Fertil Steril* 1988;49:544–6.

227. **Corenblum B, Donovan L.** The safety of physiological estrogen plus progestin replacement therapy and with oral contraceptive therapy in women with pathological hyperprolactinemia. *Fertil Steril* 1993;671–3.

228. **Scheithauer BW, Kovacs KT, Randall RV, Ryan N.** Effects of estrogen on the human pituitary: a clinicopathologic study. *Mayo Clin Proc* 1989;64:1077–84.

229. **Krupp P, Monka C.** Bromocriptine in pregnancy: safety aspects. *Klin Wochenschr* 1987;65:823–7.

230. **Raymond JP, Golstein E, Konopka P.** Follow-up of children born of bromocriptine-treated mothers. *Horm Res* 1985;22:239–46.

231. **Ruiz-Velasco V, Tolis G.** Pregnancy in hyperprolactinemic women. *Fertil Steril* 1984;41:793–805.

232. **Turkalj I, Braun P, Krupp P.** Surveillance of bromocriptine in pregnancy. *JAMA* 1982;247:1589–91.

233. **Tunbridge WM, Evered DC, Hall R, Appleton D, Brewis M, Clark F.** The spectrum of thyroid disease in a community: the Whickham survey. *Clin Endocrinol* 1977;7:481–93.

234. **Whartona T.** Adenographia: sive glandularum totius corporis descripto. London, 1659.

235. **Portmann L, Hamada N, Heinrich G, DeGroot LJ.** Antithyroid peroxidase antibody in patients with autoimmune thyroid disease: possible identity with antimicrosomal antibody. *J Clin Endocrinol Metab* 1985;61:1001–3.

236. **Czarnocka B, Ruf J, Ferrand M, Carayon P, Lissitzky S.** Purification of the human thyroid peroxidase and its identification as the microsomal antigen involved in autoimmune thyroid disease. *FEBS Lett* 1985;190:147–52.

237. **Norman AW, Litwack G.** Thyroid hormones. In: **Norman AW, Litwack G,** eds. *Hormones.* San Diego: Academic Press, 1987:221.

238. **Boukis MA, Koutrar DA, Souvatzoglou A, Evangelopoulou A, Vrontakis M, Moulopoulos SD.** Thyroid hormone and immunological studies in endemic goiter. *J Clin Endocrinol Metab* 1983;57:859–62.

239. **Asamer H, Riccabona G, Holthaus N.** Immunohistochemical findings in thyroid disease in an endemic goiter area. *Arch Klin Med* 1968;215:270–5.

240. **Greer MA.** Antithyroid drugs in the treatment of thyrotoxicosis. *Thyroid Today* 1980;3:1.

241. **McGregor MA, Weetman AP, Ratanchaiyavong S, Owen GM, Ibbertson HK, Hall R.** Iodine: an influence on the development of autoimmune thyroid disease. In: **Hall R, Kobberling J,** eds. *Thyroid Disorders Associated with Iodine Deficiency and Excess.* New York: Raven Press, 1985:209–16.

242. **Weetman AP, McGregor AM, Campbell H, Lazarus JH, Ibbertson KH, Hall R.** Iodide enhances Ig synthesis by human peripheral blood lymphocytes in vitro. *Acta Endocrinol (Copenh)* 198;103:210–5.

243. **Allen EM, Appel MC, Braverman LM.** The effect of iodide ingestion on the development of spontaneous lymphocytic thyroiditis in the diabetes prone BB/W rat. *Endocrinology* 1986; 118:1977–81.

244. **Sundick RS, Herdegen D, Brown TR.** Thyroiditis induced by dietary iodine may be due to the increased immunogenicity of highly iodinated thyroglobulin. In: **Drexhage HA, Wiersinga WM,** eds. *The Thyroid and Autoimmunity.* Amsterdam: Elsevier, 1986:213.

245. **Bahn AK, Mills JL, Snyder PJ, Gann PH, Houten L, Bialik O, et al.** Hypothyroidism in workers exposed to polybrominated biphenols. *N Engl J Med* 1980;302:31–3.

246. **Gaitan E, Cooksey RC, Legan J.** Simple goiter and autoimmune thyroiditis: environmental and genetic factors. *Clin Ecol* 1985;3:158–62.

247. **Wenzel BE, Hessemann J.** Antigenic homologies between plasmid encoded proteins from enteropathogenic Yersinia and thyroid autoantigen. *Horm Metab Res* 1987;17:77–8.

248. **Caldwell G, Kellett HA, Gow SM, Beckett GJ, Sweeting VW, Seth J, et al.** A new strategy for thyroid function testing. *Lancet* 1985;1:1117–9.

249. **DelPozo E, Wyss H, Tolis G, Alcaniz J, Campana A, Naftolin F.** Prolactin and deficient luteal function. *Obstet Gynecol* 1979;53:282–6.

250. **Van Hearle AJ, Uller RP, Matthews NL, Brown J.** Radioimmunoassay for measurement of thyroglobulin in human serum. *J Clin Invest* 1973;52:1320–27.

251. **Nyle L, Pontes de Carvalho LC, Roitt IM.** Restrictions in the response to autologous thyroglobulin in the human. *Clin Exp Immunol* 1980;56:129.

252. **Permachandra BN, Blumenthal HT.** Abnormal binding of thyroid hormone in sera of patients with Hashimoto's thyroiditis. *J Clin Endocrinol Metab* 1967;27:931–6.

253. **Drexhage HA, Bottazzo GF, Bitensky L, Chayen J, Doniach D.** Thyroid growth-blocking antibodies in primary myxedema. *Nature* 1981;239:594–5.

254. **Konishi J, Iida Y, Endo K, Misaki T, Nohara Y, Matsuura N, et al.** Inhibition of thyrotropin-induced adenosine 3'5'-monophosphate increase by immunoglobulins from patients with primary myxedema. *J Clin Endocrinol Metab* 1983;57:544–9.

255. **Steel NR, Bingle JP, Ramsey ID.** Myxedema followed by TS Ab induced hyperthyroidism-report of two cases. *Postgrad Med J* 1985;61:25–7.

256. **Drexhage HA, Bottazzo GF, Doniach D, Bitensky L, Chayen J.** Evidence for thyroid-growth-stimulating immunoglobulins in some goitrous thyroid disease. *Lancet* 1980;2:287–92.

257. **Valente WA, Vitti P, Rotella CM, Vaughan MM, Aloj SM, Grollman EF.** Antibodies that promote thyroid growth: a distinct population of thyroid stimulating auto-antibodies. *N Engl J Med* 1983;309:1028–34.

258. **McMullan NM, Smyth PPA.** In vitro generation of NADPH as an index of thyroid stimulating immunoglobulin (TGI) in goiterous disease. *Clin Endocrinol (Oxf)* 1984;20:269–80.

259. **Schatz H, Beckman FH, Floren M.** Radioassay for thyroid growth stimulating immunoglobulins (TGI) with cultured porcine thyroid follicles. *Horm Metab Res* 1983;15:626–7.

260. **Niswander RR, Gordon M, Berendes HW.** The women and their pregnancies: the collaborative perinatal study of the National Institute of Neurologic Disease and Stroke. Philadelphia: WB Saunders, 1972:246.

261. **Albright F.** Metropathia hemorrhagica. *Maine MJ* 1938;29:235–8.

262. **Lao TTH, Chin RKH, Panesar NS.** Observations on thyroid hormones in hyperemesis gravidarum. *Asia Oceania J Obstet Gynaecol* 1988;14:449–52.

263. **Morimoto C, Reinherz EL, Schlossman SF.** Alterations in immunoregulator: cell subsets in active systemic lupus erythematosus. *J Clin Invest* 1990;66:1171.

264. **Grodstein F, Goldman MB, Ryan L, Cramer DW.** Self reported use of pharmaceuticals and primary ovulatory infertility. *Epidemiology* 1993;4:151–65.

265. **Wilansky DL, Greisman B.** Early hypothyroidism in patients with menorrhagia. *Am J Obstet Gynecol* 1989;160:673–7.

266. **Honbo KS, Van Herle AJ, Kellet KA.** Serum prolactin in untreated primary hypothyroidism. *Am J Med* 1978;64:782–7.

267. **Kleinberg DL, Noel G, Frantz AG.** Galactorrhea: a study of 235 cases. *N Engl J Med* 1977; 296:589–601.

268. **Yamada T, Tsukui T, Ikejiri K, Yukmura Y, Kotani M.** Volume of sella turcica in normal patients and in patients with primary hypothyroidism. *J Clin Endocrinol Metab* 1976; 42:817–22.

269. **Feek CM, Sawers JSA, Brown NS, Seth J, Irvine WJ, Toft AD.** Influence of thyroid status on dopaminergic inhibition of thyrotropin and prolactin secretion. *J Clin Endocrinol Metab* 1980;51:585–89.

270. **Kramer M, Kauschansky A, Genel M.** Adolescent secondary amenorrhea: association with hypothalamic hypothyroidism. *Pediatrics* 1979;94:300–3.

271. **Scanlon MF, Chan V, Heath M, Pourmand M, Rodriquez-Arnao MD, Weightman DR.** Dopaminergic control of thyrotropin α-subunit, thyrotropin β-subunit and prolactin in euthyroidism and hypothyroidism. *J Clin Endocrinol Metab* 1981;53:360–5.

272. **Thomas R, Reid RL.** Thyroid disease and reproductive dysfunction. *Obstet Gynecol* 1987; 70:789–98.

273. **Bohnet HG, Fieldler K, Leidenberger FA.** Subclinical hypothyroidism and infertility. *Lancet* 1981;2:1278.

274. **DelPozo E, Wyss H, Tolis G, Alcaniz J, Campana A, Naftolin F.** Prolactin and deficient luteal function. *Obstet Gynecol* 1979;53:282–6.

275. **Warfel W.** Thyroid regulation pathways and its effect on human luteal function. *Gynakol GeburtshilFliche Rundsch* 1992;32:145–8.

276. **Frantz AG.** Hyperprolactinemia. In: **Collu R, Brown Gm, Van Loon GR,** eds. *Clinical Neuroendocrinology.* Cambridge: Blackwell Scientific Publications, 1986:311–32.

277. **Keye WR, Ho Yuen B, Knopf R, Jaffe RB.** Amenorrhea, hyperprolactinemia, and pituitary enlargement secondary to primary hypothyroidism. *Obstet Gynecol* 1976;48:697–702.

278. **Natari S, Karashima T, Koga S.** A case report of idiopathic myxedema with secondary amenorrhea and hyperprolactinemia: effect of thyroid hormone replacement on reduction of pituitary enlargement and restoration of fertility. *Fukuoka Igako Zasshi* 1991;82:461–2.

279. **Volpe R.** The immunologic basis of Graves' disease. *N Engl J Med* 1972;287:463.

280. **Bottazzo GF, Dean BM.** Autoimmune thyroid disease. *Annu Rev Med* 1986;37:353–4.

281. **Hanafusa T, Pujol-Borrell R, Chiovato L, Russell RC, Doniach D, Bottazzo GF.** Aberrant expression of HLA-DR antigen on thyrocytes in Graves' disease; relevance for auto-immunity. *Lancet* 1983;2:1111–4.

282. **Londei M, Lamb JR, Bottazzo GF, Feldmann M.** Epithelial cells expressing aberrant MHC class II determinants can present antigen to cloned human T cells. *Nature* 1984;312:639–41.

283. **Todd I, Pujol-Borrell R, Hammond LJ, Bottazzo GF, Feldmann M.** Interferon-gamma induced HLA-DR expression by thyroid epithelium. *Clin Exp Immunol* 1985;61:265–73.

284. **Wenzel BE, Gutekunst R, Schultek, Scriba PC.** In vitro induction of class II and autoantigen expression of human thyroid monolayers stimulates autologous T-lymphocytes in co-cultures. *Ann Endocrinol* 1986;47:15–8.

285. **Pinchera A, Fenzi GF, Bartalena L.** Thyroid antigens involved in autoimmune thyroid disorders. In: **Klein E, Horster J,** eds. *Auto-immunity in Thyroid Diseases.* Stuttgart: Schattauer, 1979:49.

286. **Belfiore A, Pujol-Borell R, Mauerhoff R, Mirakian R, Bottazzo GF.** Effect of SV-40 transformation of HLA expression by thyroid follicular cells: arise of a population of DR positive thyrocytes. *Ann Endocrinol* 1986;47:17–21.

287. **LeClere J, Bene MC, Faure G.** Experimental in vivo induction of class II antigens in the thyroid. *Ann Endocrinol* 1986;47:17–20.

288. **Burrow CN.** Thyroid disease. In: **Burrow GN, Ferris TF,** eds. *Medical Complications During Pregnancy.* Philadelphia: WB Saunders, 1982:205.

289. **Stoffer SS, Hamberger JI.** Inadvertent ^{131}I therapy for hyperthyroidism in the first trimester of pregnancy. *J Nucl Med* 1976;17:146–8.

290. **McKenzie JM, Zakarija M.** Hyperthyroidism. In: **DeGroot LJ, Cahill GF, Martini L,** eds. *Endocrinology.* New York: Grune & Stratton, 1979:647.

291. **Zakarija M, Garcia M, McKenzie JM.** Studies on multiple thyroid cell membrane directed antibodies in Graves' disease. *J Clin Invest* 1985;76:1885–98.

292. **Zakarija M, McKenzie JM.** Pregnancy associated changes in the thyroid stimulating antibodies of Graves' disease and the relationship to neonatal hyperthyroidism. *J Clin Endocrinol Metab* 1983;57:1036–40.

293. **Akande E, Hockaday T.** Plasma luteinizing hormone levels in women with thyrotoxicosis. *J Endocrinol* 1972;53:173–5.

294. **Greenman GW, Gabrielson MA, Howard-Flanders J, Wessel MA.** Thyroid dysfunction in pregnancy, fetal loss and followup evaluation of surviving infants. *N Engl J Med* 1962;267:426–31.

295. **Tanaka T, Tamai H, Kuma K, Matsuzuka F, Hidaka H.** Gonadotropin response to luteinizing hormone releasing hormone in hyperthyroid patients with menstrual disturbances. *Metabolism* 1981;30:323–5.

296. **Goldsmith RE, Sturgis SH, Lerman J, Stanbury JB.** The menstrual pattern in thyroid disease. *J Clin Endocrinol Metab* 1952;12:846–55.

297. **Thomas R, Reid RL.** Thyroid disease and reproductive dysfunction. *Obstet Gynecol* 1987; 70:789–98.

298. **Roger J.** Menstruation and systemic disease. *N Engl J Med* 1958;259:676–81.

299. **Mussey RD.** Hyperthyroidism complicating pregnancy. *Mayo Clin Proc* 1939;14:205–8.

300. **Amino N, Mori H, Iwatani Y, Tanizawa O, Kawashima M, Tsuge I.** High prevalence of transient postpartum thyrotoxicosis and hypothyroidism. *N Engl J Med* 1982;306:849–52.

301. **Jansson R, Dahlberg PA, Karlsson FA.** Postpartum thyroiditis. *Baillieres Clin Endocrinol Metab* 1988;2:619–35.

302. **Amino N.** Autoimmunity and hypothyroidism. *Baillieres Clin Endocrinol Metab* 1988;2: 591–617.

303. **Freeman R, Rosen H, Thysen B.** Incidence of thyroid dysfunction in an unselected postpartum population. *Arch Intern Med* 1986;146:1361–4.

304. **Nikolai TF, Turney SL, Roberts RC.** Postpartum lymphocytic thyroiditis: prevalence, clinical course, and long term follow up. *Arch Intern Med* 1987;147:221–4.

305. **Fung HYM, Kologlu M, Collison K, John R, Richards CJ, Hall R, et al.** Postpartum thyroid dysfunction in Mid Glamorgan. *BMJ* 1988;196:241–4.

306. **Hayslip CC, Fein HG, O'Donnell VM, Friedman DS, Klein TA, et al.** The value of serum antimicrosomal antibody testing in screening for symptomatic postpartum thyroid dysfunction. *Am J Obstet Gynecol* 1988;159:203–9.

307. **Iwatani Y, Amino N, Tamaki H, Aozasa M, Kabutomori O, Mori M, et al.** Increase in peripheral large granular lymphocytes in postpartum autoimmune thyroiditis. *Endocrinol Jpn* 1988;35:447–53.

308. **Vargas MT, Briones-Urbina R, Gladman D, Papsin FR, Walfish PG.** Antithyroid microsomal autoantibodies and HLA-DR5 are associated with postpartum thyroid dysfunction: evidence supporting an autoimmune pathogenesis. *J Clin Endocrinol Metab* 1988;67:327–33.

309. **Jansson R, Karlson A.** Autoimmune thyroid disease in pregnancy and the postpartum period. In: **McGregory AM,** ed. *Immunology of Endocrine Disease.* Lancaster, UK: MTP Press, 1986:181–8.

310. **Walfish PG, Chan JYC.** Post-partum hyperthyroidism. *J Clin Endocrinol Metab* 1985;14: 417–47.

311. **Glinoer D, Soto MF, Bourdoux P, Lejeune B, Delange F, Lemme M, et al.** Pregnancy in patients with mild thyroid abnormalities: maternal and neonatal repercussions. *J Clin Endocrinol Metab* 1991;73:421–7.

312. **Pratt D, Novotny M, Kaberlein G, Dudkiewicz A, Gleicher N.** Antithyroid antibodies and the association with non-organ-specific antibodies in recurrent pregnancy loss. *Am J Obstet Gynecol* 1993;168:837–41.

313. **Stagnaro-Green A, Roman SH, Cobin RH, el-Haranz E, Alvarez-Marfany M, Davies TF.** Detection of at-risk pregnancy by means of highly sensitive assays for thyroid autoantibodies. *JAMA* 1990;264:1422–5.

314. **Cowchock S, Smith RJ.** Gocial B antibodies to phospholipids and nuclear antigens in patients with repeated abortion. *Am J Obstet Gynecol* 1986;155:1002–10.

315. **Gleicher N, El-Roeiy A, Confino E, Friberg J.** Reproductive failure because of autoantibodies: unexplained infertility and pregnancy wastage. *Am J Obstet Gynecol* 1989;160:1376–85.

316. **Maier DB, Parke A.** Subclinical autoimmunity and recurrent aborters. *Fertil Steril* 1989;51:280–85.

317. **Magaro M, Zoli A, Altomonte L, Mirone L, LaSala L, Barini A, et al.** The association of silent thyroiditis and active systemic lupus erythematosus. *Clin Exp Rheumatol* 1992;10:67–70.

318. **LaBarbera A, Miller MM, Ober C, Rebar RW.** Autoimmune etiology in premature ovarian failure. *Am J Reprod Immunol* 1988;16:114–18.

319. **Peterson CM.** Thyroid disease and fertility. In: **Gleicher N,** ed. Autoimmunity in reproduction. Immunol Allergy Clin NA 1995;14:725–38.

320. **Ezzat S, Sarti DA, Cain DR, Braunstein GD.** Thyroid incidentalomas: prevalence by palpitation and ultrasonography. *Arch Intern Med* 1994;154:1838–40.

321. **McHenry CR, Walfish PG, Rosen IB.** Non-diagnostic fine needle aspiration biopsy: A dilemma in management of nodular thyroid disease. *Am Surg* 1993;59:415–9.

26

Endometriosis

Thomas M. D'Hooghe
Joseph A. Hill

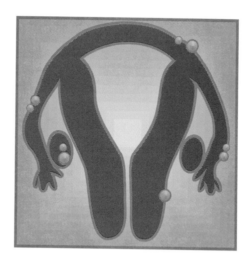

Endometriosis is defined as the presence of endometrial tissue (glands and stroma) outside the uterus. The most frequent sites of implantation are the pelvic viscera and the peritoneum. Endometriosis varies in appearance from a few minimal lesions on otherwise intact pelvic organs to massive ovarian endometriotic cysts that distort tubo-ovarian anatomy and extensive adhesions often involving bowel, bladder, and ureter. It is estimated to occur in 7% of reproductive age women in the U.S. and may be associated with pelvic pain and infertility. Considerable progress has been made in understanding the pathogenesis, spontaneous evolution, diagnosis, and treatment of endometriosis.

Etiology

Although endometriosis has been described since the 1800s, its widespread occurrence was acknowledged only during this century. Endometriosis is an estrogen-dependent disease. Three theories have been proposed to explain the histogenesis of endometriosis:

1. Ectopic transplantation of endometrial tissue

2. Coelomic metaplasia

3. The induction theory

No single theory can account for the location of endometriosis in all cases.

Transplantation Theory The transplantation theory, originally proposed by Sampson in the mid-1920s, is based on the assumption that endometriosis is caused by the seeding or implantation of endometrial cells by transtubal regurgitation during menstruation (1). Substantial clinical and experimental data support this hypothesis (2, 3). Retrograde menstruation occurs in 70–90% of women (4, 5), and it may be more common in women with endometriosis than in those without the disease (5). The presence of endometrial cells in the peritoneal fluid, indicating retrograde menstruation, has been reported in 59–79% of women

887

during menses or in the early follicular phase (6, 7), and these cells can be cultured *in vitro* (7). Evidence supporting retrograde menstruation is the presence of endometrial cells in the dialysate of women undergoing peritoneal dialysis during menses (8). Also, endometriosis is most often found in dependent portions of the pelvis—on the ovaries, the anterior and posterior cul-de-sac, the uterosacral ligaments, the posterior uterus, and the posterior broad ligaments (9).

Endometrium obtained during menses can grow when injected beneath abdominal skin or into the pelvic cavity of animals (10, 11). Endometriosis has been found in 50% of Rhesus monkeys after surgical transposition of the cervix to allow intra-abdominal menstruation (12). Increased retrograde menstruation by obstruction of the outflow of menstrual fluid from the uterus is associated with a higher incidence of endometriosis in women (13, 14) and in baboons (15). Women with shorter intervals between menstruation and longer duration of menses are more likely to have retrograde menstruation and have a higher risk of developing endometriosis (16).

Ovarian endometriosis may be caused by either retrograde menstruation or by lymphatic flow from the uterus to the ovary (17). Extrapelvic endometriosis, although rare (1–2%), potentially may result from vascular or lymphatic dissemination of endometrial cells to many gynecologic (vulva, vagina, cervix) and nongynecologic sites. The latter include bowel (appendix, rectum, sigmoid colon, small intestine, hernia sacs), lungs and pleural cavity, skin (episiotomy or other surgical scars, inguinal region, extremities, umbilicus), lymph glands, nerves, and brain (18).

Coelomic Metaplasia   The transformation (metaplasia) of coelomic epithelium into endometrial tissue has been proposed as a mechanism for the origin of endometriosis. This theory has not been supported by either strong clinical or experimental data, however.

Induction Theory   The induction theory is, in principle, an extension of the coelomic metaplasia theory. It proposes that an endogenous (undefined) biochemical factor can induce undifferentiated peritoneal cells to develop into endometrial tissue. This theory has been supported by experiments in rabbits (19, 20), but has not been substantiated in women and primates.

Genetic Factors

The risk of endometriosis is seven times greater if a first-degree relative has been affected by endometriosis (21). Because no specific Mendelian inheritance pattern has been identified, multifactorial inheritance has been postulated. A relative risk for endometriosis of 7.2 has been found in mothers and sisters, and a 75% (six of eight) incidence has been noted in homozygotic twins of patients with endometriosis (22). A relationship has been shown between endometriosis and other autoimmune diseases (e.g., systematic lupus erythematosus) (23), as well as between endometriosis and individual human leukocyte antigens (24–26).

Immunologic Factors

Although retrograde menstruation appears to be a common event in women, not all women who have retrograde menstruation develop endometriosis. The immune system may be altered in women with endometriosis, and the disease may develop as a result of reduced immunologic clearance of viable endometrial cells from the pelvic cavity (27, 28). Decreased cell-mediated cytotoxity toward autologous endometrial cells has been reported to be associated with endometriosis (29–33). However, these studies used techniques that have considerable variability in target cells and methods (34, 35). It is unlikely that autologous endometrial cells provide a natural target for a woman's immune system because autologous transplantation of other autologous tissues has generally been successful (30–32). Whether natural killer (NK) cell activity is lower in endometriosis patients than in women without endometriosis is controversial. Some reports demonstrate reduced NK activity (32, 36–39), whereas others have found no increase in NK activity, even in women with moderate to severe disease (31–33, 40). There is also great variability in NK cell activity among normal individuals that may be related to variables such as smoking, drug use, and exercise (34).

A higher basal activation status of peritoneal macrophages in women with endometriosis may impair fertility by reducing sperm motility, increasing sperm phagocytosis, or interfering with fertilization (41, 42), possibly by increased secretion of cytokines such as tumor necrosis factor (α-TNF) (43–45). α-TNF may also facilitate the pelvic implantation of ectopic endometrium. The adherence of human endometrial stromal cells to mesothelial cells *in vitro* has been shown to be increased by the pretreatment of mesothelial cells with physiological doses of α-TNF (46). Macrophages or other cells may promote the growth of endometrial cells (47, 48) by secretion of growth and angiogenetic factors such as epidermal growth factor (EGF) (46), macrophage-derived growth factor (MDGF) (49), fibronectin (50), and adhesion molecules such as integrins (51).

Future Research

The study of endometriosis is compounded by the need to exclude other causes and to assess symptoms within the context of the pelvic condition (i.e., the presence or absence of pathology). The pathogenesis of endometriosis, the pathophysiology of related infertility, and its spontaneous evolution are still being investigated. At the time of diagnosis, most patients with endometriosis have had the disease for an unknown period, making it difficult to initiate any clinical experiments that would determine definitely the etiology or progression of the disease (3). Because endometriosis occurs naturally in only humans and nonhuman primates and invasive experiments cannot be performed easily, it is difficult to undertake properly controlled studies. Thus, there is a need for the development of a good animal model with spontaneous endometriosis.

The main advantage of the rat and rabbit animal models used to study endometriosis is their low cost relative to nonhuman primates. The disadvantages are numerous, however. Rodents lack a menstrual cycle comparable to that of primates and do not have spontaneous endometriosis. While the rat ovulates spontaneously, it has a shorter luteal phase than humans. The reproductive pattern of the rabbit lacks a luteal phase. There is a wide phylogenetic gap between these two species and the human, and in both rodent models, the type of lesions appear to be quite different from the variety of pigmented and nonpigmented lesions observed in women (52–54).

Nonhuman primates, on the other hand, are phylogenetically close to the human, have a comparable menstrual cycle, are afflicted with spontaneous endometriosis, and induced endometriosis results in macroscopic lesions that are similar to those found in the human disease (12, 55–59). While the great apes are closest to humans in many anatomic and physiologic aspects of reproduction, they are not practical models for study; therefore, Rhesus and cynomolgus monkeys have been used. Baboons may be a better choice for study because they are continuous breeders, are phylogenetically very close to humans, and have similar reproductive anatomy and physiology with regard to menstrual cycle characteristics and regularity, embryo implantation, and fetal development (55). In addition, spontaneous endometriosis in the baboon has been found to be both minimal and disseminated, similar to the different stages of endometriosis in women (55, 60, 61).

Prevalence

Endometriosis is predominantly found in women of reproductive age but has been reported in adolescents and in postmenopausal women receiving hormonal replacement (62). It is found in women from all ethnic and social groups. In women with pelvic pain or infertility, a high prevalence of endometriosis (from a low of 20% to a high of 90%) has been reported (2, 63). In asymptomatic women having tubal ligation (women of proven fertility), the prevalence of endometriosis ranges from 3% to 43% (5, 64–68). This great variation in the reported prevalence may be explained by several factors. First, it may vary with the diagnostic method used: laparoscopy, the operation of choice for diagnosis, is generally accepted to be a better method than laparotomy for diagnosing minimal to mild endometriosis. Second, minimal or mild endometriosis may be more thoroughly noted in a symptomatic patient being given general anesthesia than in an asymptomatic patient during tubal sterilization. Third, the experience of the surgeon is important because there is a wide variation in the appearance of subtle endometriosis implants, cysts, and adhesions. Most studies that evaluate the prevalence of endometriosis in women of reproductive age lack histologic confirmation (5, 64, 65, 68–73).

Diagnosis

Clinical Presentation

Endometriosis should be suspected in women with subfertility, dysmenorrhea, dyspareunia, or chronic pelvic pain. However, endometriosis may be asymptomatic.

Pain

In adult women, dysmenorrhea may be especially suggestive of endometriosis if it begins after years of pain-free menses. The dysmenorrhea often starts before the onset of menstrual bleeding and continues throughout the menstrual period. In adolescents, the pain may be present without an interval of pain-free menses after menarche. The distribution of pain is variable but most often is bilateral.

Local symptoms can arise from rectal, ureteral, and bladder involvement. Lower back pain can occur. Most studies have failed to detect a correlation between the degree of pelvic pain and the severity of endometriosis (66). Some women with extensive disease have no pain, whereas others with only minimal disease may experience severe pelvic pain. Severe pelvic pain and dyspareunia may be associated with deep infiltrating subperitoneal endometriosis (63, 73). Possible mechanisms causing pain in patients with endometriosis include local peritoneal inflammation, deep infiltration with tissue damage, adhesion formation, fibrotic thickening, and collection of shed menstrual blood in endometriotic implants, resulting in painful traction with the physiologic movement of tissues (73, 74).

Subfertility

An association between endometriosis and subfertility is generally accepted, but most of the studies suggesting this link have been based on retrospective or cross-sectional analysis. When endometriosis is moderate or severe, involving the ovaries and causing adhesions that block tubo-ovarian motility and ovum pickup, it is associated with subfertility (75). This effect has also been shown in nonhuman primates (58) and baboons (76). Although numerous mechanisms (ovulatory dysfunction, luteal insufficiency, luteinized unruptured follicle syndrome, recurrent abortion, altered immunity, and intraperitoneal inflammation) have been proposed (77), the association between fertility and minimal or mild endometriosis remains controversial (75).

Infertility **Based on the number of asymptomatic women who are found to have endometriosis during tubal ligation, it would seem that the prevalence of endometriosis is not necessarily higher in infertile than in fertile women with endometriosis (5). In fertile women, endometriosis has been reported to be minimal or mild in 80% and moderate or severe in 20% (5, 64–68).**

In women with mild disease, some studies have reported a lower spontaneous *monthly fecundity rate (MFR)*, which is the total number of pregnancies divided by the number of months of pregnancy exposure (i.e., 5–11% compared to 25% in a normally fertile population) (77). Other studies using artificial insemination with donor semen have reported

890

that the MFR in women with minimal and mild endometriosis is either reduced (4%) or normal (20%) (78–81). Fertility is not reduced in baboons with spontaneous minimal endometriosis (76, 82). Because of the lack of prospective controlled studies in women, it is unclear whether the mere presence of peritoneal endometriosis directly correlates with infertility.

Spontaneous Abortion   In uncontrolled, retrospective studies, endometriosis has been associated with an increased rate of spontaneous abortion—up to 40% compared with a normal spontaneous abortion rate of 15–25% (83–87). The spontaneous abortion rate has been reported to be decreased after surgical treatment (85, 86, 88) as well as after no (expectant) treatment (89), but no correlation was found between the stage of disease and the abortion rate. In another study using fertile and infertile women without endometriosis as controls, an increased abortion rate in infertile endometriosis patients was found before evaluation but not after treatment (90). This finding suggests that the higher abortion rate observed before evaluation in patients who have endometriosis occurs primarily as a result of selection bias because infertile women with endometriosis are more likely to seek care than fertile women with endometriosis (90). Other retrospective studies using infertile women without endometriosis or women with adenomyosis who habitually abort as controls have not demonstrated an increased abortion rate in patients who have endometriosis (91, 92). Similarly, a retrospective cohort study determining the preclinical abortion rate (using a sensitive assay for serum human chorionic gonadotropin) failed to demonstrate differences between infertile women with and without endometriosis (93). Thus, the association of endometriosis and spontaneous abortion is difficult to assess adequately because of the lack of prospective studies with well-defined control groups.

Endocrinologic Abnormalities

Endometriosis has been associated with anovulation, abnormal follicular development, luteal insufficiency, and premenstrual spotting (i.e., the *luteinized unruptured follicle syndrome*), and galactorrhea and hyperprolactinemia. However, no convincing data exist to conclude that the incidence of these endocrinologic abnormalities is increased in women who have endometriosis.

Extrapelvic Endometriosis

Extrapelvic endometriosis, although often asymptomatic, should be suspected when symptoms of pain or a palpable mass occur outside the pelvis in a cyclic pattern. Endometriosis involving the intestinal tract (especially colon and rectum) is the most common site of extrapelvic disease and may cause abdominal and back pain, abdominal distension, cyclic rectal bleeding, constipation, and obstruction. Ureteral involvement can lead to obstruction and result in cyclic pain, dysuria, and hematuria. Pulmonary endometriosis can manifest as pneumothorax, hemothorax, or hemoptysis during menses. Umbilical endometriosis should be suspected when a patient has a palpable mass and cyclic pain in the umbilical area (18).

Clinical Examination

In many women with endometriosis, no abnormality is detected during the clinical examination. The vulva, vagina, and cervix should be inspected for any signs of endometriosis, although the occurrence of endometriosis in these areas is rare (e.g., episiotomy scar). Other possible signs of endometriosis include uterosacral or cul-de-sac nodularity, painful swelling of the rectovaginal septum, and unilateral ovarian (cystic) enlargement. In more advanced disease, the uterus is often in fixed retroversion and the mobility of the ovaries and fallopian tubes is reduced. Evidence of deeply infiltrative endometriosis (deeper than 5 mm under the peritoneum) in the cul-de-sac and rectovaginal septum should be sought during menses (94, 95). The clinical examination may have false-negative results. Therefore, the diagnosis of endometriosis should always be confirmed by biopsy of suspicious lesions that are obtained laparoscopically. Ultrasound, computed tomography (CT), or magnetic resonance imaging (MRI) can be used to provide additional and confirmatory information but cannot be used for determining the primary diagnosis.

CA125

There is no blood test available for the diagnosis of endometriosis. Levels of CA125, a marker found on derivatives of the coelomic epithelium and common to most nonmucinous epithelial ovarian carcinomas (96), have been found to be significantly higher in women with moderate or severe endometriosis and normal in women with minimal or mild disease (97). During menstruation, an increase in CA125 levels has been shown in women with and without endometriosis (98–102). Other studies have not found an increase during menses (103, 104) or have found an increase only with moderate to severe endometriosis (105, 106). The levels of CA125 vary widely, not only in patients without endometriosis (8–22 U/ml in the nonmenstrual phase), but also in those with minimal to mild endometriosis (14–31 U/ml in the nonmenstrual phase) and in those with moderate to severe disease (13–95 U/ml in the nonmenstrual phase).

The reason CA125 levels are increased in moderate to severe endometriosis is unclear. It has been hypothesized that endometriosis lesions contain a greater amount of CA125 than normal endometrium and that the associated inflammation could lead to an increased shedding of CA125 (97).

The specificity of CA125 has been reported to be higher than 80% in most studies. This high level of specificity is achieved in selected women with infertility or pain who are known to be at risk for endometriosis. The low level of sensitivity of CA125 (20–50% in most studies) poses limitations for the clinical use of this test for diagnosis of endometriosis. Theoretically, the sensitivity might increase during the menstrual period, when the increase in CA125 levels is more pronounced in women who have endometriosis. However, studies using cutoff levels of 35 U/ml (105, 106) or 85 U/ml (107) have not found a significant improvement in sensitivity. A sensitivity of 66% was found when CA125 was determined during both the follicular phase and the menstrual phase in each patient and when the ratio of menstrual versus follicular values (>1.5) was used instead of one CA125 level (106).

Serial CA125 determinations may be useful to predict the recurrence of endometriosis after therapy (108, 109). CA125 levels decrease after combined medical and surgical therapy (110) or during medical treatment of endometriosis with *danazol* (111), gonadotropin-releasing hormone (GnRH) analogs (112), or *gestrinone* (113), but not with *medroxyprogesterone acetate (MPA)* or placebo (110). CA125 levels have been reported to increase to pretreatment levels as early as 3, 4, or 6 months after the cessation of therapy with *danazol, GnRH analogs,* or *gestrinone* (102, 111–115). Post-treatment increases in CA125 levels have been reported to correlate with endometriosis recurrence (101, 109, 116). However, other studies have not substantiated a correlation between post-treatment CA125 levels and disease recurrence (110, 113, 117). Further studies with second-look laparoscopy over a longer follow-up interval would be required to establish a correlation.

Laparoscopic Findings

At diagnostic laparoscopy, the pelvic and abdominal cavity should be systematically investigated for the presence of endometriosis. This must include an inspection and palpation with a blunt probe of the bowel, bladder, uterus, tubes, ovaries, cul-de-sac, and broad ligament (Fig. 26.1).

Characteristic findings at laparoscopy include typical ("powder-burn," "gunshot") lesions on the serosal surfaces of the peritoneum. These are black, dark-brown, or bluish nodules or small cysts containing old hemorrhage surrounded by a variable degree of fibrosis (Fig. 26.2). Endometriosis can appear as subtle lesions (Fig. 26.3), including red implants (petechial, vesicular, polypoid, hemorrhagic, red flame-like), serous or clear vesicles, white plaques or scarring, yellow-brown peritoneal discoloration of the peritoneum, and subovarian adhesions (53–55, 118, 119).

Histologic confirmation of the laparoscopic impression is essential for the diagnosis of endometriosis (120), **not only for subtle lesions but also for typical lesions reported**

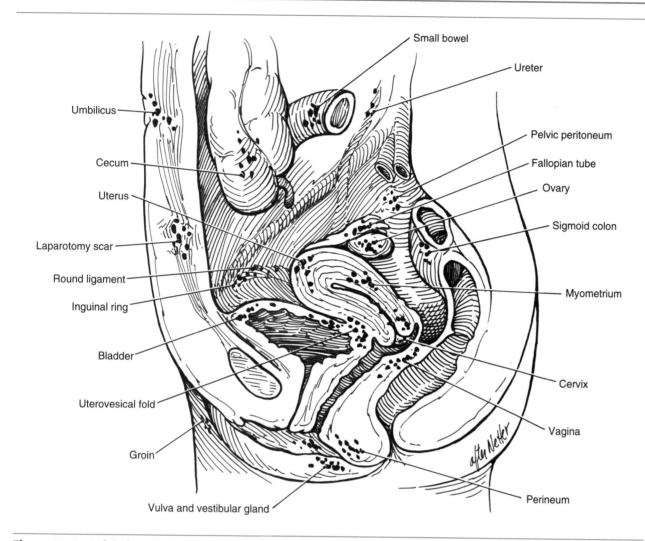

Figure 26.1   Pelvic localization of endometriosis.

to be histologically negative in 24% of cases (121). Mild forms of deep endometriosis may only be detected by palpation under an endometriotic lesion or by discovery of a palpable mass beneath visually normal peritoneum, most notably in the posterior cul-de-sac (Fig. 26.4) (95). The diagnosis of ovarian endometriosis is facilitated by careful inspection of all sides of both ovaries, which may be difficult when adhesions are present in more advanced stages of disease (Fig. 26.5). With superficial ovarian endometriosis, lesions can be both typical and subtle. Larger ovarian endometriotic cysts (endometrioma) are usually located on the anterior surface of the ovary associated with retraction, pigmentation, and adhesions to the posterior peritoneum. These ovarian endometriotic cysts often contain a thick, viscous dark-brown fluid ("chocolate fluid") composed of hemosiderin derived from previous intraovarian hemorrhage. Because this fluid may also be found in other conditions, such as a hemorrhagic corpus luteum cysts or neoplastic cysts, biopsy and preferably removal of the ovarian cyst for histologic confirmation are necessary.

Histological Confirmation

Microscopically, endometriotic implants consist of endometrial glands and stroma with or without hemosiderin-laden macrophages (Fig. 26.6). It has been suggested, however, that using these stringent and unvalidated histologic criteria may result in significant underdiagnosis of endometriosis (2). Furthermore, problems in obtaining biopsies (especially small vesicles) and variability in tissue processing (step or partial instead of serial sectioning) may contribute to false-negative reports. Endometrioid stroma may be more charac-

893

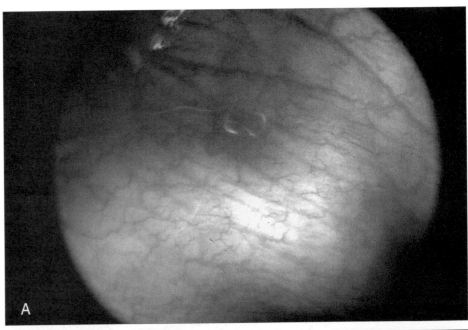

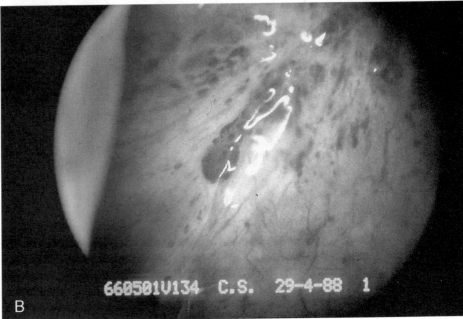

Figure 26.2   Subtle and typical endometriotic lesions. *A,* Clear translucent vesicle on pelvic peritoneum. *B,* Red polypoid lesions and petechial/hemorrhagic areas on pelvic peritoneum. *C,* Typical black-puckered lesions on uterosacral ligaments. *D,* Combination of typical black-puckered lesions on left uterosacral ligament and red polypoid lesions in cul-de-sac.

teristic of endometriosis than endometrioid glands (122). Stromal endometriosis, containing endometrial stroma with hemosiderin-laden macrophages or hemorrhage, has been reported in women (120, 121) and in baboons (61) and may represent a very early event in the pathogenesis of endometriosis. Different types of lesions may have different degrees of proliferative or secretory glandular activity (122). Vascularization, mitotic activity, and the three-dimensional structure of endometriosis lesions are key factors (123–125). Deep endometriosis has been described as a specific type of pelvic en-

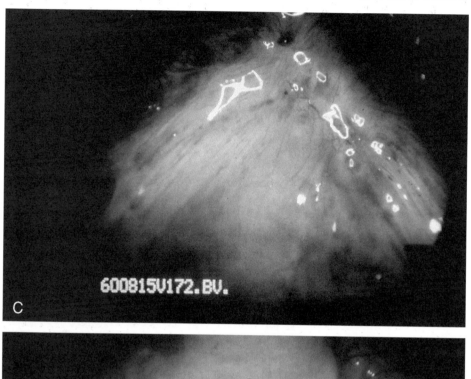

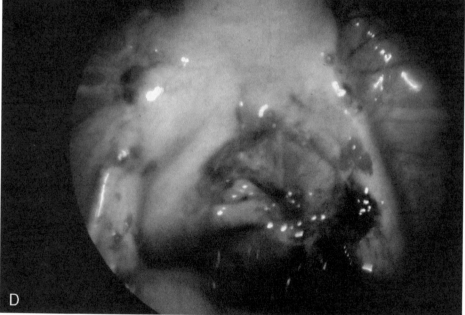

Figure 26.2—*continued*

dometriosis characterized by proliferative strands of glands and stroma in dense fibrous and smooth muscle tissue (73).

Microscopic Endometriosis   Microscopic endometriosis is defined as the presence of endometrial glands and stroma in macroscopically normal pelvic peritoneum. It is believed to be important in the histogenesis of endometriosis (126) and its recurrence after treatment (127). The clinical relevance of microscopic endometriosis is controversial because it has not been observed uniformly. Using undefined criteria for what constitutes normal peritoneum, peritoneal biopsies of 1–3 cm were obtained during laparotomy from 20 patients with moderate to severe endometriosis (127). Examination of the biopsies with low-power scanning electron microscopy (SEM) revealed unsuspected microscopic endometriosis in

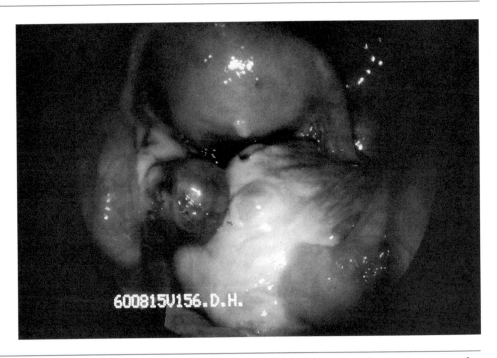

Figure 26.3   Ovarian endometriosis: endometriotic cyst (endometrioma) on the left ovary.

Figure 26.4   Laparoscopic excision of deep endometriosis from the cul-de-sac.

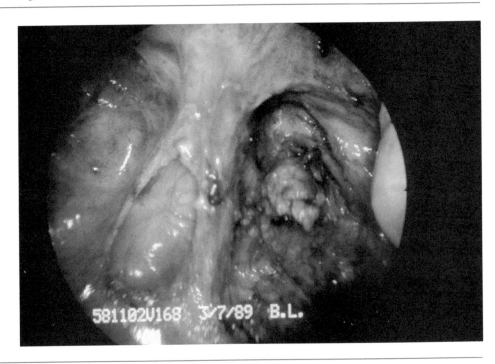

Revised American Fertility Society Classification of Endometriosis: 1985

Patient's Name _____ Date_____

Stage I (Minimal) - 1-5
Stage II (Mild) - 6-15
Stage III (Moderate) - 16-40
Stage IV (Severe) - >40
Total_____

Laparoscopy_____ Laparotomy_____ Photography_____
Recommended Treatment_____

Prognosis_____

PERITONEUM	**ENDOMETRIOSIS**	$<$1cm	1-3cm	$>$3cm
	Superficial	1	2	4
	Deep	2	4	6
OVARY	R Superficial	1	2	4
	Deep	4	16	20
	L Superficial	1	2	4
	Deep	4	16	20

	POSTERIOR CULDESAC OBLITERATION	Partial	Complete
		4	40

	ADHESIONS	$<$1/3 Enclosure	1/3-2/3 Enclosure	$>$2/3 Enclosure
OVARY	R Filmy	1	2	4
	Dense	4	8	16
	L Filmy	1	2	4
	Dense	4	8	16
TUBE	R Filmy	1	2	4
	Dense	4*	8*	16
	L Filmy	1	2	4
	Dense	4*	8*	16

*If the fimbriated end of the fallopian tube is completely enclosed, change the point assignment to 16.

Additional Endometriosis: _____

Associated Pathology: _____

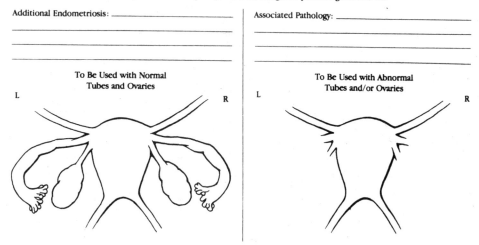

To Be Used with Normal Tubes and Ovaries

To Be Used with Abnormal Tubes and/or Ovaries

Figure 26.5   Revised American Fertility Society Classification, 1985. (Reproduced with permission from **The America Fertility Society.** Revised American Fertility Society Classification of endometriosis. *Fertil Steril* 1985;43:351–2. Reproduced, with permission of the publisher, the American Society for Reproductive Medicine.)

25% of cases not confirmed by light microscopy. Peritoneal endometriotic foci have been demonstrated by light microscopy in areas that show no obvious evidence of disease (128). In serial sections of laparoscopic biopsies of normal peritoneum, 13–15% of women were shown to have microscopic endometriosis, and endometriosis was found in 6% of those without macroscopic disease (119, 129). In contrast, other studies have been unable to detect microscopic endometriosis in 2-mm biopsies of visually normal peritoneum (52,

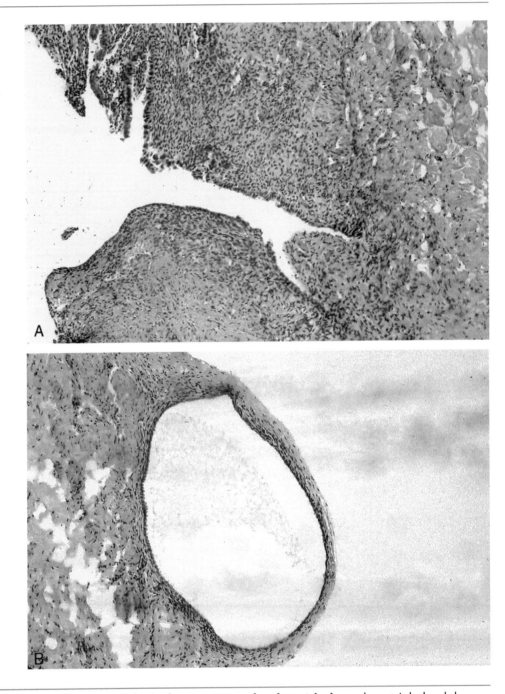

Figure 26.6   Histological appearance of endometriosis: endometrial glandular epithelium, surrounded by stroma in (*A*) typical lesion and (*B*) clear vesicle.

130–132). Examination of larger samples (5–15 mm) of visually normal peritoneum has revealed microscopic endometriosis in only one of 55 patients studied (133). Similarly, a histologic study of serial sections through the entire pelvic peritoneum of visually normal peritoneum from baboons with and without disease indicated that microscopic endometriosis is a rare occurrence (134). Therefore, it seems that macroscopically appearing normal peritoneum rarely contains microscopic endometriosis (133).

Classification   The current classification system of endometriosis is the revised American Fertility Society (AFS) system (75). It is based on appearance, size, and depth of peritoneal and ovarian implants; the presence, extent, and type of adnexal adhesions; and the degree of cul-de-sac obliteration. This system reflects the extent of endometriotic disease, but it is not based on the correlation of pain or infertility and it has considerable intraobserver and interobserver variability (135). A classification system that includes parameters of disease activity is currently being considered; however, the revised AFS classification of endometriosis is the only internationally accepted standard to evaluate spontaneous evolution and to compare therapeutic outcomes.

Spontaneous Evolution

Endometriosis appears to be a progressive disease. During serial observations, deterioration (47%), improvement (30%), or elimination (23%) was documented over a 6-month period (136). In another study, endometriosis progressed in 64%, improved in 27%, and remained unchanged in 9% over 12 months (137). However, spontaneous improvement in the scoring or staging of endometriosis has not been found in either women (138) or baboons (139) during follow-up laparoscopy 6 to 12 months after the original diagnosis was established. Several studies have reported that subtle lesions and typical implants may represent younger and older types of endometriosis, respectively. In a cross-sectional study, the incidence of subtle lesions decreased with age (140). This was recently confirmed by a 3-year prospective study that reported that the incidence, overall pelvic area involved, and volume of subtle lesions decreased with age, but in typical lesions these parameters and the depth of infiltration increased with age (63). Remodeling of endometriotic lesions (transition between typical and subtle subtypes) has been reported to occur in women (141) and in baboons (139), indicating that endometriosis is a dynamic condition. Several studies in women (142), cynomolgus monkeys (143), and rodents (144) have described that endometriosis is ameliorated after pregnancy. The characteristics of endometriosis are variable during pregnancy, and lesions tend to enlarge during the first trimester but regress thereafter (145). Studies in baboons have revealed no change in the number or surface area of endometriosis lesions during the first two trimesters of pregnancy. These results do not exclude a beneficial effect that potentially may occur during the third trimester or immediately postpartum. Establishment of a "pseudopregnant state" with exogenously administered estrogen and progestins was based on the belief that symptomatic improvement may result from decidualization of endometrial implants during pregnancy (146). This hypothesis, however, has not been substantiated.

Treatment

No strategies to prevent endometriosis have been uniformly successful. Although a reduced incidence of endometriosis has been reported in women who engaged in aerobic activity from an early age (16), the possible protective effect of exercise has not been investigated thoroughly.

Regardless of the clinical profile (subfertility, pain, asymptomatic), treatment of endometriosis may be justified because endometriosis appears to progress in two-thirds of patients within a year from diagnosis and because it is not possible to predict in which patients it will progress (137). **Unfortunately, elimination of the endometriotic implants by surgical or medical treatment often provides only temporarily relief. Therefore, the goal should be to eliminate the endometriotic lesions and, more importantly, to treat the sequelae (pain and subfertility) often associated with this disease.**

Surgical Treatment

In most women with endometriosis, preservation of reproductive function is desirable. Therefore, the least invasive and least expensive approach that is effective should be used. Laparoscopy can be used in most women, and this technique decreases cost, morbidity, and the possibility of recurrence of adhesions postoperatively. **Laparotomy should be reserved for patients with advanced stage disease and for those in whom fertility con-**

servation is no longer necessary. Endometriosis lesions can be removed during laparoscopy with bipolar coagulation, the CO_2 laser, the potassium-titany-phosphate laser, or the argon laser. The CO_2 laser appears to be the preferred method because it causes only minimal thermal damage. The goal of surgery is to excise or coagulate all visible endometriotic lesions and associated adhesions and to restore normal anatomy. Superficial ovarian lesions can be vaporized. Small ovarian endometriomata (<3 cm) can be aspirated, irrigated, and inspected with ovarian cystoscopy for intracystic lesions; their interior wall can be vaporized to destroy the mucosal lining of the cyst (147). Large (>3 cm in diameter) ovarian endometriomata should be aspirated, followed by incision and removal of the cyst wall from the ovarian cortex. To prevent recurrence, the cyst wall of the endometrioma must be removed and normal ovarian tissue must be preserved. As little as one-tenth of an ovary is enough to preserve function and fertility (148). The removal of adhesions (adhesiolysis) should be performed carefully as described in Chapter 21.

In patients with severe endometriosis, it has been recommended that surgical treatment be preceded by a 3-month course of medical treatment to reduce vascularization and nodular size (95). Radical procedures such as oophorectomy or total hysterectomy are indicated only in severe situations and can be performed either laparoscopically or, more commonly, by laparotomy. **Postoperative hormone replacement with estrogen is required after bilateral oophorectomy, and there is a negligible risk of renewed growth of residual endometriosis. To reduce this risk, hormone replacement therapy should be withheld until 3 months after surgery. The addition of progestins to this regimen protect the endometrium.** Some cases of adenocarcinoma have been reported, presumably arising from endometriosis lesions left in women treated with unopposed estrogen (148).

Results of Surgical Treatment

Pain   The outcome of surgical therapy in patients with endometriosis and pain is influenced by many psychological factors relating to personality, depression, and marital and sexual problems. There is a significant placebo response to surgical therapy: diagnostic laparoscopy without complete removal of endometriosis may alleviate pain in 50% of patients (138, 149, 150). Similar results have been reported using oral placebos (151). Although some reports have claimed pain relief with laser laparoscopy in 60–80% of patients with very low morbidity, none was prospective or controlled and, thus, did not allow a definitive conclusion regarding treatment efficacy (95, 152–155). In a prospective, controlled, randomized, double-blind study, surgical therapy has been shown to be superior to expectant management six months after treatment of mild and moderate endometriosis (138). In women with mild and moderate disease treated with laser, 74% achieved pain relief. Treatment was least effective in women with minimal disease. There were no reported operative or laser complications (138). Patients with severe disease were not included because it had previously been shown that surgery resulted in pain relief in 80% of patients who did not respond to medical therapy (156). These results suggest that laser laparoscopy may be effective for the treatment of pain associated with mild to severe endometriosis. In women with minimal endometriosis, laser treatment may limit progression of disease.

Subfertility   When endometriosis causes mechanical distortion of the pelvis, surgery should be performed if reconstruction of normal pelvic anatomy can be achieved. The success of surgery in relieving infertility is directly related to the severity of endometriosis. Treatment of moderate disease has an approximate 60% pregnancy success rate, and treatment of severe disease has a success rate of 35% (157). Preoperative medical treatment with *danazol*, GnRH agonists, or progestins may be useful to reduce the extent of endometriosis in patients with advanced disease. Postoperative medical treatment is rarely indicated because it prevents pregnancy, and the highest pregnancy rates occur during the first 6 to 12 months after conservative surgery. If pregnancy does not occur within 2 years of surgery, there is little chance of subsequent fertility (158).

Surgical management of infertile women with minimal to mild endometriosis is controversial. The cumulative pregnancy rate after 5 years without therapy is 90% in women with minimal or mild endometriosis (159). This is comparable to the 93% rate reported in women who do not have endometriosis. Laparoscopic destruction of endometriosis has been reported to improve fertility in patients with minimal to mild disease by some (160–162) but not all investigators (163–165). It is possible that the MFR is higher during the first 6 to 12 months after laparoscopic surgery than with expectant management (166, 167). Using monthly fecundity rates and life-table analysis, no study has shown an advantage for conservative surgery as opposed to expectant treatment of women with minimal to mild endometriosis. The surgical removal of peritoneal endometriosis may be important to prevent progression because the recurrence rate of endometriosis is lower after surgical than after medical therapy. However, it is not proven that this treatment will improve fertility, and it does pose the risk of the development of adhesions postoperatively.

Medical Treatment

Because estrogen is known to stimulate the growth of endometriosis, hormonal therapy has been designed to suppress estrogen synthesis, thereby inducing atrophy of ectopic endometrial implants or interrupting the cycle of stimulation and bleeding. Implants of endometriosis react to gonadal steroid hormones in a manner similar but not identical to normally stimulated ectopic endometrium. Ectopic endometrial tissue displays histologic and biochemical differences from normal ectopic endometrium in characteristics such as glandular activity (proliferation, secretion), enzyme activity (17-β-hydroxysteroid dehydrogenase), and steroid (estrogen, progestin, and androgen) hormone receptor levels. The use of diethylstilbestrol, methyltestosterone, or other androgens is no longer advocated because they lack efficacy, have significant side effects, and pose risks to the fetus if pregnancy occurs during therapy.

Oral Contraceptives

The treatment of endometriosis with low-dose monophasic combination contraceptives (one pill per day for 6 to 12 months) was originally used to induce "pseudopregnancy" caused by the resultant amenorrhea and decidualization of endometrial tissue (146). Estrogens in oral contraceptives potentially may stimulate the proliferation of endometriosis. The reduced menstrual bleeding that often occurs in women taking oral contraceptives may be beneficial to women with prolonged, frequent menstrual bleeding, which is a known risk factor for endometriosis (16). There is no convincing evidence that combination oral contraceptives provide prophylaxis against either the development or recurrence of endometriosis. Further research is warranted to assess the effect of low-dose oral contraceptives in preventing endometriosis and in treating associated pain.

Manipulation of the endogenous hormonal milieu is the basis for the medical management of endometriosis. Kistner was the first to introduce the concept of an adynamic endometrium through elimination of the normal cyclic hormonal changes characteristic of the menstrual cycle (168). This induction of a pseudopregnancy state with combination oral contraceptive pills has been shown to be effective in reducing dysmenorrhea and pelvic pain. In addition, the subsequent amenorrhea induced by oral contraceptives could potentially reduce the amount of retrograde menstruation (one of the many risk factors proposed in the etiology of endometriosis), decreasing the risk of disease progression. Pathologically, oral contraceptive pill use is associated with decidualization of endometrial tissue, necrobiosis, and possibly absorption of the endometrial tissue (169). Unfortunately, there is no convincing evidence that medical therapy with oral contraceptives offers definitive therapy. Instead, the endometrial implants survive the induced atrophy with reactivation in most patients following termination of treatment.

Any low-dose combination oral contraceptive pill containing 30–35 μg of *ethinyl estradiol* used continuously can be effective in the management of endometriosis. The objective of the treatment is the induction of amenorrhea, which should be continued for 6 to 12 months. Symptomatic relief of dysmenorrhea and pelvic pain is reported in 60–95% of patients (170, 171). Following a first-year recurrence rate of 17–18%, a 5–10% annual recurrence rate has been observed. In addition, a post-treatment pregnancy rate of up to 50% can be expected. Although oral contraceptives are effective in inducing a decidualized endometrium, the estrogenic component in oral contraceptives may potentially stimulate endometrial growth and increase pelvic pain in the first few weeks of treatment. The long-term significance of this remains to be determined. Oral contraceptives are less costly than other treatment modalities and may be helpful in the short-term management of endometriosis with potential long-term benefits in some women.

Progestins

Progestins may exert an antiendometriotic effect by causing initial decidualization of endometrial tissue followed by atrophy. They can be considered as the first choice for the treatment of endometriosis because they are as effective in reducing AFS scores and pain as *danazol* and have a lower cost and a lower incidence of side effects than *danazol*. There is no evidence that any single agent or any particular dose is preferable to another. The effective doses of several progestins are summarized in Table 26.1. In most studies, the effect of treatment has been evaluated after 3 to 6 months of therapy. *Medroxyprogesterone acetate (MPA)* has been the most studied agent and is effective in relieving pain starting at a dose of 30 mg/day and increasing the dose based on the clinical response and bleeding patterns (172, 173). *Medroxyprogesterone acetate (MPA)* (150 mg) given intramuscularly every 3 months is also effective for the treatment of pain associated with endometriosis, but it is not indicated in infertile women because it induces profound amenorrhea and anovulation, and a varying length of time is required for ovulation to resume after discontinuation of therapy. *Megestrol acetate* has been administered in a dose of 40 mg daily with good results (174). Other treatment strategies have included *dydrogesterone* (20–30 mg daily, either continuously or days 5–25) and *lynestrenol* (10 mg daily). Natural progesterone has not been evaluated.

Side effects of progestins include nausea, weight gain, fluid retention, and breakthrough bleeding due to hypoestrogenemia. Breakthrough bleeding, although common, is usually corrected by short-term (7-day) administration of estrogen. Depression and other mood disorders are a significant problem in approximately 1% of women taking these medications.

Gestrinone

Gestrinone is a 19-nortestosterone derivative with androgenic, antiprogestagenic, antiestrogenic, and antigonadotropic properties. It acts centrally and peripherally to increase

Table 26.1   Medical Treatment of Endometriosis-Associated Pain: Effective Regimens (Usual Duration: six months)

	Administration	Dose	Frequency
Progestogens			
Medroxyprogesterone acetate	PO	30 mg	daily
Megestrol acetate	PO	40 mg	daily
Lynestrenol	PO	10 mg	daily
Dydrogesterone	PO	20–30 mg	daily
Antiprogestins			
Gestrinone	PO	1.25 or 2.5 mg	twice weekly
Danazol	PO	400 (2 × 200) mg	daily
Gonodotropin-Releasing Hormone			
Leuprolide	SC	500 μg	daily
	IM	3.75 mg	monthly
Goserelin	SC	3.6 mg	monthly
Buserelin	IN	3 × 300 μg	daily
	SC	1 × 200 μg	daily
Nafarelin	IN	2 × 200 μg	daily
Tryptorelin	IM	3.75 mg	monthly

PO, oral; SC, subcutaneous; IM, intramuscular; IN, intranasal.

free testosterone and reduce sex-hormone binding globulin (SHBG) levels (androgenic effect), reduce serum estradiol values to early follicular phase levels (antiestrogenic), reduce mean luteinizing hormone (LH) levels, and obliterate the LH and follicle-stimulating hormone (FSH) surge (antigonadotropic). *Gestrinone* causes cellular inactivation and degeneration of endometriotic implants but not their disappearance (175). Amenorrhea occurs in 50–100% of women and is dose-dependent.

Resumption of menses generally occurs 33 days after discontinuing the medication (176, 177). An advantage of *gestrinone* is its long half-life (28 hours) when given orally. The standard dose has been 2.5 mg twice a week, but a recent study has shown that 1.25 mg twice weekly is equally effective (178). The clinical side effects are dose-dependent and similar but less intense than those caused by *danazol* (176). They include nausea, muscle cramps, and androgenic effects such as weight gain, acne, seborrhea, and oily hair/skin. *Gestrinone* appears to be as effective as *danazol* for treatment of pain, but it has fewer side effects and has the added advantage of twice weekly administration. Pregnancy is contraindicated while taking *gestrinone* because of the risk of masculinization of the fetus.

Danazol

Danazol is no more effective than other available medications to treat endometriosis. Recognized pharmacologic properties of *danazol* include suppression of GnRH or gonadotropin secretion, direct inhibition of steroidogenesis, increased metabolic clearance of estradiol and progesterone, direct antagonistic and agonistic interaction with endometrial androgen and progesterone receptors, and immunologic attenuation of potentially adverse reproductive effects (179, 180). The multiple effects of *danazol* produce a high-androgen, low-estrogen environment (estrogen levels in the early follicular to postmenopausal range) that does not support the growth of endometriosis, and the amenorrhea that is produced prevents new seeding of implants from the uterus into the peritoneal cavity.

The immunologic effects of *danazol* have been studied in women with endometriosis and adenomyosis and include a decrease in serum immunoglobulins (181, 182), a decrease in serum C3, a rise in serum C4 levels (182), decreased serum levels of autoantibodies against various phospholipid antigens (181, 182), and decreased serum levels of CA125 during treatment (101, 102, 112–115). *Danazol* inhibits peripheral blood lymphocyte proliferation in cultures activated by T-cell mitogens but does not affect macrophage-dependent T-lymphocyte activation of B lymphocytes (180). *Danazol* inhibits interleukin- 1 (IL1) and TNF production by monocytes in a dose-dependent manner (183) and suppresses macrophage/monocyte-mediated cytotoxicity of susceptible target cells in women with mild endometriosis (184). These immunological findings may be important in the remission of endometriosis with *danazol* treatment and may offer an explanation of the effect of *danazol* in the treatment of a number of autoimmune diseases, including hereditary angioedema (185), autoimmune hemolytic anemia (186), systemic lupus erythematosus (187), and idiopathic thrombocytopenic purpura (188, 189).

Doses of 800 mg/day are frequently used in North America, whereas ≤600 mg/day is commonly prescribed in Europe and Australia. It appears that the absence of menstruation is a better indicator of response than drug dose. A practical strategy for the use of *danazol* is to start treatment with 400 mg daily (200 mg twice a day) and increase the dose, if necessary, to achieve amenorrhea and relieve symptoms (177).

The significant adverse side effects of *danazol* are related to its androgenic and hypoestrogenic properties. The most common side effects include weight gain, fluid retention, acne, oily skin, hirsutism, hot flashes, atrophic vaginitis, reduced breast size, reduced libido, fatigue, nausea, muscle cramps, and emotional instability. Deepening of the voice is another potential side effect that is nonreversible. Although *danazol* can cause increased cholesterol and low-density lipoprotein levels and decreased high-density lipoproteins levels, it is unlikely that these short-term effects are clinically important. *Danazol* is contraindicated in patients with liver disease because it is largely metabolized in the liver and may cause hepatocellular damage. *Danazol* is also contraindicated in patients with hypertension, congestive heart failure, or impaired renal function because it can cause fluid retention. The use of *danazol* is contraindicated in pregnancy because of its androgenic effects on the fetus.

Gonadotropin-Releasing Hormone Agonists

GnRH agonists bind to pituitary GnRH receptors and stimulate LH and FSH synthesis and release. However, the agonists have a much longer biological half-life (3 to 8 hours) than endogenous GnRH (3.5 minutes), resulting in the continuous exposure of GnRH receptors to GnRH agonist activity. This causes a loss of pituitary receptors and downregulation of GnRH activity, resulting in low FSH and LH levels. Consequently, ovarian steroid production is suppressed, providing a medically induced and reversible state of pseudomenopause. Various GnRH agonists have been developed and used in treating endometriosis. These include *leuprolide, buserelin, nafarelin, histrelin, goserelin, deslorelin,* and *tryptorelin.* These drugs are inactive orally and must be administered intramuscularly, subcutaneously, or by intranasal absorption. The best therapeutic effect is often associated with an estradiol dose of 20–40 pg/ml (75–150 pmol/l). These so-called "depo" formulations are attractive because of the reduced frequency of administration and because nasal administration can be complicated by variations in absorption rates and problems with patient compliance (177). The results with GnRH agonists are similar to those with *danazol* or progestin therapy. While GnRH agonists do not have an adverse effect on serum lipids and lipoproteins, their side effects are caused by hypoestrogenism and include hot flashes, vaginal dryness, reduced libido, and osteoporosis (6–8% loss in trabecular bone density after 6 months of therapy). Reversibility of bone loss is equivocal and therefore of concern (190, 191), especially because treatment periods of longer than 6 months may be required. The goal is to suppress endometriosis and maintain serum estrogen levels of 30–45 pg/ml. More extreme estradiol suppression will induce bone loss (190). The dose of daily GnRH agonist can be regulated by monitoring estradiol levels or by the addition of low-dose progestin or estrogen/progestin "*add-back regimen.*" The addition of 1.2 mg of *norethisterone* daily during therapy with *nafarelin* (400 mg daily) for an additional 6 months, followed by daily administration of *norethisterone* 1.2 mg for 6 months, will produce similar subjective and objective improvements in endometriosis compared with those achieved with *nafarelin* alone. A combined add-back regimen with conjugated estrogens 0.625 mg administered daily concomitantly with 2.5 mg of *medroxyprogesterone acetate* is effective for treating most cases of endometriosis without concomitant bone loss (191, 192).

Efficacy of Medical Therapy

Pain   Medical treatment with *progestins, danazol, gestrinone,* or *GnRH agonists* is effective in treating pain associated with endometriosis as shown in several prospective, randomized, placebo-controlled double-blind studies (136, 150, 193, 194). Based on published studies, *medroxyprogesterone acetate, danazol, gestrinone,* and *GnRH agonists* have similar efficacy in resolution of the laparoscopically documented disease and in pain alleviation (176). Postoperative medical therapy may be required in patients with incomplete surgical resection and persistent pain. Treatment should last at least 3 to 6 months and pain relief may be of short duration, presumably because endometriosis recurs. Disadvantages of medical therapy over surgical therapy include the high cost of hormone preparations, the high prevalence of side effects, and the higher recurrence rate of endometriosis.

Subfertility   Conception is either impossible or contraindicated during medical treatment of endometriosis. **There is no evidence that medical treatment of minimal to mild endometriosis leads to better chances of pregnancy than expectant management** (136, 159, 193–199).

Recurrence

Endometriosis tends to recur unless definitive surgery is performed. The recurrence rate is approximately 5–20% per year, reaching a cumulative rate of 40% after 5 years. The recurrence rates reported in women five years after therapy with various *GnRH agonists* were 37% for minimal disease and 74% for severe disease (200). In women treated with *GnRH agonists* or *danazol* for endometriosis associated with pelvic pain, the recurrence rates of endometriosis were similar, and associated pain symptoms usually return after cessation of therapy (201). Pain will recur within 5 years in about one in five patients with pelvic pain treated by complete laparoscopic excision of visible endometriotic lesions (202).

Assisted Reproductive Technology

Infertility in patients with minimal to mild endometriosis can be treated by nonspecific cycle fecundity enhancement (77), including controlled ovarian hyperstimulation with intrauterine insemination, gamete intrafallopian transfer (GIFT), and *in vitro* fertilization (IVF). *In vitro* fertilization is the method of choice when distortion of the tubo-ovarian anatomy contraindicates the use of superovulation with intrauterine insemination or GIFT. It is not certain that the pregnancy rate per cycle after *in vitro* fertilization is decreased in women with minimal to mild endometriosis when compared with those who do not have the disease. The pregnancy rate after IVF treatment has been reported to be decreased (203–207) or normal (203) in infertile women with endometriosis (not staged by the AFS classification system) when compared with infertile patients who do not have endometriosis. The reduced pregnancy rate has been explained by a reduced oocyte recovery rate (205), oocyte fertilization rate (203, 205), and embryo implantation rate (205) caused by abnormalities in either embryo quality or endometrial receptivity. When endometriosis was assigned a stage, the pregnancy rate after IVF was decreased in patients with stage IV endometriosis but normal in women with less advanced disease (208–214). However, some studies have been unable to demonstrate a significant negative correlation between either the presence or stage of endometriosis and the pregnancy rate per cycle (215, 216). The use of *danazol, gestrinone,* or *GnRH agonists* in women with endometriosis prior to IVF has been reported to improve the pregnancy rate by some (206, 214) but not all (216) investigators.

The use of GIFT in patients with endometriosis is reported to result in a higher monthly fecundity rate (25%) than IVF (14%), but this difference may be related to selection bias because less severe forms of endometriosis may have been more likely to be treated with GIFT, reserving IVF for more advanced stages of disease (167). In one study, the GIFT pregnancy rate in patients with a primary diagnosis of endometriosis (32.5%) was lower than in matched controls (217).

Prevention of Infertility

The incidental finding of minimal to mild endometriosis in a young woman without immediate interest in pregnancy is a common clinical problem. Mild disease can be treated by surgical removal of implants at the time of diagnosis, followed by administration of cyclic low-dose combination oral contraceptives to prevent recurrence. More advanced disease can be treated medically for 6 months, followed by cyclic or continuous oral contraceptives to prevent progression of disease.

References

1. **Sampson JA.** Peritoneal endometriosis due to menstrual dissemination of endometrial tissue into the pelvic cavity. *Am J Obstet Gynecol* 1927;14:422–69.

2. **Haney AF.** Endometriosis: pathogenesis and pathophysiology. In: **Wilson EA,** ed. *Endometriosis.* New York: AR Liss, 1987:23–51.

3. **Ramey JW, Archer DF.** Peritoneal fluid: its relevance to the development of endometriosis. *Fertil Steril* 1993;60:1–14.

4. **Halme J, Becker S, Hammond MG, Raj SG, Talbert LM.** Retrograde menstruation in healthy women and in patients with endometriosis. *Obstet Gynecol* 1984;64:151–4.

5. **Liu DTY, Hitchcock A.** Endometriosis: its association with retrograde menstruation, dysmenorrhoea and tubal pathology. *Br J Obstet Gynaecol* 1986;93:859–62.

6. **Koninckx PR, De Moor P, Brosens IA.** Diagnosis of the luteinized unruptured follicle syndrome by steroid hormone assays in peritoneal fluid. *Br J Obstet Gynaecol* 1980b;87:929–34.

7. **Kruitwagen RFPM, Poels LG, Willemsen WNP, de Ronde IJY, Jap PHK, Rolland R.** Endometrial epithelial cells in peritoneal fluid during the early follicular phase. *Fertil Steril* 1991b; 55:297–303.

8. **Blumenkrantz MJ, Gallagher N, Bashore RA, Tenckhoff H.** Retrograde menstruation in women undergoing chronic peritoneal dialysis. *Obstet Gynecol* 1981;57:667–70.

9. **Jenkins S, Olive DL, Haney AG.** Endometriosis: pathogenetic implications of the anatomic distribution. *Obstet Gynecol* 1986;67:355–8.

10. **Scott RB, TeLinde RW, Wharton LR Jr.** Further studies on experimental endometriosis. *Am J Obstet Gynecol* 1953;66:1082–99.

11. **D'Hooghe TM, Bambra CS, Isahakia M, Koninckx PR.** Intrapelvic injection of menstrual endometrium causes endometriosis in baboons (Papio cynocephalus, Papio anubis). *Am J Obstet Gynecol* 1995;173:125–34.

12. **TeLinde RW, Scott RB.** Experimental endometriosis. *Am J Obstet Gynecol* 1950;60:1147–73.

13. **Olive DL, Henderson DY.** Endometriosis and müllerian anomalies. *Obstet Gynecol* 1987;69: 412–5.

14. **Pinsonneault O, Goldstein DP.** Obstructing malformations of the uterus and vagina. *Fertil Steril* 1985;44:241–7.

15. **D'Hooghe TM, Bambra CS, Suleman MA, Dunselman GA, Evers HL, Koninckx PR.** Development of a model of retrograde menstruation in baboons (Papio anubis). *Fertil Steril* 1994:62:635–8.

16. **Cramer DW, Wilson E, Stillman RJ, Berger MJ, Belisle S, Schiff I, et al.** The relation of endometriosis to menstrual characteristics, smoking and exercise. *JAMA* 1986;355:1904–8.

17. **Ueki M.** Histologic study of endometriosis and examination of lymphatic drainage in and from the uterus. *Am J Obstet Gynecol* 1991;165:201–9.

18. **Rock JA, Markham SM.** Extra pelvic endometriosis. In: **Wilson EA,** ed. *Endometriosis.* New York: AR Liss, 1987:185–206.

19. **Levander G, Normann P.** The pathogenesis of endometriosis: an experimental study. *Acta Obstet Gynecol Scand* 1955;34:366–98.

20. **Merrill JA.** Endometrial induction of endometriosis across millipore filters. *Am J Obstet Gynecol* 1966;94:780–9.

21. **Simpson JL, Elias S, Malinak LR, Buttram VC.** Heritable aspects of endometriosis. I. Genetics studies. *Am J Obstet Gynecol* 1980;137:327–31.

22. **Moen MH, Magnus P.** The familial risk of endometriosis. *Acta Obstet Gynecol Scand* 1993; 72:560–4.

23. **Grimes DA, LeBolt SA, Grimes KR, Wingo PA.** Systemic lupus erythematosis and reproductive function: a case-control study. *Am J Obstet Gynecol* 1985;153:179–86.

24. **Simpson JL, Malinak LR, Elias S, Carson S, Radvany RA.** HLA associations in endometriosis. *Am J Obstet Gynecol* 1984;148:395–7.

25. **Moen M, Bratlie A, Moen T.** Distribution of HLA-antigens among patients with endometriosis. *Acta Obstet Gynecol Scand* 1984;123(Suppl):25–7.

26. **Maxwell C, Kilpatrick DC, Haining R, Smith SK.** No HLA-DR specificity is associated with endometriosis. *Tissue Antigens* 1989;34:145–7.

27. **D'Hooghe TM, Hill JA.** Immunobiology of endometriosis. In: **Bronston R, Anderson DJ,** eds. *Immunology of Reproduction.* Cambridge, MA: Blackwell Scientific, 1996:322–56.

28. **Dmowski WP, Steele RN, Baker GF.** Deficient cellular immunity in endometriosis. *Am J Obstet Gynecol* 1981;141:377–83.

29. **Steele RW, Dmowski WP, Marmer DJ.** Immunologic aspects of endometriosis. *Am J Reprod Immunol* 1984;6:33–6.

30. **Oosterlynck D, Cornillie FJ, Waer M, Vandeputte M, Koninckx PR.** Women with endometriosis show a defect in natural killer cell activity resulting in a decreased cytotoxicity to autologous endometrium. *Fertil Steril* 1991;56:45–51.

31. **Vigano P, Vercillini P, Di Blasio AM, Colombo A, Candiani GB, Vignali M.** Deficient antiendometrium lymphocyte-mediated cytotoxicity in patients with endometriosis. *Fertil Steril* 1991; 56:894–9.

32. **Melioli G, Semino C, Semino A, Venturini PL, Ragni N.** Recombinant interleukin-2 corrects in vitro the immunological defect of endometriosis. *Am J Reprod Immunol* 1993;30:218–77.

33. **D'Hooghe TM, Scheerlinck JP, Koninckx PR, Hill JA, Bambra CS.** Anti-endometrial lymphocytotoxicity and natural killer activity in baboons with endometriosis. *Hum Reprod* 1995; 10:558–62.

34. **Hill JA.** Immunology and endometriosis. *Fertil Steril* 1992;58:262–4.

35. **Hill JA.** "Killer cells" and endometriosis. *Fertil Steril* 1993;60:928–9.

36. **Oosterlynck DJ, Meuleman C, Waer M, Vandeputte M, Koninckx PR.** The natural killer activity of peritoneal fluid lymphocytes is decreased in women with endometriosis. *Fertil Steril* 1992;58:290–5.

37. **Iwasaki K, Makino T, Maruyama T, Matsubayashi H, Nozawa S, Yokokura T.** Leukocyte subpopulations and natural killer activity in endometriosis. *Int J Fertil Menopausal Stud* 1993; 38:229–34.

38. **Garzetti GG, Ciavattini A, Provinciali M, Fabris N, Cignitti M, Romanini C.** Natural killer activity in endometriosis: correlation between serum estradiol levels and cytotoxicity. *Obstet Gynecol* 1993;81:665–8.

39. **Tanaka E, Sendo F, Kawagoe S, Hiroi M.** Decreased natural killer activity in women with endometriosis. *Gynecol Obstet Invest* 1992;34:27–30.

40. **Hirata J, Kikuchi Y, Imaizumi E, Tode T, Nagata I.** Endometriotic tissues produce immunosuppressive factors. *Gynecol Obstet Invest* 1993;37:43–7.

41. **Zeller JM, Henig I, Radwanska E, Dmowski WP.** Enhancement of human monocyte and peritoneal macrophage chemiluminescence activities in women with endometriosis. *Am J Reprod Immunol Microbiol* 1987;13:78–82.

42. **Halme J, Becker S, Haskill S.** Altered maturation and function of peritoneal macrophages: possible role in pathogenesis of endometriosis. *Am J Obstet Gynecol* 1987;156:783–9.

43. **Hill JA, Haimovici F, Politch JA, Anderson DJ.** Effects of soluble products of activated macrophages (lymphokines and monokines) on human sperm motion parameters. *Fertil Steril* 1987;47:460–5.

44. **Halme J.** Release of tumor necrosis factor-α by human peritoneal macrophages in vivo and in vitro. *Am J Obstet Gynecol* 1989;161:1718–25.

45. **Hill JA, Cohen J, Anderson DJ.** The effects of lymphokines and monokines on human sperm fertilizing ability in the zona-free hamster egg penetration test. *Am J Obstet Gynecol* 1989;160: 1154–9.

46. **Zhang R, Wild RA, Ojago JM.** Effect of tumor necrosis factor-alpha on adhesion of human endometrial stromal cells to peritoneal mesothelial cells: an in vitro system. *Fertil Steril* 1993; 59:1196–201.

47. **Olive DL, Montoya I, Riehl RM, Schenken RS.** Macrophage-conditioned media enhance endometrial stromal cell proliferation in vitro. *Am J Obstet Gynecol* 1991;164:953–8.

48. **Sharpe KL, Zimmer RL, Khan RS, Penney LL.** Proliferative and morphogenic changes induced by the coculture of rat uterine and peritoneal cells: a cell culture model for endometriosis. *Fertil Steril* 1992;58:1220–9.

49. **Halme J, White C, Kauma S, Estes J, Haskill S.** Peritoneal macrophages from patients with endometriosis release growth factor activity in vitro. *J Clin Endocrinol Metab* 1988;66:1044–9.

50. **Kauma S, Clark MR, White C, Halme J.** Production of fibronectin by peritoneal macrophages and concentration of fibronectin in peritoneal fluid from patients with or without endometriosis. *Obstet Gynecol* 1988;72:13–8.

51. **van der Linden PJQ, de Goeij APFM, Dunselman GAJ, van der Linden EPM, Ramaekers FCS, Evers JHL.** Expression of integrins and E-cadherin in cells from menstrual effluent, endometrium, peritoneal fluid, peritoneum, and endometriosis. *Fertil Steril* 1994;61:85–90.

52. **Jansen RPS, Russell P.** Nonpigmented endometriosis: clinical, laparoscopic and pathologic definition. *Am J Obstet Gynecol* 1986;155:1160–3.

53. **Stripling MC, Martin DC, Chatman DL, Vander Zwaay R, Poston WM.** Subtle appearance of pelvic endometriosis. *Fertil Steril* 1988;49:427–31.

54. **Martin DC, Hubert GD, Vander Zwaag R, El-Zeky FA.** Laparoscopic appearances of peritoneal endometriosis. *Fertil Steril* 1989;51:63–7.

55. **D'Hooghe TM, Bambra CS, Cornillie FJ, Isahakia M, Koninckx PR.** Prevalence and laparoscopic appearances of endometriosis in the baboon (Papio Cynocephalyus, Papio anubis). *Biol Reprod* 1991;45:411–6.

56. **Schenken RS, Williams RF, Hodgen GD.** Experimental endometriosis in primates. *Ann NY Acad Sci* 1991;622:242–55.

57. **Dizerega GS, Barber DL, Hodgen GD.** Endometriosis: role of ovarian steroids in initiation, maintenance and suppression. *Fertil Steril* 1980;649–53.

58. **Schenken RS, Asch RH, Williams RF, Hodgen GD.** Etiology of infertility in monkeys with endometriosis: luteinized unruptured follicles, luteal phase defects, pelvic adhesions, and spontaneous abortions. *Fertil Steril* 1984;41:122–30.

59. **Mann DR, Collins DC, Smith MM, Kessler MJ, Gould KG.** Treatment of endometriosis in Rhesus monkeys: effectiveness of a gonadotropin-releasing hormone agonist compared to treatment with a progestational steroid. *J Clin Endocrinol Metab* 1986;63:1277–83.

60. **Da Rif CA, Parker RF, Schoeb TR.** Endometriosis with bacterial peritonitis in a baboon. *Lab Anim Sci* 1984;34:491–93.

61. **Cornillie FJ, D'Hooghe TM, Lauweryns JM, Bambra CS, Isahakia M, Koninckx PR.** Morphological characteristics of spontaneous pelvic endometriosis in the baboon (Papio anubis and Papio cynocephalus). *Gynecol Obstet Invest* 1992;34:225–8.

62. **Sanfilippo JS, Williams RS, Yussman MA, Cook CL, Bissonnette F.** Substance P in peritoneal fluid. *Am J Obstet Gynecol* 1992;166:155–9.

63. **Koninckx PR, Meuleman C, Demeyere S, Lesaffre E, Cornillie FJ.** Suggestive evidence that pelvic endometriosis is a progressive disease, whereas deeply infiltrating endometriosis is associated with pelvic pain. *Fertil Steril* 1991;55:759–65.

64. **Moen MH.** Endometriosis in women at interval sterilization. *Acta Obstet Gynecol Scand* 1987;66:451–4.

65. **Kirshon B, Poindexter AN, Fast J.** Endometriosis in multiparous women. *J Reprod Med* 1989;215–7.

66. **Mahmood TA, Templeton A.** Prevalence and genesis of endometriosis. *Hum Reprod* 1991;6:544–9.

67. **Moen MH, Muus KM.** Endometriosis in pregnant and non-pregnant women at tubal sterilization. *Hum Reprod* 1991;6:699–702.

68. **Waller KG, Lindsay P, Curtis P, Shaw RW.** The prevalence of endometriosis in women with infertile partners. *Eur J Obstet Gynecol Reprod Biol* 1993;48:135–9.

69. **Strathy JH, Molgaard CA, Coulam CB, Melton LJ III.** Endometriosis and infertility: a laparoscopic study of endometriosis among fertile and infertile women. *Fertil Steril* 1982;38:667–72.

70. **Fakih HN, Tamura R, Kesselman A, DeCherney AH.** Endometriosis after tubal ligation. *J Reprod Med* 1985;30:939–41.

71. **Dodge ST, Pumphrey RS, Miyizawa K.** Peritoneal endometriosis in women requesting reversal of sterilization. *Fertil Steril* 1986;45:774–7.

72. **Trimbos JB, Trimbos-Kemper GCM, Peters AAW, van der Does CD, van Hall EV.** Findings in 200 consecutive asymptomatic women having a laparoscopic sterilization. *Arch Gynecol Obstet* 1990;247:121–4.

73. **Cornillie FJ, Oosterlynck D, Lauweryns JM, Koninckx PR.** Deeply infiltrating pelvic endometriosis: histology and clinical significance. *Fertil Steril* 1990;53:978–83.

74. **Barlow DH, Glynn CJ.** Endometriosis and pelvic pain. *Baillieres Clin Obstet Gynaecol* 1993;7:775–90.

75. **American Fertility Society:** Revised American Fertility Society Classification of Endometriosis. *Fertil Steril* 1985;43:351–2.

76. **D'Hooghe TM, Bambra CS, Raeymaekers BM, Riday AM, Suleman MA, Koninckx PR.** A prospective controlled study over 2 years shows a normal monthly fertility rate (MFR) in baboons with stage I endometriosis and a decreased MFR in primates with stage II-IV disease. *Fertil Steril* 1994;5(Suppl):1–113.

77. **Haney AF.** Endometriosis-associated infertility. *Baillieres Clin Obstet Gynaecol* 1993;7: 791–812.

78. **Jansen RPS.** Minimal endometriosis and reduced fecundability: prospective evidence from an artificial insemination by donor program. *Fertil Steril* 1986;46:141–3.

79. **Hammond MG, Jordan S, Sloan CS.** Factors affecting pregnancy rates in a donor insemination program using frozen semen. *Am J Obstet Gynecol* 1986;155:480–5.

80. **Portuondo JA, Echanojauregui AD, Herran C, Alijarte I.** Early conception in patients with untreated mild endometriosis. *Fertil Steril* 1983;39:22–5.

81. **Rodriguez-Escudero FJ, Negro JL, Corcosstegui B, Benito JA.** Does minimal endometriosis reduce fecundity? *Fertil Steril* 1988;50:522–4.

82. **D'Hooghe TM, Bambra CS, Koninckx PR.** Cycle fecundity in baboons of proven fertility with minimal endometriosis. *Gynecol Obstet Invest* 1994;37;63–5.

83. **Naples JD, Batt RE, Sadigh H.** Spontaneous abortion rate in patients with endometriosis. *Obstet Gynecol* 1981;57:509–12.

84. **Olive DL, Franklin RR, Gratkins LV.** The association between endometriosis and spontaneous abortion. A retrospective clinical study. *J Reprod Med* 1982;27:333–6.

85. **Wheeler JM, Johnston BM, Malinak LR.** The relationship of endometriosis to spontaneous abortion. *Fertil Steril* 1983;39:656–60.

86. **Groll M.** Endometriosis and spontaneous abortion. *Fertil Steril* 1984;44:933–5.

87. **Damewood MD.** The association of endometriosis and repetitive early spontaneous abortions. *Semin Reprod Endocrinol* 1989;7:155–60.

88. **Malinak LR, Wheeler JM.** Association of endometriosis with spontaneous abortion, prognosis for pregnancy and risk for recurrence. *Semin Reprod Endocrinol* 1986;3:361–6.

89. **Metzger DA, Olive DL, Stohs GF, Franklin RR.** Association of endometriosis and spontaneous abortion: effect of control group selection. *Fertil Steril* 1986;45:18–22.

90. **Pittaway DE, Ellington CP, Klimek M.** Preclinical abortions and endometriosis. *Fertil Steril* 1988;49:221–3.

91. **FitzSimmons J, Stahl R, Gocial B, Shapiro SS.** Spontaneous abortion and endometriosis. *Fertil Steril* 1987;47:696–8.

92. **Ando K, Koike K, Hirata O.** Clinical observations on endometriosis as related to sterility and habitual abortions. *Jpn J Fertil Steril* 1975;20:34–9.

93. **Pittaway DE, Vernon C, Fayez JA.** Spontaneous abortions in women with endometriosis. *Fertil Steril* 1988;50:711–5.

94. **Koninckx PR, Martin DC.** Deep endometriosis: a consequence of infiltration or retraction or possibly adenomyosis externa? *Fertil Steril* 1992;58:924–8.

95. **Koninckx PR, Oosterlynck D, D'Hooghe TM, Meuleman C.** Deeply infiltrating endometriosis is a disease whereas mild endometriosis could be considered a non-disease. *Ann NY Acad Sci* 1994;734:333–41.

96. **Bast RC, Klug TL, St. John E, Jenison E, Niloff JM, Lazarus H, et al.** A radio-immunoassay using a monoclonal antibody to monitor the course of epithelial ovarian cancer. *N Engl J Med* 1983;309:883–7.

97. **Barbieri RL, Niloff JM, Bast RC Jr, Schaetzl E, Kistner RW, Knapp RC.** Elevated serum concentrations of CA125 in patients with advanced endometriosis. *Fertil Steril* 1986;45:630–4.

98. **Pittaway DE, Fayez JA.** The use of CA125 in the diagnosis and management of endometriosis. *Fertil Steril* 1986;46:790–5.

99. **Pittaway DE, Fayez JA.** Serum CA125 levels increase during menses. *Am J Obstet Gynecol* 1987;156:75–6.

100. **Masahashi T, Matsuzawa K, Ohsawa M, Narita O, Asai T, Ishihara M.** Serum CA125 levels in patients with endometriosis: changes in CA125 levels during menstruation. *Obstet Gynecol* 1988;72:328–31.

101. **Takahashi K, Yoshino K, Kusakari M, Katoh S, Shibukawa T, Kitao M.** Prognostic potential of serum CA125 levels in danazol-treated patients with external endometriosis: a preliminary study. *Int J Fertil* 1990;35:226–9.

102. **Franssen AMHW, van der Heijden PFM, Thomas CMG, Doesburg WH, Willemsen WNP, Rolland R.** On the origin and significance of serum CA125 concentrations in 97 patients with endometriosis before, during, and after buserelin acetate, nafarelin, or danazol. *Fertil Steril* 1992;57:974–9.

103. **Moloney MD, Thornton JG, Cooper EH.** Serum CA125 antigen levels and disease severity in patients with endometriosis. *Obstet Gynecol* 1989;73:767–9.

104. **Nagamani M, Kelver ME, Smith ER.** CA125 levels in monitoring therapy for endometriosis and in prediction of recurrence. *Int J Fertil* 1992;37:227–31.

105. **Hornstein M, Thomas PP, Gleason RE, Barbieri RL.** Menstrual cyclicity of CA125 in patients with endometriosis. *Fertil Steril* 1992;58:279–83.

106. **O'Shaughnessy A, Check JH, Nowroozi K, Lurie D.** CA125 levels measured in different phases of the menstrual cycle in screening for endometriosis. *Obstet Gynecol* 1993;81:99–103.

107. **Pittaway DE, Douglas JW.** Serum CA125 in women with endometriosis and chronic pain. *Fertil Steril* 1989;51:68–70.

108. **Pittaway DE.** CA125 in women with endometriosis. *Obstet Gynecol Clin North Am* 1989;16:237–52.

109. **Pittaway DE.** The use of serial CA125 concentrations to monitor endometriosis in infertile women. *Am J Obstet Gynecol* 1990;163:1032–7.

110. **Kauppila A, Telimaa S, Ronnberg L, Vuori J.** Placebo-controlled study on serum concentrations of CA125 before and after treatment with danazol or high-dose medroxyprogesterone acetate alone or after surgery. *Fertil Steril* 1988;49:37–41.

111. **Dawood MY, Khan-Dawood FS, Wilson L Jr.** Peritoneal fluid prostaglandins and prostanoids in women with endometriosis, chronic pelvic inflammatory disease, and pelvic pain. *Am J Obstet Gynecol* 1984;148:391–5.

112. **Bischof P, Galfetti MA, Seydoux J, von Hospenthal JU, Campana A.** Peripheral CA125 levels in patients with uterine fibroids. *Hum Reprod* 1992;7:35–8.

113. **Ward BG, McGuckin MA, Ramm L, Forbes KL.** Expression of tumour markers CA125, CASA and OSA in minimal/mild endometriosis. *Aust N Z J Obstet Gynaecol* 1991;31:273–5.

114. **Fraser IS, McCarron G, Markham R.** Serum CA125 levels in women with endometriosis. *Aust N Z J Obstet Gynecol* 1989;29:416–20.

115. **Acien P, Shaw RW, Irvine L, Burford G, Gardner R.** CA125 levels in endometriosis patients before, during and after treatment with danazol or LHRH agonists. *Eur J Obstet Gynecol* 1989;32:241–6.

116. **Takahashi K, Abu Musa A, Nagata H, Kitao M.** Serum CA125 and 17-β-estradiol in patients with external endometttriosis on danazol. *Gynecol Obstet Invest* 1990;29:301–4.

117. **Fedele L, Arcaini L, Vercellini P, Bianchi S, Candiani GB.** Serum CA125 measurements in the diagnosis of endometriosis recurrence. *Obstet Gynecol* 1988;72:19–22.

118. **Vasquez G, Cornillie F, Brosens IA.** Peritoneal endometriosis: scanning electron microscopy and histology of minimal pelvic endometriotic lesions. *Fertil Steril* 1984;42:696–703.

119. **Nisolle M, Paindaveine B, Bourdin A, Berliere M, Casanas-Roux F, Donnez J.** Histological study of peritoneal endometriosis in infertile women. *Fertil Steril* 1990;53:984–8.

120. **Clement PB.** Pathology of endometriosis. *Pathol Annu* 1990;245–95.

121. **Moen MH, Halvorsen TB.** Histologic confirmation of endometriosis in different peritoneal lesions. *Acta Obstet Gynecol Scand* 1992;71:337–42.

122. **Czernobilsky B.** Endometriosis. In: **Fox H,** ed. *Obstetrical and Gynecological Pathology*. New York: Churchill Livingstone, 1987:763–77.

123. **Cornillie FJ, Vasquez G, Brosens IA.** The response of human endometriotic implants to the anti-progesterone steroid R2323: a histologic and ultrastructural study. *Pathol Res Pract* 1990;180:647–55.

124. **Donnez J, Nisolle M, Casanas-Roux F.** Three-dimensional architectures of peritoneal endometriosis. *Fertil Steril* 1992;57:980–3.

125. **Nisolle M, Casanas-Roux F, Anaf V, Mine J, Donnez J.** Morphometric study of the stromal vascularization in peritoneal endometriosis. *Fertil Steril* 1993;59:681–4.

126. **Wardle PG, Hull MGR.** Is endometriosis a disease? *Baill Clin Obstet Gynecol* 1993;7: 673–85.

127. **Murphy AA, Green WR, Bobbie D, de la Cruz ZC, Rock JA.** Unsuspected endometriosis documented by scanning electron microscopy in visually normal peritoneum. *Fertil Steril* 1986;46:522–4.

128. **Steingold KA, Cedars M, Lu JKH, Randle D, Hudd GL, Meldrum DR.** Treatment of endometriosis with a long-acting gonadotropin-releasing hormone agonist. *Obstet Gynecol* 1987;69:403–11.

129. **Nezhat F, Allan CJ, Nezhat F, Martin DC.** Nonvisualized endometriosis at laparoscopy. *Int J Fertil* 1991;36:340–3.

130. **Hayata T, Matsu T, Kawano Y, Matsui N, Miyikawa I.** Scanning electron microscopy of endometriotic lesions in the pelvic peritoneum and the histogenesis of endometriosis. *Int J Gynecol Obstet* 1992;39:311–9.

131. **Murphy AA, Guzick DS, Rock JA.** Microscopic peritoneal endometriosis. *Fertil Steril* 1989;51:1072–4.

132. **Redwine DB.** Is "microscopic" peritoneal endometriosis invisible? *Fertil Steril* 1988;50: 665–6.

133. **Redwine DB, Yocom LB.** A serial section study of visually normal pelvic peritoneum in patients with endometriosis. *Fertil Steril* 1990;54:648–51.

134. **D'Hooghe TM, Bambra CS, De Jonge I, Machai PN, Korir R, Koninckx PR.** A serial section study of visually normal posterior pelvic peritoneum from baboons with and without spontaneous endometriosis. *Fertil Steril* 1995;63:1322–5.

135. **Hornstein MD, Gleason RE, Orav J, Haas ST, Friedman AJ, Rein MS, et al.** The reproducibility of the revised American Fertility Society classification of endometriosis. *Fertil Steril* 1993;59:1015–21.

136. **Thomas EJ, Cooke ID.** Impact of gestrinone on the course of asymptomatic endometriosis. *BMJ* 1987;294:272–4.

137. **Mahmood TA, Templeton A.** The impact of treatment on the natural history of endometriosis. *Hum Reprod* 1990;5:965–70.

138. **Sutton CJG, Ewen SP, Whitelaw N, Haines P.** Prospective, randomized, double-blind, controlled trial of laser laparoscopy in the treatment of pelvic pain associated with minimal, mild, and moderate endometriosis. *Fertil Steril* 1994;62:696–700.

139. **D'Hooghe TM, Bambra CS, Isahakia M, Koninckx PR.** Evolution of spontaneous endometriosis in the baboon (Papio anubis, Papio Cynocephalus) over a 12-month period. *Fertil Steril* 1992;58:409–12.

140. **Redwine DB.** Age-related evolution in color appearance of endometriosis. *Fertil Steril* 1987;48:1062–3.

141. **Wiegerinck MAHM, Van Dop PA, Brosens IA.** The staging of peritoneal endometriosis by the type of active lesion in addition to the revised American Fertility Society classification. *Fertil Steril* 1993;60:461–4.

142. **Hanton EM, Malkasian GD Jr, Dockerty MB, Pratt JH.** Endometriosis associated with complete or partial obstruction of menstrual egress. *Obstet Gynecol* 1966;28:626–9.

143. **Schenken RS, Williams RF, Hodgen G.** Effect of pregnancy on surgically induced endometriosis in cynomolgus monkeys. *Am J Obstet Gynecol* 1987;157:1392–6.

144. **Vernon MW, Wilson EA.** Studies on the surgical induction of endometriosis in the rat. *Fertil Steril* 1985;44:684–94.

145. **McArthur JW, Ulfelder H.** The effect of pregnancy upon endometriosis. *Obstet Gynecol Surv* 1965;20:709–33.

146. **Kistner RW.** The treatment of endometriosis by inducing pseudopregnancy with ovarian hormones: a report of fifty-eight cases. *Fertil Steril* 1959;10:539–56.

147. **Brosens IA, Puttemans PJ.** Double-optic laparoscopy. Salpingoscopy, ovarian cystoscopy, and endoovarian surgery with the argon laser. *Baillieres Clin Obstet Gynaecol* 1989;3:595–608.

148. **Heaps JM, Berek JS, Nieberg RK.** Malignant neoplasms arising in endometriosis. *Obstet Gynecol* 1990;75:1023–8.

149. **Candiani GB, Fedele L, Vercellini P, Bianchi S, Di Nola G.** Presacral neurectomy for the treatment of pelvic pain associated with endometriosis: a controlled study. *Am J Obstet Gynecol* 1992;167:100–3.

150. **Fedele L, Bianchi S, Bocciolone L, Nola GD, Franchi D.** Buserelin acetate in the treatment of pelvic pain associated with minimal and mild endometriosis: a controlled study. *Fertil Steril* 1993;59:516–21.

151. **Overton CE, Lindsay PC, Johal B, Collins SA, Siddle NC, Shaw RW, Barlow DH.** A randomized, double-blind, placebo-controlled study of luteal phase dydrogesterone (Duphaston) in women with minimal to mild endometriosis. *Fertil Steril* 1994;62:701–7.

152. **Feste JR.** Laser laparoscopy: a new modality. *J Reprod Med* 1985;30:413–7.

153. **Nezhat C, Winer W, Crowgey S, Nezhat F.** Videolaparoscopy for the treatment of endometriosis associated with infertility. *Fertil Steril* 1989;51:237–40.

154. **Sutton CJG, Hill D.** Laser laparoscopy in the treatment of endometriosis. A 5 year study. *Br J Obstet Gynaecol* 1990;97:181–5.

155. **Daniell JF.** Fiberoptic laser laparoscopy. *Baillieres Clin Obstet Gynaecol* 1989;3:545–62.

156. **Sutton CJG, Hill D.** Laser laparoscopy in the treatment of endometriosis. A 5 year study. *Br J Obstet Gynaecol* 1990;97:181–5.

157. **Sutton CJG, Nair S, Ewen SP, Haines P.** A comparison between the CO_2 and KTP lasers in the treatment of large ovarian endometriomas. *Gynaecol Endoscopy* 1993;2:113–8.

158. **Olive DL, Lee KL.** Analysis of sequential treatment protocols for endometriosis-associated infertility. *Am J Obstet Gynecol* 1986;154:613–9.

159. **Badawy SZA, El Bakry MM, Samuel D, Dizer M.** Cumulative pregnancy rates in infertile women with endometriosis. *J Reprod Med* 1988;33:757–60.

160. **Nowroozi K, Chase JS, Check JH, Wu CH.** The importance of laparoscopic coagulation of mild endometriosis in infertile women. *Int J Fertil* 1987;32:442–4.

161. **Paulson JD, Asmar P, Saffan DS.** Mild and moderate endometriosis. Comparison of treatment modalities for infertile couples. *J Reprod Med* 1991;36:151–5.

162. **Tulandi T, Mouchawar M.** Treatment-dependent and treatment-independent pregnancy in women with minimal and mild endometriosis. *Fertil Steril* 1991;56:790–1.

163. **Schenken RS, Malinak LR.** Conservative versus expectant management for the infertile patient with mild endometriosis. *Fertil Steril* 1982;37:183–6.

164. **Arumugam K, Urquhart R.** Efficacy of laparoscopic electrocoagulation in infertile patients with minimal or mild endometriosis. *Acta Obstet Gynecol Scand* 1991;70:125–7.

165. **Adamson S, Edwin SS, LaMarche S, Mitchell MD.** Actions of interleukin-4 on prostaglandin biosynthesis at the chorion-decidual interface. *Am J Obstet Gynecol* 1993;169:1442–7.

166. **Olive DL, Martin DC.** Treatment of endometriosis-associated infertility with CO_2 laser laparoscopy: the use of one- and two-parameter exponential models. *Fertil Steril* 1987;48:18–23.

167. **Rosen GF.** Treatment of endometriosis-associated infertility. *Infert Reprod Med Clin North Am* 1992;3:721–30.

168. **Kistner RW.** The use of progestins in the treatment of endometriosis. *Am J Obstet Gynecol* 1958;75:264–78.

169. **Moghissi KS.** Pseudopregnancy induced by estrogen-progestogen or progestogens alone in the treatment of endometriosis. *Prog Clin Biol Res* 1990;323:221–32.

170. **Dawood MY.** Endometriosis. In: **Gold JJ, Josimovich JB,** eds. *Gynecologic Endocrinology.* New York: Plenum, 1987:387–404.

171. **Dmowski WP.** Endometriosis. In: **Glass RH,** ed. *Office Gynecology.* Baltimore: Williams & Wilkins, 1987:317–36.

172. **Moghissi KS, Boyce CR.** Management of pelvic endometriosis with oral medroxyprogesterone-acetate. *Obstet Gynecol* 1976;47:265–7.

173. **Luciano AA, Turksoy RN, Carleo J.** Evaluation of oral medroxyprogesterone acetate in the treatment of endometriosis. *Obstet Gynecol* 1988;72:323–7.

174. **Schlaff WD, Dugoff L, Damewood MD, Rock JA.** Megestrol acetate for treatment of endometriosis. *Obstet Gynecol* 1990;75:646–8.

175. **Brosens IA, Verleyen A, Cornillie FJ.** The morphologic effect of short-term medical therapy of endometriosis. *Am J Obstet Gynecol* 1987;157:1215–21.

176. **Fedele L, Bianchi S, Viezzoli T, Arcaini L, Candiani GB.** Gestrinone versus danazol in the treatment of endometriosis. *Fertil Steril* 1989;51:781–5.

177. **Wingfield M, Healy DL.** Endometriosis: medical therapy. *Baillieres Clin Obstet Gynecol* 1993;7:813–38.

178. **Hornstein MD, Gleason RE, Barbieri RL.** A randomized double-blind prospective trial of two doses of gestrinone in the treatment of endometriosis. *Fertil Steril* 1990;53:237–41.

179. **Barbieri RL, Ryan KJ.** Danazol: endocrine pharmacology and therapeutic applications. *Am J Obstet Gynecol* 1981;141:453–63.

180. **Hill JA, Barbieri RL, Anderson DJ.** Immunosuppressive effects of danazol in vitro. *Fertil Steril* 1987;48:414–8.

181. **El-Roeiy A, Dmowski WP, Gleicher N, Radwanska E, Harlow L, Binor Z, et al.** Danazol but not gonadotropin-releasing hormone agonists suppresses autoantibodies in endometriosis. *Fertil Steril* 1988:50;864–71.

182. **Ota H, Maki M, Shidara Y, Kodama H, Takahashi H, Hayakawa M, et al.** Effects of danazol at the immunologic level in patients with adenomyosis, with special reference to autoantibodies: a multi-center cooperative study. *Am J Obstet Gynecol* 1992;167:481–6.

183. **Mori H, Nakagawa M, Itoh N, Wada K, Tamaya T.** Danazol suppresses the production of interleukin-1β and tumor necrosis factor by human monocytes. *Am J Reprod Immunol* 1990;24:45–50.

184. **Braun DP, Gebel H, Rotman C, Rana N, Dmowski WP.** The development of cytotoxicity in peritoneal macrophages from women with endometriosis. *Fertil Steril* 1992;1203:1203–10.

185. **Gelfand JA, Sherins RJ, Alling DW, Frank MM.** Treatment of hereditary angioedema with danazol. *N Engl J Med* 1976;295:1444–8.

186. **Ahn YS, Harrington WJ, Mylvaganam R, Ayub J, Pall LM.** Danazol therapy for autoimmune hemolytic anemia. *Ann Intern Med* 1985;102:298–301.

187. **Agnello V, Pariser K, Gell J, Gelfand J, Turksoy RN.** Preliminary observations on danazol therapy of systemic lupus erythematosus: effect on DNA antibodies, thrombocytopenia and complement. *J Rheumatol* 1983;10:682–7.

188. **Schreiber AD, Chien P, Tomaski A, Cines DB.** Effect of danazol in immune thrombocytopenic purpura. *N Engl J Med* 1987;316:503–8.

189. **Mylvaganam R, Ahn YS, Harrington WJ, Kim CI.** Immune modulation by danazol in autoimmune thrombocytopenia. *Clin Immunol Immunopathol* 1987;42:281–7.

190. **Barbieri RL.** Hormone treatment of endometriosis: the estrogen threshold hypothesis. *Am J Obstet Gynecol* 1992;166:740–5.

191. **Riis BJ, Christiansen C, Johansen JS, Jacobson J.** Is it possible to prevent bone loss in young women treated with luteinizing hormone-releasing agonists? *J Clin Endocrinol Metab* 1990;70:920–4.

192. **Friedman AJ, Hornstein MD.** Gonadotropin-releasing hormone agonist plus estrogen-progestin "add-back" therapy for endometriosis-related pelvic pain. *Fertil Steril* 1993;60:236–41.

193. **Telimaa S, Puolakka J, Ronnberg L, Kaupilla A.** Placebo-controlled comparison of danazol and high-dose medroxyprogesterone acetate in the treatment of endometriosis. *Gynecol Endocrinol* 1987;1:13–23.

194. **Dlugi AM, Miller JD, Knittle J, Lupron Study Group.** Lupron depot (leuprolide acetate for depot suspension) in the treatment of endometriosis: a randomized, placebo-controlled, double-blind study. *Fertil Steril* 1990;54:419–27.

195. **Evers JLH.** The pregnancy rate of the no-treatment group in randomized clinical trials of endometriosis therapy. *Fertil Steril* 1989;52:906–9.

196. **Bayer SR, Seibel MM, Saffan DS, Berger MJ, Taymor ML.** Efficacy of danazol treatment for minimal endometriosis in infertile women: a prospective randomized study. *J Reprod Med* 1988;33:179–83.

913

197. **Fedele L, Bianchi S, Marchini M, Villa L, Brioschi D, Parazzini F.** Superovulation with human menopausal gonadotrophins in the treatment of infertility associated with minimal or mild endometriosis: a controlled randomized study. *Fertil Steril* 1992;58:28–31.

198. **Thomas EJ, Cooke ID.** Successful treatment of asymptomatic endometriosis: does it benefit infertile women? *BMJ* 1987;294:1117–9.

199. **Fedele L, Parazzini F, Radici E, Bocciolone L, Bianchi S, et al.** Buserelin acetate versus expectant management in the treatment of infertility associated with endometriosis: a randomized clinical trial. *Am J Obstet Gynecol* 1992;166:1345–50.

200. **Fedele L, Bianchi S, DiNola G, Landiani M, Busacca M, Vignali M.** The recurrence of endometriosis. *Am NY Acad Sci* 1994;734:358–64.

201. **Vercellini P, Trespidi L, Colombo A, Vendola N, Marchini M, Crosignani PG.** A gonadotropin-releasing hormone agonist versus a low-dose oral contraceptive for pelvic pain associated with endometriosis. *Fertil Steril* 1993;60:75–9.

202. **Redwine DB.** Conservative laparoscopic excision of endometriosis by sharp dissection: life table analysis of reoperation and persistent of recurrent disease. *Fertil Steril* 1991;56:628–34.

203. **Wardle PG, McLaughlin EA, McDermott A, Mitchell JD, Ray BD, Hull MGR.** Endometriosis and ovulatory disorder: reduced fertilisation in vitro compared with tubal and unexplained infertility. *Lancet* 1985;236–9.

204. **O'Shea RT, Chen C, Weiss T, Jones WR.** Endometriosis and in vitro fertilization. *Lancet* 1985;2:723.

205. **Yovich JL, Yovich JM, Tuvik AI, Matson PL, Willcox DO.** In vitro fertilisation for endometriosis. *Lancet* 1985;2:552.

206. **Wardle PG, Foster PA, Mitchell JD, McLaughlin EA, Sykes JAC, et al.** Endometriosis and IVF: effect of prior therapy. *Lancet* 1986:276–7.

207. **Jones HW Jr, Acosta AA, Andrews MC, Garcia JE, Jones GS, Mayer J, et al.** Three years of in vitro fertilization at Norfolk. *Fertil Steril* 1984;42:826–34.

208. **Chillik CF, Acosta AA, Garcia JE, Perera S, Van Uem JFHM, et al.** The role of in vitro fertilization in infertile patients with endometriosis. *Fertil Steril* 1985;44:56–9.

209. **Matson PL, Yovich JL.** The treatment of infertility associated with endometriosis by in vitro fertilization. *Fertil Steril* 1986;46:432–434.

210. **Molloy D, Martin M, Speirs A, Lopata A, Clarke G, et al.** Performance of patients with a "frozen pelvis" in an in vitro fertilization program. *Fertil Steril* 1987;47:450–5.

211. **Yovich JL, Matson PL, Richardson PA, Hilliard C.** Hormone profiles and embryo quality in women with severe endometriosis treated by in vitro fertilization and embryo transfer. *Fertil Steril* 1988;50:249–56.

212. **Oehninger S, Acosta AA, Kreiner D, Muasher SJ, Jones HW Jr, Rosenwaks Z.** In vitro fertilization and embryo transfer (IVF/ET): an established and successful therapy for endometriosis. *J In Vitro Fertil Embryo Transf* 1988;5:248–56.

213. **Redwine DB.** Conservative laparoscopic excision of endometriosis by sharp dissection: life table analysis of reoperation and persistent of recurrent disease. *Fertil Steril* 1991;56:628–34.

214. **Dicker D, Goldman JA, Levy T, Feldberg D, Ashkenazi J.** The impact of long-term gonadotrophin-releasing hormone analogue treatment on preclinical abortions in patients with severe endometriosis undergoing in vitro fertilization-embryo transfer. *Fertil Steril* 1992;57:597–600.

215. **Inoue M, Kobayashi Y, Honda I, Awaji H, Fujii A.** The impact of endometriosis on the reproductive outcome of infertile patients. *Am J Obstet Gynecol* 1992;167:278–82.

216. **Tummon IS, Colwell KA, Mackinnon CJ, Nisker JA, Yuzpe AA.** Abbreviated endometriosis-associated infertility correlates with in vitro fertilization success. *J In Vitro Fertil Embryo Transf* 1991;8:149–53.

217. **Guzick DS, Yao YAS, Berga SL, Krasnow JS, Stovall DW, et al.** Endometriosis impairs the efficacy of gamete intrafallopian transfer: results of a case-control study. *Fertil Steril* 1994;62:1186–91.

27

Infertility

Mark D. Hornstein
Daniel Schust

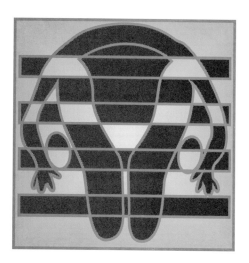

Infertility is defined as 1 year of unprotected intercourse without pregnancy. This condition may be further classified as *primary infertility,* in which no previous pregnancies have occurred, and *secondary infertility,* in which a prior pregnancy, although not necessarily a live birth, has occurred. *Fecundability* is the probability of achieving pregnancy within a single menstrual cycle, and *fecundity* is the probability of achieving a live birth within a single cycle. The fecundability of a normal couple has been estimated at 20–25% (1). **On the basis of this estimate, approximately 90% of couples should conceive after 12 months.**

Infertility affects approximately 10–15% of reproductive-age couples in the U.S. Despite the relatively stable prevalence of infertility in the U.S., the use of infertility services has increased significantly in recent years. Between 1968 and 1984, the number of office visits for infertility increased nearly threefold—to the current level of 1.6 million visits annually (2). There are several reasons for this increase: recent media coverage of assisted reproductive technologies (ARTs) and other fertility treatments has heightened awareness of the problem and its treatment; the aging of the post-World War II "baby boomers" has led to an increase in the number of reproductive-age women; and sociologic changes have led to delayed marriage with a consequent postponement of childbearing. Despite an increase in awareness of available therapies, only 43% of infertile couples seek treatment and only 24% seek specialized care. Fewer than 2% use *in vitro* fertilization (IVF) or other ARTs. The women most likely to have obtained specialized treatment are 30 years of age or older, white, married, and of relatively high socioeconomic status (3).

Epidemiology

Although the use of infertility services has increased over the past few decades, the prevalence of infertility has remained virtually the same. Data from the U.S. National Survey of Family Growth indicate that the prevalence of infertility among women who had not been surgically sterilized was 13.3% in 1965, 13.9% in 1982, and 13.7% in 1988 (4). In 1990, approximately one in three women in the U.S. reported 12 consecutive months of unprotected coitus without pregnancy at some time in her life (5).

A number of demographic variables, including age and socioeconomic status, have been associated with infertility. The delay in childbearing the U.S. population has led to attempts to conceive by a higher percentage of women in the older reproductive age groups. **Although the prevalence of infertility has not changed in the U.S. since 1965, the percentage of women with primary infertility has increased significantly.** In 1965, only one of six infertile females was nulliparous, whereas in 1988, more than one-half of infertile women had never been pregnant. This apparent decline in secondary infertility is probably the result of the increase in the number of surgical sterilizations performed (6).

The prevalence of infertility does not differ significantly among racial and ethnic groups. Although patients seeking treatment for infertility are predominantly of high socioeconomic status, infertility is more common among groups of relatively low socioeconomic status (6). Improved familiarity with and access to infertility services among the affluent and better educated patients probably accounts for their greater use of these medical resources.

Infertility and Age

An association between the age of the woman and reduced fecundability has been well documented. This decline in fecundability begins in the early thirties and accelerates in the late thirties and early forties. Approximately 30% of couples in which the female partner is aged 35–44 years are infertile (4). Data from rural Senegal, in which each female gives birth to an average of 7.9 children, show declining fertility rates with a peak of fertility at 25 years of age and a steep decline after 35 years of age (Fig. 27.1) (7). In a fe-

Figure 27.1   Age pattern of male and female fertility in a transitional society (Senagal).

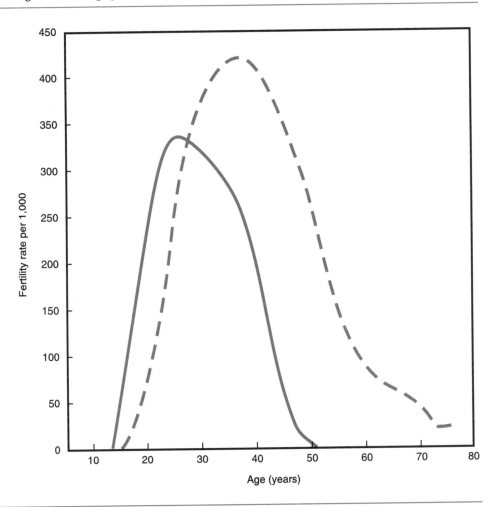

cundity study involving the Hutterites, a communal sect living in the Dakotas and Montana that practices no contraception and has large families, fertility peaks by 25 years of age, and one-third of women are no longer fertile by 40 years of age (8). The fecundability of women undergoing donor insemination whose husbands are azoospermic provides insight into the effects of age on the fertility of the female alone. A French group that studied women enrolled in artificial insemination programs found that fertility rates begin to drop after 30 years of age. The pregnancy rate after 1 year of inseminations was 74% in women aged 30 years and younger, 62% in women aged 30–35 years, and 54% in women older than 35 years of age (9). Data from the U.S. National Survey of Family Growth verify the age-related loss of female fecundity; however, the age-specific rate of impaired fecundity does not appear to be changing (6).

Oocyte Depletion

The age-related decline in fertility appears to be attributable to oocyte depletion. For women in their late thirties, a small increase in follicle-stimulating hormone (FSH) correlates with subtle changes in oocyte number and perhaps oocyte competence, translating into reduced fertility. As FSH levels rise and a woman approaches menopause, the chances of successful pregnancy decline further. The data that correlate FSH levels with poor reproductive outcome show that women with FSH levels of >15 mIU/ml on cycle day 3 have reduced pregnancy rates in IVF, and women with higher FSH levels have even lower pregnancy rates (10). There is, however, a considerable variation in FSH assays, so the results depend on the method used.

The physiology of declining fertility in older women is better understood in light of data from oocyte donation programs. When embryos produced from oocytes retrieved from younger women are transferred into older women, the pregnancy rates among the older women approximate those of the younger women (11). In addition, pregnancy rates remain relatively constant among recipients of donor oocytes up to 50 years of age (12). These observations strongly suggest that **it is the age of the oocyte, rather than the age of the endometrium, that accounts for the age-related decline in female fertility.**

Spontaneous Abortion

Another factor contributing to decreased fecundity in older reproductive-age women is the increased risk of spontaneous abortion. The rate of clinically recognized spontaneous abortion more than doubles between 20 and 40 years of age (13). This increased loss rate, coupled with the reduced conception rate, significantly reduces the chance of a live birth for women older than 40 years of age.

Male Factor

There is little doubt that increasing age is accompanied by reduced female fecundity; however, the age-related decline for men is more controversial. Male fertility peaks at about 35 years of age and declines sharply after 45 years of age; however, men have reportedly fathered children into their eighties (6). Also, the risk of chromosomal trisomies appears to be related in part to increased paternal age. Recent observations have shown an increase in rates of autosomal recessive disorders among the progeny of men over 35 years of age (14, 15). These findings suggest an age-related decline in gamete quality in men, albeit a more subtle decline than that experienced by women.

The Infertile Couple

Initial Visit

The physician's initial encounter with the infertile couple is the most important one because it sets the tone for subsequent evaluation and treatment. The male partner should be present at this first visit because his history is a key component in the selection of a diagnostic and therapeutic plan. **It cannot be overemphasized that infertility is a problem of the couple. The presence of the male partner beginning with the initial evaluation involves him in the therapeutic process;** this demonstrates that the physician is receptive to the male partner's needs as well as to those of the female partner and gives the male partner an opportunity to ask questions and to verbalize his concerns.

The physician should obtain a complete medical, surgical, and gynecologic history from the woman. Specifically, information regarding menstrual cyclicity, pelvic pain, and obstetric history are important. Risk factors for infertility, such as a history of pelvic inflammatory disease, intrauterine device use, or pelvic surgery, should be reviewed. A history of intrauterine exposure to diethylstilbestrol (DES) is significant. In addition, questions should be asked about pituitary, adrenal, and thyroid function. Information regarding genital surgery, infections, trauma, and history of mumps should be obtained from the male partner. A history of occupational exposures that might affect reproductive function is important. The interviewer should also obtain information about coital frequency, dyspareunia, and sexual dysfunction.

The initial interview provides the physician with the opportunity to assess the emotional impact of infertility on the couple. It gives the physician a chance to emphasize the emotional support available to the couple as they proceed with the diagnostic evaluation and suggested treatments. In some cases, referral to a trained social worker or psychologist may be beneficial.

The physical examination of the female should be thorough, with particular attention given to height, weight, body habitus, hair distribution, thyroid gland, status with regard to galactorrhea, and findings of the pelvic examination. Referral of the male to a urologist for examination is often beneficial if historic information or subsequent evaluation suggests an abnormality. The initial encounter also gives the doctor the opportunity to outline the general causes of infertility and to discuss subsequent diagnostic testing.

Causes of Infertility

The main causes of infertility include the following:

1. Abnormalities in the semen (male factor infertility)

2. Ovulatory disorders (ovulatory factor)

3. Tubal injury, blockage, paratubal adhesions, or endometriosis (tubal/peritoneal factor)

4. Abnormalities in cervical mucus-sperm interaction (cervical factor)

5. Rarer conditions, such as uterine abnormalities, immunologic aberrations, and infections

In some cases, no specific cause is detected despite an extensive and complete evaluation. The relative prevalence of the different causes of infertility varies widely among patient populations (Table 27.1).

Male Factor

Abnormalities of the semen, or male factor infertility, probably represent the most common cause of infertility. Semen analysis is the basic laboratory study assessing such abnormalities. Because this test is inexpensive and noninvasive, it should be a part of every infertility workup. Assessment of semen parameters, however, is confounded by controversies regarding the proper range of normal values. Semen parameters in normal fertile men vary considerably over time and may even drop below established norms; this situa-

Table 27.1   Causes of Infertility

The relative prevalence of the etiologies of infertility

	Prevalence
Male factor	25–40%
Both	10%
Female factor	40–55%
Unexplained infertility	10%

The approximate prevalence of the causes of infertility in the female

	Prevalence
Ovulatory dysfunction	30–40%
Tubal/periotoneal factor	30–40%
Unexplained infertility	10–15%
Miscellaneous causes	10–15%

tion makes evaluation of the male patient more difficult. Before the value and interpretation of the semen analysis and other tests for male infertility are considered, a brief review of male reproductive physiology is in order.

Physiology

The male reproductive tract consists of the testis, epididymis, vas deferens, prostate, seminal vesicles, ejaculatory duct, bulbourethral glands, and urethra. The testes contain two cell types: the Sertoli cells, which line the seminiferous tubules (the site of spermatogenesis), and the Leydig cells (the site of androgen synthesis). In the male, the pituitary gland secretes luteinizing hormone (LH) and FSH, which act on the testes. Luteinizing hormone stimulates the synthesis and secretion of testosterone by the Leydig cells, and FSH stimulates the Sertoli cells to secrete inhibin. FSH and testosterone act on the seminiferous tubules to stimulate spermatogenesis. In humans, the process of transforming spermatogonia into mature sperm cells lasts 74 days. The immature spermatogonia undergo mitotic division, giving rise to spermatocytes, which subsequently undergo meiosis, or reduction division, ultimately producing spermatozoa containing 23 (rather than 46) chromosomes. The spermatozoa then enter the epididymis, which they traverse in 12–21 days as they mature and become progressively more motile.

During ejaculation, the mature spermatozoa are released from the vas deferens along with fluid from the prostate, seminal vesicles, and bulbourethral glands. The semen released is a gelatinous mixture of spermatozoa and seminal plasma; however, liquefaction generally occurs in 20–30 minutes because of the presence of proteolytic enzymes within the prostatic fluid. The released spermatozoa are not usually capable of fertilization. Instead, a series of poorly understood biochemical and electrical events, termed capacitation, must take place within the sperm's outer surface membrane before fertilization can occur. Normally, capacitation occurs in the cervical mucus; however, it can occur in physiologic media *in vitro*. Lastly, as part of fertilization, the sperm must undergo the acrosome reaction, in which the release of enzymes of the inner acrosomal membrane results in the breakdown of the outer plasma membrane and its fusion with the outer acrosomal membrane (16). Several of the enzymes within the acrosome appear to be important to the sperm's penetration of the egg's zona pellucida. As the sperm penetrates the egg, it initiates a hardening of the zona pellucida (cortical reaction), which prevents penetration by additional sperm (17).

Semen Analysis

The basic semen analysis measures semen volume, sperm concentration, sperm motility, and sperm morphology. In addition, many laboratories measure pH, fructose, and white blood cells. Normal values suggested by the World Health Organization (WHO) are listed in Table 27.2 (18). It should be emphasized that these values represent only general guidelines and normal values should be established by individual andrology laboratories.

Specimen Collection   The method of semen specimen collection is important to achieving accurate results. The optimal period of abstinence prior to semen collection is unknown; however, because a decrease in sperm concentration is associated with frequent ejaculation, a period of 2–3 days is usually recommended. The specimens should be obtained by masturbation and collected in a clean container. Because of the presence of spermicidal agents, collection into condoms is generally unacceptable; however, special sheaths that do not contain spermicides are available for semen collection. The specimens should be taken to the laboratory within 1–2 hours of collection. Proper interpretation of the semen analysis is complicated by wide differences in normal semen parameters (19), seasonal variability (20), variations among laboratories or technicians (21), and inconsistent correlation with fertility outcome. Semen parameters may also vary widely from one man to another and between men with proven fertility. In many circumstances, several specimens are necessary to verify an abnormality.

Sperm Volume   The normal semen volume ejaculated is 2–6 ml. Volumes may be abnormally low in cases of retrograde ejaculation, and high volumes usually reflect relatively long periods of abstinence or inflammation of the accessory glands. Absence of fructose or high pH may be associated with ejaculatory tract obstruction or seminal vesicle dysfunction.

Sperm Concentration   **Sperm concentration or density is defined as the number of sperm per milliliter in the total ejaculate.** Establishing a lower limit of normal for sperm concentration is difficult. Historically, cutoffs of 60 million sperm per milliliter for normal fertility have been advocated, but most WHO laboratories recognize the value of 20 million sperm per milliliter as a lower limit of normal (22). Some have advocated concentrations of 5 million sperm per milliliter as a lower limit of normal (23, 24).

Sperm Motility   **An equally important parameter in the semen analysis is sperm motility, which is defined as the percentage of progressive motile sperm in the ejaculate.** Lower limits of normal vary considerably and depend on the local laboratory's experience. The WHO and many laboratories use a cutoff of 50% motility as the lower limit of normal; however, the Society for Assisted Reproductive Technology requires motilities of 40% as a criterion for defining male factor infertility (25). Using computer-assisted semen analysis, in which computer-generated images of sperm specimens quantitate both sperm counts and sperm motilities, may yield results very different from those of nonautomated semen analyses. As in the case of sperm concentration, interpretation of motility is hampered by significant variability in successive samples from one individual as well as by poor correlation of motility with fertility.

Assessment of sperm morphology has become more complicated in recent years with the introduction of "strict criteria" (26). Using these criteria, most sperm from normal men have minor abnormalities; **men with as few as 15% normal sperm have normal rates of fertilization in IVF programs. When a man has fewer than 4% normal sperm, rates**

Table 27.2   Normal Values for a Semen Analysis

Volume	<2.0 ml
Sperm concentration	<20 million/ml
Motility	<50%
Morphology	<30% normal forms

World Health Organization. *Laboratory Manual for the Examination of Human Semen and Sperm-Cervical Interaction.* Cambridge, England: Cambridge University Press, 1992.

of fertilization and pregnancy in IVF are greatly reduced; at 4–14% normal sperm, fertilization rates are intermediate (27). The clinician must understand the methodology used by the local andrology laboratory to properly interpret semen analysis results.

White Cells   Although measurements of semen volume, sperm concentration, sperm motility, and sperm morphology make up the standard semen analysis, some laboratories also report numbers of round cells. These cells, which may be lymphocytes, can signify the presence of prostatitis or, alternatively, they can be immature germ cells. The WHO views ejaculates with more than 5 million round cells per milliliter or more than 1 million leukocytes per milliliter as abnormal (18). These two cell types can be distinguished by an immunoperoxidase staining technique that identifies leukocytes (Endtz test) (28). The prognostic significance of leukocytes in the semen is controversial, however. The presence of immature sperm cells in the ejaculate suggests a defect in spermatogenesis and, therefore, may signify a relatively poor prognosis for fertilization (29). Although the standard semen analysis and associated tests provide a fairly good picture of semen quality, they yield little information about sperm function. Consequently, several tests of sperm function have been devised in an effort to assess the physiologic properties of sperm and thereby predict the likelihood of fertilization of normal oocytes.

Sperm Penetration Assay   The most commonly used test of sperm function is the *sperm penetration assay* (SPA), or hamster egg penetration test (30). This test attempts to measure the ability of an individual patient's sperm to undergo capacitation (i.e., the acrosome reaction), to fuse with and penetrate the oocyte membrane, and to undergo nuclear decondensation. In the SPA, golden hamsters are superovulated, and their eggs are collected and treated with enzymes to remove the cumulus and zona pellucida. The sperm are placed in a protein-rich environment, which promotes capacitation. Sperm from normal fertile men are used as positive controls. After incubation, the zona-free eggs are exposed to sperm. The presence of one or more swollen sperm heads within the oocyte demonstrates penetration. Most laboratories report the percentage of eggs successfully penetrated; however, some laboratories count the number of penetrations per egg (usually two or more is considered normal). Cutoff values for the lower limit of normal in the SPA differ remarkably among laboratories.

The prognostic value of the SPA has been controversial almost since its inception. On the basis of a meta-analysis of the SPA, the test does not discriminate between fertile and infertile men (31). The value of the test as a predictor of success in IVF has been no less controversial. In most evaluations of the male partner, the SPA offers little definitive information; however, it may uncover sperm abnormalities in couples with otherwise unexplained infertility.

Several other tests attempt to correlate sperm function with fertility prognosis. The *human zona-binding assay* (the *Hemizona test*) examines the ability of the sperm to bind to zona. In this assay, human zona are bisected; one-half of the zona is exposed to the patient's sperm and one-half is exposed to sperm from a known fertile donor control (32). The hypoosmotic swelling test examines the normality of the sperm tail. When placed in a hypo-osmotic solution of sodium citrate and fructose, the normal sperm tail swells and coils; when there is an abnormality in fluid transport across the tail membrane, the sperm tail fails to swell (33). To detect the acrosome reaction, some investigators have utilized monoclonal antibodies (34); others have measured adenosine triphosphate (ATP) content in the semen (35). These tests should be considered experimental until more definitive evidence demonstrates their utility in clinical settings.

Further Evaluation

If abnormalities in the semen are detected, further evaluation by a urologist is indicated to diagnose the defect. Several groups have attempted to assess the distribution of male diagnoses; two such distributions are shown in Table 27.3. The first is the result of a WHO

Table 27.3   Male Factor Causes of Infertility

Cause	Percentage	Cause	Percentage
No demonstrable cause	48.5%	Varicocele	37.4%
Idiopathic abnormal semen	26.4%	Idiopathic	25.4%
Varicocele	12.3%	Testicular failure	9.4%
Infectious factors	6.6%	Obstruction	6.1%
Immunologic factors	3.1%	Cryptorchidism	6.1%
Other acquired factors	2.6%	Low semen volume	4.7%
Congenital factors	2.1%	Semenagglutination	3.1%
Sexual factors	1.7%	Semen viscosity	1.9%
Endocrine disturbances	0.6%	Other	5.9%
Total	103.9%*		100%

The ESHRE CAPRI Workshop Group. Male sterility and subfertility: guidelines for management. *Hum Reprod* 1994;9:1260–4.
Burkman LJ, Cobbington CC, Franken DR, Kruger TF, Rosenwaks Z, Hodgen GD. The hemizona assay (HZA): development of a diagnostic test for the binding of human spermatozoa to the human hemizona pellucida to predict fertilization potential. *Fertil Steril* 1988;49:688–97.
*>100% because of multiple factors.

study of 7057 men with complete diagnoses based on the WHO standard investigation of the infertile couple (36). The figures include data from cases in which the male partner was normal and the presumed cause of the couple's infertility was a female factor. The second distribution is the result of a study of 425 subfertile male patients (37). Although the two studies offer somewhat different incidences of male infertility diagnoses (one is from a study of couples, the other from a urologic practice), idiopathic male factor and varicocele predominate. Other anatomic and endocrine causes are less frequent.

Varicocele   A varicocele is an abnormal dilation of the veins within the spermatic cord. Varicoceles nearly always occur on the left side, presumably because of the direct insertion of the spermatic vein into the renal vein on that side. The pathophysiologic effects of varicocele on testicular function are uncertain but appear to be mediated by an associated rise in testicular temperature or a reflux of toxic metabolites from the left adrenal or renal veins (38). In either event, the effect on sperm production is bilateral. An understanding of the role of varicocele in infertility is complicated by two issues: the prevalence of varicocele in the normal male population and the efficacy of varicocele repair in infertile men. A WHO study found a varicocele in 25.4% of men with abnormal semen as opposed to 11.7% of men with normal semen (39). This study failed to demonstrate a difference in the frequency of spontaneous pregnancies in couples in which the men did and did not have varicoceles. Nonetheless, varicoceles were associated with decreased testicular volume, impaired semen quality, and a reduction in serum testosterone levels.

Anatomic Abnormalities   Congenital abnormalities, such as hypospadias or cryptorchidism, may be associated with infertility. Congenital absence or obstruction of the vas deferens or ejaculatory ducts may be detected by the absence of fructose in the semen and confirmed by vasography. In addition, testicular biopsy may be indicated to differentiate between primary testicular damage and outflow obstruction. Some men with reduced semen volume may have retrograde ejaculation, in which sperm are propelled into the bladder rather than through the urethra. This diagnosis can be confirmed by examination of a postejaculatory voided or catheterized urine specimen. This condition occurs in rare cases of patients with diabetes mellitus, in certain neurologic conditions, and after bladder or prostatic surgery.

Endocrine Abnormalities   Although rare, the diagnosis of an endocrine disorder in an infertile man may be amenable to efficacious therapy. A full endocrine history, including information on puberty and growth and a review of endocrine systems, should guide the physician in the evaluation. Impotence may be associated with hyperprolactinemia and, in such cases, is readily treatable. Men with histories suggestive of hypogonadotropic hypogonadism, such as *Kallmann's syndrome,* have low levels of gonadotropins (LH and FSH) and low serum levels of testosterone and often respond to treatment. Men with hypergonadotropic hypogonadism (elevated levels of LH and FSH with low serum levels of testosterone) generally have primary gonadal failure. A karyotype should be obtained in such cases to detect chromosomal abnormalities such as *Klinefelter's syndrome* (47XXY). If the diagnosis of gonadal failure is confirmed on biopsy, endocrine therapy is contraindicated.

Environmental Toxins and Drug Exposure   The mean sperm concentration and mean sperm volume in normal males have dropped substantially over the past 50 years (19). This decline in semen quality has been suggested to be associated with increased levels of environmental toxins in the last half of the 20th century. The nature of such toxins, however, remains speculative. Heavy marijuana and cocaine use can reduce sperm concentration. Certain drugs, such as anabolic steroids, chemotherapeutic agents, *cimetidine, erythromycin, nitrofurans, spironolactone, sulfasalazine,* and *tetracycline,* may reduce semen parameters. In addition, cigarette smoking and heavy coffee consumption diminish semen quality (40).

Ovulatory Factor

Disorders of ovulation account for approximately 30–40% of all cases of female infertility. These disorders are generally among the most easily diagnosed and most treatable causes of infertility. The normal length of the menstrual cycle in reproductive-age women varies from 25 to 35 days; most women have cycle lengths of 27–31 days. Women who have regular monthly menses (approximately every 4 weeks) with moliminal symptoms, such as premenstrual breast swelling and dysmenorrhea, almost invariably have ovulatory cycles. Because ovulation is an obvious prerequisite to conception, ovulation must be documented as part of the basic assessment of the infertile couple.

The initial diagnoses may be anovulation (complete absence of ovulation) or oligo-ovulation (infrequent ovulation). The differential diagnosis includes hypothalamic and pituitary abnormalities, thyroid disease, adrenal disorders, and hyperandrogenic oligo-ovulation.

Methods to Document Ovulation

Basal Body Temperature   The easiest and least expensive method of detecting ovulation is for the patient to record her temperature each morning on a basal body temperature (BBT) chart. The temperature should be determined orally before the patient arises, eats, or drinks. Smoking is forbidden. Use of a basal body thermometer is preferred because of its precision in the temperature range under consideration. The patient records her temperature daily and also records the times when coitus takes place. The principle of temperature charting is simple. Significant progesterone secretion by the ovary generally occurs only after ovulation. Progesterone is a thermogenic hormone; the secretion of progesterone leads to temperature increases of approximately 0.5°F over the base line temperature in the follicular phase, which is generally in the range of 97–98°F. The difference between the two phases of the cycle produces the characteristic biphasic pattern indicative of ovulation. Frequently, there is a nadir around the time of the LH surge, but this finding is inconsistent. The luteal phase is characterized by a temperature elevation lasting at least 10 days.

The BBT, although simple, has several drawbacks. Presumptive ovulation can be identified only retrospectively; i.e., the test merely confirms rather than predicts ovulation. Also, in a small percentage of patients, the BBT charts are monophasic despite the documentation of ovulation by other methods. The exact time of ovulation is difficult to predict, but in most instances, it is probably 1 day before temperature elevation. The unequivocal temperature rise generally occurs 2 days after the LH surge and correlates with serum progesterone levels of >4 ng/ml (41). The correlation between BBT rise and LH surge may be more reliable than correlations with progesterone levels (42).

Despite its limitations, BBT charting is a simple way to document ovulation. Unequivocal biphasic cycles are almost certainly ovulatory, but monophasic cycles require the confirmation of the patient's ovulatory status.

Midluteal Serum Progesterone   Elevations in serum levels of progesterone constitute indirect evidence of ovulation. The lower limit of progesterone levels in the luteal phase varies among laboratories, but a level of >3 ng/ml (10 nmol/l) confirms ovulation. The measurement should be made as progesterone secretion peaks in the midluteal phase (typically on days 21–23 of an ideal 28-day cycle). Typically, ovulatory levels are considerably higher than 3 ng/ml. Interpretation of a single measurement of the progesterone level is complicated by the pulsatile nature of the secretion of this hormone (43); therefore, low levels are not necessarily diagnostic of anovulation, but appropriate concentrations in the luteal phase confirm prior ovulation.

Numerous investigators have attempted to correlate elevated midluteal progesterone levels with adequate corpus luteum function (44, 45). Others have tried to correlate progesterone levels with findings on endometrial biopsy (46, 47). A single progesterone measurement is not a substitute for an endometrial biopsy in the assessment of adequacy in the luteal phase.

Luteinizing Hormone Monitoring   **Documentation of the LH surge is a reproducible method of predicting ovulation. Ovulation occurs 34–36 hours after the onset of the LH surge and approximately 10–12 hours after the LH peak** (48, 49). Because LH is a pulsatile hormone, the detection of a true elevation may be difficult. A two- to threefold elevation of serum LH levels over base line, however, is sufficient to document an LH surge. A number of manufacturers have developed self-administered home kits to detect the LH surge in the urine. The kits are generally accurate, quick, convenient, and relatively inexpensive enzyme-linked immunoabsorbent assays (50). Unlike assays that measure serum LH levels, these tests detect urinary LH levels above a certain threshold.

Endometrial Biopsy   Another method of confirming ovulation is the endometrial biopsy; the finding of secretory endometrium confirms ovulation. Because this procedure is more invasive than other methods and may be somewhat uncomfortable for some patients, its major role in the infertility evaluation is not in documentation of ovulation but rather in diagnosis of luteal phase defects. Generally, the biopsy is performed 2–3 days before the expected onset of menses. The patient may be offered a sensitive serum pregnancy test prior to biopsy, but the risk that the biopsy will interrupt an early pregnancy is small (51). The biopsy is interpreted by dating of the endometrium according to the criteria of Noyes, Hertig, and Rock (52). Despite widespread agreement on the pathologic criteria, there may be significant variability in the dating of the specimen (53).

Ultrasound Monitoring   Ovulation can be documented by monitoring the development of the dominant follicle by ultrasound until ovulation takes place. Ovulation is characterized by a decrease in follicular size and the appearance of fluid in the cul-de-sac (54). Ovulation is reported to occur when follicular size reaches 21–23 mm, although it may occur with follicles as small as 17 mm or as large as 29 mm (55, 56). Because of the inconvenience and expense of serial ultrasound measurements, use of this method for documenting ovulation is discouraged; instead, it is recommended that its use be confined to the monitoring of ovulation induction in ART patients.

Luteal Phase Defect   There are probably few areas of greater controversy in the field of infertility than that surrounding the existence, diagnosis, and treatment of luteal phase defect (LPD) or inadequate luteal phase. The controversy has been fueled by disagreements over the definition of this entity and the efficacy of its treatment. Although variously defined, **most agree that LPD occurs when two endometrial biopsies show a delay of more than 2 days beyond the actual cycle day in the histologic development of the en-**

dometrium as assessed by the criteria of Noyes et al. (52). In calculating the day of the cycle, the convention is to count the onset of the next menses after the biopsy as day 28. If a luteal-phase lag is found on the initial biopsy, it must be confirmed on a subsequent biopsy to meet criteria for the diagnosis of LPD. Some physicians have diagnosed a short luteal phase from BBT charts alone in cases in which the temperature elevation is sustained in the luteal phase for fewer than 11 days. In cases in which LPD is hypothesized, the presumed cause is a reduction in progesterone production by the corpus luteum. In cases in which LPD is presumed to be a cause of infertility, inadequate progesterone secretion is believed to lead to poor secretory endometrial development manifest by a delay in endometrial maturation. This set of circumstances, hypothetically, could cause a failure of implantation or a very early abortion—even prior to a missed menses. The underlying causes of LPD may include inadequate follicular development, inadequate FSH secretion, abnormal LH secretion, or an abnormal effect of progesterone on the endometrium (57). In addition, LPD may be associated with hyperprolactinemia and may occur in women at the extremes of reproductive age whose menstrual cycles fluctuate accordingly.

Perhaps the crucial question is whether LPD exists at all. Davis and colleagues conducted multiple biopsies of normally fertile women; their documentation of out-of-phase biopsies in 31.4% and of sequential out-of-phase biopsies in 6.6% suggested that normal women often have out-of-phase endometria (58). Other authors have suggested that the frequency of out-of-phase biopsies in infertile patients is no greater than the rate that would occur by chance alone (59, 60).

Because of the discomfort and inconvenience associated with the multiple endometrial biopsies needed to confirm the diagnosis of LPD, several investigators have attempted to identify a luteal phase serum progesterone level that correlates sufficiently with biopsy results to serve as a substitute. Although some studies have advocated the use of a single mid-luteal-phase serum progesterone level (above which LPD is ruled out), data that convincingly correlate these single-value cutoffs with data from normal women are lacking. The pulsatile secretion of progesterone further reduces the utility of a single progesterone measurement (61). Other investigators have attempted to "fine-tune" the use of the endometrial biopsy, suggesting that examination of a midluteal-phase serum sample may detect more patients with an abnormal luteal phase, but this approach has been controversial (62, 63). Given the uncertainties about the diagnosis and treatment of LPD, attempts to diagnose LPD should be confined to infertile patients who are at high risk for this diagnosis or lack another diagnosis.

Tubal/Peritoneal Factors

Tubal and peritoneal factors account for 30–40% of cases of female infertility. Tubal factors include damage or obstruction of the fallopian tubes, usually associated with previous pelvic inflammatory disease (PID) or previous pelvic or tubal surgery. Peritoneal factors include peritubal and periovarian adhesions, which generally result from PID or surgery, and endometriosis. The risk of infertility after a single bout of PID is high. The incidence of tubal infertility has been reported to be 12%, 23%, and 54% after one, two, and three episodes of PID, respectively (64). Approximately 50% of patients with documented tubal damage have no identifiable risk factors for tubal disease (65). Most of these women are presumed to have subclinical chlamydial infections.

Hysterosalpingography (HSG) is the initial test of tubal patency. The test should be performed between cycle days 6 and 11. To reduce the chance of infection associated with the procedure, ideally HSG should follow the cessation of menstrual flow; to avoid possible fetal irradiation, HSG should precede ovulation. It is estimated that infection follows 1–3% of HSG procedures and occurs almost exclusively in women with current or prior pelvic infection. In cases of suspected chronic PID, the erythrocyte sedimentation rate should be determined before HSG is performed; if this rate is elevated, antibiotic therapy should be considered. Also, a careful bimanual examination should be performed just

925

before the test to identify adnexal masses or tenderness, which could signal current infection. In cases in which these conditions are identified, the procedure should be postponed. Hysterosalpingography often causes cramping; prophylaxis with a nonsteroidal anti-inflammatory drug may minimize discomfort. The issue of universal antibiotic prophylaxis for HSG is controversial. Although PID infrequently develops after HSG and mainly involves women with hydrosalpinx, routine prophylaxis should be given with *doxycycline* 100 mg twice daily, beginning the day before HSG and continuing for 3 to 5 days.

After a bimanual examination, an acorn (Jarcho) cannula, a pediatric Foley catheter, or some other injection device is introduced into the uterus. A paracervical anesthetic block is not routinely needed but may be used in selected patients. Either a water-soluble contrast medium, such as meglumine diatrizoate (*Renografin-60*), or a low-viscosity oil-based dye, such as ethiodized oil (*Ethiodol*), may be used. Each contrast material has its advantages. Water-soluble contrast material is more rapidly absorbed than oil-based dyes and does not carry the risk of lipid embolism due to dye extravasation or lipid granuloma formation. Oil-based dyes are associated with less cramping, better resolution of tubal architecture, and a higher postprocedure pregnancy rate (66). The procedure should be performed under fluoroscopy, with minimal x-ray exposure of the ovaries. Slow injection of 3–4 ml of media should give a clear outline of the uterine cavity. A sufficient volume of dye, usually a total of 10–20 ml, should demonstrate bilateral tubal patency or tubal obstruction. Generally, only two radiographic views are needed, one demonstrating the filling of the uterine cavity and the other (at the completion of the procedure) showing tubal findings.

Laparoscopy   **The "gold standard" for diagnosing tubal and peritoneal disease is laparoscopy.** It allows visualization of all the pelvic organs and permits detection of intramural and subserosal uterine fibroids, peritubal and periovarian adhesions, and endometriosis. Although the results of HSG may suggest adhesions, the aggregate sensitivity and specificity of HSG are only 76% and 83%, respectively, for this condition (67). Abnormal findings on HSG should be confirmed by direct visualization with laparoscopy. Tubal patency may be confirmed at laparoscopy by observation of the passage of a dye, such as methylene blue or indigo carmine, through the fimbrial openings of the tubes. Laparoscopy allows a careful assessment of the architecture of the tubes and, in particular, visualization of the fimbria. It also provides an opportunity to treat as well as to detect abnormalities—the enhanced optics and magnification and the improved instrumentation now permit surgical treatment of tubal obstruction, pelvic adhesions, and endometriosis at the time of diagnosis.

Falloposcopy   Based on techniques derived from coronary angioplasty, a system has been developed that uses small guide wires to permit direct observation of the lumen of the fallopian tube. Such direct visualization of the internal tubal architecture may be accomplished via laparoscopy (68) or hysteroscopy (69). Falloposcopy can define normal tubal appearance and has identified abnormal mucosal tubal patterns, tubal ostial spasm, and the presence of intraluminal debris as a cause of tubal obstruction. This technique, used in association with radiologic methods for the treatment of proximal tubal obstruction, holds promise as a less invasive procedure that can facilitate the diagnosis and treatment of tubal-factor infertility.

Cervical Factor

Cervical factor is the cause of infertility in no more than 5% of cases. The classic test for evaluation of the potential role of cervical factor in infertility is the postcoital test (PCT). The PCT is designed to assess the quality of cervical mucus, the presence and number of motile sperm in the female reproductive tract after coitus, and the interaction between cervical mucus and sperm. The PCT does not yield sufficient information on sperm count, motility, or morphology to allow assessment of semen quality.

The PCT should be performed just before ovulation because its proper interpretation requires the examination of cervical mucus at a time of sufficient estrogen exposure. Serum estrogen levels peak just before ovulation, providing optimal stimulation to the estrogen-sensitive, mucus-producing cervical glands. The PCT should be performed 1 or 2 days before the anticipated time of ovulation. The patient's urinary LH surge may be helpful in scheduling the test for patients with irregular cycles. One area of controversy concerns the timing of coitus preceding examination of the cervical mucus. Although an optimal interval may be less than 2 hours from intercourse to PCT, an adequate test can be performed within 24 hours of intercourse. Although the data are not definitive, intercourse after 2 days of abstinence, or approximately 2–12 hours before the PCT is performed, should yield adequate information. Couples should be reminded not to use lubricants that may contain spermicidal agents.

The PCT is performed easily. A small amount of cervical mucus is withdrawn by means of long oval forceps with small apertures at the tip. Alternatively, an angiocatheter syringe or tuberculin syringe may be used to withdraw mucus from the endocervical canal. The mucus is placed on a glass slide and covered with a cover slip. A small trail of mucus may be left outside the cover slip to dry so that ferning can be assessed. Many infertility specialists also take a "vaginal pool" specimen from the posterior vaginal fornix to document the presence of sperm in the vagina.

The mucus is rapidly evaluated for *spinnbarkeit* (i.e., stretchability), ferning, and clarity. The presence, number, and motility of sperm per high-power field should be carefully assessed by the examination of several microscopic fields. Normal estrogen-stimulated mucus should stretch 8–10 cm when it is pulled from the cervix with forceps or when the cover slip is lifted off the slide, should demonstrate a highly characteristic ferning pattern similar to that seen on examination of amniotic fluid, and should be clear and watery. The characteristics of cervical mucus change under the influence of progesterone after ovulation; at that time, the mucus appears thick and opaque and lacks ferning.

The number of motile sperm per high-power field should be counted; however, the number considered normal has not been established. Some authors suggest that virtually any number of motile sperm seen on the PCT is normal (70), while others advocate more than 20 sperm per high-power field as the cutoff for a normal test (71).

There are several potential causes for an abnormal PCT result. The most common cause is poor timing within the menstrual cycle. If the mucus is of poor quality, the test should be repeated in a subsequent cycle, with careful documentation of its timing in relation to ovulation. The causes of repeated poor PCT results include hormonal abnormalities (i.e., oligo-ovulation), the production of poor-quality cervical mucus, anatomic factors (e.g., prior cervical conization or cryotherapy), and infection. Also, some medications may alter the quality of the cervical mucus. The most prominent example is *clomiphene citrate,* which may have detrimental effects on cervical mucus through its antiestrogenic action on the cervical glands. The PCT may reveal poor mucus-sperm interaction or may uncover abnormalities in sperm concentration or sperm motility; the latter findings must be confirmed by semen analysis. The observation of shaking sperm or uniformly dead sperm suggests the presence of antisperm antibodies and warrants further evaluation.

In recent years, the PCT has come under attack from several investigators who challenge its benefit as a prognostic test in the diagnosis of infertility. Collins et al. found no difference in pregnancy rates in groups of women whose cervical mucus contained 0–11 motile sperm per high-power field (72). Another study showed that 20% of fertile couples had less than one motile sperm per high-power field (71). Griffith and Grimes challenged the validity of the PCT by reviewing the world's English-language literature and finding that the sensitivity and specificity of the test ranged from 0.09 to 0.71 and from 0.62 to 1.00, respectively (73). These authors concluded that the test suffers from a lack of standard methodology, a lack of uniform definition of normal, and an unknown degree of reproducibility. Glatstein and co-workers prospectively assessed the reproducibility of the PCT and concluded that the characteristics of the test exhibit only poor to fair reproducibility, even among trained observers using a standard scoring system (74). Thus, the role of this single test has come into question, although its value seems greatest as a screening mechanism for antisperm antibodies or for poor cervical mucus due to hormonal, anatomic, or infectious factors.

Uterine Factor

Whereas uterine abnormalities are generally associated with recurrent pregnancy loss rather than with infertility, certain anatomic abnormalities of the uterus have been proposed as causes of infertility. Uterine fibroids, especially submucous leiomyomas, may be associated with pregnancy loss. Some researchers have speculated that the location of fibroids within the endometrial cavity may interfere with sperm transport or implantation. The abnormal bleeding associated with such fibroids may not permit proper preparation of the endometrium for successful implantation. The association of intramural and submucous fibroids with infertility is probably even more tenuous than that with pregnancy loss. However, **fibroids are an infrequent cause of infertility (75), and abdominal myomectomy may even cause infertility through the formation of postoperative adhesions** (76). Congenital uterine malformations, such as unicorneate uterus, uterine septum, and uterine didelphys, are more often associated with spontaneous abortion than with infertility.

The association of *in utero* DES exposure with infertility remains controversial. Abnormalities of the uterus, such as the classical T-shaped endometrial cavity as well as cervical and tubal abnormalities, seem clearly associated with DES exposure. The relationship of these abnormalities to infertility, however, is less clear; some reports show an increased incidence of infertility (77) and others reveal no significant difference in infertility rates between DES-exposed women and women who were not exposed to DES (78). However, there is no effective surgery to aid women with DES-related uterine malformations.

Patients with intrauterine adhesions, or *Asherman's syndrome,* may be infertile. In its severe forms, *Asherman's syndrome* is associated with amenorrhea, menstrual irregularities, and spontaneous abortion. Like submucous myomas, intrauterine adhesions may hypothetically interfere with embryo implantation.

In the evaluation of uterine factors, HSG is used to visualize the contours of the endometrial cavity. Endometrial polyps, submucous fibroids, congenital abnormalities, and intrauterine synechiae usually are readily apparent. Hysteroscopy should be used to further define and treat abnormalities detected by HSG.

Immunologic Factor

Injection of sperm from one animal into another can elicit an antibody response (79). Spermatozoa can also be autoantigenic; thus, it is possible that an antibody response to sperm could reduce fertility. Antisperm antibodies have been detected in human males and females and are known to be of the IgG or IgM class. Systemically produced IgG molecules may be found in serum as well as in cervical mucus and semen. Agglutinating antibodies of the IgA class are typically found in cervical mucus and seminal plasma. The larger IgM antibodies have difficulty traversing the genital tract mucosa and therefore are found exclusively in serum.

The etiology of antisperm antibodies is not well defined and may be multifactorial (80). During intercourse, a woman is repeatedly exposed to billions of spermatozoa but very rarely exhibits an immune response. In women who do exhibit such a response, the development of antisperm antibodies may be associated with trauma resulting in breaks in the vaginal epithelium. In males, the blood-testis barrier normally shields the serum from exposure to sperm or their antigens. Conditions that cause breaks in this barrier could activate the immune system. Testicular trauma or torsion, vasectomy reversal, and genital tract infection have all been implicated as causes of antisperm antibody formation.

928

Assessment of the significance of antibodies is complicated by the variety of locations at which antibodies bind to sperm cells. For example, antibodies binding to the sperm head may interfere with sperm binding to the zona pellucida, whereas tail-binding antibodies could reduce sperm motility. Thus, antisperm antibodies may interfere with fertilization by disrupting sperm transport, by obstructing gamete interaction, or by promoting sperm phagocytosis.

Another confusing aspect of the evaluation of immunologic infertility is the myriad tests available for the detection of antisperm antibodies. *Sperm agglutination tests* (Kibrick's or Franklin-Dukes) and sperm *complement-dependent immobilization tests* (Isojoma's) have been replaced by the *immunobead* or *mixed agglutination tests* (Fig. 27.2). The immunobead test uses commercially available anti-IgG-, anti-IgA-, or anti-IgM-coated polyacrylamide beads. Washed spermatozoa are exposed to the labeled beads, and sperm binding is assessed. The test yields specific information on both the immunoglobulin class of the antisperm antibody and the site of binding to the involved sperm (81). In the mixed agglutination reaction, human red blood cells sensitized with human IgG are mixed with "pa-

Figure 27.2   The mixed agglutination reaction (MAR) to evaluate immunologic infertility by assessment of antisperm antibodies. (Redrawn and adapted from **Garenne ML, Frisch RE.** Natural fertility. *Infert Reprod Med Clin North Am* 1994;5:259–82.)

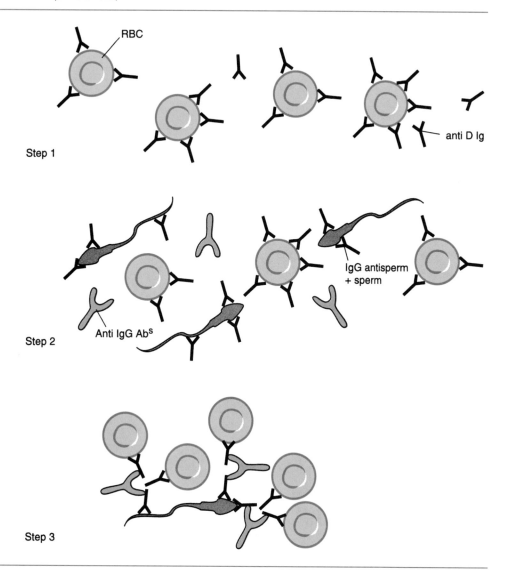

tient" semen. The presence of antibody-coated spermatozoa will result in the formation of mixed agglutinates with the red blood cells (82). A comparison of these two methods demonstrates good correlation of results; however, the latter test is easier to perform (83).

Despite the recent improvement in techniques for the identification of antisperm antibodies, the case for these antibodies as a cause of infertility is not clear. A number of older studies demonstrate an association between reduced fertility and antisperm antibodies in the male and female. However, these studies have been criticized for their use of various methods to detect antibodies, for lack of proper control groups, and for the retrospective analysis of data (84). A prospective double-blind cohort analysis comparing conception in antibody-positive and antibody-negative couples failed to identify a less-favorable prognosis for conception in antibody-positive couples, thus calling into question the utility of antisperm antibody testing (84). At present, the proper role of such testing in the evaluation of infertility is unclear. Physicians may wish to use antibody testing in selected cases in which risk factors for antisperm antibodies are documented or the cause of infertility remains elusive.

Infections

The relationship between subclinical infection and fertility has received considerable attention. Particular interest has focused on two potential pathogens: *Chlamydia trachomatous* and *Mycoplasma species*. The association of chlamydia with PID is well established. *Chlamydia* is the predominant pathogen in approximately 20% of cases of acute salpingitis in the U.S. *Chlamydia* may produce an asymptomatic infection in the female genital tract, presumably associated in some women with silent tubal infection and perhaps tubal damage. Several studies have suggested that serologic evidence of chlamydial infection is related to an increased risk of asymptomatic tubal disease (85, 86). Moreover, the prevalence of positive chlamydial cultures may be higher among infertile patients than among controls (87). Whether the diagnosis and treatment of asymptomatic *Chlamydia*-positive patients improves fecundity remains unresolved.

Mycoplasmas are pleuropneumonia-like organisms. Both *Mycoplasma hominis* and *Ureaplasma urealyticum* have been recovered from the cervical mucus and semen of infertile couples. There are higher rates of mycoplasma infection among infertile couples than among fertile controls. In one study, 60% of infertile males who were culture-positive for *Ureaplasma* and whose infection was subsequently cleared by antibiotic treatment impregnated their partners; the rate was only 5% among men whose infection was not cleared (88). In contrast, a double-blind study of *doxycycline* treatment for mycoplasma infection failed to show an effect on conception rates (89). Mycoplasmas have been isolated from the cervix of the female partner in 47% of previously infertile couples who conceived and 53% of couples who remained infertile (89). Thus, **these studies do not support a role for genital mycoplasma in infertility.**

Unexplained Infertility

The laboratory assessment of the infertile couple is relatively simple and should be performed rapidly in order to establish a diagnosis and initiate appropriate therapy (Fig. 27.3). Evaluation of the male by semen analysis in an accredited laboratory skilled in andrology testing is essential. In the female, ovulation should be documented by BBT charting or midluteal serum progesterone measurement. Home urine LH detection is convenient but relies on the patient for interpretation. Blood LH testing, ultrasound, and endometrial biopsy are expensive, invasive tests that should be reserved for cases in which the initial testing yields equivocal results. Some test of tubal patency—either HSG or laparoscopy—is necessary. In fact, no evaluation of infertility can be considered complete unless laparoscopy is performed. This is not to say that in some patients treatment up to and including IVF may not be undertaken without laparoscopy, but the proper diagnosis of endometriosis, pelvic adhesions, and nonobstructive tubal disease requires laparoscopy.

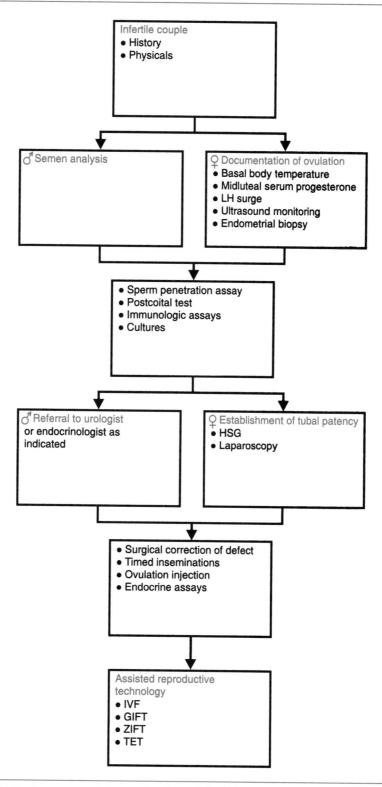

Figure 27.3   Summary of the evaluation of the infertile couple.

The European Society for Human Reproduction and Embryology workshop on unexplained infertility suggested that other tests, such as the PCT, the hamster-egg penetration test, and antisperm antibody testing, are more controversial. In addition, abnormal results in these tests frequently are followed by fertility, even without treatment (90). The workshop further suggested that the results of several tests (i.e., endometrial dating, varicocele assessment, and chlamydia testing) are not correlated with fertility. For these specific tests, data confirming a correlation between test results and pregnancy are lacking, and proper follow-up studies do not exist.

Following is a reasonable approach to the assessment of unexplained infertility:

1. A semen analysis should be performed, ovulation should be documented, and an HSG should be performed. All previous studies should be reviewed and repeated if the results are in doubt, particularly in the case of the semen analysis.

2. If the results of these tests are normal, a laparoscopy should be performed.

3. If the etiology of infertility remains enigmatic, further endocrine evaluation should be undertaken with measurements of thyroid-stimulating hormone, FSH, and prolactin levels.

4. Cervical factor infertility should be assessed with PCT and chlamydia cultures.

5. The evaluation of sperm function with the hamster-egg test and endometrial maturation by endometrial biopsy may be considered.

Contemporary treatment of unexplained infertility has increasingly included empiric therapy with ovulation induction and intrauterine insemination or the use of ART. A more focused workup followed by a more aggressive approach to therapy may prove more cost-effective and expedient.

Treatment Options

Very few couples who are unable to conceive are diagnosed with absolute infertility. Instead, most couples are faced with reduced fertility or subfertility and can achieve pregnancy without treatment if attempts are continued for a prolonged period. In 1983, Collins et al. (91) evaluated treatment-independent fecundity in 1145 infertile couples; these couples were followed for 2 to 7 years. Treatment-independent pregnancies were defined as those occurring in untreated patients or those occurring more than 3 months after the last medical treatment or more than 12 months after adnexal surgery. In patients with ovulatory factor infertility, 44% of the pregnancies were treatment-independent. Likewise, 61% of patients with infertility related to endometriosis, tubal factor, or male factor and 96% of patients with cervical-factor or unexplained infertility achieved pregnancy independent of treatment. This impressive rate of "spontaneous cure" illustrates why it is best to view the treatment of infertility as an attempt to improve fertility efficacy. Thus, **most infertility therapy is directed toward decreasing the time it would take to conceive without intervention. Such therapy is often undertaken in an effort to achieve pregnancy before or during the natural age-related decline in female fecundity.**

Male Factor Infertility

Medical Therapy

With few exceptions, options for medical therapy of male infertility are of questionable benefit. One exception is the use of gonadotropin-releasing hormone (GnRH) in hypogonadotropic hypogonadal males, which has been shown conclusively to be efficacious. Pulsatile GnRH therapy is conceptually indicated and effective in infertile men with hypothalamic dysfunction (92), including those with *Kallmann's syndrome.* Infertile males with hypogonadotropic hypogonadism secondary to panhypopituitarism may also respond to GnRH therapy (93). For subfertile males with retrograde ejaculatory dysfunction, α-adrenergic agonists such as *phenylephrine* have been used effectively to strengthen internal urethral sphincter tone (94). Sperm may also be isolated from the neutralized urine of men with retrograde ejaculation and processed for insemination or for ART (95).

Clomiphene citrate, an estrogen agonist and partial antagonist, has often been used to treat male infertility of idiopathic origin. *Clomiphene citrate* acts on the hypothalamic-pituitary axis and, in men, increases serum levels of LH, FSH, and testosterone (96). Although efficacy of *clomiphene* for male factor infertility is controversial, most studies have shown little improvement in semen parameters and no improvement in pregnancy rates (97). Severe idiopathic male factor infertility has been treated with pure FSH with no notable improvement in semen parameters but a significant increase in fertilization rates during ART (98).

If antisperm antibodies in the cervical mucus or attached to the sperm cell itself are a factor in some cases of infertility, it is probably related to their effects on sperm motility and sperm-oocyte interaction (99). Medical therapy for infertility associated with antisperm antibodies, including the use of condoms and glucocorticoids, has been used for many years but has never been proven effective.

Surgical Therapy

Surgical therapy for male factor infertility includes varicocele-corrective procedures, surgical reversal of vasectomy, artificial insemination, and ART (e.g., IVF, gamete intrafallopian tubal transfer [GIFT], and micromanipulation). Varicocele repair involves interruption of the internal spermatic vein and is commonly performed in the 40% of infertile men with clinically evident varicoceles. Currently, it is performed as an outpatient procedure and may involve laparoscopy, open surgery, or the injection of embolizing agents. Despite its widespread use, the therapeutic benefits of varicocele repair have remained controversial. A large nonrandomized study from Australia showed only minimal improvement in sperm motility following surgical repair. The group that did not undergo surgery had a similar small improvement in sperm motility, and the pregnancy rate was no higher in the group that underwent surgery than in the group that did not (100). Another report, however, described improved sperm parameters and fertility rates for infertile men treated by high spermatic vein ligation than for men who were not treated (101).

The most common cause of obstructive azoospermia in infertile men is prior vasectomy. The reversal of vasectomy by microsurgical vasovasostomy is quite effective; vas deferens patency was obtained in 86% and pregnancy was achieved in 52% of cases after primary procedures (102). Rates of patency and pregnancy vary inversely with the length of time from vasectomy. For patients with azoospermia 3 months after the reversal procedure, either the reanastomosis has failed or the epididymis is obstructed. Repeat vasovasostomy is associated with patency rates of 75% and pregnancy rates of 43% (102). Epididymal obstruction is best diagnosed via vasography or documentation of normal spermatogenesis on testicular biopsy. Epididymal aspiration proximal to the obstruction may be used in cases of epididymal or vas deferens obstruction to obtain sperm for use in ART. Microsurgical vasoepididymostomy is associated with patency rates of 70% and postoperative pregnancy rates of 44% at 1 year if no other infertility factor is present (103).

Artificial Insemination

Artificial insemination encompasses a variety of procedures involving placement of whole semen or processed sperm into the female reproductive tract, which permits sperm-oocyte interaction in the absence of intercourse. The placement of whole semen into the vagina as a mode of fertility treatment is of historical interest and is not currently performed, except in cases of severe coital dysfunction, including those involving severe hypospadias, retrograde ejaculation, erectile abnormalities, and psychosocial dysfunction precluding intercourse. Currently, the more common forms of artificial insemination use processed sperm from the male partner or a donor.

Types of Insemination   Types of insemination performed include intracervical, intrauterine, intraperitoneal, and intrafollicular insemination and fallopian-tube sperm perfusion. *Intrauterine insemination* (IUI) is the best studied and most widely practiced of the techniques. It involves placement of approximately 0.3 ml of washed, processed, and concentrated sperm into the intrauterine cavity via transcervical catheterization. Male factor infertility is one of the most common indications for IUI; however, its effectiveness for this indication, even when combined with ovulation induction, has yet to be defined (103). *Intracervical insemination* may be performed with unwashed or processed specimens. The success rates with intracervical insemination are consistently lower than those with IUI (104, 105). *Fallopian tube sperm perfusion,* which has been used for artificial insemination, differs from IUI in that a large volume of washed sperm (approximately 4 ml) is injected into the intrauterine cavity. In combination with ovulation induction with human menopausal gonadotropin/human chorionic gonadotropin (hMG/hCG), fallopian tube sperm perfusion has been shown to be superior to conventional IUI for unexplained infertility, with pregnancy rates reported as 29% per cycle (106). Direct *intraperitoneal insemination* may be indicated in selected cases of male factor infertility. This procedure involves the injection of washed, processed sperm into the intraperitoneal cavity via puncture of the posterior vaginal cul-de-sac. Used in combination with superovulation, direct intraperitoneal insemination has been reported to be as effective as IUI for couples with unexplained infertility, male factor infertility, or infertility related to mild endometriosis (107). *Intrafollicular insemination* as a treatment for male factor infertility has also been reported (108).

Processing Semen   Two important issues regarding the use of artificial insemination procedures are the mode of processing of semen samples and the number and timing of inseminations. Many protocols have been developed for sperm preparation. Seminal fluid is usually prevented from reaching the intrauterine cavity and intra-abdominal space by the cervical barrier. The introduction of seminal fluid past this barrier may be associated with severe uterine cramping or anaphylactoid reactions, possibly mediated by seminal factors such as prostaglandins. Thus, protocols for processing whole semen include the washing of specimens in order to isolate pure sperm preparations. Some semen preparation methods attempt to enhance sperm motility or morphology in the final specimen through separation procedures. These include centrifugation through density gradients, sperm migration protocols, and differential adherence procedures. Finally, phosphodiesterase inhibitors, such as pentoxiphylline, have been used in an attempt to enhance sperm motility, fertilization capacity, and acrosome reactivity for IVF procedures (109).

Sperm retain their fertilizing capacity for 24–48 hours after ejaculation if they are able to escape the intravaginal environment. Oocytes can be fertilized for approximately 12–24 hours after ovulation. The timing of insemination procedures in the infertile couple is important; however, too much emphasis on precision is artificial. Although the data refer to IUI in conjunction with ovulation induction, fecundity is greater with two IUIs 18 and 42 hours after hCG administration than with a single procedure at 34 hours (110). The extrapolation of these findings to male infertility and nonstimulated cycles is difficult, particularly in light of the findings that 1) semen parameters may be significantly impaired in second-day specimens from consecutive-day collections (111) and 2) the best results are achieved when IUI is performed 18–30 hours after the spontaneous onset of the LH surge (112).

Donor Insemination   For males with azoospermia, couples with significant male factor infertility who do not desire ART, or women seeking pregnancy without a male partner, therapeutic donor insemination offers an effective option. A number of important issues surround the use of this form of artificial insemination. First, despite reports that the use of fresh donor semen is associated with higher pregnancy rates than the use of frozen specimens (113), both the Centers for Disease Control and Prevention (CDC) and the American Society for Reproductive Medicine recommend the use of frozen samples (114). This recommendation stems from the increasing incidence of human immunodeficiency virus (HIV) infection in the general population and the lag between HIV infection and seroconversion. Currently, semen donors are screened for HIV infection, hepatitis B, hepatitis C, syphilis, gonorrhea, chlamydial infection, and cytomegalovirus infections, all of which may be transmitted through the semen vector. All cryopreserved samples are quarantined for 6 months, and the donor is retested for HIV prior to clinical use of the specimen. Donors are likewise questioned concerning a family history of genetically transmitted disorders, both Mendelian (e.g., hemophilia, Tay-Sachs disease, thalassemia, cystic fibrosis, congenital adrenal hyperplasia, Huntington's disease) and polygenic/multifactorial (e.g., mental retardation, diabetes, heart malformation, spina bifida). Those with positive family histories are eliminated as donor candidates.

A second issue surrounding the use of therapeutic donor insemination—that which is most important to the patient—is the success rate of treatment. **In patients under 30 years of age who have no other infertility factors, conception rates approach 62% after 12 cycles of treatment with frozen sperm** (115).

The length of recommended treatment is a third factor to be addressed. When frozen semen is used, more than 80% of consequent pregnancies will occur during the first 12 months of treatment (116). Thus, patients should be encouraged to terminate treatment or move to alternative forms of therapy after 1 year of unsuccessful efforts at donor insemination.

In addition, one must consider the psychosocial aspects of pregnancies involving donor gametes. In patients without a male partner, the potential repercussions of becoming a single mother and the issue of telling others about the father of the child must be discussed. It is imperative that the husband of a couple using donor gametes be aware of the process, and most programs require that the husband sign a consent form. A skilled infertility social worker or psychologist can be immeasurably helpful in addressing these concerns.

Ovulatory Factor

Patients with ovulatory factor infertility have the greatest success rates with infertility therapy. Therapeutic choices for ovulatory factor infertility include various medical modes of ovulation induction and surgical treatment for polycystic ovaries. Table 27.4 presents the success rates and side effects of the various medical therapies for ovulation induction.

Table 27.4   Success Rates and Side Effects of Various Agents for Induction of Ovulation (in appropriately selected patients)

Agent	Ovulation Rates	Pregnancy Rates	Multiple Pregnancy Rates	Common Side Effects
Clomiphene citrate	≤80%	≤40%	≤8%	Hot flashes, visual symptoms, nausea, breast tenderness
Bromocriptine	≤95%	≤85%	<1%	Gastrointestinal irritation, orthostatic hypotension, nasal congestion, headache
Gonadotropins	30–100%*	10–90%*	≤30%	Local (injection related), hyperstimulation syndrome
Gonadotropin-releasing hormone	30–100%*	10–90%*	≤12%	Local (injection related)

*Patients with low levels of estrogen and gonadotropins are likely to fare much better than those with normal levels.
Reproduced with permission from ACOG Technical Bulletin. Managing the anovulatory state: medical induction of ovulation. American College of Obstetricians and Gynecologists. Washington, DC. 1994;197:1–7.

Clomiphene Citrate

The first-line regimen for medical induction of ovulation in most patients with ovulatory infertility is *clomiphene citrate (Clomid, Serophene)*. In light of its mechanism of action, all patients treated with this agent have a functional hypothalamic-pituitary-ovarian axis. *Clomiphene citrate* is a weak synthetic estrogen, but it acts clinically as an estrogen antagonist for ovulation induction at typical pharmacologic doses. Although *clomiphene citrate* has antiestrogenic effects in the hypothalamus that induce ovulation, its effect on other estrogen-sensitive tissues may be primarily agonistic or antagonistic. In the hypothalamus, *clomiphene citrate* binds to and blocks the estrogen receptor for prolonged periods, functionally decreasing the normal ovarian-hypothalamic estrogen feedback loop (117). This effect has recently been shown to increase GnRH pulse amplitude in some anovulatory women (118). Increased GnRH then feeds forward from the hypothalamus to the pituitary, resulting in increased gonadotropin secretion. *Clomiphene citrate* may also affect ovulation through direct action on the pituitary (119) or the ovary (120, 121). Antiestrogenic effects of *clomiphene citrate* at the level of the endometrium (122) or the cervix (123) may be involved in some failures of therapy; however, the existence and significance of these effects have been questioned (124, 125).

Success rates with the use of *clomiphene citrate* for ovulation induction are excellent, with ovulation rates of 80–85% and conception rates of 40% (126, 127). The discrepancy between ovulatory rates and conception rates is most likely secondary to the presence of additional, nonovulatory infertility factors. Most pregnancies occur during the first 6 months of therapy (126). Side effects of *clomiphene citrate* therapy include infrequent ovarian hyperstimulation syndrome, vasomotor flushes, nausea, pelvic discomfort, breast pain, and visual abnormalities (119). Use of *clomiphene citrate* is associated with a 35–60% incidence of multiple follicular recruitment (128); however, the incidence of multiple gestations with this agent is only approximately 5–8%, and most of these gestations are twin pregnancies. Rates of spontaneous abortion and teratogenicity in humans are not increased with the use of *clomiphene citrate* (129).

Clomiphene citrate is typically used for ovulation induction in the following manner (Fig. 27.4):

1. The drug is supplied in 50-mg tablets; the usual starting dosage is 50 mg/day. Therapy is typically begun on the fifth day after the onset of a spontaneous or progesterone-induced menses and is continued through day 9 of the menstrual cycle. Some practitioners begin treatment on day 2, 3, or 4 after onset of menses, and some patients respond to as low a dosage as 25 mg/day.

2. Ovulation can be documented by BBT charting, luteal-phase progesterone measurement, or timed endometrial biopsy. If ovulation does not occur at the initial dosage, the dosage is increased in each subsequent cycle by 50 mg/day. The Food and Drug Administration recommends a maximum dosage of 100 mg/day; however, in patients who ovulate as a result of *clomiphene citrate* treatment, 11.8% do so only at dosages of >150 mg/day (126). Considerable clinical experience with *clomiphene citrate* indicates that it is safe up to a dosage of 250 mg/day.

3. Ovulation is expected to occur 5–10 days after the last day of therapy; thus, with standard *clomiphene citrate* regimens, intercourse every other day for 1 week beginning on day 14 of the menstrual cycle is recommended. If IUI is to be used with *clomiphene citrate* induction of ovulation, timing of the LH surge must be documented precisely.

4. Patients in whom *clomiphene citrate* therapy fails may respond to ultrasound monitoring of follicular development and hCG for the induction of ovulation or to an appropriate individualized combination of *clomiphene citrate* with glucocorticoids or bromocriptine.

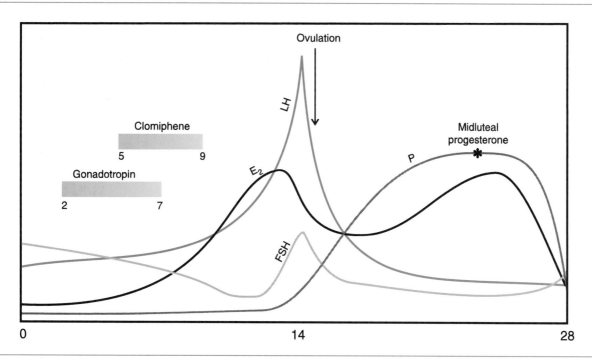

Figure 27.4   Ovulation induction: the time of administration of clomiphene citrate and gonadotropin.

Gonadotropins

Induction of ovulation with gonadotropins is the treatment of choice for women in whom *clomiphene citrate* therapy has failed and for women with ovulatory dysfunction secondary to hypogonadotropic hypogonadism. The drug used most often for this indication is hMG. Human menopausal gonadotropins (*Pergonal, Humegon*) are a mixture of FSH and LH purified from the urine of postmenopausal women (130) and supplied for intramuscular injection as a mixture of 75 IU of FSH and 75 IU of LH. The mechanism of action of hMG is much less controversial than that of *clomiphene citrate*. Functional ovarian tissue is necessary for successful therapy, because hMG supplements or replaces the woman's own gonadotropins, stimulating ovarian follicular development. As in spontaneous ovulatory cycles, FSH and LH act in concert to simulate folliculogenesis; FSH acts primarily on the granulosa cells and LH acts on the thecal lutein cells. Treatment with hCG is typically used in hMG-stimulated cycles to promote oocyte maturation, induce ovulation, and allow appropriate corpus luteum formation and function.

Therapy with hMG is most successful in patients with hypogonadotropic hypogonadism, with cumulative pregnancy rates of 91.2% after six treatment cycles of hMG alone (131). In patients with other indications for ovulation induction with gonadotropins, cumulative pregnancy rates of 50% were achieved after 12 treatment cycles (131). In clinical practice, however, other treatment modalities are usually selected after 3–6 unsuccessful cycles of hMG therapy. The two most important adverse effects of hMG therapy are ovarian hyperstimulation syndrome and multiple gestation. Both of these phenomena have significant long-term sequelae that must be discussed in detail with patients before the outset of therapy.

Ovarian hyperstimulation syndrome is a completely iatrogenic disease with an incompletely described physiology. It may present with varying degrees of severity; its onset typically comes 7–12 days after the administration of hCG. Mild hyperstimulation, characterized by ovarian enlargement and minimal symptoms, is seen in 8.4–23% of stimulated cycles. Moderate hyperstimulation occurs in 6–7% of cycles and severe hyperstimulation in 0.8–2% (132). Severe ovarian hyperstimulation syndrome can be a devastating disorder,

937

with significant ovarian enlargement, ascites, pleural effusions, hemoconcentration and hypercoagulability, ovarian torsion or rupture, severe electrolyte disturbances, seizures, respiratory compromise, renal failure, and even death.

The incidence of *multiple gestation* is reported to vary from 11 to 44%, most of which are twin pregnancies, among patients treated with gonadotropins for ovulation induction (133). Multifetal pregnancy reduction is presently a viable, safe, and effective option for patients with high-order multiple pregnancies (134); however, the choice to terminate a pregnancy for a patient with longstanding infertility may be emotionally harrowing. Use of hMG does not appear to be associated with an increased incidence of spontaneous abortion (135) or fetal malformation (129), but it is linked to an increase in rates of ectopic pregnancy (136).

As with ovulation induction with *clomiphene citrate,* ovulation induction with hMG must be determined on an individual basis. Multiple regimens have been proposed, and a typical treatment regimen is as follows:

1. Patients begin therapy 2, 3, or 4 days after the onset of a spontaneous or induced menses.

2. Patients with evidence of endogenous estrogenic activity begin therapy by taking 1 or 2 ampules of hMG (75–150 IU) per day; those with hypogonadotropic hypogonadism take 1 ampule per day.

3. The daily dosage is maintained until cycle day 6 or 7, when the serum estradiol level is measured to document ovarian response.

4. If no such response has occurred, the hMG dosage is increased by 1 or 2 ampules per day every 3 or 4 days until a response is evidenced by rising estradiol levels or until a protocol-determined maximal dosage is reached.

5. Once an ovarian response is obtained, treatment is typically continued without a further increase in dose.

6. Vaginal ultrasonography and serum estradiol measurements are performed every 2 or 3 days to evaluate follicular size, number, and quality. Follicular development is believed to be adequate when maximal follicular diameter exceeds 16–18 mm, with a corresponding serum estradiol level of 150–250 pg/ml per mature follicle. Serum estradiol levels associated with adequate folliculogenesis and oocyte maturation vary with follicular number and are laboratory specific but should be >600 pg/ml and should not exceed 1500–2000 pg/ml.

7. When appropriate follicular size and estradiol levels have been attained, 5000–10,000 IU of hCG is administered intramuscularly. Ovulation is expected 36 hours later, so timing of intercourse or insemination may be planned accordingly. The targeted window for completion of folliculogenesis is approximately 10–15 days.

In the absence of conception, the hMG dosage for subsequent cycles may be modified to improve the response documented in previous cycles.

In an attempt to both improve pregnancy rates and lower the significant costs and adverse effects of ovulation induction with hMG, alternative regimens consisting of combination or substitute medications have been proposed. Combination therapy with *clomiphene citrate* and hMG for ovulation induction has been termed "minimal stimulation." Initial study of the use of minimal stimulation protocols for ART has shown promise, with no difference in rates of pregnancy, implantation, or cancellation but a significant decrease in cost when compared with conventional hMG protocols (137). Ovulation induction protocols entailing the addition of growth hormone to the hMG regimen in patients with a poor response to hMG alone have recently received much attention. The efficacy rates of growth hormone use have not been consistent (138, 139).

Patients with polycystic ovarian (PCO) syndrome in whom therapy with *clomiphene citrate* fails present a very difficult management problem. These patients tend to be either unresponsive or hyperresponsive to gonadotropin therapy and have a correspondingly increased incidence of multiple pregnancy and ovarian hyperstimulation syndrome (140). Use of GnRH agonists has been proposed as potentially beneficial in the treatment of infertile patients with PCO syndrome because the downregulation of the hypothalamic-pituitary-ovarian axis blocks the hormonal feedback loops involved in the disorder. The use of GnRH agonists in the absence of ovulation induction in PCO patients has been associated with the resumption of spontaneous ovulation (141). Treatment with GnRH agonists in conjunction with hMG ovulation induction has not been consistently associated with improved rates of pregnancy (141, 142) but has been related to decreased rates of spontaneous abortion (143).

Purified human FSH (*Metrodin*) has also been isolated from human urine and is presently being used by some practitioners in place of hMG for ovulation induction. Purified preparations contain <1 IU of LH and 75 IU of FSH. Ovulation requires the presence of both FSH and LH; thus, patients with hypogonadotropic hypogonadism, who have minimal endogenous LH, typically are not appropriate candidates for induction of ovulation with purified FSH. Most studies investigating purified FSH for ovulation induction have concentrated on its use in infertile patients with PCO syndrome. Because the secretion of LH is inappropriately elevated in these patients, the use of purified FSH to reduce alteration in the LH/FSH ratio seems logical. In fact, purified FSH has been used successfully for ovulation induction in patients with PCO syndrome (144), although pregnancy rates may be lower than with standard hMG therapy (145). Most recently, recombinant FSH has been utilized successfully for ovulation induction (146).

Pulsatile GnRH Therapy

Patients with hypothalamic failure and subsequent ovulatory factor infertility are the best candidates for ovulation induction with GnRH. To mimic physiologic hypothalamic-pituitary interactions, GnRH must be administered in a pulsatile fashion, avoiding downregulation and associated hypothalamic-pituitary-ovarian downregulation. Because GnRH is rapidly degraded and thus ineffective when administered orally, pulsatile GnRH is administered either intravenously or subcutaneously with a mini-pump delivery system. Adverse effects of pulsatile GnRH therapy are mainly related to pump function and route of delivery (i.e., phlebitis at the needle site). It is therefore recommended that women with a history of bacterial endocarditis be offered only subcutaneous therapy.

Normal pituitary negative and positive feedback mechanisms remain intact in patients treated with pulsatile GnRH. In this situation, pulsatile GnRH offers some advantages over hMG as treatment for ovulatory infertility. More than two dominant follicles are seen in 18.9% of patients with hypogonadotropic infertility who are treated with pulsatile GnRH and more than three follicles are seen in only 5.4% of patients (147). Because hyperstimulation is a rare occurrence, less intensive monitoring is required during treatment cycles. Moreover, the risk of multiple pregnancies is similar to that associated with *clomiphene citrate* therapy—approximately 8% (147). Cumulative pregnancy rates among women with hypothalamic hypogonadotropism approach 80% after six treatment cycles and 93% after 12 cycles (148). There appears to be no increase in the rate of spontaneous abortion with pulsatile GnRH therapy (149). The association of a lower incidence of ovarian hyperstimulation with pulsatile GnRH therapy than with hMG therapy led to trials of GnRH induction of ovulation in patients with polycystic ovary syndrome. Using prior GnRH agonist downregulation in conjunction with pulsatile GnRH therapy, Filicori et al. (150) documented a cumulative pregnancy rate of 60% in such patients.

Various regimens of pulsatile GnRH have been investigated. A recent review of these studies concludes that 1) the intravenous route is superior to the subcutaneous route, 2) the best dosing interval is 60–90 minutes, and 3) the optimal dosage is 75 ng/kg/pulse (151). With typical regimens of pulsatile GnRH, ovulation occurs on day 14 and can be documented by standard LH testing. Patients treated with pulsatile GnRH usually benefit from luteal-phase support through continuation of the GnRH pump, administration of hCG, or progesterone supplementation.

Bromocriptine and Dexamethasone Supplementation

In selected patients with ovulatory factor infertility, the addition of *bromocriptine* or *dexamethasone* to standard ovulation-induction regimens may be of benefit. Hyperprolactinemia can be associated with ovulatory factor infertility. Correction of the hyperprolactinemic state with *bromocriptine* is followed by restoration of ovulation in 90% of patients (152). More controversial is the use of *bromocriptine* alone or the addition of *bromocriptine* to *clomiphene citrate* therapy in patients with normal or minimally elevated prolactin levels. Such therapy has been associated with improved pregnancy rates among normoprolactinemic women with unexplained infertility and galactorrhea (153).

The addition of *dexamethasone* to ovulation induction regimens for women with hyperandrogenism and ovulatory factor infertility is less controversial. Glucocorticoid administration suppresses adrenally derived androgens in women with or without hyperandrogenism. Rates of ovulation and pregnancy with the addition of *dexamethasone* to *clomiphene citrate* regimens than with standard *clomiphene citrate* treatment among patients with elevated serum levels of dehydroepiandrosterone sulfate (>200 mg/dl) (154) and among patients with polycystic ovary syndrome (155). A standard glucocorticoid-*clomiphene citrate* regimen uses 0.5 mg of *dexamethasone* taken at bedtime each day beginning either in the follicular phase of the *clomiphene citrate* treatment cycle or in the luteal phase cycle preceding the outset of *clomiphene citrate* therapy. Treatment is continued until menses or pregnancy occurs. *Dexamethasone* therapy at this dosage is associated with minimal adverse effects.

Surgical Treatment

The pathophysiologic changes in the polycystic ovary have been the subject of many years of intense investigation. As early as 1935, with the initial description of the syndrome, ovarian surgical treatment was considered (156). Initial surgical management involved ovarian wedge resection in an effort to reduce the volume of androgen-producing tissue and thereby alleviate hyperandrogenic abnormalities. In fact, ovarian wedge resection does decrease circulating levels of testosterone (157) and is associated with a resumption of menses in 91% of patients (158). Unfortunately, many patients suffer from postoperative adhesions leading to iatrogenic tubal factor infertility (158, 159). Practitioners have attempted to perform partial ovarian tissue destruction without significant postoperative adhesion formation by using laparoscopic methods such as ovarian wedge resection, ovarian electrocautery, ovarian diathermy, and ovarian laser vaporization.

Laparoscopic techniques appear to be associated with less pelvic adhesion formation than is noted after ovarian wedge resection by laparotomy (160, 161) and seem to result in similar improvements in hormonal profile (162, 163). Compared with controls, patients undergoing laparoscopic ovarian tissue destruction have higher rates of ovulation and lower resistance to standard ovulation induction agents (164, 165). Improved pregnancy rates are also reported for this difficult-to-treat population (165). No single laparoscopic technique has proven unequivocally superior.

Luteal Phase Defect

The diagnosis and significance of LPD in infertile patients are controversial. Nevertheless, there are well-described therapeutic modalities to address LPD. The efficacy of such treatment depends on the importance the disorder plays in infertility. The two most commonly

940

employed treatments for LPD are luteal phase progesterone supplementation and follicular phase clomiphene citrate use.

Luteal-phase progesterone can be administered by either intramuscular injection or vaginal suppository. Treatment regimens vary, but most begin on the third day after the mid-cycle temperature rise or on the second or third day after the onset of the LH surge. It is administered in dosages of 25–50 mg twice a day for vaginal suppositories and 50–100 mg each day for intramuscular injection. Some practitioners administer progesterone through approximately 10 weeks of gestation; others terminate supplementation with the first positive pregnancy test. Pregnancy rates in studies of progesterone treatment for LPD are 50–80% (166); however, many of these studies are small and poorly controlled.

Clomiphene citrate has also been used successfully in the treatment of LPD with regimens similar to those used for ovulation induction (59). This agent is given orally at a dosage of 50 mg/day on days 5–9 of the menstrual cycle. Endometrial biopsy is performed in the late luteal phase of the treatment cycle to assess efficacy, and the dosage is increased by 50 mg/day per cycle until LPD correction is noted. The maximal dosage is typically 150–250 mg/day. Use of *clomiphene citrate* has been shown to be as effective as progesterone supplementation in therapy for LPD (167, 168). Ironically, *clomiphene citrate* may also cause LPD when used for ovulation induction (169). Luteal phase support is often used in IVF/GIFT and zygote intrafallopian tubal transfer (ZIFT) procedures.

Tubal and Peritoneal Factor

As success rates continue to improve for ART, the indications for surgical therapy for tubal factor infertility may become increasingly limited, but various approaches to tubal infertility remain important. Therapy for tubal factor infertility is entirely surgical and includes correction of periadnexal disease; correction of proximal, distal, or combined tubal disease; and correction of iatrogenic tubal abnormalities (e.g., tubal sterilization). Treatment of periadnexal disease—via both laparotomy (170) and laparoscopy (171)—has been proven effective in the management of tubal factor patients. Adhesion prevention is integral to the treatment of adhesive periadnexal disease. The relative value of laparotomy versus laparoscopy for the treatment of tubal infertility and the respective effects of these methods on postoperative adhesion formation have received considerable attention. In a recent study comparing laparoscopy and laparotomy for the treatment of ectopic pregnancy, adhesion formation occurred more frequently after laparotomy, even when meticulous technique was maintained during all procedures (172). Many other adjuncts for postoperative adhesion prevention have been proposed, including the use of anti-inflammatory agents, barrier agents, fibrinolytic substances, and anticoagulants. No data have revealed consistent significant improvement with these other methods. Thus, careful hemostatic surgical technique and judicious use of the laparoscopic approach are generally recommended for the treatment of tubal factor infertility.

Proximal Tubal Occlusion   Treatment of proximal tubal occlusion has received much recent attention. However, success rates for corrective procedures can be difficult to confirm because diagnosis of proximal tubal obstruction by hysterosalpingography is notoriously inaccurate. Until the mid-1970s, tubal implantation was considered the standard of care for proximal tubal obstruction. Since that time, tubocornual anastomosis has become the preferred technique and has shown notable improvement in outcome (173). Rates of term pregnancy after tubocornual reanastomosis have reached 44% in some series (174). Adhesion formation after pelvic surgery has led some investigators to explore methods of correcting proximal tubal occlusion with techniques that avoid peritoneal entry. These minimally invasive transcervical techniques may involve the use of ultrasonography, fluoroscopy, hysteroscopy, or recanalization falloposcopy. A postoperative pregnancy rate of 31% has been reported for fluoroscopic recanalization (175), and a 34% clinical pregnancy rate has been noted after transcervical balloon tuboplasty (176).

Distal Tubal Occlusion   **Treatment of distal tubal disease involves surgical correction via fimbrioplasty or neosalpingostomy.** By definition, fimbrioplasty is the lysis of fimbrial adhesions or dilatation of fimbrial phimosis, whereas neosalpingostomy involves the creation of a new tubal opening in an occluded fallopian tube (177). Distal tubal disease can be treated with conventional microsurgical techniques, although laparoscopic management can be equally efficacious. The resurgence of the minilaparotomy in gynecologic surgery, however, has called this practice into question. Recent evidence suggests that neosalpingostomy can be performed via laparotomy with very brief postoperative hospital stays (<24 hours) and subsequent pregnancy rates equivalent to those obtained with laparoscopic management (178).

Regardless of the method used, the efficacy of neosalpingostomy or fimbrioplasty as treatment for distal tubal occlusion rests largely on the extent of tubal and peritubal disease, as assessed by hysterosalpingography and laparoscopy. **The poor prognostic factors for a successful pregnancy after neosalpingostomy include hydrosalpinx >30 mm in diameter, absence of visible fimbriae, and dense pelvic or adnexal adhesions** (179). The appearance of the tubal mucosa has added prognostic significance for the fertility outcome of laparoscopic tuboplasty for distal tubal occlusion (180). In one study, laparoscopic distal tuboplasty has produced an overall pregnancy rate of 27% and an ectopic pregnancy rate of 4.5% among 44 patients (181). Fimbrioplasty appeared to be more successful than neosalpingostomy; however, the choice of surgery may have been influenced by the extent of disease. **Patients with both proximal and distal tubal disease represent the poorest candidates for surgical management of infertility.** Studies of surgical treatment for these patients have had small numbers of patients but have universally yielded dismal results (182). This select group of patients should benefit most from IVF.

Sterilization Reversal   **Approximately 0.2% of women who chose surgical tubal sterilization will request reversal procedures** (183, 184). The success of tubal reanastomosis is dependent on the method of sterilization, the site of anastomosis, and the presence of other infertility factors. **Pregnancy rates are lowest (49%) after the reversal of sterilization procedures involving unipolar electrocautery.** In contrast, pregnancy rates are 67% when the mode of sterilization uses the Fallope ring or spring-loaded clip and 75% after Pomeroy tubal ligation. The prognosis is best when anastomotic sites had no significant discrepancy in diameter (e.g., isthmic-isthmic or cornual-isthmic anastomoses). Fimbriectomy cases were excluded from this study; however, pregnancy rates higher than 40% have been reported after microsurgical fimbriectomy correction (185). Tubal length is an important prognostic consideration: final anastomosed tubal lengths of less than 4 cm are associated with low pregnancy rates (186). Laparoscopy is often utilized before laparotomy and microsurgical fallopian tubal reanastomosis to assess surgical prognostic factors such as potential final tubal length, site of reanastomosis, method of sterilization (if not previously known), and presence or absence of associated pelvic pathology. Those patients with the poorest prognosis should not undergo surgical reanastomosis and may be more appropriate candidates for IVF. Finally, some practitioners are performing tubal anastomoses after sterilization entirely through the laparoscope, with postprocedure pregnancy rates of 50% (187). Studies of animals are underway to examine the use of fibrin glue in lieu of sutures for tubal reanastomoses (188).

Peritoneal Factor   Peritoneal factor infertility and tubal factor infertility often occur concurrently, and the approaches to their treatment are similar. Like tubal adhesions, peritoneal adhesions may be the result of pelvic inflammatory processes or abdominal or pelvic surgical procedures. If significant peritoneal adhesive disease is believed to be affecting tubal motility or the access of ova to tubal fimbriae, microsurgical adhesiolysis is the treatment of choice. The other major cause of peritoneal factor infertility not discussed under tubal disorders is endometriosis. Data on the treatment of endometriosis-associated infertility show that there is no conclusive evidence that minimal or mild endometriosis causes infertility (189). The role of more severe endometriosis may be largely related to accompanying adhesive disease. In a recent review of the literature on the treatment of endometriosis-associated infertility (190), the following conclusions and general recommendations can be made:

1. Suppression of ovulation with *danazol, gestrinone, medroxyprogesterone acetate,* GnRH agonists, and oral contraceptive pills is not effective for this indication; further trials evaluating their efficacy are unwarranted.

2. Laparoscopic destruction of endometriotic implants may be effective; larger, well-designed trials are warranted to determine the effectiveness of this procedure.

3. *Danazol* therapy does not improve upon the results derived from laparoscopy alone.

4. Conservative surgical therapy via laparotomy may be of benefit, particularly in cases of severe endometriosis, but further studies are mandatory.

5. *Danazol* therapy offers no advantages over conservative laparotomy alone.

Cervical Factor Infertility

Anatomic patency and the production of adequate amounts of hospitable mucus are the two cervical characteristics necessary for normal reproduction. Treatment of cervical factor infertility is directed to abnormalities in these areas. A history of exposure to DES, previous cone biopsy or cauterization of the cervix, congenital anomalies, cervicitis, anovulation, and use of *clomiphene citrate* for ovulation induction are all associated with the potential for cervical stenosis or poor mucus quality (191). The presence of antisperm antibodies in cervical mucus is likewise associated with poor sperm-cervical mucus interactions.

Abnormalities not amenable to surgical therapy may be bypassed by IUI alone or by ovulation induction combined with IVF, GIFT, or ZIFT. If inhospitable cervical mucus is associated with cervicitis, cervical cultures for bacteria such as *Chlamydia trachomatous* and *Neisseria gonorrhoea* should be performed, along with evaluations for yeast infection, bacterial vaginosis, and trichomoniasis. Specific therapy for diagnosed conditions should lead to improved sperm survival and transport through the cervix. Anovulation, with its associated high progesterone:estrogen ratio, is associated with inhospitable cervical mucus. It follows, therefore, that ovulation induction should reverse poor cervical mucus parameters. Ovulation induction with either hMG (192) or pure FSH (193) has been reported to ameliorate mucus hostility and possibly enhance fecundity in patients with cervical factor infertility. *Clomiphene citrate,* in contrast, appears to exert primarily antiestrogenic effects on the cervical mucus, and its use is associated with a worsening of cervical mucus status (194).

The treatment of antisperm antibodies in cervical mucus is a topic of considerable controversy (see Chapter 28). Both ART and IUI have been suggested as potentially beneficial in patients with antisperm antibodies, but relevant data remain inconclusive (195, 196). Similarly, although IUI is widely practiced for cervical factor infertility in the absence of humoral immunity abnormalities, data on subsequent fertility rates are inconsistent (112).

Uterine Factor

Treatment of uterine factor infertility is predominantly surgical. Traditionally, therapy for intrauterine polyps and leiomyomas has been performed hysteroscopically, although some pedunculated submucous fibroids and intrauterine polyps may be removed in the physician's office. The role of these abnormalities in uterine factor infertility and the mechanism through which they operate have been questioned; however, restoration of normal intrauterine anatomy prior to ART is routine practice (75). Postoperative hormonal supplementation may be employed for adhesion prevention in cases of extensive intrauterine resection. Intramural leiomyomas of the uterus have also been reported to be associated with infertility, although the mechanism of this relationship is even more tenuous than that of intrauterine neoplasms. A recent reevaluation of abdominal myomectomy in patients with uterine fibroids and otherwise unexplained infertility supports this procedure as an effective therapeutic measure (197). This treatment, however, remains controversial. Patients undergoing myomectomy as infertility therapy are encouraged to attempt pregnancy as soon as is appropriate after surgery.

Prenatal exposure to diethylstilbestrol has been linked to an increased incidence of müllerian tract abnormalities, and both DES exposure and müllerian anomalies have been linked to infertility (198–200). Treatment of müllerian anomalies necessitates surgery; thus, the relationship between this uterine characteristic and infertility needs close critical evaluation. Reports addressing the role of uterine anomalies in subfertility have been questioned, and it is generally held that surgery is rarely indicated for the treatment of infertility in affected patients (201–202). A much clearer association exists between recurrent fetal wastage and müllerian tract anomalies such as septate uteri. Hysteroscopic resection of septate uteri is appropriate treatment.

In some third world countries, tuberculous endometritis may be the cause of uterine factor infertility (203). Tuberculous endometritis differs from most other types of chronic bacterial or viral endometritis in that its treatment is followed by low pregnancy rates (204). Fibrotic endometritis, commonly known as Asherman's syndrome, can follow tuberculous endometritis but is typically iatrogenic. The first description of this condition in 1948 noted an association with infertility that has since been confirmed (205). Intrauterine synechiae can be treated with lysis of adhesions via either dilation and curettage or hysteroscopic resection. Postsurgical therapy with estrogen is often employed to help prevent the reformation of scar tissue. A typical regimen consists of *conjugated estrogen* at a dosage of 2.5 mg/day for 1–2 months. To prevent adhesions, some practitioners insert an intrauterine device or an intrauterine pediatric Foley catheter to be retained for 1 week postoperatively. Treatment of intrauterine synechiae can yield very satisfying results; pregnancy rates above 80% have been reported among patients with mild to moderate disease (206). As with müllerian tract anomalies, a strong association exists between Asherman's syndrome and recurrent fetal wastage.

Unexplained Infertility

In the treatment of unexplained infertility, it is essential to consider the rate of spontaneous pregnancy among untreated patients with this diagnosis. This point is not insignificant: up to 65% of "normal" infertile patients will become pregnant during 3 years of expectant management (207). Reports of efficacious therapy for unexplained infertility, therefore, must be examined closely for appropriate control populations and study design. Of the multiple empiric therapies that have been tried, the most often used and potentially helpful include ovulation induction with or without IUI, IUI alone, and ART (particularly GIFT).

Both *clomiphene citrate* and hMG have been used in empiric treatment of unexplained infertility. *Clomiphene citrate* alone (208) and in conjunction with IUI (209) have been associated with improved pregnancy rates; hMG, however, is more often used. Used alone, IUI alone has not been consistently associated with improvement in pregnancy rates for patients with unexplained infertility (210), but the addition of hMG ovulation induction to IUI does appear to provide consistently superior results (211, 212). ART, including standard IVF, ZIFT, and GIFT, have also been used successfully in the treatment of unexplained infertility (213–215). One study comparing GIFT with controlled ovarian hyperstimulation (COH) alone in patients with unexplained infertility demonstrated no difference in pregnancy rates (216). This result suggests that the effectiveness of ART regimens may rest mainly on the use of ovulation induction.

Assisted Reproductive Technologies

Assisted reproductive technologies include IVF, GIFT, ZIFT, use donor oocytes, and cryopreserved embryo transfers. The success rates of these techniques are summarized in Table 27.5.

944

Table 27.5   Comparison of Reported Outcomes for All ART Procedures

	IVF	GIFT	ZIFT	Donor*	Cryopreserved Embryo Transfers[†]
Cycles/procedures[‡]	29,404	5,767	1,993	1,802	5,354
Cancellation (%)	15.4	16.2	15.0	5.2	NA[§]
Retrievals	24,996	4,837	1,696	1,708	NA
Transfers	21,870	4,712	1,497	1,699	5,354
Transfers per retrieval (%)	87.5	97.4	88.3	99.4	NA
Pregnancies	5,279	1,621	488	625	820
Pregnancy loss (%)	20.0	16.9	21.1	14.9	23.8
Deliveries	4,206	1,273	386	534	619
Deliveries per retrieval (%)	16.8	26.7	22.8	31.3	NA
Singleton (%)	67.3	67.3	64.2	63.3	77.9
Ectopic pregnancy	272	61	20	14	32
Ectopic per transfer (%)	1.2	1.3	1.3	0.8	0.6
Birth defects per neonates delivered (%)	1.9	2.4	2.5	1.7	1.3

*Donor includes known or anonymous, but not surrogate.
[†]Cryopreserved embryo transfer cycles not done in combination with fresh Embryo Transfers and not with donor egg/embryo.
[‡]Includes all cycles, regardless of age or diagnosis.
[§]NA, not available.
||Birth defect reporting did not account for all neonatal outcomes.
Reproduced with permission from **American Fertility Society, Society for Assisted Reproductive Technology.** Assisted reproductive technology in the United States and Canada: 1992 results generated from the American Fertility Society/Society for Assisted Reproductive Technology Registry. *Fertil Steril* 1994;62:1121–8.

In unassisted ovulation, the cohort of follicles destined to begin folliculogenesis in any particular menstrual cycle are recruited in the previous cycle's luteal phase. By approximately the middle of the next follicular phase, one of these follicles becomes dominant, and further development of this dominant follicle suppresses maturation of other follicles in the selected cohort. Follicular-phase growth of a single dominant follicle in nonstimulated cycles induces an intricate series of hormonally regulated feedback loops, resulting in the midcycle LH surge and ovulation. Because hCG is structurally similar to and has a longer half-life than LH, its use in gonadotropin stimulation of ovulation is now standard. Gonadotropin-releasing hormone agonists have also been used as a substitute for hCG in inducing follicular maturation and triggering ovulation (217).

Gonadotropins

Gonadotropins (hMG or purified FSH) are presently the standard agents used for the induction of ovulation for ART. Their use overrides physiologic ovarian-hypothalamic-pituitary feedback and follicular suppression, allowing multiple follicles to develop simultaneously in the stimulated cycle. The goal of controlled ovarian hyperstimulation with gonadotropins is to obtain mature oocytes in high numbers and thereby improve the likelihood of obtaining adequate numbers of embryos for subsequent transfer. At times, additional embryos may remain after an appropriate number have been transferred. These embryos can be cryopreserved for use in future nonstimulated cycles, and the overall cost of ART per pregnancy can thus be reduced.

The removal of granulosa cells during aspiration of each developing follicle is believed to lower risk of ovarian hyperstimulation syndrome among patients treated with gonadotropin stimulation plus intercourse or insemination (218). Thus, higher serum estradiol levels and larger follicular sizes are typically allowed prior to hCG administration. Still, even with ART, increases in the number of follicles, in follicular size, and in serum estradiol levels are associated with ovarian hyperstimulation syndrome (219). Reasonable parameters must therefore be established for the timing of hCG administration, even when follicular aspiration is to be undertaken. In general, **10,000 USP units of hCG are administered when at least two follicles have reached an average diameter of 18 mm (as documented by ultrasound) and estradiol levels are >600 pg/ml.** In certain cases, these parameters may be exceeded, but this precaution should be taken to avoid ovarian hyperstimulation and close clinical follow-up is required.

GnRH Agonists

The addition of GnRH agonists to ovulation induction regimens for ART is now common. The major advantage consists of the downregulation of the physiologic hypothalamic-pituitary-ovarian feedback mechanisms and the subsequent effective suppression of spontaneous ovulation. The result should be the elimination of premature follicular luteinization and the cancellation of ART cycles secondary to premature ovulation (spontaneous ovulation prior to oocyte retrieval).

Protocols   Many regimens have been suggested for the administration of GnRH agonists in gonadotropin-stimulated cycles (Fig. 27.5):

1. The *ultra-long protocol,* with long-term suppression via depot agents prior to stimulation

2. The *long protocol,* with treatment beginning in the previous luteal phase

Figure 27.5   Ovulation induction: regimens for the administration of GnRH agonists in gonadotropin-stimulated cycles.

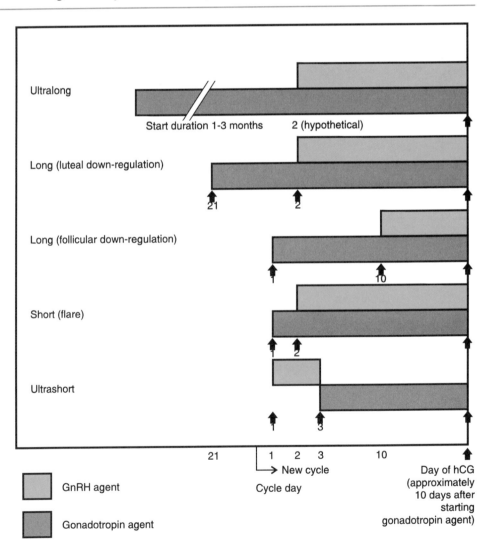

3. The *short protocol,* in which treatment begins just before or simultaneously with the initiation of gonadotropin stimulation in the follicular phase (flare)

4. The *ultra-short protocol,* in which GnRH agonist is given for only 3 days at the beginning of the follicular phase

5. The *follicular-phase protocol,* in which downregulation begins in the follicular phase of the cycle prior to gonadotropin stimulation

Efficacy   In a meta-analysis reviewing the efficacy of various GnRH agonist regimens, the authors concluded that the addition of GnRH agonist downregulation to ovulation induction regimens for ART was advantageous (220). Improvement in pregnancy rates and a decrease in cancellation rates without an associated increase in spontaneous abortion rates were noted. No single GnRH agonist regimen was shown conclusively to be superior to the others. One additional significant difference between the ovulation induction protocols for IUI and intercourse and those for ART is the common use of luteal phase support in the latter. Following are two typical regimens:

1. The intramuscular administration of hCG (2500 IU) every 3 days for three doses, beginning 5 days after the ovulatory dose of hCG

2. The intramuscular administration of progesterone (100 mg/day) for 14 days, beginning the evening after embryo transfer

In vivo fertilization of the human oocyte by human sperm requires the interaction of capacitated spermatozoa with ovulated oocytes and most often occurs in the ampullary portion of the fallopian tube. Under the influence of incompletely described factors, capacitation of sperm naturally takes place in the female reproductive tract and involves changes in the sperm cell membrane that allow the acrosome reaction as well as changes in sperm motility. Acrosome-reacted sperm are able to penetrate the oocyte's cumulus oophorus and zona pellucida, binding to the cell membrane and promoting fertilization. The interaction of spermatozoa and oocyte is now believed to be more than a chance occurrence, with complex oocyte-sperm intercommunication playing an important role in the process (221).

Reproductive endocrinologists attempt to recreate precisely the processes known to occur in unassisted conception. For all ART procedures, semen specimens are collected via masturbation, processed, and incubated in protein-supplemented media for 3–4 hours prior to use for fertilization. This incubation allows for sperm capacitation. Before fertilization, retrieved oocytes are cultured in protein-supplemented media for approximately 6–8 hours. For IVF purposes, 50,000–100,000 capacitated sperm are placed in culture with a single oocyte; 16–18 hours later, fertilization is documented by the presence of two pronuclei within the developing embryo. One advantage of most ART procedures is the opportunity they afford to assess a patient's fertilizing capability. A single failure must not be viewed as an immediate indication for therapeutic change. Many patients experiencing such an initial failure have no difficulties in subsequent cycles (222).

Micromanipulation

Until recently, patients in whom ART failed more than twice had few remaining therapeutic options. Such couples with male-factor infertility or with semen parameters too poor to permit IVF (i.e., <1 million total motile sperm) can now be referred for micromanipulation. Micromanipulation is a broad term encompassing a number of prefertilization gamete-processing techniques, most of which are intended to enhance fertilization capability. These techniques include assisted hatching, partial zona dissection, zona drilling, subzonal sperm injection, and intracytoplasmic sperm injection. Of these modalities, the last has proven most effective for the treatment of severe male-factor infertility and of previous fertilization failure. Intracytoplasmic sperm injection involves the direct insertion of a single sperm cell into the cytoplasm of a single oocyte by micropuncture. Because only a single spermatozoon is required, even very poor quality specimens, including those obtained after epididymal aspiration, may be used successfully. Van Steirteghem et al. report fertilization rates of 61% and clinical pregnancy rates of 31% (223).

In unassisted conception, the fertilized oocyte must make its way through the major portion of the fallopian tube and into the uterus for implantation. This transport is largely dependent on directional ciliary movement within the fallopian tube, although tubal muscular contractions may be involved. Transport through the tube requires approximately 2–3 days (224). The embryo reaches the uterine cavity when it is at the morular or early blastocyst stage of development. By this time, the endometrium has undergone decidual changes under the influence of luteal-phase levels of progesterone and is thereby prepared for implantation. In a 28-day cycle, the period of maximal endometrial receptivity is from cycle day 16 to cycle day 19 (225). The embryo resides in the intrauterine cavity for 2–3 days and during this period loses its zona pellucida—an event that allows implantation. Implantation typically begins 5–7 days after fertilization.

With assisted reproduction, fertilized embryos typically remain in culture for a total of 48 hours after oocyte retrieval. In an attempt to more closely simulate physiologic conditions, a prolonged pretransfer culture period and alternative culture conditions have been investigated. For example, some ART programs are now supporting a 72-hour embryo culture period after oocyte retrieval and prior to transfer. A serum-free medium has been developed for this purpose, with initial results suggesting improved implantation rates (226). Similarly, in an effort to recreate the fallopian tubal microenvironment, other researchers have investigated the growth of embryos in coculture with a monolayer of fallopian tubal cells prior to transfer. Improved pregnancy rates have been reported with such coculture techniques (227).

The period of *in vitro* embryo culture is now recognized as an important window for embryonic evaluation by micromanipulation. One application of embryonic micromanipulation that has received a significant amount of attention is preimplantation genetic diagnosis, in which one or more blastomeres are removed from the developing embryo at the blastocyst stage. DNA is extracted from these cells and analyzed for the presence of chromosomal abnormalities. At present, genetic analysis allows the detection of numerous X-linked and autosomal disorders. Detection is limited only by the molecular geneticist's ability to identify and sequence genetic alterations associated with a particular disorder. The clinical application of this technology is important for couples known to carry a genetically transmissible disease. Embryos from these couples may be analyzed, and, if the results for carriage are positive, transfer of the embryos may be deferred. Thus, the couple can avoid the birth of an affected child or the termination of a pregnancy at the time of diagnosis via chorionic villous sampling, amniocentesis, or ultrasonography.

In Vitro Fertilization

The rate of reproductive success decreases with age, regardless of the fertility treatment regimens used. The impact of age is especially pronounced for ART. Patients deemed candidates for IVF include those with primary indications and those in whom alternative (and often less costly and less invasive) therapies have failed. Some authorities propose that the primary indications for IVF may now include nearly all infertility diagnoses. Certainly, patients with no fallopian tubes or with previous tubal damage and a poor prognosis for effective repair are candidates for primary IVF. Some patients with prior tubal sterilization may also be served best by primary referral for IVF. Patients who fail to conceive within 18 months after tubal repair are appropriate candidates for ART. Patients in whom three to six cycles of ovulation induction in combination with inseminations have failed should be offered ART.

IVF Protocol   A typical protocol for standard IVF is as follows:

1. GnRH agonist downregulation is performed prior to ovulation induction with gonadotropins.

2. Follicular maturation and ovulation are effected with combined hMG/hCG administration.

3. Oocyte retrieval is performed transvaginally, under ultrasonographic guidance.

4. Analgesia for oocyte retrieval is provided on an individualized basis but most commonly involves intravenous sedation or spinal nerve block.

5. Embryo transfer is undertaken 48 hours after oocyte retrieval, when most embryos have reached the four- to six-cell stage. For standard IVF procedures, transfer is accomplished via transcervical cannulation and injection of embryos into the intrauterine cavity.

6. Luteal phase support is provided until menses or pregnancy is documented. The initial evaluation for pregnancy during IVF cycles consists of quantitative β-hCG measurement 16 days after embryo transfer.

Embryo Transfer   The number and selection of embryos to transfer are difficult decisions. The assessment of embryo quality has been the subject of intense investigation and considerable controversy. At present, morphologic criteria, including such parameters as cell number, symmetry, fragmentation, and granularity, are utilized in most centers. This method of embryo quality assessment, however, is inadequate for the detection of developmental potential (228). The overall pregnancy rate and the incidence of multiple gestation depend on the number of embryos transferred (typically, four to eight) (229). The lack of association with pregnancy at more than four transferred embryos may reflect a tendency to transfer more embryos when embryo quality is poor. In view of the increase in the rate of success and complications with increasing numbers of transferred embryos, it is incumbent on the reproductive endocrinologist to balance and discuss these factors when counseling patients prior to embryo transfer. The increase in maternal morbidity with high-order multiple gestation and the psychosocial (and often ethical) dilemma presented by selective reduction have led countries such as Great Britain to mandate that no more than three embryos be transferred.

The success of modern ovulation induction and fertilization regimens allows the creation of embryos in excess of the number appropriate for transfer in a single cycle. Cryopreservation of these embryos permits embryo transfer to the same patient in future nonstimulated cycles. Some patients receive cryopreserved embryos during "natural" cycles; others undergo endometrial preparation with sequential exogenous estrogen and progesterone. Either regimen is significantly less expensive than a gonadotropin-stimulated cycle. Therefore, pregnancies resulting from transfer of a cryopreserved embryo effectively reduce the cost of pregnancy per ovulation stimulation.

Success Rates   Success rates for IVF vary from program to program; within a program, the rate of success varies with patients' diagnosis and age. The most accurate assessment of the efficacy of North American ART programs comes from the database of the Society for Assisted Reproductive Technology (Table 27.5). The society's collection of data began in 1985, and its yearly summaries are published in an effort to improve the quality of statistical reporting on ART. The database effectively eliminates the effects of interprogram variation. The most recently published report of the society summarizes the results of ART in the U.S. and Canada for 1992 (230). A 16.8% rate of delivered pregnancies was reported per oocyte retrieval for standard IVF, with a cancellation rate of 15.4%, a pregnancy loss rate of 20%, and an ectopic pregnancy rate of 1.2% per transfer. The delivered-pregnancy rate for cryopreserved embryo transfer was 11.6%. Rates of birth defects were no higher than in the general population. A female older than 40 years of age and male-factor infertility were associated with a decreased rate of treatment success.

949

GIFT/ZIFT/TET

Compared with standard IVF transfer regimens, the transfer of gametes or embryos to the fallopian tube may better mimic physiologic reproductive processes. Techniques such as GIFT, ZIFT, and tubal embryo transfer (TET) all utilize the tubal microenvironment as the initial point of contact after transfer. **Patients considered appropriate candidates for these techniques must have functional fallopian tubes.** As in standard IVF, all regimens typically involve ovulation induction with hMG/hCG after GnRH agonist downregulation. The point at which the techniques first differ is the time of transfer.

For the *GIFT procedure,* oocyte retrieval is performed either transvaginally or laparoscopically and is followed immediately by laparoscopic placement of the recovered oocytes and processed sperm into the fallopian tubes. The disadvantages of GIFT include both the requirement for laparoscopy and the inability to document fertilization prior to gamete transfer. An alternative to the laparoscopic approach is the transcervical placement of gametes into the fallopian tube. Attempts at transcervical GIFT have been plagued by low rates of success and reproducibility (231). Patients selected for primary GIFT who fail to conceive should be assessed to determine their capability of fertilization.

In the *ZIFT procedure,* retrieved oocytes are fertilized and cultured overnight. Zygote-stage embryos are then transferred to the fallopian tubes laparoscopically 24 hours after oocyte retrieval.

Tubal embryo transfer involves either the culture of embryos longer than 24 hours before laparoscopic tubal transfer or the laparoscopic transfer of cryopreserved embryos to the fallopian tubes. All tubal transfer procedures are followed by standard luteal phase support.

Donor Oocytes

Women with ovarian failure have very limited reproductive options. The use of donor oocytes appears to be the sole method by which most of these patients can become pregnant. Other patients appropriate for donor oocyte technology are those with a history of failed fertilization, particularly in association with "oocyte factor" infertility. Donor oocyte programs involving anonymous and directed donors are now available in multiple centers. The most common type of donor oocyte program requires the infertile patient to provide her own fertile donor—typically a sister or friend, but occasionally a volunteer secured by the patient through monetary compensation. Other programs use compensated anonymous volunteers or a combination of anonymous and directed donors.

Screening Oocyte Donors   Like semen donors, potential oocyte donors must be stringently assessed, including for transmissible infectious or genetic diseases. However, unlike semen, oocytes cannot presently be cryopreserved and quarantined, so the risk of transmission of infectious agents may be problematic. Moreover, oocyte donation involves the use of intensive monitoring and of medications with significant potential side effects. Thus, in addition to undergoing medical screening, oocyte donors are provided with detailed educational information and are subjected to a comprehensive psychosocial evaluation before being accepted as program participants. Even with such extensive screening and preparation, there is a significant dropout rate for both anonymous and directed oocyte donors (232). It is advisable to obtain legal counsel in the development of any ovum donation center, as many potentially litigious issues arise in the administration of such a program.

Because oocyte cryopreservation is not generally available, considerable coordination is required if the retrieved donated oocytes are to be fertilized and returned to an appropriately receptive uterus (233). The regimen of ovulation induction and oocyte retrieval for the oocyte donor follows that of standard IVF protocols (Fig. 27.6). The oocyte donor is therefore exposed to some of the adverse effects associated with ovulation induction protocols. To virtually eliminate the risk of ovarian hyperstimulation syndrome, multiple ges-

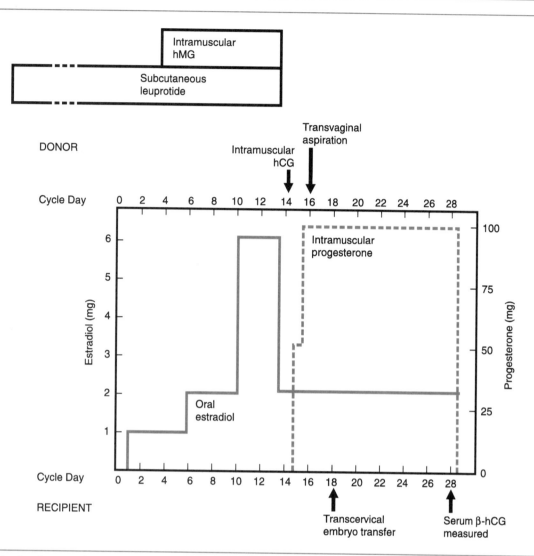

Figure 27.6   Regimens of ovarian stimulation and hormone replacement used to synchronize the development of ovarian follicles in the ooycte donor and the endometrial cycle in the recipient. hMG denotes human menopausal gonadotropin, hCG human chorionic gonadotropin, and β-hCG the beta subunit of hCG.

tation, and ectopic pregnancy, oocyte donors are instructed to either abstain from intercourse or use barrier contraception during their stimulation cycle.

Method of Oocyte Donation   To ensure adequate endometrial preparation, most recipients of donor oocytes are taken through a "mock" cycle prior to the donation cycle. During this cycle, all hormonal agents are administered, and endometrial adequacy is documented by timed endometrial biopsy. Many regimens for endometrial preparation have been described, all of which involve the administration of exogenous estrogen and the addition of supplemental progesterone near the time of embryo transfer. One typical regimen for ovulatory or oligoovulatory patients begins with luteal-phase GnRH agonist downregulation. For patients with ovarian function, estrogen therapy is begun with the onset of menses, and GnRH agonist downregulation is confirmed by the documentation of serum estradiol levels of <50 pg/ml and progesterone levels of <1.0 ng/ml. GnRH agonist treatment is then continued, but at a reduced dose. Patients with ovarian failure begin estrogen therapy without downregulation or hormonal monitoring. All patients first receive transdermal estradiol (*Estraderm,* 0.2 mg every 48 hours or *Estrace* 1.0 mg twice a day). Serum estradiol levels are monitored every 3–7 days, and the estrogen dosage is adjusted to maintain serum levels of 150–300 pg/ml. After approximately 21 days of adequate estrogen treatments, patients who have been taking GnRH agonists stop doing so; at this time, all patients continue to take estrogen and begin treatment with intramuscular injections of progesterone (25 mg for the first injection and 50 mg/day for subsequent injections). Endometrial biopsy to document endometrial adequacy is scheduled 10–12 days after the initiation of progesterone therapy. Regimens used in the actual donor cycle are the same as those used to prepare the endometrium in the mock cycle, except that progesterone treatment is timed to begin on the day of donor egg retrieval. Ovulation induction in the donor is begun only after the recipient has maintained serum estradiol levels higher than 150 pg/ml more than 5 days.

Adoption

One of the most important aspects of the treatment of patients with subfertility or infertility is the process of deciding when no further treatment is indicated. This crucial topic must be addressed early in infertility therapy. Patients must be accurately informed of estimated success rates and reasonable expectations for all therapeutic interventions. It is equally important to identify an end point for intervention at the outset of treatment. This end point offers patients a mental time frame in which they can make both medical and personal decisions. One viable alternative for many couples is adoption. The process of adoption has recently become increasingly complex. Many patients may want to simultaneously explore infertility therapy and adoption. Which course to pursue is a very difficult decision that may be facilitated by both physician input and strong psychosocial counseling and support.

References

1. **Cramer DW, Walker Am, Schiff I.** Statistical methods in evaluating the outcome of infertility therapy. *Fertil Steril* 1979;32:80–6.

2. **Office of Technology Assessment, U.S. Congress.** Infertility: medical and social choices. Publication No. OTA-BA-358. Washington, DC: U.S. Government Printing Office, May 1988.

3. **Wilcox LS, Mosher WD.** Use of infertility services in the United States. *Obstet Gynecol* 1993; 82:122–7.

4. **Mosher WD, Pratt WF.** The demography of infertility in the United States. In: **Asch RH, Stubb JWW,** eds. *Annual Progress in Reproductive Medicine.* Park Ridge, NJ: The Parthenon Publishing Group, Inc., 1993:37–43.

5. **Cates W Jr, Rolfs AT, Arel SO.** Sexually transmitted diseases, pelvic inflammatory disease and infertility: an epidemiologic update. *Epidemiol Rev* 1990;12:199–220.

6. **Chandra A, Mosher WD.** The demography of infertility and the use of medical care for infertility. *Infert Reprod Med Clin North Am* 1994;5:283–96.

7. **Garenne ML, Frisch RE.** Natural fertility. *Infert Reprod Med Clin North Am* 1994;5:259–82.

8. **Tietze C.** Reproductive span and role of reproduction among Hutterite women. *Fertil Steril* 1957;8:89–97.

9. **Federation CECOS, Schwartz D, Mayaux MJ.** Female fecundity as a function of age: results of artificial insemination in 2193 nulliparous women with azoospermic husbands. *N Engl J Med* 1982;306:404–6.

10. **Toner JP, Philput CB, Jones GS.** Basal follicle stimulating hormone level is a better mediator of in vitro fertilization performance than age. *Fertil Steril* 1991;55:784–91.

11. **Navot D, Drews MR, Bergh PA, Guzman I, Karstoedt A, Scott RT Jr, et al.** Age-related decline in female fertility is not due to diminished capacity of the uterus to sustain embryo implantation. *Fertil Steril* 1994;61:97–101.

12. **Sauer MV, Paulson RJ, Lobo RA.** Reversing the natural decline in human fertility: an extended clinical trial of oocyte-donation to women of advanced reproductive age. *JAMA* 1992;268:1275–9.

13. **Warburton D.** Reproductive loss: how much is preventable? *N Engl J Med* 1987;316:158–60.

14. **Stene J, Fischer G, Stene E, Mikhelson M, Petersen E.** Paternal age affect in Down's syndrome. *Ann Hum Genet* 1977;40:299–306.

15. **Bedford JM.** Sperm capacitation and fertilization in mammals. *Biol Reprod* 1970;2(Suppl): 128–58.

16. **Barros C, Yanagimachi R.** Induction of the zona reaction in golden hamster eggs by cortical granule material. *Nature* 1971;233:268–9.

17. **Bordson BL, Leonardo VS.** The appropriate upper age limit for semen donors: a review of the genetic effects of potential age. *Fertil Steril* 1991;56:397–401.

18. **World Health Organization.** *Laboratory Manual for the Examination of Human Semen and Sperm-Cervical Mucus Interaction.* Cambridge, England: Cambridge University Press, 1992.

19. **Carlsen E, Giwercman A, Keiding N, Skakkebaek NE.** Evidence for decreasing quality of semen during the past 50 years. *BMJ* 1992;305:609–13.

20. **Politoff L, Birkhausen M, Almendral A, Zorn A.** New data confirming a circannual rhythm in spermatogenesis. *Fertil Steril* 1989;52:486–9.

21. **Jequier AM, Ukombre EB.** Errors inherent in the performance of a routine semen analysis. *Br J Urol* 1983;55:434–6.

22. **MacLeod J.** The semen examination. *Clin Obstet Gynecol* 1965;8:115–27.

23. **Smith KD, Rodriguez-Rigau LJ, Steinberger E.** Relation between indices of semen analysis and pregnancy rate in infertile couples. *Fertil Steril* 1977;28:1314–9.

24. **Bostofte E, Serup J, Rebbe H.** Relation between number of immobile spermatozoa and pregnancies obtained during a twenty-year follow-up period. *Int J Androl* 1982;5:379–86.

25. **The American Fertility Society and Society for Assisted Reproductive Technology.** *Clinic-Specific Outcome Assessment for the Year 1992.* Birmingham, Alabama: The American Fertility Society, 1994.

26. **Kruger TF, Menkveld R, Stander FS, Lombard CJ, Van der Merwe JP, van Zyl JA, et al.** Sperm morphologic features as a prognostic factor in in vitro fertilization. *Fertil Steril* 1986; 46:1118–23.

27. **Kruger TF, Acosta AA, Simmons KF, Swanson RJ, Matta JF, Oehninger S.** Predictive value of abnormal sperm morphology in in vitro fertilization. *Fertil Steril* 1988;49:112–7.

28. **Wolff H, Anderson DJ.** Immunohistologic characterization and quantitation of leukocyte subpopulations in human semen. *Fertil Steril* 1988;49:497–504.

29. **Tomlinson MJ, Barratt CLR, Bolton AE, Lenton EA, Roberts HB, Cooke ID.** Round cells and sperm fertilizing capacity: the presence of immature germ cells but not seminal leukocytes are associated with reduced success of in vitro fertilization. *Fertil Steril* 1992;58:1257–9.

30. **Yanagimachi R, Yanagimachi H, Rogers BJ.** The use of zone-free animal ova as a test for assessment of fertilizing capacity of human spermatozoa. *Biol Reprod* 1976;15:471–6.

31. **Mao C, Grimes DA.** The sperm penetration assay: can it discriminate between fertile and infertile men? *Am J Obstet Gynecol* 1988;159:279–86.

32. **Burkman LJ, Cobbington CC, Franken DR, Kruger TF, Rosenwaks Z, Hodgen GD.** The hemizona assay (HZA): development of a diagnostic test for the binding of human spermatozoa to the human hemizona pellucida to predict fertilization potential. *Fertil Steril* 1988;49:688–97.

33. **Jeyrendran RS, Van der Ven HH, Perez-Pelaez M, Crabo BG, Zaneveld LJ.** Development of an assay to assess the functional integrity of the human sperm membrane and its relationship to other semen characteristics. *J Reprod Fertil* 1984;70:219–28.

34. **Wolf D, Boldt J, Byrd W, Bechtol RB.** Acrosomal status evaluation in normal ejaculated sperm with monoclonal antibodies. *Biol Reprod* 1985;32:1157–62.

35. **Comhaire FH, Vermeolen L, Schoonjans F.** Reassessment of the accuracy of traditional sperm characteristics and adenosine triphosphate (ATP) in estimating the fertilizing potential of human semen in vivo. *Int J Androl* 1987;10:653–62.

36. **The ESHRE CAPRI Workshop Group.** Male sterility and subfertility: guidelines for management. *Hum Reprod* 1994;9:1260–4.

37. **Greenberg SH, Lipshultz LI, Wein AJ.** Experience with 425 subfertile male patients. *J Urol* 1978;119:507–10.

38. **Takihara H, Sakatoku J, Cockett ATK.** The pathophysiology of varicocele male infertility. *Fertil Steril* 1991;55:861–8.

39. **World Health Organization.** The influence of varicocele on parameters of fertility in a large group of men presenting to infertility clinics. *Fertil Steril* 1992;57:1289–93.

40. **Marshburn PB, Sloan CS, Hammond MG.** Semen quality and association with coffee drinking, cigarette smoking, and ethanol consumption. *Fertil Steril* 1989;52:162–5.

41. **Luciano AA, Peluso J, Koch EI, Maier D, Kuslis S, Davison E.** Temporal relationship and reliability of the clinical, hormonal, and ultrasonographic indices of ovulation in infertile women. *Obstet Gynecol* 1990;75:412–6.

42. **Quagliarello J, Arny M.** Inaccuracy of basal body temperature charts in predicting urinary luteinizing hormone surges. *Fertil Steril* 1986;45:334–7.

43. **Filcori M, Butler JP, Crowley WF.** Neuroendocrine regulation of the corpus luteum in the human: evidence for pulsatile progesterone secretion. *J Clin Invest* 1984;73:1638–47.

44. **Rosenfeld DC, Chudnow S, Bronson RA.** Diagnosis of luteal phase inadequacy. *Obstet Gynecol* 1980;56:193–6.

45. **Cumming DC, Honore LH, Scott JZ, Williams KP.** The late luteal phase in infertile women: comparison of simultaneous endometrial biopsy and progesterone levels. *Fertil Steril* 1985; 43:715–40.

46. **Shepard MK, Senturia YD.** Comparison of serum progesterone and endometrial biopsy for confirmation of ovulation and evaluation of luteal function. *Fertil Steril* 1977;28:541–8.

47. **Shangold M, Berkley A, Gray J.** Both midluteal serum progesterone levels and late luteal endometrial histology should be assessed in all infertile women. *Fertil Steril* 1983;40:627–30.

48. **World Health Organization.** Temporal relationships between ovulation and defined changes in the concentration of plasma estradiol 17β luteinizing hormone, follicle stimulating hormone and progesterone. *Am J Obstet Gynecol* 1980;138:383–90.

49. **Hoff JD, Quigley ME, Yen SSC.** Hormonal dynamics at midcycle: a reevaluation. *J Clin Endocrinol Metab* 1987;57:792–6.

50. **Elkind-Hirsch K, Goldzieher JW, Gibbons WE, Besch PK.** Evaluation of the Ovu-Stick urinary luteinizing hormone kit in normal and stimulated menstrual cycles. *Obstet Gynecol* 1986;67:450–3.

51. **Wentz AC, Herbert CM III, Maxon WS, Hill GA, Pittaway DE.** Cycle of conception endometrial biopsy. *Fertil Steril* 1986;46:196–9.

52. **Noyes RW, Hertig A, Rock J.** Dating the endometrial biopsy. *Fertil Steril* 1950;1:3–25.

53. **Scott RT, Snyder RR, Bagnell JW, Reed KD, Adair CF, Hensley SD.** Evaluation of the impact of intraobserver variability on endometrial dating and the diagnosis of luteal phase defects. *Fertil Steril* 1993;60:652–7.

54. **Katz E.** The luteinized unruptured follicle and other ovulatory dysfunctions. *Fertil Steril* 1988;50:839–50.

55. **Kerin JF, Edmonds DK, Warner GM, Cox LW, Seamark RF, Mathews CD, et al.** Morphological and functional relations of Graafian follicle growth to ovulation in women using ultrasonic, laparoscopic and biochemical measurements. *Br J Obstet Gynaecol* 1981;88:81–90.

56. **O'Herlihy C, de Crespigny LC, Lopata A, Johnston I, Hoult I, Robinson H.** Preovulatory follicle size: comparison of ultrasound and laparoscopic measurements. *Fertil Steril* 1980;34: 24–6.

57. **Soules MR, McLachlan RI, Ek M, Dahl KD, Cohen NL, Bremner WJ.** Luteal phase deficiency: characterization of reproductive hormones over the menstrual cycle. *J Clin Endocrinol Metab* 1989;69:804–12.

58. **Davis OK, Berkeley AS, Naus GJ, Cholst IN, Freedman KS.** The incidence of luteal phase defect in normal fertile women determined by serial endometrial biopsies. *Fertil Steril* 1989;51:582–6.

59. **Wentz AC, Kossoy LR, Parker RA.** The impact of luteal phase inadequacy in an infertile population. *Am J Obstet Gynecol* 1990;162:937–45.

60. **Balasch J, Fabregues F, Creus M, Vanrell JA.** The usefulness of endometrial biopsy for luteal phase evaluation in infertility. *Hum Reprod* 1992;7:973–7.

61. **Soules MR, Clifton DK, Steiner RA, Cohen NL, Bremner WJ.** The corpus luteum: determinants of progesterone secretion in the normal menstrual cycle. *Obstet Gynecol* 1988;71:659–6.

62. **Castelbaum AJ, Wheeler J, Coutifaris CB, Mastroianni L Jr, Lessey BA.** Timing of the endometrial biopsy may be critical for the accurate diagnosis of luteal phase deficiency. *Fertil Steril* 1994;61:443–7.

63. **Batista MC, Cartledge TP, Merino MJ, Axiotis C, Platia MP, Merriam GR, et al.** Midluteal phase endometrial biopsy does not accurately predict luteal function. *Fertil Steril* 1993;59:294–300.

64. **Westrom L.** Incidence, prevalence and trends of acute pelvic inflammatory disease and its consequences in industrialized countries. *Am J Obstet Gynecol* 1980;138:880–92.

65. **Rosenfeld DL, Seidman SM, Bronson RA, Scholl GM.** Unsuspected chronic pelvic inflammatory disease in the infertile female. *Fertil Steril* 1983;39:44–8.

66. **Watson A, Vanderkerckhove P, Lilford R, Vail A, Brosens I, Hughes E.** A meta-analysis of the therapeutic role of oil-soluble contrast media at hysterosalpingography: a surprising result? *Fertil Steril* 1994;61:470–7.

67. **Collins JA.** Diagnostic assessment of the infertile female partner. *Curr Probl Obstet Gynecol Fertil* 1988;11:6–42.

68. **Shapiro BS, Diamond MP, DeCherney AH.** Salpingoscopy: an adjunctive technique for evaluation of the fallopian tube. *Fertil Steril* 1988;49:1076–9.

69. **Kerin JF, Williams DB, San Roman GA, Pearlstone AC, Grundfest WS, Surrey ES.** Falloscopic classification and treatment of fallopian tube lumen disease. *Fertil Steril* 1992;57:731–41.

70. **Kovacs GT, Newman GB, Henson GL.** The postcoital test: what is normal? *BMJ* 1978;1:818.

71. **Jette NT, Glass RH.** Prognostic value of the postcoital test. *Fertil Steril* 1972;23:29–32.

72. **Collins JA, So Y, Wilson EH, Wrixon W, Casper RF.** The postcoital test as a predictor of pregnancy among 355 infertile couples. *Fertil Steril* 1984;41:703–8.

73. **Griffith CS, Grimes DA.** The validity of the postcoital test. *Am J Obstet Gynecol* 1990;162:615–20.

74. **Glatstein IZ, Best CL, Palumbo A, Sleeper LA, Friedman AJ, Hornstein MD.** The reproducibility of the postcoital test: a prospective study. *Obstet Gynecol* 1995;85:396–400.

75. **Buttram VC, Reiter RC.** Uterine leiomyomata: etiology, symptomatology, and management. *Fertil Steril* 1981;36:433–45.

76. **Berkeley AS, DeCherney AH, Polan ML.** Abdominal myomectomy and subsequent fertility. *Obstet Gynecol* 1983;156:319–22.

77. **Senekjian EK, Potlkul RK, Frey K, Herbst AL.** Infertility among daughters either exposed or not exposed to diethylstilbestrol. *Am J Obstet Gynecol* 1988;158:493–8.

78. **Barnes AB, Colton T, Gunderson J, Noller KL, Tilley BC, Strama T, et al.** Fertility and outcome of pregnancy of women exposed in utero to diethylstilbestrol. *N Engl J Med* 1990;302:609–13.

79. **Bronson R, Cooper G, Rosenfeld D.** Sperm antibodies: their role in infertility. *Fertil Steril* 1984;42:171–83.

80. **Bronson R, Cooper GW, Rosenfeld DL.** Complement-mediated effects of sperm head-directed human antibodies on the ability of human spermatozoa to penetrate zona-free hamster eggs. *Fertil Steril* 1983;40:91–5.

81. **Jager S, Kermer J, van Slochteren-Draeisma T.** A simple method of screening for antisperm antibodies in the human male: detection of spermatozoan surface IgG with the direct mixed agglutination reaction carried out on untreated fresh human semen. *Int J Fertil* 1978;23:12–21.

82. **Kremer J, Jager S.** The significance of antisperm antibodies for sperm-cervical mucus interaction. *Hum Reprod* 1992;7:781–4.

83. **Collin JA, Burrows EA, Yeo J, YoungLai EV.** Frequency and predictive value of antisperm antibodies among infertile couples. *Hum Reprod* 1993;8:592–8.

84. **Moore DE, Spadoni LR, Foy HM, Wang SP, Daling JR, Kuo CL, et al.** Increased frequency of serum antibodies to Chlamydia trachomatis in infertility due to distal tubal disease. *Lancet* 1982;2:574–7.

85. **Henry-Suchet J, Catalan F, Loffredo V, Sanson MJ, Debache C, Pigeau F, et al.** Chlamydia trachomatis associated with chronic inflammation in abdominal specimens from women selected for tuboplasty. *Fertil Steril* 1981;36:599–605.

86. **Fedele L, Acaia B, Ricciardiello O, Marchini M, Benzi-Cipelli R.** Recovery of Chlamydia trachomatic from the endometria of women with unexplained infertility. *J Reprod Med* 1989; 34:393–6.

87. **Toth A, Lesser ML, Brooks C, Labriola D.** Subsequent pregnancies among 161 couples treated for T-mycoplasma genital tract infection. *N Engl J Med* 1983;308:505–7.

88. **Harrison RF, de Louvois J, Blades M, Hurley R.** Doxycycline treatment and human infertility. *Lancet* 1975;1:605–7.

89. **Gump DW, Gibson M, Ashikaga T.** Lack of association between genital mycoplasmas and infertility. *N Engl J Med* 1984;310:937–41.

90. **Crosignami PG, Collins J, Cooke ID, Diezfalusy E, Rubin E.** Unexplained infertility. *Hum Reprod* 1993;8:977–80.

91. **Collins JA, Wrixon W, Janes LB, Wilson EH.** Treatment-independent pregnancy among infertile couples. *N Engl J Med* 1983;309:1201–6.

92. **Whitcomb RW, Crowley WF Jr.** Male hypogonadotropic hypogonadism. *Endocrinol Metab Clin North Am* 1993;22:125–43.

93. **Van de Berk D, Wijnberg M, Van Dop PA.** Initiation of spermatogenesis and successful in vitro fertilization in an infertile male with panhypopituitarism; superiority of pulsatile LH-RH over gonadotropins? A case report. *Eur J Obstet Gynecol Reprod Biol* 1991;40:153–7.

94. **Stockamp K, Schreiter F, Altwein JE.** α-adrenergic drugs in retrograde ejaculation. *Fertil Steril* 1974;25:817–20.

95. **Shangold GA, Cantor B, Schreiber JR.** Treatment of infertility due to retrograde ejaculation: a simple, cost-effective method. *Fertil Steril* 1990;54:175–7.

96. **Sokol RZ, Steiner BS, Bustillo M, Peterson G, Swerdloff RS.** A controlled comparison of the efficacy of clomiphene citrate in male infertility. *Fertil Steril* 1988;49:865–70.

97. **World Health Organization.** A double-blind trial of clomiphene citrate for the treatment of idiopathic male infertility. *Int J Androl* 1992;7:1067–72.

98. **Acosta AA, Khalifa E, Oehninger S.** Pure human follicle stimulating hormone has a role in the treatment of severe male factor infertility by assisted reproduction: Norfold's total experience. *Hum Reprod* 1992;7:1067–72.

99. **Marshburn PB, Kutteh WH.** The role of antisperm antibodies in infertility. *Fertil Steril* 1994;61:799–811.

100. **Baker HWG, Burger HG, de Kretser DM, Hudson B, Rennie GC, Straffon WGE.** Testicular vein ligation and fertility in men with varicoceles. *BMJ* 1985;291:1678–80.

101. **Madgar I, Weissenberg R, Lunnenfeld B, Karasik A, Goldwasser B.** Controlled trial of single spermatic vein ligation for varicocele in infertile men. *Fertil Steril* 1995;63:120–4.

102. **Belker AM, Thomas AJ Jr, Fuchs EF, Konnak JW, Sharlip ID.** Results of 1469 microsurgical vasectomy reversals by the Vasovasostomy Study Group. *J Urol* 1991;145:505–11.

103. **Schlegel PN, Goldstein M.** Microsurgical vasoepididymostomy: refinements and results. *J Urol* 1993;150:1165–8.

104. **Urry RL, Poulson M, Middleton RG, Worley R, Jones K, Keye W.** Artificial insemination: a comparison of pregnancy rates with intrauterine versus cervical insemination and washed sperm versus swim-up sperm preparations. *Fertil Steril* 1988;49:1036–8.

105. **Patton PE, Novy MJ, Burry KA, Wolf DP, Thurmond A.** Intrauterine insemination out performs intracervical insemination in a randomized, controlled study with frozen, donor semen. *Fertil Steril* 1992;57:559–64.

106. **Kahn JA, Sunde A, Koskemies A, von During V, Sordal T, Christensen F, et al.** Fallopian tube sperm perfusion (FTSP) versus intrauterine insemination (IUI) in the treatment of unexplained infertility: a prospective randomized study. *Hum Reprod* 1993;8:890–4.

107. **Hovatta O, Kurunmaki H, Tiitinen A, Lahteenmaki P, Koskimies AI.** Direct intraperitoneal insemination and superovulation in infertility treatment: a randomized study. *Fertil Steril* 1990;54:339–41.

108. **Abella EA, Tarantino S, Wade R.** Intrafollicular insemination for male factor infertility. *Fertil Steril* 1992;58:442–3.

109. **Yovich JL.** Pentoxifylline: actions and applications in assisted reproduction. *Hum Reprod* 1993;8:1786–91.

110. **Silverberg KM, Johnson JV, Burns WN, Schenken RS, Olive DL.** A prospective, randomized trial comparing two different intrauterine insemination regimens in controlled ovarian hyperstimulation cycles. *Fertil Steril* 1992;57:357–61.

111. **Hornstein MD, Gleason RE, Cohen JN, Friedman AG, Thomas PP, Mutter GL.** The effect of consecutive day inseminations on semen characteristics in an intrauterine insemination program. *Fertil Steril* 1992;58:433–5.

112. **Martiniez AR, Bernardus RE, Vermeiden JPW, Schoemaker J.** Basic questions on intrauterine inseminations: an update. *Obstet Gynecol Surv* 1993;48:811–28.

113. **Subak LL, Adamson GD, Boltz NL.** Therapeutic donor insemination: a prospective, randomized trial of fresh versus frozen sperm. *Am J Obstet Gynecol* 1992;166:1597–1604.

114. **The American Fertility Society.** Guidelines for gamete donation: 1993. *Fertil Steril* 1993;59 (Suppl 1):1S–9S.

115. **Shenfield F, Doyle P, Valentine A, Steele SJ, Tan SL.** Effects of age, gravidity, and male infertility status on cumulative conception rates following artificial insemination with cryopreserved donor semen: analysis of 2998 cycles of treatment in one center over 10 years. *Hum Reprod* 1993;8:60–4.

116. **Speroff L, Glass RH, Kase N.** *Clinical Gynecologic Endocrinology and Fertility.* 5th ed. Baltimore: Williams & Wilkins, 1994:890.

117. **Clark JH, Markaverich BM.** The agonist-antagonist properties of clomiphene. *Pharmacol Ther* 1981;15:467–519.

118. **Kettel LM, Roseff SH, Berga SL, Mortola JF, Yen SSC.** Hypothalamic-pituitary-ovarian response to clomiphene citrate in women with polycystic ovarian syndrome. *Fertil Steril* 1993;59:532–8.

119. **Adashi EY.** Clomiphene citrate-initiated ovulation: a clinical update. *Semin Reprod Endocrinol* 1986;4:255–76.

120. **Kessel B, Hsueh AJW.** Clomiphene citrate augments follicle-stimulating hormone-induced luteinizing hormone receptor content in cultured rat granulosa cells. *Fertil Steril* 1987;47:334–40.

121. **Hammerstein J.** Mode of action of clomiphene. *Acta Endocrinol* 1969;60:635–44.

122. **Eden JA, Place J, Carter GD, Jones J, Alaghband-Zadeh J, Pawson ME.** The effect of clomiphene citrate on follicular phase increase in endometrial thickness and uterine volume. *Obstet Gynecol* 1989;73:187–990.

123. **Van Campenhout J, Simiard R, Leduc B.** Antiestrogenic effects of clomiphene in the human being. *Fertil Steril* 1968;19:700–6.

124. **Li TC, Warren MA, Murphe C, Sargent S, Cooke ID.** A prospective, randomized, crossover study comparing the effects of clomiphene citrate and cyclofenil on endometrial morphology in the luteal phase of normal, fertile women. *Br J Obstet Gynaecol* 1992;99:10008–13.

125. **Thompson LA, Barrett CLR, Thornton SJ, Bolton AE, Cooke ID.** The effects of clomiphene citrate and cyclofenil on cervical mucus volume and receptivity over the periovulatory period. *Fertil Steril* 1993;59:125–9.

126. **Gysler M, March CM, Mishell DR Jr, Bailey EJ.** A decade's experience with an individualized clomiphene treatment regimen including its effects on the postcoital test. *Fertil Steril* 1982;37:161–7.

127. **Hammond MG, Halme JK, Talbert LM.** Factors affecting pregnancy rate in clomiphene citrate induction of ovulation. *Obstet Gynecol* 1983;62:196–202.

128. **Ritchie WGM.** Ultrasound in the evaluation of normal and induced ovulation. *Fertil Steril* 1985;43:167–81.

129. **Shoham Z, Zosmer A, Insler V.** Early miscarriage and fetal malformation after induction of ovulation (by clomiphene citrate and/or human menotropins), in vitro fertilization, and gamete intrafallopian transfer. *Fertil Steril* 1991;55:1051–6.

130. **Donini P, et al.** Purification of gonadotropin from human menopausal urine. *Acta Endocrinol* 1964;45:321–8.

131. **Dor J, Itzkowic DH, Mashiach S, Lunenfeld B, Serr DM.** Cumulative conception rates following gonadotropin therapy. *Am J Obstet Gynecol* 1980;136:102–5.

132. **Shenker JG, Weinstein D.** Ovarian hyperstimulation syndrome: a current survey. *Fertil Steril* 1978;30:255–68.

133. **Bettendorf G, Braendle W, Sprotte CH, Weise CH, Zimmerman R.** Overall results of gonadotropin therapy. In: **Insler B, Bettendorf G,** eds. *Advances in Diagnosis and Treatment of Infertility.* New York: Elsevier/North Holland, 1981:21–6.

134. **Timor-Tritsch IE, Peisner DB, Monteagudo A, Lerner JP, Sharma S.** Multifetal pregnancy reduction by transvaginal puncture: evaluation of the technique used in 134 cases. *Am J Obstet Gynecol* 1993;68:799–804.

135. **Kurachi K, Aono T, Suzuki M, Hirano M, Kobayashi T, Kaibara M.** Results of hMG (Humegon)-hCG therapy in 6096 treatment cycles of 2166 Japanese women with anovulatory infertility. *Eur J Obstet Gynecol Reprod Biol* 1985;19:43–51.

136. **Lam SY, Baker HW, Evans JH, Pepperell RJ.** Factors affecting fetal loss in induction of ovulation with gonadotropins: increased abortion rates related to hormonal profiles in conceptual cycles. *Am J Obstet Gynecol* 1989;160:621–8.

137. **Corfman RS, Milad MP, Bellavance TL, Ory SJ, Erickson LD, Ball GC.** A novel ovarian stimulation protocol for use with the assisted reproductive technologies. *Fertil Steril* 1993;60:864–70.

138. **Hughes SM, Huang ZH, Morris ID, Matson PL, Buck P, Lieberman BA.** A double-blind, cross-over, controlled study to evaluate the effect of human biosynthetic growth hormone on ovarian stimulation in previous poor responders to in vitro fertilization. *Hum Reprod* 1994;9:13–8.

139. **Ibrahim ZH, Matson PL, Buck P, Lieberman BA.** The use of biosynthetic human growth hormone to augment ovulation induction in with buserelin acetate/human menopausal gonadotropin in women with a poor ovarian response. *Fertil Steril* 1991;55:202–4.

140. **MacDougall MJ, Tan SH, Balen A, Jacobs HS.** A controlled study comparing patients with and without polycystic ovaries undergoing in vitro fertilization. *Hum Reprod* 1993;8:233–7.

141. **MacLeod AF, Wheeler MH, Gordon P, Lowry C, Sonksen PH, Conaglen JV.** Effect of long-term inhibition of gonadotropin secretion by the gonadotropin-releasing hormone agonist, buserelin, on sex steroid secretion and ovarian morphology in polycystic ovary syndrome. *J Endocrinol* 1990;125:317–25.

142. **Dodson WC, Hughes CL Jr, Yancy SE, Haney AF.** Clinical characteristics of ovulation induction with human menopausal gonadotropins with and without leuprolide acetate in polycystic ovary syndrome. *Fertil Steril* 1989;52:915–8.

143. **Homberg R, Feldberg D, Levy T, Ashkenazi J, Berkovitz D, Ben-Rafael Z, et al.** Gonadotropin-releasing hormone agonist reduces the miscarriage rate for pregnancies achieved in women with polycystic ovarian syndrome. *Fertil Steril* 1993;59:527–31.

144. **Kim J-H, Richards CH, Seibel MM.** Proper selection of patients for intermediate-dose pure follicle stimulating hormone. *J Reprod Med* 1994;39:1–5.

145. **Farhi J, Homburg R, Lerner A, Ben-Rafael Z.** The choice of treatment for anovulation associated with polycystic ovary syndrome following failure to conceive with clomiphene. *Hum Reprod* 1993;8:1367–71.

146. **Donderwinkel PFJ, Schoot DC, Coelingh Bennink HJT, Fauser BEHM.** Pregnancy after induction of ovulation with recombinant human FSH in polycystic ovary syndrome. *Lancet* 1992;340:983.

147. **Martin KA, Hall JE, Adams JM, Crowley WF Jr.** Comparison of exogenous gonadotropins and pulsatile gonadotropin-releasing hormone for the induction of ovulation in hypogonadotropic amenorrhea. *J Clin Endocrinol Metab* 1993;77:125–9.

148. **Braat DD, Schoemaker R, Schoemaker J.** Life table analysis of fecundity of intravenously gonadotropin-releasing hormone-treated patients with normogonadotropic and hypogonadotropic amenorrhea. *Fertil Steril* 1991;55:266–71.

149. **Skarin G, Ahlgren M.** Pulsatile gonadotropin releasing hormone (GnRH)-treatment for hypothalamic amenorrhea causing infertility. *Acta Obstet Gynecol Scand* 1994;73:482–5.

150. **Filcori M, Flamigni C, Campaniello E, Meiggiola MC, Michelacci L, Valdiserri A, et al.** Polycystic ovary syndrome: abnormalities and management with pulsatile gonadotropin-re-

leasing hormone and gonadotropin-releasing hormone analogs. *Am J Obstet Gynecol* 1990; 163:1737–42.

151. **Jansen RP.** Pulsatile intravenous gonadotropin releasing hormone for ovulation induction: determinants of follicular and luteal phase response. *Hum Reprod* 1993;8:193–6.

152. **Blacker CM.** Ovulation stimulation and induction. *Endocrinol Metab Clin North Am* 1992; 21:57–84.

153. **Devane GW, Guzick DS.** Bromocriptine therapy in normoprolactinemic women with unexplained infertility and galactorrhea. *Fertil Steril* 1986;46:1026–31.

154. **Daly DC, Walters CA, Soto-Albors CE, Tohan N, Riddick DH.** A randomized study of dexamethasone in ovulation induction with clomiphene citrate. *Fertil Steril* 1984;41:844–8.

155. **Singh KB, Dunniho DR, Mahajan DK, Bairnsfaterh LE.** Clomiphene-dexamethasone treatment of clomiphene resistant women with and without the polycystic ovary syndrome. *J Reprod Med* 1992;37:215–8.

156. **Stein IF, Leventhal ML.** Amenorrhea associated with bilateral polycystic ovaries. *Am J Obstet Gynecol* 1935;29:181–91.

157. **Judd HL, Rigg LA, Anderson DC, Yen SS.** The effects of ovarian wedge resection on circulating gonadotropin and ovarian steroid levels in patients with polycystic ovarian syndrome. *J Clin Endocrinol Metab* 1976;43:347–55.

158. **Adashi EY, Rock JR, Guzick D, Wentz AC, Jones GS, et al.** Fertility following bilateral ovarian wedge resection: a critical analysis of 90 consecutive cases of the polycystic ovarian syndrome. *Fertil Steril* 1981;36:320–5.

159. **Weinstein D, Polishuk WZ.** The role of wedge resection of the ovary as a cause for mechanical sterility. *Surg Gynecol Obstet* 1975;141:417–23.

160. **De Waart MJ, Boeckx W, Brosens I.** Pelvic adhesions following microsurgical wedge resection compared to laparoscopic electrocoagulation of the rabbit ovaries. *Infert* 1987;10: 33–9.

161. **Naether OGJ, Fischer R.** Adhesion formation after laparoscopic electrocoagulation of the ovarian surface in the polycystic ovary patients. *Fertil Steril* 1993;60:95–8.

162. **Campo S, Felli A, Lamanna MA, Barini A, Garcea N.** Endocrine changes and clinical outcome after laparoscopic ovarian resection in patients with polycystic ovaries. *Human Reprod* 1993;8:359–63.

163. **Aakvaag A, Gjonnaess H.** Hormonal response to electrocautery of the ovary in patients with polycystic ovarian disease. *Br J Obstet Gynaecol* 1985;92:1258–64.

164. **Daniell JF, Miller W.** Polycystic ovaries treated by laparoscopic laser vaporization. *Fertil Steril* 1989;51:232–6.

165. **Armar NA, McGarrigle HHG, Honour J, Holownia P, Hacobs HS, Lachelin GCL.** Laparoscopic ovarian diathermy in the management of anovulatory infertility in women with polycystic ovaries; endocrine changes and clinical outcome. *Fertil Steril* 1990;53:45–9.

166. **Wentz AC, Herbert CM, Maxson WS, Garner CH.** Outcome of progesterone treatment of luteal phase insufficiency. *Fertil Steril* 1984;41:856–62.

167. **Huang K.** The primary treatment of luteal phase inadequacy: progesterone versus clomiphene citrate. *Obstet Gynecol* 1986;155:824–8.

168. **Murray DL, Reich L, Adashi EY.** Oral clomiphene citrate and vaginal progesterone suppositories in the treatment of luteal phase dysfunction: a comparative study. *Fertil Steril* 1989;51:35–41.

169. **Garcia JE, Jones GS, Wentz AC.** The use of clomiphene citrate. *Fertil Steril* 1977;28:707.

170. **Tulandi T, Collins JA, Burrows E, Jarrell JF, McInnes RA, Wrixon W, et al.** Treatment-dependent and treatment-independent pregnancy among women with periadnexal adhesions. *Am J Obstet Gynecol* 1992;162:354–7.

171. **Gomel V.** Salpingoovariolysis by laparoscopy in infertility. *Fertil Steril* 1983;40:607–11.

172. **Lundroff P, Hahlini P, Kallfelt B, Thornburn J, Lindblom B.** Adhesion formation after laparoscopic surgery in tubal pregnancy: a randomized trial after laparotomy. *Fertil Steril* 1991; 55:911–5.

173. **McComb P.** Microsurgical tubocornual reanastomosis for occlusive cornual disease: reproducible results without the need for tubouterine implantation. *Fertil Steril* 1986;46:571–7.

174. **Donnez J, Casanas-Roux F.** Prognostic factors influencing the pregnancy rate after microsurgical cornual reanastomosis. *Fertil Steril* 1986;46:1089–92.

175. **Thurmond AS, Rosch J.** Nonsurgical fallopian tube recanalization for treatment of infertility. *Radiology* 1990;174:371–4.

176. **Confino E, Tur-Kaspa I, DeCherney A, Corfman R, Coulam C, Robinson E, et al.** Transcervical balloon tuboplasty: a multicenter study. *JAMA* 1990;264:2079–82.

177. **Rock JA.** Infertility: surgical aspects. In: **Yen SSC, Jaffe RB,** eds. *Reproductive Endocrinology: Physiology and Clinical Management.* 3rd ed. Philadelphia: WB Saunders, 1991.

178. **Fayez JA, Dempsey RA.** Short hospital stay for gynecologic reconstructive surgery via laparotomy. *Obstet Gynecol* 1993;81:598–600.

179. **Schlaff WD, Hassiakos DK, Damewood MD, Rock JA.** Neosalpingostomy for distal tubal obstruction: prognostic factors and impact of surgical technique. *Fertil Steril* 1990;54:984–90.

180. **Dobuisson JB, Chapron C, Morice P, Aubriot FX, Foulot H, Bouquet de Joliniere J.** Laparoscopic salpingostomy: fertility results according to the tubal mucosal appearance. *Hum Reprod* 1994;9:334–9.

181. **Eyraud B, Erny R, Vergnet F.** Chirugie tubaire distale par coelioscopie. *J Gynecol Obstet Biol Reprod (Paris)* 1993;22:9–14.

182. **Singhal V, Li TC, Cooke ID.** An analysis of factors influencing the outcome of 232 consecutive tubal microsurgery cases. *Br J Obstet Gynaecol* 1991;98:628–36.

183. **Wilcox LS, Chu SY, Peterson HB.** Characteristics of women who considered or obtained tubal reanastomosis: results from a prospective study of tubal sterilization. *Obstet Gynecol* 1990;75:661–5.

184. **TeVelde ER, Boer ME, Looman CWN, Habbema JDF.** Factors influencing success or failure after reversal of sterilization. *Fertil Steril* 1990;54:270–7.

185. **Novy MJ.** Reversal of Kroener fimbriectomy sterilization. *Am J Obstet Gynecol* 1980;137:198–206.

186. **Silber SH, Cohen R.** Microsurgical reversal of female sterilization; the role of tubal length. *Fertil Steril* 1980;33:598–601.

187. **Katz E, Donesky BW.** Laparoscopic tubal anastomosis: a pilot study. *J Reprod Med* 1994;39:497–8.

188. **Gauwerky JF, Kloss RP, Forssman WG.** Fibrin glue for anastomosis of the fallopian tube-morphology. *Hum Reprod* 1993;8:2108–14.

189. **Wheeler JM, Malinak LR.** Does mild endometriosis cause infertility? *Semin Reprod Endocrinol* 1988;6:239–49.

190. **Hughes EG, Fedorkow DM, Collins JA.** A quantitative overview of controlled trials in endometriosis-associated infertility. *Fertil Steril* 1993;59:963–70.

191. **Schmidt G, Fowler WF.** Cervical stenosis following minor gynecologic procedures in DES-exposed women. *Obstet Gynecol* 1980;56:333–5.

192. **Soto-Albors C, Daly DC, Ying YK.** Efficacy of human menopausal gonadotropins as therapy for abnormal cervical mucus. *Fertil Steril* 1989;51:58–62.

193. **Nicotra M, Muttinelli C, Rolfi G, Amato P.** Purified FSH as a treatment for cervical hostility. *Acta Eur Fertil* 1993;24:19–21.

194. **Gelety TJ, Buyalos RP.** The effect of clomiphene citrate and menopausal gonadotropins on cervical mucus in ovulatory cycles. *Fertil Steril* 1993;60:471–6.

195. **van der Merwe JP, Gruger TF, Windt ML, Hulme VA, Menkveld R.** Treatment of male sperm autoimmunity by using the gamete intrafallopian transfer procedure with washed spermatozoa. *Fertil Steril* 1990;53:682–7.

196. **Margollath EJ, Sauter E, Bronson RA, Rosenfeld DL, Scholl GM, Cooper GW.** Intrauterine insemination as treatment for antisperm antibodies in the female. *Fertil Steril* 1988;50:441–6.

197. **Verkauf BS.** Myomectomy for fertility enhancement and preservation. *Fertil Steril* 1992;58:1–15.

198. **Kaufman RH, Adam E, Noller K, Irwin JF, Gray M.** Upper genital tract changes and infertility in diethylstilbestrol-exposed women. *Am J Obstet Gynecol* 1986;154:1312–8.

199. **Berger MJ, Goldstein DP.** Impaired reproductive performance in DES-exposed women. *Obstet Gynecol* 1980;55:25–7.

200. **Tulandi T, Arronet GH, McInnes RA.** Arcuate and bicornuate uterine anomalies and infertility. *Fertil Steril* 1980;34:362–4.

201. **Heinonen PK, Pystnen PP.** Primary infertility and uterine anomalies. *Fertil Steril* 1983;40:311–6.

202. **Georgakopoulos PA, Gogas CG.** Zur Fertilitat bei Uterusmissbildungen. *Geburtshilfe Frauenheilkd* 1982;42:533–6.

203. **Oosthuizen AP, Wessels PH, Hefer JN.** Tuberculosis of the female genital tract in patients attending an infertility clinic. *S Afr Med J* 1990;77:562–4.

204. **Varma TR.** Genital tuberculosis and subsequent fertility. *Int J Gynecol Obstet* 1991;35:1–11.

205. **Asherman JG.** Amenorrhea traumatica (atretica). *J Obstet Gynaecol Br Comm* 1948;55:23–30.

206. **Isamjovich B, Lindor A, Confino E, David MP.** Treatment of minimal and moderate intrauterine adhesions (Asherman's syndrome). *J Reprod Med* 1985;30:769–72.

207. **Rousseau S, Lord J, Lepage Y, Van Campenhout J.** The expectancy of pregnancy for "normal" infertile couples. *Fertil Steril* 1983;40:768–72.

208. **Glazener CMA, Coulson C, Lambert PA, Watt EM, Hinton RA, Kelley NG, et al.** Clomiphene treatment for women with unexplained infertility: placebo-controlled study of hormonal responses and conception rates. *Gynecol Endocrinol* 1990;4:75–83.

209. **Deaton JL, Gibson N, Blackmer KM, Nakajima ST, Badger GJ, Brumsted JR.** A randomized, controlled trial of clomiphene citrate and intrauterine insemination in couples with unexplained infertility or with surgically corrected endometriosis. *Fertil Steril* 1990;54:1083–8.

210. **Kirby CA, Flaherty SP, Godfrey BM, Warnes GM, Matthews CD.** A prospective trial of intrauterine insemination of motile spermatozoa versus timed intercourse. *Fertil Steril* 1991;56:102–7.

211. **Aboulghar MA, Mansour RT, Serour GI, Amin Y, Abbas AM, Salah IM.** Ovarian superstimulation and intrauterine insemination for the treatment of unexplained infertility. *Fertil Steril* 1993;60:303–6.

212. **Dimarzo SH, Kennedy JF, Young PE, Hervert SA, Rosenberg DC, Villanueva B.** Effect of controlled ovarian hyperstimulation on pregnancy rates after intrauterine insemination. *Am J Obstet Gynecol* 1992;166:1607–13.

213. **Navot D, Muasher SH, Oehninger S, Liu HC, Veeck LL, Kreiner D, et al.** The value of in vitro fertilization for the treatment of unexplained infertility. *Fertil Steril* 1988;49:854–7.

214. **Devroey P, Staessen C, Camus M, DeGrauwe E, Wisanto A, Van Streiteghem AC.** Zygote intrafallopian transfer as a successful treatment for unexplained infertility. *Fertil Steril* 1989;52:246–9.

215. **Murdoch AP, Harris M, Mahroo M, Williams M, Dunlop W.** Is GIFT (gamete intrafallopian transfer) the best treatment for unexplained infertility? *Br J Obstet Gynaecol* 1991;98:643–7.

216. **Hogerzeil HV, Speikerman JC, de Bries JW, de Schepper G.** A randomized trial between GIFT and ovarian stimulation in the treatment of unexplained infertility and failed artificial insemination by donor. *Hum Reprod* 1992;7:1235–9.

217. **Segal S, Casper RF.** Gonadotropin-releasing hormone agonist versus human chorionic gonadotropin for triggering follicular maturation in in vitro fertilization. *Fertil Steril* 1992;57:1254–8.

218. **Gonen Y, Powell WA, Casper RF.** Effect of follicular aspiration on hormonal parameters in patients undergoing ovarian stimulation. *Hum Reprod* 1991;6:356–8.

219. **Forman RG, Frydman R, Egan D, Roos C, Barlow DH.** Severe ovarian hyperstimulation using agonists of gonadotropin-releasing hormone for in vitro fertilization: European series and a proposal for prevention. *Fertil Steril* 1990;53:502–9.

220. **Hughes EG, Fedorkow DM, Daya S, Sagle MA, Van de Koppel P, Collins JA.** The routine use of gonadotropin-releasing hormone agonists prior to in vitro fertilization and gamete

intrafallopian transfer: a meta-analysis of randomized, controlled trials. *Fertil Steril* 1992; 58:888–96.

221. **Eisenbach M, Ralt D.** Pre-contact mammalian sperm-egg communication and role in fertilization. *Am J Physiol* 1992;262:C1095–1101.

222. **Molloy D, Harrison K, Breen T, Hennessey J.** The predictive value of idiopathic failure to fertilize on the first in vitro fertilization attempt. *Fertil Steril* 1991;56:285–9.

223. **Van Steirteghem A, Nagy Z, Liu J, Joris H, Verheyen G, Smitz, et al.** Intracytoplasmic sperm injection. *Baillieres Clin Obstet Gynecol* 1994;8:85–93.

224. **Croxatto HB, Ortiz MS.** Egg transport in the fallopian tube. *Gynecol Invest* 1975;6:215–25.

225. **Rosenwaks Z.** Donor eggs: their application in modern reproductive technologies. *Fertil Steril* 1987;47:859–909.

226. **Bertheussen K.** Embryo culture techniques in the IVF laboratory. *Hum Reprod* 1992;7:56–7.

227. **Bongso A, Ng SC, Fong CY, Anandakumar C, Marshall B, Edirisinghe R, et al.** Improved pregnancy rate after the transfer of embryos grown in human fallopian tubal cell coculture. *Fertil Steril* 1992;58:568–74.

228. **Plachot M, Mandelbaum J, Junca AM, de Grouchy J, Salat-Baroux J, Cohen J.** Cytogenic analysis and developmental capacity of normal and abnormal embryos after IVF. *Hum Reprod* 1989;4:99–103.

229. **Medical Research International and the Society for Assisted Reproductive Technology, the American Fertility Society.** In vitro fertilization/embryo transfer in the United States: 1987 results from the National IVF-ET Registry. *Fertil Steril* 1989;51:13–9.

230. **The American Fertility Society, Society for Assisted Reproductive Technology.** Assisted reproductive technology in the United States and Canada: 1992 results generated from the American Fertility Society/Society for Assisted Reproductive Technology Registry. *Fertil Steril* 1994;62:1121–8.

231. **Bauer O, Diedrich K.** Transcervical tubal transfer of gametes and embryos. *Curr Opin Obstet Gynecol* 1994;6:178–83.

232. **Quigley MM, Collins RL, Schover LR.** Establishment of an oocyte donor program. Donor screening and selection. *Ann N Y Acad Sci* 1991;626:445–51.

232. **Toth TI, Baka SG, Veeck LL, Jones HW Jr, Muasher S, Lazendorf SE.** Fertilization and in vitro development of cryopreserved human prophase I oocytes. *Fertil Steril* 1994;61:891–4.

28 Recurrent Spontaneous Early Pregnancy Loss

Joseph A. Hill

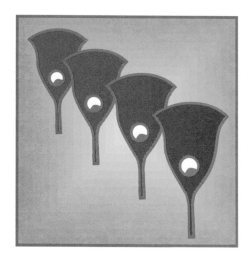

Spontaneous abortion is the most common complication of pregnancy and is responsible for significant emotional distress to couples desiring children. Approximately 70% of human conceptions fail to achieve viability, and an estimated 50% are lost before the first missed menstrual period (1). Most of these pregnancy losses are unrecognized. Recent studies using sensitive assays for human chorionic gonadotropin (hCG) have indicated that the actual rate of pregnancy loss after implantation is 31% (2). Of pregnancies that are clinically recognized, loss occurs in 15% prior to 20 weeks of gestation (from last menstrual period) (3, 4).

Traditionally, recurrent abortion has been defined as the occurrence of three or more clinically recognized pregnancy losses before 20 weeks from the last menstrual period. It occurs in approximately one in 300 pregnancies (2). Clinical investigation of pregnancy loss, however, should be initiated after two consecutive spontaneous abortions, especially when fetal heart activity had been identified prior to the pregnancy loss, when the women is older than 35 years of age, or when the couple has had difficulty conceiving. Epidemiologic surveys indicate that after four spontaneous abortions, the risk is 40–50% (5). These data should be considered when assessing results of studies that claim therapeutic efficacy for various treatments.

Etiology

Parental chromosomal abnormalities are the only undisputed cause of recurrent abortion. Such abnormalities occur in 5% of couples who experience recurrent pregnancy loss. Other associations have been made with anatomic abnormalities (12%), endocrinologic problems (17%), infections (5%), and immunologic factors (50%). Other miscellaneous factors have been implicated and account for 10% of cases. After a thorough evaluation, the potential cause in 60% of cases remains unexplained (Table 28.1).

Genetic Factors

The most common inborn parental chromosomal abnormality contributing to recurrent abortion is balanced translocation, often giving rise to trisomic conceptions (6).

963

Table 28.1   Proposed Etiologies for Recurrent Spontaneous Abortion

Etiology	Proposed Incidence
Genetic factors Chromosomal Multifactorial	5%

Anatomic factors
 1. Congenital
   a. Incomplete Müllerian fusion or septum reabsorption
   b. Diethylstilbestrol exposure
   c. Uterine artery anomalies
   d. Cervical incompetence
 2. Acquired
   a. Cervical incompetence
   b. Synechiae
   c. Leiomyomas
   d. Endometriosis, adenomyosis
	12%

Endocrine factors 1. Luteal phase insufficiency, including luteinizing hormone disorders 2. Thyroid disorders 3. Diabetes mellitus 4. Androgen disorders 5. Prolactin disorders	17%
Infectious factors 1. Bacteria 2. Viruses 3. Parasites 4. Zoonotic 5. Fungal	5%

Immunologic factors
 1. Humoral Mechanisms
   a. Antiphospholipid antibodies
   b. Antisperm antibodies
   c. Antitrophoblast antibodies
   d. Blocking antibody deficiency
 2. Cellular Mechanisms
   a. TH1 cellular immune response to reproductive antigens (embryo/trophoblast–toxic factors/cytokines)
   b. TH2 cytokine, growth factor, and oncogene deficiency
   c. Supressor cell and factor deficiency
   d. Major histocompatibility antigen expression
	50%

Miscellaneous factors
 1. Environmental
 2. Drugs
 3. Placental abnormalities
   a. Circumvallate
   b. Marginate
 4. Medical illnesses
   a. Cardiac
   b. Renal
   c. Hematological
 5. Male factors
 6. Dyssynchronous fertilization
 7. Coitus
 8. Exercise
	10%

Neither family history alone nor history of prior term births is sufficient to rule out a potential parental chromosomal abnormality. The chance of detecting a parental chromosomal abnormality is higher in couples who have not experienced a live birth; however, a history of spontaneous abortions interspersed with stillbirths and live births with or without congenital anomalies also may disclose parental chromosomal abnormalities on karyotype analysis. Other structural chromosome anomalies, including mosaicism, single gene defects, and inversions, may contribute to recurrent abortion. Single gene disorders may be recognized either through analysis of detailed family histories or by identification of a pattern of anomalies that make up a syndrome with a known inheritance pattern. Rarely, X-linked disorders may result in recurrent abortion of only male conceptions. New diagnostic capabilities using molecular cytogenetic techniques will undoubtedly provide insight into new parental genetic abnormalities that contribute to recurrent pregnancy loss.

Anatomic Anomalies

Anatomic causes may be either congenital or acquired. Congenital anomalies include incomplete müllerian duct fusion or septum resorption defects, diethylstilbestrol (DES) exposure, and uterine cervical anomalies. Women with an intrauterine septum may have a 60% risk for spontaneous abortion (7). Second-trimester losses are most common. First-trimester losses may occur, however, if the embryo becomes implanted on the septum because the endometrium overlying the septum is poorly developed, potentially causing abnormal placentation (8). *In utero* diethylstilbestrol (DES) exposure can cause uterine anomalies, most commonly hypoplasia contributing to first- and second-trimester spontaneous abortion, incompetent cervix, and premature labor (9). Uterine artery anomalies may contribute to pregnancy loss related to compromised blood flow to the implanted blastocyst and developing placenta (10). Acquired anatomic anomalies potentially contributing to pregnancy loss include intrauterine adhesions, leiomyomas that distort the intrauterine cavity, and endometriosis. The association of these conditions to recurrent pregnancy loss is tenuous, but theoretic mechanisms include interference with the blood supply in cases of adhesions and leiomyomas (11) and immunologic phenomena potentially involved with endometriosis (12).

Endocrinologic Abnormalities

Endocrinologic factors associated with recurrent abortion include luteal phase insufficiency, with or without disorders in which luteinizing hormone (LH) is hypersecreted, diabetes mellitus, and thyroid disease. Early pregnancy maintenance depends on progesterone production by the corpus luteum until sufficient amounts are produced by the developing trophoblast, which occurs at 7–9 weeks of gestation (13). Spontaneous abortion before 10 weeks of gestation could occur if the corpus luteum fails to produce sufficient quantities of progesterone, if progesterone delivery to the uterus is impaired, or if progesterone utilization within the endometrium and decidua is compromised. Early pregnancy failure may also ensue if the trophoblast is unable to produce biologically active progesterone following demise of the corpus luteum. Abnormal LH secretion may have a direct effect on the developing oocyte, causing premature aging, and on the endometrium, causing dyssynchronous maturation. Alternatively, abnormal LH secretion may contribute to abortion indirectly by elevating testosterone levels (14). The potential mechanism of abortion in women with diabetes mellitus may be compromised blood flow to the uterus, especially in cases of advanced disease, although elevated hemoglobin A_{1c} levels prior to conception have been associated with spontaneous abortion. There is no conclusive evidence, however, that either unsuspected or overt diabetes mellitus is a cause of spontaneous abortion (15).

Hypothyroidism is another endocrinologic disorder that has been associated with recurrent abortion, most likely as a result of ovulation or corpus luteum dysfunction, which often accompanies thyroid disease. Recently, antithyroid antibodies have been associated with recurrent abortion (16), which may be related to generalized autoimmunity. Alternatively, because in early pregnancy the body needs higher levels of thyroid hormones, antithyroid antibodies may provide a marker for individuals who are at increased risk for developing thyroid abnormalities that can culminate in pregnancy loss if this increased demand is not met.

Maternal Infections

The association of infection with recurrent abortion is among the most controversial and poorly explored of potential causes for pregnancy loss. Reproductive tract infection with bacterial, viral parasitic, zoonotic, and fungal organisms have been proposed, but mycoplasma, ureaplasma, chlamydia, and β-streptococcus are the most commonly reported

965

pathogens (17). A theoretic possibility warranting study is that early pregnancy loss results from immunologic activation in response to pathologic organisms. A large body of evidence supports the role of this mechanism in adverse events later in gestation, such as intrauterine growth retardation (18), premature rupture of membranes, and preterm parturition (19).

Immunologic Phenomena

Immunologic responses are regulated by genes of the major histocompatibility complex (MHC), located on chromosome 6. MHC class I antigens (human leukocyte antigens (HLA)-A, HLA-B, and HLA-C) and MHC class II antigens (HLA-DR, HLA-DP, and HLA-DQ) determine immunologic compatibility of tissues. Immunologic recognition of classical MHC antigens on allografts can lead to rejection. Class I MHC antigens are important recognition structures in rejection responses mediated by cytotoxic T lymphocytes. Class II MHC antigens present antigens to T lymphocytes and initiate immunity. Class II MHC genes, called immune response genes, are genetically regulated and are believed to affect susceptibility to certain diseases. Recently, a nonclassical truncated class I MHC antigen, termed HLA-G, has been described in human cytotrophoblast and the trophoblast cell lines JEG-3 and BeWo but not in Jar (20, 21). The significance of HLA-G remains speculative, however, because it is unique to trophoblast, an intriguing hypothesis is that HLA-G could be necessary for successful gestation and that aberrant responses to HLA-G may lead to abortion.

Cellular Immunity Abnormalities

As discussed in Chapter 6, immunity is more specifically regulated by CD4(+) T cells, which can be divided into T helper 1 (TH1) and T helper 2 (TH2) cells based on their production of cytokines. TH1 cells primarily secrete interferon (IFN)-γ, as well as interleukin (IL)-2, and tumor necrosis factor (TNF)-β; TH2 cells secrete primarily IL-10, IL-4, IL-5, and IL-6 (22–24). Although TNF-α can be secreted by both TH1 and TH2 cells, it is most often characteristic of a TH1 response (25, 26). A reciprocal regulating relationship exists between TH1 and TH2 cells and cytokines (27–34).

The human endometrium and decidua are replete with immune and inflammatory cells capable of cytokine secretion (35–41). An abnormal TH1 cellular immune response involving the cytokines IFN-γ and TNF is the most recent hypothesis proposed for immunologic reproductive failure (42–46). This hypothesis states that the conceptus may be a target of local cell-mediated immune responses culminating in abortion. In affected women, trophoblast antigens activate macrophages and lymphocytes, causing a cellular immune response mediated by the TH1 cytokines, IFN-γ, and TNF (42), which have been shown to inhibit *in vitro* embryo development and trophoblast growth and function (47–50). Higher levels of TNF and IL-2 have been reported in peripheral serum of women having a miscarriage compared with women having a normal pregnancy (51). However, cause-versus-effect mechanisms for this association have not been elucidated. Depending on the individual series, 60–80% of nonpregnant women with a history of otherwise unexplained recurrent spontaneous abortion have been found to have evidence of an abnormal TH1 cellular immune response to trophoblast antigens, whereas fewer than 3% of women with normal reproductive histories have cellular immunity to these same trophoblast antigens (42, 46, 52–54). In contrast to TH1 immunity to trophoblasts in women with unexplained recurrent abortion, recent evidence also indicates that most women with normal pregnancies have a TH2 immune response to trophoblast antigens (54). These data provide evidence for a new non-MHC-related mechanism for reproductive failure involving TH1 immunity to trophoblast. Cytokines may affect reproductive events either directly or indirectly, depending on the specific cytokines secreted, their concentrations, and the differentiation stage of potential reproductive target tissues.

Other cellular immune mechanisms have been implicated in recurrent abortion. Suppressor cell deficiency and macrophage activation have been associated with fetal loss, although cause-versus-effect mechanisms for these observations have not been established (17). Aberrant expression of class II MHC determinants, or enhanced expression of MHC class I on syncytiotrophoblast occurring in response to IFN-γ could mediate abortion by enhancing cytotoxic T cell attack (45). This theory appears unlikely, however, because recent data indicate that classical MHC antigens are not expressed on aborted tissues from women experiencing either their first miscarriage or their fourth or more miscarriages (55).

Humoral Immunity Abnormalities

The most scientifically credible humoral immune (antibody-mediated) mechanism implicated in recurrent abortion involves *antiphospholipid antibodies* to either cardiolipin or phosphatidylserine. These are either immunoglobulin (Ig) G or IgM directed against negatively charged phospholipid. Antiphospholipid antibodies were originally characterized by prolonged phospholipid dependent coagulation tests *in vitro* (activated partial thromboplastin time (aPTT), Russell Viper Venum Time) and thrombosis *in vivo*. The association of these antiphospholipid antibodies with obstetric complications—including spontaneous abortion, premature labor, premature rupture of membranes, stillbirth, intrauterine growth retardation, and preeclampsia—has been termed the *antiphospholipid syndrome* (56). The presence of these antiphospholipid antibodies during pregnancy is a major risk factor for adverse pregnancy outcome (57). In large series of couples with recurrent abortion, the incidence of the antiphospholipid syndrome is between 3–5% (17). **The proposed mechanism for antiphospholipid antibodies' mediation of pregnancy loss is increased thromboxane and decreased prostacycline synthesis leading to platelet adhesion within placental vessels** (58–60). *In vitro* evidence in trophoblast cell lines indicates that IgM action against phosphatidylserine can inhibit syncytial trophoblast formation (61). The pathologic evidence of the antiphospholipid antibody syndrome is often equivocal, because the characteristic lesions for this syndrome (placental infarction, abruption and hemorrhage) are often missing in women with antiphospholipid antibodies (62), and these same pathologic lesions can be found in placentae from women with recurrent abortion who do not have biochemical evidence of antiphospholipid antibodies (63).

Other antibody-mediated mechanisms for recurrent abortion have been proposed, including *antisperm* **and** *antitrophoblast antibodies* **and** *blocking antibody deficiency,* **but the relevance of these hypotheses to recurrent abortion have been disproven** (17, 45). Historically, the blocking antibody deficiency hypothesis has historically received the most attention in the literature. This hypotheses was based on the supposition that blocking factors (presumably antibodies) were required to prevent an antifetal, maternal cell-mediated immune response that was believed to occur in all pregnancies. In the absence of blocking antibodies, abortion occurred (64). This supposition has not been substantiated (65). Maternal hyporesponsiveness in mixed lymphocyte culture with paternal stimulator cells was originally proposed to identify women with deficient blocking activity (64). This work was continued by others (66, 67) who proposed that parental HLA sharing resulted in a predisposition to blocking antibody deficiency. These reports were of limited sample size, were retrospective in nature, and lacked population-based controls. More recent prospective, population-based control studies have conclusively demonstrated that HLA heterogeneity is not essential for successful pregnancy (68). Further evidence refuting the blocking antibody hypothesis for recurrent abortion comes from reports of successful pregnancies in women who do not produce serum factors capable of mixed lymphocyte culture inhibition (69) and who do not produce antipaternal cytotoxic antibodies and yet have successful pregnancies (70). These mixed lymphocyte culture results are believed to represent the effect of abortion rather than the cause of recurrent abortion (65, 70, 71).

A novel HLA-linked alloantigen system based on polyclonal rabbit antisera cross-reactive with trophoblast and lymphocytes called TLX was proposed to produce maternal blocking antibody deficiency (72). This theory was later invalidated when TLX was found to be identical to CD46, a complement receptor that is theorized to protect the placenta from complement-mediated attack (73). CD46 is found on a wide variety of cells, thus explaining the cross-reactive nature of the original antisera, which lead to the misconception that it represented a new alloantigen system.

967

Pregnancy is not dependent on an intact maternal immune system because agammaglobulinemic animals and women can successfully reproduce (74). Viable births also occur despite severe immune deficiencies and in knockout, scid, and nude mice (genetically altered mice with immune deficits). Immune mechanisms, however, such as those described for TH1-type cytokines, may be involved in pregnancy failure (54). Further work will be necessary to validate these hypotheses.

Other Factors

Other factors associated with recurrent pregnancy loss include environmental toxins, especially heavy metal toxicity and prolonged exposure to organic solvents (75); drugs such as antiprogestogens, antineoplastic agents, inhalation anesthetics, nicotine, and ethanol; ionizing radiation; and chronic medical illnesses that could interfere with uterine blood flow. Thrombocytosis (platelet counts >1 million) has also been associated with spontaneous abortion. Exposure to video display terminals and microwave ovens does not cause spontaneous abortion. The association of spontaneous abortion with living under high-energy electric power lines also has not been substantiated (76). Coffee consumption of less than 300 mg/day is not associated with spontaneous abortion (77), although there may be a risk of intrauterine growth retardation (78). There is no evidence that moderate exercise during pregnancy is associated with spontaneous abortion. Coitus has been associated with preterm birth loss (79), but this association has not been unequivocally confirmed (80).

Preconception Evaluation

Investigative measures that are potentially useful in the evaluation of recurrent spontaneous abortion include obtaining a thorough history from both partners and performing a physical assessment of the woman with attention to the pelvic examination and laboratory testing (Table 28.2).

History

A description of all prior pregnancies and their sequence as well as whether histologic assessment and karyotype determinations were performed are important aspects of the his-

---

Table 28.2   Investigative Measures Potentially Useful in the Evaluation of Recurrent Early Pregnancy Loss

History
1. Pattern, trimester, and characteristics of prior pregnancy losses
2. Exposure to environmental toxins and drugs
3. Gynecologic or obstetric infections
4. Features associated with antiphospholipid syndrome (i.e., thrombosis, autoimmune phenomena, false-positive tests for syphilis)
5. Genetic relationship between reproductive partners (consanguinity)
6. Family history of recurrent spontaneous abortion of syndrome associated with embryonic or fetal loss
7. Previous diagnostic tests and treatments

Physical
1. General physical examination, including gynecologic examination

Laboratory
1. Parental periphereal blood karyotype
2. Hysterosalpingogram followed by hysteroscopy/laparoscopy, if indicated
3. Luteal phase endometrial biopsy
4. Thyroid-stimulating hormone, antithyroid antibodies
5. Antiphospholipid antibodies (cardiolipin, phosphatidylserine)
6. Lupus anticoagulant (a partial thromboplastin time or Russell Viper Venom)
7. Compete blood count with platelets
8. Cervical cultures (mycoplasma, ureaplasma, chlamydia), if necessary

tory. Approximately 60% of abortuses lost before 8 weeks of gestation have been reported to be chromosomally abnormal (81); most of these pregnancies are affected by a type of trisomy, especially trisomy 16 (82). The most common single chromosomal abnormality is monosome X (45X), especially in anembryonic conceptuses (83). Aneuploidy may be less likely in recurrent abortions when the couple is euploidic, although this hypothesis is controversial. Most women tend to have spontaneous abortion at approximately the same time (fetal size) in sequential pregnancies. Gestational age when pregnancy loss occurred, as determined by last menstrual period, may not be informative because there is often a 2- to 3-week delay between fetal demise and signs of expulsion (84). The designation of couples experiencing recurrent abortion into either primary or secondary categories is not helpful in either the diagnosis or management of women with recurrent abortion. Also, approximately 10–15% of couples cannot be classified in either the primary or secondary categories because their first pregnancy resulted in a loss followed by a term delivery and subsequent losses. Information concerning conception ability should be obtained because approximately one-third of couples with recurrent abortion also have subfertility (attempted conception for more than 1 year). This subfertility may indicate preclinical losses. Menstrual cycle history may also provide information about the possibility of oligo-ovulation or other endocrine abnormalities. Timing of intercourse relative to ovulation should be reviewed to detect dyssynchronous fertilization that could contribute to pregnancy loss (85). Detailed family histories and drug histories should also be obtained.

Physical Examination

A general physical examination should be performed to detect signs of metabolic illness, including hyperandrogenism. During pelvic examination, signs of infection, DES exposure, and previous trauma should be ascertained. The size and shape of the uterus should also be determined.

Laboratory Assessment

Laboratory assessment includes the following:

1. Parental peripheral blood karyotyping with banding techniques

2. Assessment of the intrauterine cavity with either office hysteroscopy or hysterosalpingography, followed by operative hysteroscopy if a potentially correctable anomaly is found

3. A well-timed luteal phase endometrial biopsy, ideally 10 days after the LH surge or after cycle day 24 of an idealized 28-day cycle (if the cycle is abnormal by 3 or more days, the assessment should be repeated in a subsequent cycle; in out-of-phase biopsies, serum prolactin and androgen profile should be obtained)

4. Thyroid function testing, including thyroid-stimulating hormone and antithyroid antibodies

5. Anticardiolipin, antiphosphatidylserine, and a lupus anticoagulant test (aPTT or Russell Viper Venom)

6. Platelet assessment

7. Cervical culture for mycoplasma, ureaplasma, and chlamydia should be considered.

There is no place in the clinical care of couples with recurrent abortion for testing of the following:

1. Antinuclear antibodies

2. Antipaternal cytotoxic antibodies

3. Parental HLA profiles

4. Mixed lymphocyte culture reactivities

Likewise, other immunologic tests are necessary unless they are performed, with informed consent, under a specific study protocol in which the costs of these experimental tests are not borne by the couple or their third-party payers. Further work is necessary before suppressor cell/factor determinations, cytokine, oncogene, and growth factor measurements or embryotoxic factor assessment can be clinically justified and available.

Postconception Evaluation

Following conception, close monitoring is advised to provide psychologic support and to confirm intrauterine viability. The incidence of ectopic pregnancy and complete molar gestation is increased in women with a history of recurrent spontaneous abortion. Preliminary data suggest that the risk of pregnancy complications other than spontaneous abortion is not significantly different between women with and without a history of spontaneous abortion. An exception is women who have antiphospholipid antibodies or who have an intrauterine infection.

Determining the β-hCG may also be helpful in monitoring early pregnancy until an ultrasonographic examination can be performed. Not all investigators have found inadequate hCG levels in pregnancies ultimately aborting, however (86). Other hormonal determinations are rarely of benefit, because levels are often normal until fetal death or abortion occurs (87).

The "gold standard" for monitoring early pregnancy is ultrasonography. β-hCG should be serially monitored from the time of a missed menstrual period until the level is approximately 1500 mIu/ml, at which time an ultrasonographic scan is performed and blood sampling is discontinued. Ultrasonographic assessment is performed every 2 weeks until the time of gestation at which previous pregnancies were aborted. In the absence of fetal cardiac activity, intervention is recommended to expedite removal and to obtain tissue for karyotype analysis.

Maternal serum is obtained for α-fetoprotein assessment at 16–18 weeks of gestation. Amniocentesis is recommended to assess the fetal karyotype after the pregnancy has progressed past the time of prior losses. In the future, fetal karyotype assessment may be performed through DNA isolation from nucleated fetal erythrocytes in maternal blood (88), but this technique is not yet a clinical reality.

Therapy

Therapeutic options include the use of donor oocytes or sperm, repair of anatomic anomalies, the correction of any endocrine abnormalities, the treatment of infections, and a variety of immunologic interventions and drug treatments. Psychologic counseling and support should be recommended.

Advances in transplantation biology and molecular immunology will undoubtedly enable the formulation and utilization of new, more effective treatment modalities for recurrent abortion. Before any therapy can be clinically advocated, however, the scientific rationale for its use must be established and its safety and efficacy must be substantiated in appropriately controlled clinical trials.

Chromosomal Aberrations

No therapy is available for parental chromosomal anomalies that potentially contribute to recurrent abortion, except when a Robersonian translocation involving homologous chromosomes is detected. In such cases, either donor oocyte or donor sperm, depending on the affected partner, is recommended because this anomaly always results in aneuploidy. In other cases, synchronization of intercourse with ovulation may be of benefit, and in all cases, genetic counseling is warranted.

Anatomic Anomalies

Hysteroscopic resection of intrauterine filling defects represents state-of-the-art therapy for submucous leiomyomas, intrauterine adhesions, and intrauterine septa. Ultrasonographically guided transcervical metroplasty has also been reported to be safe and effective (89).

Cervical cerclage should be considered after the first trimester for women with DES-associated uterine anomalies. If endometriosis is encountered during a diagnostic evaluation, it should be resected laparoscopically.

Endocrine Abnormalities

Stimulating folliculogenesis with ovulation induction or luteal phase support with progesterone should be considered for women with luteal phase insufficiency. The effect of therapy, however, has not been substantiated (90). Ovulation induction may be beneficial for women with hyperandrogen and LH hypersecretion disorders, especially following pituitary desensitization with gonatropin-releasing hormone (GnRH) agonist therapy (17), although well-designed prospective, randomized control studies have not been performed. There is no evidence that assisted reproductive technologies are beneficial in preventing recurrent abortion in women who can conceive without difficulty.

Thyroid hormone replacement with synthroid may be helpful in cases of hypothyroidism. There is no place in the medical management of recurrent abortion for either thyroid medication or bromocriptine for women who do not have a thyroid or prolactin disorder.

Infections

Empiric antibiotic treatment has been used for couples with recurrent abortion. Such use is not justified unless an infection has been documented. For cases in which an infectious organism has been identified, appropriate antibiotics should be administered to both partners, followed by posttreatment culture to verify eradication of the infectious agent before attempting repeat conception.

Immunologic Factors

Because the developing conceptus contains paternally inherited gene products and tissue-specific differentiation antigens, speculation has arisen that recurrent abortion may result from maternal immunologic rejection of the semiallogenic conceptus. As a consequence of this reaction, both immunostimulating and immunosuppressive therapies have been proposed.

Leukocyte Immunization

Clinical trials addressing the efficacy of leukocyte immunization have reported conflicting results for this therapy (90–94). Despite an unsubstantiated rationale for this therapy and controversial reports concerning efficacy, paternal leukocyte transfusion has been widely used, often in response to patient demand that some form of therapy be initiated. Several meta-analyses have not established consensus regarding therapy (95–97). One published analysis reported that approximately 11 women with unexplained recurrent abortion needed to be immunized before one additional live birth was achieved (97). Approximately 92% of successful pregnancy outcomes in this study were not attributable to leukocyte immunization. Whether the 8% successful pregnancy rate achieved in leukocyte-immunized women is clinically relevant remains uncertain. Unfortunately, an entrepreneurial atmosphere has clouded the rational assessment of couples experiencing recurrent abortion, resulting in a growing number of financially lucrative leukocyte immunization clinics. However, there is no credible clinical or laboratory method to identify a specific individual who may benefit from such therapy. Leukocyte immunization is also not without significant risk to both the mother and her fetus (98–99). Several cases of graft-versus-host disease, severe intrauterine growth retardation, autoimmune and isoimmune complications, and potentially fatal thrombocytopenia in the fetus resulting from alloimmunization to platelets contained in the paternal leukocyte preparation have been reported (17, 78–102). The routine use of this therapy for recurrent abortion (that, at best, will only be efficacious in one of 11 women treated) cannot be justified clinically at this time. The procedure should be performed only as part of an appropriately controlled trial using informed consent and the costs are borne by the investigators.

Immunoregulatory Therapies

Other immunostimulating therapies have been proposed and abandoned. Intravenous preparations consisting of syncytiotrophoblast microvillus plasma membrane vesicles have been used to mimic the fetal cell contact with maternal blood that normally occurs in pregnancy (103). However, the efficacy of this approach has not been established (103). The use of third-party seminal plasma suppositories has also been attempted (104), based on the misconception that TLX was part of an idiotype-antiidiotype control system (105). Third-party seminal plasma suppositories for recurrent abortion have no scientifically credible rationale and should not be used.

Immunosuppressive and other immunoregulating therapies have been advocated for cases in which abortion was believed to be due to antiphospholipid antibodies or cellular immunity. Study design problems, including small numbers of recruited patients, lack of prestratification by maternal age and number of prior losses before randomization, and other methodological and statistical inaccuracies preclude definitive statements regarding therapeutic efficacy.

Aspirin and Heparin

A combination of low-dose *aspirin* (80 mg/day) and subcutaneous *heparin* (5000–10,000 units twice daily) has been advocated during pregnancy in women with antiphospholipid antibody syndrome (106). This therapy is not without potential risks, including gastric bleeding, osteopenia, and abruptio placenta. *Prednisone* has also been advocated but has not been found to offer any advantage over *aspirin* and *heparin* (106).

For women with antiphospholipid antibody syndrome, *aspirin* (80 mg every day) is recommended. After pregnancy has been confirmed, 10,000 IU sodium *heparin* should be administered subcutaneously twice daily throughout gestation. A PTT should be obtained weekly and the dose of heparin should be adjusted until anticoagulation is achieved. These patients should be treated by a perinatologist because of the risk of premature labor, premature rupture of the membranes, intrauterine growth retardation, intrauterine fetal demise, and preeclampsia.

Immunoglobulin

Intravenous *immunoglobulin* and plasmapheresis have also been used to treat women with recurrent abortion suspected to be caused by antiphospholipid antibodies (107, 108), although these approaches have not been substantiated. Intravenous immunoglobulin administration has also been advocated to treat women with unexplained recurrent abortion, although in studies promoting this therapy, patients were neither prestratified by age or number of prior losses before randomization nor included in sufficient numbers to achieve meaningful results (109–113). The specific rationale for this therapy is unclear, although immunoglobulin has a number of immunoregulating actions, including T cell and Fc receptor regulation, complement inactivation, enhanced T cell suppressor function, and down-regulation of TH1 cytokine synthesis (114). Therefore, intravenous immunoglobulin administration may be of benefit in treating women with recurrent abortion related to TH1 immunity to trophoblast.

Other Therapies

Other immunoregulating therapies theoretically useful in treating recurrent abortion include *cyclosporine, pentoxifylline,* and *nifedipine,* although maternal and fetal risks with these agents preclude their clinical use. *Progesterone* also has immunosuppressive effects in doses approaching 10^{-5} mmol/l concentrations of *progesterone* can inhibit in vitro TH1 immunity to trophoblast (117).

Psychological Support

A caring, empathetic attitude is prerequisite to healing. The acknowledgement of the pain and suffering couples have experienced as a result of recurrent abortion can be a cathartic catalyst enabling them to incorporate their experience of loss into their lives rather than their lives into their experience of loss (17). Referrals to support groups and counselors should be offered. Self-help measures, including meditation, yoga, exercise, and biofeedback, may also be helpful.

Prognosis

The prognosis for successful pregnancy depends on the potential underlying etiology of pregnancy loss and epidemiologically on the number of prior losses (Table 28.3). As previously discussed, epidemiologic surveys indicate that the chance of a viable birth even after four prior losses may be as high as 60%. Depending on the study, the prognosis for successful pregnancy in couples with a cytogenetic etiology for reproductive loss varies from 20 to 80% (118–120). Women with corrected anatomical anomalies may expect a successful pregnancy in 60–90% of cases (118, 119, 121, 122). A success rate higher than 90% has been reported for women with corrected endocrinologic abnormalities (118). Between 70 and 90% of viable pregnancies have been reported for women receiving therapy for antiphospholipid antibodies (123, 124). Assessment of TH1 immunity to trophoblast in early pregnancy has been reported to be useful in predicting successful pregnancy outcome. Of 85 women determined to be negative for embryotoxic TH1 cytokines in early pregnancy, only 11 (13%) subsequently aborted whereas 74 (87%) had a successful pregnancies. Of 56 women determined to be positive for these embryotoxic cytokines, 40 (71%) aborted and only 16 (29%) subsequently had a viable pregnancies (46).

Ultrasonography may also be useful in predicting pregnancy outcome. In one study, the live birth rate following documentation of fetal cardiac activity between 5 and 6 weeks from the last menstrual period was approximately 77% in women with two or more unexplained spontaneous abortions (125).

Table 28.3   Prognosis for Viable Birth

Following:	
One abortion	76%
Two abortions	70%
Three abortions	65%
Four abortions	60%
With:	
Genetic factors	20–80%
Anatomic factors	60–90%
Endocrine factors	>90%
Infectious factors	70–90%
Antiphospholipid antibodies	70–90%
TH1 cellular immunity	70–87%
Unknown factors	40–90%
Following:	
Ultrasound detected fetal cardiac activity at 6 weeks of gestation	77%

References

1. **Edmonds DK, Lindsay KI, Miller JF.** Early embryonic mortality in women. *Fertil Steril* 1982;38:447–53.

2. **Wilcox AJ, Weinberg CR, O'Connor JF, Baird DD, Schlatterer JP, Canfield RE, et al.** Incidence of early loss of pregnancy. *N Engl J Med* 1988;319:189–94.

3. **Alberman E.** The epidemiology of repeated abortion. In: **Beard RW, Sharp F,** eds. *Early Pregnancy Loss: Mechanisms and Treatment.* New York: Springer-Verlag, 1988:9–17.

4. **Warburton D, Fraser FC.** Spontaneous abortion rate in man: data from reproductive histories collected in a medical genetics unit. *Am J Hum Genet* 1963;16:1–25.

5. **Regan L, Braude PR, Trembath PL.** Influence of post reproductive performance on risk of spontaneous abortion. *BMJ* 1989;299:541–5.

6. **Daniel A, Hook EB, Wolf G.** Risks of unbalanced progeny at amniocentesis of carriers of chromosome rearrangements: data from United States and Canadian laboratories. *Am J Hum Genet* 1989;33:14–53.

7. **Buttram VC, Gibbons WE.** Müllerian anomalies: a proposed classification on analysis of 144 cases. *Fertil Steril* 1979;32:40–6.

8. **Mizuno K, Koske K, Ando K.** Significance of Jones operation on double uterus: vascularity and dating of endometrium in uterine septum. *Jpn J Fertil Steril* 1978;29:9.

9. **Barnes AB, Colton T, Gundersen J, Noller KL, Tilley BC, Strama T, et al.** Fertility and outcome of pregnancy in women exposed in utero to diethylstilbestrol. *N Engl J Med* 1980;302:609–13.

10. **Burchell RC, Creed F, Rasoulpour M, Whitcomb M.** Vascular anatomy of the human uterus and pregnancy wastages. *Br J Obstet Gynaecol* 1978;85:698–706.

11. **Buttram VC, Reiter RC.** Uterine leiomyomata: etiology symptomology and management. *Fertil Steril* 1981;76:433–55.

12. **Hill JA.** Endometriosis: immune cells and their products. In: **Hunt JS,** ed. *Immunobiology of Reproduction.* Serono Symposium, USA. New York: Springer-Verlag, 1994:23–33.

13. **Csapo AI, Pulkkinen MO, Ruttner B, Sauvage JB, Wiest WG.** The significance of the corpus luteum in pregnancy maintenance. I - Preliminary studies. *Am J Obstet Gynecol* 1972;112:1061–7.

14. **Watson H, Kiddy DS, Hamilton-Fairley D, Scanlon MJ, Barnard C, Collins WP, et al.** Hypersecretion of luteinizing hormone and ovarian steroids in women with recurrent early miscarriages. *Hum Reprod* 1993;8:829–33.

15. **Kalter H.** Diabetes and spontaneous abortion: a historical review. *Am J Obstet Gynecol* 1987;156:1243–53.

16. **Stagnaro-Green A, Roman SH, Cobin RH, el-Harazy E, Alvarez-Marfany M, Davies TF.** Detection of at risk pregnancy by means of highly sensitive assays for thyroid auto-antibodies. *JAMA* 1990;264:1422–5.

17. **Hill JA.** Sporadic and recurrent spontaneous abortion. *Curr Probl Obstet Gynecol Fertil* 1994;17:114–62.

18. **Heyborne KD, Wilkin SS, McGregor JA.** Tumor necrosis factor-α in midtrimester amniotic fluid is associated with impaired intrauterine fetal growth. *Am J Obstet Gynecol* 1992;167:920–5.

19. **Romero R, Mazor M, Sepulueda W, Auila C, Copeland D, Williams J.** Tumor necrosis factor in preterm and term labor. *Am J Obstet Gynecol* 1992;166:1576–87.

20. **Kovats S, Main EK, Librach C, Stubblebine M, Fisher SJ, DeMars R, et al.** A class I antigen HLA-G expressed in human trophoblasts. *Science* 1990;248:220–3.

21. **Feinman MA, Kliman JH, Main EK.** HLA antigen expression and induction by α-interferon in cultured human trophoblast. *Am J Obstet Gynecol* 1987;157:1429–34.

22. **Mosmann TR, Cherminski HM, Bond MW, Griedlin MA, Coffman RL.** Two types of murein helper T cell clones I. Definition according to profiles of lymphokine activities and secreted proteins. *J Immunol* 1986;2348–57.

23. **Kurt-Jones EA, Hamberg S, Ohara J, Paul WE, Abbas AK.** Heterogeneity of helper/inducer T lymphocytes. I. Lymphokine production and lymphokine responsiveness. *J Exp Med* 1987;166:1774–87.

24. **Romagnani S.** Human TH1 and TH2 subsets: doubt no more. *Immunol Today* 1991;8:256–7.

25. **Mosmann TR, Coffman RL.** Heterogeneity of cytokine secretion patterns and functions of helper T cells. *Adv Immunol* 1989;46:111–47.

26. **Ramagnani S.** Human TH1 and TH2 subsets: regulation of differentiation and role in protection and immunopathology. *Int Arch Allergy Immunol* 1992;4:279–85.

27. **Cher DJ, Mosmann TR.** Two types of murine helper T cell clones II. Delayed type hypersensitivity is mediated by TH1 clones. *J Immunol* 1987;138:3688–94.

28. **Mosmann TR, Coffman RL.** TH1 and TH2 cells: different patterns of lymphokine secretion lead to different functional properties. *Annu Rev Immunol* 1989;7:145–73.

29. **Maggi E, Parronchi P, Monetti R, Simonell C, Piccinni MP, Rugiu FS, et al.** Reciprocal regulatory effects of IFN-α and IL-4 in *in vitro* development of human TH1 and TH2 clones. *J Immunol* 1992;148:2142–7.

30. **Fiorentino DF, Bond MW, Mosmann TR.** Two types of mouse T helper cell IV. TH2 clones secrete a factor that inhibits cytokine production by TH1 clones. *J Exp Med* 1989;170:2081–95.

31. **Mosmann TR, Moore KW.** The role of IL-10 in cross regulation of TH1 and TH2 responses. *Immunol Today* 1991;12:A49–53.

32. **Oswald IP, Wynn TA, Sher A, James SL.** Interleukin-10 inhibits macrophage microbicidal activity by blocking the endogenous production of tumor necrosis factor-α required as a costimulating factor for interferon-α activation. *Proc Natl Acad Sci U S A* 1992;88:8676–80.

33. **Cunha FQ, Moncada S, Lieu FY.** Interleukin-10 inhibits the induction of nitric oxide synthase by interferon-α in murine macrophages. *Biochem Biophys Res Commun* 1992;182:1155–9.

34. **Fraser EJ, Grines DA, Schulz KF.** Immunizations as therapy for recurrent spontaneous abortion: a review and meta-analysis. *Obstet Gynecol* 1993;82:854–9.

35. **Sen DR, Fox H.** The lymphoid tissue of the endometrium. *Gynecol Pathol* 1967;163:371.

36. **Kearns M, Lala PH.** Bone marrow origin of decidual cell precursors in the pseudopregnant mouse uterus. *J Exp Med* 1982;155:1537.

37. **Bulmer JN, Sunderland CA.** Immunohistological characterization of lymphoid cell populations in the early human placental bed. *Immunology* 1984;52:349–57.

38. **Kabawat SE, Mostaoufi-Zedeh M, Driscoll SG, Bhan AK.** Implantation site in normal pregnancy: a study with monoclonal antibodies. *Am J Pathol* 1985;118:76–84.

39. **Morris H, Edwards J, Tiltman A, Emms M.** Endometrial lymphoid tissue: an immunohistological study. *J Clin Pathol* 1985;38:644–52.

40. **Tabibzadeh S.** Human endometrium: an active site of cytokine production and action. *Endocr Rev* 1991;12:272–90.

41. **Klentzeris LD, Bulmer JN, Warren A, Morrison L, Li TC, Cooke ID.** Endometrial lymphoid tissue in the timed endometrial biopsy: morphometric and immunohistochemical aspects. *Am J Obstet Gynecol* 1992;167:667–74.

42. **Hill JA, Polgar K, Harlow BL, Anderson DJ.** Evidence of embryo- and trophoblast-toxic cellular immune response(s) in women with recurrent spontaneous abortion. *Am J Obstet Gynecol* 1992;166:1044–52.

43. **Hill JA.** Sporadic and recurrent spontaneous abortion. *Curr Probl Obstet Gynecol Fertil* 1994; 17:113–64.

44. **Hill JA, Anderson DJ.** Cell-mediated immune mechanisms in recurrent spontaneous abortion. In: **Talwar GP,** ed. *Contraceptive Research for Today and the Nineties.* New York: Springer-Verlag, 1988:171–80.

45. **Hill JA.** Immunological mechanisms of pregnancy maintenance and failure: a critique of theories and therapy. *Am J Reprod Immunol* 1990;22:33–42.

46. **Ecker JL, Laufer MR, Hill JA.** Measurement of embryotoxic factors is predictive of pregnancy outcome in women with a history of recurrent abortion. *Obstet Gynecol* 1993;81:84–7.

47. **Berkowitz RS, Hill JA, Kurtz CB, Anderson DJ.** Effects of products of activated leukocytes (lymphokines and monokines) on the growth of malignant trophoblast cells in vitro. *Am J Obstet Gynecol* 1988;158:199–204.

48. **Hunt JS, Soales MJ, Lei MG, Smith RN, Weaton D, Atherton RA, et al.** Products of lipopolysaccharide-activated macrophages (tumor necrosis factor-α, transforming growth factor-β) but not lipopolysaccharide modify DNA synthesis by rat trophoblast cells exhibiting the 80-KDa LPS-binding protein. *J Immunol* 1989;143:1606–13.

49. **Hill J, Haimovici F, Anderson DJ.** Products of activated lymphocytes and macrophages inhibit mouse embryo development in vitro. *J Immunol* 1987;139:2250–4.

50. **Drasner K, Epstein CJ, Epstein LB.** The antiproliferative effects of interferon on murine embryonic cells. *Proc Soc Exp Biol Med* 1979;160:46–9.

51. **Mallmann P, Werner A, Krebs D.** Serum levels of interleukin-2 and tumor necrosis factor-α in women with recurrent abortion. *Am J Obstet Gynecol* 100;163:1367.

52. **Laufer MR, Ecker JL, Hill JA.** Pregnancy outcome following ultrasound detected fetal cardiac activity in women with a history of multiple spontaneous abortions. *J Soc Gynecol Invest.* 1994;1:138–42.

53. **Yamada H, Polgar K, Hill JA.** Cell-mediated immunity to trophoblast antigens in women with recurrent spontaneous abortion. *Am J Obstet Gynecol* 1994;170:1339–44.

54. **Hill JA, Polgar K, Anderson DJ.** T Helper 1-type immunity to trophoblast antigens in women with recurrent spontaneous abortion. *JAMA* 1995;273:1933–6.

55. **Hill JA, Melling GC, Johnson PM.** Immunohistochemical studies of human uteroplacental tissues from first trimester spontaneous abortion. *Am J Obstet Gynecol* 1995;173:90–6.

56. **Harris EN.** Syndrome of the black swan. *Br J Rheumatol* 1986;26:324–6.

57. **Out HJ, Bruinse HW, Christians CML, van Vliet M, de Groot PG, Nieuwenhuis HU, et al.** A prospective, controlled multicenter study of the obstetric risks of pregnant women with antiphosphalipid antibodies. *Br J Obstet Gynaecol* 1992;167:26–32.

58. **Harris EN, Asherson RA, Gharavi AE, Morgan SH, Derue G, Hughes GR.** Thrombocytopenia in SLE and related disorders: association with anticardiolipin antibodies. *Br J Haematol* 1985;59:227–30.

59. **Cariou R, Tobelem G, Soria C, Caen J.** Inhibition of protein C activation by endothelial cells in the presence of lupus anticoagulant. *N Engl J Med* 1986;314:1193–4.

60. **Freyssinet JM, Wiesel ML, Gauchy J, Boneu B, Cazenave JP.** An IgM lupus anticoagulant that neutralizes the enhancing effect of phospholipid on purified endothelial thrombomodulin activity: a mechanism for thrombosis. *Thromb Haemost* 1986;55:309–13.

61. **Lyden TW, NG AK, Rote NJ.** Modulation of phosphatidyl-serine epitope expression on BeWo cells during forskolin treatment. *Am J Reprod Immunol* 1992;27:24.

62. **Hanly JG, Gladman DD, Rose TH, Laskin CA, Urowitz MB, et al.** Lupus pregnancy: a prospective study of placental changes. *Arthritis Rheum* 1988;31:358–66.

63. **Lockshin MD, Druzin ML, Goei S, Qamar T, Magid MS, Jovanovic L, et al.** Antibody to cardiolipin as a predictor of fetal distress or death in pregnant patients with systemic lupus erythematosus. *N Engl J Med* 1985;313:152–6.

64. **Rocklin RE, Kitzmiller JL, Garvey MR.** Maternal-fetal relation: further characterization of an immunologic blocking factor that develops during pregnancy. *Clin Immunol Immunopathol* 1982;22:305–15.

65. **Sargent IL, Wilkins T, Redman CWG.** Maternal immune responses to the fetus in early pregnancy and recurrent miscarriage. *Lancet* 1994;2:1099–104.

66. **Beer AE, Quebbeman JF, Ayers JW, Haines RF.** Major histocompatibility complex antigens, maternal and paternal immune responses and chronic habitual abortion in humans. *Am J Obstet Gynecol* 1981;141:987–99.

67. **McIntyre JA, Faulk WP.** Recurrent spontaneous abortion in human pregnancy: results of immunogenetical, cellular and humoral tests. *Am J Reprod Immunol* 1983;4:165–70.

68. **Ober CL, Martin AO, Simpson JL, Hauck WW, Amos DB, Kostyu DD, et al.** Shared HLA antigens and reproductive performance among Hutterites. *Am J Hum Genet* 1983;35:994–1004.

69. **Rocklin RE, Kitzmiller JL, Garvey MR.** Maternal-fetal relation: further characterization of an immunologic blocking factor that develops during pregnancy. *Clin Immunol Immunopathol* 1982;22:305–15.

70. **Amos DB, Kostyn DD.** HLA: a central immunological agency of man. *Adv Hum Genet* 1980; 10:137–41.

71. **Coulam CB.** Immunological tests in the evaluation of reproductive disorders: a critical review. *Am J Obstet Gynecol* 1992;167:1844–51.

72. **McIntyre JA, Faulk WP, Verhulst ST, Colliver JA.** Human trophoblast-lymphocyte cross-reactive (TLX) antigens define a new alloantigen system. *Science* 1983;222:1135–7.

73. **Purcell DF, McKenzie IF, Lublin DM, Johnson PM, Atkinson JP, Oglesby TJ, et al.** The human cell surface glycoproteins Hu Ly-M5, membrane co-factor protein (MCP) of the complement system, and trophoblast leukocyte common (TLX) antigen are CD46. *Immunology* 1990;70:155–61.

74. **Rodger C.** Lack of a requirement for a maternal humoral immune response to establish and maintain successful allogenic pregnancy. *Transplantation* 1985;40:372–5.

75. **Polifka JE, Friedmann JM.** Environmental toxins and recurrent pregnancy loss. *Infert Reprod Med Clin North Am* 1991;2:195–213.

76. **Schnorr TM, Grajewski BA, Hornung RW, Thun MJ, Egeland GM, Murray WE, et al.** Video display terminals and the risk of spontaneous abortions. *N Engl J Med* 1991;324:727–33.

77. **Mills JL, Holmes LB, Aarons JH, Simpson JL, Brown ZA, Jovanic-Peterson LG, et al.** Moderate caffeine use and the risk of spontaneous abortion and intrauterine growth retardation. *JAMA* 1993;269:593–7.

78. **Dlugosz L, Bracken MB.** Reproductive effects of caffeine: a review and theoretical analysis. *Epidemiol Rev* 1992;4:83–100.

79. **Naeye RL.** Coitus and associated amniotic-fluid infections. *N Engl J Med* 1979;301:1198–200.

80. **Kwki T, Ylikorkala O.** Coitus during pregnancy is not related to bacterial vaginosis or preterm birth. *Am J Obstet Gynecol* 1993;169:1130–4.

81. **Boue J, Bove A, Laser P.** Retrospective and prospective epidemiologic studies of 1,500 karyotyped spontaneous abortions. *Teratology* 1975;11:11–26.

82. **Stein Z.** Early fetal loss. *Birth Defects* 1981;17:95–111.

83. **Hook EB, Warburton D.** The distribution of chromosomal genotypes associated with Turner's syndrome: live birth prevalence rates and evidence for administered fetal mortality and severity in genotypes associated with structural X abnormalities of mosaicism. *Hum Genet* 1983; 64:24–7.

84. **Miller JF, Williamson E, Glue J, Gordon YB, Grudzinskas JG, Sykes A.** Fetal loss after implantation: a prospective study. *Lancet* 1980;2:554–6.

85. **Boue J, Boue A.** Increased frequency of chromosomal anomalies in abortions after induced ovulation. *Lancet* 1973;7804:679–80.

86. **Lird T, Whittaker PG.** The endocrinology of early pregnancy failure. In: **Huisjes HJ, Lird T,** eds. *Early Pregnancy Failure*. New York: Churchill Livingstone, 1990:39–54.

87. **Westergaard JG, Teisner B, Sinosich MJ, Madsen LT, Grudzinskas JG.** Does ultrasound examination render biochemical tests obsolete in the predicting of early pregnancy failure? *Br J Obstet Gynaecol* 1985;92:77–83.

88. **Bianchi DW, Flint AF, Pizzimenti MF, Knoll JH, Latt SA.** Isolation of fetal DNA from nucleated erythrocytes in maternal blood. *Proc Natl Acad Sci U S A* 1990;87:3279–83.

89. **Querlen D, Brasme TL, Parmentier D.** Ultrasound-guided transcervical metroplasty. *Fertil Steril* 1990;54:995–8.

90. **Karamardin LM, Grimes DA.** Luteal phase deficiency: effect of treatment on pregnancy rates. *Am J Obstet Gynecol* 1992;167:1391–8.

91. **Mowbray JF, Gibbings C, Liddell H, Reginald PW, Underwood JL, Beard RW.** Controlled trial of treatment of recurrent spontaneous abortion by immunostimulation with paternal cells. *Lancet* 1985;1:941–3.

92. **Ho HN, Gill TJ 3rd, Hsieh HJ, Jiang JJ, Lee TY, Hsieh CY, et al.** Immunotherapy for recurrent spontaneous abortion in a Chinese population. *Am J Reprod Immunol* 1991;25:10–5.

93. **Cuchi MN, Lim D, Yong DE, Kloss M, Pepperell RJ.** The treatment of recurrent aborters by immunization with paternal cells: controlled trials. *Am J Reprod Immunol* 1991;25:16–7.

977

94. **Gatenby PA, Cameron K, Simes RJ, Adelstein S, Bennett MJ, Jansen RP, et al.** Treatment of recurrent spontaneous abortion by immunization with paternal lymphocytes: results of a controlled trial. *Am J Reprod Immunol* 1993;29:88–94.

95. **Fraser EJ, Grimes DA, Schulz KF.** Immunization as therapy for recurrent spontaneous abortion: a review and meta-analysis. *Obstet Gynecol* 1993;82:854–9.

96. **Scott JS, Prendiville W, Jeny G.** Recurrent miscarriage and early pregnancy failure immunotherapy. In: **Liliford R, Ddrife J, Jarvis G,** eds. *The Oxford Trials in Gynecology: Effective Core in Gynecology.* London: 1994.

97. **The Recurrent Miscarriage Immunotherapy Trialist Group.** Worldwide collaborative observational study and meta-analysis of allogenic leukocyte immunotherapy for recurrent spontaneous abortion. *Am J Reprod Immunol* 1994;32:55–72.

98. **Hill JA, Anderson DJ.** Blood transfusions for recurrent abortion? Is the treatment worse than the disease? *Fertil Steril* 1986;46:152–3.

99. **Hormeyr GJ, Jaffe MI, Bezwoda WR, VanIdekinge B.** Immunologic investigation of recurrent pregnancy loss and consequences of immunization with husbands leukocytes. *Fertil Steril* 1987;48:681–4.

100. **Katz I, Fisch B, Amit S, Ovadia J, Tadir Y.** Cutaneous graft-versus host-like reaction after paternal lymphocyte immunization for prevention of recurrent abortion. *Fertil Steril* 1992; 57:927–9.

101. **Menge A, Beer AE.** The significance of human leukocyte antigen profiles in human infertility, recurrent abortion and pregnancy disorders. *Fertil Steril* 1985;43:693–4.

102. **Christiansen OB, Mathiesen O, Husth M, Lahsitsen JG, Giannet N.** Placebo controlled trial of active immunization with third party leukocytes in recurrent miscarriage. *Acta Obstet Gynecol Scand* 1994;73:261–8.

103. **Johnson PM, Ramsden GH.** Recurrent miscarriage. *Baillieres Clin Immunol Allergy* 1992; 2:607–24.

104. **Coulam CB, Stern JJ.** Seminal plasma treatment of recurrent spontaneous abortion. In: **Dondero F, Johnson PM,** eds. *Reproductive Immunology.* Serono Symposia 97. New York: Raven Press, 1993:205–16.

105. **Thaler CJ.** Immunologic role for seminal plasma in insemination and pregnancy. *Am J Reprod Immunol* 1989;21:147.

106. **Lubbe WF, Butler WS, Palmer SJ, Liggins GC.** Fetal survival after prednisone suppression of maternal lupus-anticoagulant. *Lancet* 1983;1:1361–3.

107. **Bernstein RM, Crawford RJ.** Intravenous IgG therapy for anticardiolipin syndrome: a case report. *Clin Exp Rheumatol* 1988;6:198.

108. **Ferro D, Quintarelli C, Russo G, Valesini G, Bonavita MS, Violi F.** Successful removal of antiphospholipid antibodies using repeated plasma exchanges and prednisone. *Clin Exp Rheumatol* 1989;7:103–4.

109. **Müeller-Eckhardt G, Heine O, Neppert J, Kunzel W, Müeller-Eckhardt C.** Prevention of recurrent spontaneous abortion by intravenous immunoglobulin. *Vox Sang* 1989;56:151–4.

110. **Coulam CB.** Immunotherapy with intravenous immunoglobulin for the treatment of recurrent pregnancy loss: American experience. *Am J Reprod Immunol* 1994;32:286–9.

111. **Müeller-Eckhart G, Huni O, Poltrin B.** IVIG to prevent recurrent spontaneous abortion. *Lancet* 1991;1:424–5.

112. **Christiansen OB, Mathiesen O, Lauristien JG.** Intravenous immunoglobulin treatment of women with multiple miscarriages. *Hum Reprod* 1992;7:718–22.

113. **Coulam CB, Stern JJ, Bustillo M.** Ultrasonic findings of pregnancy losses after treatment of recurrent pregnancy loss: intravenous immunoglobulin versus placebo. *Fertil Steril* 1994;61: 248–51.

114. **Dwyer JM.** Manipulating the immune system with immunoglobulin. *N Engl J Med* 1992; 326:107–16.

115. **Siiteri PK, Febres F, Clemens LE, Chang RJ, Gondos B, Stites D.** Progesterone and maintenance of pregnancy. Is progesterone nature's immunosuppressant? *Ann N Y Acad Sci* 1977; 286:384–97.

978

116. **Hill JA, Barbieri RL, Anderson DJ.** Immunosuppressive effects of danazol *in vitro. Fertil Steril* 1987;48:414–18.

117. **Polgar K, Hill JA.** Progesterone inhibits *in vitro* embryotoxic factor production in women with recurrent spontaneous abortion. *Proc Soc Gynecol Invest* 1994;41:22–26.

118. **Tho PT, Byrd JR, McDonough PG.** Etiologic and subsequent reproductive performance of 100 couples with a prior history of habitual abortion. *Fertil Steril* 1979;32:389–95.

119. **Harger JH, Archer DF, Marchese SG, Muracca-Clemens M, Garver KL.** Etiology of recurrent pregnancy loss and outcome of subsequent pregnancies. *Obstet Gynecol* 1983;62: 574–81.

120. **Vlaadneren W, Treffers PE.** Prognosis of subsequent pregnancies after recurrent spontaneous abortion in first trimester. *BMJ* 1987;295;92–3.

121. **March CM, Israel R.** Hysteroscopic management of recurrent abortion caused by septate uterus; with discussion. *Am J Obstet Gynecol* 1987;156:834–42.

122. **DeCherney AH, Russell JB, Graebe RA, Polan ML.** Resectoscopic management of müllerian fusion defects. *Fertil Steril* 1986;45:726.

123. **Lubbe WF, Liggins GC.** Role of lupus anticoagulant and autoimmunity in recurrent pregnancy loss. *Semin Reprod Endocrinol* 1988;6:161–90.

124. **Branch DW, Silver RM, Blackwell JL, Reading JC, Scott JR.** Outcome of treated pregnancies in women with antiphospholipid syndrome: an update of the Utah experience. *Obstet Gynecol* 1992;80:614–20.

125. **Laufer MR, Ecker JL, Hill JA.** Pregnancy outcome following ultrasound detected fetal cardiac activity in women with history of multiple spontaneous abortion. *J Soc Gynecol Invest* 1994;1:138–42.

29 Menopause

William W. Hurd

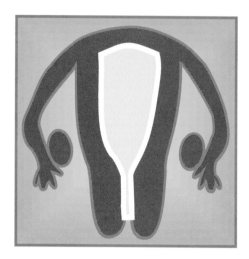

More than 30% of the female population of the United States is postmenopausal, and this percentage is increasing (1). Despite the universality of "the change of life," the importance of its medical and psychological implications only recently has been appreciated. Because each woman's response to menopause may be different, the management of conditions during this midlife period must be based on the individual.

Although menopause, defined as the permanent cessation of menses that occurs after the cessation of ovarian function, is the most identifiable event during this period, the years immediately before and the decades afterward are of much greater clinical significance. The perimenopause encompasses the time before, during, and after menopause. The period of hormonal transition before menopause, also known as the menopausal transition, can be uneventful or a time of significant symptoms. This period may have an insidious or relatively abrupt onset, usually in the mid- to late forties. The symptoms that begin with the menopausal transition usually continue into the postmenopausal period.

The postmenopausal period is associated with a significant increase in the incidence of age-related medical conditions. It is becoming increasingly clear, however, that some of the conditions, specifically osteoporosis and cardiovascular disease, are related to estrogen deficiency as well as to age. For this reason, gynecologic care of postmenopausal women should address the issue of hormonal replacement therapy.

Perimenopausal Phases

Menopausal Transition **The period that precedes menopause is characterized by a varying degree of somatic and psychological changes that reflect alterations in the normal cyclic functioning of the ovary.** Early recognition of the symptoms and the use of appropriate screening tests can minimize the impact of this potentially disruptive period.

981

The menopausal transition begins gradually and may be heralded in the mid- to late forties with subtle symptoms. These symptoms may be ignored or discounted by both the patient and the physician. It is often difficult to differentiate stress-related symptoms from those that could be related to lower levels of estrogen. For this reason, both stress and relative estrogen deficiency should be considered when managing the problems associated with menopausal transition.

The most significant symptom of menopausal transition in some women is menstrual irregularity (2). This symptom occurs in 90% of women during the 4 years of transition prior to menopause. Because abnormal bleeding is one of the most common indications for hysterectomy, menstrual irregularity during the menopausal transition should be evaluated carefully to determine whether it is the result of lower levels of estrogen or underlying pathology (3).

Menopause

The cessation of menses resulting from the loss of ovarian function is an event rather than a period of time. Menopause occurs at a median age of 51 years (2–4). The age of menopause appears to be determined genetically and does not seem to be related to race or nutritional status. Menopause occurs earlier in cigarette smokers (4), in some women who have had hysterectomies (5), and in nulliparous women (4).

With the depletion of ovarian follicles that are able to respond to gonadotropins, follicular development and cyclic estrogen production cease. Traditionally, menopause has been diagnosed retrospectively. Using modern laboratory tests, however, menopause may be defined more precisely as amenorrhea in the presence of signs of hypoestrogenemia and a serum follicle-stimulating hormone (FSH) level higher than 40 IU/l. Menopause can also be diagnosed on the basis of subjective symptoms, such as hot flushes or flashes, or the results of a provocative test such as progesterone withdrawal. Some of the more acute symptoms of menopause, such as hot flashes, become most intense near menopause, when the level of circulating estrogen may drop suddenly. This is especially true with women who experience premature ovarian failure.

Postmenopausal Period

Following menopause is a period of relative ovarian quiescence that lasts more than one-third of the average woman's life. Menopause is a natural event—a part of the normal process of aging.

Hormone replacement therapy is one of the primary concerns of women's health care after menopause. Even though the long-term health impact of estrogen deficiency may be similar to that of thyroid or adrenal deficiencies, relatively little attention has been paid to this problem. This may be because the health problems associated with estrogen deficiency tend to be chronic rather than acute. For example, osteoporosis is usually not clinically apparent until decades after menopause, when it is harder to treat. The impact of estrogen deficiency on cardiovascular disease is often confused with age-related changes.

Another factor that may obscure the impact of menopause is that the loss of ovarian function does not result in an absolute estrogen deficiency. Because of peripheral conversion of androgens of both ovarian and adrenal origin, some women are less affected by estrogen deficiency than others.

Premature Ovarian Failure

Loss of ovarian function is usually a gradual process that occurs over a number of years and culminates in menopause. In some women, however, ovarian function is lost earlier and more suddenly than expected as a result of natural causes, chemotherapy, or surgery.

Premature ovarian failure is defined as when menopause occurs spontaneously before 40 years of age (6). Because of the relatively young age and the unexpected nature of the event, both psychological and hormonal support may be necessary. Although most practitioners are not adequately prepared to offer comprehensive psychological support, asking appropriate questions and making support services available can be helpful. The possibility of associated endocrine abnormalities should be considered in women who develop premature ovarian failure (see Chapter 24).

In more than 40% of hysterectomies, both ovaries are removed (3). The young age of these women compared with those undergoing natural menopause, and the abrupt onset of associated symptoms create special problems (7).

Usually, estrogen replacement is needed immediately. The most obvious problem is the acute onset of hot flashes (8). After several months, hot flashes may be followed by signs of vaginal atrophy. Long-term, surgical menopause has been associated with significantly higher risk for both osteoporosis and cardiovascular disease than with natural menopause (9, 10). These risks can be decreased with estrogen replacement therapy. Because long-term replacement may expose women to some risks, the relative risks and benefits of oophorectomy and estrogen replacement therapy should be thoroughly discussed with any woman considering bilateral oophorectomy at the time of hysterectomy.

Hormonal Changes of Menopause

Changes in hormone production and metabolism occur gradually during the menopausal transition. After almost 4 decades of cyclic production of estrogen and progesterone by the ovaries, these organs decrease their production of estrogen production and eventually cease any cyclic activity. However, the ovaries continue to indefinitely produce some level of hormones postmenopausally.

Menopausal Transition

During the menopausal transition, ovarian follicles become increasingly resistant to FSH stimulation while estradiol levels remain relatively constant. This process is most clearly demonstrated by the relative resistance to gonadotropins in women undergoing ovulation stimulation for *in vitro* fertilization. In the average women younger than 30 years of age, levels of estradiol higher than 1000 pg/ml are attainable using stimulation of approximately 225 IU FSH per day. In contrast, most women older than 40 years of age rarely attain estradiol levels this high, despite stimulation with up to three times as much FSH per day. This degree of ovarian resistance to stimulation may explain the hot flashes experienced by some women, despite what appear to be normal levels of estradiol as evidenced by monthly menstruation. Hot flashes may be the result of gonadotropin surges related to low estradiol levels.

Progesterone, the hormone of ovulation, is produced almost exclusively by granulosa cells during the luteal phase. During the menopausal transition, ovulation becomes less frequent in most women (11). In some women, ovulation continues to occur, but the luteal levels of progesterone are lower than in younger women (12).

Menopause

During menopause, the levels of hormones, the way they are produced, and their roles change. The hormones most affected include those produced by the ovaries: estrogen, progesterone, and androgens.

Estrogen

At the time of menopause, ovarian estrogen secretion becomes negligible (13). Although the amount of estrogen secreted by the ovaries after menopause appears to be insignificant, all women continue to have measurable levels of circulating estradiol and estrone throughout their lifetimes. The answer to this apparent paradox lies in the ability of peripheral tissue to aromatize adrenal and ovarian androgens.

Assessment of the postmenopausal levels of peripheral circulating estrogens illustrates the role of peripheral conversion of androgens to estrogens. Prior to menopause, estradiol levels range from 50 to 300 pg/ml. After menopause, when ovarian estrogen secretion is negligible, levels of both estradiol and estrone can be as high as 100 pg/ml (14). **For the most part, these estrogens are the result of peripheral conversion (aromatization) of androstenedione, an androgen produced primarily by the adrenal gland as well as by the ovary postmenopausally** (15). **Aromatization of androgens to estrogens occurs primarily in muscle and adipose tissue** (16). For this reason, obese women often have an increased level of circulating estrogens and the unopposed estrogen places them at an increased risk of endometrial cancer (17). In contrast, thin women have a decreased level of circulating estrogens, thus explaining their increased risk for osteoporosis (18). Surprisingly, the increased levels of estrogen often seen in obese women do not appear to protect them from menopausal symptoms (19).

Progesterone

After menopause, progesterone production ceases (20). The absence of cyclic increases and decreases in progesterone is usually associated with the absence of premenstrual symptoms (21). Decreased progesterone levels affect organs, such as endometrium and breast, that are responsive to gonadal steroids. Progesterone protects the endometrium from excess estrogen stimulation during the reproductive years. Progesterone primarily regulates estrogen receptors, but it also exerts direct intranuclear effects that inhibit the tropic effects of estrogen on the endometrium (22). Because circulating levels of estrogen remain high enough to stimulate the endometrium prior to menopause and, in many women, postmenopausally (12), unopposed stimulation of the endometrium may be a relatively common phenomenon. This probably explains the higher risk of endometrial hyperplasia and cancer found just prior to and after menopause (23).

Breast tissue is known to be extremely sensitive to gonadal hormones. Although the relationship is less clear than with endometrial tissue, unopposed estrogen stimulation of the breast in the absence of progesterone has been hypothesized to play a role in the development of breast cancer (24). Although there are data that suggest that the use of combined estrogen and progestin replacement therapy may decrease the risk of breast cancer (25), a more recent large study does not support this (24).

Androgens

The third class of steroids produced by the ovaries are androgens, most notably testosterone and androstenedione. The potential role of the ovaries in androgen production, especially after menopause, has only recently been appreciated (11).

Prior to menopause, the ovary produces approximately 50% of the circulating androstenedione and 25% of the testosterone. This results in a circulating concentration of testosterone of less than one-tenth that in men (0.50 ng/ml vs. 6 ng/ml). Also, the free (unbound and thus biologically active) testosterone is only one-third that in men, because the relative amount of sex hormone binding globulin is relatively higher in women.

After menopause, total androgen production decreases, mainly because ovarian production decreases but also because adrenal production decreases (11). The circulating levels of androstenedione and testosterone during the quiescence are approximately 0.53 and 0.23 ng/ml, respectively (26). Of this total production, the ovaries are responsible for 20% of the androstenedione and 40% of the testosterone, primarily as a result of gonadotropin stimulation of the stromal cells (27). Because of the role of the ovaries before and after menopause, oophorectomy results in a sharp decrease in androgen levels (12).

The significance of this decrease is uncertain because the physiologic role of circulating androgens in women is not well defined.

Patient Concerns about Menopause

As women go through changes in their hormone levels and bodies, they may experience emotions ranging from mild concern to frank denial (28). The physician should be aware that a patient's concerns may differ from the physician's medical concerns (29). A patient's response to menopause may be affected by other factors, such as lifestyle and genetic regulation of the aging process.

The loss of fertility and menstrual function that accompany natural or surgical menopause may have an impact on a woman's sense of well-being. The physician should be sensitive to the potentially significant emotional distress faced by these women and be prepared to offer psychological support.

Menopause may be viewed as a transition from middle age to old age by many women. Although some may look upon this with pleasant anticipation as a time of relative freedom from such worries as undesired pregnancies and the stress of childbearing, many women fear this period because of the anticipated losses. Thus, the subtle signs of the menopausal transition may be ignored as a means of denial. Because of denial, a woman may be hesitant to report unusual and potentially hormonally related symptoms to her physician. Unless directly asked, many symptoms may go undetected, resulting in a delay in diagnosis and treatment.

Loss of Childbearing Capacity

The effect of the loss of the ability to have children may depend on the role childbearing has played in a woman's life. For some women, childbearing and childrearing have been a major source of status and self-esteem; thus, loss of fertility may cause great distress (29). Some women have delayed childbearing for various reasons, and if they have tried to become pregnant too late to be successful, the onset of menopausal symptoms may represent tangible evidence of their "failure" to have children. However, the results of one study suggest that single and childless women are less likely to be depressed than other women (30).

The loss of fecundity may not be a problem for all women. For some, unwanted fertility has been a concern for many of their reproductive years. For them, the ultimate birth control, menopause, may be a welcome occurrence. An individual's response to the loss of childbearing capacity may not even be readily apparent to the patient, and thus, all potential reactions to this loss should be understood by the physician.

Loss of Youth

Regardless of the effect of the loss of childbearing capacity, the distress produced by the loss of youth symbolized by menopause may be subtle yet disturbing (31). In our society, youth is highly prized whereas maturity often is not; thus, tangible evidence of aging may be traumatic. The degree to which this may affect a woman may be related to the value she places on personal appearance. Aging may not be important to many women, but the possibility that this may cause anxiety or depression should be considered.

Skin Changes

The apparent acceleration of the skin changes associated with aging, especially after menopause, is a concern for many women. Increasing evidence suggests that estrogen deficiency plays a significant role in these changes. Estrogen therapy during the quiescence has been shown to maintain skin thickness (32). Although mechanisms underlying this effect are ill-understood, a major factor may be the ability of estrogen to both prevent and restore age-related loss of skin collagen (33). Because changes in collagen may be the major determinant in skin aging, these effects of estrogen may be important (34).

Certainly, estrogen therapy cannot completely prevent the effects of aging on skin, nor can it counteract the effects of environmental stresses on skin, such as sun exposure and cigarette smoking. However, estrogen therapy during the quiescence appears to have beneficial effects on the skin.

Changes in Mood or Behavior

Depression

Depression is one of the most frequent medical disorders seen in patients by primary care providers (35). More than 20% of patients who seek medical care for any symptoms suffer from clinical depression. This is a particular problem for women and older patients. It is a widely held belief that depression occurs more often during the perimenopausal period. Studies have failed to show a relationship between clinical depression and hormonal status, however, suggesting that many psychiatric symptoms that occur during this period may be more related to psychosocial events such as changes in relationships with children, marital status, and other life events (36).

Anxiety and Irritability

Many women report an increased level of anxiety and irritability during the perimenopausal period; thus, these symptoms have become a prominent part of what is sometimes termed the "climacteric syndrome" (37). Although the incidence of overt psychiatric disorders may not be increased, these complaints become more frequent. It is commonly accepted by the lay public that anxiety and irritability are the result of estrogen deficiency (29). Despite this, multiple studies have found no evidence that most psychological symptoms experienced during the menopausal transition are related to estrogen deficiency or that they resolve with estrogen replacement therapy (38, 39). The increased anxiety and irritability associated with the perimenopausal period is more clearly associated with psychosocial factors than with estrogen status (40). It is important to investigate and treat the constellation of symptoms that occur during the menopausal transition. Psychological intervention may be helpful for some women.

Loss of Libido

A major concern is a decrease in libido or in sexual satisfaction that may occur with natural or surgical menopause. However, sexual activity remains relatively stable in women before and after menopause (41). Although only one-half of menopausal women report being sexually active (42), this may be related to the relative decrease in the number of men in the aging population (1).

Vaginal atrophy is a factor that can contribute to a decrease in sexual satisfaction. Approximately one-third of postmenopausal woman who are not taking estrogen therapy will experience vaginal atrophy (43). The discomfort that results from a lack of vaginal lubrication may decrease sexual satisfaction. Atrophy can easily be treated with oral or vaginal estrogen therapy. Vaginal lubricants, especially those that are water soluble, can also be useful.

The role that androgens play in libido before and after menopause is uncertain. Levels of circulating androgen decrease after menopause, and this decrease may be accentuated by oophorectomy (11). In men, the relationship of androgens and libido is well established. For this reason, androgen therapy for women experiencing decreased libido has been advocated (44). Libido is a complex cerebral phenomenon that is dependent on input from multiple sources, and the decrease in androgens associated with menopause has not been shown to consistently alter libido. Available evidence suggests that sexual satisfaction among postmenopausal women is not decreased over time (45).

Diagnostic Approaches

Beginning at about 40 years of age, routine health maintenance should include screening for problems related to hormonal changes. Questions concerning changes in menstrual function, abnormal bleeding, hot flashes, sleep disturbances, and sexual function should be asked routinely. Early detection of perimenopausal problems and appropriate intervention is important.

Abnormal Bleeding

During the menopausal transition, it has been estimated that menstrual irregularity occurs in more than half of all women (46). Bleeding can be irregular, heavy, or prolonged. In most cases, uterine bleeding is related to anovulatory cycles. This disruption of menstrual patterns has been attributed to a gradual decrease in the number of normally functioning follicles reflected by gradually increasing follicular-phase FSH levels (47).

Although anovulation is one of the most common causes of abnormal uterine bleeding, it is not the only or the most important cause. Pregnancy always should be considered in any menstruating woman, because pregnancies are still reported in the late forties. Many of these women do not consider themselves to be fertile; thus, abnormal bleeding may be the first indicator of an unexpected pregnancy.

As pregnancy rates decline, the incidence of endometrial cancer increases. Endometrial cancer should be suspected in perimenopausal women with abnormal uterine bleeding. After menopause, the overall incidence of endometrial cancer is approximately 0.1% women per year (48), but in women with abnormal uterine bleeding, it is about 10% (49–51). This risk is increased at least fivefold in women with a history of unopposed estrogen use (50, 51) and decreased by more than two-thirds in women taking a combination of estrogen and a progestin (48).

Malignant precursors such as complex endometrial hyperplasia become more common during the menopausal transition. Because early diagnosis is the most effective way to improve prognosis, perimenopausal women who have abnormal uterine bleeding should undergo endometrial biopsy. Other causes of abnormal bleeding that should be considered are cervical cancer, polyps, or leiomyomas.

Evaluation

Endometrial Sampling   **The importance of endometrial biopsy cannot be overemphasized for women with abnormal uterine bleeding during the menopausal transition and after menopause. Although dilation and curettage was formerly the sampling method of choice, it is now well accepted that an office endometrial biopsy is just as accurate (52). For this reason, office endometrial biopsy should be the initial approach to the management of abnormal uterine bleeding (in the perimenopausal patient) (Fig. 29.1) (53). Endocervical curettage should also be performed to exclude endocervical pathology. If endometrial biopsy is hindered by cervical stenosis, dilation and curettage should be performed with adequate anesthesia in the operating room.**

Vaginal Ultrasound   In 15% of cases, the results of endometrial biopsy are reported as "tissue insufficient for diagnosis" (54). In the past, when few diagnostic options were available, this situation was an indication for uterine curettage (52). With newer diagnostic modalities available, however, uterine curettage is not usually necessary. In general, the most likely diagnosis is endometrial atrophy, especially in women taking monthly progestin therapy. **If the amount of tissue obtained on endometrial biopsy is insufficient for diagnosis, vaginal ultrasonography can be performed to obtain additional information. Preliminary studies suggest that if the endometrial stripe is less than 5 mm thick, the risk of endometrial hyperplasia or cancer is extremely small** (55, 56). A thickened endometrial lining or an obvious intrauterine lesion is an indication for more thorough evaluation.

Hysteroscopy   Another evaluation that may be helpful in selected cases is hysteroscopy (57). This technique, which has been adapted for use as an office procedure, allows visual inspection of the endometrial cavity with directed biopsy when indicated (58). Hysteroscopy allows the identification of endometrial polyps or submucosal leiomyomas. Like many high-

987

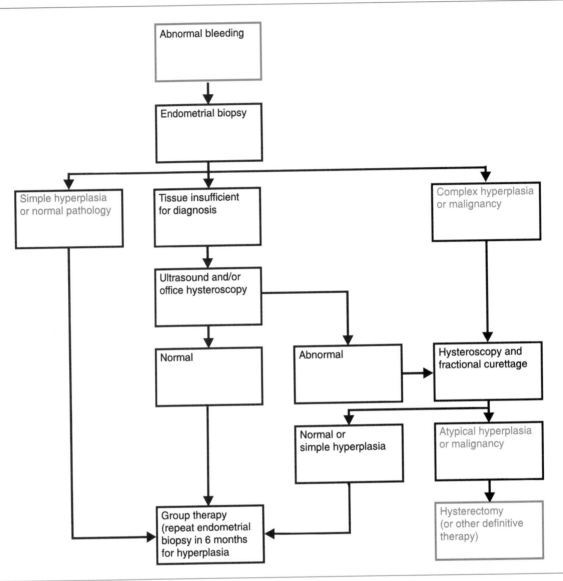

Figure 29.1   Management of perimenopausal abnormal uterine bleeding.

technology approaches, hysteroscopy requires appropriate training and equipment to ensure patient safety. If the diagnosis is in doubt, dilation and curettage is the most widely accepted method for evaluation of the endometrium (52) (see Chapter 13).

Treatment   Treatment of perimenopausal abnormal uterine bleeding is either hormonal or surgical, depending on the patient's symptoms and diagnosis. Because anovulation is one of the most common causes of abnormal uterine bleeding during menopause, hormonal therapy is the first approach after intrauterine pathology has been excluded.

Hormonal   *Oral Contraceptives*   In low-risk premenopausal women with hormone-related symptoms who are not using any form of contraception, modern low-dose (<35 μg *ethinyl estradiol*) oral contraceptives offer many advantages with minimal risk (59). New formulations contain as little as 20 μg of *ethinyl estradiol* and 1 mg of *norethindrone acetate*. In addition to preventing undesired pregnancies, these formulations are associated with a high degree of menstrual regularity and can be used to treat symptoms associated with relative estrogen deficiency. **The use of oral contraceptives until menopause has been found to be safe in women with no risk factors for cardiovascular disease** (60). Before starting the administration of oral contraceptives in this age group, patients should be free of the following risk factors: hypertension, hypercholesterolemia, cigarette smoking, previous thromboembolic disorders, cerebral vascular disease, or coronary artery disease. **Because the estrogen dose in these pills is approximately four times the dose used after the menopause, women taking this therapy should be switched to traditional estrogen therapy by the 50 years of age, or sooner if symptoms occur.**

Cyclic Progestins   Some women may not be candidates for oral contraceptives because their use is contraindicated or unacceptable based on the presence of other symptoms or because of fear of complications. In these patients, alternative methods of hormonal therapy can be used. A standard approach is cyclic progestin therapy (*medroxyprogesterone* 10 mg daily for 10 days each month) to induce withdrawal bleeding and to decrease the risk of endometrial hyperplasia. It may be difficult to control abnormal uterine bleeding with cyclic progestin use during the menopausal transition because the ovaries continue to cycle intermittently. Progestin administration may be difficult to synchronize with spontaneous ovulation.

Surgical

During the menopausal transition, surgery may be required for abnormal uterine bleeding, pelvic relaxation, or pelvic masses.

Dilation and Curettage   When endometrial polyps are determined to be the cause of abnormal uterine bleeding, curettage can be both therapeutic and diagnostic. Because polyps can be missed by curettage alone, it has been recommended that diagnostic hysteroscopy be performed prior to uterine curettage for abnormal uterine bleeding (57). **With the exception of endometrial polyps, uterine curettage has not been shown to have any long-term benefit in the treatment of abnormal uterine bleeding.**

Hysterectomy   Although removal of the uterus is the most common and effective surgical treatment for abnormal uterine bleeding (61), hysterectomy is associated with a certain degree of morbidity and cost. Prior to recommending hysterectomy, an adequate preoperative evaluation must include endometrial sampling and an adequate trial of hormonal therapy to control the bleeding.

A special consideration is whether normal ovaries should be removed (see Chapter 22). It is now standard practice for postmenopausal women undergoing hysterectomy to have their ovaries removed to avoid the subsequent risk of ovarian cancer (62). Oophorectomy has been recommended in women older than 40–45 years of age for the same reason. In premenopausal women, however, there are some disadvantages to oophorectomy. First, immediate hormonal replacement is necessary and may be somewhat more difficult to manage because of the sudden and precipitous drop in estrogen levels. In addition, oophorectomy also results in a decrease in androgen production, which may have as yet unknown long-term effects (11). **After 40 years of age, the decision to remove normal ovaries during hysterectomy should be discussed carefully and the patient should be made aware of the potential known advantages and disadvantages.**

Endometrial Ablation   A relatively new and potentially advantageous approach to dysfunctional uterine bleeding during the menopausal transition is endometrial ablation. This relatively minor surgical procedure involves destroying the functioning endometrium with electrical energy using a hystero-resectoscope, as discussed in Chapter 21. The risks of uterine perforation, bowel injury, and fluid overload related to the nonconducting distention media are low if the correct technique is used (61). However, the long-term risks remain uncertain, although this technique has been used for several years in high-risk patients.

The risk of uterine malignancy is unknown. The concern is that as the injured endometrial lining remodels, glandular tissue may be buried under scar tissue. Theoretically, this situation could delay uterine bleeding, which is the earliest sign of endometrial cancer. However, subsequent endometrial cancer after endometrial ablation has been reported only in women who had preexisting endometrial hyperplasia (63). For this reason, a thorough fractional curettage should be performed prior to the procedure. Monthly progestin therapy could be used thereafter in an attempt to decrease the risk in these potentially anovulatory women. Until long-term data become available, women considering this therapy should be informed about this potential risk of endometrial ablation.

Estrogen Deficiency

Most women experience some effects of estrogen deficiency during menopause. Other symptoms often associated with menopause may not be directly related to estrogen deficiency but rather are multifactorial. Effects can range from short-term discomfort to long-term changes that can have a profound effect on a woman's health. Both short-term and chronic effects respond to estrogen replacement therapy.

Diagnosis

The determination of ovarian function is based primarily on clinical criteria. If a woman's body is producing enough hormones for regular menstruation, her estrogen level is sufficient to protect against osteoporosis and heart disease. If a woman who is almost 50 years old stops menstruating completely, a presumptive diagnosis of estrogen insufficiency can be made without further testing. In a younger woman who has oligomenorrhea or amenorrhea or who is experiencing subtle symptoms, however, hormonal assays may be necessary to confirm the diagnosis.

The progestin challenge test is a frequently used bioassay for estrogen status (64). If a nonpregnant woman has amenorrhea but no other symptom of estrogen deficiency, administration of *medroxyprogesterone* (10 mg orally for 10 days) will produce withdrawal bleeding in women who have levels of circulating estrogen adequate to produce endometrial proliferation.

Estradiol

In women who have amenorrhea with other symptoms of estrogen deficiency or in whom progestin withdrawal bleeding does not occur, a measurement of serum estradiol can be helpful. In a menstruating woman, normal estradiol levels range from 40 to 300 pg/ml. In an oligo-ovulatory woman, an estradiol level >30 pg/ml usually indicates some degree of residual ovarian function. Women older than 70 years of age occasionally have levels this high, presumably as a result of peripheral conversion (29). For this reason, the absolute estradiol level should not be the deciding factor when considering hormonal replacement therapy. During the menopausal transition, relative ovarian resistance may result in hot flashes and related symptoms despite relatively normal serum estradiol levels. Because many of the symptoms of the menopausal transition are central nervous system in origin, treatment is sometimes indicated for symptoms alone and should not be withheld simply because the serum estradiol levels are in the normal range.

Follicle-Stimulating Hormone

The most consistent finding in the menopausal transition is an elevation of serum FSH levels. In menstruating women, FSH on cycle day 3 should be 5–10 IU/l with normally functioning ovaries (65). Elevated FSH levels (10–25 IU/l) suggest relative ovarian resistance consistent with the menopausal transition, even if estradiol levels are in the normal range. Physiologically, this is believed to be the result of decreased inhibin production by the ovarian follicles during the last decade of menstrual function. FSH

levels >40 IU/l are consistent with complete cessation of ovarian function. However, ovarian function can wax and wane over several years. Therefore, women with amenorrhea and FSH >40 IU/l may resume menstruating for a short time in the future and occasionally may achieve pregnancy (66).

Luteinizing Hormone

Evaluation of luteinizing hormone (LH) levels appears to be of somewhat less value than other hormone assessments during the menopausal transition. Prior to menopause, LH levels are usually in the range of 5–20 IU/l. Although LH levels increase in the menopausal transition in a manner similar to FSH, LH is also significantly elevated during the midcycle surge and in cases of chronic anovulation. Because individuals rarely may present with amenorrhea as a result of gonadotropin-secreting pituitary adenomas, it is reasonable to check both LH and FSH in women, especially young patients, with apparent loss of ovarian function (67).

Symptoms

Amenorrhea

The most obvious symptom of cessation of cyclic ovarian function is prolonged amenorrhea. The cessation of menstruation indicates that the amount of estrogen produced by the ovaries is no longer enough to promote endometrial proliferation, and the absence of cyclic progesterone production is accompanied by the absence of withdrawal bleeding.

This is an advantageous situation for several reasons. First, the sometimes disabling discomfort and anemia suffered by many women as a result of cyclic bleeding is no longer a problem. Second, any abnormal bleeding that may occur later serves as a warning for potential malignancy and is obvious to both the patient and her physician.

Unfortunately, estrogen replacement therapy results in vaginal bleeding in most women (68). Not only is this effect a common reason for discontinuing estrogen replacement therapy, but bleeding that would normally be interpreted as a warning sign is attributed to the hormonal therapy, potentially delaying diagnosis of a malignancy.

Hot Flashes

The classic symptom associated with estrogen deficiency is the hot flash, also known as a "hot flush." This symptom is described as "recurrent, transient periods of flushing, sweating, and a sensation of heat, often accompanied by palpitations, feelings of anxiety, and sometimes followed by chills" (69). The entire episode usually lasts no more than 1–3 minutes and may recur as many as 30 times per day, although 5–10 times per day is probably more common (8). Hot flashes are experienced by at least one-half of all women during natural menopause and by even more women after surgical menopause (69, 70).

Although most women do not report these events as particularly disturbing, as many as 25% complain of severe or frequent hot flashes, especially after surgical menopause. In these cases, hot flashes may be accompanied by fatigue, nervousness, anxiety, irritability, depression, and memory loss (71). These sensations may result in part from hot flashes that occur at night, referred to as "night sweats," which are believed to exert their effect by the interruption of sleep patterns. Early in the menopausal transition, vasomotor instability may manifest as an intermittent sleep disturbance in the absence of obvious hot flashes.

Physiologically, hot flashes correspond to marked, episodic increases in the frequency and intensity of gonadotropin-releasing hormone (GnRH) pulses from the hypothalamus. Although it has not been firmly established, it is believed that these symptoms are not the result of increased GnRH secretion. Instead, the increased pulsatile activity is a marker for the same central disturbance of the body temperature regulation center that is responsible for the hot flashes (72).

991

Estrogen replacement therapy results in the resolution of hot flashes in most women in a matter of days. In some women, especially after oophorectomy, a higher dose of estrogen is commonly needed. In the case of women without risk factors for cardiovascular disease, low-dose oral contraceptives can be used with excellent results. Alternatively, the daily estrogen dose can be increased stepwise to as high as the equivalent of 2.5 mg of *conjugated estrogens* to resolve persistent hot flashes. The estrogen dose should be tapered slowly down over a period of months to no more than 1.25 mg of conjugated estrogen per day, because the risk of cardiovascular disease actually may be increased in women taking larger doses (73).

In women for whom estrogen replacement is contraindicated, multiple alternate treatments for hot flashes have been developed. The most effective alternatives may be progestins such as *medroxyprogesterone* (10–30 mg daily orally) (74) or *megestrol acetate* (20–40 mg daily orally) (75). If either of these progestins result in intolerable side effects, the use of alternative progestins may be given, although few data exist regarding their efficacy.

In addition to the progestins, other nonsteroidal treatment for hot flashes have been developed. One of the best studied is the α_2-adrenergic agonist, *clonidine*. This drug probably works through both central and peripheral mechanisms and can be given either orally (0.05 mg twice daily) or by transdermal patch (0.1 mg weekly) (76).

In the past, night sweats were treated with a formulation that contained a combination of *phenobarbital, ergotamine,* and *belladonna (Bellergal)*. However, this combination has a marked sedative effect and potentially can be habit-forming. In addition, controlled studies show little long-term effectiveness of this treatment (77). For these reasons, this formulation is not currently recommended as a treatment for hot flashes.

Many women have mild hot flashes that they do not feel require therapy. If estrogen therapy is not prescribed for other medical indications (e.g., osteoporosis or cardiovascular prophylaxis), the patient can be advised that without treatment, the symptoms usually slowly subside over 3–5 years (69).

Sleep Disturbances

Changes in sleep patterns occur in both sexes with age. However, during the menopausal transition, many women experience increasing difficulties with sleep and insomnia that appear to be related to estrogen deficiency (37). Hot flashes may disrupt sleep and sleep patterns, a problem that may be markedly improved by estrogen therapy (78).

Long-Term Health Problems

Low estrogen levels have a cumulative effect on many tissues. Prolonged estrogen deficiency may contribute to the development of potentially reversible conditions, such as genitourinary atrophy, or more life-threatening and irreversible conditions, such as cardiovascular disease and osteoporosis. Prevention and early detection remain the cornerstones of health maintenance in this age group.

Vaginal and Urinary Tract Changes

Vaginal tissue and the tissues of the urethra and bladder base are known to be estrogen-sensitive. Within 4–5 years of menopause, approximately one-third of women who are not taking estrogen therapy develop symptomatic atrophy (79). Vaginal symptoms include dryness, dyspareunia, and recurrent vaginal infections. Fortunately, these symptoms are reversible with estrogen therapy (80).

Urinary symptoms may include dysuria, urgency, and recurrent urinary tract infections (43). In addition, genuine stress urinary incontinence may be related to estrogen deficiency. Urethral shortening associated with postmenopausal atrophic changes may result in urinary incontinence. Estrogen therapy may improve or cure stress urinary incontinence in more than 50% of treated women, presumably by exerting a direct effect on urethral mucosa (81). A trial of estrogen therapy should be undertaken prior to a surgical approach in any woman with vaginal atrophy.

Central Nervous System

Estrogen deficiency appears to have effects on the central nervous system that have only recently been appreciated. Perimenopausal women often experience difficulty in concentrating and loss of short-term memory. These symptoms have been attributed either to the effects of aging alone or to subtle sleep deprivation associated with hot flashes (82). Estrogen appears to have direct effects on mental function, and replacement therapy has been shown to improve both short-term memory and psychological function in postmenopausal women (83, 84).

One of the most intriguing areas of research is the potential role of estrogen therapy in the prevention or treatment of Alzheimer's disease. **Evidence suggests that the risk of developing Alzheimer's disease can be decreased by estrogen therapy** (85, 86). Although the precise role of estrogen deficiency in Alzheimer's disease has yet to be defined, the implications of this finding for the aging population are readily apparent.

Cardiovascular Disease

Cardiovascular disease, including coronary artery disease and cerebrovascular disease, continues to be the leading public health problem in this country. Combined, these diseases account for more than 50% of all deaths in women older than 50 years of age (87).

Cardiovascular disease has been associated with multiple causes, the most important of which may be age. The risk of cardiovascular disease throughout their lifetimes increases for men and women (87). Although the risk of death from coronary artery disease is at least three times as great for men as for women before menopause, the relative risk for women increases significantly after menopause. It is essential to be aware of preventable risk factors for cardiovascular disease and to encourage women to minimize these risk factors.

One of the most pervasive and treatable risk factors after the menopause is hypoestrogenemia. In the past, it was believed that age alone explained the increased risk of cardiovascular disease observed after menopause (88). Recent data have indicated that estrogen deficiency significantly increases the risk of cardiovascular disease and that this risk can be reduced by estrogen replacement therapy (89). Postmenopausal women taking estrogen replacement therapy have less than one-half the risk of either myocardial infarction or stroke as women who are not taking estrogen therapy (73, 87, 90). This substantial and well-documented benefit of estrogen therapy should be made known to patients, especially those who may be reluctant to take estrogens for other reasons.

Although hypoestrogenemia is apparently a major contributing factor to cardiovascular disease in women, other risk factors that are amenable to change may be equally as important. Probably the most significant risk factors are hypertension and cigarette smoking (53). Studies suggest that hypertension increases the risk of cardiovascular disease by 10-fold and cigarette smoking increases the risk by at least threefold (91). Other risk factors include diabetes mellitus, hypercholesterolemia, and a sedentary lifestyle. To decrease cardiovascular disease in postmenopausal women, screening for these risk factors must be performed and lifestyle changes must be recommended.

Osteoporosis

The association between both natural and surgical menopause and osteoporosis has been clearly established. **By definition, osteoporosis is the reduction in the quantity of bone. Because this definition may be too broad to be clinically useful, some authors have narrowed the definition to include only bone loss that has progressed to a point that** specific parts of the skeleton are so thin that they have an enhanced susceptibility to fractures or that fractures are actually present (92). The degree of cortical and trabecular bone loss necessary to meet this criterion is uncertain in those who have not yet had a bone fracture. The numbers of elderly women who have osteoporosis-related crush fractures of spinal vertebrae or fractures of either the radius or the neck of the femur have reached epidemic proportions (93). With the aging of the population, the problem is likely to increase in the future.

Although the rate of bone loss significantly increases at the time of menopause, the maximum incidence of osteoporosis-related fractures appears to occur several decades later. It is estimated that more than 30% of all women older than 90 years of age will experience hip fractures (94) and approximately 20% of these women will die within 3 months, most commonly from complications related to prolonged immobilization (95). By the time signs of osteoporosis become apparent, treatment is difficult.

Pathophysiology   The cause of osteoporosis is multifactorial. The primary factors associated with osteoporosis include heredity, age, estrogen status, and dietary calcium intake.

Age is the most important factor associated with bone loss (96). All women begin losing bone mass in their early thirties, and this loss continues throughout their lives. Before menopause, the rate of loss is less than 1% of total bone tissue per year. After menopause, the rate of bone loss increases to as high as 5% per year in estrogen-deficient women. Evidence suggests that this may be related to the gradual decrease in growth hormone levels associated with age (97).

Heredity plays a role primarily by determining the peak bone mass that a woman will attain during her life and the subsequent rate of bone loss. On average, African-American women have a much higher bone mass than white women, and this may explain the low risk of osteoporotic bone fractures observed in African-Americans (98). A family history of osteoporosis is a strong risk factor (99).

A third factor associated with bone loss is estrogen status. For women not taking estrogen replacement, bone loss after menopause is accelerated to a rate of 3–5% per year (100). This loss is most rapid during the first 5 years after menopause, when up to 20% of the expected lifetime loss from the femoral neck may occur (101). Depending on the age at surgery, surgical menopause poses a higher risk than natural menopause because of the longer period with low estrogen (102). Hypoestrogenemia has a direct effect on osteoblast function and appears to exert its adverse effects by altering calcium balance (103, 104).

A fourth factor is dietary calcium. Dietary calcium, primarily in the form of dairy products, has been shown to be associated with decreased bone loss in premenopausal women (105). In postmenopausal women taking estrogen therapy, calcium supplementation of 1000 mg/day appears to be sufficient to decrease bone loss (106). However, the average dietary intake of calcium in the U.S. is only 500 mg/day for adults (105). Calcium therapy can be given as calcium carbonate (oyster shell) tablets or as calcium citrate. Fortunately, this amount of calcium supplementation does not appear to increase the risk of kidney stones (107). However, it may be associated with gastrointestinal complaints such as constipation or increased flatus.

Other factors that preserve bone density and decrease the risk of osteoporosis include physical activity (108) and avoidance of cigarette smoking (109). There have been no controlled studies of these factors to determine their impact on osteoporosis-related fractures in later life.

Methods for Detection   After a prolonged period of hypoestrogenemia, bone loss is only partially reversible. For these reasons, it is more practical and effective in most women to implement therapy to prevent bone loss at the time of menopause than to screen for early signs of osteoporosis.

In some women, estrogen replacement therapy may be contraindicated or not desired by the patient. In these women, an alternative approach would be to screen for bone loss at set intervals and institute therapy if a defined threshold of osteopenia is reached (Table 29.1). No standard guideline for significant osteopenia has been established, and the indications for the use of these techniques, e.g., densitometry, are not yet established.

Estrogen Replacement Therapy

Estrogen deficiency has been considered by many to be a physiologic rather than a pathologic condition, probably because ovarian failure is genetically programmed. With the increased life expectancy of women, however, the negative impact of prolonged estrogen deficiency becomes more significant. Although estrogen deficiency is treatable, fewer than 20% of postmenopausal women take estrogen (110). Although estrogen replacement therapy is not completely risk-free, the health benefits appear to outweigh the risks.

Benefits

Estrogen replacement therapy is indicated for any woman with signs or symptoms of hypoestrogenemia (Table 29.2). Because of the health risks associated with estrogen deficiency, replacement therapy should be offered to all postmenopausal woman who do not have a contraindication. Women with known risk factors for cardiovascular disease or osteoporosis should be encouraged to take estrogen to minimize their risks. Some of the ben-

Table 29.1   Radiographic Techniques to Screen for Osteoporosis

Test	Advantages	Disadvantages
Standard x-ray	Lowest total radiation exposure	Detects only bone losses of >30–40%
Single photon absorptiometry, hand		Does not closely correlate with vertebral bone density
Duel energy x-ray absorptiometry	Measures radius, hip, and spine	
Quantitative computed tomography		Highest total radiation exposure

Table 29.2   Indications and Contraindications for Estrogen Replacement Therapy

Indications	Contraindications
Menopause	**Absolute**
Hot flashes	Pregnancy
Vaginal atrophy	Undiagnosed uterine bleeding
Urinary tract symptoms	Active thrombophlebitis
High risk for osteoporosis	Current gallbladder disease
Family history	Liver disease
Cigarette smoker	
Low body weight	**Relative**
Radiographic evidence	History of breast cancer
High risk for cardiovascular disease	History of recurrent thrombophlebitis
Previous myocardial infarction/angina	or thromboembolic disease
Hypertension	
Family history	
Cigarette smoker	

efits of estrogen are felt immediately, but the long-term benefits may not be apparent for several decades.

Hot Flashes

Hot flashes are the most common factors motivating women to start and continue hormonal replacement. Hot flashes may interfere with the normal sleep cycle resulting in insomnia (82), and in severe cases, they may also interfere with concentration (69). Although oral estrogen therapy usually is effective in reducing the severity and frequency of hot flashes within a few days, patients should be advised that it may be several weeks before maximal relief is achieved.

Osteoporosis

Estrogen replacement therapy helps maintain bone mass and skeletal integrity, thereby protecting against osteoporosis (111). Estrogen conserves calcium by both enhancing the efficiency of intestinal absorption and by improving renal calcium conservation (103). In addition, estrogen appears to have a direct effect on osteoblast function (104). Although estrogen can effectively slow bone loss, it can reverse, to a limited degree, the bone loss associated with osteoporosis (112). For this reason, estrogen replacement therapy should be initiated at menopause and should be given for a long term, although the optimal duration is unclear.

Recent evidence has suggested that progesterone also has a role in maintaining bone density (113). Progesterone appears to promote bone formation by increasing osteoblast activity either directly or indirectly, by inhibiting the glucocorticoid effect on osteoblasts. This finding supports the use of a progestin alone in women who are unable to take estrogen therapy.

Cardiovascular Disease

Estrogen replacement therapy protects against cardiovascular disease, including coronary artery disease and stroke. Multiple cohort and case-control studies have shown that estrogen decreases the risk of both myocardial infarction and stroke by 50% (73, 87, 90). Even when there is angiographic evidence of coronary artery disease, estrogen enhances survival (114).

There are several mechanisms by which estrogen protects the heart. The most important mechanism appears to be the effect of estrogen on serum lipids and lipoproteins. Estrogen decreases circulating levels of low-density lipoproteins (115, 116) and increases high-density lipoproteins. Both the absolute decrease in total cholesterol and the increase in the high-density/low-density lipoprotein ratio appear to retard progression of coronary artery disease. Although these effects are attenuated by concomitant progestin use, this effect appears to decrease over time (117). It has been estimated that estrogen accounts for 20–50% of the total protective effect for cardiovascular disease. The degree to which progestins may diminish this effect, if any, is unknown.

Estrogen also exerts an anti-atherosclerosis effect on blood vessels (118). This appears to result, in part, from a direct effect on blood vessels that is not reversed by progestin. Estrogen appears to be an antioxidant that decreases the formation of lipid peroxidases, which may decrease atherosclerosis by minimizing the oxidation of low-density lipoprotein cholesterol, a potent inducer of plaque formation in vessels (119).

A third beneficial effect is that of vasodilation (120). There appears to be a direct effect on blood vessel endothelial cells that results in immediate vasodilatation, perhaps mediated by estrogen receptors (121).

A final effect is on coagulation. Low doses of estrogen (i.e., 0.625 mg daily of *conjugated estrogens*) results in a subclinical decrease in coagulability by decreasing platelet aggregation and fibrinogen and by inhibiting plasminogen formation (122). This effect appears to be lost with higher doses of estrogen (i.e., 1.25 mg of conjugated estrogens). At even higher doses, equivalent to those used in oral contraceptives, there is an increase in coagulability. Therefore, doses of estrogen equivalent to 0.625 mg of *conjugated estrogens* should be used for long-term therapy.

Potential Health Risks

The risks of estrogen therapy appear to be dose-related. Many of the side effects of high-dose oral contraceptives have not occurred with the lower doses of estrogen used for estrogen replacement therapy. Because of the sensitivity of some tissues to estrogen, the potential risks of estrogen for postmenopausal women must be considered.

Breast Cancer

Numerous retrospective studies have evaluated whether endogenous estrogens in the form of either oral contraceptives or estrogen replacement therapy have an impact on the incidence of breast cancer. Although some recent meta-analyses have concluded that there is no increased risk of this malignancy among women who receive hormone replacement (123, 124), others have demonstrated a significant increase in breast cancer risk that may be related to the duration of estrogen use (24, 125, 126). One of these studies showed a relative risk for the development of breast cancer of 1.46 in women who took postmenopausal estrogens for 5 years or longer (24). However, the benefits of hormone replacement may outweigh this theoretic risk in some patients.

Endometrial Cancer

A well-established risk of estrogen replacement therapy is endometrial hyperplasia and endometrial cancer. Early studies found that women who used estrogen alone were four to seven times more likely to develop endometrial cancer than women who did not (51). The simultaneous use of progestins effectively prevents this problem in most cases (127). However, it should be kept in mind that even women taking progestin therapy can develop endometrial cancer, especially if they have used unopposed estrogens in the past (128). Therefore, endometrial evaluation remains an important part of management for all women with irregular vaginal bleeding.

Gallbladder Disease

The risk of symptomatic gallbladder disease is increased by the use of oral contraceptives (129). In a recent questionnaire study of postmenopausal women, estrogen replacement therapy doubled the risk of gallbladder disease compared with women taking no hormones (130). However, in two case-control studies, no increased risk could be appreciated (129, 131).

Thrombophlebitis

There is no increased risk of thrombophlebitis associated with estrogen replacement therapy, despite the well-established association with the use of oral contraceptives. With the standard doses of conjugated estrogens normally used, there is no increased risk of either venous thrombosis or pulmonary embolism (132). Estrogen replacement therapy does not significantly alter clotting factors (133).

History of Thrombophlebitis

No study has specifically addressed the risk of recurrent thrombophlebitis for women taking estrogen. Therefore, women who have a history of thrombophlebitis should be offered estrogen therapy with the understanding that it is unlikely, but uncertain, that this therapy alters the risk of recurrent thrombophlebitis (134).

Hypertension

Hypertension has been one of the relative contraindications to oral contraceptives because the higher-dose formulations were found to further increase blood pressure (135). In contrast, the dose of conjugated estrogens used for estrogen replacement therapy have little effect on blood pressure (136). Because chronic hypertension is a well-established risk factor for both myocardial infarction and stroke, women with this disorder should be encouraged to maintain low blood pressure levels and to take advantage of the protective effect of estrogen replacement therapy for cardiovascular disease.

Side Effects

Vaginal Bleeding Any vaginal bleeding may be distressing; therefore, hormonal replacement regimens associated with amenorrhea are therefore preferable. Daily use of estrogen and cyclic progestin produces cyclic bleeding in most women. In an effort to avoid cyclic bleeding, the daily use of estrogen and progestin has been advocated. After several months, daily progestin therapy will result in amenorrhea in more than one-half of women with minimal risk of hyperplasia (68).

Irregular bleeding may be an early warning sign of endometrial hyperplasia or malignancy. More commonly, it is a sign of endometrial atrophy or dyssynchronous shedding. Because of the known association of estrogen replacement therapy with endometrial neoplasia, endometrial biopsy is indicated when irregular uterine bleeding occurs postmenopausally.

Breast Tenderness Breast tenderness can occur with estrogen replacement therapy (137). This may be related to both estrogen and progesterone stimulation of breast tissue. The symptoms of fibrocystic breast changes may be increased (137, 138). The initial approach to relieving breast symptoms is to decrease the daily estrogen dose to the equivalent of 0.625 mg of *conjugated equine estrogen,* and reduce progestin to the equivalent of 2.5 mg of *medroxyprogesterone.* If this is ineffective, the type of estrogen may be changed.

Mood Changes Progestins are known to cause mood disturbances similar to those of premenstrual syndrome, including anxiety, irritability, or depression (139, 140). Because of the significant protective effect of progestins against endometrial cancer, a dose or formulation of progestin that has the fewest side effects should be sought.

Weight Gain and Water Retention Some women are extremely sensitive to exogenous estrogens and experience symptoms such as weight gain or water retention (141). Although few data are available regarding these problems, alternate doses and formulations of both estrogen and progestins should be used to find the combination with the fewest side effects.

Special Cases

In some women, the standard approach to estrogen replacement therapy may not be appropriate or sufficient. Despite the benefits of estrogen administration after menopause, for some, this therapy is contraindicated (Table 29.2).

History of Breast Cancer

One of the most controversial subjects concerning estrogen replacement therapy is whether a woman with a history of successfully treated breast cancer can receive estrogen. Because it appears that estrogen replacement therapy may increase the risk of breast cancer, there has been a fear that estrogen may increase the risk of recurrent breast cancer. The limited data available suggest no increased risk of recurrent breast cancer among postmenopausal estrogen users (142, 143). Until more long-term data are available, estrogen should be used with caution in women with a history of breast cancer. In a woman with nonmetastatic (node-negative) estrogen receptor-negative breast cancer, particularly if she has a strong family history of osteoporosis and heart disease, the benefits of estrogen may outweigh the low theoretic risk that the hormone will predispose her to the development of recurrent cancer.

History of Endometrial Cancer

Although, theoretically, estrogen and progestin therapy should not increase the risk of recurrent endometrial cancer, there are few data regarding estrogen or progestin therapy in women who have been treated for endometrial cancer (144). Progestins have been used to treat recurrent endometrial cancer (145). One study of women successfully treated for Stage I endometrial cancer revealed that a combination of estrogen and progestin therapy does not increase the risk of recurrence (146). Because of the limited information available, any woman with a history of endometrial cancer should be informed of the unknown risk of recurrence with hormonal therapy.

Endometriosis

There have been anecdotal reports of recurrent endometriosis (147, 148) or malignant transformation of endometriosis in women with endometriosis who take estrogen replacement therapy following bilateral oophorectomy (149). Therefore, these women should be treated with continuous estrogen and a progestin. In women with severe endometriosis, especially when the bowel, bladder, or ureter is involved, a hormone-free period for up to 6 months immediately after surgery may also be advisable prior to instituting combined estrogen and progestin therapy.

Liver Disease

Estrogen replacement therapy has not been associated with the development of liver disease. However, estrogens are metabolized in the liver, and women with normal ovarian function and chronic liver disease are known to have significantly elevated levels of circulating estrogens (150). Likewise, normal doses of conjugated estrogens could lead to a substantially higher level of circulating estrogens than expected in these women. Therefore, estrogen replacement therapy should be avoided in women with active or chronic liver disease.

Replacement Hormones and Regimens

The mainstay of hormonal replacement in the absence of ovarian function is estrogen, usually with the addition of a progestin. Standard replacement therapy has consisted of 3 weeks of estrogen and 1 week of added progestin in anyone with an intact uterus. Estrogen only was given to women who had hysterectomies. Better understanding of the effects hormones have on the body has altered these classic approaches to therapy.

Types of Estrogen and Progesterone

Estrogens are available in oral and parenteral forms (Table 29.3). The basic oral estrogen preparation is conjugated equine estrogen, a combination of estrone (50%), equilin (23%), 17-α dihydroequilin (13%), and various other estrogens extracted from the urine of pregnant mares (151). This formulation has been available in the U.S. for more than 50 years; thus, most of the data regarding the safety and efficacy of estrogen replacement therapy have been gathered from women taking conjugated estrogens. Several other estrogen preparations have been developed, and data are accumulating regarding their comparable effectiveness. There is, at present, no compelling reason to recommend one preparation over others based on risks or side effects. If side effects become a problem with one formulation, a woman should be encouraged to try a different dose or estrogen formulation rather than abandon estrogen replacement altogether.

Estrogens are used orally as the first line of therapy in most women. Transdermal estradiol patches have also been found to be an effective method for hormone administration. However, there are several potential drawbacks to this approach. On a physiologic level, it is uncertain whether the same benefit is achieved in terms of reduction of cardiovascular disease risks, because changes in lipoprotein profiles do not occur as rapidly as with oral therapy (152). Transdermal patches are more expensive than oral preparations and result in some skin irritation at the site of placement in one-third of users (153). In women in whom oral estrogen therapy does not alleviate symptoms or is poorly tolerated or in whom oral

Table 29.3   Standard Dosages of Commonly Used Estrogens and Progestins

Estrogens	Dosage range
Oral	
Conjugated estrogens	0.625–1.25 mg daily
Ethinyl estradiol	5–10 μg daily
Piperazine estrone sulfate	1.0 mg daily
Micronized 17β-estradiol	0.5–2.0 mg daily
Parenteral	
Transdermal estradiol	0.05–0.10 mg patch twice weekly
Vaginal conjugated estrogens	0.2–0.625 mg, 2–7 times per week
Vaginal 17β-estradiol	1.0 mg, 1–3 times per week
Progestins (Oral)	
Medroxyprogesterone	2.5–5.0 mg daily, or 10 mg 12–14 days/month
Norethindrone	5 mg daily
Norethindrone acetate	1.25–5 mg daily
Norgestrel	0.15 mg daily
Micronized progesterone	100–300 mg daily

preparations create a problem with hypertriglyceridemia, estrogen patches may offer some advantage (115).

A special situation is the vaginal use of conjugated estrogens. Apparently, the rate of vaginal absorption of estrogen is similar to that of oral absorption (154). This has two important implications. First, when women who have contraindications to oral estrogen therapy use vaginal estrogen for atrophic vaginitis, the amount of systemically absorbed estrogen must be considered. In these women, it is recommended that the smallest dose needed to maintain the vaginal tissue effect be used. This is usually approximately one-third applicator (0.2 mg) used 2–3 times weekly. Second, women who desire estrogen therapy but are unable to take oral estrogen for any reason can try vaginal administration. This route of administration appears to be less effective in resolving symptoms of estrogen deficiency (155) and may not alter serum lipids to the same degree as oral estrogens (156).

Progestins are also available in several different formulations (Table 29.3). The most common progestin used is *medroxyprogesterone* given orally. In the doses prescribed to protect the endometrium (2.5–10 mg daily), some women experience psychological effects such as anxiety, irritability, or depression (136, 137). Although these problems may be associated to some degree with all progestins, few studies have evaluated them. Many progestin formulations have been evaluated for the treatment of irregular bleeding and have been found to be effective. No single progestin is clearly superior to another. If a woman has significant side effects with one progestin dose, a lower dose or a different progestin formulation should be given.

Estrogen Only

Whenever possible, unopposed estrogen therapy should be avoided in women with a uterus (157). However, some women experience intolerable side effects from progestin therapy. If no dose or formulation of progestin can be found that has acceptable side effects, unopposed estrogens may be given. A reasonable approach is the use of the lowest effective dose of estrogen daily coupled with yearly surveillance of the endometrium by endometrial biopsy. The use of vaginal ultrasonography for endometrial surveillance may prove ultimately to be effective for this use.

Daily estrogen alone has been recommended for women after hysterectomy. Progestins have been avoided because they may partially reverse the beneficial effects of oral estrogens on serum lipids. However, the effects of progestins on lipids appear to be short term (117), and only part of the protective effect of estrogens on the cardiovascular system are derived from lipid effects. Therefore, it is controversial whether progestins should be used in combination with estrogen for these women (24).

Estrogen Plus Cyclic Progesterone

Methods have been sought to avoid the risks of estrogen therapy while retaining the benefits. The addition of a progestin to estradiol minimizes the risk of endometrial hyperplasia and cancer (158). **The use of 12–14 days per month of** *medroxyprogesterone* **results in a risk of endometrial cancer less than that for the population at large.**

Initially, in the U. S., estrogen was given for only 21–25 days per month and progestins were given for the last 7–10 days of the estrogen therapy (158), followed by a monthly period of 6–8 days when no hormones were given. Although this had the theoretic advantage of giving all hormonally responsive tissue "a rest," no study has ever shown a benefit to this hormone-free period. However, **data from Great Britain suggest that 10 days of progestin therapy per month may not be enough to prevent endometrial hyperplasia in some women (159). Therefore, when cyclic progestins are used, they should be given for 12–14 days per month. With 14 days of therapy (10 mg** *medroxyprogesterone* **or equivalent), endometrial hyperplasia is uncommon** (160).

Estrogen Plus Continuous Progesterone

Although cyclic progestins given at appropriate doses can protect the endometrium from hyperplasia, this approach also results in cyclic endometrial shedding and menstruation in most women (161). Vaginal bleeding is one of the most common reasons that women discontinue estrogen replacement therapy (162). In addition, the relatively high dose of progestin used may result in significant symptoms in some women (136). These may include physical symptoms such as breast tenderness, fluid retention, and edema and psychological symptoms such as anxiety, irritability, or depression. Therefore, regimens using lower daily doses of progestins have been developed (158, 163). Daily progestin therapy (2.5–5.0 mg *medroxyprogesterone acetate* or equivalent) protects against endometrial hyperplasia to a degree similar to that of cyclic administration at higher doses (Fig. 29.2) (160).

More than 50% of women who take a daily combination of estrogen and progestin will experience irregular bleeding, even after 1 year of therapy (68). This group of women may be better served by continuous estrogen accompanied by cyclic progesterone. For many women, regular bleeding may be preferable to unpredictable bleeding.

Testosterone

Testosterone has been used in women, especially after surgical menopause, to alleviate specific symptoms (164). In the U.S., testosterone is available in an injectable form (*testosterone enanthate* 75–150 mg intramuscular every month), and as a combined oral formulation (*methyltestosterone* 2.5–5 mg, plus *conjugated* or *esterified estrogens* 0.625–1.25 mg). In Great Britain, a subcutaneous *testosterone implant* is also available.

The most common indication for androgens is loss of libido (164). Studies of testosterone administration have shown mixed results in terms of libido improvement (164–169). One 6-month study of the oral preparation showed an adverse effect on the estrogen-induced changes in lipoproteins (170). Because of a lack of long-term studies of any of these agents, the effects on heart disease and other organ systems are unknown. Until studies establish a benefit for this type of therapy, androgens should be prescribed with caution. For women who experience decreased sexual responsiveness, appropriate counseling appears to be the most effective therapy (167, 171).

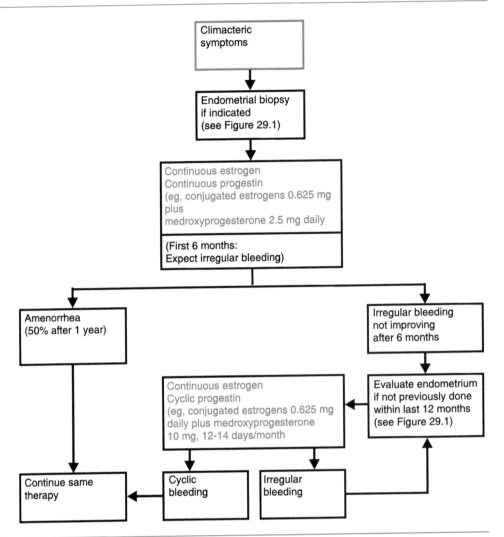

Figure 29.2   Administration of hormone replacement therapy.

Patient Surveillance

Continued monitoring of patients taking estrogen replacement relies heavily on self-reporting of symptoms and bleeding patterns. Postmenopausal women also should undergo routine assessments that should include evaluation and counseling regarding risk factors.

Symptoms

In women for whom the standard doses of estrogen do not seem to be sufficient to control hot flashes, doses as high as 2.5 mg of *conjugated estrogens* per day can be used. In premenopausal women who have undergone oophorectomy, oral contraceptives may offer relief in difficult cases (62), but they have increased side effects compared with estrogen replacement therapy (59).

Vaginal dryness responds somewhat slower than hot flashes to estrogen replacement therapy. However, even at the lowest therapeutic doses, complete resolution of vaginal dryness is usually seen after 3–6 weeks (172). Any symptoms of atrophic vaginitis will decrease over the same amount of time.

Vaginal Bleeding

The bleeding patterns associated with estrogen therapy depend on the type of hormonal protocol used. The most common pattern with unopposed estrogen is amenorrhea (68). If breakthrough bleeding occurs, endometrial biopsy should be performed. Even with no vaginal bleeding, yearly endometrial evaluation is recommended for women taking unopposed estrogen because of the risk of endometrial cancer.

With continuous estrogen and cyclic *medroxyprogesterone,* cyclic estrogen withdrawal bleeding almost always occurs monthly (161). If irregular or intermenstrual bleeding occurs, endometrial biopsy should be performed (Fig. 29.2). Although endometrial hyperplasia or cancer occur only rarely, risk is not completely eliminated with progestin therapy.

When continuous estrogen and continuous progestins are used, the bleeding pattern is more variable. Many women taking this therapy will develop amenorrhea (68). One-half of women will have some degree of irregular bleeding even after 1 year. The best method for evaluation of the endometrium has not been determined. Although the bleeding is almost always light, the significance of it cannot be determined without endometrial evaluation. It is reasonable to consider a base line endometrial biopsy for anyone on this protocol who has irregular bleeding. If irregular bleeding persists for 6 months, further evaluation with ultrasound and possibly hysteroscopy may be of benefit.

Nonhormonal Drugs

In addition to estrogen, calcium, fluoride, *calcitrol,* and *calcitonin,* the biphosphates, especially *etidronate* and *alendronate,* have been used for the treatment of postmenopausal osteoporosis. Calcium can slow bone loss but does not increase bone mass (173). Fluoride is the only known agent that can stimulate bone formation and substantially increase bone density (174). *Calcitronin* is probably less effective than estrogen and is relatively expensive (175). *Calcitrol,* a vitamin D analog, can increase lumbar bone mass and decrease the rate of vertebral fractures (176).

Of the biphosphates, *alendronate* is approximately 1000 times more potent than *etidronate* in terms of the inhibition of bone resorption. Newer biphosphates, *tiludronate* and *residronate,* are being evaluated. In a randomized study, *alendronate* was given orally 5–20 mg/day for 3 years or 20 mg/day for 2 years followed by 5 mg/day for the third year, along with 500 mg/day of calcium (177). Compared with placebo, the rate of vertebral fracture was approximately one-half: 3.2% for those receiving *alendronate* versus 6.2% for the placebo group.

References

1. **Kingkade WW, Torrey BB.** The evolving demography of aging in the United States of American and the former USSR. *World Health Stat Q* 1992;45:15–28.

2. **McKinlay SM, Brambilla DJ, Posner JG.** The normal menopause transition. *Maturitas* 1992;14:103–15.

3. **Whelan EA, Sandler DP, McConnaughey DR, Weinberg CR.** Menstrual and reproductive characteristics and age at natural menopause. *Am J Epidemiol* 1990;131:625–8.

4. **Brambrilla DJ, McKinlay SM.** A prospective study of factors affecting age at menopause. *J Clin Epidemiol* 1989;42:1031–9.

5. **Siddle N, Sarrel P, Whitehead M.** The effect of hysterectomy on the age at ovarian failure: identification of a subgroup of women with premature loss of ovarian function and literature review. *Fertil Steril* 1987;47:94–100.

6. **Coulam CB, Anderson SC, Annegan JF.** Incidence of premature ovarian failure. *Obstet Gynecol* 1986;67:604–6.

7. **Wilcox LS, Koonin LM, Pokras R, Strauss LT, Xia Z, Peterson HB.** Hysterectomy in the United States, 1988–1990. *Obstet Gynecol* 1994;83:549–55.

8. **Feldman BM, Voda A, Gronseth E.** The prevalence of hot flash and associated variables among perimenopausal women. *Res Nurs Health* 1985;8:261–8.

9. **Hreshchyshyn MM, Hopkins A, Zylstra S, Anbar M.** Effects of natural menopause, hysterectomy, and oophorectomy on lumbar spine and femoral neck bone densities. *Obstet Gynecol* 1988;72:631–8.

10. **Centerwall BS.** Premenopausal hysterectomy and cardiovascular disease. *Am J Obstet Gynecol* 1981;139:58–61.

11. **Hee J, MacNaughton J, Bangah M, Burger HG.** Perimenopausal patterns of gonadotrophins, immunoreactive inhibin, oestradiol and progesterone. *Maturitas* 1993;18:9–20.

12. **Reyes FI, Winter JS, Faiman C.** Pituitary-ovarian relationships preceding the menopause. I. A cross-sectional study of serum follicle-stimulating hormone, luteinizing hormone, prolactin, estradiol, and progesterone levels. *Am J Obstet Gynecol* 1977;129:557–64.

13. **Adashi EY.** The climacteric ovary as a functional gonadotropin-driven androgen-producing gland. *Fertil Steril* 1994;62:20–7.

14. **Judd HL.** Hormonal dynamics associated with the menopause. *Clin Obstet Gynecol* 1976;19:775–88.

15. **Grodin JM, Siiteri PK, MacDonald PC.** Source of estrogen production in postmenopausal women. *J Clin Endocrinol Metab* 1973;36:207–14.

16. **MacDonald PC, Edman CD, Hemsell DL, Porter JC, Siiteri PK.** Effect of obesity on conversion of plasma androstenedione to estrone in postmenopausal women with and without endometrial cancer. *Am J Obstet Gynecol* 1978;130:448–55.

17. **Harlap S.** The benefits and risks of hormone replacement therapy: an epidemiologic overview. *Am J Obstet Gynecol* 1992;166:1986–92.

18. **Daniell HW.** Osteoporosis of the slender smoker. Vertebral compression fractures and loss of metacarpal cortex in relation to postmenopausal cigarette smoking and lack of obesity. *Arch Intern Med* 1976;136:298–304.

19. **Sherman BM, Wallace RB, Bean JA, Chang Y, Schlabaugh L.** The relationship of menopausal hot flushes to medical and reproductive experience. *J Gerontol* 1981;36:306–9.

20. **Dennefors BL, Janson PO, Knutson F, Hamberger L.** Steroid production and responsiveness to gonadotropin in isolated stromal tissue of human postmenopausal ovaries. *Am J Obstet Gynecol* 1980;136:997–1002.

21. **Gath D, Osborn M, Bungay G, Iles S, Day A, Bond A, et al.** Psychiatric disorder and gynaecological symptoms in middle aged women: a community survey. *BMJ* 1987;294:213–8.

22. **Gambrell R Jr, Bagnell CA, Greenblatt RB.** Role of estrogens and progesterone in the etiology and prevention of endometrial cancer: review. *Am J Obstet Gynecol* 1983;146:696–707.

23. **de Aloysio D, Rocca G, Miliffi L.** Cyto-histologic evaluation of the endometrium in climacteric women at risk for endometrial carcinoma. *Tumori* 1986;72:431–7.

24. **Colditz GA, Hankinson SE, Hunter AJ, Willett WC, Manson JE, Stampfer MJ, et al.** The use of estrogens and progestins and the risk of breast cancer in postmenopausal women. *N Engl J Med* 1995;332:1589–93.

25. **Nachtigall MJ, Smilen SW, Nachtigall RD, Nachtigall RH, Nachtigall LE.** Incidence of breast cancer in a 22-year study of women receiving estrogen-progestin replacement therapy. *Obstet Gynecol* 1992;80:827–30.

26. **Meldrum DR, Davidson BJ, Tataryn IV, Judd HL.** Changes in circulating steroids with aging in postmenopausal women. *Obstet Gynecol* 1981;57:624–8.

27. **Deutsch S, Benjamin F, Seltzer V, Tafreshi M, Kocheril G, Frank A.** The correlation of serum estrogens and androgens with bone density in the late postmenopause. *Int J Gynaecol Obstet* 1987;25:217–22.

28. **Sheehy G.** *The Silent Passage: Menopause.* New York: Simon & Schuster Inc., 1991.

29. **Nadelson CC.** Psychosomatic aspects of obstetrics and gynecology. *Psychosomatics* 1983;24:878–80.

30. **Hunter MS.** Psychological and somatic experience of the menopause: a prospective study. *Psychosom Med* 1990;52:357–67.

31. **Harris MB.** Growing old gracefully: age concealment and gender. *J Gerontol* 1994;49:149–58.

32. **Maheux R, Naud F, Rioux M, Grenier R, Lemay A, Guy J, et al.** A randomized, double-blind, placebo-controlled study on the effect of conjugated estrogens on skin thickness. *Am J Obstet Gynecol* 1994;170:642–9.

33. **Brincat M, Versi E, Moniz CF, Magos A, de Trafford J, Studd JW.** Skin collagen changes in postmenopausal women receiving different regimens of estrogen therapy. *Obstet Gynecol* 1987;70:123–7.

34. **Imayama S, Braverman IM.** A hypothetical explanation for the aging of skin. Chronologic alteration of the three-dimensional arrangement of collagen and elastic fibers in connective tissue. *Am J Pathol* 1989;134:1019–25.

35. **Zung WW, Broadhead WE, Roth ME.** Prevalence of depressive symptoms in primary care. *J Fam Pract* 1993;37:337–44 (erratum, 1989;11:169).

36. **Ballinger SE.** Psychosocial stress and symptoms of menopause: a comparative study of menopause clinic patients and nonpatients. *Maturitas* 1985;7:315–27.

37. **de Aloysio D, Fabiani AG, Mauloni M, Bottiglioni F.** Analysis of the climacteric syndrome. *Maturitas* 1989;11:43–53 (erratum, 1989;11:169).

38. **Holte A, Mikkelsen A.** The menopausal syndrome: a factor analytic replication. *Maturitas* 1991;13:193–203.

39. **Strickler RC, Borth R, Cecutti A, Cookson BA, Harper JA, Potvin R, et al.** The role of oestrogen replacement in the climacteric syndrome. *Psychol Med* 1977;7:631–9.

40. **Hunter M, Battersby R, Whitehead M.** Relationships between psychological symptoms, somatic complaints and menopausal status. *Maturitas* 1986;8:217–28.

41. **Traupmann J.** Does sexuality fade over time? A look at the question and the answer. *J Geriatr Psychiatry* 1984;17:149–59.

42. **Traupmann J, Eckels E, Hatfield E.** Intimacy in older women's lives. *Gerontologist* 1982;22:493–8.

43. **Notelovitz M.** Estrogen replacement therapy: indications, contraindications, and agent selection. *Am J Obstet Gynecol* 1989;161:1832–41.

44. **Greenblatt RB, Karpas A.** Hormone therapy for sexual dysfunction. The only "true aphrodisiac." *Postgrad Med* 1983;74:78–80.

45. **Bachmann GA.** Correlates of sexual desire in postmenopausal women. *Maturitas* 1985;7:211–6.

46. **Treloar AE.** Menstrual cyclicity and the pre-menopause. *Maturitas* 1981;3:249–64.

47. **Buckler HM, Evans CA, Mamtora H, Burger HG, Anderson DC.** Gonadotropin, steroid, and inhibin levels in women with incipient ovarian failure during anovulatory and ovulatory rebound cycles. *J Clin Endocrinol Metab* 1991;72:116–24.

48. **Gambrell R Jr.** Clinical use of progestins in the menopausal patient: dosage and duration. *J Reprod Med* 1982;27:531–8.

49. **Lidor A, Ismajovich B, Confino E, David MP.** Histopathological findings in 226 women with post-menopausal uterine bleeding. *Acta Obstet Gynecol Scand* 1986;65:41–3.

50. **Jick H, Watkins RN, Hunter JR, Dinan BJ, Madsen S, Rothman KJ, et al.** Replacement estrogens and endometrial cancer. *N Engl J Med* 1979;300:218–22.

51. **Ernster VL, Bush TL, Huggins GR, Hulka BS, Kelsey JL, Schottenfeld D.** Benefits and risks of menopausal estrogen and or progestin hormone use. *Prev Med* 1988;17:301–23.

52. **Feldman S, Berkowitz RS, Tosteson AN.** Cost-effectiveness of strategies to evaluate postmenopausal bleeding. *Obstet Gynecol* 1993;81:968–75.

53. **Grimes DA.** Prevention of cardiovascular disease in women: role of the obstetrician-gynecologist. *Am J Obstet Gynecol* 1988;158:1662–8.

54. **Stovall TG, Solomon SK, Ling FW.** Endometrial sampling prior to hysterectomy. *Obstet Gynecol* 1989;73:405–9.

55. **Castelo-Branco C, Puerto B, Duran M, Gratacos E, Torne A, Fortuny A, et al.** Transvaginal sonography of the endometrium in postmenopausal women: monitoring the effect of hormone replacement therapy. *Maturitas* 1994;19:59–65.

56. **Cacciatore B, Ramsay T, Lehtovirta P, Ylostalo P.** Transvaginal sonography and hysteroscopy in postmenopausal bleeding. *Acta Obstet Gynecol Scand* 1994;73:413–6.

57. **Loffer FD.** Hysteroscopy with selective endometrial sampling compared with D&C for abnormal uterine bleeding: the value of a negative hysteroscopic view. *Obstet Gynecol* 1989;73:16–20.

58. **Goldrath MH, Sherman AI.** Office hysteroscopy and suction curettage: can we eliminate the hospital diagnostic dilatation and curettage? *Am J Obstet Gynecol* 1985;152:220–9.

59. **Mishell D Jr.** Use of oral contraceptives in women of older reproductive age. *Am J Obstet Gynecol* 1988;158:1652–7.

60. **Trussell J, Vaughan B.** Contraceptive use projections: 1990 to 2010. *Am J Obstet Gynecol* 1992;167:1160–4.

61. **Lalonde A.** Evaluation of surgical options in menorrhagia. *Br J Obstet Gynaecol* 1994;11:8–14.

62. **Hartge P, Whittemore AS, Itnyre J, McGowan L, Cramer D.** Rates and risks of ovarian cancer in subgroups of white women in the United States. The Collaborative Ovarian Cancer Group. *Obstet Gynecol* 1994;84:760–4.

63. **Ramey JW, Koonings PP, Given FT Jr, Acosta AA.** The process of carcinogenesis for endometrial adenocarcinoma could be short: development of a malignancy after endometrial ablation. *Am J Obstet Gynecol* 1994;170:1370–1.

64. **Nakano R, Hashiba N, Washio M, Tojo S.** Diagnostic evaluation of progesterone. Challenge test in amenorrheic patients. *Acta Obstet Gynecol Scand* 1979;58:59–64.

65. **MacNaughton J, Banah M, McCloud P, Hee J, Burger H.** Age related changes in follicle stimulating hormone, luteinizing hormone, oestradiol and immunoreactive inhibin in women of reproductive age. *Clin Endocrinol* 1992;36:339–45.

66. **Tang L, Sawers RS.** Twin pregnancy in premature ovarian failure after estrogen treatment: a case report. **Am J Obstet Gynecol** 1989;161:172–3.

67. **Okuda K, Yoshikawa M, Ushiroyama T, Sugimoto O, Maeda T, Mori H.** Two patients with hypergonadotropic ovarian failure due to pituitary hyperplasia. *Obstet Gynecol* 1989;74:498–501.

68. **Archer DF, Pickar JH, Bottiglioni F.** Bleeding patterns in postmenopausal women taking continuous combined or sequential regimens of conjugated estrogens with medroxyprogesterone acetate. Menopause Study Group. *Obstet Gynecol* 1994;83:686–92.

69. **Kronenberg F.** Hot flashes: epidemiology and physiology. *Ann N Y Acad Sci* 1990;592:52–86.

70. **Weinstein L.** Hormonal therapy in the patient with surgical menopause. *Obstet Gynecol* 1990; 75:47S–50S.

71. **Utian WH.** Biosynthesis and physiologic effects of estrogen and pathophysiologic effects of estrogen deficiency: review. *Am J Obstet Gynecol* 1989;161:1828–31.

72. **Ravnikar V.** Physiology and treatment of hot flushes. *Obstet Gynecol* 1990;75:3S–8S.

73. **Stampfer MJ, Colditz GA, Willett WC, Manson JE, Rosner B, Speizer FE, et al.** Postmenopausal estrogen therapy and cardiovascular disease: ten-year follow-up from the Nurses' Health Study. *N Engl J Med* 1991;325:756–62.

74. **Cedars MI, Lu JK, Meldrum DR, Judd HL.** Treatment of endometriosis with a long-acting gonadotropin-releasing hormone agonist plus medroxyprogesterone acetate. *Obstet Gynecol* 1990;75:641–5.

75. **Erlik Y, Meldrum DR, Lagasse LD, Judd HL.** Effect of megestrol acetate on flushing and bone metabolism in post-menopausal women. *Maturitas* 1981;3:167–72.

76. **Edington RF, Chagnon JP, Steinberg WM.** Clonidine (Dixarit) for menopausal flushing. *Can Med Assoc J* 1980;123:23–6.

77. **Bergmans MG, Merkus JM, Corbey RS, Schellekens LA, Ubachs JM.** Effect of Bellergal Retard on climacteric complaints: a double-blind, placebo-controlled study. *Maturitas* 1987;9:227–34.

78. **Erlik Y, Tataryn IV, Meldrum DR, Lomax P, Bajorek JG, Judd HL.** Association of waking episodes with menopausal hot flushes. *JAMA* 1981;245:1741–4.

79. **Notelovitz M.** Gynecologic problems of menopausal women: part 1. Changes in genital tissue. *Geriatrics* 1978;33:24–30.

80. **Raz R, Stamm WE.** A controlled trial of intravaginal estriol in postmenopausal women with recurrent urinary tract infections. *N Engl J Med* 1993;329:753–6.

81. **Bhatia NN, Bergman A, Karram MM.** Effects of estrogen on urethral function in women with urinary incontinence. *Am J Obstet Gynecol* 1989;160:176–81.

82. **Dennerstein L, Burrows GD, Hyman GJ, Sharpe K.** Hormone therapy and affect. *Maturitas* 1979;1:247–59.

83. **Ditkoff EC, Crary WG, Cristo M, Lobo RA.** Estrogen improves psychological function in asymptomatic postmenopausal women. *Obstet Gynecol* 1991;78:991–5.

84. **Kampen DL, Sherwin BB.** Estrogen use and verbal memory in healthy postmenopausal women. *Obstet Gynecol* 1994;83:979–83.

85. **Henderson VW, Paganini-Hill A, Emanuel CK, Dunn ME, Buckwalter JG.** Estrogen replacement therapy in older women. Comparisons between Alzheimer's disease cases and nondemented control subjects. *Arch Neurol* 1994;51:896–900.

86. **Paganini-Hill A, Henderson VW.** Estrogen deficiency and risk of Alzheimer's disease in women. *Am J Epidemiol* 1994;140:256–61.

87. **Bush TL.** The epidemiology of cardiovascular disease in postmenopausal women. *Ann N Y Acad Sci* 1990;592:263–71.

88. **Colditz GA, Willett WC, Stampfer MJ, Rosner B, Speizer FE, Hennekens CH.** Menopause and the risk of coronary heart disease in women. *N Engl J Med* 1987;316: 1105–10.

89. **Lobo RA.** Cardiovascular implications of estrogen replacement therapy. *Obstet Gynecol* 1990;75:18S–25S.

90. **Henderson BE, Paganini-Hill A, Ross RK.** Decreased mortality in users of estrogen replacement therapy. *Arch Intern Med* 1991;151:75–8.

91. **Perlman JA, Wolf PH, Ray R, Lieberknecht G.** Cardiovascular risk factors, premature heart disease, and all-cause mortality in a cohort of northern California women. *Am J Obstet Gynecol* 1988;158:1568–74.

92. **Kanis JA.** Editorial: osteoporosis and osteopenia. *J Bone Miner Res* 1990;5:209–11.

93. **Phillips S, Fox N, Jacobs J, Wright WE.** The direct medical costs of osteoporosis for American women aged 45 and older, 1986. *Bone* 1988;9:271–9.

94. **Resnick NM, Greenspan SL.** Senile osteoporosis reconsidered. *JAMA* 1989;261:1025–9.

95. **Riggs BL, Melton LJ III.** Involutional osteoporosis. *N Engl J Med* 1986;314:1676–86.

96. **Riggs BL.** Pathogenesis of osteoporosis. *Am J Obstet Gynecol* 1987;156:1342–6.

97. **Rubin CD.** Southwestern internal medicine conference: growth hormone-aging and osteoporosis. *Am J Med Sci* 1993;305:120–9.

98. **Kellie SE, Brody JA.** Sex-specific and race-specific hip fracture rates. *Am J Public Health* 1990;80:326–8.

99. **Seeman E, Hopper JL, Bach LA, Cooper ME, Parkinson E, McKay J, et al.** Reduced bone mass in daughters of women with osteoporosis. *N Engl J Med* 1989;320:554–8.

100. **Peck WA.** Estrogen therapy (ET) after menopause. *J Am Med Wom Assoc* 1990;45:87–90.

101. **Hedlund LR, Gallagher JC.** The effect of age and menopause on bone mineral density of the proximal femur. *J Bone Miner Res* 1989;4:639–42.

102. **Richelson LS, Wahner HW, Melton LJ, Riggs BL.** Relative contributions of aging and estrogen deficiency to postmenopausal bone loss. *N Engl J Med* 1984;311:1273–5.

103. **Heaney RP, Recker RR, Saville PD.** Menopausal changes in calcium balance performance. *J Lab Clin Med* 1978;92:953–63.

104. **Emans SJ, Grace E, Hoffer FA, Gundberg C, Ravnikar V, Woods ER.** Estrogen deficiency in adolescents and young adults: impact on bone mineral content and effects of estrogen replacement therapy. *Obstet Gynecol* 1990;76:585–92.

105. **Baran D, Sorensen A, Grimes J, Lew R, Karellas A, Johnson B, et al.** Dietary modification with dairy products for preventing vertebral bone loss in premenopausal women: a three-year prospective study. *J Clin Endocrinol Metab* 1990;70:264–70.

106. **Reid IR, Ames RW, Evans MC, Gamble GD, Sharpe SJ.** Effect of calcium supplementation on bone loss in postmenopausal women. *N Engl J Med* 1993;328:460–4.

107. **Levine BS, Rodman JS, Wienerman S, Bockman RS, Lane JM, Chapman DS.** Effect of calcium citrate supplementation on urinary calcium oxalate saturation in female stone formers: implications for prevention of osteoporosis. *Am J Clin Nutr* 1994;60:592–6.

108. **Chow RK, Harrison JE, Brown CF, Hajek V.** Physical fitness effect on bone mass in post-menopausal women. *Arch Phys Med Rehabil* 1986;67:231–4.

109. **Jensen J, Christiansen C, Rodbro P.** Cigarette smoking, serum estrogens, and bone loss during hormone-replacement therapy early after menopause. *N Engl J Med* 1985;313:973–5.

110. **Cauley JA, Cummings SR, Black DM, Mascioli SR, Seeley DG.** Prevalence and determinants of estrogen replacement therapy in elderly women. *Am J Obstet Gynecol* 1990;165:1438–44.

111. **Genant HK, Baylink DJ, Gallagher JC.** Estrogens in the prevention of osteoporosis in post-menopausal women. *Am J Obstet Gynecol* 1989;161:1842–6.

112. **Lindsay R, Tohme JF.** Estrogen treatment of patients with established postmenopausal osteoporosis. *Obstet Gynecol* 1990;76:290–5.

113. **Prior JC, Vigna YM, Barr SI, Rexworthy C, Lentle BC.** Cyclic medroxyprogesterone treatment increases bone density: a controlled trial in active women with menstrual cycle disturbances. *Am J Med* 1994;96:521–30.

114. **Sullivan JM, Vander Zwaag R, Hughes JP, Maddock V, Kroetz FW, Ramanathan KB, et al.** Estrogen replacement and coronary artery disease. Effect on survival in postmenopausal women. *Arch Intern Med* 1990;150:2557–62.

115. **Walsh BW, Schiff I, Rosner B, Greenberg L, Ravnikar V, Sacks FM.** Effects of post-menopausal estrogen replacement on the concentrations and metabolism of plasma lipoproteins. *N Engl J Med* 1991;325:1196–204.

116. **Egeland GM, Kuller LH, Matthews KA, Kelsey SF, Cauley J, Guzick D.** Hormone replacement therapy and lipoprotein changes during early menopause. *Obstet Gynecol* 1990;76:776–82.

117. **Fletcher CD, Farish E, Dagen MM, Hart DM.** A comparison of the effects of lipoproteins of two progestogens used during cyclical hormone replacement therapy. *Maturitas* 1987;9:253–8.

118. **Wagner JD, Clarkson TB, St. Clair RW, Schwenke DC, Shively CA, Adams MR.** Estrogen and progesterone replacement therapy reduces low density lipoprotein accumulation in the coronary arteries of surgically postmenopausal cynomolgus monkeys. *J Clin Invest* 1991;88:1995–2002.

119. **Sack MN, Rader DJ, Cannon R.** Oestrogen and inhibition of oxidation of low-density lipoproteins in postmenopausal women. *Lancet* 1994;343:269–70.

120. **Williams JK, Adams MR, Herrington DM, Clarkson TB.** Short-term administration of estrogen and vascular responses of atherosclerotic coronary arteries. *J Am Coll Cardiol* 1992;20:452–7.

121. **Karas RH, Patterson BL, Mendelsohn ME.** Human vascular smooth muscle cells contain functional estrogen receptor. *Circulation* 1994;89:1943–50.

122. **Bar J, Tepper R, Fuchs J, Pardo Y, Goldberger S, Ovadia J.** The effect of estrogen replacement therapy on platelet aggregation and adenosine triphosphate release in post-menopausal women. *Obstet Gynecol* 1993;81:261–4.

123. **Armstrong BK.** Oestrogen therapy after the menopause—boon or bane? *Med J Aust* 1988;148:213–4.

124. **Dupont WD, Page DL.** Menopausal estrogen replacement therapy and breast cancer. *Arch Intern Med* 1991;151:67–72.

125. **Sillero-Arenas M, Delgado-Rodriguez M, Rodigues-Canteras R, Bueno-Cavanillas A, Galvez-Vargas R.** Menopausal hormone replacement therapy and breast cancer: a meta-analysis. *Obstet Gynecol* 1992;79:286–94.

126. **Steinberg KK, Thacker SB, Smith SJ, Stroup DF, Zack MM, Flanders WD, et al.** A meta-analysis of the effect of estrogen replacement therapy on the risk of breast cancer. *JAMA* 1991;265:1985–90.

127. **Persson I, Adami HO, Bergkvist L, Lindgren A, Pettersson B, Hoover R, et al.** Risk of endometrial cancer after treatment with oestrogens alone or in conjunction with progestogens: results of a prospective study. *BMJ* 1989;298:147–51.

128. **Leather AT, Savvas M, Studd JW.** Endometrial histology and bleeding patterns after 8 years of continuous combined estrogen and progestogen therapy in postmenopausal women. *Obstet Gynecol* 1991;78:1008–10.

129. **Scragg RK, McMichael AJ, Seamark RF.** Oral contraceptives, pregnancy, and endogenous oestrogen in gall stone disease-a case-control study. *BMJ* 1984;288:1795–9.

130. **Grodstein F, Colditz GA, Stampfer MJ.** Postmenopausal hormone use and cholecystectomy in a large prospective study. *Obstet Gynecol* 1994;83:5–11.

131. **Kakar F, Weiss NS, Strite SA.** Non-contraceptive estrogen use and the risk of gallstone disease in women. *Am J Public Health* 1988;78:564–6.

132. **Devor M, Barrett-Connor E, Renvall M, Feigal D Jr, Ramsdell J.** Estrogen replacement therapy and the risk of venous thrombosis. *Am J Med* 1992;92:275–82.

133. **de Aloysio D, Mauloni M, Roncuzzi A, Altieri P, Bottiglioni F, Trossarelli GF, et al.** Effects of an oral contraceptive combination containing 0.150 mg desogestrel plus 0.020 mg ethinyl estradiol on healthy premenopausal women. *Arch Gynecol Obstet* 1993;253:15–9.

134. **Young RL, Goepfert AR, Goldzieher HW.** Estrogen replacement therapy is not conducive of venous thromboembolism. *Maturitas* 1991;13:189–92.

135. **Spellacy WN, Birk SA.** The development of elevated blood pressure while using oral contraceptives: a preliminary report of a prospective study. *Fertil Steril* 1970;21:301–6.

136. **Pfeffer RI, Kurosaki TT, Charlton SK.** Estrogen use and blood pressure in later life. *Am J Epidemiol* 1979;110:469–78.

137. **McNicholas MM, Heneghan JP, Milner MH, Tunney T, Hourihane JB, MacErlaine DP.** Pain and increased mammographic density in women receiving hormone replacement therapy: a prospective study. *AJR Am J Roentgenol* 1994;163:311–5.

138. **Pastides H, Najjar MA, Kelsey JL.** Estrogen replacement therapy and fibrocystic breast disease. *Am J Prev Med* 1987;3:282–6.

139. **Dennerstein L, Burrows G.** Psychological effects of progestogens in the postmenopausal years. *Maturitas* 1986;8:101–6.

140. **Sherwin BB.** The impact of different doses of estrogen and progestin on mood and sexual behavior in postmenopausal women. *J Clin Endocrinol Metab* 1991;72:336–43.

141. **Studd J.** Complications of hormone replacement therapy in post-menopausal women [editorial]. *J R Soc Med* 1992;85:376–8.

142. **Cobleigh MA, Berris RF, Bush T, Davidson NE, Robert NJ, Sparano JA, et al.** Estrogen replacement therapy in breast cancer survivors. A time for change. Breast Cancer Committees of the Eastern Cooperative Oncology Group. *JAMA* 1994;272:540–5.

143. **Wile AG, Opfell RW, Margileth DA.** Hormone replacement therapy in previously treated breast cancer patients. *Am J Surg* 1993;165:372–5.

144. **Baker DP.** Estrogen-replacement therapy in patients with previous endometrial carcinoma. *Compr Ther* 1990;16:28–35.

145. **Lentz SS.** Advanced and recurrent endometrial carcinoma: hormonal therapy. *Semin Oncol* 1994;21:100–6.

146. **Creasman WT, Henderson D, Hinshaw W, Clarke-Pearson DL.** Estrogen replacement therapy in the patient treated for endometrial cancer. *Obstet Gynecol* 1986;67:326–30.

147. **Kapadia SB, Russak RR, O'Donnell WF, Harris RN, Lecky JW.** Postmenopausal ureteral endometriosis with atypical adenomatous hyperplasia following hysterectomy, bilateral oophorectomy, and long-term estrogen therapy. *Obstet Gynecol* 1984;64:60S–63S.

148. **Lam AM, French M, Charnock FM.** Bilateral ureteric obstruction due to recurrent endometriosis associated with hormone replacement therapy. *Aust N Z J Obstet Gynaecol* 1992;32:83–4.

149. **Reimnitz C, Brand E, Nieberg RK, Hacker NF.** Malignancy arising in endometriosis associated with unopposed estrogen replacement. *Obstet Gynecol* 1988;71:444–7.

150. **Pentikainen PJ, Pentikainen LA, Azarnoff DL, Dujovne CA.** Plasma levels and excretion of estrogens in urine in chronic lever disease. *Gastroenterology* 1975;69:20–7.

151. **Lyman GW, Johnson RN.** Assay for conjugated estrogens in tablets using fused-silica capillary gas chromatography. *J Chromatogr* 1982;234:234–9.

152. **Stanczyk FZ, Shoupe D, Nunez V, Macias-Gonzales P, Vijod MA, Lobo RA.** A randomized comparison of nonoral estradiol delivery in postmenopausal women. *Am J Obstet Gynecol* 1988;159:1540–6.

153. **Fraser DI, Parsons A, Whitehead MI, Wordsworth J, Stuart G, Pryse-Davies J.** The optimal dose of oral norethindrone acetate for addition to transdermal estradiol: a multicenter study. *Fertil Steril* 1990;53:460–8.

154. **Englund DE, Johansson ED.** Plasma levels of oestrone, oestradiol and gonadotrophins in postmenopausal women after oral and vaginal administration of conjugated equine oestrogens (Premarin). *Br J Obstet Gynaecol* 1978;85:957–64.

155. **Dickerson J, Bressler R, Christian CD, Hermann HW.** Efficacy of estradiol vaginal cream in postmenopausal women. *Clin Pharmacol Ther* 1979;26:502–7.

156. **Mandel FP, Geola FL, Meldrum DR, Lu JH, Eggena P, Sambhi MP, et al.** Biological effects of various doses of vaginally administered conjugated equine estrogens in postmenopausal women. *J Clin Endocrinol Metab* 1983;57:133–9.

157. **Ettinger B, Golditch IM, Friedman G.** Gynecologic consequences of long-term, unopposed estrogen replacement therapy. *Maturitas* 1988;10:271–82.

158. **Whitehead MI, Hillard TC, Crook D.** The role and use of progestogens. *Obstet Gynecol* 1990;75:59S–76S.

159. **Whitehead MI, King RJ, McQueen J, Campbell S.** Endometrial histology and biochemistry in climacteric women during oestrogen and oestrogen/progestogen therapy. *J R Soc Med* 1979;72:322–7.

160. **Woodruff JD, Pickar JH.** Incidence of endometrial hyperplasia in postmenopausal women taking conjugated estrogens (Premarin) with medroxyprogesterone acetate or conjugated estrogens alone. The Menopause Study Group. *Am J Obstet Gynecol* 1994;170:1213–23.

161. **MacLennan AH, MacLennan A, O'Neill S, Kirkgard Y, Wenzel S, Chambers HM.** Oestrogen and cyclical progestogen in postmenopausal hormone replacement therapy. *Med J Aust* 1992;157:167–70.

162. **Ravnikar VA.** Compliance with hormone therapy. *Am J Obstet Gynecol* 1987;156:1332–4.

163. **Marslew U, Riis BJ, Christiansen C.** Bleeding patterns during continuous combined estrogen-progestrogen therapy. *Am J Obstet Gynecol* 1991;164:1163–8.

164. **Sherwin BB, Gelfand MM.** The role of androgen in the maintenance of sexual functioning in oophorectomized women. *Psychosom Med* 1987;49:397–409.

165. **Sherwin BB, Gelfand MM.** Sex steroids and affect in the surgical menopause: a double-blind, cross-over study. *Psychoneuroendocrinology* 1985;10:325–35.

166. **Sherwin BB, Gelfand MM.** Differential symptom response to parenteral estrogen and/or androgen administration in the surgical menopause. *Am J Obstet Gynecol* 1985;151:153–60.

167. **Dow MG, Gallagher J.** A controlled study of combined hormonal and psychological treatment for sexual unresponsiveness in women. *Br J Clin Psychol* 1989;28:201–12.

168. **Dow MG, Hart DM, Forrest CA.** Hormonal treatments of sexual unresponsiveness in postmenopausal women: a comparative study. *Br J Obstet Gynaecol* 1983;90:361–6.

169. **Myers LS, Dixen J, Morrissette D, Carmichael M, Davidson JM.** Effects of estrogen, androgen, and progestin on sexual psychophysiology and behavior in postmenopausal women. *J Clin Endocrinol Metab* 1990;70:1124–31.

170. **Hickok LR, Toomey C, Speroff L.** A comparison of esterified estrogens with and without methyltestosterone: effects on endometrial histology and serum lipoproteins in postmenopausal women. *Obstet Gynecol* 1993;82:919–24.

171. **Whitehead A, Mathews A.** Factors related to successful outcome in the treatment of sexually unresponsive women. *Psychol Med* 1986;16:373–8.

172. **Semmens JP, Tsai CC, Semmens EC, Loadholt CB.** Effects of estrogen therapy on vaginal physiology during menopause. *Obstet Gynecol* 1985;66:15–8.

173. **Reid IR, Ames RW, Evans MC, Gamble GD, Sharpe SJ.** Long-term effects of calcium supplementation on bone loss and fractures in postmenopausal women: a randomized controlled trial. *Am J Med* 1995;98:331–5.

174. **Riggs BL, O'Fallon WM, Lane A, Hodgson SF, Wahner HW, Muhs J, et al.** Clinical trial of fluoride therpy in postmenopausal osteoporotic women: extended observations and additional analysis. *J Bone Miner Res* 1994;9:265–75.

175. **Overgaard K, Hansen MA, Jensen SB, Christiansen C.** Effect of calcitonin given intranasally on bone mass and fracture rates in established osteoporosis: a dose-response study. *BMJ* 1992;305:556–61.

176. **Tilyard MW, Spears GFS, Thomson J, Dovey S.** Treatment of postmenopausal osteoporosis with calcitrol or calcium. *N Engl J Med* 1992;326:357–62.

177. **Liberman UA, Weiss ST, Broll J, Minne HW, Qua H, Bell NH, et al.** Effect or oral alendronate on bone mineral density and the incidence of fractures in postmenopausal osteoporosis. *N Engl J Med* 1995;333:1437–43.

GYNECOLOGIC ONCOLOGY

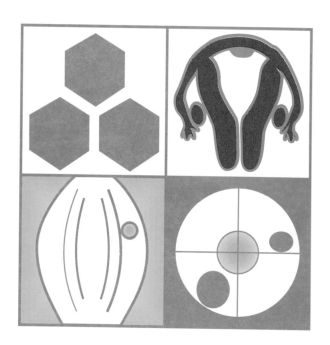

30 General Principles of Cancer Therapy

Robert C. Young
Gillian M. Thomas

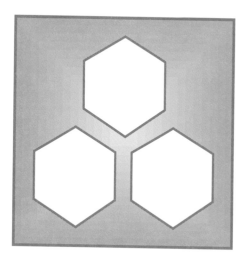

Drugs capable of the relatively selective destruction of malignant cells are used routinely to treat patients with cancer (1, 2). A wide variety of such agents is available, and the selection of the most appropriate is often difficult. Furthermore, because most antineoplastic agents have a narrower therapeutic index than drugs of other types, careful consideration should be given to the factors outlined in Table 30.1 before antineoplastic chemotherapy is instituted.

Radiation therapy has an important role in the treatment of primary and recurrent gynecologic malignancies. In some circumstances, chemotherapy and radiation therapy are combined in an attempt to improve the outcome.

Biologic Factors

Cell Kinetic Concepts

Both normal and tumorous cells have a certain growth capacity and are influenced and regulated by various internal and external forces. The differential growth and regulatory influences occurring in both normal and tumorous tissues form the basis of effective cancer treatment. The exploitation of these differences forms the basis for the effective use of both radiation therapy and chemotherapy in cancer management (1).

Patterns of Normal Growth All normal tissues are capable of cellular division and growth. Normal tissues grow in three general patterns, which are classified as *static, renewing,* and *expanding.*

1. The *static* cells consist of relatively well-differentiated cells that, after initial proliferative activity in the embryonic and neonatal period, rarely undergo cell division (e.g., striated muscle and neurons).

2. The *expanding* cells are characterized by the capacity to proliferate under special stimuli (e.g., tissue injury). Under those circumstances, the normally quiescent tissue (e.g., liver or kidney) undergoes a surge of proliferation with regrowth.

1015

Table 30.1   Issues To Be Considered Before Using Antineoplastic Drugs

1. *Natural History of the Particular Malignancy*
   a. Diagnosis of a malignancy made by biopsy
   b. Rate of disease progression
   c. Extent of disease spread

2. *Patient's Circumstances and Tolerance*
   a. Age, general health, underlying diseases
   b. Extent of previous treatment
   c. Adequate facilities to evaluate, monitor, and treat potential drug toxicities
   d. The patient's emotional, social, and financial situation

3. *Likelihood of Achieving a Beneficial Response*
   a. Cancers in which chemotherapy is curative in some patients, e.g., ovarian germ cell tumors
   b. Cancers in which chemotherapy has demonstrated improvement in survival, e.g., epithelial ovarian cancer
   c. Cancers that respond to treatment but in which improved survival has not been clearly demonstrated, e.g., cervical cancer
   d. Cancers with marginal or no response to chemotherapy, e.g., melanoma

3. The *renewing* cells are in a constantly proliferative state. There is constant cell division, a high degree of cell turnover, and constant cell loss (e.g., bone marrow, epidermis, and gastrointestinal mucosa).

Understanding these patterns of normal tissue growth partially explains some of the most common types of toxicity that occur with cancer treatments. Normal tissues with a static pattern of growth are rarely seriously injured by drug therapy, whereas renewing cell populations, such as bone marrow, gastrointestinal mucosa, and spermatozoa, are usually injured.

Cancer Cell Growth   Tumor cell growth represents a disruption in normal cellular brake mechanisms; consequently, continued proliferation and eventual death of the host result. Although cell proliferation occurs continuously in human tumors, there is evidence that it does not take place more rapidly in cancers than in normal tissue. It is not the speed of cell proliferation but the failure of the regulated balance between cell loss and cell proliferation that differentiates tumorous tissues from normal tissues.

Gompertzian Growth   The characteristics of cancer growth have been assessed by multiple studies in animals and more limited studies in humans. When tumors are extremely small, growth follows an exponential pattern but later seems to slow. Such a growth pattern is known as *Gompertzian growth*. More simply, **Gompertzian growth means that as a tumor mass increases, the time required to double the tumor's volume also increases.**

Doubling Time   The doubling time of a human tumor is the time that it takes for the mass to double in size. There is considerable variation in doubling times of human tumors. For example, embryonal tumors, lymphomas, and some malignant mesenchymal tumors have relatively fast doubling times (20–40 days), whereas adenocarcinomas and squamous cell carcinomas have relatively slow doubling times (50–150 days). Metastases generally have faster doubling times than primary lesions.

If it is assumed that exponential growth occurs early in a tumor's history and that a tumor starts from a single malignant cell, then a 1-mm mass will have undergone approximately 20 tumor doublings, a 5-mm mass (a size that might be first visualized on x-ray film) will have undergone 27 doublings, and a 1-cm mass will have undergone 30 doublings. If such a lesion were discovered clinically, the physician would assume that the tumor had been detected early. The reality is that it would have already undergone 30 doublings or would have been present approximately 60% of its life span. Our current clinical techniques recognize most tumors late in their growth, and metastasis may well have occurred long before there is evidence of the primary lesion. The second implication of kinetic concepts is that in late stages of tumor growth, a very few doublings in tumor mass have a dramatic impact on the size of the tumor. Once a tumor becomes palpable (1 cm in diameter), only three more doublings would produce an enormous tumor mass (8 cm in diameter).

Cell Cycle   Growth patterns and doubling times relate to the growth of the tumor mass as a whole. The kinetic behavior of individual tumor cells has been well described and a classic cell cycle model has been produced, as discussed in Chapter 6. **The generation time is the duration of the cycle from M phase to M phase.** Variation occurs in all phases of the cell cycle, but the variation is greatest during the G_1 period. The events controlling this variation are not well understood.

These cell cycle events have important implications for cancer therapy (2). Different sensitivities to chemotherapy and radiotherapy are associated with different proliferative states. Dividing cancer cells that are actively traversing the cell cycle are very sensitive to chemotherapeutic agents. Cells in a resting state (G_0) are relatively insensitive to chemotherapeutic agents, although they occupy space and contribute to the bulk of the tumor.

In cell kinetic studies of human tumors, the duration of the S phase (DNA synthesis phase) is relatively similar for most human tumors, ranging from a low of 10 hours to a high of approximately 31 hours. The length of the cell cycle in human tumors varies from slightly more than 1/2 day to perhaps 5 days. With cell cycle times in the range of 24 hours and doubling times in the range of 10–1000 days, it is clear that only a small proportion of tumor cells are in active cell division at any one time.

Two major factors that affect the rate at which tumors grow are the *growth fraction* and *cell death*. **The growth fraction is the number of cells in the tumor mass that are actively undergoing cell division.** There is a marked variation in the growth fraction of tumors in human beings, ranging from 25 to 95%. In the past, it was believed that human tumors contained billions of cells, all growing slowly. In actuality, only a small fraction of cells within a tumor mass are rapidly proliferating; the remainder are out of the cell cycle and quiescent.

Tumor growth may be altered by the following factors:

1. *Cytotoxic chemotherapy,* which alters both the generation time and the growth fraction of tumors.

2. *Hormones,* which appear to alter the growth fraction without changing the generation time.

3. *X-ray therapy,* which alters both the generation time and the growth fraction.

4. *Alterations in oxygen tension and vascular supply,* which alter the growth fraction without altering generation time.

5. *Immunologic therapies,* which seem to alter both generation time and growth fraction.

Chemotherapy

The natural history of each patient's malignancy has a bearing on therapy. The use of chemotherapeutic agents should be restricted to patients in whom the presence of a malignancy has been confirmed by biopsy. In some instances, second opinions regarding definitive histologic diagnoses should be obtained before instituting chemotherapy. When doubt exists concerning the diagnosis, it is preferable to delay initial therapy and not to use response to chemotherapy as a diagnostic trial.

The decision to use chemotherapy also depends on a thorough knowledge of the extent of the patient's disease as well as the rate of progression of that disease. Limited evidence of metastatic spread or documented slow disease progression may warrant withholding chemotherapy for a period. Because all chemotherapeutic agents produce toxicity, a tumor that can be evaluated to assess response should be present. It is inappropriate, in general, to administer antineoplastic agents unless one can objectively determine a benefit to the patient. Thus, except in rare instances, the ability to determine tumor response to chemotherapy is an important factor in treatment decisions.

The patient's circumstances may play a major role in decisions regarding chemotherapy. The extent of previous therapy and the patient's age, general health, and the presence of other complicating illnesses form an important part of the physician's decision and may affect substantially the patient's tolerance of antineoplastic drug treatment. In addition, the patient's emotional, social, and even financial status must be respected and evaluated before a final decision is made.

Chemotherapy should only be used when facilities are available for careful monitoring and treatment of the resulting toxicities. If such facilities are not available and chemotherapy clearly is required, the patient should be referred to a physician or another facility that has the necessary capabilities.

Differential Sensitivity

For any antineoplastic agent to be effective, it must have greater toxicity for the malignant cells than for the patient's normal cells. In that sense, all useful chemotherapeutic agents have greater activity against tumors than against normal tissues. The window between antitumor effect and normal tissue toxicity may be narrow because most chemotherapeutic agents work by disrupting DNA or RNA synthesis, affecting crucial cellular enzymes, or by altering protein synthesis.

Normal cells also use these vital cellular processes in ways similar to those of malignant cells, particularly fetal or regenerating tissue or normal cell populations in which constant cell proliferation is required (e.g., bone marrow, gastrointestinal epithelium, and hair follicles). As a result, the differential effect of antineoplastic drugs on tumors as compared with normal tissues is quantitative rather than qualitative, and some degree of injury to normal tissue is produced by every chemotherapeutic agent. The normal tissue toxicity produced by most chemotherapeutic agents correlates with the intrinsic cellular proliferation of the target tissue. This explains why toxicities, such as blood count suppression, mucosal injury, and alopecia, are often seen with most chemotherapeutic regimens.

Therapeutic Index

The net effect of a chemotherapeutic agent on the patient is often referred to as the drug's therapeutic index (i.e., a ratio of the doses at which therapeutic effect and toxicity occur). Cancer chemotherapy requires a balance of therapeutic effect and toxicity to optimize the therapeutic index. Because the window of toxicity is narrow for most chemotherapeutic agents, successful chemotherapy depends on careful attention to pharmacologic and biologic factors that influence treatment.

Cell Cycle-Specific Versus Cycle-Nonspecific Drugs

Antineoplastic agents have complex mechanisms of action and alter cells in a wide variety of ways. Different drugs have different sites of action in the cell cycle, and their effectiveness is also a function of the proliferative capacity of the tissue involved. By applying kinetic concepts, it is possible to classify chemotherapeutic agents on the basis of their cell cycle specificity and their site of maximal drug action within the cell cycle (Table 30.2). Cell cycle-nonspecific agents kill in all phases of the cell cycle and are not too dependent on proliferative capacity. At the other end of the spectrum, the action of cell cycle-specific agents, such as *hydroxyurea,* depends on the proliferative capacity of the cell and on the phase of the cell cycle. These agents kill in only one portion of the cell cycle, and cells not in that phase will not be injured. They tend to be most effective against tumors with relatively long S phases and those tumors in which there is a relatively high growth fraction and a rapid proliferation rate. Between these two broad classifications, there is a spectrum of drugs with variable degrees of cell cycle and proliferation dependence (Table 30.3).

Log Kill Hypothesis

From knowledge of basic cellular kinetics, there have emerged certain concepts of chemotherapy that have proven useful in the design of chemotherapeutic regimens. In experimental tumor systems in animals, the survival of an animal is inversely proportional to the number of cells implanted or to the size of the tumor at the time treatment is initiated (3). Treatment immediately after tumor implantation or when the tumor is subclinical in size results in better cure rates than when the tumor is clinically obvious and large.

Chemotherapeutic agents appear to work by first-order kinetics (i.e., they kill a constant fraction of cells rather than a constant number). This concept has important conceptual implications in cancer treatment. For instance, a single exposure of tumor cells to an antineoplastic drug might be capable of producing 2–5 logs of cell kill. With typical body tumor burdens of 10^{12} cells (1 kg), a single dose of chemotherapy is unlikely to be curative. This explains the need for intermittent courses of chemotherapy to achieve the magnitude of cell kill necessary to produce tumor regression and cure. It also provides a rationale for multiple drug or combination chemotherapy. The cure rate would be significantly improved if small tumors were present, but cell masses of $10^{1}-10^{4}$ cells are too small for clinical detection. This is the basis for using *adjuvant chemotherapy* in early stages of disease when subclinical numbers of cancer cells are suspected.

Table 30.2   Cell Cycle-Specificity of Chemotherapeutic Agents

Classification	Examples
Cell cycle specific, proliferation dependent	*Hydroxyurea, Ara-C*
Cell cycle specific, less proliferation dependent	*5-FU, methotrexate*
Cell cycle nonspecific, proliferation dependent	*Cytoxan, actinomycin D, cisplatin*
Cell cycle nonspecific, less proliferation dependent	*Nitrogen mustard*

Ara-C, cytosine arabinoside; 5-FU, 5-fluorouracil.

Table 30.3   Site of Action in the Cell Cycle

Portion of Cell Cycle	Drugs
G$_1$	*Actinomycin D*
Early S	*Hydroxyurea, Ara-C, 5-FU, methotrexate*
Late S	*Doxorubicin, daunomycin*
G$_2$	*Bleomycin, etoposide, teniposide*
M	*Vincristine, vinblastine*

Ara-C, cytosine arabinoside; 5-FU, 5-fluorouracil.

Drug Resistance and Tumor Cell Heterogeneity

The clinical utility of a chemotherapeutic agent or drug combination may be compromised severely when *drug resistance* develops. Chemotherapeutic agents often are active when used initially in cancer treatment, but tumors commonly become resistant during chemotherapy. Hence, patients often have an initial remission followed by a recurrence that is no longer responsive to the drugs that were effective initially.

A variety of cellular mechanisms is involved in drug resistance. Resistant tumor cells may display increased deactivation or decreased activation of drugs; they may be associated with increased drug efflux; or they may resist normal drug uptake. In some instances, drug resistance occurs as a result of altered specificity to an inhibiting enzyme or increased production of the target enzyme.

Dose Intensity

For many years, it has been taught that full doses of chemotherapy were necessary to obtain optimal clinical results. Substantial laboratory and clinical evidence now exists to support this concept. Studies in human solid tumors *in vitro* frequently demonstrate steep dose-response curves, suggesting the importance of full drug dosage. In clinical trials, higher doses of certain chemotherapeutic agents often produce responses after conventional doses have failed. In ovarian cancer, for example, twofold or threefold increases in *cisplatin* dosage can produce clinical responses in patients who experienced relapses after receiving conventional doses.

A systematic analysis of dose intensity has been performed for breast and ovarian cancer (6), and it is now possible to compare different chemotherapeutic regimens by converting the drug dosage within individual programs to milligrams per meter squared per week:

$$\text{Dose Intensity} = \text{Drug (mg)/Surface Area (M}^2\text{)/Time (week)}$$

When results of chemotherapy trials are analyzed and compared, it is important that maximum dose intensity be used and that drug intensity be reported. Most of the data on the clinical impact of dose intensity come from retrospective analyses, but several prospective trials of dose intensity in ovarian cancer have produced mixed results (7, 8). Other approaches are now being explored to increase the intensity of drug regimens in an attempt to increase remission rates and durations. These approaches have included intensifying chemotherapy with the use of bone marrow or stem cell transplantation or hematopoietic growth factors to enhance marrow recovery.

Bone marrow transplantation is being used on an experimental basis in cases of advanced, refractory ovarian cancer in which the prognosis is poor. Although higher response rates are often achieved, the toxicity of these regimens often are severe (mortality 10–35%), and as yet no survival benefit has been documented. Peripheral stem cell transplantations are also being studied and offer the advantage of not requiring marrow harvest under general anesthesia.

Attempts are being made to reduce dose-limiting myelotoxicity by using *granulocyte-macrophage colony-stimulating factor (GM-CSF),* or *G-CSF*. Although these therapies accelerate the recovery of granulocytes after treatment and often reduce the duration of hospitalization after bone marrow transplantation, they are expensive and have yet to be shown to alter the therapeutic outcome. There is no study that documents any benefit from the routine prophylactic use of these hematopoietic growth factors during conventional chemotherapy. Furthermore, none of the growth factors currently available has any significant impact on platelet recovery, which is often the toxicity limiting the dose of platinum-based chemotherapy.

Pharmacologic Factors Influencing Treatment

Pharmacologically, it is useful to describe effective chemotherapy as concentration (C) of the active agent or its metabolite over time (T) at the primary site of antitumor action:

Drug Effect = Drug Concentration × Duration of Exposure = C × T

Although it is not possible to determine exact pericellular pharmacokinetics, information can be obtained from analysis of plasma concentration × time (C × T) (9). A number of important factors influence this pharmacokinetic result, including route of administration, drug absorption, drug transport, distribution, biotransformation, inactivation, excretion, and interactions with other drugs.

Route of Administration and Absorption	Traditionally, drugs have been given *orally, intravenously, intramuscularly,* or *intra-arterially.* More recently, considerable attention has been given to the *intraperitoneal* administration of chemotherapeutic agents, particularly in ovarian cancer (10). The intraperitoneal approach is based on the concept that the pleural or peritoneal clearance of the agent is slower than its plasma clearance. As a result, an increased concentration of the drug in the pleural or peritoneal cavity is maintained while plasma concentrations remain low. Studies of a wide variety of chemotherapeutic agents have demonstrated a differential concentration of 30- to 500-fold, depending on the molecular weight, charge, and lipid solubility of the particular drug. Clinical trials have been performed to study the effects of *cisplatin and paclitaxel (Taxol)* and drug combinations in ovarian cancer. In clinical trials using intraperitoneal *cisplatin* second-line, third-look laparotomies have been negative in 30% of patients with minimal residual disease (10). Recent clinical trials in previously untreated women with optimal stage III ovarian cancer show that the use of intraperitoneal *cisplatin* is associated with a longer survival than intravenous *cisplatin* (11).
Principles of Combination Chemotherapy	Antineoplastic agents are often used in combinations (12, 13). Combination chemotherapy has become the standard approach to management of ovarian germ cell tumors as well as many other adult solid tumors. The enthusiasm for combinations results from several significant limitations inherent to single-agent chemotherapy. In addition, there is a solid theoretic basis for combination chemotherapy, which is derived from knowledge of cellular kinetics, drug metabolism, drug resistance, and tumor heterogeneity.
Limitations of Single-Drug Therapy	One of the major limitations of single-agent chemotherapy is that toxicity limits the dose and duration of drug administration and thus restricts the tumor cell kill achievable. Adoptive mechanisms allow cell survival and eventual regrowth of resistant tumor cells despite the lethal effects produced in the bulk of the tumor. This leads to the development of spontaneous and multiple (pleiotropic) drug resistance. Several different mechanisms of resistance are seen with antineoplastic agents. Most problems inherent to single-drug therapy cannot be corrected by simply altering the dose or schedule of that single drug. As a result, increasing use has been made of multidrug combination chemotherapy.
Combination Chemotherapy Mechanisms	Different chemotherapeutic agents may act in different phases of the tumor cell cycle. Use of multiple drugs with different cellular kinetic characteristics reduces the tumor mass more completely than any individual chemotherapeutic agent while minimizing the impact of single-drug resistance. For instance, if a cell cycle-nonspecific agent is administered, producing a 2 log cell kill in a tumor mass with 10^9 cells and no further therapy is given, a minor tumor response will occur, followed by tumor regrowth and no impact on survival. If a cell cycle-specific agent produces a similar degree of cell kill, only the cells coming into cell cycle will be affected by such an agent. By using combinations or sequences of cell cycle-specific and cycle-nonspecific agents, log kill can be enhanced in tumors. With identification of appropriate combinations and proper sequencing, sufficient log kill may be achieved to produce a cure.

Drug Resistance

Combination chemotherapy can help circumvent spontaneous mutations to drug resistance. After initial cell kill, the residual tumor may contain drug-resistant cells. **The probability of the emergence of drug-resistant cells in any given population is reduced if two or more agents with different mechanisms of action can be used in a tightly sequenced treatment scheme.**

Drug Interaction

Drug interactions may be additive, synergistic, or antagonistic. Combinations that result in improved therapy because of increased antitumor activity or decreased toxicity are said to be *synergistic*. *Additive* therapies produce enhanced antitumor activity equivalent to the sum of both agents acting singly. Finally, using multiple antitumor agents may actually *antagonize* the effect of each agent, producing a lesser therapeutic effect than when used singly. For example, *5-fluorouracil (5-FU)* prevents the antifolate action of *methotrexate* when used before *methotrexate* administration. The general principles that allowed the development of successful combinations are shown in Table 30.4. Although these principles do not apply to every regimen and some overlap in toxicities is common, they are a central feature of most of the regimens currently being used successfully in cancer treatment.

Remission

Once a treatment regimen has been selected, it is necessary to have some standardized way to evaluate the response to drug treatment. The terms "complete remission" and "partial remission" are used frequently and provide a convenient way to describe responses and compare various published regimens.

Complete Remission   **Complete remission is the complete disappearance of all objective evidence of tumor as well as the resolution of all signs and symptoms referable to the tumor.** Complete regressions of cancer are generally those associated with significant prolongation of survival.

Partial Remission   **Partial remission is a $\geq 50\%$ reduction in the size of all measurable lesions along with some degree of subjective improvement and the absence of any new lesions during therapy.** Partial remissions generally translate into improved well-being for the patient but only occasionally are associated with longer overall survival. Finally, various terms indicate lesser responses, such as "objective response" or "minor response," but such responses rarely result in any significant improvement in survival.

Dose Adjustment

Patients vary in their tolerance to chemotherapy; therefore, it is necessary to have some mechanism for tailoring the treatment to the patient. One convenient method involves the use of a "sliding scale." A typical scheme for adjusting chemotherapy based on myelosuppression is presented in Table 30.5. Doses of myelosuppressive agents are reduced if

---

Table 30.4   Important Factors in the Design of Drug Combinations

1. The drugs used must be active as single agents against the particular tumor.

2. The drugs should have different mechanisms of action to minimize emergence of drug resistance.

3. The drugs should have a biochemical basis of at least additive and preferably synergistic effects.

4. The drugs chosen should have a different spectrum of toxicity so they can be used for maximum cell kill at full doses.

5. The drugs chosen should be administered intermittently so that cell kill is enhanced and prolonged immunosuppression is minimized.

Table 30.5   Drug Dose Adjustments for Combination Chemotherapy (Sliding Scale Based on Bone Marrow Toxicity)

If White Blood Count Before Starting the Next Course Is:	Then Dosage Is:
>4000/mm³	100% of all drugs
3999–3000/mm³	100% of nonmyelotoxic agents and 50% of each myelotoxic agent
2999–2000/mm³	100% of nonmyelotoxic agents and 25% of each myelotoxic agent
1999–1000/mm³	50% of nonmyelotoxic agents and 25% of myelotoxic agents
999–0/mm³	No drug until blood counts recover

If the Platelet Count Before Starting Next Course Is:	Then Dosage Is:
>100,000/mm³	100% of all drugs
50,000–100,000/mm³	100% of nonmyelotoxic drugs and 50% of myelotoxic drugs
<50,000/mm³	No drug until blood counts recover

the patient is very sensitive to the regimen but can be returned to full levels if tolerance improves in subsequent courses.

Many experimental protocols provide for an escalation of drug dose if no significant toxicity is experienced with initial courses of therapy. A sliding scale offers the best opportunity to give the maximum amount of therapy possible. The sliding scale presented is based only on bone marrow toxicity. If the drugs used in any particular combination have other serious toxicities, such as renal or hepatic toxicity, sliding scales based on the other toxicities are used to minimize toxicity but maximize therapeutic effect.

For example, carboplatin is generally given intravenously at 300 mg/M² every 4 weeks to patients with good bone marrow reserves. Because the drug is cleared renally and occasional severe marrow toxicity occurs, dose-adjustment scales based on renal function have been developed, i.e., the Calvert formula (14). Dose adjustments are based on the glomerular filtration rate (GFR) or creatinine clearance and the target serum concentration multiplied by the "area under curve" (AUC) for the drug's antitumor activity:

$$\textbf{Dose (mg)} = \textbf{Target AUC} \times (\textbf{GFR} + \textbf{25})$$

The desired target AUC is 4–6 mg/ml for previously treated patients and 6–8 mg/ml for those previously untreated. The use of these dose-adjustment schemes tailored to a particular toxicity allows safer administration of chemotherapeutic agents.

Drug Toxicity

Antineoplastic drugs are among the most toxic agents used in modern medicine. Many of the toxic side effects, particularly those to organ systems with a rapidly proliferating cell population, are dose related and predictable. Usually, the mechanism of toxicity is similar to the mechanism that produces the desired cytotoxic effect on tumors. Even organs with limited cell proliferation can be damaged by chemotherapeutic agents in either a dose-related or an idiosyncratic fashion. In almost all instances, chemotherapeutic agents are used in doses that produce some degree of toxicity to normal tissues.

Severe systemic debility, advanced age, poor nutritional status, or direct organ involvement by primary or metastatic tumor can result in unexpectedly severe side effects of chemotherapy. Idiosyncratic drug reactions also can have severe and unexpected consequences. As a result, patients receiving cancer chemotherapy should be monitored carefully and closely (15, 16).

Hematologic Toxicity

The proliferating cells of the erythroid, myeloid, and megakaryocytic series of the bone marrow are highly susceptible to damage by many commonly employed antineoplastic agents. Granulocytopenia and thrombocytopenia are predictable side effects of most antitumor agents and occur with all effective regimens of combination chemotherapy. The severity and duration of these side effects are variable and depend on the drugs used, the dose, the schedule, and whether the patient has had previous irradiation therapy or chemotherapy.

In general, acute granulocytopenia occurs 6–12 days after administration of most myelosuppressive chemotherapeutic agents and recovery occurs in 21–24 days; platelet suppression occurs 4–5 days later, and recovery occurs after white cell count returns to base line.

Granulocytopenia   **Patients with an absolute granulocyte count less than 500/mm³ for 5 days or longer are at high risk of rapidly fatal sepsis.** The widespread prophylactic and empiric use of broad-spectrum antibiotics in patients with febrile cancer and granulocytopenia has significantly decreased the incidence of life-threatening infections. Temperature should be checked every 4 hours in patients with granulocytopenia; these patients should also be examined frequently for evidence of infection. Recent availability of hematopoietic growth factors such as G-CSF and GM-CSF has enabled physicians to reduce the duration of granulocytopenia in certain patients. However, thrombocytopenia is not reversed.

Thrombocytopenia   **Patients with sustained thrombocytopenia who have platelet counts less than 20,000/mm³ are at risk of spontaneous hemorrhage, particularly gastrointestinal or acute intracranial hemorrhage.** Routine platelet transfusions for platelet counts less than 20,000/mm³ have significantly reduced the risk of spontaneous hemorrhage. It is customary to transfuse 6–10 units of random donor platelets to the patient with a platelet count less than 20,000/mm³. Repeated transfusions at intervals of 2–3 days for the duration of the severe thrombocytopenia are indicated. Although patients with platelet counts greater than 50,000/mm³ do not usually experience severe bleeding, transfusion at this level is indicated if active bleeding manifests or if active peptic ulcer disease is present before and during surgical procedures. A posttransfusion platelet count performed 1 hour after platelet administration should show an appropriate incremental increase. If the platelet count does not increase after transfusion, it is likely that there has been previous sensitization to random donor platelets and the patient will require single-donor human leukocyte antigen (HLA) matched platelets for future transfusions.

Gastrointestinal Toxicity

The gastrointestinal tract is a frequent site of serious toxicity to antineoplastic drug treatment. Mucositis caused by a direct effect on the rapidly dividing epithelial mucosal cells is common; concomitant granulocytopenia allows the injured mucosa to become infected and serves as a portal of entry for bacteria and fungi into the bloodstream. The onset of mucositis frequently occurs 3–5 days earlier than the myelosuppression. Lesions of the mouth and pharynx are difficult to distinguish from those caused by candidiasis and herpes simplex virus infection. Esophagitis resulting from direct drug toxicity can be confused with radiation esophagitis or infections with bacteria, fungi, or herpes simplex virus, all of which produce dysphagia and retrosternal burning pain. Oral candidiasis (thrush) responds to oral administration of *chlortrimazole* (10 mg five times daily). Esophageal or severe oral candidiasis usually responds to a 7-day course of intravenous *amphotericin B* (0.5 mg/kg/day). Mucocutaneous herpes simplex infection clears more rapidly with intravenous use of *acyclovir* (750 mg/m²/day). Symptomatic management of painful upper gastrointestinal inflammation includes warm saline mouth rinses and topical anesthetics such as viscous *lidocaine*. Intravenous fluids or hyperalimentation may be required.

Mucositis in the lower gastrointestinal tract is invariably associated with diarrhea. Serious complications include bowel perforation, hemorrhage, and necrotizing enterocolitis. *Necrotizing enterocolitis* includes a spectrum of severe diarrheal illnesses that can be fatal in a patient with granulocytopenia. Broad-spectrum antibiotic therapy may predispose the patient to necrotizing enterocolitis. Symptoms of necrotizing enterocolitis include watery or bloody diarrhea, abdominal pain, sore throat, nausea, vomiting, and fever. Physical examination usually reveals abdominal tenderness and distention. Most cases of necrotizing enterocolitis are seen in patients who are treated with *clindamycin* and are caused by the anaerobic bacteria *Clostridium difficile*. The treatment for a *C. difficile* infection is oral administration of *vancomycin,* 125 mg four times daily for 10–14 days.

Immunosuppression

Most anticancer drugs are capable of suppressing cellular and, to a lesser extent, humoral immunity. The magnitude and duration of the immunosuppression vary with the dose and schedule of drug administration and have been inadequately characterized for most chemotherapeutic agents. However, most of the acute immunosuppressive side effects do not persist after completion of drug treatment. Laboratory studies suggest that there is a marked decrease in host defenses during treatment and that a rebound to complete or nearly complete restoration occurs 2–3 days after treatment is completed.

Dermatologic Reactions

Drug toxicities can involve skin reactions, including alopecia, local necrosis from drug extravasation, and allergic or hypersensitivity reactions. Skin necrosis and sloughing may result from extravasation of certain particularly irritating chemotherapeutic agents such as *doxorubicin* and *actinomycin D*. The extent of necrosis depends on the quantity of drug extravasated and can vary from local erythema to chronic ulcerative necrosis. Management often includes immediate removal of the intravenous line, local infiltration of corticosteroids, ice pack therapy four times a day for 3 days, and elevation of the affected limb.

Alopecia is the most common side effect of many anticancer drugs. Although not intrinsically injurious, it has major emotional consequences for patients. Agents commonly associated with severe hair loss include *paclitaxel* and *cyclophosphamide,* but most commonly used drug combinations produce variable degrees of alopecia. Alopecia is virtually always reversible once chemotherapy is discontinued. Generally, hair regrowth begins 10 days to several weeks after treatment is completed. Attempts to minimize alopecia by using "cold caps" have been variably effective.

Generalized allergic skin reactions can occur with chemotherapeutic agents, as with other drugs, and sometimes can be severe. Other skin reactions occasionally seen with chemotherapeutic agents include increased skin pigmentation (*bleomycin*), photosensitivity reactions, transverse banding or nail loss, folliculitis (*actinomycin D, methotrexate*), and radiation recall reactions (*doxorubicin*).

Hepatic Toxicity

Modest elevations in transaminase, alkaline phosphatase, and bilirubin levels are frequently seen with many anticancer agents, but they resolve soon after treatment is completed. Nevertheless, more severe reactions do occur. Long-term administration of *methotrexate* induces hepatic fibrosis, which can progress to frank cirrhosis. Cirrhosis and drug-induced hepatitis should be managed by withdrawal of the toxic agent, with the same supportive measures that are used for hepatitis or cirrhosis of any cause.

Pulmonary Complications

Patients with cancer have a wide variety of problems that can manifest as pulmonary complications. Respiratory compromise resulting from lung metastases, pulmonary emboli, radiation pneumonitis, tumor-induced neuromuscular dysfunction, and pneumonia all may be significant complications. In addition, some anticancer drugs can cause direct pulmonary toxicity. Interstitial pneumonitis with pulmonary fibrosis is the usual pattern of lung damage associated with cytotoxic drugs. Agents likely to cause such an effect are *bleomycin*, alkylating agents, and the *nitrosoureas*. The physical and chest x-ray findings are not easily distinguishable from those of interstitial pneumonitis resulting from infectious agents, viruses, or lymphangitic spread of cancer. Management of drug-induced interstitial pneumonitis includes discontinuation of the suspected agent and supportive care.

Cardiac Toxicity

Cardiac toxicity occurs with several important cancer chemotherapeutic agents. Although the myocardium consists of largely nondividing cells, drugs of the anthracycline antibiotic class, specifically *doxorubicin*, can cause severe cardiomyopathy. **The risk of cardiac toxicity increases with the total cumulative dose of *doxorubicin*.** For this reason, a cumulative dose of 500 mg/m² of ideal body surface area is now widely used as the maximum tolerable dose of *doxorubicin*. With careful and frequent monitoring of left ventricular function by means of ejection fraction studies, therapy can be continued to higher doses if no satisfactory alternative exists. More infrequently, anthracyclines and *paclitaxel* can cause acute arrhythmias that generally disappear within a few days of drug treatment. They appear to be unrelated to total drug dose. Anthracycline cardiac toxicity is potentiated by radiation. Rarely, *cyclophosphamide* has been reported to produce cardiotoxicity, particularly in the massive doses used in conjunction with bone marrow transplantation. With conventional doses of *cyclophosphamide*, this complication is unlikely.

The medical management of cardiomyopathy induced by anthracyclines is supportive, but results are generally unsatisfactory. Radionuclide cardiac scintigraphy should be performed for early detection of cardiac compromise before the clinical manifestations of congestive heart failure appear. Discontinuation of the drug at the first indication of decreasing left ventricular function will minimize the risk of cardiovascular decompensation.

Genitourinary Toxicity

In addition to chemotherapeutic agents, various other cancer-related complications may produce chronic azotemia or acute renal failure. Such complications include fluid depletion, infection, tumor infiltration of the kidney, ureteral obstruction by tumor, radiation damage, and tumor lysis syndrome.

Drugs that cause kidney damage include *cisplatin*, which produces renal tubular toxicity associated with azotemia and magnesium wasting, and *methotrexate*, which can precipitate in the renal tubules, causing oliguric renal failure. *Methotrexate* toxicity can be prevented by maintenance of a high urine volume and alkalinization of the urine. Metabolites of *cyclophosphamide* are irritants to the bladder mucosa and cause *chronic hemorrhagic cystitis*, particularly during high-dose or prolonged treatment. Vigorous hydration and diuresis can reduce the risk of this complication.

Drug-related genitourinary toxicity should be treated by discontinuation of the possibly nephrotoxic drugs and volume expansion to increase glomerular filtration. Specific metabolic abnormalities, such as hyperuricemia and hypomagnesemia, should be corrected. If oliguria develops or if medical management is unsuccessful in restoring acceptable kidney function, short-term peritoneal dialysis or hemodialysis may be required. Daily administration of 3 l of fluid containing 100–150 mEq of sodium bicarbonate per liter will maintain the urinary pH level above 7. Because *methotrexate* is poorly dialyzed, prolonged toxic levels can result if *leucovorin* rescue therapy is not continued until the *methotrexate* concentration is less than 5×10^{-8} M.

N-acetylcysteine or *mesna* (sodium mercaptoethanesulfonate) has been used in conjunction with very high doses of *cyclophosphamide* or *iphosphamide* to prevent bladder toxicity by inactivating the toxic metabolite *acrolein*. Persistent hemorrhagic cystitis that does not respond to conservative management may be treated with υ-*aminocaproic acid*.

Neurotoxicity

Many antineoplastic drugs are associated with some central or peripheral neurotoxicity. Generally, these neurologic side effects are mild, but occasionally they can be severe. *Cisplatin* produces ototoxicity, peripheral neuropathy, and, rarely, retrobulbar neuritis and blindness. High doses of *cisplatin,* such as those often used in ovarian cancer therapy, are particularly likely to produce a progressive and somewhat delayed peripheral neuropathy. This defect is characterized by sensory impairment and loss of proprioception, whereas motor strength generally is preserved. Progression of this neuropathy 1–2 months after cessation of high-dose *cisplatin* therapy has been reported. *Paclitaxel* can also produce a peripheral neuropathy; therefore, when used in combination with *cisplatin,* this toxicity can be potentiated. Rarely, *5-FU* is associated with an acute cerebellar toxicity, apparently related to its metabolism to fluorocitrate, a neurotoxic metabolite of the parent compound. *Hexamethylmelamine* has been reported to produce peripheral neuropathy and encephalopathy. Some improvement in peripheral neuropathy has been reported with administration of B vitamin supplements, but therapeutic effectiveness may be reduced.

Vascular and Hypersensitivity Reactions

Occasionally, severe hypersensitivity reactions in the form of anaphylaxis develop with the use of chemotherapeutic agents. In rare cases, this has been associated with the use of *cyclophosphamide, doxorubicin, cisplatin,* intravenous *melphalan,* and high doses of *methotrexate. Bleomycin* administration may be associated with marked fever reactions, anaphylaxis, Raynaud's phenomenon, and a chronic scleroderma-like reaction. Hypersensitivity reactions have been seen with *paclitaxel* and are believed to be caused by hypersensitivity to the *cremophor* vehicle. These reactions can be ameliorated with intravenous infusions of *dexamethasone* (20 mg), *diphenhydramine* (50 mg), and *cimetidine* (300 mg) 30 minutes before *paclitaxel* is administered.

Second Malignancies

Many antineoplastic agents in current use are mutagenic and teratogenic. The potential of these agents to induce second malignancies appears to vary with the class of agent (17). Alkylating agents (especially *melphalan*) seem to be the major offenders. The cumulative 7-year risk of acute nonlymphocytic leukemia (ANL) developing in patients treated primarily with oral *melphalan* for ovarian cancer is as high as 9.6% in patients receiving therapy for more than 1 year (17). Antimetabolite use, in contrast, seems to pose less risk. Evidence from long-term studies of patients with Hodgkin's disease suggests a major risk with combined chemotherapy and radiation therapy. In such patients, there is a risk of acute leukemia as well as an increase in solid tumors, which is seen particularly in the radiation ports. An increase in the frequency of acute leukemia has been reported in patients treated for Hodgkin's disease, multiple myeloma, and ovarian cancer.

The second malignancy commonly occurs 4–7 years after successful therapy. Encouragingly, recent evidence suggests that after 11 years, the risk of acute leukemia in patients treated for Hodgkin's disease decreases to that of the normal population. Also encouraging are the long-term follow-up studies in women in whom choriocarcinoma was cured, primarily with antimetabolite therapy. In such patient populations, there is no evidence of an increased risk of second malignancy. Radiation therapy alone appears to produce a relatively low risk of late leukemia. Chemotherapeutic regimens alone, particularly those in which alkylating agents are not used, are also associated with relatively little risk. Combination chemotherapy and limited-field radiation therapy increase the risk only slightly. Particularly high risks are associated with extensive radiation therapy plus combination chemotherapy, prolonged alkylating agent therapy (longer than 1 year), prolonged maintenance therapy, and age at initial treatment older than 40 years.

Gonadal Dysfunction   Many cancer chemotherapeutic agents have profound and lasting effects on testicular and ovarian function. Chemotherapeutic agents, particularly alkylating agents, can cause azoospermia and amenorrhea. Secondary sexual characteristics related to hormonal function are generally less disturbed. Prolonged intensive combination chemotherapy commonly produces azoospermia in males, and recovery is uncommon.

The onset of amenorrhea and ovarian failure is accompanied by an elevation of the serum follicle-stimulating hormone (FSH) and luteinizing hormone (LH) and a decrease in the serum estradiol level. Occasionally, this hormonal pattern occurs before the onset of amenorrhea. In the presence of this characteristic pattern, patients should be advised to consider conception, because these findings predict premature ovarian failure and early menopause.

When short-term intensive chemotherapy is used, particularly with antimetabolites, vinca alkaloids, or antitumor antibiotics, injury to the reproductive system is less common. For example, males treated for testicular cancer, children with acute leukemia, and women cured of gestational trophoblastic disease or ovarian germ cell malignancies generally recover reproductive capacity after therapy.

Chemotherapy in Pregnancy   The risk of congenital abnormalities from chemotherapeutic agents is highest during the first trimester of pregnancy, especially when antimetabolites (e.g., *methotrexate*) and alkylating agents are used. Chemotherapy administered during the second or third trimesters is generally not associated with an increase in fetal abnormalities, although the number of patients studied is relatively small.

Metabolic Abnormalities   Inappropriate antidiuretic hormone (ADH) secretion is characterized by hyponatremia, high urine osmolality, and high urinary sodium values and is associated with several malignancies, most commonly small cell carcinoma of the lung. It can also be seen as a complication of vinca alkaloid chemotherapy. Symptoms are primarily neurologic and include altered mental status, confusion, lethargy, seizures, and coma. The severity of symptoms is related to the rapidity of development of hyponatremia. The diagnosis rests on the documentation of hyponatremia, the presence of urine that is hypertonic to plasma, and the exclusion of hypothyroidism or adrenal insufficiency.

Hyperuricemia may be a complication of effective cancer chemotherapy in certain tumors, particularly hematologic malignancies in which rapid tumor lysis occurs in response to initial treatment. Rapid tumor lysis produces release of predominant intracellular ions and uric acid and can result in life-threatening hyperkalemia, hyperphosphatemia, hypocalcemia, and hyperuricemia. Renal failure associated with hyperuricemia can be severe. Prevention of the *tumor lysis syndrome* requires maintenance of a high urinary output, maintenance of high urinary pH (above 7.0), and prophylactic use of the xanthine oxidase inhibitor, *allopurinol*.

Antineoplastic Drugs   The characteristics of commonly used chemotherapeutic agents in gynecologic cancers are presented in Table 30.6.

Alkylating Agents   Alkylating agents act primarily by interacting chemically with DNA (18). These drugs form extremely unstable alkyl groups that react with nucleophilic (electron-rich) sites on many important organic compounds, such as nucleic acids, proteins, and amino acids. These interactions produce the primary cytotoxic effects.

Alkylating agents usually bind to the N-7 position of guanine and to other key DNA sites. In doing so, they interfere with accurate base pairing, cross-link DNA, and produce single-

Table 30.6   Chemotherapeutic Drugs Used in Gynecologic Cancers

Drug	Route of Administration	Common Treatment Schedules	Common Toxicities	Diseases Treated
Alkylating agents				
Cyclophosphamide (Cytoxan)	Oral, I.V.	1.5–3.0 mg/kg/day p.o. 10–50 mg/kg I.V. every 1–4 weeks	Myelosuppression, cystitis ± bladder fibrosis, alopecia, hepatitis, amenorrhea, azoospermia	Breast, ovary, soft tissue sarcomas
Melphalan (Alkeran, L-PAM)	Oral	0.2 mg/kg/day × 5 days every 4–6 weeks	Myelosuppression, nausea and vomiting (rare), mucosal ulceration (rare), second malignancies	Ovary, breast
Triethylene thiophosphoramide (TSPA, Thiotepa)	I.V. Intracavitary	I.V.: 0.8 mg/kg every 4–6 weeks Intracavitary: 45–60 mg	Myelosuppression, nausea and vomiting, headaches, lever (rare)	Ovary, breast; intracavitary for malignant effusions
Iphosphamide (Ifex)	I.V.	1.0 or 1.2 g/m²/day × 5 days With mesna: 200 mg/m² immediately before and 4 and 8 hr after iphosphamide	Myelosuppression, bladder toxicity, CNS dysfunction, renal toxicity	Cervix, ovary
Alkylating-Like Agents				
Cis-dichlorodiamino-platinum (cisplatin)	I.V.	10–20 mg/m²/day × 5 every 3 weeks or 50–75 mg/m² every 1–3 weeks	Nephrotoxicity, tinnitis and and hearing loss, nausea and vomiting, myelosuppression, peripheral neuropathy	Ovarian and germ cell carcinomas, cervical cancer
Carboplatin	I.V.	300–400 mg/m² × 6 every 3–4 weeks	Less neuropathy, ototoxicity, and nephrotoxicity than cisplatin; more hemato-poeitic toxicity, especially thrombocytopenia, than cisplatin	Ovarian and germ cell carcinomas
Decarbazine (DTIC)	I.V.	2–4.5 mg/kg/day × 10 days every 4 weeks	Myelosuppression, nausea and vomiting, flulike syndrome, hepatotoxicity	Uterine sarcomas, soft tissue sarcomas
Antitumor Antibiotics				
Actinomycin D (dactinomycin, Cosmegen)	I.V.	0.3–0.5 mg/m² I.V. × 5 days every 3–4 weeks	Nausea and vomiting, skin necrosis, mucosal ulceration, myelosuppression	Germ cell ovarian tumors, choriocarcinoma, soft tissue sarcoma
Bleomycin (Blenoxane)	I.V., S.C., I.M., I.P.	10–20 units/m² 1–2 times/week to total dose of 400 units; for effusions: 60–120 units	Fever, dermatologic reactions, pulmonary toxicity, anaphylactic reactions	Cervix, germ cell ovarian tumors, malignant effusions
Mitomycin-C (Mutamycin)	I.V.	10–20 mg/m² every 6–8 weeks	Myelosuppression, local vesicant, nausea and vomiting, mucosal ulcerations, nephrotoxicity	Breast, cervix, ovary
Doxorubicin (Adriamycin)	I.V.	60–90 mg/m² every 3 weeks or 20–35 mg/m² every day × 3 every 3 weeks	Myelosuppression, alopecia, cardiotoxicity, local vesicant, nausea and vomiting, mucosal ulcerations	Ovary, breast, endometrium

Table 30.6—continued

Drug	Route of Administration	Common Treatment Schedules	Common Toxicities	Diseases Treated
Mithramycin (Mithracin)	I.V.	20–50 mg/kg/day every 4–6 weeks; Hypercalcemia: 25 mg/kg every 3–4 days	Nausea and vomiting, hemorrhagic diathesis, hepatotoxicity, renal toxicity, fever, myelosuppression, facial flushing	Hypercalcemia of malignancy
Antimetabolites				
5-Fluorouracil (Fluorouracil, 5-FU)	I.V.	10–15 mg/kg/week	Myelosuppression, nausea and vomiting, anorexia, alopecia	Breast, ovary
Methotrexate (MTX, amethopterin)	P.O., I.V., Intrathecal	Oral: 15–40 mg/day × 5 days; I.V.: 240 mg/m^2 with leucovorin rescue; Intrathecal: 12–15 mg/m^2/week	Mucosal ulceration, myelosuppression, hepatotoxicity, allergic pneumonitis; with intrathecal: meningeal irritation	Choriocarcinoma, breast, ovary
Hydroxyurea (Hydrea)	P.O., I.V.	1–2 gm/m^2/daily for 2–6 weeks	Myelosuppression, nausea and vomiting, anorexia	Cervix
Plant Alkaloids				
Vincristine (Oncovin)	I.V.	0.01–0.03 mg/kg/week	Neurotoxicity, alopecia, myelosuppression, cranial nerve palsies, gastrointestinal	Ovarian germ cell, sarcomas, cervical cancer
Vinblastine (Velban)	I.V.	5–6 mg/m^2 every 1–2 weeks	Myelosuppression, alopecia, nausea and vomiting, neurotoxicity	Ovarian germ cell, choriocarcinoma
Epipodophyllotoxin (Etoposide, VP-16)	I.V.	300–600 mg/m^2 divided over 3–4 days every 3–4 weeks	Myelosuppression, alopecia, hypotension	Ovarian germ cell, choriocarcinoma
Paclitaxel (Taxol)	I.V.	135–250 mg/m^2 as a 3- to 24-hour infusion every 3 weeks	Myelosuppression, alopecia, allergic reactions, cardiac arrhythmias	Ovarian cancer, breast cancer
Taxotere	I.V.	50–100 mg/m^2	Myelosuppression, alopecia, derratologic reactins	Ovarian cancer, breast cancer
Miscellaneous Agent				
Hexamethylmelamine, Altretamine (Hexalen)	Oral	120 mg/m^2/day × 14 days every 4 weeks	Nausea and vomiting myelosuppression, neurotoxicity, skin rashes	Ovary, breast

I.V., intravenous; S.C., subcutaneous; I.M., intramuscular; I.P., intraperitoneal; CNS, central nervous system, P.O., postoperative.

and double-stranded breaks. This results in the inhibition of DNA, RNA, and protein synthesis. Because alkylating agents share some effects of irradiation, they are often called *radiomimetic*. Most of the effective alkylating agents are bifunctional or polyfunctional and have two or more potentially unstable alkyl groups per molecule. These bifunctional alkylating agents allow cross-linkage of DNA, which results in cellular disruption. Because all alkylating agents have similar mechanisms of action, cross-resistance to other agents of the same class tends to occur.

In addition, several antineoplastic agents of different types are generally classified as alkylating-like agents, although their precise mechanism of action is less well understood and is probably not exclusively alkylation (19). These agents include the platinum analogs *cisplatin* and *carboplatin*.

Antitumor Antibiotics

Antitumor antibiotics are antineoplastic drugs that, in general, have been isolated as natural products from fungi found in the soil (20). These natural products generally have extremely complex and diverse chemical structures, although they generally function by forming complexes with DNA.

The interaction between these drugs and DNA often involves intercalation, in which the compound is inserted between DNA base pairs. A second mechanism believed to be important in their antitumor action is the formation of free radicals capable of damaging DNA, RNA, and vital proteins. Other effects include metal ion chelation and alteration of tumor cell membranes. This class of antineoplastic agents generally is believed to be *cell cycle nonspecific*.

The anthracyclines are antibiotics isolated from the fungi, *Streptomyces*. These pigmented compounds have an anthraquinone nucleus attached to an amino sugar and have multiple mechanisms of action. Because of the planar structure of the anthraquinone moiety, these agents act as intercalators in the DNA double helix. In addition, they are known to chelate divalent cations and are avid calcium binders. These agents cause single-stranded DNA breaks, inhibit DNA repair, and actively generate free radicals that are capable of producing DNA damage. Recent evidence suggests that anthracyclines are capable of reacting directly with cell membranes, disrupting membrane structure, and altering membrane function.

Bleomycin is also isolated from the *Streptomyces* fungus. Its structure contains a DNA-binding fragment and an ion-binding unit. It appears to produce its antitumor action primarily by producing single- and double-stranded breaks in DNA, mainly at sites of guanine bases. The drug is excreted primarily in urine, and increased toxicity may be seen in patients with impaired renal function.

Antimetabolites

The antimetabolite family of antineoplastic agents interacts with vital intracellular enzymes, leading to their inactivation or to the production of fraudulent products incapable of normal intracellular function (21, 22). In general, their structures resemble analogs of normal purines and pyrimidines or they resemble normal substances that are vital for cell function. Some antimetabolites are active as intact drugs, and others require biotransformation to active agents in order to be effective.

Although many of these agents act at different sites in biosynthetic pathways, they appear to exert their antitumor activity by disruption of functions crucial to the viability of the cell. These effects are generally more disruptive to actively proliferating cells; therefore, the antimetabolites are generally classed as *cell cycle-specific* agents.

Although hundreds of antimetabolites have been investigated in cancer treatment, those used most often in gynecology include the folate antagonist *methotrexate*, which inhibits the enzyme dihydrofolate reductase, the pyrimidine antagonists *5-FU*, and the ribonucleotide reductase inhibitor *hydroxyurea (Hydrea)*. In most instances, the antimetabolites are used not as single drugs but in combinations because of their cell cycle specificity and their capacity for complementary inhibition.

Plant Alkaloids

The most common plant alkaloids in use are the vinca alkaloids, natural products derived from the common periwinkle plant (*Vinca rosea*), although the epipodophyllotoxins and, recently, *paclitaxel* are used frequently in gynecologic malignancies (23). Like most natural products, these compounds are large and complex molecules, but *vincristine* and *vinblastine* differ only by a single methyl group on one side chain.

Vincristine and *vinblastine* act primarily by binding to vital intracellular microtubular proteins, particularly tubulin. Tubulin binding produces inhibition of microtubule assembly and destruction of the mitotic spindle, causing cells to be arrested in mitosis. Generally, this class of antineoplastic agent is believed to be *cell cycle specific*. At high concentrations, these drugs also have effects on nucleic acid and protein synthesis.

Paclitaxel has a unique mechanism of action; it binds preferentially to microtubules and results in their polymerization and stabilization. *Paclitaxel*-treated cells contain large numbers of microtubules, free and in bundles, that disrupt microtubule function and, ultimately, cause cell death. Renal clearance is minimal (5%).

Vinblastine is used primarily in the treatment of breast cancer and ovarian germ cell tumors. Its primary toxicity is myelosuppression. In contrast, *vincristine* causes little myelosuppression. Its primary dose-limiting toxicity is peripheral neuropathy. *Vincristine* is used primarily in cervical carcinoma and genital tract sarcomas.

A new family of plant alkaloids known as the *epipodophyllotoxins* has been shown to have significant antitumor properties. Members of this family are extracts from the mandrake plant. Although the primary plant extracts had tubulin-binding properties similar to those of the vinca alkaloids, active derivatives such as *etoposide (VP-16)* do not seem to function either by inhibiting mitotic spindle formation or by tubulin binding. They appear to function by causing single-stranded DNA breaks. Unlike many of the other compounds that act primarily by DNA, these agents appear to be *cell cycle specific* and *schedule dependent*. The drugs are poorly water soluble and thus are administered intravenously. The dose-limiting toxicity is myelosuppression. Other toxicities include an infusion rate-limited hypotension, nausea, vomiting, anorexia, and alopecia.

Paclitaxel (Taxol) is an extract from the bark of the Pacific yew tree. Its chemical formula is complex, and it has not yet been synthesized. Toxic effects of *paclitaxel* include bone marrow suppression, alopecia, myalgias, arthralgias, and hypersensitivity reactions. The most common dose-limiting toxic effect is granulocytopenia.

Taxotere is the first semisynthetic taxoid compound that is an analog of *paclitaxel*. Its molecular structure differs only slightly from *paclitaxel,* although it is somewhat more water soluble. *Taxotere* has been approved for clinical use and appears to be active in ovarian cancer. Comparative trials are being conducted and toxicities are comparable.

Other Agents

Another group of drugs used for chemotherapy does not fall into any particular class. They have unique or poorly understood mechanisms. The only agent commonly used in gynecologic malignancies is *hexamethylmelamine (Hexalen)*.

New Drug Trials

A number of chemotherapeutic agents have been studied experimentally but are not commercially available. Many of these agents have demonstrated activity against human tumors, but sufficient evidence to allow human experimentation has not yet been acquired. In addition, many investigational agents are currently being studied in phase I and phase II trials.

Phase I Trials   These studies define the spectrum of toxicity of a new chemotherapeutic agent and are complete when the dose-limiting toxicity of any particular dose and schedule has been defined.

Phase II Trials   These studies generally use the dose established from phase I trials and apply this dose and schedule to selected tumor types of importance.

Phase III Trials   These studies compare one effective treatment with another in a randomized fashion.

Radiation Therapy

Radiation therapy plays a major role in the management of gynecologic malignancies. Its specific curative role has been established for cervical cancer (24, 25); when surgery is not possible, radiation therapy also may be curative for localized endometrial cancer (26). For selected patients with ovarian cancer, postoperative adjuvant radiation therapy may be curative (27, 28). It improves pelvic control when used as adjuvant therapy after surgery for high-risk endometrial cancer (29) and has an expanding role in the management of carcinomas of the vagina and vulva (30, 31).

Our understanding of the principles of radiation biology has improved. Although the clinical practice of radiation therapy has evolved empirically, new concepts of radiobiology, particularly the significance of radiation *dose fractionation schedules* (32) and the use of *combined modality therapy* (33), have allowed a better understanding of the usefulness of radiation therapy for the treatment of gynecologic cancer. The basic principles of radiation therapy, including physics and radiobiology, and the specific use of radiation therapy in gynecologic malignancies are presented.

Radiobiology

Ionizing Radiation

Cell death in the context of radiation biology is defined as the loss of clonogenic capacity (i.e., the ability of the cell to undergo continued reproduction). Ionizing radiation in sufficient dosage will produce cell death, which is the basis for its use in treating malignancies. The critical target for radiation injury for most cell types is DNA. Thus, the damage caused by ionizing radiation is expressed when cells attempt to undergo mitosis. Ionizing radiation produces free radical formation, which disrupts the reproductive integrity of DNA and produces mitotic death. After DNA damage, the cell may undergo a limited number of mitoses, but cellular death ultimately ensues because the cell can no longer reproduce indefinitely. Although the cell may appear normal morphologically, it may have lost its reproductive capacity. Disruption of plasma membranes is another form of cell damage that may result from ionizing radiation, and it is not linked to cell division.

The effect of ionizing radiation of any type is not selective for neoplastic cells, and this interaction with matter occurs in both the normal and neoplastic tissues in the path of the radiation beam. Interaction with the normal tissues and cells is responsible for both the acute and chronic complications associated with radiation therapy.

Rad and Gray

The rad is the unit commonly used to measure the amount of energy absorbed per unit mass of tissue. **The new standard nomenclature for measuring absorbed dose is the Gray (1 joule/kg); 1 Gray = 100 rad. Current practice uses the term *centigray (cGy)*, because 1 cGy = 1 rad.**

Fractionation

Conventional radiation therapy usually is given in a fractionated course using daily doses of 180–200 cGy per fraction. The resultant survival curve after fractionated radiation therapy has a smaller gradient than that seen after a single dose of therapy (Fig. 30.1). Comparison of these curves reveals that a single dose of radiation (e.g., 600 cGy) will result in

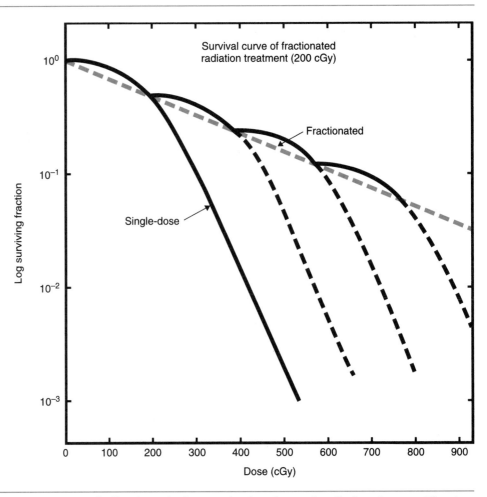

Figure 30.1   Idealized survival curve for fractionated radiation therapy. The time interval between fractions is sufficient to allow repair of sublethal damage, and the shoulder is repeated with each fraction. The resultant slope of the survival curve with *fractionated* radiation is more shallow than that of the *single dose*. Reduction of the surviving fraction *to* 10^{-1} requires 350 cGy in a single fraction or 600 cGy in three fractions. (Reproduced from **Berek JS, Hacker NF.** *Practical Gynecologic Oncology.* 2nd ed. Baltimore: Williams & Wilkins, 1994:38.)

fewer surviving cells than the same total dose given in several smaller fractions (e.g., three fractions of 200 cGy each). This "sparing" effect results from repetition of the shoulder region of the curve with each fraction of radiation. The shoulder region has been interpreted to represent the presence of *repair of sublethal damage* in an irradiated cell population (34, 35).

Radiosensitivity

Many factors can modify the biologic effect of ionizing radiation on the cellular radiosensitivity. Therefore, the amount of cell kill produced by a given dose of radiation may vary, depending on the following factors:

1. The "four Rs of radiobiology," which are (*a*) repair, (*b*) reoxygenation, (*c*) repopulation, and (*d*) redistribution

2. The quality of radiation

3. The temperature of the tissues

4. The presence of various drugs.

Different doses of radiation can achieve the same biologic effect on tumor by adjusting fractionation schedules. A typical "isoeffect" curve (34) is shown in Figure 30.2. For example, 90% of squamous cell cancers of the skin measuring 2 cm or less in diameter will be controlled with 2800 cGy in one fraction or 4100 cGy in 10 fractions. The magnitude of the dose required to produce a given level of biologic damage depends on the manner in which the radiation is fractionated. The explanation for this isoeffect phenomenon is related to cellular repair (35), cellular repopulation (36), redistribution of cells in the cell cycle (37), and reoxygenation (38).

Oxygen Enhancement Ratio   The dose of radiation required under hypoxic conditions is approximately three times greater than the dose required under fully oxygenated conditions. The ratio of these doses is referred to as the oxygen enhancement ratio (OER). Most of the changes in radiosensitivity occur as the oxygen concentration increases from 0–30 mm Hg, well below the PO_2 of venous blood. Nevertheless, clinically significant hypoxia does exist in human solid tumors, and the hypoxic cells are relatively radioresistant when compared with fully oxygenated ones. During a fractionated course of radiation therapy, relatively hypoxic cells may become more oxygenated and, therefore, more sensitive to the effects of ionizing radiation; thus, fractionation may allow reoxygenation and, therefore,

Figure 30.2   Isoeffect curves relating the total radiation dose to the overall treatment time for normal tissue end points (erythema, desquamation, necrosis) and 90% cure of skin cancer. (Redrawn from **Strandquvist M.** *Acta Radiol* 1994;55(Suppl):1; reproduced from **Berek JS, Hacker WF.** *Practical Gynecologic Oncology.* 2nd ed. Baltimore: Williams & Wilkins, 1994:39.)

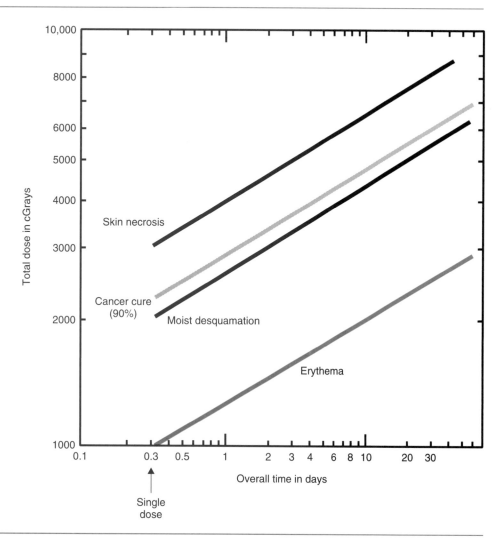

effects of ionizing radiation; thus, fractionation may allow reoxygenation and, therefore, increased tumor destruction (38).

Treatment Strategies   Because of the importance of the oxygen effect, many treatment strategies have been used to try to overcome the relative radioresistance of hypoxic cells in solid human tumors (39–42). These strategies include the use of modifications of fractionation schedules, carbogen breathing during radiation therapy, selective vasoconstriction of normal tissues by tourniquet application, various pharmacologic agents (e.g., *misonidasole*) that can act as hypoxic cell radiation sensitizers, hyperbaric oxygen, and high linear energy transfer radiation. Tumor hypoxia continues to be a probable cause of the failure of radiation to control some tumors (e.g., advanced cervical cancers with a significant population of hypoxic tumor cells) (43, 44).

Radiation Effects and Drugs

Some drugs can modify the response to radiation. This may result from the independent cytotoxicity of the two modalities or from the direct interaction between the drug and the radiation (45). Four terms are used to describe the types of possible interactions.

Independent Action   Drugs and radiation may act independently when their mechanisms of action are different. As a result, the total effect of the combination is equal to that of each agent separately.

Additivity   Agents may act at the same site in the cell. Therefore, sublethal damage inflicted by each agent interacts to cause greater cell kill than that which occurs with either agent alone.

Synergism (Superadditivity)   The interaction between two agents can result in greater cell kill than that seen with additivity. An example is the interaction of actinomycin-D and radiation.

Antagonism (Subadditivity)   The cell kill that results from the use of the two agents is less than that expected by independent action. Clinically, it is difficult to determine which mode of interaction occurs when two agents are used. When an increased reaction is observed, the term *synergism* often is used, but the mechanism of interaction may be simply independent action or additivity.

The addition of a cytotoxic drug to radiation may be useful if the dose-limiting tissue toxicity of the drug is different from that of radiation therapy (i.e., it may provide an improvement in the therapeutic index). The addition of the two agents can separate the dose-response curves for cure and toxicity. The drug may be independently cytotoxic or act additively to increase tumor cell kill without increasing the toxicity to normal tissues that would require reduction in the radiation dose. Clinical trials are being conducted with a combination of radiation and cytotoxic drugs (e.g., *5-FU* and *cisplatin*) in advanced carcinomas of the cervix and vulva (33).

Therapeutic Ratio

All cells in the path of radiation, including those of the normal tissues, suffer radiation injury. If the dose of radiation given is plotted against the likelihood of cure for a given tumor, a sigmoid curve is generated (Fig. 30.3).

Figure 30.3   Theoretical sigmoid dose-response curves for tumor control and severe complications. The farther apart the two curves, the higher the therapeutic ratio. *Top,* Dose A produces cure in 80% with 5% complications. *Dose B* falls on the steep part of the complication curve and produces a much higher rise in the complication rate than in the cure rate. *Bottom,* This shows a shift to the left in the dose-cure curve (e.g., by the addition of sensitizing drugs). *Dose A* produces 95% cure with 5% complications. (Reproduced from **Berek JS, Hacker WF.** *Practical Gynecologic Oncology.* 2nd ed. Baltimore: Williams & Wilkins, 1994:44.)

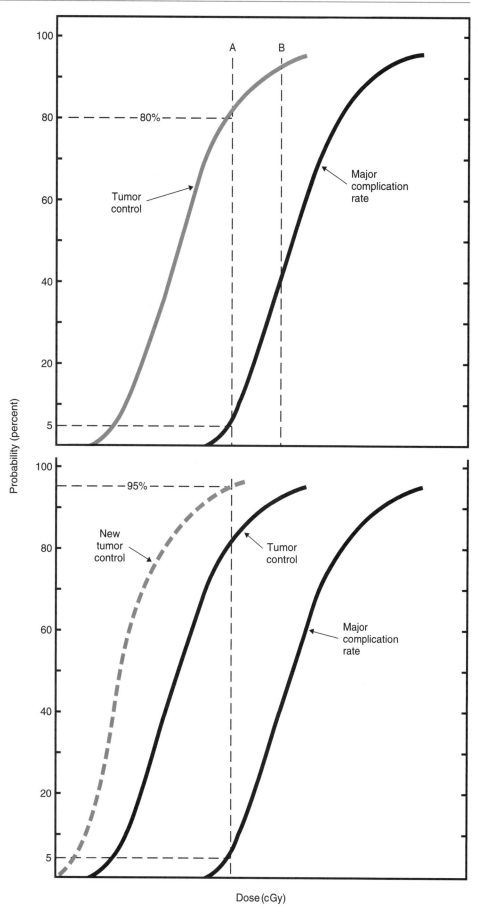

At low radiation doses, there is insufficient cell kill to produce tumor cure. As the dose is increased, the likelihood of cure rises rapidly and plateaus. The shape and steepness of the dose-response curve vary for different tumors (46, 47). A similar sigmoid relationship is seen when the likelihood of complications is plotted against the dose of radiation. A simultaneous plot of the dose-control curve for tumor and the dose-complication curve for the normal tissues allows an examination of the therapeutic ratio. This term indicates that for a given dose of radiation there is an expected rate of tumor control and an expected complication rate. In the optimistic situation, the complication curve is placed to the right of the cure curve, and the difference between these curves is a measure of the therapeutic gain of a given dose of radiation. Research efforts are directed to improving the therapeutic ratio by separating these curves.

The extent of radiation damage to normal tissues depends on the rate of division of the irradiated cells (48). Tissues that are turning over rapidly (i.e., whose functional activity requires constant cell renewal) manifest acute radiation injury soon after exposure. Examples of *acutely reacting* tissues include most epithelia (e.g., the skin, the gastrointestinal mucosa, bone marrow, and reproductive tissues). In contrast, tissues in which the cells are characterized by low cellular turnover rates and functional activity does not require rapid cell renewal do not manifest any early radiation injury. Examples of *late-reacting* tissues are the connective tissues, muscle, and neural tissues.

Acute Reactions

With pelvic irradiation, acute reactions, such as diarrhea, are usually associated with denudation of the intestinal mucosa, which in turn causes an increased regenerative response (49). The regenerative response usually can keep pace with weekly doses of 900–1000 cGy in five fractions. This empirically derived weekly dose continues to be in common use because it minimizes acute complications. If an increased dose is given over shorter periods, the regenerative capacity of the epithelium may be overwhelmed (50), and the acute reaction may be so severe that it may be necessary to introduce a *split-treatment course* to enable the epithelial regeneration to catch up before therapy is resumed. The severity of the acute reactions also depends on the *volume* of the normal tissues irradiated and the specific *nature* of the tissues.

Late Reactions

The sensitivity of late-reacting tissues is markedly dependent on the size of the dose per fraction of radiation used. **The larger the dose per fraction used, the greater the risk of late complications.** Therefore, if a few fractions of large size are used rather than a greater number of smaller fractions, there is an increased risk of overdosage for the late-reacting tissues if the doses are adjusted to equalize the acute reactions (32, 48, 49, 51, 52).

If the overall treatment time is constant and the dose per fraction is increased, there will be a relatively greater effect on the late-reacting tissues than on the acutely reacting tissues. If the overall time of treatment is varied while the number of fractions is held constant, the effect is different. If treatment time is extended, the acute reactions may be spared preferentially because of the regenerative capacity of the acutely reacting tissues. Therefore, a total dose of radiation that produces an equal effect on acutely reacting tissues may lead to excessive late effects. Thus, radiation schemes that produce similar acute reactions but use larger-than-normal doses per fraction or protracted treatment times may produce excessive late normal-tissue reactions.

Fractionation Schedules

Two possible nonconventional fractionation schedules—hyperfractionation and accelerated fractionation—offer theoretic improvements in the therapeutic ratio for tumor control versus late normal injury (39, 53).

Hyperfractionation   The term *hyperfractionation* refers to an altered fractionation scheme in which (54) the size of the dose per fraction is reduced, the number of dosage fractions is increased, the total dose is increased, and the overall time is relatively unchanged.

With hyperfractionation, treatment usually is given two or more times daily with at least 4–6 hours between fractions to allow repair. The rationale behind anticipating an improvement in the therapeutic ratio with hyperfractionation is that an increase in the total dose may be given without exceeding the tolerance of the late-reacting normal tissues. The increased dose can be given because a smaller dose per fraction is used, which allows preferential sparing of the late-reacting normal tissues.

Accelerated Fractionation   In an accelerated fractionation scheme, the overall time of treatment is shortened, whereas the number of dose fractions is unchanged (39). Treatment is given two or more times daily, using fraction sizes that are unchanged or only slightly reduced and a total dose that is unchanged or slightly reduced. The result of accelerated fractionation is the delivery of the same dose of radiation in a shorter overall time. The theoretic benefits of an accelerated fractionation scheme are that a decrease in the overall time reduces the chance of tumor cell repopulation during treatment, which may increase the likelihood of tumor control for a given total dose.

Combination of Surgery and Radiation

There are theoretic reasons why the combination of surgery and radiation therapy may provide better tumor control. The two modalities may be complementary in some situations, because the mechanisms of failure for the two techniques are different. Surgery may remove gross tumor masses, but the extent of surgical dissection may be limited. Even when all gross tumor is resected, tumor regrowth may occur because of residual microscopic tumor in the periphery of the lesion. Radiation therapy, on the other hand, is more likely to control microscopic disease at the periphery of tumors, where the cell numbers are small and the vascularity is good (25). When radiation fails, it is often because of the inability to control bulky central tumor masses in which the number of clonogenic cells and the probability of hypoxia are high. The choice of sequence of radiation and surgery depends on the specific tumor and the clinical situation. The potential advantages and disadvantages of preoperative and postoperative irradiation are presented in Table 30.7.

When surgery and radiation are combined, the initial plan of treatment must exploit the complementary features of the two modalities. Following are some examples of the usefulness of combined surgery and radiation in gynecologic malignancies:

Table 30.7   Preoperative and Postoperative Radiation

Advantages	*Disadvantages*
Preoperative	
1. Surgically undisturbed tumor bed: intact vascularity (good oxygenation)	1. Precludes accurate pretreatment staging
2. May facilitate surgical dissection, allowing a lesser procedure	2. May be given unnecessarily to patients with limited disease with high likelihood of cure with surgery alone
3. May decrease the risk of implantation or dissemination of viable tumor cells by surgery, e.g., tumor marginally resectable or cut-through	3. Delays wound healing
Postoperative	
1. Extent of locoregional disease accurately defined	1. Surgery may change tumor proliferation kinetics
2. Radiation therapy may be used more selectively or omitted in some patients	2. Surgery may disturb vascularity and increase risk of hypoxia

1. *Vulvar Cancer*—The addition of postoperative pelvic and groin irradiation provides a survival advantage to patients with multiple positive inguinal nodes over that achieved with pelvic node dissection (30).

2. *Endometrial Cancer*—Postoperative pelvic irradiation reduces the incidence of pelvic recurrence in patients with high-risk stage I disease, presumably by sterilizing microscopic residual tumor cells in the pelvis and pelvic lymph nodes (29, 55).

3. *Cervical Cancer*—In patients with "bulky" or "barrel-shaped" stage Ib disease, hysterectomy may be required to remove residual central disease that has not been eradicated by radiation therapy (25).

Radiation Techniques

Radiation therapy is delivered in three ways:

1. *Teletherapy* (i.e., external beam)

2. *Brachytherapy*, in which the radiation device is placed either within or close to the target volume (i.e., interstitial and intracavitary irradiation)

3. *Intracavitary radioisotopes*

Teletherapy

Many factors influence the deposition of external radiation into deep tissues (56). The beam energy is defined by its voltage; the higher the beam energy, the more deeply it penetrates into tissues. In modern radiation therapy, external beam treatment is largely given with megavoltage or supervoltage equipment.

Photons **A photon is a quantum of high-energy electromagnetic radiation that travels at the speed of light, and its interaction with tissues causes ionization. Photons may be x-rays or gamma rays: x-rays are produced by bombardment of an anode by a high-speed electron beam; gamma rays result from the decay of radioactive isotopes.** The average energy of the photons produced by the decay of radioactive cobalt is 1.2 million electron volts (MeV). Higher-energy x-ray beams in the 2–35 MeV range are produced mainly from linear accelerators. High-energy electron beams also can be generated from linear accelerators. Comparative isodose distributions for typical beams of varying energies are presented in Figure 30.4.

Under ideal conditions, external radiation therapy maximizes the dose of radiation delivered to the target while minimizing the dose delivered outside the target. It will also pro-

Figure 30.4 *Top,* **Depth-dose curves for x-ray and *y*-ray beams of increasing energy.** As the energy increases, the depth of maximum dose (100%) increases; thus, for 100 keV and 250 keV, it is at the skin surface. With ^{60}Co and 25 MeV, it moves below the surface, minimizing the skin reactions; as the energy increases, the beam penetrates more deeply. At a depth of 10 cm from the surface, the depth dose is approximately 25% for 250 kV, 60% for ^{60}Co, and 80% for 25 MeV. Thus, deep pelvic tumors are treated more approximately with higher-energy beams. *Bottom,* **Depth-dose curves for various electron energies.** The depth of maximum dose increases with increasing energy. At depths just beyond the maximum, the dose falls off rapidly and therefore may spare deeper underlying tissues. An approximate way to choose optimal electron energy is to determine the depth of the tumor from the surface and use an electron energy of three times the depth (e.g., with a tumor at 2 cm, choose electron energy of 6 to 7 MeV). (Reproduced from **Berek JS, Hacker WF.** *Practical Gynecologic Oncology.* 2nd ed. Baltimore: Williams & Wilkins, 1994:50.)

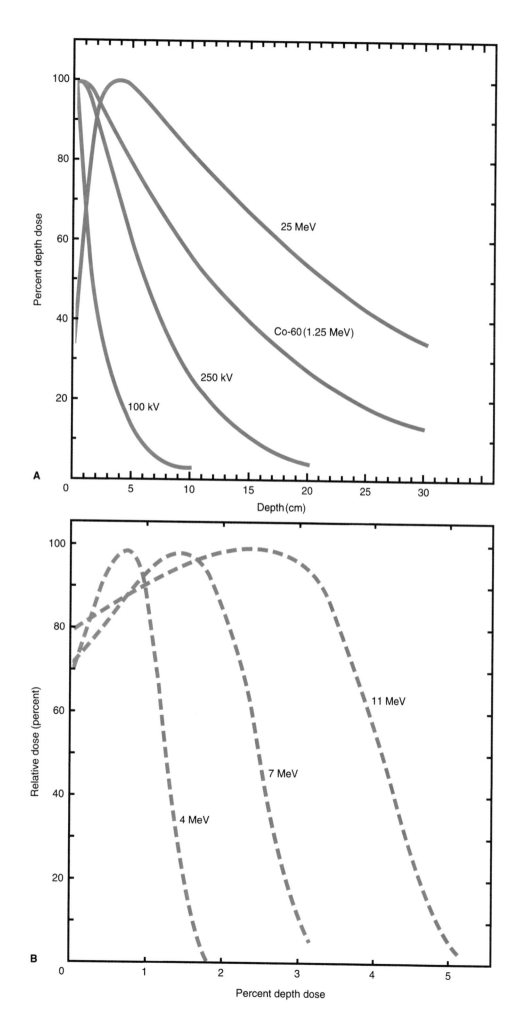

duce a relatively homogeneous dose within the volume of interest. This is important because wide variation of dose within the volume (>5–10%) can result in either low-dose areas that could lead to tumor recurrence or high-dose areas that increase the risk of complications. For irradiation of tumor volumes in this homogeneous fashion, multiple external fields are usually required. The use of multiple beams may tend to decrease the dose to the normal tissues in transit toward the tumor. The isodose distributions for two opposing parallel portals and a four-field technique used for the treatment of cervical cancer are presented in Figure 30.5.

Figure 30.5   Isodose distribution for external radiation using 25 MeV. *A,* Parallel pair (anterior-posterior) fields; *B,* box field arrangement superimposed on a computed tomography scan showing a large cervical cancer. The parallel pair essentially treats the bladder and rectum to full tumor dose. The positioning and size of the lateral beams in the box technique determine where the high-dose volume is located. In this arrangement, the dose to the rectum (*dark shadow*) is significantly reduced. The isodose distribution may be tailored to almost any desired by varying the beam angles, numbers, energies, and arrangements. (Reproduced from **Berek JS, Hacker WF.** *Practical Gynecologic Oncology.* 2nd ed. Baltimore: Williams & Wilkins, 1994:52.)

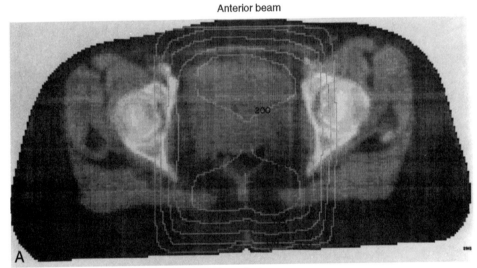

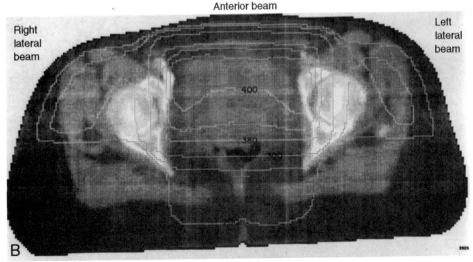

The radiation beam may be modified to conform better to a specific tumor while protecting normal tissues by shielding or blocking part of the beam. Specific anatomic volumes may be treated with surrounding vital structures protected by means of individually fashioned blocks that are made to conform to the patient's tumor (56).

Electrons   Electron beams also can be used for external radiation therapy. These beams usually are generated from betatrons or high-energy accelerators, and the depth dose characteristics differ substantially from those of photon or x-ray beams. Electron beams may be much less skin sparing. The maximum dose is reached at a depth that depends on the energy of the beam, after which there is a rapid falloff.

Electron beams are most useful in the treatment of superficially placed tumors in which it is desirable to spare the deeper tissues (e.g., irradiation of the inguinal nodes in vulvar cancer). The choice of beam energy is tailored to the estimated depth of the nodes. This technique allows considerably more sparing of the underlying femoral heads than other techniques while permitting an adequate dose of radiation to be delivered to a superficially placed tumor.

Brachytherapy

Intracavitary

The intrauterine and intravaginal *intracavitary* devices used in the treatment of cervical and endometrial cancer are examples of brachytherapy used for gynecologic malignancies. These devices vary in their appearance and configuration, but their general construction is similar despite the great number and variety of applicators used. These devices usually consist of a hollow stem, such as the classic intrauterine tandem, which often carries the name of the designer of the applicator (e.g., Fletcher-Delclos and Fletcher-Suit) (25) (Fig. 30.6).

These intrauterine tandems may be placed within the uterine cavity, and the hollow center may be afterloaded with radioactive material such as radium or cesium. Similarly, various afterloading applicators (e.g., vaginal ovoids or colpostats) have been designed for placement in the vaginal vault. Other applicators that hold line sources of radioactivity may be used to treat varying lengths of the vagina.

To minimize the exposure of personnel to radiation, most applicators currently used are *afterloaded* with radioactive sources once they have been shown by x-ray to be satisfactorily

Figure 30.6   Itrauterine stem and vaginal colpostats used for intracavity irradiation in cervical cancer. Reproduced from **Berek JS, Hacker WF.** *Practical Gynecologic Oncology,* 2nd ed. Baltimore: Williams & Wilkins, 1994:53.

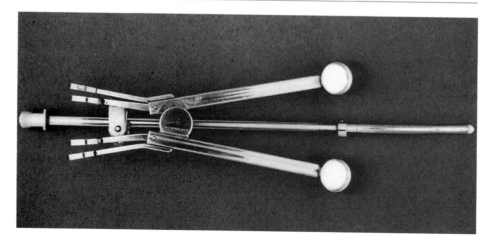

positioned. The more recent use of *remote afterloading devices* (e.g., the Selectron) can further protect personnel from radiation exposure. With these remote afterloading devices, radioactive sources are stored in a lead-lined safe in the patient's room and connected to the intrauterine or intravaginal devices by hollow tubes. The sources then may be remotely afterloaded after the personnel caring for the patient have left the room. Although these devices do offer further protection of personnel, the intermittent automatic removal of sources may prolong the intracavitary radiation treatment time.

Inverse Square Law

The inverse square law states that the dose of radiation at a given point is inversely proportional to the square of the distance from the source of radiation (56). Therefore, with brachytherapy, the dose at a distance from the source is determined largely by the inverse square law.

A typical isodose distribution around a line source and colpostats loaded with radioactive *cesium-137* used for the treatment of cervical cancer are shown in Figure 30.7. The dose decreases rapidly as the distance from the applicator increases. Because of this rapid change of dose over short distances, accurate positioning of intracavitary sources is very important. The advantage of intracavitary therapy is that a very high dose of radiation can be achieved in a very small volume. Thus, in the treatment of cervical cancer, high doses of radiation can be delivered centrally within the tumor and also within the adjacent paracervical tissues. However, the rapid falloff of dose means that many of the sensitive normal tissues within the pelvis, particularly the rectum and bladder, may be spared an excessive radiation dose.

Interstitial Implants

Interstitial sources are another form of brachytherapy. The term *interstitial* implies the placement of radioactive sources within tissues. Various sources of radiation, such as *iridium-192, iodine-125,* and *tantalum-182,* may be available as radioactive wires or seeds. Hollow guide needles are placed in a specified geometric pattern that will deliver a known, relatively uniform dose of radiation to a target volume. The position of these guides is checked radiologically and, when satisfactory, they can be threaded with the radioactive sources that are left in the tissues; the hollow guides then are removed.

The interstitial therapy used in gynecologic malignancies usually involves a temporary implant. The implant will be left in the tissues for a period determined by the strength of the sources and the radiation dose required. Interstitial therapy has the advantage of delivering a relatively high dose of radiation to a relatively small volume (the tumor) and therefore offers a theoretic advantage over external beam therapy. The disadvantage is the greater potential damage to normal tissues in or near the tumor, especially if it is difficult to accurately place the needles. This damage may cause an increased incidence of severe late complications. Interstitial implants in the parametrial areas have been used with some success in the treatment of advanced or recurrent carcinoma of the cervix (57) (Fig. 30.8).

The use of interstitial implants is increasing, particularly for patients with advanced pelvic malignancy. Clinical experience and refinements in templates for transperineal applications have contributed to an apparent decrease in serious morbidity (58). The radiation oncology community remains polarized regarding the appropriateness of interstitial therapy, and as yet no randomized trials have been conducted to compare the therapeutic ratio of conventional intracavitary irradiation with interstitial parametrial treatment.

Recurrence after conventional radical therapy cannot be retreated with external beam radiation because of the limited tolerance of the surrounding normal tissues. Limited parametrial implants have controlled tumors in some patients and resulted in occasional cures of recurrent disease (25), but vesicovaginal and rectovaginal fistula rates may be excessive.

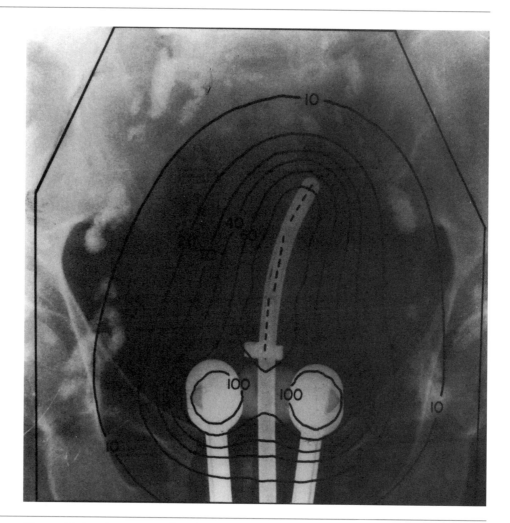

Figure 30.7   Treatment plan for cervical carcinoma showing a radiograph of the intracavitary irradiation *in situ* with its isodose distribution in cGy per hour. The stem is loaded with ^{137}Cs sources of radium equivalent strengths of 15 mg, 10 mg, and 10 mg from proximal to distal. Each of the colpostats contains 5 mg radium equivalent sources. The dose to point A is 50 cGy per hour. The duration of the application is determined by the dose required. The usual external beam edges are superimposed on the x-ray and include the pelvic nodes as visualized on lymphography. (Reproduced from **Berek JS, Hacker WF.** *Practical Gynecologic Oncology.* 2nd ed. Baltimore: Williams & Wilkins, 1994:54.)

Interstitial implants also may be used to treat selected vaginal or vulvar malignancies, either primarily or secondarily. Interstitial radiation may be used in combination with external beam radiation to achieve a high-tumor dose while sparing the surrounding normal tissues from unnecessary irradiation.

Intracavitary Radioisotopes

Radioisotopes have been used to treat epithelial ovarian cancer because of the pattern of dissemination throughout the peritoneal cavity (59). Theoretically, if the tumor remains confined to this body cavity, the even distribution of a radioisotope in the peritoneum could irradiate all structures within the cavity. The pattern of energy deposition and the depth of penetration from the surface that the isotope contacts depend on many factors, including the physical characteristics of the particular isotope used, the energies of the decay products, and the distribution of the isotope within the peritoneal cavity.

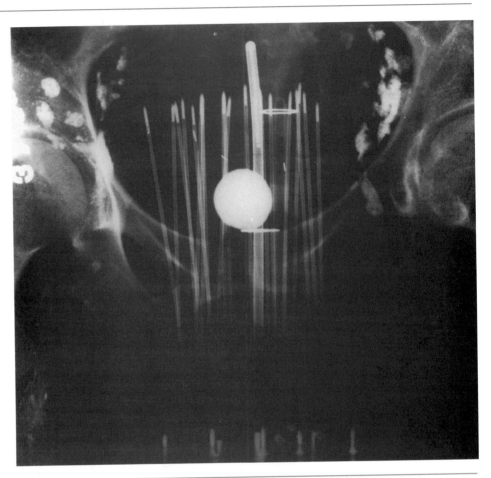

Figure 30.8 Interstitial implant for an advanced cervical cancer. (Reproduced with permission from Dr. Mark Schray, Division of Radiation Oncology, Mayo Clinic, Rochester, MN.)

Radioactive *chromic phosphate* (^{32}P) has largely replaced *colloidal gold* (^{198}Au) for intracavitary irradiation. Its longer half-life (14.3 days) and its pure β decay with a mean energy of 0.698 MeV allow deeper penetration into tissues (8 mm compared with 3.8 mm for ^{198}Au), a slightly longer exposure, and fewer radiation protection problems. After instillation, most of the isotope is adsorbed onto the peritoneal surface, but some is phagocytosed by macrophages and taken up by lymphatics (60).

Although theoretically sound, studies reveal that, in practice, the isotope seldom is delivered uniformly to the peritoneal and omental surfaces (60). Postsurgical adhesions may limit the free flow of colloid, and this nonuniform distribution may result in significant underdosage of some tumor sites and significant overdosage of some normal tissues, resulting in unacceptable complications. **The curative potential of radiocolloid in the treatment of ovarian cancer has not been established.**

The most commonly employed radioisotopes in gynecologic oncology and their half-lives are presented in Table 30.8.

Clinical Uses

Cervical Cancer

Radiation therapy for the treatment of cervical cancer usually combines both external pelvic irradiation and brachytherapy (25). Because of the wide variation in radiation tech-

Table 30.8   Isotopes

Isotope		Half-Life	γ-Ray Energy (MeV)	β-Ray Average Energy at 1 cm	γ-Factor* R/mc/hr
Phosphorus	^{32}P	14.3 days		0.698	
Technesium	^{99}Tc	6.0 hours	0.14	0.014	0.56
Iodine	^{131}I	8.07 days	Many 0.08–0.72	0.188	2.24
Cesium	^{137}Cs	30 years	0.662	0.242	3.2
Iridium	^{192}Ir	74 days	Several 0.32–0.61		5.0
Gold	^{198}Au	2.7 days	Several 0.41–1.1	0.328	2.43
Radium	^{226}Ra	1620 years	Several 0.19–0.6		8.25

*γ(gamma) factor: Dose rate from a γ-emitting isotope expressed as the exposure rate in roentgens per hour at 1 cm from a point source of 1 mc.

niques, it is sometimes difficult to understand the basic principles on which the radiation treatment is formulated.

Radiation therapy, like surgery, is local therapy and, therefore, influences cancer only within the applied radiation volume. Thus, radiation will not be curative for those with disease outside the volume treated, although it may provide worthwhile control of disease that would otherwise cause pelvic symptoms. Curative doses of radiation therapy may be applied to treat the pelvic tissues and also to treat involved para-aortic nodes.

The principle of radiation therapy for cervical cancer is the delivery of curative doses of radiation to the primary tumor and its local extensions, as well as to the regional lymph nodes (i.e., the obturator nodes and the internal, external, and common iliac nodes). The tolerance of the normal tissues within the pelvis limits the dose that can be applied to the described volume. The dose-limiting normal tissues in the pelvis are the rectum posteriorly, the bladder anteriorly, and any loops of small bowel within the pelvic radiation fields. Because the bulk of tumor usually lies centrally within the pelvis, higher central tumor doses can be achieved by the judicious application of brachytherapy.

Treatment Dosage

The doses of radiation prescribed usually are tailored to the volume of cancer present in the primary tumor and regional nodes (25). Local control of microscopic or occult tumor deposits from epithelial cancers requires 4000–5000 cGy, whereas for a clinically obvious tumor, more than 6000 cGy is required (46, 47).

Reference Points   Two reference points in the pelvis are used to describe the dose prescription:

1. *Point A*—This point is 2 cm lateral and 2 cm superior to the external cervical os.

2. *Point B*—This point is 3 cm lateral to point A and corresponds to the pelvic sidewall.

Although the cGy doses from intracavitary and external radiation therapy may not be biologically equivalent, it is common practice to use the sum of these doses to express the dose prescription for points A and B.

1. The summated dose to point A believed to be adequate for central control is usually between 7500 and 8500 cGy.

2. The prescribed dose to point B is 4500–6500 cGy, depending on the bulk of parametrial and sidewall disease.

Milligram-Hours   Some centers continue to express the dose of radiation by intracavitary application in "milligram-hours." This term does not express the radiation prescription well: it refers to the number of milligrams of radium or radium equivalent present and the duration over which the insertion is left *in situ.* For purposes of communication between various centers, the term "milligram-hours" to express radiation dose is transferable only if the geometry and volume of the intracavitary system used are identical. The dose that any given system of radiation delivers to various points in the pelvis should be expressed in terms of the Gray (cGy) and can be derived from the appropriate isodose distributions related to the specific intracavitary or interstitial techniques used.

Treatment Volume   **The term** *treatment volume* **describes the volume receiving the prescribed tumor dose ± 5%.** It is not coincident with the marked borders of the field on check films. The treatment volume is usually smaller than those borders, and the degree of constriction of the high-dose volume is related to the number of beams used, the energy of the beams, and various other technical factors. The treatment volume is designed to encompass the primary tumor in the pelvis and its possible adjacent extensions, in addition to the appropriate first- and sec;ond-echelon draining lymph nodes. The pelvis is usually treated to within acceptable tolerance of the normal tissues.

The borders of the treatment field used to achieve the appropriate treatment volumes are as follows:

1. *Inferior Border*—This usually lies at the inferior aspect of the obturator foramina and thus encompasses the obturator nodes. If vaginal extension has occurred, the border is moved inferiorly to 2 cm below the visible and palpable tumor. Usually, no attempt is made to encompass the entire vaginal tube unless disease extends into the lower one-third of the vagina.

2. *Superior Border*—This is usually between L4 and L5 or in the midvertebral level of L5. The only reason to treat up to this level is to provide some dose to the common iliac nodes, although it is unclear whether there is additional therapeutic benefit in taking the fields up to this level as opposed to the L5/S1 junction.

3. *Lateral Borders*—These are 1 cm lateral to the pelvic lymph nodes as visualized on lymphography or at least 1 cm lateral to the margins of the bony pelvis. Appropriate shielding along the common iliac nodes decreases the volume of normal tissue irradiated.

The incidence of late complications depends on the specific tolerance of the normal tissues irradiated, the dose that they receive, and the volume of radiation (62). Every effort should be made to minimize the high-dose treatment volume while adequately encompassing the tumor and its regional lymph nodes. The volume is significantly less using a *box technique* rather than an anterior and posterior parallel opposed pair of beams (Fig. 30.5). If there is no tumor extension along the uterosacral ligaments, a box technique may spare some of the rectum and sigmoid colon posteriorly. Even when there is posterior tumor extension and the rectum cannot be spared, a box technique may allow significant sparing of anteriorly placed small bowel if an anterior/superior corner shield is used to exclude structures in front of the external iliac lymph nodes.

In general, particularly for bulky lesions, external radiation therapy is given first to decrease the size of the primary tumor. One or two applications of intracavitary irradiation are performed after external radiation therapy to achieve the desired radiation dose levels.

The amount of radiation delivered by each technique is determined by the extent of the tumor (25). Where disease is mainly central (e.g., in the cervix only or in the medial parametria), a higher proportion of the total dose will be prescribed for the intracavitary radiation; less external radiation will be used, because the lateral disease will be microscopic. Where bulky lateral parametrial or sidewall disease is present, a greater proportion of the dose will be delivered with the external beam.

Complications   Late complications of radical irradiation for cervical cancer occur in 5–15% of patients and are related to the size of the daily dose per fraction, the total dose administered, and the volume irradiated (63). The positioning of the intracavitary system also may influence complications. Late effects that may be seen in the bladder include hematuria, fibrosis and contraction, or fistulas. Similar effects may occur in the rectosigmoid or terminal ileum with bleeding, stricture, obstruction, or perforation. Although late effects may increase with time, 75% of the late complications develop within 30 months of radiation therapy (64).

Interstitial Implants   Interstitial therapy with iridium-192 is being used increasingly in the management of cervical cancer, despite the lack of controlled clinical trials. It has been used to provide a small volume boost in patients with bulky cervical stump carcinomas after external therapy. Both central and pelvic sidewall implants have been used in the management of recurrent pelvic cancer after radiation therapy (65, 66). This treatment is being used more frequently in a number of centers for patients with bulky primary cervical cancer, stages Ib to III (65). The Syed-Neblett template has been used as a guide for afterloading interstitial sources to deliver a relatively uniform dose to the implanted volume. The risk of complications is considerably higher than with conventional external and intracavitary therapy, particularly in the hands of inexperienced operators. However, recent reports claim high local control rates with acceptable morbidity (58).

Palliation   Because cervical cancer is generally a radioresponsive lesion, radiation therapy has an important role in the palliation of metastatic disease. Short courses of palliative radiation, such as 2000 cGy in five fractions or 3000 cGy in 10 fractions, usually will alleviate symptoms related to bony metastases or para-aortic nodal disease. It also may relieve symptoms related to pressure from enlarging mediastinal or supraclavicular nodal disease. In rare circumstances, disease recurrent in the pelvis after initial radiation therapy may be palliated with further external beam radiation. Such circumstances may include the patient who has a late recurrence years after primary radiation therapy or the patient in whom inadequate initial doses of radiation were used.

Endometrial Cancer

The role of radiation therapy in the treatment of endometrial carcinoma is discussed in Chapter 31, but its use may be summarized as follows:

1. As an adjunct to surgery to prevent pelvic recurrence after bilateral salpingo-oophorectomy and hysterectomy.

2. With curative intent in some patients whose preexisting medical problems preclude surgery.

3. With curative intent in patients with isolated vaginal or vaginal and pelvic recurrence. Therapy is directed to the whole pelvis and the entire vagina with the use of both external and intracavitary or interstitial radiation.

4. For palliative treatment of nonresectable intrapelvic or metastatic disease.

In the past, disease confined to the uterus often was treated with the routine application of preoperative irradiation with tumor doses of 40–60 Gy. An intracavitary line source was placed in the uterus, or the uterus was packed with multiple radioactive capsules (Heyman's capsules) in an attempt to distribute the dose more uniformly throughout the myometrium (67). If routine preoperative intracavitary irradiation was not used, routine postoperative vault irradiation was given. **The use of preoperative or postoperative irradiation decreases the overall incidence of recurrence at the vaginal vault, but no significant survival benefit has been demonstrated** (29, 67–69).

Approximately 75–80% of patients with stage I disease fall into a low-risk category in which the chance of recurrence is in the order of 5% after surgery alone. In this group, it is unlikely that adjuvant radiation therapy will provide measurable improvement in pelvic control or survival rates. **At present, the role of adjuvant pelvic radiation therapy appears to be in the reduction of pelvic recurrences in high-risk patients** (29, 55). Previously, this treatment included both whole pelvic irradiation to 4500–5000 cGy and vault colpostats to boost the dose to the vaginal cuff. The additional benefit of the vault boost has been questioned, but its usefulness has not been tested formally. Many have abandoned its routine use.

Ovarian Cancer

A therapeutic role for whole abdominal radiotherapy has been shown for some patients with epithelial ovarian cancer (70–74). Because most studies of radiotherapy use in ovarian cancer include patients with no macroscopic residual disease after primary surgery, reports do not indicate in how many patients disease was controlled by the radiotherapy; some may have been cured by surgery alone. Approximately 40–50% of patients with minimal residual lesions have long-term survival; most of these patients are those with stage II disease in whom the residual tumor was confined to the pelvis, where a higher radiation dose can be delivered. With larger residual lesions, the probability of survival after radiotherapy is only 5–15%.

Techniques of radiation encompassing the whole peritoneal cavity are more likely to be effective than those that treat the pelvis alone or the lower abdomen (Fig. 30.9). The dose of radiation that can be given to the upper abdomen is 2200–3000 cGy.

The incidence of bowel complications after initial abdominal surgery and irradiation is low—fewer than 2% required operative correction of bowel obstruction. The frequency of bowel complications will increase if higher total doses or larger fraction sizes are used. The extent and number of previous abdominal operations, especially para-aortic lymphadenectomy may add to the risk of bowel damage (75).

Postoperative whole abdominal irradiation should be limited to patients who are most likely to benefit, i.e., those with microscopic residual disease only (74–80). In addition, abdominal radiotherapy is most effective in patients with low-grade and low-stage disease.

Vulvar Cancer

The role of radiation therapy in the treatment of vulvar cancer has remained largely unexplored until recently (31, 81). Historically, radiation therapy was delivered with nonskin-sparing orthovoltage equipment in relatively high doses per fraction. This technique produced extensive acute morbidity with desquamation of the skin of the vulva and groins. Vulvar irradiation thus fell into disrepute.

The curative value of radiation therapy in the control of squamous cell cancers of other sites, including the head and neck and anal canal, is well established. Because the radiosensitivity of squamous cell carcinomas of the vulva should be the same as that of other squamous cell cancers, the use of radiation in this disease is being redefined with newer techniques (81–84). Current concepts in the integration of more limited surgery and adjunctive or primary radiation therapy in vulvar cancer are discussed in Chapter 34.

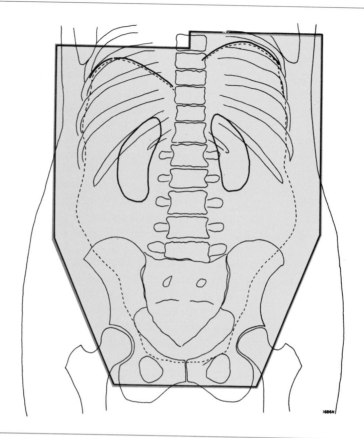

Figure 30.9   Treatment portals for carcinoma of the ovary. The entire peritoneal cavity is encompassed by the field. Reproduced from **Berek JS, Hacker WF.** *Practical Gynecologic Oncology.* 2nd ed. Baltimore: Williams & Wilkins, 1994.

The aims of integrated multimodality therapy, including surgery, radiation, and possibly concurrent chemoradiation therapy, are to reduce the risks of postoperative locoregional failure in patients with advanced primary or nodal disease and to obviate the need for exenteration in patients with disease involving the anus or proximal urethra (83). When radiation is used in vulvar cancer, the following guidelines with respect to radiation technique and dosage should be followed:

1. The total dose of radiation should be tailored to the volume of tumor with doses in the order of 4500–5000 cGy for microscopic disease and 6000–6400 cGy for macroscopic disease.

2. When the vulva is irradiated, the fraction size should be limited to 160–175 cGy to minimize late radiation sequelae.

3. When disease is macroscopic, vulvar or nodal, concurrent "sensitizing" chemotherapy (e.g., with infusional *5-FU* or *cisplatin*) may be a useful adjunct.

4. When concurrent infusional chemotherapy is used, two radiation fractions per day may be advantageous to maximize drug-radiation interaction and shorten the overall treatment time.

5. Treatment interruptions (split) should be kept to a minimum to avoid possible tumor proliferation during rests in radiation therapy.

6. A perineal port should be used when technically feasible. It is recommended that the vulvar lesion be encompassed with an adequate margin. No attempt should be made to include the entire vulva in the radiation field if disease is unifocal and can be included in smaller fields. The beam energies to be used for treatment of the primary tumor by direct fields should be cobalt or 4–6 MeV photons. Appropriate energy electrons may be used, tailored to the thickness of the lesion, but the dose from electrons to the primary lesion should probably be limited to 30–50% of the dose in view of the subcutaneous fibrosis that is commonly seen when all electron therapy is given. Advanced or very bulky disease may require whole vulvar irradiation using anterior-posterior parallel opposed fields.

7. Inguinopelvic nodal irradiation should be delivered with the use of energies greater than 6 MeV photons. Appropriate use of bolus or mixed beams should be employed to ensure that the inguinal nodal regions lying 0–4 cm below the skin receive full tumor dosage.

Acute moist desquamation of the skin of the inguinal creases and vulva is expected. The severity and duration of this acute reaction may be minimized by the choice of daily fraction sizes of 150–175 cGy. Late complications may include lymphedema, atrophy, and fibrosis of the skin and subcutaneous tissues in the treatment field. The risk of hip fracture in elderly women may be increased. Fractures have been reported in four of 13 women older than 50 years of age who have been treated with cobalt irradiation in doses of 2600–4500 cGy (83).

References

1. **Silver RT, Young RC, Holland J.** Some new aspects of modern cancer chemotherapy. *Am J Med* 1977;63:772–87.

2. **Young RC.** Principles of chemotherapy in gynecologic cancer. In: **Hoskins WJ, Perez CA, Young RC,** eds. *Principles and Practices of Gynecologic Oncology.* Philadelphia: JB Lippincott, 1992:333–49.

3. **Skipper HE, Schabel FM Jr, Mullett LB.** Implications of biochemical, cytokinetic, pharmacologic, and toxicologic relationships in the design of optimal therapeutic schedules. *Cancer Chemother Rep* 1950;54:431.

4. **Goldie JH, Coldman AJ.** A mathematical model for relating the drug sensitivity of tumors to their spontaneous mutation rate. *Cancer Treat Rep* 1979;63:1727–33.

5. **Ling V.** Drug resistance and membrane mutants of mammalian cells. *Can J Genet Cytol* 1975;17:503–15.

6. **Hryniuk W, Bush H.** The importance of dose intensity in chemotherapy of metastatic breast cancer. *J Clin Oncol* 1984;2:1281–8.

7. **McGuire WP, Hoskins WJ, Brady MS, Homesley HD, Creasman WT, Berman ML, et al.** Assessment of dose-intensive therapy in suboptimally debulked ovarian cancer: A Gynecologic Oncology Group study. *J Clin Oncol* 1995;13:1589–99.

8. **Kaye SB, Lewis CR, Paul J, Duncan ID, Gordon HK, Kitchener HC, et al.** Randomised study of two doses of cisplatin with cyclophosphamide in epithelial ovarian cancer. *Lancet* 1992;340:329–33.

9. **Chabner BA.** Clinical strategies for cancer treatment: the role of drugs. In: **Chabner BA, Collins JM,** eds. *Cancer Chemotherapy: Principles and Practice.* Philadelphia: JB Lippincott, 1990:1–16.

10. **Markman M.** Intraperitoneal chemotherapy. In: **Rubin SC, Sutton GP,** eds. *Ovarian Cancer.* New York: McGraw-Hill, 1993:325.

11. **Alberts DS, Liu PY, Hannigan EV, O'Toole R, Williams SD, Young J, et al.** Phase III study of intraperitoneal cisplatin/IV cyclophosphamide versus IV cisplatin/IV cyclophosphamide in patients with optimal disease stage III ovarian cancer: a SWOG-GOG-ECOG intergroup study (INT DO51). *Proc Am Soc Clin Oncol* 1995;14:273 (abstract).

12. **Haskell CM.** Principles and practice of cancer chemotherapy. In: **Haskell CM,** ed. *Cancer Treatment.* 4th ed. Philadelphia: WB Saunders, 1995.

13. **Frei E III.** Combination cancer therapy. Presidential Address. *Cancer Res* 1972;32:2593–607.

14. **Calvert AH, Newell DR, Gumbrell LA, O'Reilly S, Barnell M, Boxall FE, et al.** Carboplatin dosage: prospective evaluation of a simple formula based on renal function. *J Clin Oncol* 1989; 7:1748–56.

15. **Calabresi P, Parks RE Jr.** Chemotherapy of neoplastic diseases. In: **Goodman LS, Gilman A,** ed. *Goodman and Gilman's The Pharmacological Basis of Therapeutics.* 6th ed. New York: Macmillan, 1980:1249.

16. **Kaufman D, Rosen N, Young RC.** Clinical consequences and management of antineoplastic agents. In: **Parrillo JE, Masur H,** eds. *The Critically Ill Immunosuppressed Patient: Diagnosis and Management.* Rockville, Maryland: Aspen Press, 1986.

17. **Schilsky RL, Erlichman C.** Late complications of chemotherapy: infertility and carcinogenesis. In: **Chabner BA,** ed. *Pharmacologic Principles of Cancer Treatment.* Philadelphia: WB Saunders, 1982:109–31.

18. **Greene MH, Boice JD, Greer BE, Blessing JA, Dembo AJ.** Acute nonlymphocytic leukemia after therapy with alkylating agents for ovarian cancer. *N Engl J Med* 1982;307:1416–21.

19. **Colvin M, Chabner BA.** Alkylating agents. In: **Chabner BA, Collins JM,** eds. *Cancer Chemotherapy: Principles and Practice.* Philadelphia: JB Lippincott, 1990:276–314.

20. **Chabner BA, Myers CE.** Clinical pharmacology of cancer chemotherapy. In: **DeVita VT, Hellman S, Rosenberg SA,** eds. *Cancer: Principles and Practice of Oncology.* 3rd ed. Philadelphia: JB Lippincott, 1989:349–96.

21. **Chabner BA.** Cytadine analogues. In: **Chabner BA,** ed. *Cancer Chemotherapy: Principles and Practice.* Philadelphia: JB Lippincott, 1990:154–80.

22. **McCormick JJ, Johns DG.** Purine and purine nucleoside antimetabolites. In: **Chabner BA, Collins JM,** eds. *Cancer Chemotherapy: Principles and Practice.* Philadelphia: JB Lippincott, 1990:234–53.

23. **Bender RA, Hamel E, Hande KR.** Plant alkaloids. In: **Chabner BA, Collins JM,** eds. *Cancer Chemotherapy: Principles and Practice.* Philadelphia: JB Lippincott, 1990:253–76.

24. **Perez CA, Breaux S, Madoc-Jones H, Bedwinek JM, Camel HM, Purdy JA, et al.** Radiation therapy alone in the treatment of carcinoma of the uterine cervix. *Cancer* 1983;51:1393–402.

25. **Fletcher GH.** *Textbook of Radiotherapy.* Philadelphia: Lea & Febiger, 1980:720–89.

26. **Landgren RC, Fletcher GH, Delclos L, Wharton JT.** Irradiation of endometrial cancer in patients with medical contraindications to surgery or with unresectable lesions. *Am J Roentgenol Radium Ther Nucl Med* 1976;126:148–54.

27. **Dembo AJ, Bush RS, Beale FA, Bean HA, Pringle JF, Sturgeon J, et al.** Ovarian carcinoma: improved survival following abdominopelvic irradiation in patients with a completed pelvic operation. *Am J Obstet Gynecol* 1979;134:793–800.

28. **Dembo AJ.** Radiotherapeutic management of ovarian cancer. *Semin Oncol* 1984;11:238–50.

29. **Aalders J, Abeler V, Kolstad P, Onsrud M.** Postoperative external irradiation and prognostic parameters in Stage I endometrial carcinoma. *Obstet Gynecol* 1980;55:419–27.

30. **Homesley HD, Bundy BN, Sedlis A, Adcock L.** Radiation therapy versus pelvic node resection for carcinoma of the vulva with positive groin nodes. *Obstet Gynecol* 1986;68:733–40.

31. **Boronow RC.** Combined therapy as an alternative to exenteration for locally advanced vulvovaginal cancer. *Cancer* 1982;49:1085–91.

32. **Peters LJ, Ang KK.** Unconventional fractionation schemes in radiotherapy. In: *Important Advances in Oncology 1986.* Philadelphia: JB Lippincott, 1986:269–85.

33. **Thomas GM, Dembo AJ, Beale F, Bean H, Bush R, Herman J, et al.** Concurrent radiation, mitomycin-C and 5-fluorouracil in poor prognosis carcinoma of the cervix: preliminary results of a Phase I-II study. *Int J Radiat Oncol Biol Phys* 1984;10:1785–90.

34. **Hall EJ.** *Radiobiology for the Radiologist.* 2nd ed. Philadelphia: Harper & Row, 1978.

35. **Elkind MM, Sutton H.** Radiation response of mammalian cells grown in culture: 1. Repair of x-ray damage in surviving Chinese hamster cells. *Radiat Res* 1960;13:556–93.

36. **Parsons JT, Bova FJ, Million RR.** A re-evaluation of split-course technique for squamous carcinoma of the head and neck. *Int J Radiat Oncol Biol Phys* 1980;6:1645–52.

37. **Terasima R, Tolmach LJ.** X-ray sensitivity and DNA synthesis in synchronous population of HeLa cells. *Science* 1963;140:490–2.

38. **Kallman RF.** The phenomenon of reoxygenation and its implications for fractionated radiotherapy. *Radiology* 1972;105:135–42.

39. **Thames HD Jr, Peters LJ, Withers HR, Fletcher GH.** Accelerated fractionation vs. hyperfractionation: rationales for several treatments per day. *Int J Radiat Oncol Biol Phys* 1985;11:87.

40. **Adams GE, O'Neill P, Ahmed I, Fielden EM, Stratford EM, Fielden EM.** The development of some mitronidazoles as hypoxic cell sensitizers. *Cancer Clin Trials* 1980;3:37–42.

41. **Watson ER, Halnan KE, Dische S, Saunders MI, Cade IS, McEwen JB, et al.** Hyperbaric oxygen and radiotherapy: a Medical Research Council trial in carcinoma of the cervix. *Br J Radiol* 1978;51:879–87.

42. **Barendsen GW.** Response of cultured cells, tumors and normal tissues to radiations of different linear energy transfer. *Curr Top Radiat Res* 1968;4:293–356.

43. **Bush RS, Jenkin RP, Allt WE, Beaule FA, Bean H, Dembo AJ, et al.** Definitive evidence for hypoxic cells influencing cure in cancer therapy. *Br J Cancer* 1978;37:302–6.

44. **Steel GG, Peckham MJ.** Exploitable mechanisms in combined radiotherapy and chemotherapy: the concept of additivity. *Int J Radiat Oncol Biol Phys* 1979;5:85–91.

45. **Manning MR, Cetas TC, Miller RC, Oleson JR, Connor WG, Gerner EW.** Clinical hyperthermia: results of a Phase I trial employing hyperthermia alone or in combination with external beam or interstitial radiotherapy. *Cancer* 1982;49:205–16.

46. **Fletcher GH.** Clinical dose-response curves of human malignant epithelial tumours. *Br J Radiol* 1973;46:1–12.

47. **Shukovsky LJ.** Dose, time volume relationships in squamous cell carcinoma of the supraglottic larynx. *Am J Roentgenol Radium Ther Nucl Med* 1970;108:27–9.

48. **Rubin P, Casarett GW.** *Clinical Radiation Pathology.* Philadelphia: WB Saunders, 1968.

49. **Withers HR, Mason KA.** The kinetics of recovery in irradiated colonic mucosa in the mouse. *Cancer* 1974;34:896–903.

50. **Reinke U, Hannon EC, Rosenblatt M, Hellman S.** Proliferative capacity of murine hematopoietic stem cells in vitro. *Science* 1982;215:1619–22.

51. **Withers HR, Peters LJ, Kogelnik HD.** The pathobiology of late effects of irradiation. In: **Meyn RE, Withers HR,** eds. *Radiation Biology in Cancer Research.* New York: Raven Press, 1980:439–48.

52. **Peters LJ.** Biology of radiation therapy. In: **Thawley S, Panje W,** eds. *Comprehensive Management of Head and Neck Tumours.* Philadelphia: WB Saunders, 1985:132–52.

53. **Thames HD, Withers HR, Peters LJ, Fletcher GH.** Changes in early and late radiation response with altered dose fractionation: implications for dose-survival relationships. *Int J Radiat Oncol Biol Phys* 1982;8:219–26.

54. **Withers HR, Peters LJ, Thames HD, Fletcher GH.** Hyperfractionation. *Int J Radiat Oncol Biol Phys* 1982;8:1807–9.

55. **Onsrud M, Kolstad P, Normann T.** Postoperative external pelvic irradiation in carcinoma of the corpus Stage I: a controlled clinical trial. *Gynecol Oncol* 1976;4:222–31.

56. **Johns HE, Cunningham JR.** *The Physics of Radiology.* Springfield, IL: Charles C Thomas, 1977.

57. **Orton GG, Seyedsadr M, Somnay A.** Comparison of high and low dose rate remote afterloading for cervix cancer and the importance of fractionation. *Int J Radiat Oncol Biol Phys* 1992;21:1425–34.

58. **Martinez A, Edmundson GK, Cox RS, Gunderson LL, Howes AE.** Combination of external beam irradiation and multiple-site perineal applicator (MUPIT) for treatment of locally advanced or recurrent prostatic, anorectal and gynecologic malignancies. *Int J Radiat Oncol Biol Phys* 1985;11:391–8.

59. **Rosenshein NB.** Radioisotopes in the treatment of ovarian cancer. *Clin Obstet Gynecol* 1983; 10:279–95.

60. **Reed GW, Watson ER, Chesters MS.** A note on the distribution of radioactive colloidal gold following intraperitoneal injection. *Br J Radiol* 1961;34:323.

61. **Tewfik HH, Gruber H, Tewfik FA, Lifshitz SG.** Intraperitoneal distribution of ^{32}P chromic phosphate suspension in the dog. *Int J Radiat Oncol Biol Phys* 1979;5:1907–13.

62. **Allt WEC.** Supervoltage radiation treatment in advanced cancer of the uterine cervix. *Can Med Assoc J* 1969;100:792–7.

63. **Hamberger AD, Ural A, Gershenson DM, Fletcher GH.** Analysis of the severe complications of irradiation of the carcinoma of the cervix. Whole pelvis irradiation and intracavitary radium. *Int J Radiat Oncol Biol Phys* 1983;9:367–71.

64. **Covens A, Thomas GM, DePetrillo A, Jamieson C, Myhr T.** The prognostic importance of site and type of radiation-induced bowel injury in patients requiring surgical management. *Gynecol Oncol* 1991;43:270–4.

65. **Prempree T.** Parametrial implant in Stage IIIb cancer of the cervix. A five-year study. *Cancer* 1983;52:748–50.

66. **Randall ME.** Results of interstitial reradiation for recurrent gynecologic malignancies. *Proc Int Gynecol Cancer Soc* 1991;3:266.

67. **Heyman J, Reuterwell O, Benner S.** The Radiumhemmet experience with radiotherapy in cancer of the corpus of the uterus. *Acta Radiol* 1941;22:14–98.

68. **Piver SM, Yazigi R, Blumenson L, Tsukada Y.** A prospective trial comparing hysterectomy, hysterectomy plus vaginal radium, and uterine radium plus hysterectomy in Stage I endometrial carcinoma. *Obstet Gynecol* 1979;54:85–9.

69. **Boronow RC, Morrow CP, Creasman WT, Pisaia PJ, Silverberg SG, Miller A, et al.** Surgical staging in endometrial cancer: clinical-pathological findings of a prospective study. *Obstet Gynecol* 1984;63:825–32.

70. **Dembo AJ.** Abdominopelvic radiotherapy in ovarian cancer: a 10 year experience. *Cancer* 1985;55:2285–90.

71. **Martinez A, Schray MF, Howes AE, Bagshaw MA.** Postoperative radiation therapy for epithelial ovarian cancer: the curative role based on a 24-year experience. *J Clin Oncol* 1985;3:901–11.

72. **Fuller DB, Sause WT, Plenk H, Menlove RL.** Analysis of post-operative radiation therapy in Stage I through III epithelial ovarian carcinoma. *J Clin Oncol* 1987;5:897–905.

73. **Weiser EB, Burke TW, Heller PB, Woodward J, Hoskins WJ, Park RC.** Determinants of survival of patients with epithelial ovarian carcinoma following whole abdominal irradiation (WAR). *Gynecol Oncol* 1988;30:201–8.

74. **Goldberg N, Peschel RE.** Postoperative abdominopelvic radiation therapy for ovarian cancer. *Int J Radiat Oncol Phys* 1988;14(3):425–9.

75. **van Bunnigen B, Bouma J, Kooijman C, Warlam-Rodenhuis CC, Heintz AP, Lindert A.** Total abdominal irradiation in stage I and II carcinoma of the ovary. *Radiother Oncol* 1988;11:305–10.

76. **Dembo AJ, Bush RS, Brown TC.** Clinico-pathological correlates in ovarian cancer. *Bull Cancer* (Paris) 1982;69:292–7.

77. **Carey MS, Dembo AJ, Simm JE, Fyles AW, Treger T, Bush RS.** Testing the validity of a prognostic classification in patients with surgically optimal ovarian carcinoma: a 15-year review. *Int J Gynecol Cancer* 1993;3:24–35.

78. **Dembo AJ, Bush RS.** Current concepts in cancer: ovary—treatment of stages III and IV. Choice of postoperative therapy based on prognostic factors. *Int J Radiat Oncol Biol Phys* 1982;8:893–7.

79. **Sell A, Bertelsen K, Anderson JE, Stroyer I, Pandur J.** Randomized study of whole abdomen irradiation versus pelvic irradiation plus cyclophosphamide in treatment of early ovarian cancer. *Gynecol Oncol* 1990;37:367–73.

80. **Lindner H, Willich H, Atzinger A.** Primary adjuvant whole abdominal irradiation in ovarian carcinoma. *Int J Radiat Oncol Biol Phys* 1990;19:1203–6.

81. **Pirtoli L, Rottoli ML.** Results of radiation therapy for vulvar carcinoma. *Acta Radiol Oncol* 1982;21:45–8.

82. **Prempree T, Amornmarn R.** Radiation treatment of recurrent carcinoma of the vulva. *Cancer* 1984;54:1943–9.

83. **Thomas GM, Dembo AJ, Bryson SCO, Osborne R, DePetrillo AD.** Changing concepts in the management of vulvar cancer. *Gynecol Oncol* 1991;42:9–21.

84. **Guarishi A, Keane TJ, Elhakim T.** Metastatic inguinal nodes from an unknown primary neoplasm. *Cancer* 1987;59:572–7.

Modified from **Berek JS, Hacker WF.** *Practical Gynecologic Oncology.* 2nd ed. Baltimore: Williams & Wilkins, 1994:1–73.

31

Uterine Cancer

John R. Lurain

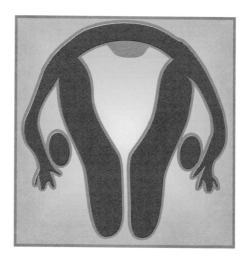

Endometrial carcinoma is the most common malignancy of the female genital tract, accounting for almost one-half of all gynecologic cancers in the U.S. Approximately 34,000 new cases are diagnosed annually, resulting in over 6000 deaths. Endometrial carcinoma is the fourth most common cancer, ranking behind breast, bowel, and lung cancers, and the seventh leading cause of death from malignancy in women. Overall, about 2–3% of women will develop endometrial cancer during their lifetimes (1).

Recently, certain factors have led to an increasing awareness of and emphasis on diagnosis and treatment of endometrial cancer. These factors include the declining incidence of cervical cancer and related deaths in the U.S., prolonged life expectancy, postmenopausal use of hormone replacement therapy, and earlier diagnosis. The availability of easily applied diagnostic tools and a clearer understanding of premalignant lesions of the endometrium have led to an increase in the diagnosis of endometrial cancer as well. Although endometrial carcinoma usually presents as early-stage disease and can generally be managed without radical surgery or radiation therapy, deaths from endometrial carcinoma now exceed those from cervical carcinoma in the U.S. **Endometrial cancer is a disease that occurs primarily in postmenopausal women and is increasingly virulent with advancing age. The role of estrogen in the development of most endometrial cancers has been established clearly; any factor that increases exposure to unopposed estrogen increases the risk of endometrial cancer.**

During the past several decades, the histopathology, spread patterns, and prognostic factors of endometrial cancers have been better defined. During this time, management of endometrial cancer has evolved from a program of preoperative intrauterine radium packing or external pelvic irradiation followed in 6 weeks by hysterectomy, to a single brachytherapy session using an intrauterine tandem and colpostats followed immediately by hysterectomy, to an individualized approach using hysterectomy as primary therapy and employing additional postoperative treatment depending on surgical and pathologic findings. Further analysis and investigation are needed to determine whether this initial operative approach to treatment and staging followed by targeted postoperative therapy will translate into improved survival rates.

Epidemiology and Risk Factors

There appear to be two different pathogenetic types of endometrial cancer (2). The most common type occurs in younger, perimenopausal women with a history of exposure to unopposed estrogen, either endogenous or exogenous. In these women, tumors begin as hyperplastic endometrium and progress to carcinoma. These *"estrogen-dependent" tumors* tend to be better differentiated and have a more favorable prognosis than tumors that are not associated with hyperestrogenism. The other type of endometrial carcinoma occurs in women with no source of estrogen stimulation of the endometrium. These spontaneously occurring cancers are not associated pathologically with endometrial hyperplasia but may arise in a background of atrophic endometrium. They are lees differentiated and associated with a poorer prognosis than estrogen-dependent tumors. These *"estrogen-independent" tumors* tend to occur in older, postmenopausal, thin women and are present disproportionately in African-American and Asian women.

Several risk factors for the development of endometrial cancer have been identified (Table 31.1) (3–8). Most of these risk factors are related to prolonged, unopposed estrogen stimulation of the endometrium.

1. Nulliparous women have 2–3 times the risk of parous women.

2. Infertility and a history of irregular menses, as a result of anovulatory cycles (prolonged exposure to estrogen without sufficient progesterone) increases the risk.

3. Natural menopause occurring after 52 years of age increases the risk of endometrial cancer 2.4 times compared with women in whom menopause occurred before 49 years of age, probably as a result of prolonged exposure of the uterus to progesterone-deficient menstrual cycles.

4. The risk of endometrial cancer is increased three times for women who are 21–50 pounds overweight and 10 times for those who are more than 50 pounds overweight (excess estrone as a result of peripheral conversion of adrenally derived androstenedione by aromatization in fat).

5. Other factors leading to long-term estrogen exposure, such as polycystic ovary syndrome and functioning ovarian tumors, also are associated with an increased risk of endometrial cancer.

6. Menopausal use of estrogen replacement therapy without progestins increases the risk of endometrial cancer four to eight times. This risk is greater with higher doses and prolonged use and can be reduced to essentially base line levels by the addition of progestin (7).

Table 31.1   Risk Factors for Endometrial Cancer

Characteristic	*Relative Risk*
Nulliparity	2–3
Late menopause	2.4
Obesity	
21–50 lbs	3
>50 lbs	10
Diabetes mellitus	2.8
Unopposed estrogen therapy	4–8
Tamoxifen	2–3
Atypical endometrial hyperplasia	8–29

7. It has been noted that use of the antiestrogen *tamoxifen* for treatment of breast cancer is associated with a two- to threefold increased risk for the development of endometrial cancer (8).

8. Diabetes mellitus increases a woman's risk of endometrial cancer by 1.3 to 2.8 times. Other medical conditions such as hypertension and hypothyroidism have been associated with endometrial cancer, but a causal relationship has not been confirmed.

Endometrial Hyperplasia

Endometrial hyperplasia represents a spectrum of morphologic and biologic alterations of the endometrial glands and stroma, ranging from an exaggerated physiologic state to carcinoma *in situ*. Clinically significant hyperplasias usually evolve within a background of proliferative endometrium as a result of protracted estrogen stimulation in the absence of progestin influence. Endometrial hyperplasias are important clinically because they may cause abnormal uterine bleeding, may be associated with estrogen-producing ovarian tumors, may result from hormonal therapy, and may precede or occur simultaneously with endometrial cancer.

The most recent classification scheme endorsed by the International Society of Gynecological Pathologists is based on both architectural and cytologic features as well as long-term studies that reflect the natural history of the lesions (Table 31.2) (9). Architecturally, hyperplasias are either simple or complex; the major differing features are complexity and crowding of the glandular elements. *Simple hyperplasia* is characterized by dilated or cystic glands with round to slightly irregular shapes, an increased glandular-to-stromal ratio without glandular crowding, and no cytologic atypia. *Complex hyperplasia* has architecturally complex (budding and infolding), crowded glands with less intervening stroma without atypia. *Atypical hyperplasia* refers to cytologic atypia and can be categorized as simple or complex, depending on the corresponding glandular architecture. Criteria for cytologic atypia include large nuclei of variable size and shape that have lost polarity, increased nuclear-to-cytoplasmic ratios, prominent nucleoli, and irregularly clumped chromatin with parachromatin clearing (Fig. 31.1).

The risk of endometrial hyperplasia progressing to carcinoma is related to the presence and severity of cytologic atypia. Kurman et al. retrospectively studied endometrial curettings from 170 patients with untreated endometrial hyperplasia followed for a mean of 13.4 years. They found that **progression to carcinoma occurred in 1% of patients with simple hyperplasia, 3% of patients with complex hyperplasia, 8% of patients with atypical simple hyperplasia, and 29% of patients with atypical complex hyperplasia.** Most of the hyperplasias seemed to remain stable (18%) or regress (74%) (10). The premalignant potential of hyperplasia is influenced by age, underlying ovarian disease, endocrinopathy, obesity, and exogenous hormone exposure (11, 12). **In patients with atypical hyperplasia detected during endometrial biopsy or in a curettage specimen, approximately 25% will have an associated, usually well-differentiated, endometrial carcinoma if a hysterectomy is performed.** Marked cytologic atypia, a high mitotic rate, and marked cellular stratification are features of atypical endometrial hyperplasia most of-

Table 31.2   Classification of Endometrial Hyperplasias

Type of Hyperplasia	Progression to Cancer (%)
Simple (cystic without atypia)	1
Complex (adenomatous without atypia)	3
Atypical	
Simple (cystic with atypia)	8
Complex (adenomatous with atypia)	29

Reproduced with permission from **Kurman RJ, Kaminski PF, Norris HJ.** The behavior of endometrial hyperplasia: a long term study of "untreated" hyperplasia in 170 patients. *Cancer* 1985;56:403–12.

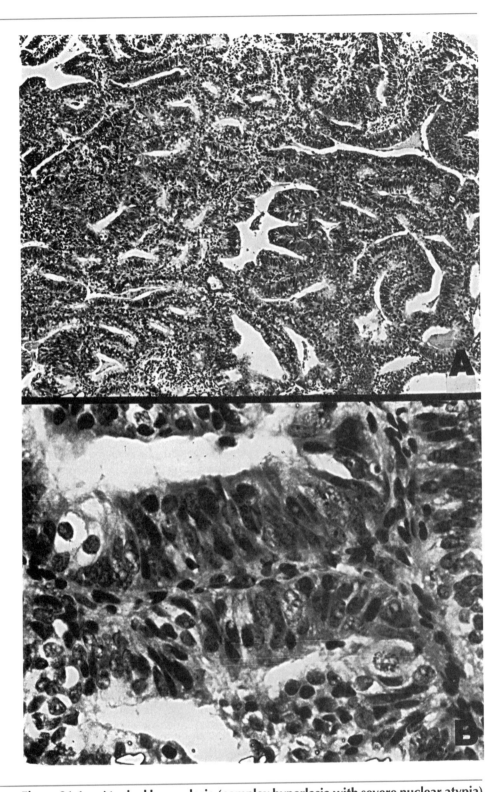

Figure 31.1.   Atypical hyperplasia (complex hyperlasia with severe nuclear atypia) of endometrium. *A,* The proliferative endometrial glands reveal considerable crowding and papillary infoldings. The endometrial stroma, although markedly diminished, can still be recognized between the glands. *B,* Higher magnification demonstrates disorderly nuclear arrangement and nuclear enlargement and irregularity. Some contain small nucleoli. (Figures 31.1–31.10 Reproduced or modified from **Berek JS, Hacker WF.** *Practical Gynecologic Oncology.* 2nd ed. Baltimore: Williams & Wilkins, 1994.)

and marked cellular stratification are features of atypical endometrial hyperplasia most often associated with the finding of an undiagnosed carcinoma at hysterectomy.

Ferenczy and Gelfand reported on 85 postmenopausal women with endometrial hyperplasia treated with progestin (13). Of 65 patients without cytologic atypia, complete reversal of the lesions in 84% when treated with *medroxyprogesterone acetate* 10–20 mg daily; recurrent hyperplasia developed in 6% but cancer developed in none of the patients, with a mean follow-up of 7 years. By contrast, of 20 patients with cytologic atypia, only 50% responded to progestin, recurrent hyperplasia developed in 25%, and adenocarcinoma developed in 25%. In another study, lesions were resolved in 94% of 32 patients with atypical endometrial hyperplasia who were treated with *megestrol acetate* 20–40 mg daily; however, relapse occurred in all seven patients who discontinued progestin therapy (14).

Progestin therapy is very effective in reversing endometrial hyperplasia without atypia but is less effective for endometrial hyperplasia with atypia. For women with endometrial hyperplasia without atypia, ovulation induction, cyclical progestin therapy (e.g., *medroxyprogesterone acetate* 10–20 mg/day for 14 days per month), or continuous progestin therapy (e.g., *megesterol acetate* 20–40 mg daily) all seem to be effective therapies. Continuous progestin therapy with *megestrol acetate* (40 mg daily) is probably the most reliable treatment for reversing complex or atypical hyperplasia. Therapy should be continued for 2–3 months, and endometrial biopsy should be performed at the completion of therapy to assess response. Periodic endometrial biopsy, transvaginal ultrasound, or both is advisable (especially in patients treated for atypical hyperplasia) because of the presence of undiagnosed cancer in 25% of cases, the 29% progression rate to cancer, and the high recurrence rate after treatment with progestins.

Endometrial Cancer Screening

Screening for endometrial cancer should not be undertaken because of the lack of an appropriate, cost-effective, and acceptable test that reduces mortality (15–17). **Routine Papanicolaou (Pap) testing is inadequate and endometrial cytologic assessment is too insensitive and nonspecific to be useful in screening for endometrial cancer, even in a high-risk population.** A progesterone challenge test will reveal whether the endometrium has been primed by estrogen, but it will not identify abnormal endometrial pathology. Transvaginal ultrasound examination of the uterus and endometrial biopsy are too expensive to be employed as screening tests.

Although many risk factors for endometrial cancer have been identified, screening of high-risk individuals could at best detect only 50% of all cases of endometrial cancer. Furthermore, no controlled trials have been carried out to evaluate the effectiveness of screening in endometrial cancer. Fortunately, most patients who have endometrial cancer present with abnormal perimenopausal or postmenopausal uterine bleeding early in the development of the disease, when the tumor is still confined to the uterus. Endometrial biopsy performed in this situation usually results in early diagnosis, timely treatment, and a high cure rate.

Endometrial Cancer

Symptoms

Endometrial carcinoma most often occurs in women in the sixth and seventh decades of life, at an average age of 60 years; 75% of cases occur in women older than 50 years of age. **Approximately 90% of women with endometrial carcinoma have vaginal bleeding or discharge as their only presenting complaint.** Most women recognize the importance of this symptom and seek medical consultation within 3 months. Some women present with pelvic pressure or discomfort indicative of uterine enlargement or extrauterine disease spread. Bleeding may not have occurred because of cervical stenosis, especially in older patients, and may be associated with hematometra or pyometra, causing a purulent vaginal discharge. This finding is often associated with a poor prognosis (18). **Less than**

5% of women diagnosed with endometrial cancer are asymptomatic. In the absence of symptoms, endometrial cancer usually is detected as the result of investigation of abnormal Pap test results, discovery of cancer in a uterus removed for some other reason, or evaluation of an abnormal finding on a pelvic ultrasound or computed tomography (CT) scan obtained for an unrelated reason. Women who are found to have malignant cells on Pap test are more likely to have a more advanced stage of disease (19).

Abnormal perimenopausal and postmenopausal bleeding should always be taken seriously and should be investigated no matter how minimal or nonpersistent. Causes may be nongenital, genital, extrauterine, or uterine (20). Nongenital tract sites should be considered based on the history or examination, including testing for blood in the urine and stool. Invasive tumors of the cervix, vagina, and vulva are usually evident on examination, and any tumors discovered should undergo biopsy. Traumatic bleeding from an atrophic vagina may account for up to 15% of all causes of postmenopausal bleeding. **Endometrial atrophy is the most common endometrial finding in women with postmenopausal bleeding, accounting for 60–80% of such bleeding.** This diagnosis can be considered if inspection reveals a thin, friable vaginal wall, but the possibility of a uterine source of bleeding must first be eliminated.

Possible uterine causes of peri- or postmenopausal bleeding include endometrial atrophy, endometrial polyps, estrogen replacement therapy, hyperplasia, and cancer or sarcoma (Table 31.3) (21–24). Uterine leiomyomas should never be accepted as a cause of postmenopausal bleeding. Women with endometrial atrophy have usually been menopausal for about 10 years. Endometrial biopsy often yields insufficient tissue or only blood and mucus, and there is usually no additional bleeding after biopsy. Endometrial polyps account for 2–12% of postmenopausal bleeding. Polyps are often difficult to identify with office endometrial biopsy or curettage. Hysteroscopy, transvaginal ultrasound, or both may be useful adjuncts in identifying endometrial polyps. Unrecognized and untreated polyps may be a source of continued or recurrent bleeding, leading eventually to unnecessary hysterectomy. Estrogen therapy is an established risk factor for endometrial hyperplasia and cancer. Endometrial biopsy should be performed as indicated to assess unscheduled bleeding or annually in women not taking progestin. **Endometrial hyperplasia occurs in 5–10% of patients with postmenopausal uterine bleeding.** The source of excess estrogen should be considered, including obesity, exogenous estrogen, or an estrogen-secreting ovarian tumor. **Only approximately 10% of patients with postmenopausal bleeding have endometrial cancer.**

Premenopausal women with endometrial cancer invariably have abnormal uterine bleeding, which is often characterized as menometrorrhagia or oligomenorrhea or cyclical bleeding that continues past the usual age of menopause. The diagnosis of endometrial cancer must be considered in premenopausal women when abnormal bleeding is persistent or recurrent or if obesity or chronic anovulation are present.

Signs

Physical examination seldom reveals any evidence of endometrial carcinoma, although obesity and hypertension are associated constitutional factors. Special attention should be given to the more common sites of metastasis. Peripheral lymph nodes and breasts should

Table 31.3   Causes of Postmenopausal Uterine Bleeding

Cause of Bleeding	Frequency (%)
Endometrial atrophy	60–80
Estrogen replacement therapy	15–25
Endometrial polyps	2–12
Endometrial hyperplasia	5–10
Endometrial cancer	10

be assessed carefully. Abdominal examination usually is unremarkable, except in advanced cases in which ascites or hepatic or omental metastases may be palpable. The vaginal introitus and suburethral area, as well as the entire vagina and cervix, should be carefully inspected and palpated. Bimanual rectovaginal examination should specifically evaluate the uterus for size and mobility, the adnexa for masses, the parametria for induration, and the cul-de-sac for nodularity.

Diagnosis

Office endometrial aspiration biopsy is the first step in evaluating a patient with abnormal uterine bleeding or suspected endometrial pathology (25). **The diagnostic accuracy of office-based endometrial biopsy is 90–98% when compared with subsequent findings of dilation and curettage (D&C) or hysterectomy** (26, 27). The narrow plastic cannulas now available are relatively inexpensive; they can often be used without a tenaculum, cause less uterine cramping (resulting in increased patient acceptance), and are successful in obtaining adequate tissue samples in more than 95% of cases. If cervical stenosis is encountered, a paracervical block can be performed and the cervix can be dilated. Premedication with an antiprostaglandin agent can reduce uterine cramping. Complications following endometrial biopsy are exceedingly rare; uterine perforation occurs in only one to two cases per 1000. Endocervical curettage may also be performed at the time of endometrial biopsy if cervical pathology is suspected. **A Pap test is an unreliable diagnostic test, because only 30–50% of patients with endometrial cancer will have abnormal Pap test results** (28).

Hysteroscopy and D&C should be reserved for situations in which cervical stenosis or patient tolerance does not permit adequate evaluation by aspiration biopsy, bleeding recurs after a negative endometrial biopsy, or the specimen obtained is inadequate to explain the abnormal bleeding. Hysteroscopy is more accurate in identifying polyps and submucous myomas than endometrial biopsy or D&C alone (29, 30).

Transvaginal ultrasound may be a useful adjunct to endometrial biopsy for evaluating abnormal uterine bleeding and selecting patients for additional testing (31–33). Transvaginal ultrasound, with or without endometrial fluid instillation (ultrasonohysterography), may be helpful in distinguishing between patients with minimal endometrial tissue whose bleeding is caused by perimenopausal anovulation or postmenopausal atrophy and patients with significant amounts of endometrial tissue or polyps who are in need of further evaluation. The findings of an endometrial thickness greater than 5 mm, a polypoid endometrial mass, or a collection of fluid within the uterus require further evaluation. Although most studies agree that an endometrial thickness of 5 mm or less in a postmenopausal woman is consistent with atrophy, more data are needed before ultrasound findings can be considered to eliminate the need for endometrial biopsy in a symptomatic patient.

Pathology

The histologic classification of carcinoma arising in the endometrium is shown in Table 31.4 (9, 34).

Endometrioid Adenocarcinoma

The endometrioid type accounts for approximately 80% of endometrial carcinomas. These tumors are composed of glands that resemble normal endometrial glands; they have columnar cells with basally oriented nuclei, little or no intracytoplasmic mucin, and smooth intraluminal surfaces (Fig. 31.2). As tumors become less differentiated, they contain more solid areas, less glandular formation, and more cytologic atypia. The well-differentiated lesions may be difficult to separate from atypical hyperplasia.

Criteria that indicate the presence of invasion and are used to diagnose carcinoma are desmoplastic stroma, glands back-to-back without intervening stroma, extensive papillary pattern, and squamous epithelial differentiation.

Table 31.4   Classification of Endometrial Carcinomas

Endometrioid adenocarcinoma

  Usual type

  Variants

    Villoglandular/papillary

    Secretory

  With squamous differentiation

Mucinous carcinoma

Papillary serous carcinoma

Clear cell carcinoma

Squamous carcinoma

Undifferentiated carcinoma

Mixed carcinoma

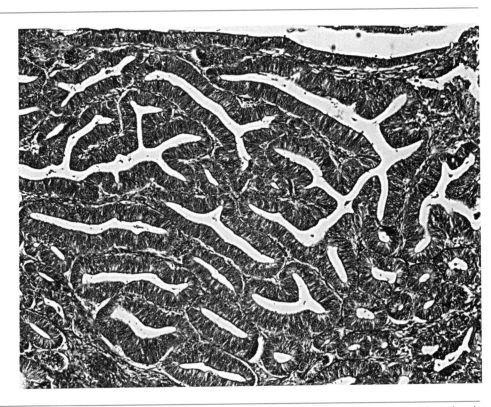

Figure 31.2.   Well-differentiated adenocarcinoma of endometrium. The glands and complex papillae are in direct contact with no intervening endometrial stroma, the so-called back-to-back pattern.

These changes, with the exception of the infiltrating pattern with desmoplastic reaction, require an area of involvement equal to or exceeding one-half of a low-power microscopic field ($\geq$ ½ LPF; 4.2 mm in diameter) (35, 36).

The differentiation of a carcinoma, expressed as its grade, is determined by architectural growth pattern and nuclear features (Table 31.5). **In the FIGO grading system proposed in 1989, tumors are grouped into three grades:**

Table 31.5   FIGO Definition for Grading of Endometrial Carcinoma

Histopathologic degree of differentiation:

G1: ≤5% nonsquamous or nonmorular growth pattern
G2: 6–50% nonsquamous or nonmorular growth pattern
G3: >50% nonsquamous or nonmorular growth pattern

Notes on pathologic grading:

1. Notable nuclear atypia, inappropriate for the architectural grade, raises the grade of a grade 1 or grade 2 tumor by one grade.
2. In serous adenocarcinoma, clear cell adenocarcinoma and squamous cell carcinoma, nuclear grading takes precedence.
3. Adenocarcinomas with squamous differentiation are graded according to the nuclear grade of the glandular component.

FIGO, International Federation of Gynecology and Obstetrics.

1. *Grade 1 (G1) — 5% or less of the tumor shows a solid growth pattern*

2. *Grade 2 (G2) — 6 to 50% of the tumor shows a solid growth pattern*

3. *Grade 3 (G3) — more than 50% of the tumor shows a solid growth pattern.*

In addition, notable nuclear atypia that is inappropriate for the architectural grade increases the tumor grade by one. Adenocarcinomas with squamous differentiation are graded according to the nuclear grade of the glandular component. This FIGO system is applicable to all endometrioid carcinomas, including its variants, and to mucinous carcinomas. In serous and clear cell carcinomas, nuclear grading takes precedence; however, most investigators believe that these two carcinomas should always be considered high-grade lesions, making grading unnecessary.

Approximately 15–25% of endometrioid carcinomas have areas of squamous differentiation (Fig. 31.3). In the past, tumors with benign-appearing squamous areas were called "adenoacanthomas," and tumors with malignant-looking squamous elements were called "adenosquamous carcinomas." It is now recommended that the term "endometrial carcinoma with squamous differentiation" be used to replace these two designations because the degree of differentiation of the squamous component parallels that of the glandular component and the behavior of the tumor is largely dependent on the grade of the glandular component (37, 38).

A *villoglandular* configuration is present in approximately 2% of endometrioid carcinomas (39, 40). In these tumors, the cells are arranged along fibrovascular stalks, giving a papillary appearance but maintaining the characteristics of endometrioid cells. The villoglandular variants of endometrioid carcinomas are always well-differentiated lesions that behave like the regular endometrioid carcinomas and should be distinguished from papillary serous carcinomas.

Secretory carcinoma is a rare variant of endometrioid carcinoma that accounts for approximately 1% of cases (41, 42). It occurs mostly in women in the early postmenopausal years. The tumors are composed of well-differentiated glands with intracytoplasmic vacuoles similar to early secretory endometrium. These tumors behave as regular well-differentiated endometrioid carcinomas and generally have an excellent prognosis. Secretory carcinoma may be an endometrioid carcinoma that exhibits progestational changes, but a history of progestational therapy is rarely elicited. Secretory carcinoma must be differentiated from clear cell carcinoma, because both tumors have predominantly clear cells. These two tumors can be distinguished because secretory carcinomas have uniform glan-

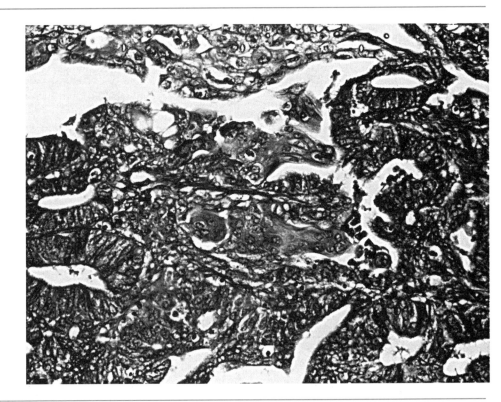

Figure 31.3.   Adenocarcinoma with squamous differentiation of endometrium. This lesion is also classified as adenoacanthoma. Squamous cells with eosinophilic cytoplasm and distinct cell borders form solid clusters in the lumina of neoplastic glands.

dular architecture, uniform cytology, and low nuclear grade, whereas clear cell carcinomas have more than one architectural pattern and a high nuclear grade.

Mucinous Carcinoma	**Approximately 5% of endometrial carcinomas have a predominant mucinous pattern in which more than 50% of the tumor is composed of cells with intracytoplasmic mucin** (43, 44). Most of these tumors have a well-differentiated glandular architecture; their behavior is similar to common endometrioid carcinomas and the prognosis is good. It is important to recognize mucinous carcinoma of the endometrium as an entity and to differentiate it from endocervical adenocarcinoma. Features that favor a primary endometrial carcinoma are the merging of the tumor with areas of normal endometrial tissue, presence of foamy endometrial stromal cells, presence of squamous metaplasia, or the presence of areas of typical endometrioid carcinoma. Positive perinuclear immunohistochemical staining with vimentin suggests an endometrial origin (45).

Papillary Serous Carcinoma	**Approximately 3–4% of endometrial carcinomas resemble serous carcinoma of the ovary and fallopian tube** (46–49). Most often, these tumors are composed of fibrovascular stalks lined with highly atypical cells with tufted stratification (Fig. 31.4). Psammoma bodies frequently are observed. Uterine papillary serous carcinomas (UPSC) are all considered high-grade lesions. They are commonly admixed with other histologic patterns, but mixed tumors behave as aggressively as pure serous carcinomas. Serous carcinomas are often associated with lymph-vascular space and deep myometrial invasion. Even when these tumors appear to be confined to the endometrium or the endometrial polyps behave without myometrial or vascular invasion, they behave more aggressively than endometri-

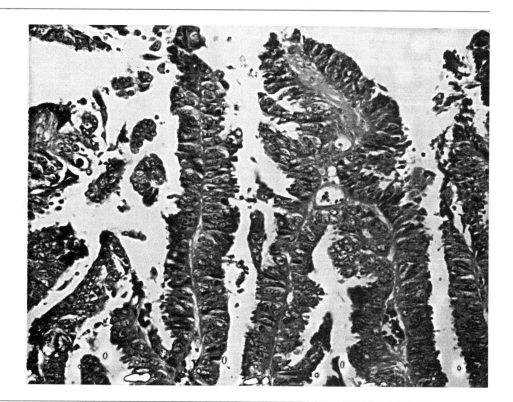

Figure 31.4.   Papillary serous carcinoma of endometrium. Branching papillae are supported by delicate fibrovascular cores and lined with columnar cells with moderate nuclear atypism, multiple nucleoli, and mitotic figures.

oid carcinomas and have a propensity to spread intra-abdominally, simulating the behavior of ovarian carcinoma. Of patients with clinical stage I disease, deep myometrial invasion occurs in more than 50% and lymph-vascular space invasion is manifest in 75%. In approximately 50% of patients, extrauterine disease is detected during surgery.

Hendrickson et al. first described UPSC in 1982, noting that this entity usually occurred in elderly, hypoestrogenic women who presented with advanced stage disease, accounting for up to 50% of deaths from endometrial carcinoma (46). Since that time, several reports have documented the aggressive nature and poor prognosis of UPSC. Silva et al. (47) and Sherman et al. (48) pointed out that even when the disease was confined to an endometrial polyp without other evidence of spread, recurrence occurred in more than 50% of patients. More recently, Goff et al. reported on 50 patients surgically staged with UPSC. Extrauterine disease was found in 72%. Presence of lymph node metastases, positive peritoneal cytology, and intraperitoneal tumor did not correlate with increasing myometrial invasion (49).

Clear Cell Carcinoma

Clear cell carcinoma accounts for less than 5% of all endometrial carcinomas (41, 50). Clear cell carcinoma usually has a mixed histologic pattern, including papillary, tubulocystic, glandular, and solid types. The cells have highly atypical nuclei and abundant clear or eosinophilic cytoplasm. Often, the cells have a hobnail configuration arranged in papillae with hyalinized stalks.

Clear cell carcinoma characteristically occurs in older women and is a very aggressive type of endometrial cancer; the prognosis is similar to or worse than papillary serous carcinoma. Overall survival rates of 33–64% have been reported. Myometrial invasion and lymph-vascular space invasion are important prognostic indicators.

Squamous Carcinoma

Squamous carcinoma of the endometrium is rare. Some tumors are pure, but most have a few glands. In order to establish primary origin within the endometrium, there must be no connection with or spread from cervical squamous epithelium. Squamous carcinoma is often associated with cervical stenosis, chronic inflammation, and pyometra at the time of diagnosis. This tumor has a poor prognosis with an estimated 36% survival rate in clinical stage I disease (51).

Simultaneous Tumors of the Endometrium and Ovary

Synchronous endometrial and ovarian cancers are the most frequent simultaneously occurring genital malignancies, with a reported incidence of 1.4–3.8% (52–56). Most commonly, both the ovarian and endometrial tumors are well-differentiated endometrioid adenocarcinomas of low stage that have an excellent prognosis. Patients are often premenopausal and present with abnormal uterine bleeding. The ovarian cancer is usually discovered as an incidental finding and diagnosed at an earlier stage because of the symptomatic endometrial tumor, leading to a more favorable outcome. As many as 29% of patients with endometrioid ovarian adenocarcinomas will have associated endometrial cancer. If more poorly differentiated, nonendometrioid histologic subtypes are present or if the uterine and ovarian tumors are histologically dissimilar, the prognosis is less favorable. Immunohistochemical studies, flow cytometry, and molecular assessment of DNA patterns to detect loss of heterogyzosity may be helpful for distinguishing between metastatic and independent tumors, but the differential diagnosis usually can be determined by conventional clinicopathologic criteria.

Pretreatment Evaluation

After establishing the diagnosis of endometrial carcinoma, the next step is to thoroughly evaluate the patient in order to determine the best and safest approach to management of the disease. A complete history and physical examination is of utmost importance. Patients with endometrial carcinoma are often elderly and obese and have a variety of medical problems, such as diabetes mellitus and hypertension, which affect surgical management. Any abnormal symptoms, such as bladder or intestinal complaints, should be evaluated.

On physical examination, attention should be given to enlarged or suspicious-looking lymph nodes, abdominal masses, and possible areas of cancer spread within the pelvis. Evidence of distant metastasis or locally advanced disease in the pelvis, such as gross cervical involvement or parametrial spread, may alter the treatment approach. Stool should be tested for occult blood.

A chest x-ray should be performed to rule out pulmonary metastasis and to evaluate the cardiorespiratory status of the patient. Other routine preoperative studies should include electrocardiography, complete blood and platelet counts, serum chemistry studies (including renal and liver function tests), blood type and screen, and urinalysis. Other preoperative or staging studies are neither required nor necessary for most patients with endometrial cancer. **Other studies such as cystoscopy, proctosigmoidoscopy, intravenous pyelography, barium enema, and CT scanning of the abdomen and pelvis are not indicated unless dictated by patient symptoms, physical findings, or other laboratory tests.** Ultrasonography and magnetic resonance imaging (MRI) can be used to preoperatively assess myometrial invasion with a fairly high degree of accuracy (57). This information may be of use in planning the surgical procedure with regard to whether lymph node sampling should be undertaken.

Serum CA125, which is elevated in 80% of patients with advanced epithelial ovarian cancers, is also elevated in most patients with advanced or metastatic endometrial cancer (58). Patsner et al. reported that 23 of 81 patients with apparently localized disease preoperatively had elevated CA125 levels. At surgery, 20 (87%) of these 23 patients with elevated CA125 were found to have extrauterine disease, whereas only one of 58 patients with a normal CA125 level had disease spread outside the uterus (59). Preoperative measurement of serum CA125 may, therefore, help determine the extent of surgical staging and, if elevated, may be useful as a tumor marker in assessing response to subsequent therapy.

Clinical Staging

Clinical staging, according to FIGO 1971 (Table 31.6), **should be performed in patients who are deemed not to be candidates for surgery, either because of their poor medical condition or the spread of their disease** (60). A small percentage of patients will not be candidates for surgery because of gross cervical involvement, parametrial spread, invasion of the bladder or rectum, or distant metastasis. With improvements in preoperative and postoperative care, anesthesia administration, and surgical techniques, almost all patients are medically suitable for operative therapy. Marziale et al. (1989) reported an operability rate of 87% in a series of 595 consecutive patients with clinical early-stage endometrial cancer (61).

Surgical Staging

Most patients with endometrial cancer should undergo surgical staging based on the 1988 FIGO system (Table 31.7) (62–64). **At a minimum, the surgical procedure should include sampling of peritoneal fluid for cytologic evaluation, exploration of the abdomen and pelvis with biopsy or excision of any extrauterine lesions suggestive of**

Table 31.6   1988 FIGO Surgical Staging for Endometrial Carcinoma

Stage Ia	**G123**	Tumor limited to endometrium
Ib	**G123**	Invasion to less than one-half of the myometrium
Ic	**G123**	Invasion to more than one-half of the myometrium
Stage IIa	**G123**	Endocervical glandular involvement only
IIb	**G123**	Cervical stromal invasion
Stage IIIa	**G123**	Tumor invades serosa and/or adnexa and/or positive peritoneal cytology
IIIb	**G123**	Vaginal metastases
IIIc	**G123**	Metastases to pelvic and/or para-aortic lymph nodes
Stage IVa	**G123**	Tumor invasion of bladder and/or bowel mucosa
IVb		Distant metastases including intra-abdominal and/or inguinal lymph nodes

FIGO, International Federation of Gynecology and Obstetrics.

Table 31.7   1971 FIGO Clinical Staging for Endometrial Carcinoma

Stage 0	Carcinoma *in situ*.
Stage I	The carcinoma is confined to the corpus.
Stage Ia	The length of the uterine cavity is 8 cm or less.
Stage Ib	The length of the uterine cavity is more than 8 cm.
Stage 1 cases should be subgrouped with regard to the histologic grade of the adenocarcinoma as follows:	
Grade 1	Highly differentiated adenomatous carcinoma.
Grade 2	Moderately differentiated adenomatous carcinoma with partly solid areas.
Grade 3	Predominantly solid or entirely undifferentiated carcinoma.
Stage II	The carcinoma has involved the corpus and the cervix but has not extended outside the uterus.
Stage III	The carcinoma has extended outside the uterus but not outside the true pelvis.
Stage IV	The carcinoma has extended outside the true pelvis or has obviously involved the mucosa of the bladder or rectum. A bullous edema as such does not permit a case to be allocated to State IV.
Stage IVa	Spread of the growth to adjacent organs.
Stage IVb	Spread to distant organs.

metastatic cancer, extrafascial hysterectomy, and bilateral salpingo-oophorectomy. The uterine specimen should be opened and the tumor size (65), depth of myometrial involvement (66, 67), and cervical extension should be assessed. Any suspicious pelvic and para-aortic lymph nodes should be removed for pathologic examination.

Additionally, clinically negative retroperitoneal lymph nodes should be sampled in all patients with one or more of the risk factors noted in Table 31.8. Tumor histology and depth of myometrial invasion seem to be the two most important factors in determining the risk of lymph node metastasis (63, 64). The overall incidence of lymph node metastasis in clinical stage I endometrial cancer is approximately 3% in grade 1, 9% in grade 2, and 18% in grade 3 tumors (Table 31.9). Less than 5% of patients with no myometrial invasion or with superficial (<½) myometrial invasion have lymph node metastasis, compared with about 20% of patients with deep (>½) myometrial invasion (Table 31.10). Pelvic lymph node metastases are present in less than 5% of grade 1 and 2 tumors with superficial myometrial invasion, approximately 15% of grade 1 and 2 tumors with deep myometrial invasion or grade 3 tumors with superficial invasion, and more than 40% of grade 3 tumors with deep myometrial invasion (Fig. 31.5). Approximately one-half to two-thirds of patients with positive pelvic lymph nodes will also have para-aortic lymph node metastases, but the aortic nodes are seldom involved in the absence of pelvic nodal disease. Cervical involvement is associated with about a 15% risk of pelvic or para-aortic

Table 31.8   Indications for Selective Pelvic and Para-aortic Lymph Node Dissection in Endometrial Cancer

Tumor histology clear cell, serous, squamous, or grade 3 endometrioid

Myometrial invasion ≥½

Isthmus-cervix extension

Tumor size >2 cm

Extrauterine disease

Table 31.9   Relationship of Grade to Lymph Node Metastasis in Clinical Stage I Endometrial Carcinoma

Grade	No.	Pelvic Nodes		Aortic Nodes	
		No.	Percentage	No.	Percentage
1	180	5	3	3	2
2	288	25	9	14	5
3	153	28	18	17	11

Reproduced with permission from **Creasman WT, Morrow CP, Bundy BN, Homesley HD, Graham JE, Heller PB.** Surgical pathologic spread patterns of endometrial cancer. *Cancer* 1987;60:2035–41.

Table 31.10   Relationship of Myometrial Invasion to Lymph Node Metastasis in Clinical Stage I Endometrial Carcinoma

Myometrial Invasion	No.	Pelvic Nodes		Aortic Nodes	
		No.	Percentage	No.	Percentage
None	87	1	1	1	1
Inner one-third	279	15	5	8	3
Middle one-third	116	7	6	1	1
Outer one-third	139	35	25	24	17

Reproduced with permission from **Creasman WT, Morrow CP, Bundy BN, Homesley HD, Graham JE, Heller PB.** Surgical pathologic spread patterns of endometrial cancer. *Cancer* 1987;60:2035–41.

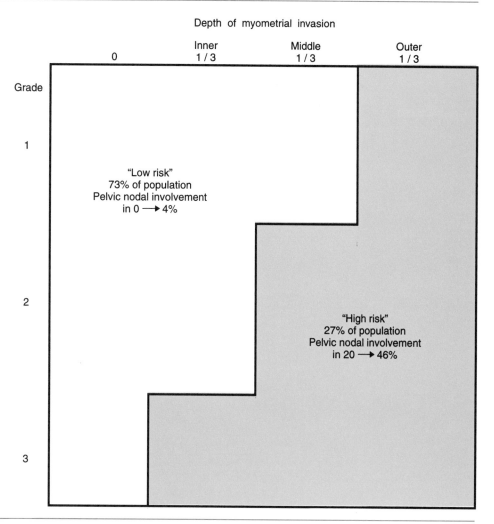

Figure 31.5.   The risk of pelvic lymph node metastasis with grade and depth of myometrial penetration in clinical Stage I endometrial cancer. Adjuvant pelvic irradiation is recommended for the high-risk group but not for the low-risk group. (Reproduced with permission from **DiSaia PJ, Creasman WT.** Management of endometrial adenocarcinoma, stage I with surgical staging followed by tailored adjuvant radiation therapy. *Clin Obstet Gynecol* 1986;13:751.)

node metastasis (64). The incidence of lymph node metastasis also correlates with tumor size ($\leq$2 cm = 4%; >2 cm = 15%; entire cavity = 35%) (65). Extrauterine spread of disease increases the risk of lymph node metastasis. Adnexal metastasis increases the risk of pelvic and para-aortic nodal metastasis to 32% and 20%, respectively. Of patients with positive peritoneal cytology, 25% have positive pelvic nodes and 19% have positive para-aortic nodes (64).

At a minimum, high common iliac/para-aortic lymph node dissections should be performed in the presence of adnexal or cervical involvement, a large tumor (>2 cm), deep (>½) myometrial invasion, or a poorly differentiated endometrioid, papillary serous, or clear cell tumor. Pelvic lymph node biopsy may not be as important in patients with these risk factors, because most of these patients will be treated postoperatively with whole pelvis irradiation.

Because fewer than 10% of patients with lymphatic metastasis have grossly enlarged nodes, palpation is not an acceptable alternative to biopsy. Conversely, because almost all patients with lymph node metastases have one or more of the aforementioned risk factors, lymph node biopsies are not required in patients at very low risk for lymphatic metastasis (i.e., patients with small (<2 cm) grade 1 and 2 endometrial cancers with only superficial myometrial invasion). In addition, partial omentectomy should be considered in some high-risk patients, especially those with papillary serous and mixed müllerian tumors, which have a propensity for intra-abdominal spread and upper abdominal recurrence.

Extended surgical staging, including selective pelvic and para-aortic lymphadenectomy in patients with endometrial cancer, does not add significantly to the morbidity from hysterectomy, which is primarily related to other factors such as patient weight, age and race, operating time, and surgical technique. The complication rate with this type of surgery is approximately 20%; about 6% of these complications are serious. The most common complications are wound infection, embolic phenomena, excess blood loss, gastrointestinal injury or obstruction, and lymphocyst formation (68–72).

Surgical staging is extremely important when one considers the poor correlation between preoperative evaluation and clinical staging with surgical and pathologic findings. Cowles et al. (1985), comparing preoperative findings with surgical pathology, noted that tumor histology was changed in 27% of patients, tumor grade was changed in 34% of patients, and stage was changed in 51% of patients (73). In the Gynecologic Oncology Group series (144), 22% of 621 patients with clinical stage I endometrial cancer had evidence of extrauterine spread, including lymph node metastasis, adnexal spread, peritoneal implants, and positive peritoneal cytology discovered at staging laparotomy (Table 31.11) (64). Chen found extrauterine spread in clinical stages I (19%) and II (40%), with an overall incidence of 23.4% (74). Vardi et al. determined that 30 (19%) of 154 clinical stage I and II patients had extrauterine disease (75). Wolfson et al. retrospectively compared clinical and surgical stage with respect to survival in 156 patients with endometrial cancer. Surgery resulted in an increase in the stage in 12.4% of clinical stage I patients

Table 31.11   Surgical-Pathologic Findings in Clinical Stage I Endometrial Cancer

Surgical-Pathologic Finding	*Percentage*
Histology	
Adenocarcinoma	80
Adenosquamous	16
Other (papillary serous, clear cell)	4
Grade	
1	29
2	46
3	25
Nyometrial invasion	
None	14
Inner one-third	45
Middle one-third	19
Outer one-third	22
Lymph-vascular space invasion	15
Isthmic tumor	16
Adnexal involvement	5
Positive peritoneal cytology	12
Pelvic lymph node metastasis	9
Aortic lymph node metastasis	6
Other extrauterine metastasis	6

Modified from **Creasman WT, Morrow CP, Bundy BN, Homesley HD, Graham JE, Heller PB.** Surgical pathologic spread patterns of endometrial cancer. *Cancer* 1987;60:2035–41.

and 27.3% of clinical stage II patients. Surgical stage was found to be the most important factor affecting prognosis (76).

Surgical staging identifies most patients with extrauterine disease and has a significant impact on treatment decisions. Surgical staging also identifies patients with uterine risk factors, including deep myometrial invasion, cervical extension, and lymph-vascular space invasion. The identification of these factors allows a more rational approach to the use of postoperative adjuvant radiation therapy and hopefully will improve survival and spare many patients unnecessary exposure to radiation (77–84).

Prognostic Variables

Although the stage of disease is the most significant variable affecting survival, a number of other individual prognostic factors for disease recurrence or survival have been identified, including tumor grade, histopathology, depth of myometrial invasion, patient age, and surgical and pathologic evidence of extrauterine disease spread (Table 31.12). Other factors such as tumor size, peritoneal cytology, hormone receptor status, flow cytometric analysis, and oncogene perturbations have also been implicated as having prognostic importance.

Age

In general, younger women with endometrial cancer have a better prognosis than older women. Crissman et al. (85) and Christopherson et al. (77) observed no deaths related to disease in patients with endometrial cancer diagnosed before 50 years of age. Nilson and Koller demonstrated a 60.9% 5-year survival rate for patients who were older than 70 years of age compared with a 92.1% survival rate for patients younger than 50 years of age (86). Decreased survival was associated with an increased risk of extrauterine spread (38% vs. 21%) and deep myometrial invasion (57% vs. 24%) for these two age groups.

Increased risk of recurrence in older patients has also been related to a higher incidence of grade 3 tumors or unfavorable histologic subtypes. Lurain et al. found increasing patient age to be independently associated with disease recurrence in endometrial cancer (82). The mean age at diagnosis of patients who had recurrence or died of disease was 68.6 years (range 53–88 years) compared with 60.3 years (range 27–83 years) for patients without recurrence. For every 1-year increase in age, the estimated rate of recurrence increased 7%. None of the patients under 50 years of age developed recurrent cancer, compared with 12% of patients aged 50–75 years and 33% of patients older than 75 year of age. Other authors have noted similar findings.

Histologic Type

Nonendometrioid histologic subtypes account for approximately 10% of endometrial cancers and carry an increased risk of recurrence and distant spread (87, 88). In a retrospective review of 388 patients treated at the Mayo Clinic for endometrial cancer, 52 (13%) were uncommon histologic subtypes, including 20 adenosquamous, 14 papillary serous, 11 clear cell, and seven undifferentiated carcinomas. In contrast to the 92% survival

Table 31.12   Prognostic Variables in Endometrial Carcinoma

Age	Lymph node metastasis
Histologic type	Intraperitoneal tumor
Histologic grade	Tumor size
Myometrial invasion	Peritoneal cytology
Lymph-vascular space invasion	Hormone receptor status
Isthmus-cervix extension	DNA ploidy/proliferative index
Adnexal involvement	oncogene amplification/expression

rate among patients with endometrioid tumors, the overall survival for patients with one of these more aggressive subtypes was only 33%. At the time of surgical staging, 62% of the patients with an unfavorable histologic subtype had extrauterine spread of disease (87).

Histologic Grade

Histologic grade of the endometrial tumor is strongly associated with prognosis (64, 69, 79–84). Lurain et al. noted that recurrences developed in 7.7% of grade 1 tumors, 10.5% of grade 2 tumors, and 36.1% of grade 3 tumors. Patients with grade 3 tumors were over 5 times more likely to have a recurrence than were patients with grade 1 and 2 tumors. The 5-year disease-free survival rates for patients with grades 1 and 2 tumors were 92% and 86%, respectively, compared with 64% for patients with grade 3 tumors (82). Sutton et al. reported similar results, noting recurrences in 9% of patients with grade 1 and 2 tumors compared with 39% of patients with grade 3 lesions (80). Increasing tumor anaplasia is associated with deep myometrial invasion, cervical extension, lymph node metastasis, and both local recurrence and distant metastasis.

Myometrial Invasion

Because access to the lymphatic system increases as cancer invades into the outer one-half of the myometrium, increasing depth of invasion has been associated with increasing likelihood of extrauterine spread and recurrence (63, 81, 84). Boronow et al. confirmed the association of depth of myometrial invasion with extrauterine disease and lymph node metastases (63). Only 1% of patients without demonstrable myometrial invasion had pelvic lymph node metastasis, compared with patients with outer one-third myometrial invasion who had 25% pelvic and 17% aortic lymph node metastases. Survival also decreases with increasing depth of myometrial invasion. In general, patients with non-invasive or superficially invasive tumors have an 80–90% 5-year survival rate, whereas those with deeply invasive tumors have a 60% survival rate. The most sensitive indicator of the effect of myometrial invasion on survival is distance from the tumor-myometrial junction to the uterine serosa. Patients with tumors that are less than 5 mm from the serosal surface are at much higher risk for recurrence and death than those with tumors more than 5 mm from the serosal surface (89, 90).

Lymph-Vascular Space Invasion

Lymph-vascular space invasion (LVSI) appears to be an independent risk factor for recurrence and death from all types of endometrial cancer (84, 91–93). The overall incidence of LVSI in early endometrial cancer is about 15%, although it increases with increasing tumor grade and depth of myometrial invasion. Hanson et al. reported LVSI in 2% of grade 1 tumors and 5% of superficially invasive tumors compared with 42% of grade 3 tumors and 70% of deeply invasive tumors (91). Aalders et al. reported deaths in 26.7% of patients with clinical stage I disease who had LVSI compared with 9.1% of patients without LVSI (84). Likewise, Abeler et al. reported an 83% 5-year survival rate for patients without demonstrable LVSI compared with a 64.5% survival rate for those in whom LVSI was present (92). Using multivariate analysis, Ambros and Kurman determined that depth of myometrial invasion, DNA ploidy, and associated with vascular invasion changes correlated significantly with survival for patients with stage I endometrial adenocarcinomas (93).

Isthmus-Cervix Extension

The location of the tumor within the uterus is important. Involvement of the uterine isthmus, cervix, or both is associated with an increased risk of extrauterine disease and lymph node metastasis as well as recurrence. DiSaia et al. reported that if the fundus of the uterus alone was involved with tumor there was a 13% recurrence rate, whereas if the lower uterine segment or cervix was involved with occult tumor, there was a 44% recurrence rate (79). In a subsequent Gynecologic Oncology Group study, Morrow et al. found that tumor involvement of the isthmus or cervix without evidence of extrauterine disease was associated with a 16% recurrence rate and a relative risk of 1.6 (69). Patients with cervical involvement also tended to have higher grade and larger and more deeply invasive tumors, undoubtedly contributing to the increased risk of recurrence.

Adnexal Involvement

Most patients with adnexal spread have other poor prognostic factors that place them at high risk for recurrence. For the 20% of patients with adnexal spread as their only high-risk factor, however, the survival rate has been reported to be as high as 85% (69).

Peritoneal Cytology

The significance of malignant peritoneal cytology in endometrial cancer is a controversial issue (94). Several reports in the literature have noted increased recurrence rates and decreased survival rates and, on this basis, have recommended treatment in the presence of positive cytology. In 1981, Creasman et al. reported positive peritoneal cytology in 26 (16%) of 167 patients with clinical stage I adenocarcinoma of the endometrium (95). Recurrent cancer developed in 10 (38%) of these 26 patients, compared with 14 (10%) of 141 patients with negative cytology. Positive peritoneal cytology was found to be associated with deep myometrial invasion, cervical involvement, adnexal spread, and lymph node metastasis as well as a propensity for intra-abdominal disease recurrence. Several subsequent reports supported the observation that positive peritoneal cytology was associated with an increased risk of cancer recurrence. Most of the reports included patients with other evidence of extrauterine disease spread without appropriate multivariate analysis of patients who were incompletely staged. The Gynecologic Oncology Group study reported by Morrow et al., however, critically analyzed 1180 patients with clinical stage I and II endometrial cancer in whom appropriate surgical and pathologic staging was performed (69). Considering only the 697 patients for whom peritoneal cytology status and adequate follow-up was available, 25 (29%) of 86 patients with positive cytology developed recurrence, compared with 64 (10.5%) of 611 patients with negative cytology. They noted, however, that 17 of the 25 recurrences in the positive cytology group were outside the peritoneal cavity.

In contrast to these reports, an equal number of studies have found no significant relationship between malignant peritoneal cytology and an increased incidence of disease recurrence in early endometrial cancer. Lurain et al. prospectively evaluated peritoneal cytology in 157 patients with clinical stage I endometrial cancer in whom primary surgical therapy was performed (96). No treatment was directed specifically to positive cytology. Positive cytology was not associated with disease recurrence. Recurrence developed in five (17%) of 30 patients with positive cytology and in 11 (9%) of 127 patients with negative cytology. Of the five patients with positive peritoneal cytology who had disease recurrence, only one recurrence arose within the peritoneal cavity. Patients with malignant washings often had other poor prognostic factors: 37% deep myometrial invasion, 37% grade 3 tumors, 17% positive lymph nodes. Disease recurrence occurred in one of the patients with positive cytology but without other poor prognostic factors. A subsequent study from the same institution confirmed by multivariate analysis that positive peritoneal cytology was not an independent prognostic factor for endometrial cancer recurrence. Only six (22%) of the 27 patients with positive cytology as the only evidence of extrauterine disease spread suffered a recurrence, despite the lack of therapy directed toward this finding (82). More recently, Kadar and colleagues found that positive peritoneal cytology had an adverse effect on survival only if the endometrial cancer had spread to the adnexa, peritoneum, or lymph nodes but not if the disease was otherwise confined to the uterus (97). They noted more grade 3 tumors (41% vs. 19%), vascular invasion (18% vs. 6%), adnexal spread (18% vs. 4%), lymph node metastasis (29% vs. 8%), and intraperitoneal spread (18% vs. 2%) in patients with positive peritoneal cytology, which contributed to the overall recurrence rate of 47% in these patients. The 5-year survival rate for patients with positive peritoneal cytology with disease otherwise confined to the uterus exceeded 90%.

The following conclusions may be reached regarding the prognostic implications of peritoneal cytology:

1. Positive peritoneal cytology is associated with other known poor prognostic factors.

2. Positive peritoneal cytology in the absence of other evidence of extrauterine disease or poor prognostic factors probably has no significant effect on recurrence and survival.

3. Positive peritoneal cytology, when associated with other poor prognostic factors and/or extrauterine disease, increases the likelihood of distant as well as intra-abdominal disease recurrence and has a significant adverse effect on survival.

4. Use of several different therapeutic modalities has not resulted in any benefit to patients with endometrial cancer and positive peritoneal cytology.

Lymph Node Metastasis

Lymph node metastasis is the most important prognostic factor in clinical early-stage endometrial cancer. Of patients with clinical stage I disease, approximately 10% will have pelvic and 6% will have para-aortic lymph node metastases. Patients with lymph node metastases have almost a sixfold higher likelihood of developing recurrent cancer than patients without lymph node metastases. Lurain et al. reported a recurrence rate of 48% with positive lymph nodes, including 45% with positive pelvic nodes and 64% with positive aortic nodes, compared with 8% with negative nodes. The 5-year disease-free survival rate for patients with lymph node metastases was 54% compared with 90% for patients without lymph node metastases (82). The Gynecology Oncology Group found that the presence or absence of para-aortic lymph node metastasis was of paramount importance in determining prognosis. Of 48 para-aortic node-positive patients, 28 (58%) developed progressive or recurrent cancer, and only 36% of these patients were alive in 5 years compared with 85% of patients without para-aortic node involvement (69).

Intraperitoneal Tumor

Extrauterine metastasis, excluding peritoneal cytology and lymph node metastasis, occurs in about 4–6% of patients with clinical stage I endometrial cancer. Creasman et al. noted that gross intraperitoneal spread correlated with lymph node metastases; 51% of patients with intraperitoneal tumor had positive lymph nodes, whereas only 7% of patients without gross peritoneal spread had positive nodes (64). Extrauterine spread other than lymph node metastasis also is associated with tumor recurrence. Lurain et al. found that 50% of patients with extrauterine disease developed recurrence, compared with 11% of patients without extrauterine disease, making recurrence almost five times more likely in patients with extrauterine disease spread. The 5-year disease-free survival rate for patients with nonlymphatic extrauterine disease was 50% compared with 88% in the other patients (82).

Tumor Size

Tumor size is a significant prognostic factor for lymph node metastasis and survival in patients with endometrial cancer (65, 98). Schink et al. determined tumor size in 142 patients with clinical stage I endometrial cancer and found lymph node metastasis in 4% of patients with tumors <2 cm, in 15% of patient with tumors ≤2 cm, and in 35% of patients with tumors involving the entire uterine cavity (65). Tumor size better defined an intermediate-risk group for lymph node metastasis (i.e., patients with grade 2 tumors with less than one-half myometrial invasion). Overall, these patients had a 10% risk of lymph node metastasis, but there was no nodal metastasis associated with tumors ≤2 cm versus 18% when tumors were >2 cm. Five-year survival rates were 98% for patients with tumors ≤2 cm, 84% for patients with tumors >2 cm, and 64% for patients with tumors involving the whole uterine cavity (98).

Hormone Receptor Status

Estrogen receptor (ER) and progesterone receptor (PR) levels have been shown to be prognostic indicators for endometrial cancer independent of grade in several studies (99–104).

Patients whose tumors are positive for one or both receptors have longer survival times than patients whose carcinomas lack the corresponding receptors. Lioa et al. noted that even patients with metastasis had an improved prognosis with receptor-positive tumors (102). Progesterone receptor levels appear to be a stronger predictor of survival than ER. The higher the absolute level of the receptors, the better the prognosis.

DNA Ploidy/Proliferative Index

About two-thirds of endometrial adenocarcinomas have a diploid DNA content as determined by flow cytometric analysis (93, 103, 105, 106). The proportion of nondiploid tumors increases with stage, lack of tumor differentiation, and depth of myometrial invasion. In several studies, DNA content has been related to clinical course of the disease, with death rates generally reported to be higher in women whose tumors contained aneuploid populations of cells. The proliferative index is related to the prognosis (103, 106).

Oncogene Amplication/ Expression

Mutations in codons 12 or 13 of the K-*ras* oncogene have been reported in 10–20% of endometrial adenocarcinomas (107). In one study, the presence of mutations of K-*ras* appeared to be an independent unfavorable prognostic factor (108). Overexpression of the HER-2/*neu* oncogene, which encodes for a cell surface glycoprotein that is similar to the human epidermal growth factor receptor, has been identified in 10–15% of endometrial adenocarcinomas. It is more frequently found in women with metastatic disease, and overexpression has been related to diminished progression-free survival (109, 110). Alteration of the tumor suppressor gene P53 has been demonstrated in about 20% of endometrial carcinomas and has been associated with papillary serous cell type, advanced stage, and poor prognosis (111, 112).

Treatment

Surgery

Total abdominal hysterectomy and bilateral salpingo-oophorectomy are the primary operative procedures for carcinoma of the endometrium. The adnexa should be removed because they may be the site of microscopic metastasis, and patients with endometrial carcinoma are at increased risk for ovarian cancer occurring either simultaneously or developing later. Removal of a segment of vagina below the cervix is not necessary. An algorithm for the management of patients with stage I and IIa endometrial cancer is presented in Figure 31.6.

Laparotomy is performed through an abdominal incision that allows thorough intra-abdominal exploration and retroperitoneal lymph node dissection, if necessary. A lower abdominal midline vertical incision is most often employed, although a lower abdominal transverse, muscle-dividing incision (e.g., Maylard) or muscle-detaching incision (e.g., Cherney) usually provides adequate exposure. After opening the abdomen, peritoneal washings are obtained from the subdiaphragmatic area, paracolic gutters, and pelvis using 50 ml of normal saline for each specimen sent to the cytology laboratory for examination. Exploration of the abdomen and pelvis is then performed, noting particularly the diaphragm, liver, omentum, and pelvic and aortic lymph nodes. The uterus should be observed for tumor on the serosal surface. Any suspicious-looking lesions should be biopsied.

Total abdominal hysterectomy and bilateral salpingo-oophorectomy are performed following exploration of the abdominal area. The pelvic lymph nodes should be visualized and palpated, and any enlarged or suspicious nodes should be removed for histologic examination. Removal of a vaginal cuff is not necessary. The uterus is opened in the operating room, and tumor size, depth of myometrial invasion, and cervical extension are assessed. This information, along with the surgical findings and knowledge of the preoperative histology, influences whether pelvic and aortic lymph node dissection is indicated. The uterus is sent to the pathology laboratory, where tissue can be obtained for measurement of steroid hormone receptors and flow cytometry.

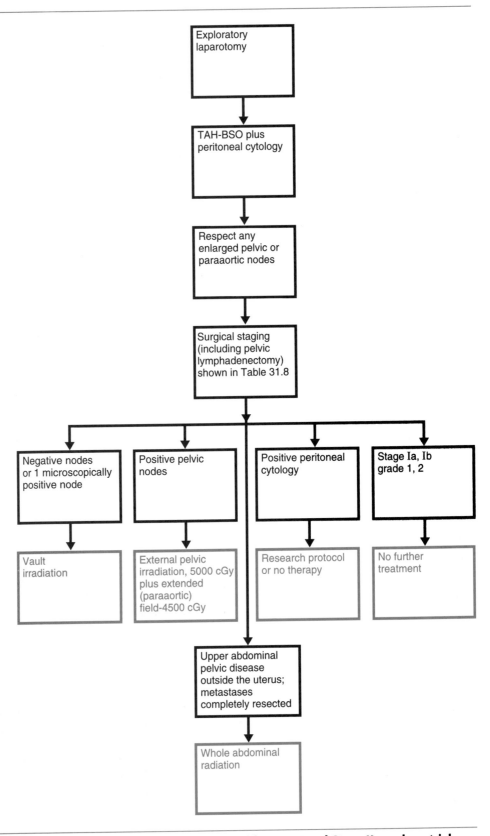

Figure 31.6   Management of patients with Stage I and Stage IIa endometrial carcinoma.

For patients in whom lymph node sampling is indicated, lower para-aortic lymph node resection can be accomplished by extending the pelvic peritoneal incisions over the common iliac arteries and lower aorta. A sample of lymph nodes along the upper common iliac vessels on either side and the fat pad overlying the vena cava are removed. Pelvic lymph node samples are obtained by removing nodes overlying the midportion of the external iliac artery and vein and within the obturator fossa above and along the obturator nerve. An omental biopsy or partial omentectomy may also be performed.

Vaginal Hysterectomy

Vaginal hysterectomy may be considered for selected patients who are extremely obese and have a poor medical status or for patients with extensive uterovaginal prolapse. The disadvantages to this approach are that bilateral salpingo-oophorectomy is often technically difficult and abdominal exploration and lymph node sampling cannot be performed. Vaginal hysterectomy is, therefore, particularly suitable for patients who are at low risk for extrauterine spread of disease, i.e., those with clinical stage I, well-differentiated tumors. Peters et al. reported a 94% survival among 56 patients with clinical stage I endometrial carcinoma treated with vaginal hysterectomy, with or without postoperative radiation therapy (mostly brachytherapy). Seventy-five percent had grade 1 lesions (113). Malkasian et al. (114) and Bloss et al. (115) reported similar good results. Vaginal hysterectomy is clearly preferable to radiation therapy alone but should generally be reserved for specific patients.

Laparoscopic Management

Recent advances in endoscopic surgery have allowed application of a laparoscopic approach to the management of endometrial cancer. Since 1992, several reports have documented the feasibility of laparoscopically assisted vaginal hysterectomy with bilateral salpingo-oophorectomy and laparoscopic retroperitoneal lymph node sampling for staging and treatment of patients with endometrial cancer (116–119). Childers et al. laparoscopically managed 59 endometrial cancer patients; 29 of these patients had retroperitoneal lymph node sampling (118). Boike et al. compared the results of laparoscopic versus traditional laparotomy management of 44 patients with endometrial cancer (119). Of 20 patients in whom laparoscopic management was successful, 15 had both pelvic and para-aortic lymph node sampling and four had pelvic node sampling only. There was no difference in the number of lymph nodes (19 vs. 17) removed in the laparoscopy and laparotomy groups, respectively. Patients undergoing laparoscopic management had shorter hospital stays (2.5 vs. 5.0 days) and a lower overall complication rate, although all serious complications (one ureteral injury and two small bowel herniations through 12-mm trocar sites) occurred in the laparoscopy group. Although it seems reasonable that many patients with endometrial cancer can undergo successful laparoscopic management, more experience with the technique and prospective studies are necessary to determine the indications for and complications of this approach.

Radical Hysterectomy

Radical hysterectomy, with removal of the parametria and upper vagina as well as bilateral pelvic lymphadenectomy, does not improve survival of patients with clinical stage I disease compared with extrafascial hysterectomy and bilateral salpingo-oophorectomy alone (120–123). Radical hysterectomy also increases both intraoperative and postoperative morbidity and should, therefore, not be performed for treatment of apparent early endometrial cancer.

Radiation Therapy

Primary surgery followed by radiation therapy has become the most widely accepted treatment for early stage endometrial cancers. However, approximately 5–15% of patients with endometrial cancer have severe medical conditions that render them unsuitable for surgery (61). These patients tend to be elderly and obese with multiple chronic or acute medical illnesses, such as hypertension, cardiac disease, and diabetes mellitus as well as pulmonary, renal, and neurologic diseases.

Several series have demonstrated that radiation therapy is effective treatment for patients with inoperable endometrial cancer (Table 31.13) (124–133). Kupelian et al. from the M.D. Anderson Cancer Center reported on the treatment of 120 patients with clinical stage I disease and 17 patients with clinical stage II endometrial cancer treated with radiation alone, 85% of whom received only intracavitary irradiation. Because of the high incidence of death caused by intercurrent illness in this group of patients, the 5- and 10-year overall survival rates were only 55% and 28% compared with disease-specific survival rates of 87% and 85%, respectively. There was no difference in disease-specific survival rates between patients with stage I and stage II disease. Intrauterine cancer recurred in 14% and extrauterine pelvic disease recurred in 3% of patients. The authors also treated 15 patients with stage III and IV disease, usually with a combination of external beam and intracavitary radiation therapy, yielding a 5-year disease-specific survival rate of 49%. Five patients (3%) had serious late complications of radiation therapy (133).

Although it is generally agreed that intracavitary irradiation is necessary to achieve adequate local control, the indications for external beam radiation therapy in the primary treatment of endometrial cancer are less well defined. Patients with cervical involvement and known or suspected extrauterine pelvic spread undoubtedly would benefit from external beam radiation therapy. Theoretically, external beam irradiation could also sterilize microscopic nodal disease and possibly increase the radiation dose to deep myometrial/subserosal uterine disease that may receive an insufficient dose from intracavitary irradiation alone. A correlation between tumor grade and recurrence has been noted by several authors. Grigsby et al. found that the 5-year progression-free survival rates for patients with medically inoperable stage I disease who were treated with radiation therapy alone was 94% for grade 1, 92% for grade 2, and 78% for grade 3 tumors (130). Therefore, patients with grade 3 tumors and a known propensity for deep myometrial invasion and lymph node metastasis may also benefit from external beam therapy.

The decision to treat a patient who has endometrial cancer with radiation alone must involve a careful analysis of the relative risks and benefits of surgery. Although radiation

Table 31.13   Review of Recent Series of Endometrial Carcinoma Treated with Radiation Alone

Authors	Ref.	Year	Stage	Number of Patients	Local Recurrence Rate (%)	Disease-Specific Survival Rate (%)	Major Complication Rate (%)
Landgren et al.	(124)	1976	I–II	124	22	68	7
			III–IV	26	42	22	
Abayomi et al.	(125)	1982	I–II	50	26	78	15
			III–IV	16	—	10	
Patanaphan et al.	(126)	1985	I–II	42	14	64	2
			III–IV	10	60	20	
Jones et al.	(127)	1986	I–II	146	22	61	4
			III	14	79	14	
Varia et al.	(128)	1987	I–II	73	21	43	10
Wang et al.	(129)	1987	I–II	41	22	76	5
Grigsby et al.	(130)	1987	I	69	9	88	16
Taghian et al.	(131)	1988	I–II	94	6	70	17
			III–IV	10	10	27	
Lehoczky et al.	(132)	1991	I	171	20	75	0
Kupelian et al.	(133)	1993	I–II	137	14	85	3
			III–IV	15	32	49	

From **Kupelian PA, Eifel PJ, Tornos C, Burke TW, Delclos L, Oswald MJ.** Treatment of endometrial carcinoma with radiation therapy alone. *Int J Radiat Oncol Biol Phys* 1993;27:817–24.

alone can produce excellent survival and local control, it should be considered for definitive treatment only if the operative risk is estimated to exceed the 10–15% risk of uterine recurrence expected with radiation treatment alone.

Postoperative Adjuvant Therapy

Postoperative therapy should be based on prognostic factors determined by surgical and pathologic staging. Patients can generally be classified into three treatment categories: those who show a low incidence of recurrence and a high rate of cure without any postoperative therapy (low risk), those who have a reduced rate of surgical cure but may or may not benefit from additional therapy (intermediate risk), and those who have a high rate of recurrence and a low survival rate without postoperative therapy (high risk) (Table 31.14). Options for postoperative management in these patients include observation, vaginal vault irradiation, external pelvic irradiation, extended field (pelvic and para-aortic) irradiation, whole abdominal irradiation, intraperitoneal ^{32}P, progestins, or systemic chemotherapy (Fig. 31.6).

Observation

Patients with grade 1 and 2 lesions without myometrial invasion (stages Ia G1, G2) have an excellent prognosis and require no postoperative therapy. In the Gynecologic Oncology Group study reported by Morrow et al., there were no recurrences and a 100% disease-free 5-year survival rate occurred in the 91 patients in this category, 72 of whom had received no additional treatment after hysterectomy (69). Other investigators have reported equally favorable results with only surgical therapy in similar patients.

Vaginal Vault Irradiation

Numerous studies have shown that **the incidence of vaginal recurrence in patients with tumors apparently confined to the uterus can be reduced from as high as 15% to**

Table 31.14   Postoperative Management of Endometrial Carcinoma Based on Surgical-Pathologic Findings and Stage

Surgical-Pathology Findings	Stage	Postoperative Treatment
Low Risk		
G1, G2, no myoinvasion	Ia G1, G2	None
No cervix/isthmus invasion		
Negative peritoneal cytology		
No lymph-vascular space invasion		
No evidence of metastasis		
Intermediate Risk		
G1, G2 less than one-half myoinvasion	Ib G1, G2	Vaginal cuff irradiation
G3, no myoinvasion	Ia G3	
G3, less than one-half myoinvasion	Ib G3	Pelvic vs. vaginal cuff irradiation
G1, G2 isthmus/cervix extension	IIa G1, G2	
G1, G2, G3, more than one-half myoinvasion	Ic G1, G2, G3	Pelvic irradiation plus vaginal cuff boost
G3 isthmus/cervix extension	IIa G3	
G1, G2, G3, cervix invasion	IIb G1, G2, G3 LVSI	
Positive peritoneal cytology	IIIa (+ cytology)	Progestin/^{32}P
High Risk		
Adnexal/serosal/parametrial spread	IIIa G1, G2, G3	Pelvic and vaginal irradiation
Vaginal metastasis	IIIb G1, G2, G3	(extended field radiation therapy if + aortic/common iliac lymph nodes)
Lymph node metastasis	IIIc G1, G2, G3	
Bladder/rectal invasion	IVa	Pelvic and vaginal irradiation
Intraperitoneal spread	IV	Whole abdomen irradiation Systemic chemotherapy

1–2% by the administration of vaginal irradiation. This find is important because vaginal vault recurrence carries a poor prognosis. Lotocki et al. reported that preoperative or postoperative vaginal vault radium use decreased the incidence of vaginal recurrence from 14 to 1.7% and improved 5-year survival rates from 75 to 90% (78). Piver et al. reported on the 10-year follow-up of a randomized trial comparing surgery alone (total abdominal hysterectomy and bilateral salpingo-oophorectomy) with preoperative or postoperative radium treatment in patients with clinical stage I endometrial adenocarcinoma. The incidence of vaginal recurrence was 7.5% with hysterectomy alone, 4.5% with preoperative intracavitary radium followed by hysterectomy, and 0% for hysterectomy followed by postoperative vaginal radium (134). In a subsequent study, Piver and Hempling treated 92 patients with surgical stage I disease who had grade 1 or 2 tumors with less than 50% myometrial invasion with total abdominal hysterectomy and bilateral salpingo-oopherectomy and postoperative vaginal cesium or radium. There were no recurrences, and the 5-year estimated disease-free survival rate was 99%. There was only one minor complication, proctitis, which responded to conservative treatment (135).

In the Gynecologic Oncology Group study of surgical and pathologic risk factors and outcomes, none of the three recurrences in the vaginal radiation implant group were vaginal or pelvic, whereas 7.4% of recurrences in the pelvic radiation therapy group were vaginal, and 18.2% of recurrences in the group receiving no adjuvant radiation were vaginal. The investigators concluded that postoperative vaginal cuff irradiation reduced local recurrence and had a therapeutic ratio superior to whole pelvis irradiation in patients at risk for isolated vaginal cuff recurrence (69).

Postoperative vaginal irradiation is most often administered using colpostats to deliver a surface dose of 6000–7000 cGy to the upper vagina. More recently, some centers have used afterloading outpatient techniques at high-dose rates (136). Morbidity is low, although vaginal stenosis and dyspareunia may be a problem for postmenopausal patients if there is no regular vaginal dilation. Patients most likely to benefit from vaginal irradiation are those who have surgical stage I grade 1 and 2 tumors with superficial (<½) myometrial invasion or grade 3 tumors with no invasion and some patients with stage IIa disease who otherwise meet the aforementioned criteria.

External Pelvic Irradiation

External pelvic irradiation decreases the risk of recurrence of pelvic disease after hysterectomy in certain high-risk groups. Patients found to benefit most from adjuvant postoperative whole pelvis irradiation are those with cervical involvement, pelvic lymph node metastases, pelvic disease outside the uterus (adnexa, parametria), and patients with clinical stage I disease who are at significant risk of nodal metastasis (grade 3 tumors with any degree of myometrial invasion, grade 1 and 2 tumors with more than one-half myometrial invasion, large (>2 cm) grade 2 tumors with superficial myometrial invasion, and any grade tumor with lymph-vascular space invasion) (137).

Piver and Hempling treated 41 endometrial cancer patients with postoperative pelvic irradiation (5000–5040 cGy) who had grade 3 tumors or deep myometrial invasion and histologically negative para-aortic lymph nodes (pelvic lymph nodes not sampled). Four patients (9.7%) developed recurrences, but only one of the recurrences (2.4%) was within the treatment field, and the 5-year estimated disease-free survival rate was 88% (135). In the Gynecologic Oncology Group study, the pelvic recurrence rate in the surgery-only group of patients (31.8%) was higher than that in the group that received postoperative external beam radiation therapy (16.8%) (69).

In 1980, Aalders et al. reported the only randomized study performed to evaluate the possible benefit of postoperative pelvic irradiation in clinical stage I endometrial cancer (84). Following total abdominal hysterectomy and bilateral salpingo-oophorectomy, all 540 patients received vaginal vault radium and were then randomized to receive either 4000 cGy whole pelvis irradiation or no further therapy. The addition of pelvic irradiation did not affect the overall 5-year survival rate. Patients receiving pelvic irradiation had a lower failure rate for pelvic disease but a higher failure rate for distant metastasis. Of note, patients with grade 3 tumors and more than one-half myometrial invasion had a lower rate of death from cancer if they received postoperative pelvic irradiation (18.2 vs. 27.5%). This study has been criticized for the lack of complete surgical staging (no lymph node biopsies were performed) and the relatively low dose of external beam irradiation (4000 cGy) is used.

Postoperative whole pelvis external beam radiation usually involves the delivery of 4500–5040 cGy in 180 cGy daily fractions over 5–6 weeks to a field encompassing the upper one-half of the vagina interiorly, the lower border of the L4 vertebral body superiorly, and 1 cm lateral to the margins of the bony pelvis (Chapter 30). The dose of radiation at the surface of the vaginal apex is usually boosted to 6000–7000 cGy by a variety of techniques. The most frequently reported side effects are gastrointestinal problems, usually abdominal cramps and diarrhea, although more serious complications such as bleeding, proctitis, bowel obstruction, and fistula can occur and may require surgical correction. The urinary system may also be affected in the form of hematuria, cystitis, or fistula. The overall complication rate ranges from 25 to 40%; however, the rate of serious complications requiring surgical intervention is much lower (about 1.5–3%).

Patients at high risk for recurrence may benefit from pelvic irradiation in two ways. The failure rate for pelvic disease is reduced and, at least in patients with grade 3 tumors and deep myometrial invasion, survival rates also seem to be improved. Patients with cervical extension and extrauterine pelvic disease, including adnexal spread, parametrial involvement, and pelvic lymph node metastases in the absence of extrapelvic disease, should also benefit from postoperative pelvic irradiation.

Extended Field Irradiation

Patients with histologically proven para-aortic node metastases who have no other evidence of disease spread outside the pelvis should be treated with extended field irradiation. The entire pelvis, common iliac lymph nodes, and para-aortic lymph nodes are included within the radiation field. The para-aortic radiation dose is limited to 4500–5000 cGy. **Extended field radiotherapy appears to improve survival in patients with endometrial cancer and positive para-aortic lymph nodes** (138–141).

Potish et al. reported 5-year survival rates of 47% and 43% for patients with surgically confirmed para-aortic lymph node metastases only and para-aortic as well as pelvic lymph node metastases, respectively, using postoperative extended field irradiation (Fig. 31.7). They reported only one case of severe enteric morbidity in 48 patients for a complication rate of 2% (138). Rose et al. compared patients with positive para-aortic nodes treated with megestrol acetate alone versus megestrol acetate and extended field irradiation. The survival rate in the patients receiving extended field irradiation was significantly better, 53% versus 12.5% (139). Feuer and Calanog treated 18 patients with positive para-aortic nodes. Five-year survival rates were 67% for microscopic nodal disease and 17% for gross nodal disease (140).

Whole Abdominal Irradiation

Whole abdominal radiation therapy is usually reserved for patients with stage III and IV endometrial cancer. It may also be considered for patients who have papillary serous or mixed müllerian tumors, which have a propensity for upper abdominal recurrence (142–146). The recommended dose to the whole abdomen is 3000 cGy in 20 daily fractions of 150 cGy with kidney shielding at 1500–2000 cGy, along with an additional 1500 cGy to the para-aortic lymph nodes and 2000 cGy to the pelvis. Gastrointestinal side effects include nausea, vomiting, and diarrhea, sometimes making it necessary to interrupt therapy, but it is rare for patients not to finish treatment because of these symptoms. Hematologic toxicity can be expected to occur during whole abdominal irradiation, but it is usu-

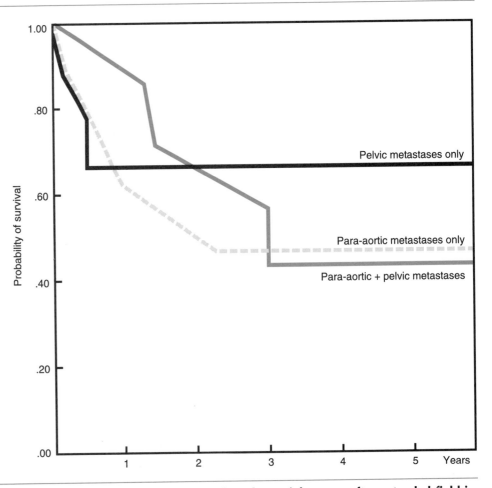

Figure 31.7   Survival of patients with endometrial cancer after extended-field irradiation for surgically confirmed para-aortic lymph node metastasis. (Reproduced with permission from **Potish RA, Twiggs LB, Adcock LL, Savage JE, Levitt SH, Prem KA.** Para-aortic lymph node radiotherapy in cancer of the uterine corpus. *Obstet Gynecol* 1985;65:251.)

ally mild. The incidence of late complications, mainly chronic diarrhea and small bowel obstruction, is generally low (5–10%).

Potish et al. treated 27 patients who had surgical stage III endometrial cancer with whole abdominal irradiation. Patients with spread to the adnexa, positive peritoneal cytology, or both had a 5-year, relapse-free survival rate of 90%, whereas all patients with macroscopic disease beyond the adnexa had recurrence (142). Similar results were reported by Greer and Hamberger (143). Martinez and colleagues have advocated the use of adjuvant whole abdominal radiation therapy for patients with high-risk stage I and II endometrial carcinoma, including those with deep myometrial invasion, high-grade tumors, and papillary serous histology, because of the high proportion of recurrences in the upper abdomen (145, 146). They reported a 5-year recurrence-free survival rate of 85%. Unfortunately, most recurrences continue to occur in the upper abdomen in all of these patients despite this type of radiation therapy. In summary, it is reasonable to use whole abdominal irradiation postoperatively to treat patients with adnexal or upper abdominal disease, such as in the omentum, that has been completely excised and in patients who are at high risk for intra-abdominal recurrence, such as those with papillary serous tumors, but it should not be used in patients with gross residual intraperitoneal disease.

Intraperitoneal ^{32}P

Creasman et al. reported apparent favorable results for the treatment of positive peritoneal cytology with intraperitoneal ^{32}P (95). In 23 patients who had positive washings, treatment with ^{32}P resulted in a lower recurrence rate than in historical controls, but the groups differed in risk factors, making conclusions regarding the efficacy of the treatment questionable. Later, Soper et al. reported that when ^{32}P was combined with external pelvic irradiation, 29% of patients suffered serious bowel complications requiring surgical intervention and two patients died of operative complications (147). At present, the role of ^{32}P in the postoperative management of endometrial cancer patients with positive cytology is limited because of the lack of evidence of therapeutic benefit and the complications that occur when this agent is combined with external pelvic irradiation, which these patients often receive for prevention of local pelvic recurrence.

Progestins

Most endometrial cancers have receptors to both estrogen and progesterone, and progestins have been used successfully to treat metastatic endometrial cancer. Because of this effect, postoperative adjuvant progestin therapy has been attempted to reduce the risk of recurrence. This therapy is attractive because it provides systemic treatment and has few side effects. Unfortunately, three large randomized, placebo-controlled studies have failed to identify a benefit for adjuvant progestin therapy (148–150).

Conversely, Piver et al. treated 25 patients with positive peritoneal cytology as their only evidence of disease spread outside the uterus with adjuvant progestin for 1 year postoperatively (151). Twenty-two patients had a second-look laparoscopy, and only one patient was found to have persistent intraperitoneal malignant cells. No patient had evidence of recurrent cancer. Therefore, progestins may have a role in treating positive peritoneal cytology in this setting.

Chemotherapy

Adjuvant cytotoxic chemotherapy has only been studied in a few trials. The Gynecologic Oncology Group treated 181 patients having poor prognostic factors with postoperative pelvic plus para-aortic irradiation and then randomly assigned patients to receive no further therapy or *doxorubicin (Adriamycin)* chemotherapy. At 5 years of observation, there was no difference in recurrence rates between the two groups (152).

Stringer and colleagues at the M.D. Anderson Cancer Center treated 33 early-stage, "high-risk" patients with postoperative adjuvant *cisplatin, doxorubicin,* and *cyclophosphamide* (PAC) chemotherapy. The presence of extrauterine disease was the only significant risk factor for recurrence, with eight of nine recurrences occurring in this group. No benefit to adjuvant chemotherapy could be demonstrated (153).

Stage II

Endometrial cancer involving the cervix either contiguously or by lymphatic spread has a poorer prognosis than disease confined to the corpus (154–169). Preoperative assessment of cervical involvement is difficult. **Endocervical curettage has relatively high false-positive (50–80%) and false-negative rates.** Histologic proof of cancer infiltration of the cervix or the presence of obvious tumor on the cervix is the only reliable means of diagnosing cervical involvement, although ultrasound, hysteroscopy, or MRI may demonstrate cervical invasion.

The relatively small number of true stage II cases in reported series and the lack of randomized, prospective studies precludes formulation of a definitive treatment plan. Three areas must be addressed in any treatment plan:

1. For optimal results, the uterus should be removed in all patients.

2. Because the incidence of pelvic lymph node metastases is about 36% in stage II endometrial cancer, any treatment protocol should include treatment of these lymph nodes.

3. Because the incidence of disease spread outside the pelvis to the para-aortic lymph nodes, adnexal structures, and upper abdomen is higher than in stage I disease, attention should be directed to evaluating and treating extrapelvic disease.

Two main approaches have usually been taken to the treatment of stage II disease:

1. Radical hysterectomy, bilateral salpingo-oophorectomy, and bilateral pelvic lymphadenectomy.

2. Combined radiation and surgery (external pelvic irradiation and intracavitary radium or cesium followed in 6 weeks by total abdominal hysterectomy and bilateral salpingo-oophorectomy).

An initial radical surgical approach to treatment of clinical stage II endometrial cancer has the advantage of allowing accurate surgical and pathologic information to be obtained. Conversely, many patients with endometrial cancer are elderly, obese, and have medical problems; therefore, this approach may be unsuitable. In addition, reported results are no better than with combined radiation and less radical surgical therapy. Rutledge recommended that the use of radical hysterectomy be limited to patients with anatomic problems that prevent optimum dosimetry or other conditions that conflict with the use of radiation therapy.

The most common approach to the management of clinical stage II endometrial cancer has been the use of external and intracavitary irradiation followed by extrafascial hysterectomy. This combined approach has resulted in 5-year survival rates of 60–80%, with severe gastrointestinal or urologic complications occurring in about 10% of patients. Patients with clinical stage II disease that is medically inoperable are usually treated with external beam irradiation and one or two intracavitary insertions. Compared with combined radiation and surgery, the results with radiation alone are diminished, but about 50% of patients will be long-term survivors (Table 31.13) (122).

Another method for management of clinical stage II endometrial cancer that is gaining favor is an initial surgical approach followed by irradiation. This method is based on the difficulty in establishing the preoperative diagnosis of cervical involvement in the absence of a gross cervical tumor, the evidence that radiation is equally effective when given following hysterectomy, and the high incidence of extrapelvic disease when the cervix is involved. Exploratory laparotomy with an extrafascial or modified radical hysterectomy, bilateral salpingo-oophorectomy, peritoneal washings for cytology, resection of grossly enlarged pelvic nodes, and selective high common iliac and lower para-aortic lymphadenectomy are performed. These procedures are followed by appropriate pelvic or extended field external and intravaginal irradiation, depending on the results of surgical staging. Excellent results have been reported using this treatment scheme (165–167).

Clinical Stages III and IV   Clinical stage III disease accounts for approximately 7–10% of all endometrial carcinomas (170–176). Patients usually have clinical evidence of disease spread to the parametria, pelvic sidewall, or adnexal structures; less frequently, there is spread to the vagina or pelvic peritoneum. Treatment for stage III endometrial carcinoma must be based on individual needs, but initial operative evaluation and treatment should be considered because of the high risk of occult lymph node metastases and intraperitoneal spread when disease is known to extend outside the uterus into the pelvis. In the presence of an adnexal mass, surgery should be performed initially to determine the nature of the mass. Surgery should also be performed to determine the extent of disease and to remove the bulk of the disease if possible. This procedure should include peritoneal washings for cytologic examination, selective para-aortic and pelvic lymphadenectomy as well as removable of any enlarged lymph nodes, biopsy or excision of any suspicious-looking areas within the peritoneal cavity, and partial omentectomy and peritoneal biopsies. Except in patients with bulky parametrial disease, total abdominal hysterectomy and bilateral salpingo-oophorectomy should be performed. Surgical eradication of all macroscopic disease should be the goal because this is of major prognostic importance in the management of patients with clinical stage III disease. Postoperative radiotherapy can then be tailored to the extent of disease.

Results of therapy depend on the extent and nature of disease. Bruckman et al. reported a 5-year survival rate of 54% for all patients with stage III disease; however, the survival was 80% when only adnexal metastases were present, compared with 15% when other extrauterine pelvic structures were involved (170). Patients with surgical and pathologic stage III disease have a much better survival rate (40%) than those with clinical stage III disease (16%) (172). Patients who are treated with combined surgery and irradiation fare better than patients who receive radiation therapy alone (176).

Stage IV endometrial adenocarcinoma, in which tumor invades the bladder or rectum or extends outside the pelvis, makes up approximately 3% of cases (176, 177). Treatment of stage IV disease depends on the individual patient but usually involves a combination of surgery, radiation therapy, and systemic hormonal therapy or chemotherapy. The objective of the surgery and radiation therapy is to achieve local disease control in the pelvis to palliate bleeding, discharge, and complications involving the bladder and rectum. Aalders et al. reported control of pelvic disease in 28% of 72 patients with stage IV disease treated with radiation alone or in combination with surgery or progestins or both (177). Pelvic exenteration may be considered in the very rare patient in whom disease is limited to the bladder or rectum (178, 179).

Recurrent Disease

Approximately one-fourth of patients treated for early endometrial cancer will develop recurrent disease. More than one-half of the recurrences will develop within 2 years, and about three-fourths will occur within 3 years of initial treatment. The distribution of recurrences is dependent in large part on the type of primary therapy-surgery alone versus surgery plus local/regional radiotherapy. In the Gynecologic Oncology Group study of 390 surgical patients with stage I disease, vaginal/pelvic recurrences were noted to make up 53% of all recurrences in the group treated with surgery alone, whereas only 30% of recurrences were vaginal/pelvic in the group treated with combined surgery-radiotherapy (69). Therefore, after combined surgery and radiotherapy (vaginal or external beam), 70% or more of patients who fail treatment will have distant metastases and most of these will not have evidence of local/pelvic recurrence. The most common sites of extrapelvic metastases are the lung, abdomen, lymph nodes (aortic, supraclavicular, inguinal), liver, brain, and bone. In general, patients with isolated vaginal recurrences fare better than those with pelvic recurrences, who have a better chance of cure than those with distant metastases. Patients who initially have well-differentiated tumors or who develop recurrent cancer more than 3 years after the primary therapy also tend to have an improved outlook.

In 1984, Aalders et al. reported on 379 patients with recurrent endometrial cancer seen at the Norwegian Radium Hospital from 1960 to 1976 (180). Site of recurrence was local/regional in 190 patients (50%), distant in 108 patients (28%), and local and distant in 81 patients (21%). The median time of recurrence was 14 months for patients with local recurrences and 19 months for patients with distant metastases. Of all recurrences, 34% were detected within 1 year and 76% were detected within 3 years of primary treatment. At the time of diagnosis of recurrence, 32% of patients had no symptoms. Vaginal bleeding was the most common symptom associated with local recurrence, and pelvic pain was most often present with pelvic recurrence. Hemoptysis was the initial symptom in 32% of patients with lung metastases, but 45% of patients with lung metastases were asymptomatic and disease was detected by routine chest x-ray. Only 9% of patients with metastases at other sites were asymptomatic; most had pain (37%) or other symptoms, such as anorexia, nausea and vomiting, or ascites related to intra-abdominal carcinomatosis, neurologic symptoms such as seizures from brain metastases, or jaundice caused by liver metastases.

Overall, only 29 (7.7%) of the 379 patients were alive without evidence of disease from 3 to 19 years. This included 22 (12%) patients with local/pelvic recurrence, five (5%) patients with distant metastases, and two (2%) patients with both local and distant recurrences. The best results were obtained in the 42 patients with vaginal vault recurrences who were treated with radiotherapy, resulting in a 24% survival. None of the 78 patients with pelvic soft tissue recurrence survived. Three patients (7%) with only lung metastases treated with progestins, two patients with lymph node metastases treated with combined radiotherapy and progestins, and two patients with local recurrence and lung metastases treated with a combination of radiation therapy, surgery, and progestins survived.

Surgery

A small subset of patients who develop recurrent endometrial cancer may benefit from surgical intervention. Pelvic or vaginal recurrence in patients who have not received prior pelvic irradiation is best treated by external irradiation plus some type of brachytherapy. Surgical resection of a metastatic vaginal nodule >2 cm in diameter prior to irradiation, however, may improve local control. Pretherapy investigation for extrapelvic metastasis in these patients may include surgical evaluation of the peritoneal cavity and retroperitoneal lymph nodes for evidence of subclinical metastases. Angel et al. found upper abdominal disease at laparotomy in three (37.5%) of eight patients with presumed localized pelvic recurrence (181). Presence of subclinical extrapelvic metastases was associated with larger pelvic tumor size (≥2 cm) and elevated serum CA125 levels. A few patients with intraperitoneal recurrence may benefit from laparotomy to relieve intestinal obstruction; tumor-reductive surgery may be performed prior to whole abdominal radiation therapy or systemic hormonal or chemotherapy.

Isolated central pelvic recurrence after irradiation is exceedingly rare. In patients with this type of recurrence, exploratory laparotomy may be performed with the plan to proceed with pelvic exenteration if there is no evidence of disease outside the pelvis and no lymph node metastases. Exenterative surgery for recurrent endometrial cancer in the pelvis has rarely been of value because of the high incidence of associated occult extrapelvic metastases. Of 36 patients reported by Barber and Brunschwig who underwent pelvic exenteration for recurrent endometrial carcinoma, 75% died of their cancer within 1 year of operation, and only 14% were alive at 5 years (179).

Radiation Therapy

Patients with isolated local and regional recurrences after initial surgical treatment of endometrial cancer should be treated with radiation therapy (182–186). The best local control and subsequent cure is usually achieved by a combination of external beam radiation therapy followed by a brachytherapy boost to deliver a total tumor dose of at least 6000 cGy. Women with low-volume disease limited to the pelvis have the best outcome. For patients with isolated vaginal recurrence treated with irradiation, reported survival rates range from 24 to 45%. For patients who have pelvic extension of disease after treatment with radiation, lower survival rates from 0 to 24% have been reported. Sears et al. noted that initial endometrial cancer grade 1, younger patient age at recurrence, recurrent tumor size ≤2 cm, time to recurrence more than 1 year, vaginal versus pelvic disease, and radiation therapy with brachytherapy boost were significant factors in determining control of pelvic disease and survival in patients with locally recurrent endometrial cancer (186).

Hormone Therapy

Kelley and Baker first described the use of progestational agents for treatment of metastatic endometrial cancer in 1961 (187). They observed an objective response rate of 29% in 21 patients. Reifenstein observed a beneficial response in 35% of 308 patients (188). Subsequent reports have noted somewhat less optimistic response rates, probably as a result of more strictly applied criteria for objective responses (Table 31.15) (189–192). Piver et al. (189) and Podratz et al. (190) noted objective responses rates of 16% and 11%, respec-

Table 31.15   Response to Progestin Therapy in Advanced or Recurrent Endometrial Cancer

Study	Progestin		Patients	Response Rate (%)
Piver et al. (1980)	HPC	1000 mg/wk IM	51	14
	MPA	1000 mg/wk IM	37	19
Podratz et al. (1985)	HPC	1–3g/wk IM	33	9
	MA	320 mg/d PO	81	11
Thigpen et al. (1986)	MPA	150 mg/d PO	219	14
		200 mg/d PO	138	26
		1000 mg/d PO	140	18

HPC, hydroxyprogesterone caproate (Delalutin; MPA, medroxyprogesterone acetate (Provera, Depo-Provera); MA, megestrol acetate (Megace); IM, intramuscular; PO, postoperative.

tively, with an additional 15–40% of patients exhibiting stable disease for at least 3 months. In 1986, the Gynecologic Oncology Group initially reported on the use of oral *medroxyprogesterone acetate* for treatment of patients with advanced or recurrent endometrial cancer (191). Of 219 patients with measurable disease, 8% had a complete response, 6% had a partial response, and 52% had stable disease; in 34%, progressive disease developed within 1 month. The mean survival for the entire group was 10.4 months. In a follow-up study comparing two different doses of oral *medroxyprogesterone acetate*, similar response rates were achieved (26% for 200 mg/d and 18% for 1000 mg/d) (192). Neither the type, dose, nor route of administration of the progestin seemed to have an effect on response in these studies.

Response of metastatic endometrial carcinoma to progestin therapy is related to several clinical and pathologic factors. Higher response rates are observed in well-differentiated tumors. Podratz et al. (190) noted a 20.5% response in low-grade tumors and only a 1.4% response in high-grade tumors. Likewise, the probability of an objective response to progestin therapy is about 70% for tumors that are positive for estrogen and progesterone receptors, compared with about 5–15% for tumors that are negative for both receptors. A longer disease-free interval is associated with higher response rates to progestins. Reifenstein (188) noted that the response rate to progestins ranged from 6% in patients with an interval from primary treatment to recurrence of less than 6 months to 65% in patients in whom disease recurred more than 5 years after initial treatment. Other observed but less well documented factors that may have an adverse effect on response to progestins are disease recurrence within a prior radiation field, large tumor burden, and advanced primary versus recurrent disease (188, 190).

Tamoxifen, a nonsteroidal antiestrogen with some estrogenic properties, has been evaluated for treatment of metastatic endometrial carcinoma based on the experience in using this agent in breast cancer treatment. Its use as either a single agent or in combination with a progestin is related to its ability to inhibit the binding of estradiol to the estrogen receptor and to increase progesterone receptors. Moore et al. reviewed eight studies using *tamoxifen* 20–40 mg/d in patients with metastatic endometrial carcinoma (193). The overall response rate was 22% (range 0–53%). Responses to *tamoxifen* were more likely to be observed in patients with low-grade, hormone-receptor-positive tumors who had a prior response to progestin therapy. In an attempt to reverse the hormone receptor down-regulation seen with progestin therapy, *tamoxifen* has been given along with progestins, but the overall responses to combined *tamoxifen*-progestin therapy have been similar to those noted for single-agent progestin therapy.

Progestins are currently recommended as initial treatment for all patients with recurrent endometrial cancer. Radiation therapy, surgery, or both should be used whenever feasible for treatment of localized recurrent cancer such as vaginal, pelvic, bone, and peripheral lymph node disease; however, these patients should also be given long-term progestin therapy unless they are known to have a progesterone-receptor-negative tumor. Patients with nonlocalized recurrent tumors, especially if progesterone receptors are known to be positive, are candidates for progestin therapy, either *megestrol acetate* 80 mg twice daily or *medroxyprogesterone acetate* 50–100 mg three times daily. Progestin therapy should be continued for at least 2–3 months before assessing response. If a response is obtained, the progestin should be continued for as long as the disease is static or in remission. In the presence of a relative contraindication to high-dose progestin therapy (e.g., prior or current thromboembolic disease, severe heart disease, or inability of the patient to tolerate progestin therapy), *tamoxifen* 20 mg twice daily is recommended. Failure to respond to hormonal therapy is an indication for initiating chemotherapy.

Chemotherapy

Although several chemotherapeutic agents or combinations of agents are capable of inducing responses and even remissions in patients with metastatic endometrial carcinoma, response and survival times are short and all cytotoxic therapy should be considered palliative (193–195). The most active chemotherapeutic agents are *doxorubicin* and the platinum compounds *cisplatin* and *carboplatin*. *Doxorubicin* in dosages of 50–60 mg/M^2 every 3 weeks has yielded response rates from 19 to 38%. *Cisplatin* (50–60 mg/M^2 every 3 weeks) and *carboplatin* (350–400 mg/M^2 every 4 weeks) have been associated with response rates of 21% and 29%, respectively. Alkylating agents, such as *cyclophosphamide* and *melphalan, 5-fluorouracil,* and *altretamine (hexamethylmelamine)* have shown activity against endometrial cancer. Most of the responses obtained with use of these agents have been partial, generally averaging only 3–6 months, with the median survival time ranging from 4 to 8 months.

Combination chemotherapy regimens using *doxorubicin* and *cisplatin* (AP) and *cyclophosphamide, doxorubicin,* and *cisplatin* (CAP) have resulted in response rates ranging from 38 to 76%. Most responses have been partial, with durations of 4–8 months. Despite these fairly impressive response rates, median survival has generally been less than 12 months.

Response to chemotherapy in patients with metastatic endometrial cancer does not seem to be affected by prior or concurrent progestin therapy. Metastatic site, age, disease-free interval, histology, and tumor grade also appear to have no effect on chemotherapy response. However, patients with long disease-free intervals and better performance status may live longer. Initial progestin therapy is advised before chemotherapy is undertaken, reserving the use of more toxic chemotherapy agents for situations in which endocrine therapy has failed. Alternatively, eligible patients should be entered into clinical trials.

Treatment Results

Comprehensive survival data for endometrial cancer, as well as results of treatment from 1987 to 1989, are available (196). Survival in relation to combined clinical and surgical stage is shown in Table 31.16; survival in relation to surgical stage and grade is shown in Table 31.17. Overall 5-year survival is 73%, including 82% for stage I and 65% for stage

Table 31.16   Carcinoma of the Corpus Uteri, 1987–1989: Stage Distribution and Actuarial Survival by Stage (Clinical and Surgical)

| | Patients Treated | | Survival (%) | |
| | No. | Percentage | 3-Year | 5-Year |
Stage				
I	8603	72.7	88	82
II	1650	13.9	70	65
III	1181	10.0	53	44
IV	399	3.4	20	15
Total	11,833	100.0	—	73

Adapted from the Annual report on the results of treatment in gynecological cancer. 1995;22:65–82.

Table 31.17   Surgically Staged Endometrial Cancer: Actuarial 5-Year Survival by Histologic Grade and Stage

Stage	Grade		
	1	2	3
Ia	96	91	83
Ib	95	89	82
Ic	90	85	73
IIa	90	81	60
IIb	77	79	55
IIIa	72	—	59
IIIc	59	42	42
IV	35	28	18

Adapted from the Annual report on the results of treatment in gynecological cancer. 1995;22:65–82.

II. Survival in surgical stage I disease ranges from more than 95% for stages Ia (grade 1) and Ib (grade 1) to less than 75% for stage Ic (grade 3).

Follow-Up After Treatment

History and physical examination remain the most effective methods of follow-up in patients treated for endometrial cancer (197). Patients should be examined every 3–4 months during the first 2–3 years and every 6 months thereafter. Approximately one-half of patients discovered to have recurrent cancer will be symptomatic, and 75–80% of recurrences will be detected initially on physical examination. Particular attention should be given to peripheral lymph nodes, the abdomen, and the pelvis.

Chest x-ray every 6–12 months is an important method of posttreatment surveillance. Almost one-half of all asymptomatic recurrences are detected by chest x-ray. Other radiologic studies, such as intravenous pyelography and CT scans, are not indicated for routine follow-up of asymptomatic patients.

Serum CA125 measurement has been suggested for posttreatment surveillance of endometrial cancer (198). Elevated CA125 levels have been documented in patients with recurrent tumor, and these levels have correlated with the clinical course of disease. However, CA125 levels may be normal in the presence of small recurrences, making the utility of CA125 measurements for follow-up of patients after treatment of early stage disease suspect.

Estrogen Replacement Therapy After Treatment of Endometrial Cancer

A history of endometrial cancer has long been considered a contraindication to estrogen replacement therapy because of the concern that occult metastatic disease might be activated by estrogen. Although this is a reasonable concern, the magnitude of this risk has never been quantified and, in fact, **there is no evidence that estrogen therapy after apparently successful treatment of endometrial cancer increases the risk of cancer recurrence.**

In 1986, Creasman et al. reported a nonrandomized, retrospective follow-up study of 221 patient with clinical stage I endometrial cancer; 47 patients who had received estrogen after treatment were compared with 174 who had not been treated with estrogen. There were no significant differences between the two groups with respect to known risk factors for cancer recurrence. There were 26 (14.9%) recurrences in the patients not treated with estrogen, compared with only one (2.1%) recurrence in the patients treated with estrogen. Moreover, in the group not receiving estrogen, there were 26 deaths (16 from cancer and 10 from intercurrent disease) compared with only one death among those taking estrogen (199). Similarly, Lee et al. reported no recurrent cancers and no intercurrent deaths in 44 women who took estrogen after treatment for endometrial cancer compared with eight recurrences and eight intercurrent deaths (five from myocardial infarction) in 99 patients who did not take estrogen (200). However, in both of these studies, estrogen replacement therapy did not commence immediately postoperatively in most patients. There was a median delay of 15 months in administering estrogen therapy in the Creasman study and a delay of more than 1 year in 43% of cases in the Lee report.

Because many women who have been successfully treated for endometrial cancer will suffer side effects of estrogen deficiency, such as vasomotor instability, vaginal dryness, and dyspareunia, as well as the long-term risks of osteoporosis and atherosclerotic heart disease, treatment with estrogen is desirable. The American College of Obstetricians and Gynecologists has stated that *"for women with a history of endometrial cancer, estrogen could be used for the same indications as for any other women, except that the selection of appropriate candidates should be based on prognostic indicators and the risk the patient is willing to assume."* A compromise between immediate postoperative estrogen replacement therapy and no hormone therapy might be to withhold estrogen for 1–3 years after treatment, the time during which most recurrences develop, thereby minimizing the chances of administering estrogen to patients with residual cancer. In the interim, symptomatic relief of hot flushes can be achieved by prescribing progestins such as *medroxyprogesterone acetate* 10 mg *orally* daily or 150 mg intramuscularly every 3 months or nonhormonal agents such as *Bellergal* and *clonidine.*

Uterine Sarcomas

Uterine sarcomas are relatively rare tumors of mesodermal origin. They constitute 2–6% of uterine malignancies (201). There is an increased incidence of uterine sarcomas, usually malignant mixed müllerian tumors, following radiation therapy to the pelvis for either carcinoma of the cervix or a benign condition. The relative risk of developing uterine sarcoma following pelvic radiation therapy has been estimated to be 5.38, usually within 10–20 years (202). Uterine sarcomas are, in general, the most malignant group of uterine tumors and differ from endometrial cancers with regard to diagnosis, clinical behavior, pattern of spread, and management.

The three most common histologic variants of uterine sarcoma are endometrial stromal sarcoma (ESS), leiomyosarcoma (LMS), and malignant mixed müllerian tumor (MMT) of both homologous and heterologous type. Other less common types include pure heterologous sarcomas, blood vessel sarcomas, and lymphosarcomas (Table 31.18) (203). Variations in the relative incidences of uterine sarcomas occur in different published series, probably related to the strictness of criteria used to classify smooth muscle and endometrial stromal tumors as sarcomas. In general, LMS and MMT each make up about 40% of tumors, followed by ESS (15%) and other sarcomas (5%), although MMT predominates in more recent reports. Staging of uterine sarcomas is based on the FIGO system for endometrial carcinoma (Tables 31.6 and 31.7).

Table 31.18   Classification of uterine Sarcomas

Type	*Homologous*	*Heterologous*
Pure	Leiomyosarcoma	Rhabdomyosarcoma
	Stromal sarcoma	Chondrosarcoma
	(i) endolymphatic stromal myosis	Osteosarcoma
	(ii) Endometrial stromal sarcoma	Liposarcoma
Mixed	Carcinosarcoma	Mixed mesodermal sarcoma

Reproduced with permission from **Hacker NF, Moore JG.** *Essentials of Obstetrics and Gynecology.* Philadelphia: WB Saunders, 1986:472.

Endometrial Stromal Tumors

Stromal tumors occur primarily in perimenopausal women between 45 and 50 years of age; about one-third of tumors occur in postmenopausal women. There is no relationship to parity, associated diseases, or prior pelvic radiotherapy. These tumors rarely occur in African-Americans. The most frequent symptom is abnormal uterine bleeding; abdominal pain and pressure due to an enlarging pelvic mass occur less often, and some patients are asymptomatic. Pelvic examination usually reveals regular or irregular uterine enlargement, sometimes associated with rubbery parametrial induration. The diagnosis may be confirmed by endometrial biopsy, but preoperatively the diagnosis usually is uterine leiomyoma. At surgery, an enlarged uterus filled with soft, gray-white to yellow necrotic and hemorrhagic tumors with bulging surfaces associated with worm-like elastic extensions into the pelvic veins suggests the diagnosis.

Endometrial stromal tumors are composed purely of cells resembling normal endometrial stroma. Based on mitotic activity, vascular invasion, and observed differences in prognosis, endometrial stromal tumors are divided into three types: 1) endometrial stromal nodule, 2) low-grade stromal sarcoma or endolymphatic stromal myosis, and 3) endometrial stromal sarcoma (Table 31.19).

Endometrial Stromal Nodule

Endometrial stromal nodule is an expansive, noninfiltrating, solitary lesion confined to the uterus with pushing margins, no lymphatic or vascular invasion, and usually less than three mitotic figures/10 high-power microscopic fields (3 MF/10 HPF). These tumors should be considered benign because there have been no recurrences or tumor deaths reported following surgery (204).

Low-Grade Stromal Sarcoma or Endolymphatic Stromal Myosis

Low-grade stromal sarcoma or endolymphatic stromal myosis is distinguished from the true endometrial stromal sarcoma microscopically by a mitotic rate of less than 10 MF/10 HPF as well as clinically by a more protracted clinical course. Recurrences typically occur late, and local recurrence is more common than distant metastases (205–209). Although low-grade stromal sarcoma often behaves in a histologically aggressive fashion, it lacks the aneuploid DNA content and high proliferative index associated with the more malignant ESS, and flow cytometric analysis can be used to differentiate the two conditions and predict response to therapy.

Low-grade stromal sarcoma has extended beyond the uterus in 40% of cases at the time of diagnosis, but the extrauterine spread is confined to the pelvis in two-thirds of the cases. Upper abdominal, pulmonary, and lymph node metastases are uncommon. Recurrence occurs in almost 50% of cases at an average interval of about 5 years after initial therapy. Prolonged survival and even cure are not uncommon, even after the development of recurrent or metastatic disease.

Optimum initial therapy for patients with low-grade stromal sarcoma consists of surgical excision of all grossly detectable tumor. Total abdominal hysterectomy and bilateral salp-

Table 31.19   AFIP Classification of Endometrial Stromal Tumors

Tumor	Malignant Potential	Cytologic Atypia	Mitoses/10 HPF
Stromal nodule	None	Mild–Moderate (pushing margins)	Less than 10; usually 1–3
Low-grade stromal sarcoma	Low to intermediate	Mild–Moderate (infiltrating margins)	Less than 10; usually 1–3
Stromal sarcoma	High	Moderate–Marked	10 or more

Reproduced with permission from **Zaloubek CJ, Norris HC.** Mesenchymal tumors of the uterus. In: Fengolio C, Wolff M, eds. *Progress in Surgical Pathology.* Vol. 3. New York: Mason Publishing, 1981:1–35.
AFIP, Armed Forces Institute of Pathology.

ingo-oophorectomy should be performed. The adnexa should always be removed because of the propensity for tumor extension into the parametria, broad ligaments, and adnexal structures as well as the possible stimulating effect on the tumor cells of estrogen from retained ovaries. A beneficial effect of radiation therapy has been reported, and pelvic irradiation is recommended for inadequately excised or locally recurrent pelvic disease (205). There is also evidence that low-grade stromal sarcoma is hormone dependent or responsive. Piver et al. noted objective responses to progestin therapy in six of 13 patients (48%) (209). Recurrent or metastatic lesions may also be amenable to surgical excision.

Endometrial stromal sarcoma is a highly lethal neoplasm exhibiting greater than 10 MF/10 HPF and having a much more aggressive course and poorer prognosis than low-grade stromal sarcoma (203, 205, 210). The 5-year disease-free survival is approximately 25%. Treatment for ESS consists of total abdominal hysterectomy and bilateral salpingo-oophorectomy. The dismal therapeutic results obtained to date suggest that radiation therapy, chemotherapy, or both should be used in combination with surgery. These tumors, unlike low-grade stromal sarcoma, are not responsive to progestin therapy.

Leiomyosarcomas

The median age for women with leiomyosarcoma (43–53 years) is somewhat lower than that for other uterine sarcomas, and premenopausal patients have a better chance of survival. This malignancy has no relationship with parity, and the incidence of associated diseases is not as high as in MMT or endometrial adenocarcinoma. There is a higher incidence and a poorer prognosis in African-Americans. A history of prior pelvic radiation therapy can be elicited in about 4% of patients with leiomyosarcoma. The incidence of sarcomatous change in benign uterine leiomyomas is reported to be between 0.13–0.81% (211–218).

Presenting symptoms that are usually of short duration (mean, 6 months) and are not specific for the disease include vaginal bleeding, pelvic pain or pressure, and awareness of an abdominal-pelvic mass. The principal physical finding is the presence of a pelvic mass. The diagnosis should be suspected if rapid uterine enlargement occurs, especially in a postmenopausal woman. Endometrial biopsy, although not as useful as in other sarcomas, may establish the diagnosis in up to one-third of cases in which the lesion is submucosal.

Survival in uterine leiomyosarcoma ranges from 20 to 63% (mean, 47%). The pattern of tumor spread is to the myometrium, pelvic blood vessels and lymphatics, contiguous pelvic structures, abdomen, and then, distantly, most often to the lungs. The number of mitoses in the tumor seems to be the most reliable microscopic indicator of malignant behavior (Fig. 31.8). **Most investigators agree that tumors with less than 5 MF/10 HPF usually behave in a benign fashion (survival, 98%), and tumors with greater than 10 MF/10 HPF are frankly malignant with a poor prognosis (survival, 15%). Tumors with 5–10 MF/10 HPF are less predictable, and many will recur or metastasize (survival, 42%).** Other histologic indicators of poor prognosis are marked anaplasia, necrosis, and blood vessel invasion. Gross presentation of the tumor at the time of surgery is also an important prognostic indicator. Tumors with infiltrating tumor margins or extension beyond the uterus are associated with poor prognosis, whereas tumors originating within myomas or with pushing margins are associated with prolonged survival.

Variants of Leiomyosarcoma

There are five other clinicopathologic variants of leiomyosarcoma that deserve special comment. These are intravenous leiomyomatosis, metastasizing uterine leiomyoma, leiomyoblastoma, leiomyomatosis peritonealis disseminata, and myxoid leiomyosarcoma.

Intravenous leiomyomatosis is characterized by the growth of histologically benign smooth muscle initially into venous channels within the broad ligament and then into uterine and iliac veins (219–221). The intravascular growth takes the form of visible, worm-like projections that extend out from a myomatous uterus into the parametria toward the

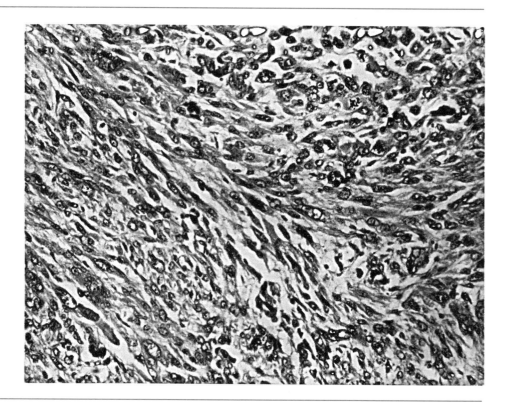

Figure 31.8.   Leiomyosarcoma of the uterus. Interlacing bundles of spindle cells have fibrillar cytoplasm, irregular and hyperchromatic nuclei, and multiple mitotic figures.

pelvic sidewalls and may be confused with endolymphatic stromal myosis. Symptoms are related to the associated uterine myomas. Most patients are in the late fifth and early sixth decades of life. The prognosis is excellent, even when tumor is left in pelvic vessels. Late local recurrences can occur, however, and deaths from extension into the inferior vena cava or metastases to the heart have been reported. Estrogen may stimulate the proliferation of these intravascular tumors. Treatment should be total abdominal hysterectomy and bilateral salpingo-oophorectomy with removal of as much of the tumor as possible.

Benign metastasizing leiomyoma is a rare condition in which a histologically benign uterine smooth muscle tumor acts in a somewhat malignant fashion and produces benign metastases, usually to the lungs or lymph nodes (222). In most instances, intravenous leiomyomatosis is not demonstrable. The metastasizing myomas are capable of growth at distant sites, whereas the intravenous tumors spread only by direct extension within blood vessels. Both experimental and clinical evidence suggests that these tumors are stimulated by estrogen. Therefore, removal of the source of estrogen, by castration or withdrawal of exogenous estrogen, or treatment with progestins, *tamoxifen,* or a gonadotropin agonist has an ameliorating effect (223). Surgical treatment should consist of total abdominal hysterectomy and bilateral salpingo-oophorectomy, as well as resection of pulmonary metastases if possible.

Leiomyoblastoma includes smooth muscle tumors designated as epithelioid leiomyomas, clear cell leiomyomas, and plexiform tumorlets (224). This group of atypical smooth muscle tumors is distinguished by the predominance of rounded rather than spindle-shaped cells and by a clustered or cord-like pattern. These lesions should be regarded as specialized low-grade leiomyosarcomas with less than 5MF/10HPF and an excellent prognosis. Standard treatment should be hysterectomy.

Leiomyomatosis peritonealis disseminata is a rare clinical entity characterized by benign smooth muscle nodules scattered throughout the peritoneal cavity on peritoneal surfaces (225). This condition probably arises as a result of metaplasia of subperitoneal mesenchymal stem cells to smooth muscle, fibroblasts, myofibroblasts, and decidual cells under the influence of estrogen and progesterone. Most reported cases have occurred in 30- to 40-year-old women who are or have recently been pregnant or who have a long history of oral contraceptive use. Intriguing features of this disease are its grossly malignant appearance, benign histology, and favorable clinical outcome. Intraoperative diagnosis requires frozen-section examination. Extirpative surgery, including total abdominal hysterectomy, bilateral salpingo-oophorectomy, omentectomy, and excision of as much gross disease as possible, may be indicated after the reproductive years. Removal of the source of excess estrogen or treatment with progestins or both has resulted in regression of unresected tumor masses. Almost all patients have responded well to therapy.

Myxoid leiomyosarcoma is characterized grossly by a gelatinous appearance and apparent circumscribed border, but microscopically, the tumors have a myxomatous stroma and extensively invade adjacent tissue and blood vessels (226). The mitotic rate is low (0–2 MF/10 HPF), which belies their aggressive behavior and poor prognosis. Surgical excision by hysterectomy is the mainstay of treatment. The low mitotic rate and abundance of intracellular myxomatous tissue suggest that these tumors would not be responsive to radiation therapy or chemotherapy.

Malignant Mixed Müllerian Tumors

Malignant mixed müllerian tumors are composed histologically of a mixture of sarcoma and carcinoma. The carcinomatous element is usually glandular, whereas the sarcomatous element may resemble the normal endometrial stroma (homologous) or the so-called carcinosarcoma or it may be composed of tissues foreign to the uterus, such as cartilage, bone, or striated muscle (heterologous) (Fig. 31.9). These tumors are most likely derived from totipotential endometrial stromal cells (227, 228).

Almost all of these tumors occur after menopause, at a median age of 62 years. There is a higher incidence in African-American women. These tumors are often found in association with other medical conditions such as obesity, diabetes mellitus, and hypertension. A history of previous pelvic irradiation can be obtained in 7–37% of patients.

The most frequent presenting symptom is postmenopausal bleeding, which occurs in 80–90% of cases. Other less common symptoms are vaginal discharge, abdominal-pelvic pain, weight loss, and passage of tissue from the vagina. The duration of symptoms is usually only a few months. On physical examination, uterine enlargement is present in 50–95% of patients, and a polypoid mass may be seen within or protruding from the endocervical canal in up to 50% of patients. Diagnosis can usually be determined by biopsy of an endocervical mass or endometrial curettage.

The tumor grows as a large, soft, polypoid mass filling and distending the uterine cavity; necrosis and hemorrhage are prominent features (Fig. 31.10). The myometrium is invaded to various degrees in almost all cases. The most frequent areas of spread are the pelvis, lymph nodes, peritoneal cavity, lungs, and liver. This metastatic pattern suggests that these neoplasms spread by local extension and regional lymph node metastasis in a manner similar to that of endometrial adenocarcinoma but behave more aggressively.

The most important single factor affecting prognosis in MMTs is the extent of tumor at the time of treatment. DiSaia et al. noted that patients with tumor apparently confined to the uterine corpus (stage I) had a 53% 2-year survival, whereas survival dropped to 8.5% when disease had extended to the cervix, vagina, or parametria (stage II and III); there were no survivors in those patients with disease outside the pelvis (stage IV) (229). Unfortunately, disease has clinically already extended outside the uterus in 40–60% of cases at the time of diagnosis, indicating the highly malignant nature of this lesion. Even when disease is

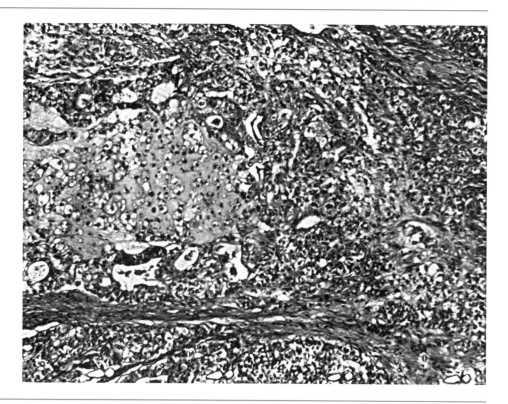

Figure 31.9.   Mixed mesodermal sarcoma of uterus. This lesion consists of poorly differentiated adenocarcinoma with rare glandular lumina (*right*) half of figure) and chondrosarcoma (*left*).

Figure 31.10   Polypoid mixed mesodermal tumor of the uterus.

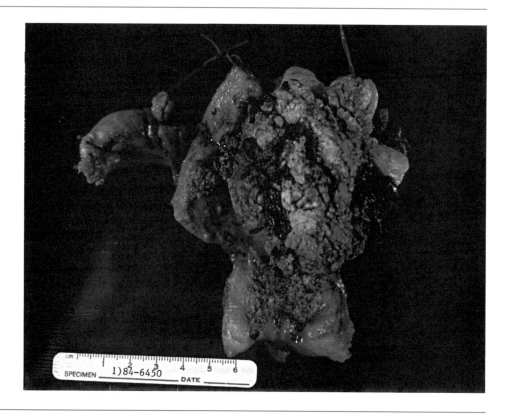

believed to be confined to the uterus preoperatively and to be potentially still curable, surgical and pathologic staging identifies extrauterine spread of disease in a significant number of cases. Macasaet et al. reported that 55% of women with clinical stage I MMT had a higher surgical and pathologic stage. In their series, only 28% of tumors were actually confined to the uterine corpus; 16% had extension to the cervix, and 56% showed extrauterine spread (230). DiSaia et al. (231) and Geszler et al. (232) also reported a significant occurrence of lymph node metastases and positive peritoneal cytology, respectively, in early stage MMTs. Deep myometrial invasion, which is present in about one-half of stage I cases, is associated with poor prognosis. Almost all patients in whom tumors involve the outer one-half of the myometrium die. Patients who die from MMT tend to have larger tumors and a higher incidence of lymph-vascular space invasion. Patients with a history of prior pelvic irradiation generally have a poorer prognosis. Overall, the 5-year survival for MMT is approximately 20–30%.

Adenosarcoma is an uncommon variant of MMT (233, 234). It consists of an admixture of benign-appearing neoplastic glands and a sarcomatous stroma. Most patients present with postmenopausal vaginal bleeding, and the disease is diagnosed or suspected based on endometrial curettage. Most adenosarcomas are well circumscribed and limited to the endometrium or superficial myometrium. The treatment is hysterectomy and bilateral salpingo-oophorectomy with or without adjuvant radiotherapy. Recurrences, mostly local pelvic or vaginal, have been reported in 40–50% of cases, leading some authors to recommend adjuvant postoperative intravaginal or pelvic irradiation.

Treatment of Uterine Sarcomas

Recurrences develop in over one-half of cases of uterine sarcoma, even when disease is apparently localized at the time of treatment (235–237). At least 50% of recurrences occur outside the pelvis; isolated pelvic failures account for less than 10% of recurrences. The most common sites of recurrence are the abdomen and the lung. These data emphasize that the major limitation to cure of uterine sarcomas is distant spread.

Based on this type of evidence, treatment of most stage I and II uterine sarcomas should include hysterectomy, bilateral salpingo-oophorectomy, and treatment of the pelvic lymphatic by irradiation or surgery. Strong consideration should also be given to the use of adjuvant chemotherapy to decrease the incidence of distant metastases. Stage III uterine sarcomas are probably best treated by an aggressive approach to combined surgery, radiation therapy, and chemotherapy. Stage IV disease must be treated with combination chemotherapy.

Surgery

The first step in the treatment of early uterine sarcoma should be exploratory laparotomy. Since extirpative survey is the most important aspect of treatment, and knowledge of the extent and spread of the disease is important for further management, one should not forego or delay surgery by using radiation therapy or chemotherapy first. At the time of surgery, the peritoneal cavity should be carefully explored and special attention should be given to the pelvic and para-aortic lymph nodes. Total abdominal hysterectomy is the standard procedure, and bilateral salpingo-oophorectomy should also be performed in all patients except premenopausal women with leiomyosarcoma. Based on the surgical and pathologic findings, additional radiation therapy or chemotherapy can then be planned more rationally. Rarely, a patient may be cured by excision of an isolated pulmonary metastasis.

Radiotherapy

Most studies have found adjuvant pre- or postoperative radiation therapy to be of value in decreasing pelvic recurrences and thereby increasing quality of life in patients with localized ESS and MMT but not LMS (238–241). Radiotherapy thus seems to have a role with surgery in the combined treatment of malignant mixed müllerian tumors and endometrial stromal sarcomas confined to the pelvis by increasing the disease-free gression interval and by increasing control of pelvic disease, thereby probably increasing the overall survival to some degree.

Chemotherapy

There is increasing interest in the role of chemotherapy in the treatment of metastatic disease, as well as adjuvant treatment of localized, uterine sarcomas. Several chemotherapeutic agents have been found to have activity in sarcomas, including *vincristine, actinomycin D, cyclophosphamide, doxorubicin, dimethyl-triazeno-imidazole carboxamide (DTIC), cisplatin,* and *ifosfamide* (242, 243). *Doxorubicin* seems to be the most active single agent in leiomyosarcoma, producing a 25% response rate. *Ifosfamide* also has some lesser activity (244). Conversely, *cisplatin* and *ifosfamide* have demonstrated clear activity in malignant mixed müllerian tumors, with responses rates of 18–42% and 32%, respectively (245–247). *Doxorubicin* has demonstrated a less than 10% response rate in MMT.

Combination chemotherapy with *doxorubicin* and *DTIC* or these two drugs plus *vincristine* (VAD) and *cyclophosphamide* (CYVADIC) has been reported to yield somewhat higher response rates (242, 243, 248). More recently, *ifosfamide* with *mesna* uroprotection, *doxorubicin,* and *DTIC* (MAID) have been combined to treat metastatic sarcomas.

Because of the relatively low survival rate in localized uterine sarcomas and the high incidence of failure due to subsequent distant metastasis, adjuvant treatment programs employing chemotherapy have been tested. Unfortunately, most reports have been unable to demonstrate a clear improvement in survival by the addition of postoperative adjuvant chemotherapy in early uterine sarcoma. The Gynecologic Oncology Group conducted a trial of postoperative adjuvant *doxorubicin* in 131 patients with stage I uterine sarcoma and 25 patients with stage II uterine sarcoma. Of the 75 patients randomized to receive *doxorubicin,* recurrence developed in 41%, compared with 53% of 81 patients receiving no adjuvant chemotherapy, but these differences were not significant (249). Other smaller, nonrandomized adjuvant chemotherapy studies using CYVADIC and *cisplatin/doxorubicin* demonstrated lower rates of recurrence (18% and 24%, respectively) than expected (250, 251).

References

1. **Parker SL, Tong T, Bolden S, Wingo PA.** Cancer statistics, 1996. *CA Cancer J Clin* 1996;46:5–28.

2. **Bokhman JV.** Two pathogenetic types of endometrial carcinoma. *Gynecol Oncol* 1983;15:10–7.

3. **MacMahon B.** Risk factors for endometrial cancer. *Gynecol Oncol* 1974;2:122–9.

4. **Parazzini F, LaVecchia C, Bocciolone L, Franceschi S.** The epidemiology of endometrial cancer. *Gynecol Oncol* 1991;41:1–16.

5. **Parazzini F, LaVecchia C, Negri E, Fedele L, Balotta F.** Reproductive factors and risk of endometrial cancer. *Am J Obstet Gynecol* 1991;64:522–7.

6. **Brinton LA, Berman ML, Mortel R, Twiggs LB, Barrett RJ, Wilbanks GD, et al.** Reproductive, menstrual and medical risk factors for endometrial cancer: results from a case control study. *Am J Obstet Gynecol* 1992;167:1317–25.

7. **Grady D, Gebretsadik T, Kerlikowske K, Ernster V, Petitti D.** Hormone replacement therapy and endometrial cancer risk: a meta-analysis. *Obstet Gynecol* 1995;85:304–13.

8. **Assikis VJ, Jordan VC.** Gynecologic effects of tamoxifen and the association with endometrial carcinoma. *Int J Gynaecol Obstet* 1995;49:241–57.

9. **Gordon MD, Ireland K.** Pathology of hyperplasia and carcinoma of the endometrium. *Semin Oncol* 1994;21:64–70.

10. **Kurman RJ, Kaminski PF, Norris HJ.** The behavior of endometrial hyperplasia: a long term study of "untreated" hyperplasia in 170 patients. *Cancer* 1985;56:403–12.

11. **Tavassoli F, Kraus FT.** Endometrial lesions in uteri resected for atypical endometrial hyperplasia. *Am J Clin Pathol* 1978;70:770–9.

12. **Hunter JE, Tritz DE, Howell MG, DePriest PD, Gallion HH, Andrews SJ, et al.** The prognostic and therapeutic implications of cytologic atypia in patients with endometrial hyperplasia. *Gynecol Oncol* 1994;55:66–71.

13. **Ferenczy A, Gelfand M.** The biologic significance of cytologic atypia in progestin-treated endometrial hyperplasia. *Am J Obstet Gynecol* 1989;160:126–31.

14. **Gal D.** Hormonal therapy for lesions of the endometrium. *Semin Oncol* 1986;13:33–6.

15. **Koss LG, Schreiber K, Oberlander SG, Moussouris HF, Lesser M.** Detection of endometrial carcinoma and hyperplasia in asymptomatic women. *Obstet Gynecol* 1984;64:1–11.

16. **Abayomi O, Dritschilo A, Emami B, Watring WG, Piro AJ.** The value of "routine tests" in the staging evaluation of gynecologic malignancies: a cost effective analysis. *Int J Radiat Oncol Biol Phys* 1982;8:241–4.

17. **Mettlin C, Jones G, Averette H, Gusberg SB, Murphy GP.** Defining and updating the American Cancer Society guidelines for the cancer-related checkup: prostate and endometrial cancers. *CA Cancer J Clin* 1993;43:42–6.

18. **Smith M, McCartney AJ.** Occult, high-risk endometrial carcinoma. *Gynecol Oncol* 1985;22:154–61.

19. **DuBeshter B, Warshal DP, Angel C, Dvoretsky PM, Lin JY, Raubertas RF.** Endometrial carcinoma: the relevance of cervical cytology. *Obstet Gynecol* 1991;77:458–62.

20. **Choo YC, Mak KC, Hsu C, Wong TS, Ma HK.** Postmenopausal uterine bleeding of nonorganic cause. *Obstet Gynecol* 1985;66:225–8.

21. **Pacheco JC, Kempers RD.** Etiology of postmenopausal bleeding. *Obstet Gynecol* 1968;32:40–6.

22. **Hawwa ZM, Nahhas WA, Copenhaver EH.** Postmenopausal bleeding. *Lahey Clin Found Bull* 1970;19:61–70.

23. **Lidor A, Ismajovich B, Confino E, David MP.** Histopathological findings in 226 women with post-menopausal uterine bleeding. *Acta Obstet Gynecol Scand* 1986;65:41–3.

24. **Fortier KJ.** Postmenopausal bleeding and the endometrium. *Clin Obstet Gynecol* 1986;29:44–5.

25. **Chambers JT, Chambers SK.** Endometrial sampling: When? Where? Why? With what? *Clin Obstet Gynecol* 1992;35:28–39.

26. **Grimes DA.** Diagnostic dilation and curettage: a reappraisal. *Am J Obstet Gynecol* 1982;142:1–6.

27. **Kaunitz AM, Masciello A, Ostrowski M, Rovira EZ.** Comparison of endometrial biopsy with the endometrial Pipelle and Vabra aspirator. *J Reprod Med* 1988;33:427–31.

28. **Zucker PK, Kasdon EJ, Feldstein ML.** The validity of Pap smear parameters as predictors of endometrial pathology in menopausal women. *Cancer* 1985;56:2256–63.

29. **Stelmachow J.** The role of hysteroscopy in gynecologic oncology. *Gynecol Oncol* 1982;14:392–5.

30. **Gimpelson RJ, Rappold HO.** A comparative study between panoramic hysteroscopy with directed biopsies and dilation and curettage: a review of 276 cases. *Am J Obstet Gynecol* 1988;158:489–92.

31. **Bourne TH, Campbell S, Steer CV, Royston P, Whitehead MI, Collins WP.** Detection of endometrial cancer by transvaginal ultrasonography with color flow imaging and blood flow analysis: a preliminary report. *Gynecol Oncol* 1991;40:253–9.

32. **Granberg S, Wikland M, Karlsson B, Norstrom A, Friberg LG.** Endometrial thickness as measured by endovaginal ultrasonography for identifying endometrial abnormality. *Am J Obstet Gynecol* 1991;164:47–52.

33. **Varner RE, Sparks JM, Cameron CD, Roberts LL, Soong SJ.** Transvaginal sonography of the endometrium in postmenopausal women. *Obstet Gynecol* 1991;78:195–9.

34. **Silverberg SG, Kurman RJ.** Tumors of the uterine corpus and gestational trophoblastic disease (3rd series). Washington, DC: Armed Forces Institute of Pathology, 1992.

35. **Hendrickson MR, Ross JC, Kempson RL.** Toward the development of morphologic criteria for well differentiated adenocarcinoma of the endometrium. *Am J Surg Pathol* 1983;7:819–38.

36. **Norris HJ, Tavassoli FA, Kurman RJ.** Endometrial hyperplasia and carcinoma. Diagnostic considerations. *Am J Surg Pathol* 1983;7:839–47.

37. **Zaino RJ, Kurman RJ.** Squamous differentiation in carcinoma of the endometrium. A critical appraisal of adenoacanthoma and adenosquamous carcinoma. *Semin Diagn Pathol* 1988;5:154–71.

38. **Zaino RJ, Kurman R, Herbold D, Gliedman J, Bundy BN, Voet R, et al.** The significance of squamous differentiation in endometrial carcinoma. *Cancer* 1991;68:2293–2302.

39. **Chen JL, Trost DC, Wilkinson EJ.** Endometrial papillary adenocarcinomas: two clinicopathologic types. *Int J Gynaecol Pathol* 1985;4:279–88.

40. **Sutton GP, Brill L, Michael H, Stehman FB, Ehrlich CE.** Malignant papillary lesions of the endometrium. *Gynecol Oncol* 1987;27:294–304.

41. **Christophenson WM, Alberhasky RC Connelly PJ.** Carcinoma of the endometrium. I. A clinicopathologic study of clear cell carcinoma and secretory carcinoma. *Cancer* 1982;49: 1511–23.

42. **Tobon H, Watkins GJ.** Secretory adenocarcinoma of the endometrium. *Int J Gynaecol Pathol* 1985;4:328–35.

43. **Ross JC, Eifel PJ, Cox RS, Kempson RL, Hendrickson MR.** Primary mucinous adenocarcinoma of the endometrium. A clinicopathologic and histochemical study. *Am J Surg Pathol* 1983;7:715–29.

44. **Melhern MF, Tobon H.** Mucinous adenocarcinoma of the endometrium: a clinicopathologic review of 18 cases. *Int J Gynaecol Pathol* 1987;6:347–55.

45. **Dabbs DJ, Geisinger KR, Norris HT.** Intermediate filaments in endometrial and endocervical carcinomas. *Am J Surg Pathol* 1986;10:568–76.

46. **Hendrickson M, Ross J, Eifel P, Martinez A, Kempson R.** Uterine papillary serous carcinoma. A highly malignant form of endometrial adenocarcinoma. *Am J Surg Pathol* 1982;6: 93–108.

47. **Silva EG, Jenkins R.** Serous carcinoma in endometrial polyps. *Mod Pathol* 1990;3:120–8.

48. **Sherman ME, Bitterman P, Rosenshein NB, Delgado G, Kurman RJ.** Uterine serous carcinoma. *Am J Surg Pathol* 1992;16:600–10.

49. **Goff BA, Kato D, Schmidt RA, Ek M, Ferry JA, Muntz HG, et al.** Uterine papillary serous carcinoma: patterns of metastatic spread. *Gynecol Oncol* 1994;54:264–8.

50. **Abeler VM, Kjorstad KE.** Clear cell carcinoma of the endometrium: a histopathological and clinical study of 97 cases. *Gynecol Oncol* 1991;40:207–17.

51. **Abeler VM, Kjorstad KE.** Endometrial squamous cell carcinoma: report of three cases and review of the literature. *Gynecol Oncol* 1990;36:321–6.

52. **Eifel P, Hendrickson M, Ross J, Ballon S, Martinez A, Kempson R.** Simultaneous presentation of carcinoma involving the ovary and the uterine corpus. *Cancer* 1982;50:163–70.

53. **Zaino RJ, Unger ER, Whitney C.** Synchronous carcinomas of the uterine corpus and ovary. *Gynecol Oncol* 1984;19:329–35.

54. **Eisner RF, Nieberg RK, Berek JS.** Synchronous primary neoplasms of the female reproductive tract. *Gynecol Oncol* 1989;33:335–9.

55. **Kline RC, Wharton JT, Atkinson EN, Burke TW, Gershenson DM, Edwards CL.** Endometrioid carcinoma of the ovary: retrospective review of 145 cases. *Gynecol Oncol* 1990; 39:337–46.

56. **Prat J, Matias-Guiu X, Barreto J.** Simultaneous carcinoma involving the endometrium and the ovary. *Cancer* 1991;68:2455–9.

57. **Gordon AN, Fleischer AC, Dudley BS, Drolshagan LF, Kalemeris GC, Partain C, et al.** Preoperative assessment of myometrial invasion of endometrial adenocarcinoma by sonography (US) and magnetic resonance imaging (MRI). *Gynecol Oncol* 1989;34:175–9.

58. **Niloff JM, Klug TL, Schaetzl E, Zurawski VR Jr, Knapp RC, Bast RC Jr.** Elevation of serum CA 125 in carcinoma of the fallopian tube, endometrium, and endocervix. *Am J Obstet Gynecol* 1984;148:1057–8.

59. **Patsner B, Mann WJ, Cohen H, Loesch M.** Predictive value of preoperative serum CA 125 levels in clinically localized and advanced endometrial carcinoma. *Am J Obstet Gynecol* 1988;158:399–402.

60. **International Federation of Obstetrics and Gynecology.** Classification and staging of malignant tumors in the female pelvis. *Int J Gynaecol Obstet* 1971;9:172–180.

61. **Marziale P, Atlante G, Pozzi M, Diotallevi F, Annunziata I.** 426 cases of Stage I endometrial carcinoma: a clinicopathological analysis. *Gynecol Oncol* 1989;32:278–81.

62. **International Federation of Obstetrics and Gynecology.** Annual report on the results of treatment in gynecologic cancer. *Int J Gynaecol Obstet* 1989;28:189–93.

63. **Boronow RC, Morrow CP, Creasman WT, Disaia PJ, Silverberg SG, Miller A, et al.** Surgical staging in endometrial cancer: clinical-pathologic findings of a prospective study. *Obstet Gynecol* 1984;63:825–32.

64. **Creasman WT, Morrow CP, Bundy BN, Homesley HD, Graham JE, Heller PB.** Surgical pathologic spread patterns of endometrial cancer. *Cancer* 1987;60:2035–41.

65. **Schink JC, Lurain JR, Wallemark CB, Chmiel JS.** Tumor size in endometrial cancer: a prognostic factor for lymph node metastasis. *Obstet Gynecol* 1987;70:216–9.

66. **Doering DL, Barnhill DR, Weiser EB, Burke TW, Woodward JE, Park RC.** Intraoperative evaluation of depth of myometrial invasion in stage I endometrial adenocarcinoma. *Obstet Gynecol* 1989;74:930–3.

67. **Goff BA, Rice LW.** Assessment of depth of myometrial invasion in endometrial adenocarcinoma. *Gynecol Oncol* 1990;38:46–8.

68. **Moore DH, Fowler WC, Walton LA, Droegemueller W.** Morbidity of lymph node sampling in cancers of the uterine corpus and cervix. *Obstet Gynecol* 1989;74:180–4.

69. **Morrow CP, Bundy BN, Kurman RJ, Creasman WT, Heller P, Homesley HD, et al.** Relationship between surgical-pathological risk factors and outcome in clinical stage I and II carcinoma of the endometrium: a Gynecologic Oncology Group study. *Gynecol Oncol* 1991;40:55–65.

70. **Orr JW Jr, Holloway RW, Orr PF, Hollman JL.** Surgical staging of uterine cancer: an analysis of perioperative morbidity. *Gynecol Oncol* 1991;42:209–16.

71. **Larson DM, Johnson K, Olson KA.** Pelvic and para-aortic lymphadenectomy for surgical staging of endometrial cancer: morbidity and mortality. *Obstet Gynecol* 1992;79:998–1001.

72. **Homesley HD, Kadar N, Barrett RJ, Lentz SS.** Selective pelvic and periaortic lymphadenectomy does not increase morbidity in surgical staging of endometrial carcinoma. *Am J Obstet Gynecol* 1992;167:1225–30.

73. **Cowles TA, Magrina JF, Masterson BJ, Capen CV.** Comparison of clinical and surgical staging in patients with endometrial carcinoma. *Obstet Gynecol* 1985;66:413–6.

74. **Chen SS.** Extrauterine spread in endometrial carcinoma clinically confined to the uterus. *Gynecol Oncol* 1985;21:23–31.

75. **Vardi JR, Tadros GH, Anselmo MT, Rafla SD.** The value of exploratory laparotomy in patients with endometrial carcinoma according to the new International Federation of Gynecology and Obstetrics staging. *Obstet Gynecol* 1992;80:204–8.

76. **Wolfson AH, Sightler SE, Markoe AM, Schwade JG, Averette HE, Ganjei P, et al.** The prognostic significance of surgical staging for carcinoma of the endometrium. *Gynecol Oncol* 1992;45:142–6.

77. **Christopherson WM, Connelly PJ, Aberhasky RC.** Carcinoma of the endometrium. V. An analysis of prognosticators in patients with favorable subtypes and stage I disease. *Cancer* 1983;51:1705–9.

78. **Lotocki RJ, Copeland LJ, DePetrillo AD, Muirhead W.** Stage I endometrial adenocarcinoma: treatment results in 835 patients. *Am J Obstet Gynecol* 1983;146:141–5.

79. **DiSaia PJ, Creasman WT, Boronow RC, Blessing JA.** Risk factors and recurrent patterns in stage I endometrial cancer. *Am J Obstet Gynecol* 1985;151:1009–15.

80. **Sutton GP, Geisler HE, Stehman FB, Young PC, Kimes TM, Ehrlich CE.** Features associated with survival and disease-free survival in early endometrial cancer. *Am J Obstet Gynecol* 1989;160:1385–93.

81. **Bucy GS, Mendenhall WM, Morgan LS, Chafe WE, Wilkinson EJ, Marcus RBJ, et al.** Clinical stage I and II endometrial carcinoma treated with surgery and/or radiation therapy: analysis of prognostic and treatment related factors. *Gynecol Oncol* 1989;33:290–5.

82. **Lurain JR, Rice BL, Rademaker AW, Poggensee LE, Schink JC, Miller DS.** Prognostic factors associated with recurrence in clinical stage I adenocarcinoma of the endometrium. *Obstet Gynecol* 1991;78:63–9.

83. **Kadar N, Malfetano JH, Homesley HD.** Determinants of survival of surgically staged patients with endometrial carcinoma histologically confined to the uterus: implications for therapy. *Obstet Gynecol* 1992;80:655–9.

84. **Aalders J, Abeler V, Kolstad P, Onsrud M.** Postoperative external irradiation and prognostic parameters in stage I endometrial carcinoma. *Obstet Gynecol* 1980;56:419–46.

85. **Crissman JD, Azoury RS, Banner ARE, Schellas HF.** Endometrial carcinoma in women 40 years of age or younger. *Obstet Gynecol* 1981;57:699–704.

86. **Nilson PA, Koller O.** Carcinoma of the endometrium in Norway 1957-1960 with special reference to treatment results. *Am J Obstet Gynecol* 1969;105:1099–1109.

87. **Wilson TO, Podratz KC, Gaffey TA, Malkasian GDJ, O'Brien PC, Naessens JM.** Evaluation of unfavorable histologic subtypes in endometrial adenocarcinoma. *Am J Obstet Gynecol* 1990;162:418–26.

88. **Fanning J, Evans MC, Peters AJ, Samuel M, Harmon ER, Bates JS.** Endometrial adenocarcinoma histologic subtypes: clinical and pathologic profile. *Gynecol Oncol* 1989;32:288–91.

89. **Lutz MH, Underwood PB, Kreutner A Jr, Miller MC.** Endometrial carcinoma: a new method of classification of therapeutic and prognostic significance. *Gynecol Oncol* 1978;6: 83–94.

90. **Kaku T, Tsuruchi N, Tsukamoto N, Hirakawa T, Kamura T, Nakano H.** Reassessment of myometrial invasion in endometrial carcinoma. *Obstet Gynecol* 1994;84:979–82.

91. **Hanson MB, Van Nagell Jr, Powell DE, Donaldson ES, Gallion H, Merhige M, et al.** The prognostic significance of lymph-vascular space invasion in stage I endometrial cancer. *Cancer* 1985;55:1753–7.

92. **Abeler VM, Kjorstad KE, Berle E.** Carcinoma of the endometrium in Norway: a histopathological and prognostic survey of a total population. *Int J Gynaecol Cancer* 1992;2:9–22.

93. **Ambros RA, Kurman RJ.** Identification of patients with stage I uterine endometrioid adenocarcinoma at high risk of recurrence by DNA ploidy, myometrial invasion, and vascular invasion. *Gynecol Oncol* 1992;45:235–9.

94. **Lurain JR.** The significance of positive peritoneal cytology in endometrial cancer. *Gynecol Oncol* 1992;46:143–4.

95. **Creasman WT, DiSaia PJ, Blessing J, Wilkinson RH Jr, Johnston W, Weed JC Jr.** Prognostic significance of peritoneal cytology in patients with endometrial cancer and preliminary data concerning therapy with intraperitoneal radiopharmaceuticals. *Am J Obstet Gynecol* 1981;141:921–9.

96. **Lurain JR, Rumsey NK, Schink JC, Wallemark CB, Chmiel JS.** Prognostic significance of positive peritoneal cytology in clinical stage I adenocarcinoma of the endometrium. *Obstet Gynecol* 1989;74:175–9.

97. **Kadar N, Homesley HD, Malfetano JH.** Positive peritoneal cytology is an adverse factor in endometrial carcinoma only if there is other evidence of extrauterine disease. *Gynecol Oncol* 1992;46:145–9.

98. **Schink JC, Rademaker AW, Miller DS, Lurain JR.** Tumor size in endometrial cancer. *Cancer* 1991;67:2791–4.

99. **Martin JD, Hahnel R, McCartney AJ, Woodings TL.** The effect of estrogen receptor status on survival in patients with endometrial cancer. *Am J Obstet Gynecol* 1983;147:322–4.

100. **Zaino RJ, Satyaswaroop PG, Mortel R.** The relationship of histologic and histochemical parameters to progesterone receptor status in endometrial adenocarcinomas. *Gynecol Oncol* 1983;16:196–208.

101. **Creasman WT, Soper JT, McCarty KS Jr, McCarty KS Sr, Hinshaw W, Clarke-Pearson DL.** Influence of cytoplasmic steroid receptor content on prognosis of early stage endometrial carcinoma. *Am J Obstet Gynecol* 1985;151:922–32.

102. **Liao BS, Twiggs LB, Leung BS, Yu WC, Potish RA, Prem KA.** Cytoplasmic estrogen and progesterone receptors as prognostic parameters in primary endometrial carcinoma. *Obstet Gynecol* 1986;67:463–7.

103. **Geisinger KR, Homesley HD, Morgan TM, Kute TE, Marshall RB.** Endometrial adenocarcinoma: a multiparameter clinicopathologic analysis including the DNA profile and sex hormone receptors. *Cancer* 1986;58:1518–25.

104. **Palmer DC, Muir IM, Alexander AI, Cauchi M, Bennett RC, Quinn MA.** The prognostic importance of steroid receptors in endometrial carcinoma. *Obstet Gynecol* 1988;72:388–93.

105. **Iverson OE.** Flow cytometric deoxyribonucleic acid index: a prognostic factor in endometrial carcinoma. *Am J Obstet Gynecol* 1986;155:770–6.

106. **Stendahl U, Strang P, Wagenius G, Bergstrom R, Tribukait B.** Prognostic significance of proliferation in endometrial adenocarcinomas: a multivariate analysis of clinical and flow cytometric variables. *Int J Gynaecol Pathol* 1991;10:271–84.

107. **Mizuuchi H, Nasim S, Kudo R, Silverberg SG, Greenhouse S, Garrett CT.** Clinical implications of K-*ras* mutations in malignant epithelial tumors of the endometrium. *Cancer Res* 1992;52:2777–81.

108. **Fujimoto I, Shimizu Y, Hirai Y, Chen JT, Teshima H, Hasumi K, et al.** Studies on *ras* oncogene activation in endometrial carcinoma. *Gynecol Oncol* 1993;48:196–202.

109. **Berchuck A, Rodriguez G, Kinney RB, Soper JT, Dodge RK, Clarke-Pearson DL, et al.** Overexpression of HER-2/*neu* in endometrial cancer is associated with advanced stage disease. *Am J Obstet Gynecol* 1991;164:15–21.

110. **Hetzel DJ, Wilson TO, Keeney GL, Roche PC, Cha SS, Podratz KC.** HER-2/*neu* expression: a major prognostic factor in endometrial cancer. *Gynecol Oncol* 1992;47:179–85.

111. **Kohler MF, Berchuck A, Davidoff AM, Humphrey PA, Dodge RK, Iglehart JD, et al.** Overexpression and mutation of p53 in endometrial carcinoma. *Cancer Res* 1992;52:1622–7.

112. **Bur ME, Perlman C, Edelmann L, Fey E, Rose PG.** p53 expression in neoplasms of the uterine corpus. *Am J Clin Pathol* 1992;98:81–7.

113. **Peters WA III, Andersen WA, Thornton N Jr, Morley GW.** The selective use of vaginal hysterectomy in the management of adenocarcinoma of the endometrium. *Am J Obstet Gynecol* 1983;146:285–9.

114. **Malkasian GD, Annegers JF, Fountain KS.** Carcinoma of the endometrium: stage I. *Am J Obstet Gynecol* 1980;136:872–83.

115. **Bloss JD, Berman ML, Bloss LP, Buller RE.** Use of vaginal hysterectomy for the management of stage I endometrial cancer in the medically compromised patient. *Gynecol Oncol* 1991;40:74–7.

116. **Childers JM, Surwit EA.** Combined laparoscopic and vaginal surgery for the management of two cases of stage I endometrial cancer. *Gynecol Oncol* 1992;45:46–51.

117. **Photopulos GJ, Stovall TG, Summitt RL Jr.** Laparoscopic-assisted vaginal hysterectomy, bilateral salpingo-oophorectomy, and pelvic lymph node sampling for endometrial cancer. *J Gynecol Surg* 1992;8:91–4.

118. **Childers JM, Brzechffa PR, Hatch KD, Surwit EA.** Laparoscopically-assisted surgical staging (LASS) of endometrial cancer. *Gynecol Oncol* 1993;51:33–8.

119. **Boike G, Lurain J, Burke J.** A comparison of laparoscopic management of endometrial cancer with traditional laparotomy. *Gynecol Oncol* 1994;52:105 (abstract).

120. **Lewis BV, Stallworthy JA, Cowdell R.** Adenocarcinoma of the body of the uterus. *J Obstet Gynecol Br Commonw* 1970;77:343–8.

121. **DeMuelenaere GFGO.** The case against Wertheim's hysterectomy in endometrial carcinoma. *J Obstet Gynaecol Br Commonw* 1973;80:728–34.

122. **Rutledge F.** The role of radical hysterectomy in adeno-carcinoma of the endometrium. *Gynecol Oncol* 1974;2:331–47.

123. **Jones HW III.** Treatment of adenocarcinoma of the endometrium. *Obstet Gynecol Surv* 1975;30:147–69.

124. **Landgren R, Fletcher G, Delclos L, Wharton T.** Irradiation of endometrial cancer in patients with medical contraindication to surgery or with unresectable lesions. *Am J Roentgenol* 1976;126:148–54.

125. **Abayomi O, Tak W, Emami B, Anderson B.** Treatment of endometrial carcinoma with radiation therapy alone. *Cancer* 1982;49:2466–9.

126. **Patanaphan V, Salazar O, Chougule P.** What can be expected when radiation therapy becomes the only curative alternative for endometrial cancer? *Cancer* 1985;55:1462–7.

127. **Jones D, Stout R.** Results of intracavitary radium treatment for adenocarcinoma of the body of the uterus. *Clin Radiol* 1986;37:169–71.

128. **Varia M, Rosenman J, Halle J, Walton L, Currie J, Fowler W.** Primary radiation therapy for medically inoperable patients with endometrial carcinoma stages I-II. *Int J Radiat Oncol Biol Phys* 1987;13:11–5.

129. **Wang M, Hussey D, Vigliotti A, Benda J, Wen BC, Doornbos JF, et al.** Inoperable adeno-carcinoma of the endometrium: Radiation therapy. *Radiology* 1987;165:561–5.

130. **Grigsby P, Kuske R, Perez C, Walz BJ, Camel MH, Kao MS, et al.** Medically inoperable stage I adenocarcinoma of the endometrium treated with radiotherapy alone. *Int J Radiat Oncol Biol Phys* 1987;13:483–8.

131. **Taghian A, Pernot M, Hoffstetter S, Luporsti E, Bey P.** Radiation therapy alone for medically inoperable patients with adenocarcinoma of the endometrium. *Int J Radiat Oncol Biol Phys* 1988;15:1135–40.

132. **Lehoczky O, Busze P, Ungar L, Tottossy B.** Stage I endometrial carcinoma: treatment of nonoperable patients with intracavitary radiation therapy alone. *Gynecol Oncol* 1991;43:211–6.

133. **Kupelian PA, Eifel PJ, Tornos C, Burke TW, Delclos L, Oswald MJ.** Treatment of endometrial carcinoma with radiation therapy alone. *Int J Radiat Oncol Biol Phys* 1993;27:817–24.

134. **Piver MS, Yazigi R, Blumenson L, Tsukada Y.** A prospective trial comparing hysterectomy, hysterectomy plus vaginal radium and uterine radium plus hysterectomy in stage I endometrial cancer. *Obstet Gynecol* 1979;54:85–9.

135. **Piver MS, Hempling RE.** A prospective trial of postoperative vaginal radium/cesium for grade 1-2 less than 50% myometrial invasion and pelvic irradiation therapy for grade 3 or deep myometrial invasion in surgical stage I endometrial adenocarcinoma. *Cancer* 1990;66:1133–8.

136. **Peschel RE, Healey GA, Smith RJ, Haffty B, Papadopoulos D, Chambers JT, et al.** High dose rate remote afterloading for endometrial cancer. *Endocurie Hyperthem Oncol* 1989;5:209–14.

137. **Stryker JA, Podczaski E, Kaminski P, Velkley DE.** Adjuvant external beam therapy for pathologic stage I and occult stage II endometrial carcinoma. *Cancer* 1991;67:2872–9.

138. **Potish RA, Twiggs LB, Adcock LL, Savage JE, Levitt SH, Prem KA.** Para-aortic lymph node radiotherapy in cancer of the uterine corpus. *Obstet Gynecol* 1985;65:251–6.

139. **Rose PG, Cha SD, Tak WK, Fitzgerald T, Peale F, Hunter RE.** Radiation therapy for surgically proven para-aortic node metastasis in endometrial carcinoma. *Int J Radiat Oncol Biol Phys* 1992;24:229–33.

140. **Feuer GA, Calanog A.** Endometrial carcinoma: treatment of positive para-aortic nodes. *Gynecol Oncol* 1987;27:104–9.

141. **Corn BW, Lanciano RM, Greven KM, Schultz DJ, Reisinger SA, Stafford PM, et al.** Endometrial cancer with para-aortic adenopathy: patterns of failure and opportunities for cure. *Int J Radiat Oncol Biol Phys* 1992;24:223–7.

142. **Potish RA, Twiggs LB, Adcock LL, Prem KA.** Role of whole abdominal radiation therapy in the management of endometrial cancer; prognostic importance of factors indicating peritoneal metastases. *Gynecol Oncol* 1985;21:80–6.

143. **Greer BE, Hamberger AD.** Treatment of intraperitoneal metastatic adenocarcinoma of the endometrial by the whole-abdomen moving-strip technique and pelvic boost irradiation. *Gynecol Oncol* 1983;16:365–73.

144. **Loeffler JS, Rosen EM, Niloff JM, Howes AE, Knapp RC.** Whole abdominal irradiation for tumors of the uterine corpus. *Cancer* 1988;61:1332–5.

145. **Martinez A, Schray M, Podratz K, Stanhope R, Malkasian G.** Postoperative whole abdomino-pelvic irradiation for patients with high-risk endometrial cancer. *Int J Radiat Oncol Biol Phys* 1989;17:371–7.

146. **Gibbons S, Martinez A, Schray M, Podratz K, Stanhope R, Garton G, et al.** Adjuvant whole abdominopelvic irradiation for high-risk endometrial carcinoma. *Int J Radiat Oncol Biol Phys* 1991;21:1019–25.

147. **Soper JT, Creasman WT, Clarke-Pearson DL, Sullivan DC, Vergadoro F, Johnson WW.** Intraperitoneal chromic phosphate P32 suspension therapy of malignant peritoneal cytology in endometrial carcinoma. *Am J Obstet Gynecol* 1985;153:191–6.

148. **Lewis GC Jr, Slack NH, Mortel R, Bross ID.** Adjuvant progestogen therapy in the primary definitive treatment of endometrial cancer. *Gynecol Oncol* 1974;2:368–76.

149. **DePalo G, Merson M, Del Vecchio M, Mangioni C, Periti P, Participants from 21 Institutions.** A controlled clinical study of adjuvant medroxyprogesterone acetate (MPA) therapy in pathologic stage I endometrial carcinoma with myometrial invasion. *Proc Am Soc Clin Oncol* 1985;4:121 (abstract).

150. **Vergote I, Kjorstad J, Abeler V, Kolstad P.** A randomized trial of adjuvant progestogen in early endometrial cancer. *Cancer* 1989;64:1011–6.

151. **Piver MS, Lele SB, Gamarra M.** Malignant peritoneal cytology in stage I endometrial adenocarcinoma: the effect of progesterone therapy (a preliminary report). *Eur J Gynaecol Oncol* 1988;9:187–90.

152. **Morrow CP, Bundy BN, Homesley H, Creasman WT, Hornback NB, Kurman R, et al.** Doxorubicin as an adjuvant following surgery and radiation therapy in patients with high-risk endometrial carcinoma, stage I and occult stage II. *Gynecol Oncol* 1990;36:166–71.

153. **Stringer CA, Gershenson DM, Burke TW, Edwards CL, Gordon AN, Wharton JT.** Adjuvant chemotherapy with cisplatin, doxorubicin, and cyclophosphamide (PAC) for early-stage high-risk endometrial cancer: a preliminary analysis. *Gynecol Oncol* 1990;38:305–8.

154. **Homesley HD, Boronow RC, Lewis JL Jr.** Stage II endometrial adenocarcinoma. Memorial Hospital for Cancer, 1949-1965. *Obstet Gynecol* 1977;49:604–8.

155. **Surwit EA, Fowler WC Jr, Rogoff EE, Jelovsek F, Parker RT, Creasman WT.** Stage II carcinoma of the endometrium. *Int J Radiat Oncol Biol Phys* 1979;5:323–6.

156. **Kinsella TJ, Bloomer WD, Lavin PT, Knapp RC.** Stage II endometrial carcinoma: a 10-year follow-up of combined radiation and surgical treatment. *Gynecol Oncol* 1980;10:290–7.

157. **Nahhas WA, Whitney CW, Stryker JA, Curry SL, Chung CK, Mortel R.** Stage II endometrial carcinoma. *Gynecol Oncol* 1980;10:303–11.

158. **Onsrud M, Aalders J, Abeler V, Taylor P.** Endometrial carcinoma with cervical involvement (stage II): prognostic factors and value of combined radiological-surgical treatment. *Gynecol Oncol* 1982;13:76–86.

159. **Berman ML, Afridi MA, Kanbour AI, Ball HG.** Risk factors and prognosis in stage III endometrial cancer. *Gynecol Oncol* 1982;14:49–61.

160. **Nori D, Hilaris BS, Tome M, Lewis JL Jr, Birnbaum S, Fuks Z.** Combined surgery and radiation in endometrial carcinoma: an analysis of prognostic factors. *Int J Radiat Oncol Biol Phys* 1987;13:489–97.

161. **Larson DM, Copeland LJ, Gallager HS, Wharton JT, Gershenson DM, Edwards CL, et al.** Prognostic factors in stage II endometrial carcinoma. *Cancer* 1987;60:1358–61.

162. **Larson DM, Copeland LJ, Gallager HS, Kong JP, Wharton JT, Stringer CA.** Stage II endometrial carcinoma. Results and complications of a combined radiotherapeutic-surgical approach. *Cancer* 1988;61:1528–34.

163. **Boothby RA, Carlson JA, Neiman W, Rubin MM, Morgan MA, Schultz D, et al.** Treatment of stage II endometrial carcinoma. *Gynecol Oncol* 1989;33:204–8.

164. **Podczaski ES, Kaminski P, Manetta A, Louk D, Andrews C, Larson J, et al.** Stage II endometrial carcinoma treated with external-beam radiotherapy, intracavitary application of cesium, and surgery. *Gynecol Oncol* 1989;35:251–4.

165. **Mannel RS, Berman ML, Walker JL, Manetta A, DiSaia PJ.** Management of endometrial cancer with suspected cervical involvement. *Obstet Gynecol* 1990;75:1016–22.

166. **Andersen ES.** Stage II endometrial carcinoma: prognostic factors and the results of treatment. *Gynecol Oncol* 1990;38:220–3.

167. **Lanciano RM, Curran WJ Jr, Greven KM, Fanning J, Stafford P, Randall ME, et al.** Influence of grade, histologic subtype, and timing of radiotherapy on outcome among patients with stage II carcinoma of the endometrium. *Gynecol Oncol* 1990;39:368–73.

168. **Higgins RV, van Nagell JR Jr, Horn EJ, Roberts SL, Donaldson ES, Gallion HH, et al.** Preoperative radiation therapy followed by extrafascial hysterectomy in patients with stage II endometrial cancer. *Cancer* 1991;68:1261–4.

169. **Rubin SC, Hoskins WJ, Saigo PE, Nori D, Mychalczak B, Chapman D, et al.** Management of endometrial adenocarcinoma with cervical involvement. *Gynecol Oncol* 1992;45:294–8.

170. **Bruckman JE, Bloomer WD, Marck A, Ehrmann RL, Knapp RC.** Stage III adenocarcinoma of the endometrium: two prognostic groups. *Gynecol Oncol* 1980;9:12–7.

171. **Danoff BF, McDay J, Louka M, Lewis GC, Lee J, Kramer S.** Stage III endometrial carcinoma: analysis of patterns of failure and therapeutic implications. *Int J Radiat Biol Phys* 1980;6:1491–5.

172. **Aalders JG, Abeler V, Kolstad P.** Clinical (stage III) as compared to subclinical intrapelvic extrauterine tumor spread in endometrial carcinoma: a clinical and histopathological study of 175 patients. *Gynecol Oncol* 1984;17:64–74.

173. **Genest P, Drouin P, Girard A, Gerig L.** Stage III carcinoma of the endometrium: a review of 41 cases. *Gynecol Oncol* 1987;26:77–86.

174. **Grigsby PW, Perez CA, Kuske RR, Kao MS, Galakatos AE.** Results of therapy, analysis of failures, and prognostic factors for clinical and pathologic stage III adenocarcinoma of the endometrium. *Gynecol Oncol* 1987;27:44–57.

175. **Greven K, Curran W, Whittington R, et al.** Analysis of failure patterns in stage III endometrial carcinoma and therapeutic implications. *Int J Radiat Oncol Biol Phys* 1989;17:35–9.

176. **Pliskow S, Penalver M, Averette HE.** Stage III and IV endometrial carcinoma: a review of 41 cases. *Gynecol Oncol* 1990;38:210–5.

177. **Aalders JG, Abeler V, Kolstad P.** Stage IV endometrial carcinoma: a clinical and histopathological study of 83 patients. *Gynecol Oncol* 1984;17:75–84.

178. **Rutledge FN, Smith JP, Wharton JT, O'Quinn AG.** Pelvic exenteration: analysis of 296 patients. *Am J Obstet Gynecol* 1977;129:881–92.

179. **Barber HRK, Brunschwig A.** Treatment and results of recurrent cancer of corpus uteri in patients receiving anterior and total exenteration 1947–1963. *Cancer* 1968;22:949–55.

180. **Aalders JG, Abeler V, Kolstad P.** Recurrent adenocarcinoma of the endometrium: a clinical and histopathological study of 379 patients. *Gynecol Oncol* 1984;17:85–103.

181. **Angel C, DuBeshter B, Dawson AE, Keller J.** Recurrent stage I endometrial adenocarcinoma in the nonirradiated patient: preliminary results of surgical "staging." *Gynecol Oncol* 1993;48:221–6.

182. **Phillips GL, Prem KA, Adcock LL, Twiggs LB.** Vaginal recurrence of adenocarcinoma of the endometrium. *Gynecol Oncol* 1982;13:323–8.

183. **Curran WJ, Whittington R, Peters AJ, Fanning J.** Vaginal recurrences of endometrial carcinoma: the prognostic value of staging by a primary vaginal carcinoma system. *Int J Radiat Oncol Biol Phys* 1988;15:803–8.

184. **Poulsen MG, Roberts SJ.** The salvage of recurrent endometrial carcinoma in the vagina and pelvis. *Int J Radiat Oncol Biol Phys* 1988;15:809–13.

185. **Kuten A, Grigsby PW, Perez CA, Fineberg B, Garcia DM, Simpson JR.** Results of radiotherapy in recurrent endometrial carcinoma: a retrospective analysis of 51 patients. *Int J Radiat Oncol Biol Phys* 1989;17:29–34.

186. **Sears JD, Greven KM, Hoen HM, Randall ME.** Prognostic factors and treatment outcome for patients with locally recurrent endometrial cancer. *Cancer* 1994;74:1303–8.

187. **Kelley RM, Baker WH.** Progestational agents in the treatment of carcinoma of the endometrium. *N Engl J Med* 1961;264:216–22.

188. **Reifenstein EC Jr.** The treatment of advanced endometrial cancer with hydroxyprogesterone caproate. *Gynecol Oncol* 1974;2:377–414.

189. **Piver MS, Barlow JJ, Lurain JR, Blumenson LE.** Medroxyprogesterone acetate (Depo-Provera) vs. hydroxyprogesterone caproate (Delalutin) in women with metastatic endometrial adenocarcinoma. *Cancer* 1980;45:268–72.

190. **Podratz KC, O'Brien PC, Malkasian GD Jr, Decker DG, Jefferies JA, Edmonson JH.** Effects of progestational agents in treatment of endometrial carcinoma. *Obstet Gynecol* 1985;66:106–10.

191. **Thigpen T, Blessing J, DiSaia P, et al.** Oral medroxyprogesterone acetate in advanced or recurrent endometrial carcinoma: results of therapy and correlation with estrogen and progesterone receptor levels. The Gynecologic Oncology Group experience. In: **Baulier EE, Iacobelli S, McGuire WL,** eds. *Endocrinology of Malignancy.* Park Ridge, NJ: Parthenon, 1986:446–54.

192. **Thigpen T, Blessing J, Hatch K, Barrett M, Adelson P, Disaia P, et al.** A randomized trial of medroxyprogesterone acetate (MPA) 200 mg versus 1000 mg daily in advanced or recurrent endometrial carcinoma: a Gynecologic Oncology Group study. *Proc Am Soc Clin Oncol* 1991;10:185 (abstract).

193. **Moore TD, Phillips PH, Nerenstone SR, Cheson BD.** Systemic treatment of advanced and recurrent endometrial carcinoma: current status and future directions. *J Clin Oncol* 1991;9:1071–88.

194. **Deppe G.** Chemotherapy for endometrial cancer. In: **Deppe G,** ed. *Chemotherapy of Gynecologic Cancer.* New York: Alan R. Liss, 1990:155–74.

195. **Muss HB.** Chemotherapy of metastatic endometrial cancer. *Semin Oncol* 1994;21:107–13.

196. **Pettersson F.** Annual report on the results of treatment in gynecological cancer. Stockholm, Sweden: Radiumhemmet. International Federation of Gynecology and Obstetrics, 1995:65–82.

197. **Podczaski E, Kaminski P, Gurski K, Mac Neil C, Stryker JA, Singapuri K, et al.** Detection and patterns of treatment failure in 300 consecutive cases of "early" endometrial cancer after primary surgery. *Gynecol Oncol* 1992;47:323–7.

198. **Patsner B, Orr JW, Mann WJ.** Use of serum CA125 measurement in posttreatment surveillance of early-stage endometrial carcinoma. *Am J Obstet Gynecol* 1990;162:427–9.

199. **Creasman WT, Henderson D, Hinshaw W, Clarke-Pearson DL.** Estrogen replacement therapy in the patient treated for endometrial cancer. *Obstet Gynecol* 1986;67:326–30.

200. **Lee RB, Burke TW, Park RC.** Estrogen replacement therapy following treatment for stage I endometrial carcinoma. *Gynecol Oncol* 1990;36:189–91.

201. **Harlow BL, Weiss NS, Lofton S.** The epidemiology of sarcomas of the uterus. *JNCI* 1986;76:399–402.

202. **Czesnin K, Wronkowski Z.** Second malignancies of the irradiated area in patients treated for uterine cervix cancer. *Gynecol Oncol* 1978;6:309–15.

203. **Kempson RL, Bari W.** Uterine sarcomas: classification, diagnosis and prognosis. *Hum Pathol* 1970;1:331–49.

204. **Tavassoli FA, Norris HJ.** Mesenchymal tumors of the uterus. VII. A clinicopathologic study of 60 endometrial stromal nodules. *Histopathol* 1981;5:1–10.

205. **Norris HJ, Taylor HB.** Mesenchymal tumors of the uterus. I. A clinical and pathologic study of 53 endometrial stromal tumors. *Cancer* 1966;19:755–66.

206. **Hart WR, Yoonessi M.** Endometrial stromatosis of the uterus. *Obstet Gynecol* 1977;49:393–403.

207. **Krieger PD, Gusberg SB.** Endolymphatic stromal myosis—a grade 1 endometrial sarcoma. *Gynecol Oncol* 1973;1:299–313.

208. **Thatcher SS, Woodruff JD.** Uterine stromatosis: a report of 33 cases. *Obstet Gynecol* 1982;59:428–34.

209. **Piver MS, Rutledge FN, Copeland L, Webster K, Blumenson L, Suh O.** Uterine endolymphatic stromal myosis: a collaborative study. *Obstet Gynecol* 1984;64:173–8.

210. **Yoonessi M, Hart WR.** Endometrial stromal sarcomas. *Cancer* 1977;40:898–906.

211. **Taylor HB, Norris HJ.** Mesenchymal tumors of the uterus. IV. Diagnosis and prognosis of leiomyosarcoma. *Arch Pathol* 1966;82:40–4.

212. **Gudgeon DH.** Leiomyosarcoma of the uterus. *Obstet Gynecol* 1968;32:96–100.

213. **Silverberg SG.** Leiomyosarcoma of the uterus. A clinicopathologic study. *Obstet Gynecol* 1971;38:613–28.

214. **Christopoherson WM, Williamson EO, Gray LA.** Leiomyosarcoma of the uterus. *Cancer* 1972;29:1512–7.

215. **Gallup DG, Cordray DR.** Leiomyosarcoma of the uterus: case reports and a review. *Obstet Gynecol Surv* 1979;34:300–12.

216. **Vardi JR, Tovell HMM.** Leiomyosarcoma of the uterus: clinicopathologic study. *Obstet Gynecol* 1980;56:428–34.

217. **Van Dinh TV, Woodruff JD.** Leiomyosarcoma of the uterus. *Am J Obstet Gynecol* 1982;144:817–23.

218. **Berchuck A, Rubin SC, Hoskins WJ, Saigo PE, Pierce VK, Lewis JL Jr.** Treatment of uterine leiomyosarcoma. *Obstet Gynecol* 1988;71:845–50.

219. **Norris HJ, Parmley T.** Mesenchymal tumors of the uterus. V. Intravenous leiomyomatosis: a clinical and pathologic study of 14 cases. *Cancer* 1975;36:2164–78.

220. **Scharfenberg JC, Geary WL.** Intravenous leiomyomatosis. *Obstet Gynecol* 1974;43:909–14.

221. **Evans AT III, Symmonds RE, Gaffey TA.** Recurrent pelvic intravenous leiomyomatosis. *Obstet Gynecol* 1981;57:260–4.

222. **Abell MR, Littler ER.** Benign metastasizing uterine leiomyoma: multiple lymph node metastases. *Cancer* 1975;36:2206–13.

223. **Banner AS, Carrington CB, Emory WB, Kittle F, Leonard G, Ringus J, et al.** Efficacy of oophorectomy in lymphangioleiomyomatosis and benign metastasizing leiomyoma. *N Engl J Med* 1981;305:204–9.

224. **Kurman RJ, Norris HJ.** Mesenchymal tumors of the uterus. VI. Epithelioid smooth muscle tumors including leiomyoblastoma and clear cell leiomyoma. A clinical and pathologic analysis of 26 cases. *Cancer* 1976;37:1853–65.

225. **Tavassoli FA, Norris HJ.** Peritoneal leiomyomatosis (leiomyomatosis peritonealis disseminata): a clinicopathologic study of 20 cases with ultrastructural observations. *Int J Gynaecol Pathol* 1982;1:59–74.

226. **King ME, Dickersin GR, Scully RE.** Myxoid leiomyosarcoma of the uterus. *Am J Surg Pathol* 1982;6:589–98.

227. **Norris HJ, Roth E, Taylor HB.** Mesenchymal tumors of the uterus. II. A clinical and pathologic study of 31 mixed mesodermal tumors. *Obstet Gynecol* 1966;28:57–63.

228. **Norris HJ, Taylor HB.** Mesenchymal tumors of the uterus. III. A clinical and pathologic study of 31 carcinosarcomas. *Cancer* 1966;19:1459–65.

229. **DiSaia PJ, Castro JR, Rutledge FN.** Mixed mesodermal sarcoma of the uterus. *Am J Roentgenol* 1973;117:632–6.

230. **Macasaet MA, Waxman M. Fruchter RG, Boyce J, Hong P, Nicastri AD, et al.** Prognostic factors in malignant mesodermal (müllerian) mixed tumors of the uterus. *Gynecol Oncol* 1985;20:32–42.

231. **DiSaia PJ, Morrow CP, Boronow R, Creasman W, Mittelstaedt L.** Endometrial sarcoma: lymphatic spread pattern. *Am J Obstet Gynecol* 1978;130:104–5.

232. **Geszler G, Szpak CA, Harris RE, Creasman W, Barter JF, Johnston WW.** Prognostic value of peritoneal washings in patients with malignant mixed müllerian tumors of the uterus. *Am J Obstet Gynecol* 1986;155:83–9.

233. **Clement PB, Scully RE.** Müllerian adenosarcoma of the uterus. *Cancer* 1974;34:1138–49.

234. **Zaloudek CJ, Norris HJ.** Adenofibroma and adenosarcoma of the uterus: a clinicopathologic study of 35 cases. *Cancer* 1981;48:354–66.

235. **Salazar OM, Bonfiglio TA, Patten SF, Keller BE, Feldstein ML, Dunne ME, et al.** Uterine sarcomas: analysis of failures with special emphasis on the use of adjuvant radiation therapy. *Cancer* 1978;42:1161–70.

236. **Spanos WJ, Peters LJ, Oswald MJ.** Patterns of recurrence in malignant mixed müllerian tumors of the uterus. *Cancer* 1986;57:155–9.

237. **Vongtama V, Karlen JR, Piver MS, Tsukada Y, Moore RH.** Treatment results and prognostic factors in stage I and II sarcomas of the corpus uteri. *Am J Roentgen Rad Ther Nucl Med* 1976;126:139–47.

238. **Belgrad R, Elbadawi N, Rubin P.** Uterine sarcomas. *Radiology* 1975;114:181–8.

239. **Salazar OM, Bonfiglio TA, Patten SF, Keller BE, Feldstein M, Dunne ME, et al.** Uterine sarcomas: natural history, treatment, and prognosis. *Cancer* 1978;42:1152–60.

240. **Perez CA, Askin F, Baglan RJ, Kao MS, Kraus FT, Perez BM, et al.** Effects of irradiation on mixed müllerian tumors of the uterus. *Cancer* 1979;43:1274–84.

241. **Hornback NB, Omura G, Major FJ.** Observations on the use of adjuvant radiation therapy in patients with stage I and II uterine sarcoma. *Int J Radiat Oncol Biol Phys* 1986;12:2127–30.

242. Gottlieb JA, Baker LH, O'Bryan RM, Sinkovics JG, Hoogstraten JM, Quagliana JM, et al. Adriamycin used alone and in combination for soft tissue and bony sarcomas. *Cancer Chemother Rep Part 3* 1975;6:271–82.

243. Blum RH, Corson JM, Wilson RE, Greenberger JS, Canellos GP, Frei E III. Successful treatment of metastatic sarcomas with cyclophosphamide, adriamycin, and DTIC (CAD). *Cancer* 1980;46:1722–6.

244. Omura GA, Major FJ, Blessing JA, Sedlacek TV, Thigpen JT, Creasman WT, et al. A randomized study of adriamycin with and without dimethyl triazenoimidazole carboxamide in advanced uterine sarcomas. *Cancer* 1983;52:626–32.

245. Thigpen JT, Blessing JA, Beecham J, Homesley H, Yordan E. Phase II trial of cisplatin as first-line chemotherapy in patients with advanced or recurrent uterine sarcomas: a Gynecologic Oncology Group study. *J Clin Oncol* 1991;9:1962–6.

246. Gershenson DM, Kavanagh JJ, Copeland LJ, Edwards CL, Stringer CA, Wharton JT. Cisplatin therapy for a disseminated mixed mesodermal sarcoma of the uterus. *J Clin Oncol* 1987;5:618–21.

247. Sutton GP, Blessing JA, Rosenshein N, Photopulos G, DiSaia PJ. Phase II trial of ifosfamide and mesna in mixed mesodermal tumors of the uterus. *Am J Obstet Gynecol* 1989;161:309–12.

248. Piver MS, DeEulis TG, Lele SB, Barlow JJ. Cyclophosphamide, vincristine, adriamycin, and dimethyltriazenoimidazole carboxamide (CYVADIC) for sarcomas of the female genital tract. *Gynecol Oncol* 1981;14:319–23.

249. Omura GA, Blessing JA, Major F, Litshitz S, Ehrlich CE, Mangan C, et al. A randomized clinical trial of adjuvant adriamycin in uterine sarcomas: a Gynecologic Oncology Group study. *J Clin Oncol* 1985;3:1240–5.

250. Piver MS, Lele SB, Marchetti DL, Emrich LJ. The effect of adjuvant chemotherapy on time to recurrence and survival of stage I uterine sarcomas. *J Surg Oncol* 1988;38:233–9.

251. Peters WA III, Rivkin SE, Smith MR, Tesh DE. Cisplatin and adriamycin combination chemotherapy for uterine stromal sarcomas and mixed mesodermal tumors. *Gynecol Oncol* 1989;34:323–7.

32 Cervical and Vaginal Cancer

Kenneth D. Hatch
Yao S. Fu

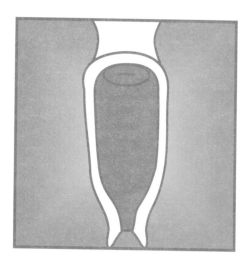

Invasive cancer of the cervix has been considered a preventable cancer because it has a long preinvasive state, because cervical cytology screening programs are available, and because the treatment for preinvasive lesions is effective. However, 15,700 new cases of invasive cervical cancer and approximately 4900 deaths were anticipated in the U.S. in 1996 (1). Although cervical cancer has not been eliminated, the incidence of invasive disease is decreasing and it is being diagnosed earlier, leading to better survival rates (1, 2). The mean age for cervical cancer is 52.2 years, and the distribution of cases is bimodal, with peaks at 35–39 years and 60–64 years (1).

Primary vaginal cancer is a relatively uncommon tumor, representing only 1–2% of malignant neoplasms of the female genital tract. Primary vaginal cancer should be differentiated from cancers metastatic to the vagina.

Cervical Cancer

Vaginal bleeding is the most common symptom occurring in patients with cancer of the cervix. Most often this is postcoital bleeding, but it may occur as irregular or postmenopausal bleeding. Patients with advanced disease may have a malodorous vaginal discharge, weight loss, or obstructive uropathy.

On general physical examination, the supraclavicular and groin lymph nodes should be palpated to exclude metastatic disease. On pelvic examination, a speculum is inserted into the vagina and the cervix is inspected for suspicious areas. The vagina is inspected for extension of disease. With invasive cancer, the cervix is usually firm and expanded, and these features should be evaluated by digital examination. Rectal examination is important to help establish cervical consistency and size, particularly in patients with endocervical carcinomas. It is the only way to determine cervical size if the vaginal fornices have been obliterated by menopausal changes or by the extension of disease. Parametrial ex-

1111

tension of disease is best determined by the finding of nodularity beyond the cervix on rectal examination.

When obvious tumor growth is present, cervical biopsy performed on an outpatient basis is usually sufficient for diagnosis. Colposcopy may be helpful in directing the examiner toward the most invasive area for biopsy. If the diagnosis cannot be established conclusively with outpatient biopsy, diagnostic conization may be necessary.

Pathology

Microinvasive Cervical Squamous Carcinoma

Cervical conization is required to assess correctly the depth and the linear extent of involvement of microinvasion. The earliest invasion is characterized by a protrusion from the stromoepithelial junction. This focus consists of cells that appear better differentiated than the adjacent noninvasive cells and have abundant pink-staining cytoplasm, hyperchromatic nuclei, and small- to medium-sized nucleoli (3). **These early invasive lesions in the form of tongue-like processes without measurable volume are classified as International Federation of Gynecology and Obstetrics (FIGO) stage Ia1.** With further progression, more tongue-like processes and isolated cells occur in the stroma (Fig. 32.1). The latter responds by a proliferation of fibroblasts (desmoplasia) and a band-like infiltration of chronic inflammatory cells. With increasing depth of invasion, invasion occurs at multiple sites, and the growth becomes measurable by depth and linear extent. **Lesions that are ≤3 mm are classified as FIGO stage Ia1. Lesions that are >3–5 mm or more in depth and ≤7 mm in linear extent are classified as FIGO stage Ia2.** (4). With increasing stromal invasion, the involvement of capillary-lymphatic spaces is increased. Foreign body multinucleated giant cells containing keratin debris, dilated capillaries, and lymphatic spaces are often seen in the stroma.

Figure 32.1 Microinvasive squamous carcinoma. Multiple irregular tonguelike processes and isolated nests of malignant cells are seen, some surrounded by clear spaces, simulating capillary lymphatic invasion. This is an artifact caused by tissue shrinkage. The depth of stromal invasion is measured from the basement membrane of the overlying cervial intraepithelial neoplasia (CIN). In this case it is 1.5 mm. (Figures 32.1–32.11 Reproduced from **Berek JS, Hacken WF.** *Practical Gynecologic Oncology,* 2nd ed. Baltimore: Williams & Wilkins, 1994.)

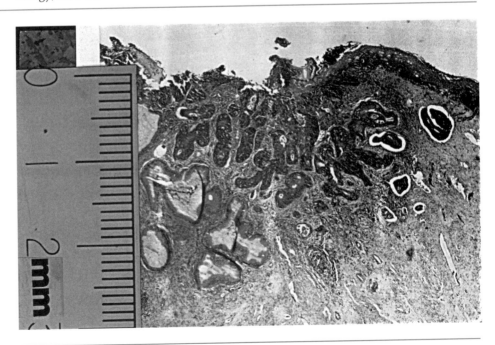

The depth of invasion should be measured with the micrometer from the base of the epithelium to the deepest point of invasion. **The depth of invasion is significant for the development of pelvic lymph node metastasis and tumor recurrence. Although lesions that have invaded 3 mm or less rarely metastasize, patients in whom lesions invade more than 3–5 mm have positive pelvic lymph nodes in 5–8% of cases** (5). Although the significance of the cutoff at 3 mm has not been identified completely, it may be postulated that capillary-lymphatic spaces are extremely small at this level and whether they can carry tumor cells beyond the specific zone is unclear. Uneven shrinkage of tissue by fixative often creates space between the tumor nests and the surrounding fibrous stroma, stimulating vascular lymphatic invasion (Fig. 32.1). **A suspected vascular involvement with invasion of less than 3 mm should be interpreted with care.** A lack of endothelial lining indicates that the space is shrinkage artifact rather than true vascular invasion.

Invasive Cervical Cancer

Squamous Cell Carcinoma   **Invasive squamous cell carcinoma is the most common variety of invasive cancer in the cervix.** Histologically, there are large cell keratinizing, large cell nonkeratinizing, and small cell types (6). Large cell keratinizing tumors are made up of tumor cells forming irregular infiltrative nests with laminated keratin pearls in the center. Large cell nonkeratinizing carcinomas reveal individual cell keratinization but do not form keratin pearls (Fig. 32.2). The category of small cell carcinoma includes poorly differentiated squamous cell carcinoma and small cell anaplastic carcinoma. If possible, these two tumors should be differentiated. The former contains cells that have small- to medium-sized nuclei, open chromatin, small or large nucleoli, and more abundant cytoplasm than those of the latter. The designation of small cell anaplastic carcinoma should be reserved for lesions resembling oat cell carcinoma of the lung. It infiltrates diffusely and consists of tumor cells that have scanty cytoplasm, round to oval small nuclei, coarsely granular chro-

Figure 32.2   Invasive squamous cell carcinoma, large cell nonkeratinizing type. Tumor cells form irregular nests and have abundant eosinophilic cytoplasm and distinct cell borders indicative of squamous differentiation.

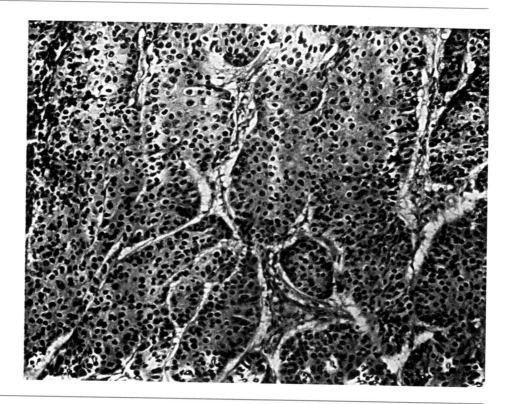

matin, and high mitotic activity. The nucleoli are absent or small. The small cell neuroendocrine tumors are differentiated by immunohistochemistry or electron microscopy.

Patients with the large cell type of carcinoma, with or without keratinization, have a better prognosis than those with the small cell variant. Furthermore, small cell anaplastic carcinomas behave more aggressively than poorly differentiated squamous carcinomas that contain small cells. The prognosis is affected adversely by the presence of vascular lymphatic invasion, deep stromal invasion, infiltration of parametrial tissue, and pelvic lymph node metastasis.

Adenocarcinoma   In recent years, there has been an increasing number of cervical adenocarcinomas affecting young women in their twenties and thirties. Adenocarcinoma *in situ* is believed to be the precursor of invasive adenocarcinoma, and it is not surprising that the two often coexist (7). In addition, squamous neoplasia, intraepithelial or invasive, also occurs in 30–50% of cervical adenocarcinomas. Adenocarcinoma may be detected by cervical sampling but less reliably so than squamous carcinomas. A definitive diagnosis may require cervical conization.

Invasive adenocarcinoma may be pure (Fig. 32.3) or mixed with squamous cell carcinoma—the adenosquamous carcinoma. Within the category of pure adenocarcinoma, the tumors are quite heterogeneous (6) with a wide range of cell types, growth patterns, and differentiation. About 80% of cervical adenocarcinomas are made up predominantly of cells of the endocervical type with mucin production. The remaining tumors are populated by endometroid cells, clear cells, intestinal cells, or a mixture of more than one cell type. By histologic examination alone, some of these tumors are indistinguishable from those arising elsewhere in the endometrium or ovary.

Figure 32.3   Invasive adenocarcinoma of the cervix, well-differentiated. Irregular glands are lined with tall columnar cells with vacuolated mucinous cytoplasm resembling endocervical cells. Nuclear stratification, mild nuclear atypism, and mitotic figures are evident.

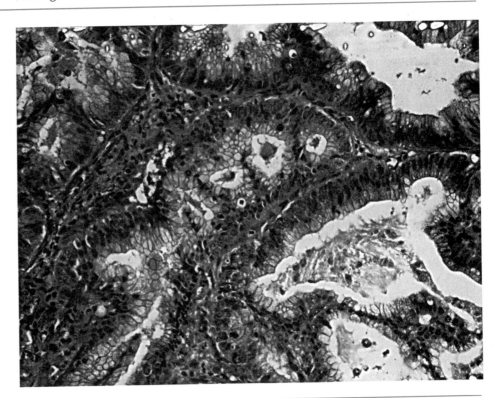

Within each tumor type, the growth patterns and nuclear abnormalities vary according to the degree of differentiation. In well-differentiated tumors, tall columnar cells line the well-formed branching glands and papillary structures, whereas pleomorphic cells tend to form irregular nests and solid sheets in poorly differentiated neoplasms. The latter may require mucicarmine and periodic acid-Schiff (PAS) stains to confirm their glandular differentiation.

There are several special variants of adenocarcinoma. *Minimal deviation adenocarcinoma (adenoma malignum)* is an extremely well-differentiated form of adenocarcinoma in which the branching glandular pattern strongly simulates that of the normal endocervical glands. In addition, the lining cells have abundant mucinous cytoplasm and uniform nuclei (8, 9). Because of this, the tumor may not be recognized as malignant in small biopsy specimens, thereby causing considerable delay in diagnosis. Earlier studies reported a dismal outcome for women with this tumor, but more recent studies have found a favorable prognosis if the disease is detected early (10). Although rare, similar tumors have also been reported in association with endometrioid, clear, and mesonephric cell types (11).

An entity recently described by Young and Scully (12) as *villoglandular papillary adenocarcinoma* also deserves special attention. It primarily affects young women, some of whom are pregnant or users of oral contraceptives. Histologically, the tumors have smooth, well-defined borders, are well differentiated, and are either *in situ* or superficially invasive. The follow-up information is encouraging, however; none of these tumors has recurred after cervical conization or hysterectomy. Among women undergoing pelvic nodal dissection, no metastases have been detected. This tumor appears to have limited risk for spread beyond the uterus.

In mature *adenosquamous carcinomas,* the glandular and squamous carcinomas are readily identified on routine histologic sections and do not cause diagnostic problems. In poorly differentiated or immature adenosquamous carcinomas, however, glandular differentiation can be appreciated only with special stains, such as mucicarmine and PAS. In the study by Benda et al. (11), 30% of squamous cell carcinomas demonstrated mucin secretion when stained with mucicarmine. These squamous cell carcinomas with mucin secretion have a higher incidence of pelvic lymph node metastases than squamous cell carcinomas without mucin secretion (11) and are similar to the signet-ring variant of adenosquamous carcinoma previously described by Glucksmann and Cherry (13).

Glucksmann and Cherry also recognized *glassy cell carcinoma* as a poorly differentiated form of adenosquamous carcinoma. Individual cells have abundant eosinophilic, granular, ground-glass cytoplasm, large round to oval nuclei, and prominent nucleoli. The stroma is infiltrated by numerous lymphocytes, plasma cells, and eosinophils. About one-half of these tumors contain glandular structures or stain positive for mucin. The poor diagnosis of this tumor is linked to understaging and resistance to radiotherapy.

Other variants of adenosquamous carcinoma include adenoid basal carcinoma and adenoid cystic carcinoma. Adenoid basal carcinoma simulates the basal cell carcinoma of the skin (14). Nests of basaloid cells extend from the surface epithelium deep into the underlying tissue. Cells at the periphery of tumor nests form a distinct parallel nuclear arrangement, the so-called "peripheral palisading." An "adenoid" pattern occasionally develops, with "hollowed-out" nests of cells. Mitoses are rare, and the tumor often extends deep into the cervical stroma.

Adenoid cystic carcinoma of the cervix behaves much like such lesions elsewhere in the body. The tumor tends to invade into the adjacent tissues and metastasize late, often 8–10 years after the primary tumor has been removed. Like other adenoid cystic tumors, they may metastasize directly to the lung. The pattern simulates that of the adenoid basal tumor, but there is a cystic component and the glands of the cervix are involved (14). Mitoses may be seen but are not numerous.

Sarcoma   The most important sarcoma of the cervix is the *embryonal rhabdomyosarcoma,* which occurs in children and young adults. The tumor has grape-like polypoid nodules, the botryoid sarcoma, and the diagnosis depends on the recognition of rhabdomyoblasts (6). Leiomyosarcomas and mixed mesodermal tumors involving the cervix may be primary but are more likely to be secondary to uterine tumors.

Malignant Melanoma   On rare occasions, melanosis has been seen in the cervix. Thus, malignant melanoma may arise *de novo* in this area. Histopathologically, it stimulates melanoma elsewhere, and the prognosis depends on the depth of invasion into the cervical stroma.

Metastatic Cancer   **The cervix is commonly involved in cancer of the endometrium and vagina. The latter is rare, and most lesions that involve the cervix and vagina are designated cervical primaries.** Consequently, the clinical classification is that of cervical neoplasia extending to the vagina, rather than vice versa. Endometrial cancer may extend into the cervix by three modes: direct extension from the endometrium, submucosal involvement by lymph vascular extension, and multifocal disease. The latter is most unusual, but occasionally a focus of adenocarcinoma may be seen in the cervix, separate from the endometrium. This lesion should not be diagnosed as metastasis but rather as "multifocal disease." Malignancies involving the peritoneal cavity (e.g., ovarian cancer) may be found in the cul-de-sac and extend directly into the vagina and cervix. Carcinomas of the urinary bladder and colon occasionally extend into the cervix. Cervical involvement by lymphoma, leukemia, and carcinoma of the breast, stomach, and kidney is usually part of the systemic spread. However, an isolated metastasis to the cervix may be the first sign of a primary tumor elsewhere in the body.

Small Cell Carcinoma   Van Nagell et al. (15) have described the aggressive nature of *small cell (neuroendocrine type) carcinoma of the cervix* and have noted its similarity to that arising from the bronchus. At the time of diagnosis, it is usually disseminated, with bone, brain, liver, and bone marrow being the most common sites of metastases. Pathologically, the diagnosis is aided by the finding of neuroendocrine granules on electron microscopy, as well as by immunoperoxidase studies that are positive for a variety of neuroendocrine proteins such as calcitonin, insulin, glucagon, somatostatin, gastrin, and adrenocorticotropic hormone (ACTH). In addition to the traditional staging for cancer of the cervix, these patients should undergo bone, liver, and brain scanning, as well as bone marrow aspiration and biopsy.

Colposcopy of the Invasive Lesion

For patients with suspected early invasive cancer based on Papanicolaou (Pap) test results and a grossly normal-appearing cervix, colposcopic examination is mandatory. Colposcopic findings that suggest invasion are 1) abnormal blood vessels, 2) irregular surface contour with loss of surface epithelium, and 3) color tone change. **Colposcopically directed biopsies may permit the diagnosis of frank invasion and thus avoid the need for diagnostic cone biopsy, allowing treatment to be administered without delay.**

Abnormal Blood Vessels   Abnormal vessels may be looped, branching, or reticular. Abnormal looped vessels are the most common and arise from the punctation and mosaic vessels present in cervical intraepithelial neoplasia (CIN). As the neoplastic growth process proceeds, the need for nutrition leads to proliferation of the blood vessels, and the punctate vessels at the surface produce double and triple loops.

These surface tufting vessels then proliferate and push out over the surface of the epithelium in an erratic fashion. Some are straight, although most have a loop, a corkscrew, or a J-shaped pattern (Fig. 32.4).

Abnormal branching vessels arise from the cervical stroma and are pushed to the surface as the underlying cancer invades and pushes upward. The normally branching cervical stromal vessels are best observed over nabothian cysts. In this area, the branches are generally at acute angles, with the caliber of vessels becoming smaller after branching, much like the arborization of a tree. The abnormal branching blood vessels seen with cancer tend to form obtuse or right angles, with the caliber sometimes enlarging after branching (Fig. 32.5). Sharp turns, dilatations, and narrowings also mark the behavior of these vessels. The surface epithelium may be lost in these areas, leading to irregular surface contour and friability.

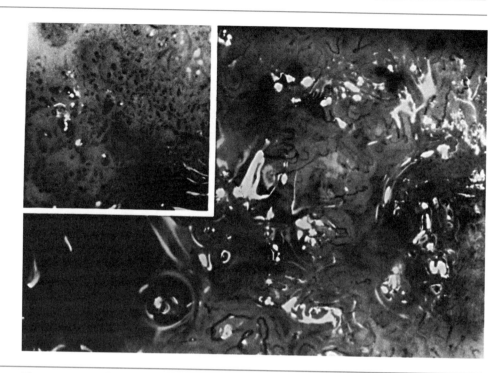

Figure 32.4   Abnormal looped vessels in invasive cervical cancer.

Abnormal reticular vessels represent the terminal capillaries of the cervical epithelium. Normal capillaries are best seen in a postmenopausal woman with atrophic epithelium. When cancer involves this epithelium, the surface is again eroded, and the capillary network is exposed. These vessels are very fine, short, and composed of small commas without an organized pattern (Fig. 32.6). They are not specific for invasive cancer; atrophic cervicitis may also have this appearance.

Irregular Surface Contour   Abnormal surface patterns are observed as the tumor growth proceeds. The surface epithelium ulcerates as the cells lose intercellular cohesiveness secondary to the loss of desmosomes. Irregular contour also may occur because of a papillary characteristic of the lesion (Fig. 32.7). **This finding sometimes can be confused with a human papillomavirus papillary growth on the cervix, and for that reason, biopsies should be performed on all papillary cervical growths.**

Color Tone Change   Color tone may change as a result of the increasing vascularity, surface epithelial necrosis, and in some cases, production of keratin. The color tone is a yellow-orange rather than the expected pink of intact squamous epithelium or the red of the endocervical epithelium.

Adenocarcinoma   Adenocarcinoma of the cervix does not have a specific colposcopic appearance. All of the aforementioned blood vessels may be seen in these lesions as well. **Because adenocarcinomas tend to develop within the endocervix, endocervical curettage is required as part of the colposcopic examination.**

Pathology

Clinical Staging

The current staging system of the International Federation of Gynecology and Obstetrics (FIGO) is presented in Table 32.1. The staging procedures allowed by FIGO are listed in Table 32.2.

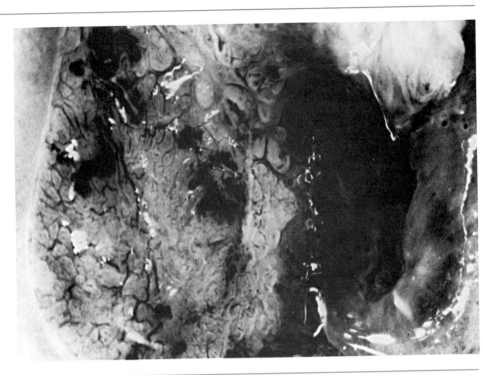

Figure 32.5   Abnormal branching vessels in invasive cervical cancer.

Figure 32.6   Abnormal reticular vessels in invasive cervical cancer.

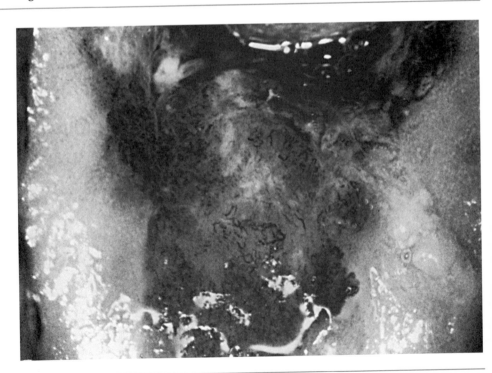

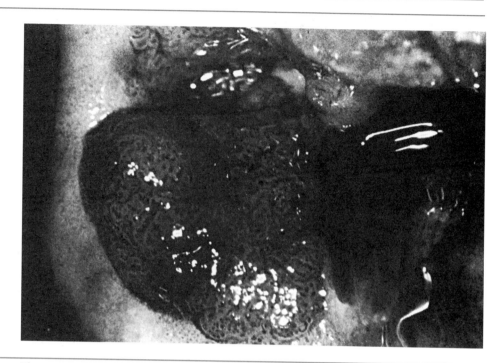

Figure 32.7   Irregular surface growth in invasive cervical cancer.

When there is doubt concerning the stage to which a cancer should be allocated, selection of the earlier stage is mandatory. After a clinical stage is assigned and treatment has been initiated, the stage must not be changed because of subsequent findings by either extended clinical staging or surgical staging. The "upstaging" of patients during treatment will produce an erroneous improvement in the results of treatment of low-stage disease. The distribution of patients by clinical stage is as follows: 38%, stage I; 32%, stage II; 26%, stage III; and 4%, stage IV (2).

Extended Clinical Staging   Lymphangiography, computerized axial tomography (CT), ultrasonography, and magnetic resonance imaging (MRI) have been used by various investigators in an attempt to improve clinical staging (16–21). Because these tests are not generally available throughout the world and because the interpretation of results is variable, the findings of these studies are not used for assigning the FIGO stage. However, they may be used in planning therapy.

Evaluation of the para-aortic lymph nodes with lymphangiography is associated with a false-positive rate of 20–40% and a false-negative rate of 10–20% (16–18). The accuracy of CT scans is 80–85%; the false-negative rate is 10–15% and the false-positive rate is 20–25% (19–21). Early MRI data are comparable (22). When abnormalities are noted by these procedures, a fine-needle aspiration (FNA) showing metastatic disease will allow the radiation treatment field to be extended and obviate the need for an exploratory laparotomy to determine the status of the lymph nodes.

Surgical Staging   The accuracy of clinical staging is somewhat limited, and surgical evaluation, which is not practical or feasible in many patients, is more accurate. The specifics of surgical staging are discussed later in this chapter.

Patterns of Spread

Cancer of the cervix spreads by 1) direct invasion into the cervical stroma, corpus, vagina, and parametrium; 2) lymphatic metastasis; 3) blood-borne metastasis; and 4) intraperitoneal implantation. The incidence of pelvic and para-aortic nodal metastasis is shown in Table 32.3.

1119

Table 32.1 FIGO Staging of Carcinoma of the Cervix Uteri

Preinvasive Carcinoma

Stage 0 Carcinoma *in situ,* intraepithelial carcinoma (cases of Stage 0 should not be included in any therapeutic statistics).

Invasive Carcinoma

Stage I* Carcinoma strictly confined to the cervix (extension to the corpus should be disregarded).

   Stage Ia Preclinical carcinomas of the cervix, that is, those diagnosed only by microscopy.

      Stage Ia1 Lesion with ≤3 mm invasion

      Stage Ia2 Lesions detected microscopically that can be measured. The upper limit of the measurement should show a depth of invasion of >3–5 mm taken from the base of the epithelium, either surface or glandular, from which it originates, and a second dimension, the horizontal spread, must not exceed 7 mm. Larger lesions should be staged as Ib.

   Stage Ib Lesions invasive >5 mm.

      Stage Ib1 Lesion less than or equal to 4 cm.

      Stage Ib2 Lesions larger than 4 cm.

Stage II† The carcinoma extends beyond the cervix but has not extended onto the wall. The carcinoma involves the vagina, but not the lower one-third.

   Stage IIa No obvious parametrial involvement.

   Stage IIb Obvious parametrial involvement.

Stage III‡ The carcinoma has extended onto the pelvic wall. On rectal examination, there is no cancer-free space between the tumor and the pelvic wall. The tumor involves the lower one-third of the vagina. All cases with hydronephrosis or nonfunctioning kidney.

   Stage IIIa No extension to the pelvic wall.

   Stage IIIb Extension onto the pelvic wall and/or hydronephrosis or nonfunctioning kidney.

Stage IV§ The carcinoma has extended beyond the true pelvis or has clinically involved the mucosa of the bladder or rectum. A bullous edema, as such, does not permit a case to be allotted to Stage IV.

   Stage IVa Spread to the growth to adjacent organs.

   Stage IVb Spread to distant organs.

---

*The diagnosis of both Stage Ia1 and Ia2 should be based on microscopic examination of removed tissue, preferably a cone, which must include the entire lesion. The depth of invasion should not be more than 5 mm taken from the base of the epithelium, either surface or glandular, from which it originates. The second dimension, the horizontal spread, must not exceed 7 mm. Vascular space involvement, either venous or lymphatic, should not alter the staging but should be specifically recorded as it may affect treatment decisions in the future. Lesions of greater size should be staged as Ib. As a rule, it is impossible to estimate clinically whether a cancer of the cervix has extended to the corpus. Extension to the corpus should therefore be disregarded.

†A patient with a growth fixed to the pelvic wall by a short and indurated, but not nodular, parametrium should be allotted to Stage IIb. At clinical examination, it is impossible to decide whether a smooth, indurated parametrium is truly cancerous or only inflammatory. Therefore, the case should be assigned to Stage III only if the parametrium is nodular to the pelvic wall or the growth itself extends to the pelvic wall.

‡The presence of hydronephrosis or nonfunctioning kidney due to stenosis of the ureter by cancer permits a case to be allotted to Stage III even if, according to other findings, it should be allotted to Stage I or II.

§The presence of the bullous edema, as such, should not permit a case to be allotted to Stage IV. Ridges and furrows into the bladder wall should be interpreted as signs of submucous involvement of the bladder if they remain fixed to the growth at palpation (i.e., examination from the vagina or the rectum during cystoscopy). A cytologic finding of malignant cells in washings from the urinary bladder requires further examination and a biopsy specimen from the wall of the bladder.

FIGO, International Federation of Gynecology and Obstetrics.

Table 32.2   Staging Procedures

Physical examination*	Palpate lymph nodes
	Examine vagina
	Bimanual rectovaginal examination
	(under anesthesia recommended)
Radiologic studies*	Intravenous pyelogram
	Barium enema
	Chest x-ray
	Skeletal x-ray
Procedures*	Biopsy
	Conization
	Hysteroscopy
	Colposcopy
	Endocervical curettage
	Cystoscopy
	Proctoscopy
Optional studies[†]	Computerized axial tomography
	Lymphangiography
	Ultrasonography
	Magnetic resonance imaging
	Radionucleotide scanning
	Laparoscopy

*Allowed by the International Federation of Gynecology and Obstetrics (FIGO).
[†]Information that is not allowed by FIGO to change the clinical stage.

Table 32.3   Incidence of Pelvic and Para-aortic Nodal Metastasis by Stage

Stage	n	% Positive Pelvic Nodes	% Positive Para-aortic Nodes
Ia1 (≤3 mm)	179[†]	0.5	0
Ia2 (>3–5 mm)	84[†]	4.8	<1
Ib	1926[††]	15.9	2.2
IIa	110[§]	24.5	11
IIb	324[§]	31.4	19
III	125[§]	44.8	30
IVa	23[§]	55	40

[†]References 14, 15, 41, 42.
[††]References 4, 23, 28, 29, 31, 33, 35, 50.
[§]References 3, 4, 23, 33, 47, 50.

Treatment

The principles of treatment for cancer of the cervix are the same as those for any other malignancy; i.e., both the primary lesion and the potential sites of spread should be treated.

The two modalities for primary treatment are surgery and radiotherapy. Whereas radiation therapy can be used in all stages of disease, surgery alone is limited to patients with stage I and IIa disease. The 5-year survival rate for stage I cancer of the cervix is approximately 85% with either radiation therapy or radical hysterectomy.

There are advantages to using surgical therapy instead of radiotherapy, particularly in younger women for whom conservation of the ovaries is important. Chronic bladder and bowel problems that require medical or surgical intervention occur in up to 8% of patients undergoing radiation therapy (23). Such problems are difficult to treat because they result from fibrosis and decreased vascularity. This is in contrast to surgical injuries, which in general are easily repairable and without long-term complications. Sexual dysfunction after radiation therapy is more likely to occur because of vaginal shortening, fibrosis, and atrophy of the epithelium. The surgical procedure shortens the vagina, but gradual lengthening is brought about by sexual activity. The epithelium does not become atrophic, because it responds either to the patient's endogenous estrogen or to exogenous estrogens if the patient is postmenopausal.

In general, radical hysterectomy is reserved for women who are in good physical condition. Chronologic age should not be a deterrent. With improvements in anesthesia, elderly patients withstand radical surgery almost as well as their younger counterparts (24).

Generally, it is prudent not to operate on lesions that are larger than 4 cm in diameter. When selected in this manner, the urinary fistula rate is <2% (25) and the operative mortality rate is <1% (26). An advantage of radiotherapy is its applicability to all stages and to most patients regardless of their age, height and weight, and medical condition.

Surgical Therapy

A summary of the surgical management of early cervical cancer is presented in Table 32.4.

Staging

Stage Ia—Microinvasive Carcinoma

Until 1985, no FIGO recommendation existed concerning the size of lesion or the depth of invasion that should be considered microinvasive (stage Ia). This led to considerable confusion and controversy in the literature. Over the years, as many as 18 different definitions have been used to describe "microinvasion." In 1974, the Society of Gynecologic Oncologists (SGO) recommended a definition that is now being accepted by FIGO: **"A microinvasive lesion is one in which neoplastic epithelium invades the stroma to a depth of ≤3 mm beneath the basement membrane and in which lymphatic or blood vascular involvement is not demonstrated." The purpose of defining microinvasion is to identify a group of patients who are not at risk of lymph node metastases or recurrence and who therefore may be treated with less than radical therapy.**

Diagnosis must be based on a cone biopsy of the cervix. Because the treatment decision rests with the gynecologist, treatment must be based on a review of the conization specimen with the pathologist. It is important that the pathologic condition be described in terms of 1) depth of invasion, 2) width and breadth of the invasive area, and 3) presence or absence of lymphatic vascular space invasion. These variables are used to determine how extensive the operation should be and whether the regional lymph nodes should be treated (4).

Stage Ia1—≤3 mm Invasion **Lesions with invasion that is ≤3 mm deep have a <1% incidence of pelvic node metastases.** Although this observation is controversial, it appears that the patients most at risk of nodal metastases or central pelvic recurrence are those with definitive evidence of tumor emboli in lymph vascular spaces (27, 28). Therefore, patients with invasion ≤3 mm and no lymph vascular space invasion may be treated

Table 32.4 Surgical management of Early Invasive Cancer of the Cervix		
Stage Ia1	≤3 mm invasion	
	No lymph-vascular space invasion	Conization
		Type I hysterectomy
	With lymph-vascular space invasion	Type I or II hysterectomy with (?) pelvic lymph node dissection
Stage Ia2	>3–5 mm invasion	Type II hysterectomy with pelvic lymphadenectomy
Stage Ib	>5 mm invasion	Type III hysterectomy with pelvic lymphadenectomy

1122

with extrafascial hysterectomy without node dissection. Therapeutic conization appears to be adequate therapy for these patients if childbearing capability is desired. Surgical margins must be free of disease. If there is lymph vascular space invasion, an alternative is a pelvic node dissection with a type I (extrafascial) or II (modified radical) hysterectomy.

Stage Ia2—>3–5 mm Invasion   **Lesions with invasion between 3–5 mm have a 3.8% incidence of pelvic node metastases** (28, 29); thus, pelvic node dissection is necessary for these lesions. The primary tumor may be treated with a modified radical hysterectomy (type II).

Stage Ib/IIa Invasive Cancer

Stage Ib lesions are subdivided into stage Ib1, which denotes lesions that are 4 cm or smaller in maximum diameter, and stage Ib2, which denotes lesions that are larger than 4 cm. Stage IIa is direct extension to the proximal vagina. **Surgical therapy of stage Ib and IIa carcinoma of the cervix involves radical hysterectomy, pelvic lymphadenectomy, and para-aortic lymph node evaluation.**

Types of Hysterectomy

Modified Radical Hysterectomy (Type II)   The hysterectomy described by Wertheim is less extensive than a radical hysterectomy and removes the medial one-half of the cardinal and uterosacral ligaments (30). This procedure is often referred to as the modified radical or type II hysterectomy. Wertheim's original operation did not include a pelvic lymph node dissection but instead included selective removal of enlarged lymph nodes.

Radical Hysterectomy (Type III)   The radical hysterectomy performed most often in the U.S. is that described by Meigs (31) in 1944. The operation includes a pelvic lymph node dissection, along with removal of most of the uterosacral and cardinal ligaments and the upper one-third of the vagina. Piver et al. (30) have referred to this operation as the type III radical hysterectomy. Radical hysterectomies can be further classified as follows.

Extended Radical Hysterectomy (Type IV)   In the type IV operation, the periureteral tissue, superior vesicle artery, and up to three-fourths of the vagina are removed (30).

Partial Exenteration (Type V)   In the type V operation, portions of the distal ureter and bladder are resected. This procedure is rarely performed because radiotherapy should be used if such extensive disease is encountered (30).

Surgical Procedure

Radical Hysterectomy and Pelvic Node Dissection

The abdomen is opened through either a midline incision or a low transverse incision after the methods of Maylard or Cherney. The low transverse incision requires division of the rectus muscles and provides excellent exposure of the lateral pelvis. It allows adequate pelvic node dissection and wide resection of the primary tumor.

Exploration   After the abdomen is entered, the peritoneal cavity is explored to exclude metastatic disease. The stomach is palpated to ensure that it has been decompressed to facilitate packing of the intestines. The liver is palpated, and the omentum is inspected for metastases. Both kidneys are palpated to ensure their proper placement and lack of congenital and other abnormalities. The para-aortic nodes are palpated transperitoneally.

During exploration of the pelvis, the fallopian tubes and ovaries are inspected for any abnormalities. In patients younger than 40 years of age, the ovaries are generally conserved. The peritoneum of the vesicouterine fold and the rectouterine pouch should be inspected for signs of tumor extension or implantation. The cervix is then palpated between the

1123

thumb anteriorly and the fingers posteriorly to determine its extent, and the cardinal ligaments are palpated for evidence of lateral tumor extension or nodularity.

Para-aortic Lymph Node Evaluation   If the patient has no evidence of disease extending beyond the cervix or vaginal fornix, i.e., "surgical stage Ib or IIa," the procedure is continued. The bowel is packed to expose the peritoneum overlying the bifurcation of the aorta. The peritoneum is incised medial to the ureter and over the right common iliac artery. A retractor is placed retroperitoneally to expose the aorta and the vena cava. Any enlarged para-aortic lymph nodes are dissected, hemaclips are applied for hemostasis, and specimens are sent for frozen section. If the lymph nodes are positive for metastatic cancer, an option is to discontinue the operation and use radiation therapy (31). If the lymph nodes are negative for disease, the left side of the aorta is palpated through the peritoneal incision with a finger passed under the inferior mesenteric artery. The lymph nodes on this side of the aorta are more lateral and nearly behind the aorta and the common iliac artery. If the left para-aortic lymph nodes appear healthy and the cervical tumor is small with no suspicious pelvic lymph nodes, these additional lymph nodes are not submitted for frozen section. If they are removed, they may be dissected through the incision made for the right para-aortic nodes, or they may be dissected after reflection of the sigmoid colon medially.

Pelvic Lymphadenectomy   Pelvic lymphadenectomy can proceed after lymph node evaluation or it can be deferred until the hysterectomy has been completed, depending on the preference of the surgeon. The pelvic lymph node dissection is begun by opening the round ligaments at the pelvic sidewall and developing the paravesical and pararectal spaces. The ureter is elevated on the medial flap by a Deaver retractor to expose the common iliac artery. The common iliac and external iliac nodes are dissected, with care taken to avoid injuring the genitofemoral nerve, which lies laterally on the psoas muscle. At the bifurcation of the common iliac artery, the external iliac node chain is divided into lateral and medial portions.

The lateral chain is stripped free from the artery to the circumflex iliac vein distally. A hemaclip is placed across the distal portion of the lymph node chain to reduce the incidence of lymphocyst formation. The medial chain is then dissected. The obturator lymph nodes are dissected next; for this procedure, the lymph nodes are grasped just under the external iliac vein and traction is applied medially. Although most patients have both the obturator artery and vein dorsal to the obturator nerve, 10% will have an aberrant vein arising from the external iliac vein. The node chain is separated from the nerve and vessels and clipped caudally. They are dissected cephalad to the hypogastric artery. The cephalad portion of the obturator space should be entered lateral to the external iliac artery and medial to the psoas muscle, where the remainder of the obturator node tissue can be dissected as far cephalad as the common iliac artery.

Development of Pelvic Spaces   The pelvic spaces are developed by sharp and blunt dissection (Fig. 32.8). The paravesical space is bordered by the following structures:

1. The obliterated umbilical artery running along the bladder medially

2. The obturator internus muscle along the pelvic sidewall laterally

3. The cardinal ligament posteriorly

4. The pubic symphysis anteriorly.

The attachments of the vagina to the tendinous arch form the floor of the paravesicle space.

The pararectal space is bordered by the following structures:

1. The rectum medially

2. The cardinal ligament anteriorly

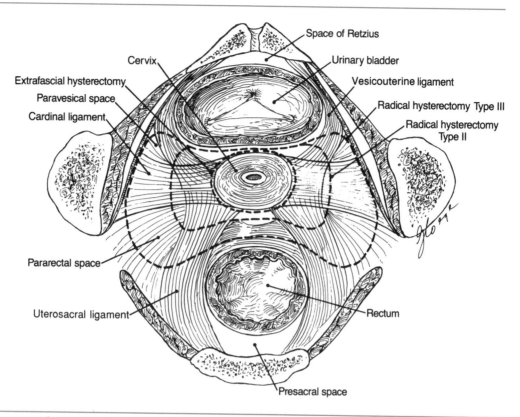

Figure 32.8   The pelvic ligaments and spaces.

3. The hypogastric artery laterally

4. The sacrum posteriorly.

The coccygeus (levator ani) muscle forms the floor of the pararectal space.

Dissection of the Bladder   A critical step is the dissection of the bladder from the anterior part of the cervix and vagina. Occasionally, tumor extension into the base of the bladder (which cannot be detected with cystoscopy) precludes adequate mobilization of the bladder flap, leading to the abandonment of the operation. Therefore, this portion of the operation should be undertaken early in the procedure.

Dissection of the Uterine Artery   The superior vesicle artery is dissected away from the cardinal ligament at a point near the uterine artery. The uterine artery, which usually arises from the superior vesicle artery, is thus isolated and divided and the vesicle arteries are preserved. The uterine vessels are then brought over the ureter by application of gentle traction. Occasionally, the uterine vein will pass under the ureter.

Dissection of the Ureter   The ureter is dissected free from its medial peritoneal flap at the level of the uterosacral ligament. As the ureter passes near the uterine artery, there is a consistent branch from the uterine artery to the ureter. This branch is sacrificed in the standard radical (type III) hysterectomy but preserved in the modified radical (type II) hysterectomy.

Dissection of the ureter from the vesicouterine ligament (ureteral tunnel) now may be accomplished. If the patient has a deep pelvis, ligation of the uterosacral and cardinal ligaments may be undertaken first in order to bring the ureteral tunnel dissection closer to the operator.

The roof of the ureteral tunnel is the anterior vesicouterine ligament. It should be ligated and divided to expose the posterior ligament. This ligament is also divided in the radical (type III) hysterectomy but conserved in the modified radical (type II) hysterectomy (Fig. 32.9).

Posterior Dissection   The peritoneum across the cul-de-sac is incised, exposing the uterosacral ligaments. The rectum is rolled free from the uterosacral ligaments, and these ligaments are divided midway to the sacrum in a radical (type III) hysterectomy and near the rectum in the modified radical (type II) operation. This allows the operator to develop the cardinal ligament separate from the rectum. A surgical clamp is placed on the cardinal ligament at the lateral pelvic sidewall in a radical hysterectomy and at the level of the ureteral bed in the modified radical procedure. A clamp is placed on the specimen side to maintain traction and is left on to ensure that the full cardinal ligament is excised with the specimen. A right-angled clamp then is placed caudad to this clamp across the paravaginal tissues. A second paravaginal clamp is usually needed to reach the vagina.

Vagina   The vagina is entered anteriorly, and the upper one-third of the vagina is removed with the specimen. More vaginal epithelium can be excised if necessary, depending on the previous colposcopic findings. The vaginal edge may be sutured in a hemostatic fashion and left open with a drain from the pelvic space or closed with a suction drain placed percutaneously. The ureteral fistula and pelvic lymphocyst rates from these two techniques are similar.

Modified Radical Hysterectomy

The modified radical hysterectomy differs from the radical hysterectomy in the following ways:

Figure 32.9   Radical hysterectomy. Uterine artery is ligated, ureter is dissected, and sites for division of the vesicouterine and uterosacral ligaments are shown.

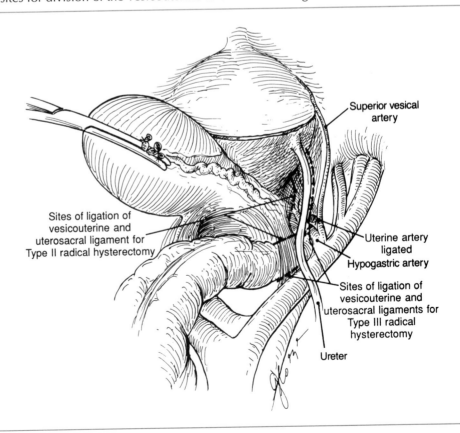

1. The uterine artery is transected at the level of the ureter, thus preserving the ureteral branch to the ureter.

2. The cardinal ligament is not divided near the sidewall but instead is divided at approximately its midportion near the ureteral dissection.

3. The anterior vesicouterine ligament is divided, but the posterior vesicouterine ligament is conserved.

4. A smaller margin of vagina is removed.

Complications of Radical Hysterectomy

Acute Complications   The acute complications of radical hysterectomy (27) include the following:

1. Blood loss (average 0.8 l)

2. Ureterovaginal fistula (1–2%)

3. Vesicovaginal fistula (<1%)

4. Pulmonary embolus (1–2%)

5. Small-bowel obstruction (1%)

6. Febrile morbidity (25–50%).

The febrile morbidity is most often pulmonary (10%) and is frequently seen with pelvic cellulitis (7%) and urinary tract infection (6%). Wound infection, pelvic abscess, and phlebitis all occur in fewer than 5% of patients (32).

Subacute Complications   The subacute effects of radical hysterectomy are postoperative bladder dysfunction and lymphocyst formation. For the first few days after radical hysterectomy, bladder volume is decreased and filling pressure is increased. The sensitivity to filling is diminished and the patient is unable to initiate voiding. The cause of this dysfunction is unclear.

It is important to maintain adequate bladder drainage during this time to prevent overdistention. Bladder drainage is best accomplished with a suprapubic catheter. It is more comfortable for the patient and allows the physician to perform cystometrography and determine residual urine volume without the need for frequent catheterization. In addition, the patient is able to accomplish trial voiding at home by clamping the catheter, voiding, and releasing to check the residual urine level. Cystometrography may be performed 3 to 4 weeks postoperatively. For use of the catheter to be discontinued, the patient must be able to sense the fullness of the bladder, initiate voiding, and void with a residual urine level of <75 ml. Otherwise, voiding trials should ensue at home until these criteria can be fulfilled.

Lymphocyst formation occurs in fewer than 5% of patients (33), and the cause is uncertain. Adequate drainage of the pelvis after radical hysterectomy may be an important step in prevention. Ureteral obstruction and partial venous obstruction and thrombosis may occur from lymphocyst formation. Simple aspiration of the lymphocyst is generally not curative, but percutaneous catheters with chronic drainage may allow healing. If this treatment is unsuccessful, operative intervention with excision of a portion of the lymphocyst wall and placement of either large bowel or omentum into the lymphocyst should be performed.

Chronic Complications   The most common chronic effect of radical hysterectomy is bladder hypotonia or, in extreme instances, atony. This condition occurs in approximately 3% of patients, regardless of the method of bladder drainage used (34, 35). It may be a result of bladder denervation and not simply a problem associated with bladder overdistention (36). Voiding every 4–6 hours, increasing intra-abdominal pressure with the Credé's maneuver, and intermittent self-catheterization may be used to manage the hypotonic bladder.

Ureteral strictures are uncommon in the absence of postoperative radiation therapy, recurrent cancer, or lymphocyst formation (25). If the stricture is associated with lymphocyst formation, treatment of the lymphocyst will usually alleviate the problem. Strictures that occur after radiation therapy should be managed with ureteral stenting. If a ureteral stricture is noted in the absence of radiotherapy or lymphocyst formation, recurrent carcinoma is the most common cause. A CT scan of the area of obstruction should be obtained and FNA cytology should be performed to exclude carcinoma if there is a target lesion. If the results of these tests are negative, a ureteral stent may be placed to relieve the stricture. Close observation for recurrent carcinoma is necessary, and diagnosis of recurrence may ultimately require laparotomy.

Results of Surgical Therapy

The survival of patients after radical hysterectomy and pelvic lymphadenectomy is dependent on several factors (27, 37–51):

1. The status of the lymph nodes

2. The size of the tumor

3. Involvement of paracervical tissues

4. The depth of invasion

5. The presence or absence of lymph vascular space invasion.

Lymph Nodes   The most dependent variable associated with survival is the status of the lymph nodes. **Patients with negative nodes will have an 85–90% 5-year survival rate (50, 52), whereas the survival rate for those with positive nodes ranges from 20 to 74%, depending on the number of nodes involved and the location and size of the metastases (46–48, 52–55).**

Other data on lymph node status can be summarized as follows:

1. When the common iliac lymph nodes are positive, the 5-year survival is about 25% versus about 65% when only the pelvic lymph nodes are involved (56–58).

2. Bilateral positive pelvic lymph nodes portend a worse prognosis (22–40% survival rate) than unilateral positive pelvic nodes (59–70%) (56, 57).

3. The presence of more than three positive pelvic lymph nodes is accompanied by a 68% recurrence rate, versus 30–50% when three or fewer lymph nodes are positive (46, 53).

4. Patients in whom tumor emboli are the only findings in the positive pelvic lymph node have an 82.5% 5-year survival rate, whereas the survival rate with microscopic invasion of the lymph nodes is 62.1% and with macroscopic disease is 54% (37).

Lesion Size   Lesion size is an independent predictor of survival. Patients with lesions smaller than 2 cm have a survival rate of approximately 90%, and patients with lesions larger than 2 cm have a 60% survival rate (40). When the primary tumor is larger than 4 cm, the survival rate drops to 40% (38, 49). An analysis of a Gynecologic Oncology Group (GOG) prospective study of 645 patients shows a 94.6% 3-year disease-free survival rate for patients with occult lesions, 85.5% for those with tumors smaller than 3 cm, and 68.4% for patients with tumors larger than 3 cm (50).

Depth of Invasion   Patients in whom depth of invasion is less than 1 cm have a 5-year survival rate around 90%, but the survival rate falls to 63–78% if the depth of invasion is more than 1 cm (27, 50, 54).

Parametrial Spread   Patients with spread to the parametrium have a 5-year survival rate of 69% versus 95% when the parametrium is negative. When the parametrium is involved and pelvic lymph nodes are also positive, the 5-year survival rate falls to 39–42% (41, 51).

Lymph Vascular Space Involvement   The significance of the finding of lymph vascular space involvement is somewhat controversial. Several reports have shown a 50–70% 5-year survival rate when lymph vascular space invasion is present and a 90% 5-year survival rate in its absence (27, 40, 44, 58–62). Others have found no significant difference in survival if the study is controlled for other risk factors (49, 50, 63–65). Lymph vascular space involvement may be a predictor of lymph node metastasis and not an independent predictor of survival.

Postoperative Radiotherapy	In an effort to improve survival rates, postoperative radiotherapy has been recommended for patients with high-risk factors such as metastasis to pelvic lymph nodes (27, 38, 52, 58), invasion of paracervical tissue (41, 42), deep cervical invasion (66), or positive surgical margins (53, 67). Although most authors agree that postoperative radiotherapy is necessary in the presence of positive surgical margins, the use of radiation in patients with other high-risk factors is controversial. Particularly controversial but best studied is the use of radiation in the presence of positive pelvic lymph nodes. The rationale for treatment is the knowledge that radiotherapy can sterilize cancer in pelvic lymph nodes and that pelvic node dissection does not remove all of the nodal and lymphatic tissue. The hesitancy to recommend postoperative radiotherapy relates to the significant rate of postradiotherapy bowel and urinary tract complications (68). A prospective randomized study has not been performed, and all data currently available are retrospective.

From retrospective studies, it appears that postoperative radiation therapy for positive pelvic nodes can decrease pelvic recurrence but does not improve 5-year actuarial survival. Morrow (53) reported a multi-institutional study that showed no difference in survival in patients with three or fewer pelvic nodes (59% vs. 60%). However, there seemed to be a benefit when radiotherapy was given to those with more than three positive nodes.

Kinney et al. (69) matched 60 pairs of irradiated and nonirradiated women for age, lesion size, and number and location of positive nodes after radical hysterectomy. They found no significant difference in projected 5-year survival rate (72% for surgery alone, 64% for surgery plus radiation). The proportion of recurrences in the pelvis only was 67% in patients treated with surgery only and 27% in patients treated with postoperative radiation (P<0.03).

Soisson et al. (46) performed a Cox regression analysis on 320 women who underwent radical hysterectomy, 72 of whom received postoperative radiation. They reported a significant decrease in pelvic recurrence but no survival benefit.

Alvarez et al. (48) performed a multi-institutional retrospective study in 185 women with positive pelvic nodes after radical hysterectomy, 103 of whom received postoperative radiotherapy. With multivariate analysis, radiotherapy was not found to be an independent predictor of survival, whereas age, lesion diameter, and number of positive nodes were found to influence survival.

These authors all conclude that additional treatment is needed to improve survival rates. Because survival is limited by distant site recurrence, the addition of chemotherapy to postoperative radiotherapy has been proposed. Lai et al. (70) reported a 75% disease-free survival rate at 3 years in 40 high-risk patients given *cisplatin, vinblastine,* and *bleomycin* after radical hysterectomy and a 46% disease-free survival in 79 comparable patients who refused treatment. Only four of 34 (11.8%) with positive pelvic nodes had recurrences, whereas disease recurred in eight of 24 (33%) untreated patients with positive nodes. Wertheim et al. (71) reported an 82% rate of disease-free survival at 2 years among 32 patients who were treated with postoperative radiation therapy plus *cisplatin* and *bleomycin.* These results have led to the prospective randomized trial of postoperative radiotherapy alone versus radiotherapy plus *5-fluorouracil (5-FU)* and *cisplatin* currently being performed by the GOG and the Southwest Oncology Group (SWOG).

The location of lymph node metastases is apparently relevant to postradiation recurrence rates. When common iliac lymph nodes are involved, the survival rate drops to 20% (58). As the number of positive pelvic nodes increases, the percentage of positive common iliac and low para-aortic nodes increases (58) (i.e., 0.6% when pelvic lymph nodes are negative, 6.3% with one positive pelvic node, 21.4% with two or three positive nodes, and 73.3% with four or more positive nodes). Inoue et al. (58) have used this information to recommend "extended-field" radiotherapy to patients with positive pelvic lymph nodes in an attempt to treat undetected extrapelvic nodal disease. They reported a 3-year disease-free survival rate of 85% in patients with positive pelvic nodes and 51% in patients with positive common iliac nodes, which is better than the survival rates of 50% and 23%, respectively, for historical control groups receiving radiotherapy to the pelvis alone.

Postoperative radiotherapy for patients with the other high-risk factors has not been shown to be effective, with the possible exception of patients with parametrial extension, in whom a 77.8% survival rate with radiotherapy versus a 72.7% survival rate without radiotherapy has been shown (37). The GOG has identified risk groups by proportional hazards modeling for patients with stage I disease and no pelvic node metastasis (50). The relative risk of recurrence was calculated for the three most important risk factors, which are 1) depth of stromal invasion, 2) clinical size of the primary tumor, and 3) capillary-lymphatic space involvement. Patients with a high risk of recurrence are being randomized to no further treatment versus pelvic radiotherapy in a current GOG protocol.

Neoadjuvant Chemotherapy	**The use of chemotherapy to shrink the tumor before radical hysterectomy or radiotherapy is termed neoadjuvant chemotherapy.** No randomized studies on the effectiveness of this technique have been reported. However, the information available from current studies suggests that, compared with historical controls, neoadjuvant therapy can achieve a 22–44% complete response rate, decrease the number of positive pelvic lymph nodes, and improve the 2- and 3-year disease-free survival rates, particularly in patients with stage I and II disease.

Kim et al. (72) used *cisplatin, vinblastine,* and *bleomycin* before radical hysterectomy in 54 patients with stage I and IIa tumors larger than 4 cm. They reported a complete response rate of 44% and a partial response rate of 50% based on evaluation of the radical hysterectomy specimen. Tumors recurred in only three patients, giving a 94% disease-free survival with a minimum of 2 years follow-up. Of the 11 patients with positive nodes, three had recurrences and all had three or more positive nodes. A comparison with historical controls for a tumor of this size revealed a 40% disease-free survival rate.

In treating 75 patients with stage I, II, and III disease whose tumors were larger than 4 cm, Panici et al. (73) administered *cisplatin, bleomycin,* and *methotrexate* before surgery or radiation therapy. A 3-year disease-free survival rate of 100%, 81%, and 66% was achieved for stages I, II, and III, respectively. Initial large tumor size and parametrial infiltration significantly correlated with a lower response to neoadjuvant therapy. Recurrence was significantly correlated with FIGO stage, parametrial infiltration, and residual cervical tumor. Eleven of the 12 recurrences involved the pelvis, indicating that additional local treatment is needed for this high-risk group.

In treating 151 patients who had stage IIb and III tumors, Sardi et al. (74) administered *cisplatin, vinblastine,* and *bleomycin* before surgery plus radiation (62.5%) or radiation alone (37.7%). They reported a 2-year disease-free survival rate in stages II and III of 79% and 50%, respectively, compared with survival rates of 47% and 26% in historical controls treated with radiation alone. For the 25 patients (22%) who experienced a complete response to the chemotherapy, there was a 96% disease-free survival rate and a 0% incidence of lymph node metastasis. To determine the efficacy of neoadjuvant chemotherapy, randomized trials have been initiated in the GOG and in other centers.

Radiation Therapy

Radiotherapy can be used to treat all stages of cervical squamous cell cancer, with cure rates of approximately 70% for stage I, 60% for stage II, 45% for stage III, and 18% for stage IV (2). A comparison of surgery and radiation for treatment of low-stage disease is shown in Table 32.5. The radiation treatment plan generally consists of a combination of external teletherapy to treat the regional nodes and to shrink the primary tumor and intracavitary brachytherapy to boost the central tumor. Intracavitary therapy alone may be used in patients with early disease when the incidence of lymph node metastasis is negligible.

The treatment sequence depends on tumor volume. Stage Ib lesions smaller then 2 cm may be treated first with an intracavitary source to treat the primary lesion, followed by external therapy to treat the pelvic nodes. Larger lesions will require external radiotherapy first to shrink the tumor and to reduce the anatomic distortion caused by the cancer. This enables the therapist to achieve better intracavitary dosimetry.

The usual dosages delivered will be 7000–8000 cGy to point A and 6000 cGy to point B, limiting the bladder and rectal dosage to <6000 cGy. To achieve this, it is necessary to have adequate packing of the bladder and bowel away from the intracavitary sources. Lo-

Table 32.5   Comparison of Surgery Versus Radiation for Stage Ib/IIa Cancer of the Cervix

	Surgery	*Radiation*
Survival	85%	85%
Serious complications	Urologic fistulas 1–2%	Intestinal and urinary strictures and fistulas 1.4–5.3%
Vagina	Initially shortened, but may lengthen with regular intercourse	Fibrosis and possible stenosis particularly in postmenopausal patients
Ovaries	Can be conserved	Destroyed
Chronic effects	Bladder atony in 3%	Radiation fibrosis of bowel and bladder in 6–8%
Applicability	Best candidates are younger than 65 years of age, <200 lb, and in good health	All patients are potential candidates
Surgical mortality	1%	1% (from pulmonary embolism during intracavitary therapy)

calization films and careful calculation of dosimetry are mandatory to optimize the dose of radiotherapy and to reduce the incidence of bowel and bladder complications. Local control depends on adequate dosage to the tumor from the intracavitary source.

Extended-Field Radiotherapy

Clinical staging fails to predict the extension of disease to the para-aortic nodes in 7% of patients with stage Ib disease, 18% with stage IIb, and 28% with stage III (75). Such patients will have "geographic" treatment failures if standard pelvic radiotherapy ports are used. Thus, these patients should be treated with extended-field radiotherapy.

Surgical "Staging" Prior to Radiation

Surgical staging procedures designed to discover the presence of positive nodes have been devised. Transperitoneal exploration was first used, but it was associated with a 16–33% mortality rate from radiotherapy-induced bowel complications and a 5-year survival rate of only 9–12% (76, 77). The radiotherapy dose to the para-aortic chain was 5500–6000 cGy, which is now known to be excessive. Postsurgical adhesions entrap the intestine in the radiotherapy field; therefore, the bowel receives the full dose of radiotherapy. In the absence of postsurgical adhesions, the small bowel would move in and out of the radiotherapy field and receive a lesser dose. To avoid these postsurgical adhesions, extraperitoneal dissection of the para-aortic nodes is now recommended, and the radiotherapy dosage should be reduced to 5000 cGy or less (78, 79).

When such an approach is used, postradiotherapy bowel complications occur in fewer than 5% of patients (80, 81), and the 5-year survival rate is 15–26% in patients with positive para-aortic nodes (21, 81). Survival appears to be related to the amount of disease in the para-aortic nodes and to the size of the primary tumor. In patients whose metastases to the para-aortic lymph nodes are microscopic and whose central tumor is not extending to the pelvic sidewall, the 5-year survival rate improves to 20–50% (82, 83).

Supraclavicular Lymph Node Biopsy   Although not standard practice, the performance of a supraclavicular lymph node biopsy has been advocated in patients with positive para-aortic lymph nodes before the initiation of extended-field irradiation as well as in patients with a central recurrence before exploration for possible exenteration. The incidence of metastatic disease in the supraclavicular lymph nodes in patients with positive para-aortic lymph nodes is 5–30% (84). FNA cytology can obviate the need for an excisional biopsy and thus should be performed if any enlarged nodes are present.

Radiation Plus Chemotherapy

Primary pelvic radiotherapy fails to control the disease in 30–82% of patients with cervical carcinoma (2). Approximately two-thirds of these failures occur in the pelvis (85).

A variety of agents has been used in an attempt to increase the effectiveness of radiation therapy in patients with large primary tumors. Hydroxyurea has produced some improvement in response rate and survival rates when compared with radiation therapy alone in a controlled series of patients (86, 87). The use *5-FU* and *mitomycin-C* has also been reported to improve response rates for advanced cervical cancer (88). *Cisplatin* has been shown to have cytotoxic activity against cervical carcinoma (89) and recently has been demonstrated to be a radiation sensitizer (90). It has produced some improvement in response and survival rates when used with radiation therapy for cervical cancer as compared with radiation therapy alone (90, 91). Currently, randomized trials are being conducted to determine the best chemotherapy to combine with radiation therapy (92) (see Chapter 30).

Complications of Radiotherapy

Perforation of the uterus may occur at the time of insertion of the uterine tandem. This is a problem particularly for elderly patients or for those who have had a previous diagnostic conization. When perforation is recognized, the tandem should be removed and the patient should be observed for bleeding or signs of peritonitis. Survival may be decreased in patients who have had uterine perforation (93), possibly because these patients have more extensive uterine disease, which predisposes them to perforation. Fever may occur after insertion of the uterine tandem and ovoids. Fever most often results from infection of the necrotic tumor and occurs 2–6 hours after insertion of the intracavitary system. If uterine perforation has been excluded by ultrasonography, intravenous broad-spectrum antibiotic coverage, usually with a cephalosporin, should be administered. If the fever does not decrease promptly or if the temperature is higher than 38.5°C, an aminoglycoside and a bacteroides-specific antibiotic should be added. If the fever persists or if the patient shows signs of septic shock or peritonitis, the intracavitary system must be removed. Antibiotics are continued until the patient has recovered and the intracavitary application is delayed for 1–2 weeks.

Acute Morbidity

The acute effects of radiotherapy occur after 2000–3000 cGy and are caused by ionizing radiation on the epithelium of the intestine and bladder. Symptoms include diarrhea, abdominal cramps, nausea, frequent urination, and occasionally bleeding from the bladder or bowel mucosa. The bowel symptoms can be treated with a low-gluten, low-lactose, and low-protein diet. Antidiarrheal and antispasmodic agents also may help. The bladder may be treated with antispasmodic medication. Severe symptoms may require a week of rest from radiotherapy.

Chronic Morbidity

The chronic effects of radiotherapy result from the induction of vasculitis and fibrosis, and they are more serious than acute effects. These complications occur several months to several years after radiotherapy has been completed. The bowel and bladder fistula rate after pelvic radiation therapy for cervical cancer is 1.4–5.3% (23, 25). Other serious toxicity (e.g., bowel bleeding, stricture, stenosis, or obstruction) occurs in 6.4–8.1% of patients (23, 25).

Proctosigmoiditis   Bleeding from proctosigmoiditis should be treated with a low-residue diet, antidiarrheal medications, and steroid enemas. In extreme cases, a colostomy may be required to rest the bowel completely, and occasionally resection of the rectosigmoid must be performed.

Rectovaginal Fistula   Rectovaginal fistulas or rectal strictures occur in fewer than 2% of patients. The successful closure of fistulas with bulbocavernosus flaps has been reported (94). Bricker and Johnston (95) have reported a technique of sigmoid colon transposition to repair rectosigmoid fistulas or rectal strictures. Occasionally, resection with anastomosis is feasible.

Small-Bowel Complications   Patients with previous abdominal surgery are more likely to have pelvic adhesions and thus sustain more radiotherapy complications in the small bowel. The terminal ileum may sustain chronic damage because of its relatively fixed position at the cecum. The patient typically has a long history of crampy abdominal pain, intestinal rushes, and distention characteristic of partial small-bowel obstruction. Often low-grade fever and anemia accompany the symptoms. Patients who have no evidence of disease should be treated aggressively with total parenteral nutrition, nasogastric suction, and early operation after the anemia has resolved and good nutritional status has been attained. The type of procedure performed depends on individual circumstances (96).

Small bowel fistulas after radiotherapy will rarely close spontaneously while total parenteral nutrition is maintained. Recurrent cancer should be excluded; then aggressive fluid replacement, nasogastric suction, and wound care should be employed. A fistulogram and a barium enema should be performed to exclude a combined large and small bowel fistula. The fistula-containing loop of bowel may be either resected or isolated and left *in situ*. In the latter case, the fistula will act as its own mucous fistula.

Urinary Tract Chronic urinary tract complications occur in 1–5% of patients and depend on the dose to the base of the bladder. Vesicovaginal fistulas are the most common complication and usually require supravesicular urinary diversion. Occasionally, a small fistula can be repaired with either a bulbocavernosus flap or an omental pedicle. Ureteral strictures are usually a sign of recurrent cancer, and FNA cytology under CT scan control should be obtained at the site of the obstruction. If the findings are negative, the patient should undergo exploratory surgery to determine disease status. If radiation fibrosis is the cause, then ureterolysis may be possible or indwelling ureteral stents may be passed through the open urinary bladder.

Posttreatment Surveillance

Patients who receive radiotherapy should be closely monitored to assess their response. Tumors may be expected to regress for up to 3 months after radiotherapy. If disease obviously progresses during this interval, however, surgical treatment should be considered.

The pelvic examination should note progressive shrinkage of the cervix and possible stenosis of the cervical os and surrounding upper vagina. The rectovaginal examination, with careful palpation of the uterosacral and cardinal ligaments for nodularity, is most important. FNA cytology of suspicious areas should be used for early diagnosis of persistent disease. In addition to the pelvic examination, the supraclavicular and inguinal lymph nodes should be carefully examined, and cervical or vaginal cytology should be performed every 3 months for 2 years and then every 6 months for the next 3 years. An endocervical curettage may be performed for patients with large central tumors.

An x-ray film of the chest may be obtained yearly in patients who have advanced disease. Metastasis to the lung has been reported in 1.5% of cases; solitary nodules are present in 25% of cases. Resection of a solitary nodule in the absence of any other persistent disease may yield some long-term survivors (97). Although intravenous pyelography (IVP) is not a part of the routine postradiotherapy surveillance, it should be performed if a pelvic mass is detected or if urinary symptoms warrant it. The finding of ureteral obstruction after radiotherapy in the absence of a palpable mass may indicate unresectable pelvic sidewall disease, but this finding should be confirmed, usually by FNA cytology (98).

Patients who have had radical hysterectomy and who are at high risk of recurrence may benefit from early recognition of recurrence because they might be saved with radiation therapy. In these patients, a routine IVP at 6–12 months may be beneficial. After radical hysterectomy, about 80% of recurrences are detected within 2 years (99). The larger the primary lesion, the shorter the median time to recurrence (100).

Special Problems

Adenocarcinoma

The incidence of adenocarcinoma of the cervix appears to be increasing relative to that of squamous cancers. Older reports indicated that 5% of all cervical cancers were adenocarcinomas (101), whereas newer reports show an incidence as high as 18.5–27% (102, 103). The FIGO annual report indicates a poorer prognosis for adenocarcinoma than for squamous cell carcinoma in every stage. This has been supported by Hopkins and Morley (103), who performed a Cox proportional hazard analysis of 203 women with adenocarcinoma and 756 women with squamous carcinoma. They reported 5-year survival rates of 90% versus 60%, 62% versus 47%, and 36% versus 8% for stages I, II, and III, respectively. Although some have attributed these rates to a relative resistance to radiation, it is more likely a reflection of the tendency of adenocarcinomas to grow endophytically and to be undetected until a larger volume of tumor is present.

The clinical features of stage I adenocarcinomas have been well studied (102, 104–106). These studies have identified size of tumor, depth of invasion, grade of tumor, and age of the patient as significant correlates of lymph node metastasis and survival. When matched with squamous carcinomas for lesion size, age, and depth of invasion, the incidence of lymph node metastases and the survival rate appear to be the same (104, 105). Patients with stage I adenocarcinomas can be selected for treatment according to the same criteria as for those with squamous cancers (105).

The proper treatment for bulky stage I and stage II tumors is controversial. Radiation alone has been advocated by some (107), but others support radiation plus extrafascial hysterectomy (108, 109). In 1975, Rutledge et al. (108) reported an 85.2% 5-year survival rate for all patients with stage I disease treated with radiation alone and an 83.8% survival rate for those who had radiation plus surgery. The central persistent disease rate was 8.3% versus 4%. In stage II disease, the 5-year survival rate was 41.9% for radiation alone and 53.7% for radiation plus surgery. A subsequent report revealed no significant difference in survival among patients treated with either radiation alone or radiation plus extrafascial hysterectomy (110).

Patients with adenosquamous carcinoma of the cervix have been reported to have a poorer prognosis than those with pure adenocarcinoma or squamous carcinoma (111). Whether this is true when corrected for size of lesion is controversial (104, 105).

The association of adenocarcinoma with squamous intraepithelial neoplasia is well documented (112). A squamous intraepithelial lesion may be observed colposcopically and treated with outpatient therapy, and the coexistent adenocarcinoma in the canal may be overlooked. Performance of an endocervical curettage at colposcopy will help prevent such an occurrence.

Cervical Cancer in Pregnancy

After a review of the literature, Hacker et al. (113) reported that the incidence of invasive cervical cancer associated with pregnancy was one in 2200. A Pap test should be performed for all pregnant patients at the initial prenatal visit, and any grossly suspicious lesions should be biopsied. Diagnosis is often delayed during pregnancy because bleeding is attributed to pregnancy-related complications. If the results of the Pap tests are positive for malignant cells and the diagnosis of invasive cancer cannot be made with colposcopy and biopsy, a diagnostic conization may be necessary. Because conization subjects the mother and fetus to complications, it should be performed only in the second trimester and only in patients with inadequate colposcopy findings and strong cytologic evidence of invasive cancer. Conization in the first trimester of pregnancy is associated with an abortion rate of up to 33% (113, 114).

Microinvasive Carcinoma   After conization, there appears to be no harm in delaying definitive treatment until fetal maturity is achieved in patients with stage Ia cervical cancer (113, 115, 116). Patients with less than 3 mm of invasion and no lymphatic-vascular space involvement may be followed to term and delivered vaginally. A vaginal hysterectomy may be performed 6 weeks postpartum if further childbearing is not desired.

Patients with 3–5 mm of invasion and those with lymph vascular space invasion may also be followed to term (113, 116). They may be delivered by cesarean birth, followed immediately by modified radical hysterectomy and pelvic lymph node dissection.

Stage Ib Carcinoma   Patients with more than 5 mm invasion should be treated as having frankly invasive carcinoma of the cervix. Treatment will depend on the stage of gestation and the wishes of the patient. Modern neonatal care affords a 75% survival rate for infants delivered at 28 weeks of gestation and 90% for those delivered at 32 weeks of gestation. Fetal pulmonary maturity can be determined by amniocentesis, and prompt treatment can be instituted when pulmonary maturity is documented. Although timing is controversial, it is probably unwise to delay therapy for longer than 4 weeks (115, 116). The recommended treatment is classic cesarean delivery followed by radical hysterectomy with pelvic lymph node dissection. There should be a thorough discussion of the risks and options with both parents before any treatment is undertaken.

Advanced-Stage Carcinoma   Patients with cervical cancer in stages II–IV should be treated with radiotherapy. If the fetus is viable, it is delivered by classic cesarean birth and therapy is begun postoperatively. If the pregnancy is in the first trimester, external radiation therapy can be started with the expectation that spontaneous abortion will occur before the delivery of 4000 cGy. In the second trimester, a delay of therapy may be entertained to improve the chances of fetal survival. If the patient wishes to delay therapy, it is important to ensure fetal pulmonary maturity before delivery is undertaken.

Prognosis   The clinical stage is the most important prognostic factor for cervical cancer during pregnancy. Overall survival is slightly better for patients with cervical cancer in pregnancy, because an increased proportion of these patients have stage I disease. For patients with advanced disease, there is evidence that pregnancy impairs the prognosis (113, 116). The diagnosis of cancer in the postpartum period is associated with a more advanced clinical stage and a corresponding decrease in survival.

Cancer of the Cervical Stump

Cancer of the cervical stump is less common today than it was several decades ago when supracervical hysterectomy was popular. Early-stage disease is treated surgically, with very little change in technique from that used when the uterus is intact (117). Advanced-stage disease may present a therapeutic problem for the radiotherapist if the length of the cervical canal is less than 2 cm. This length is necessary to allow satisfactory placement of the uterine tandem. If the uterine tandem cannot be placed, radiation therapy can be completed with vaginal ovoids or with an external treatment plan in which lateral ports are used to augment the standard anterior and posterior ports. Such a technique will reduce the dosage to the bowel and bladder and thus reduce the incidence of complications.

Coexistent Pelvic Mass

The origin of a pelvic mass must be clarified before treatment is initiated. An IVP will exclude a pelvic kidney, and a barium enema will help identify diverticular disease or carcinoma of the colon. An abdominal x-ray film may show calcifications typically associated with benign ovarian teratomas or uterine leiomyomas. Pelvic ultrasonography will differentiate between solid and cystic masses and indicate uterine or adnexal origin. Solid masses of uterine origin are most often leiomyomas and generally do not need further investigation.

Pyometra and Hematometra   An enlarged fluid-filled uterine cavity may be a pyometra or a hematometra. The hematometra can be drained by dilation of the cervical canal and will not interfere with treatment. The pyometra also should be drained and the patient should be given antibiotics to cover Bacteroides, anaerobic Staphylococcus and Streptococcus, and aerobic coliform bacteria. Placement of a large mushroom catheter through the cervix has been advocated, but the catheter itself may become obstructed and lead to further occlusion of the drainage. Repeated dilation of the cervix with aspiration of pus every 2–3 days is more effective.

If the disease is stage I, a radical hysterectomy and pelvic node dissection may be performed. However, a pyometra is usually found in patients with advanced disease, and thus radiotherapy is required. External beam therapy can begin when the pyometra has healed. Patients often have a significant amount of pus in the uterus or a tubo-ovarian abscess without signs of infection; therefore, a normal temperature and a normal white blood cell count do not necessarily exclude infection. Repeat physical examination or pelvic ultrasonography will be necessary to ensure adequate drainage.

Invasive Cancer Found During Hysterectomy

When invasive cervical cancer is found after simple hysterectomy, it may be treated with radiotherapy or reoperation involving a pelvic node dissection and radical excision of parametrial tissue, cardinal ligaments, and the vaginal stump (118).

Reoperation   Reoperation is indicated particularly for a young patient who has a small lesion and in whom preservation of ovarian function is desirable. It is not indicated for patients who have positive margins or obvious residual disease (118). Survival after radical reoperation is similar to that after radical hysterectomy for stage I disease.

Radiation Therapy   Survival after radiotherapy depends on the volume of disease, the status of the surgical margins, and the length of delay from surgery to radiotherapy. Patients with microscopic disease have a 95–100% 5-year survival rate; the 5-year survival rate is 82–84% in those with macroscopic disease and free margins, 38–87% in those with microscopically positive margins, and 20–47% in those with obvious residual cancer (119–121). A delay in treatment of more than 6 months is associated with a 20% survival rate (121).

Stage IVa Cervical Cancer

Although primary exenteration may be considered for patients with direct extension to the rectum or bladder, it is rarely performed. For patients with extension to the bladder, the survival rate with radiation therapy is as high as 30%, with a urinary fistula rate of only 3.8% (122).

The presence of tumor in the bladder may prohibit cure with radiation therapy alone; thus, consideration must be given to removal of the bladder on completion of external beam radiation. This is particularly true if the disease persists at that time and the geometry is not conducive to implant therapy. Rectal extension is less commonly observed but may require diversion of the fecal stream before therapy to avoid septic episodes from fecal contamination.

Cervical Hemorrhage

Occasionally, a large lesion can produce life-threatening hemorrhage. A biopsy of the lesion should be performed to verify neoplasia, and a vaginal pack soaked in Monsel's solution (ferric subsulfate) should be packed tightly against the cervix. After proper staging, external radiation therapy can be started with the expectation that control of bleeding may require 8–10 daily treatments at 180–200 cGy/day. Broad-spectrum antibiotics should be used to reduce the incidence of infection. If the patient becomes febrile, the pack should be removed. Rapid replacement of the pack may be necessary, and a fresh pack should be immediately available. This management of hemorrhage in the previously untreated patient is preferable to exploration and vascular ligation. Occasionally, vascular embolization under fluoroscopic control may be required in severe cases, and this procedure may obviate a laparotomy. However, vascular occlusion may lead ultimately to decreased blood flow and oxygenation of the tumor, and, because the effect of radiotherapy is dependent on tissue oxygen content, the efficacy of the radiotherapy may be compromised.

Ureteral Obstruction

Treatment of bilateral ureteral obstruction and uremia in previously untreated patients should be determined on an individual basis. Transvesicle or percutaneous ureteral catheters should be placed in patients with no evidence of distant disease, and radiotherapy with curative intent should be instituted. Patients with metastatic disease beyond curative treatment fields should be presented with the options of ureteral stenting, palliative radiotherapy, and chemotherapy for the metastatic disease. A median survival rate of 17 months for these patients may be achieved with aggressive management (123).

Barrel-Shaped Cervix

The expansion of the upper endocervix and lower uterine segment by tumor has been referred to as a barrel-shaped cervix. Patients with tumors larger than 6 cm in diameter have a 17.5% central failure rate when treated with radiotherapy alone because the tumor at the periphery of the lower uterine segment is too far from the standard intracavitary source to receive a tumoricidal dose (124). Attempts have been made to overcome this problem radiotherapeutically by means of interstitial implants into the tumor with a perineal template, but high central failure rates have also been reported with this technique (125).

Most oncologists prefer a combination of radiotherapy and surgery for these patients. The usual approach is to perform an extrafascial hysterectomy 6 weeks after the completion of radiation therapy in an effort to resect a small, centrally persistent tumor. The dose of external radiotherapy is reduced to 4000 cGy and a single intracavitary treatment is given, which is followed by an extrafascial hysterectomy (126, 127). This approach appears to result in a lower rate of central failure (2%), although it is not clear that the overall survival rate is improved. There is disagreement concerning the need for extrafascial hysterectomy, and the GOG is currently undertaking a randomized study to compare adjuvant hysterectomy with radiotherapy alone in patients who have no evidence of occult metastases in the para-aortic nodes.

Poor Vaginal Geometry

The narrow upper vaginas of older patients may preclude the use of an intracavitary source. Such patients must receive their entire course of therapy from external sources, leading to a higher central failure rate and more significant bowel and bladder morbidity. If stage I disease is present in such a patient, a radical hysterectomy with pelvic node dissection is preferable if possible according to the patient's medical condition.

Small Cell Carcinoma

Local therapy alone gives almost no chance of cure. Regimens of combination chemotherapy have improved the median survival rates in small cell bronchogenic carcinoma, and these regimens are now being used for treatment of small cell (neuroendocrine type) carcinoma of the cervix. Combination chemotherapy may consist of either *vincristine, doxorubicin,* and *cyclophosphamide*) (VAC) or *VP-16 (etoposide)* and *cisplatin* (EP) (128). Patients must be monitored carefully because they are at high risk of developing recurrent metastatic disease (129).

Recurrent Cervical Cancer

Treatment of recurrent cervical cancer depends on the mode of primary therapy and the site of recurrence. **Patients who have been treated initially with surgery should be considered for radiation therapy, and those who have had radiation therapy should be considered for surgical treatment.** Chemotherapy is palliative only and is reserved for patients who are not considered curable by the other two modalities.

Radiotherapy for recurrence after surgery consists primarily of external treatment. Vaginal ovoids also may be placed in patients with isolated vaginal cuff recurrences. Patients with a regional recurrence may require interstitial implantation with a Syed type of template in addition to the external therapy. A 25% survival rate can be expected in patients treated with radiation for a postsurgical recurrence (99).

Radiation Retreatment

Retreatment of recurrent pelvic disease by means of radiotherapy with curative intent is confined to patients who had suboptimal or incomplete primary therapy. This may allow the radiotherapist to deliver curative doses to the tumor. The proximity of the bladder and rectum to the cancer and their relative sensitivity to radiation injury are the major deterrents to retreatment with radiation.

The insertion of multiple interstitial radiation sources into the locally recurrent cancer through a perineal template may help overcome these dosimetric considerations (118, 130). However, the fistula rates are high and the consequences must be considered seriously before interstitial therapy is initiated. In general, for patients considered curable with interstitial implant therapy, pelvic exenteration is a better treatment choice.

Radiotherapy can be palliative with localized metastatic lesions. Painful bony metastases, central nervous system lesions, and severe urologic or vena caval obstructions are specific indications.

Surgical Therapy

Surgical therapy for postradiation recurrence is limited to patients with central pelvic disease. A few carefully selected patients with small-volume disease limited to the cervix may be treated with an extrafascial or radical hysterectomy. However, the difficulty of assessing tumor volume and the 30–50% rate of serious urinary complications in these previously irradiated patients lead most gynecologic oncologists to recommend pelvic exenteration as the patient's last chance for cure (131, 132).

Exenteration

The operation can be an *anterior exenteration* (removal of the bladder, vagina, cervix, and uterus), a *posterior exenteration* (removal of the rectum, vagina, cervix, and uterus), or a total *exenteration* (removal of both bladder and rectum with the vagina, cervix, and uterus). A total exenteration that includes a large perineal phase includes the entire rectum and leaves the patient with a permanent colostomy as well as a urinary conduit. In selected patients, a total exenteration may take place above the levator muscle (*supralevator*), leaving a rectal stump that may be anastomosed to the sigmoid, thus avoiding a permanent colostomy.

Preoperative Evaluation and Patient Selection   The search for metastatic disease is imperative. Physical examination includes careful palpation of the peripheral lymph nodes with FNA cytology of any nodes that appear suspicious. A random biopsy of nonsuspicious supraclavicular lymph nodes has been advocated (84, 133) but is not routinely practiced. A CT scan of the lung will detect disease missed on routine x-ray examination of the chest. Abdominal and pelvic CT scans are helpful in the detection of liver metastases and enlarged para-aortic nodes. CT-directed FNA cytologic study of any abnormality should be undertaken. If a positive cytologic diagnosis is obtained, it will obviate the need for exploratory laparotomy.

Extension of the tumor to the pelvic sidewall is a contraindication to exenteration; however, this may be difficult for even the most experienced examiner to determine because of radiation fibrosis. If any question of resectability arises, exploratory laparotomy and parametrial biopsies, the patient's last hope for cure, should be offered (134–137). **The clinical triad of unilateral leg edema, sciatic pain, and ureteral obstruction is nearly always pathognomonic of unresectable disease on the pelvic sidewall.**

Preoperatively, the patient should be prepared for a major operation. Total parenteral nutrition may be necessary to place the patient in an anabolic state for optimal healing. A bowel preparation, preoperative antibiotics, and prophylaxis for deep venous thrombosis with low-dose heparin or pneumatic calf compression should be used (138).

Surgical mortality increases with age, and the operation should rarely be considered in a patient who is older than 70 years of age. Other medical illnesses should be taken into account; when life expectancy is limited, exenterative surgery is unwise.

Anterior Exenteration   Candidates for anterior exenteration are those in whom the disease is limited to the cervix and anterior portion of the upper vagina. Proctoscopic examination should be performed because a positive finding would mandate a total exenteration.

However, a negative proctoscopic examination finding does not exclude disease in the rectal muscularis, and findings at laparotomy still must be considered. Generally, the presence of disease in the posterior vaginal mucosa directly over the rectum mandates removal of the underlying rectum.

Posterior Exenteration   A posterior exenteration is rarely performed for recurrent cervical cancer. It is indicated, however, for the patient with an isolated posterior vaginal recurrence in which dissection of the ureters through the cardinal ligaments will not be necessary.

Total Exenteration   Total exenteration with a large perineal phase is indicated when the disease extends down to the lower part of the vagina. Because distal vaginal lymphatics may empty into the inguinal node region, these nodes should be carefully evaluated preoperatively.

A supralevator total exenteration with low rectal anastomosis is indicated in the patient whose disease is confined to the upper vagina and cervix (139, 140). Frozen-section margins of the rectal edge should be obtained because occult metastases to the muscularis may occur.

The development of techniques to establish continent urinary diversion has helped improve a woman's physical appearance after exenteration (141–143). When both a rectal anastomosis and a continent diversion are performed, the patient has no permanent external appliance and the associated psychological trauma is avoided.

Every effort should be made to create a neovagina simultaneous with the exenteration (144). This procedure also helps in the reconstruction of the pelvic floor after extirpation of the pelvic viscera. Whether or not a neovagina is constructed, it is desirable to mobilize the omentum on the left gastroepiploic artery and use it to create a new pelvic floor.

Results   Surgical mortality has steadily decreased to an acceptable level of <10%. The most common causes of postoperative death are sepsis, pulmonary thromboembolism, and hemorrhage. Fistulas of the gastrointestinal and genitourinary tract are serious surgical complications, with a 30–40% mortality rate despite attempts at surgical repair. The risk of such fistulas has been decreased by the use of nonirradiated segments of bowel for formation of the urinary conduit (138).

The 5-year survival rate is 33–60% for patients undergoing anterior exenteration and 20–46% for those undergoing total exenteration (132, 134–144). Survival rates are poorer for patients with recurrent disease larger than 3 cm, invasion into the bladder, positive pelvic lymph nodes, and recurrence diagnosed within 1 year after radiotherapy (137). The 5-year survival rate of patients with positive pelvic lymph nodes is <5%. Thus, the performance of an extensive lymphadenectomy in the irradiated field is not warranted, but discontinuation of the procedure is advisable if any nodes are positive for metastatic cancer. Patients who have any disease in the peritoneal cavity have no chance of survival.

Chemotherapy

Recurrent cervical cancer is not considered curable with chemotherapy. A number of clinical trials with various drugs have shown response rates of up to 45% (145). Complete responses are unusual and are generally limited to patients with chest metastases, in whom the dose of drug delivered to the disease is stronger than that delivered to the fibrotic postirradiation pelvis (146).

Vermorken (147) has reviewed the literature on the role of chemotherapy in cervical cancer. He concludes that present data do not support the claim that toxic combination chemotherapy regimens are superior to *cisplatin* alone in terms of survival benefit, although further studies are required to determine whether combination chemotherapy may offer a benefit for certain subgroups of patients. The response rates for single agent chemotherapy in cervical cancer are about 10–25%; *cisplatin* and *carboplatin* among the most active agents. The response rate for *cisplatin* combination therapies is about 20–40% (147).

Vaginal Cancer

The FIGO staging of vaginal cancer requires that a tumor that has extended to the vagina from the cervix should be regarded as a cancer of the cervix, whereas a tumor that involves both the vulva and the vagina should be classified as a cancer of the vulva.

Pathology

Squamous cell carcinomas are the most common, occurring in 80% of the vaginal cancers, followed by adenocarcinoma, melanoma, and sarcoma. The mean age of patients with squamous cell cancer is 60 years (148, 149).

Cause

The cause of squamous cell carcinoma of the vagina is unknown. The association of cervical cancer with human papilloma virus (HPV) suggests that vaginal cancer may have a similar association (150). In addition, up to 30% of women with vaginal cancer have a history of cervical cancer treated at least 5 years earlier (151–153). Similar to cervical cancer, there appears to be a premalignant phase called vaginal intraepithelial neoplasia (VAIN) (see Chapter 16). The exact incidence of progression to invasive vaginal cancer from VAIN is not known; however, there are documented cases of invasive disease occurring despite adequate treatment for VAIN (154, 155).

By convention, any new vaginal carcinoma developing at least 5 years after the cervical cancer should be considered a new primary lesion. There are three possible mechanisms for the occurrence of vaginal cancer after cervical neoplasia:

1. Residual disease in the vaginal epithelium after treatment of the cervical neoplasia.

2. New primary disease arising in a patient with increased susceptibility to lower genital tract carcinogenesis. The role of HPV in this setting is suspected.

3. Increased susceptibility of carcinogenesis by radiation therapy.

Screening

The incidence of vaginal cancer is 0.6 per 100,000 women, making routine screening of all patients inappropriate (156). For women who have had a cervical or vulvar neoplasm, the Pap test is an important part of routine follow-up with each physician visit. This increased risk of vaginal cancer continues for the lifetime of the patient. It is recommended that Pap test surveillance for vaginal cancer be performed yearly after the patient has completed surveillance for cervix or vulvar cancer. For women who have had a hysterectomy for benign disease, Pap testing every 3–5 years has been standard practice in the U.S. When adjusted for age and prior cervical disease, the incidence of vaginal cancer is not increased for women who have had hysterectomy for benign disease (157).

Signs and Symptoms

Painless vaginal bleeding and discharge are the most common symptoms of vaginal cancer. With more advanced tumors, urinary retention, bladder spasm, hematuria, and frequency of urination may occur. Tumors developing on the posterior vaginal wall may produce rectal symptoms such as tenesmus, constipation, or blood in the stool.

Diagnosis

The diagnosis is suggested by an abnormal Pap test result or the gross appearance of a vaginal lesion. It is confirmed by a targeted biopsy using the same instruments as those used for cervical biopsies. The most common site of vaginal cancer is in the upper one-third of the vagina on the posterior wall. The developing tumor may be missed during initial inspection because the speculum blades may have obscured it (158). Colposcopy is valuable in evaluating patients with abnormal Pap test results, unexplained vaginal bleeding, or ulcerated erythematous patches in the upper vagina. A colposcopically targeted biopsy may not allow a definitive diagnosis, and a partial vaginectomy to determine invasion may be necessary. Occult invasive carcinoma may be detected by such an excision, particularly in patients who had previous hysterectomies, in whom the vaginal vault closure may bury some of the vaginal epithelium that is at risk for cancer (159).

Staging

The FIGO staging for vaginal carcinoma is shown in Table 32.6. Staging is done by clinical examination and, if indicated, cystoscopy, proctoscopy, chest radiographs and skeletal x-ray. Information derived from lymphangiography and CT and MRI scanning cannot be used to change the FIGO stage, but it can be used for planning treatment.

Unfortunately, 75% of patients present with stage II–IV disease, indicating delay in diagnosis and complicating the treatment and subsequent cure rates (151–153).

Surgical staging and resection of enlarged lymph nodes may be indicated in selected patients. FIGO staging does not include a category for microinvasive disease. Because vaginal cancer is rare and treatment is generally by radiotherapy, there is very little information concerning the spread of disease in relation to depth of invasion, lymphatic-vascular space invasion, and size of the lesion.

Patterns of Spread

Cancer of the vagina spreads most often by direct extension into the pelvic soft tissues and adjacent organs. Metastases to the pelvic and, subsequently, the para-aortic lymph nodes may occur in advanced disease (160). Lesions in the lower one-third of the vagina may spread directly to the inguinal femoral lymph nodes as well as the pelvic nodes (160). Hematogenous dissemination to the lungs, liver, or bone may occur as a late phenomenon.

Treatment

Treatment selection is based on the clinical examination, CT scan results, chest x-ray results, age, and condition of the patient. Most tumors are treated by radiation therapy; surgery is limited to highly selective cases.

Surgery

Women with stage I disease involving the upper posterior vagina may be treated by radical vaginectomy and pelvic lymphadenectomy. If the uterus is *in situ,* it would be removed as a radical hysterectomy specimen. When margins are clear and lymph nodes are negative, no additional therapy is necessary.

Table 32.6   FIGO Staging of Vaginal Cancer

Stage 0	Carcinoma *in situ,* intraepithelia carcinoma.
Stage I	The carcinoma is limited to the vaginal wall.
Stage II	The carcinoma has involved the subvaginal tissue but has not extended to the pelvic wall.
Stage III	The carcinoma has extended to the pelvic wall.
Stage IV	The carcinoma has extended beyond the true pelvis or has involved the mucosa of the bladder or rectum.
Stage IVa	Spread of the growth to adjacent organs.
Stage IVb	Spread to distant organs.

FIGO, International Federation of Gynecology and Obstetrics.

Patients with stage IV disease with either rectovaginal or vesicovaginal fistula may be candidates for primary pelvic exenteration with pelvic and para-aortic node dissection (161). Low rectal anastomosis, continent urinary diversion, and vaginal reconstruction are indicated and are more successful in these nonirradiated patients than in patients receiving prior radiation therapy (144).

Women with central pelvic recurrence after radiation therapy are candidates for pelvic exenteration similar to that for cervical cancer.

Surgical staging with resection of enlarged lymph nodes may improve the control of pelvic disease by radiotherapy techniques. Surgical exploration or laparoscopy at the time of Syed interstitial implants will more precisely define the placement of the needles as well as ensure that needles do not pass into adherent loops of bowel.

Radiation Therapy

Radiation therapy is the treatment of choice for all patients except those described previously. Small superficial lesions may be treated with intracavitary radiation alone (162). Larger, thicker lesions should be treated first with external teletherapy to decrease tumor volume and to treat the regional pelvic nodes, followed by intracavitary/interstitial therapy to deliver a high dose to the primary tumor (149, 163). If the uterus is intact and the lesion involves the upper vagina, an intrauterine tandem and ovoids can be used. If the uterus has been previously removed, a vaginal cylinder may be used for superficial irradiation. If the lesion is more than 0.5 cm thick, interstitial radiation techniques will improve the dose distribution to the primary tumor.

Extended-field radiation may be used for vaginal cancer in a manner similar to how it is used for cervical carcinoma. There is no experience reported with this technique in vaginal cancer. Likewise, there is no reported experience with combination chemotherapy/radiation. However, concurrent use of *5-FU* and *cisplatin* has been highly successful in anal and cervical cancer and should be considered.

Complications

The proximity of the rectum, bladder, and urethra leads to a major complication rate of 10–15% for both surgery and radiation treatment. For large tumors, the risk of bladder or bowel fistula is significant. Radiation cystitis and proctitis is common, as well as rectal strictures or ulcerations. Radiation necrosis of the vagina occasionally occurs, requiring debridement and often leading to fistula formation. Vaginal fibrosis, stenosis, and stricture are common following radiation therapy. Use of vaginal dilators and resumption of regular sexual relations should be encouraged, along with the use of topical estrogen to maintain adequate vaginal function.

Prognosis

The overall 5-year survival for vaginal cancer is 42% (Table 32.7). Even for patients with stage I disease, the 5-year survival rate is less than 70%, which is 15% lower than that for comparable stages of cervical or vulvar cancer (163–166). Most recurrences are in the pelvis, either from enlarged regional nodes or from large central tumors to which it is difficult to deliver an adequate dose of radiation. Radiation techniques such as interstitial implants with Syed applicator and combination chemotherapy/radiation may improve these results. Careful evaluation of the postradiation therapy patient for central recurrence may lead to some patients being salvaged by pelvic exenteration. Because of the rarity of vaginal cancer, these patients should be treated in a center that is familiar with all of the difficulties in treatment and modalities of therapy.

Adenocarcinoma

Adenocarcinoma of the vagina constitutes approximately 9% of primary tumors. In general, they affect the younger population of women, regardless of whether they were ex-

Table 32.7   Primary Vaginal Carcinoma: 5-Year Survival

Stage	No.	5-Year Survival	Percent
I	172	118	68.6
II	236	108	45.8
III	203	62	30.5
IV	114	20	17.5
Total	**725**	**308**	**42.5**

Data compiled from Benedet et al., 1983 (151); Rubin et al., 1985 (153); Kucera et al., 1985 (163); Houghton and Iversen, 1982 (164); Eddy et al, 1991 (165); and Pride et al., 1979 (166).

posed to *diethylstilbestrol (DES)* in utero (167). Adenocarcinomas may arise in Wolffian rest elements, periurethral glands, and foci of endometriosis (168). In women exposed to DES *in utero*, adenocarcinoma may develop in vaginal adenosis.

Metastatic adenocarcinoma of the vagina may originate from the colon, endometrium, ovary, or rarely, from the pancreas and stomach. Because metastatic adenocarcinoma is more common than primary adenocarcinoma, one should search for these lesions before diagnosing primary vaginal cancer.

DES Exposure *In Utero*

DES was used in the U.S. from 1940 until 1971 to maintain high-risk pregnancies in women with a history of spontaneous abortions. In 1970, Herbst and Scully reported on seven young women with clear cell adenocarcinoma of the vagina (Fig. 32.10). Later, an association between this cancer and maternal ingestion of DES during pregnancy was identified (169). Subsequently, more than 500 cases of clear cell cancer of the vagina and cervix have been reported to the Registry for Research on Hormonal Transplacental Carcinogenesis.

The estimated risk of developing clear cell adenocarcinoma from an exposed offspring is one in 1000 or less. The mean age of diagnosis is 19 years (170). Because the use of DES for pregnant women was discontinued in 1971, most of these tumors probably have been discovered. It is uncertain, however, what will happen to this cohort of women as they move into their fifth, sixth, and seventh decades of life. Continued surveillance of this cohort is indicated.

Melanoma

Malignant melanoma of the vagina is rare and extremely lethal. The average age of these patients is 58 years, and malignant melanoma occurs most often in white women (171). Most lesions are deeply invasive, corresponding to a level IV when compared to the staging for vulvar melanomas (172).

Radical excision has been the mainstay of treatment with the goal of avoiding local (vaginal) recurrence, which is the most common site of recurrence (171, 172). The need to dissect regional lymph nodes is uncertain. Because the disease is deeply invasive, hematogenous spread is the most common lethal recurrence. This finding is consistent with more conservative local excision, because there is no difference in overall survival in local versus radical excision (171). Survival is approximately 10% at 5 years.

Sarcoma

Vaginal sarcomas are usually fibrosarcomas or leiomyosarcomas. They are also extremely rare. Radical local excision followed by adjuvant chemotherapy or radiation therapy is the indicated treatment.

Embryonal Rhabdomyosarcoma

These tumors may be characterized by two structural variants: a solid form and a multicystic, grape-like form referred to as botryoid sarcoma (Fig. 32.11). Botryoid sarcoma is

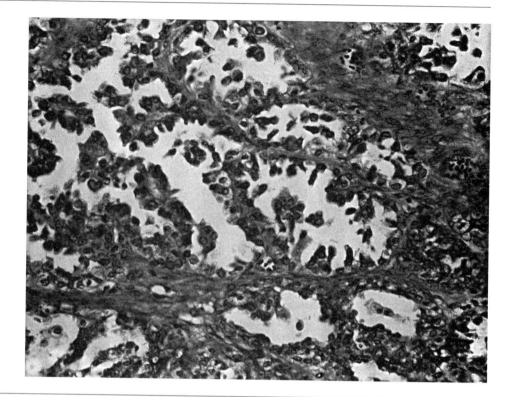

Figure 32.10 Vaginal clear cell carcinoma. Note the formation of tubules with hobnail cells lining the lumen. These cells are characterized by nuclear protrusion into the apical cytoplasm.

Figure 32.11 Embryonal rhabdomyosarcoma of the vagina (botryoid sarcoma). This lesion consists of primitive mesenchymal cells and rhabdomyoblasts, which have abundant eosinophilic cytoplasm. With further differentiation, cross striations may become evident.

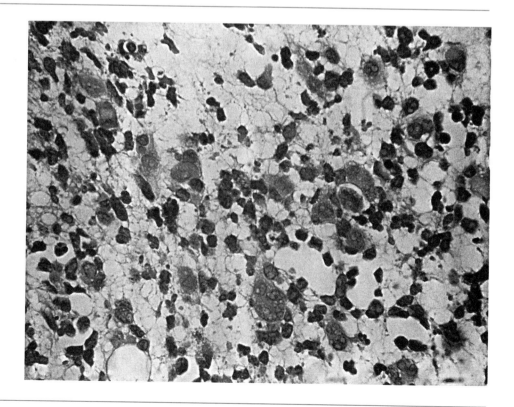

usually found in the vagina during infancy and early childhood, in the cervix during the reproductive years, and in the corpus uteri during postmenopausal years. Preoperative chemotherapy with *vincristine, actinomycin D,* and *cyclophosphamide,* followed by conservative surgery or radiation, has led to improved survival as well as organ preservation.

References

1. **Parker SL, Tong T, Bolden S, Wingo PA.** Cancer statistics, 1996. *CA Cancer J Clin* 1996; 46:5–28.

2. **Pettersson F.** *Annual Report on the Results of Treatment in Gynecological Cancer.* Radiumhemmet, Stockholm, Sweden: International Federation of Gynecology and Obstetrics (F.I.G.O.), 1994:132–68.

3. **Fu YS, Berek JS.** Minimal cervical cancer: definition and histology. In: **Grundmann E, Beck L,** eds. *Minimal Neoplasia—Diagnosis and Therapy. Recent Results in Cancer Research.* Vol. 106. Berlin: Springer-Verlag, 1988:47–56.

4. **Creasman W.** New gynecologic cancer staging. *Gynecol Oncol* 1995;58:157–8.

5. **Fu YS, Reagan, JW.** *Pathology of the Uterine Cervix, Vagina and Vulva.* Philadelphia: WB Saunders, 1989.

6. **Robert ME, Fu YS.** Squamous cell carcinoma of the uterine cervix: a review with emphasis on prognostic factors and unusual variants. *Semin Diagn Pathol* 1990;7:173–89.

7. **Fu YS, Berek JS, Hilborne LH.** Diagnostic problems of cervical in situ and invasive adenocarcinoma. *Appl Pathol* 1987:5:47–56.

8. **Kaku T, Enjoji M.** Extremely well-differentiated adenocarcinoma ("adenoma malignum"). *Int J Gynecol Pathol* 1983;2:28–41.

9. **Gilks CB, Young R, Aguirre P, DeLellis RA, Scully RE.** Adenoma malignum (minimal deviation adenocarcinoma) of the uterine cervix. *Am J Surg Pathol* 1989;13:717–29.

10. **Kaminski PF, Norris HJ.** Minimal deviation carcinoma (adenoma malignum) of the cervix. *Int J Gynecol Pathol* 1983;2:141–52.

11. **Benda JA, Platz CE, Buchsbaum H, Lifshitz S.** Mucin production in defining mixed carcinoma of the uterine cervix: a clinicopathologic study. *Int J Gynecol Pathol* 1985;4:314–27.

12. **Young RH, Scully RE.** Villoglandular papillary adenocarcinoma of the uterine cervix: a clinicopathologic analysis of 13 cases. *Cancer* 1989;63:1773–9.

13. **Glucksmann A, Cherry CP.** Incidence, histology and response to radiation of mixed carcinomas (adenoacanthomas) of the uterine cervix. *Cancer* 1956;9:971–9.

14. **Ferry JA, Scully RE.** "Adenoid cystic" carcinoma and adenoid basal carcinoma of the uterine cervix: a study of 28 cases. *Am J Surg Pathol* 1988;12:134–44.

15. **Van Nagell JR Jr, Donaldson ES, Wood EC, Maruyama Y, Utley J.** Small cell carcinoma of the cervix. *Cancer* 1979;40:2243–9.

16. **Lagasse LD, Ballon SC, Berman ML, Watring WG.** Pretreatment lymphangiography and operative evaluation in carcinoma of the cervix. *Am J Obstet Gynecol* 1979;134:219–24.

17. **Averette HE, Ford JH Jr, Dudan RC, Girtanner RE, Hoskins WJ, Lutz MH.** Staging of cervical cancer. *Clin Obstet Gynecol* 1975;18:215–32.

18. **Koehler PR.** Current status of lymphangiography in patients with cancer. *Cancer* 1976;37: 503–16.

19. **King LA, Talledo OE, Gallup DG, EL Gammal TAM.** Computed tomography in evaluation of gynecologic malignancies: a retrospective analysis. *Am J Obstet Gynecol* 1986;155:960–4.

20. **Bandy LC, Clarke-Pearson DL, Silverman PM, Creasman WT.** Computed tomography in evaluation of extrapelvic lymphadenopathy in carcinoma of the cervix. *Obstet Gynecol* 1986; 65:73–6.

21. **Hacker NF, Berek JS.** Surgical staging. In: **Surwit E, Alberts D,** eds. *Cervix Cancer.* Boston: Martinus Nijhoff, 1987:43–57.

22. **Worthington JL, Balfe DM, Lee JK, Gersell DJ, Heiker JP, Ling D, et al.** Uterine neoplasms: MR imaging. *Radiology* 1986;159:725–30.

23. **Van Nagell JR Jr, Parker JC Jr, Maruyama Y, Utley J, Luckett P.** Bladder or rectal injury following radiation therapy for cervical cancer. *Am J Obstet Gynecol* 1974;119:727–32.

24. **Lawton FG, Hacker NF.** Surgery for invasive gynecologic cancer in the elderly female population. *Obstet Gynecol* 1990;76:287–9.

25. **Hatch KD, Parham G, Shingleton HM, Orr JW Jr, Austin JM Jr.** Ureteral strictures and fistulae following radical hysterectomy. *Gynecol Oncol* 1984;19:17–23.

26. **Webb M, Symmonds R.** Wertheim hysterectomy: a reappraisal. *Obstet Gynecol* 1979;54:140–5.

27. **Boyce J, Fruchter R, Nicastri A.** Prognostic factors in stage I carcinoma of the cervix. *Gynecol Oncol* 1981;12:154–65.

28. **Simon NL, Gore H, Shingleton HM, Soong SJ, Orr JW Jr, Hatch KD.** Study of superficially invasive carcinoma of the cervix. *Obstet Gynecol* 1986;68:19–24.

29. **Delgado G, Bundy BN, Fowler WC, Stehman FB, Sevin B, Creasman WT, et al.** A prospective surgical pathological study of stage I squamous carcinoma of the cervix: a Gynecologic Oncology Group study. *Gynecol Oncol* 1989;35:314–20.

30. **Piver M, Rutledge F, Smith J.** Five classes of extended hysterectomy for women with cervical cancer. *Obstet Gynecol* 1974;44:265–72.

31. **Meigs J.** Radical hysterectomy with bilateral pelvic node dissections: a report of 100 patients operated five or more years ago. *Am J Obstet Gynecol* 1951;62:854–70.

32. **Orr JW Jr, Shingleton HM, Hatch KD.** Correlation of perioperative morbidity and conization to radical hysterectomy interval. *Obstet Gynecol* 1982;59:726–31.

33. **Potter ME, Alvarez RD, Shingleton HM, Soong SJ, Hatch KD.** Early invasive cervical cancer with pelvic lymph node involvement: to complete or not to complete radical hysterectomy? *Gynecol Oncol* 1990;37:78–81.

34. **Mann WJ Jr, Orr JW Jr, Shingleton HM, Austin JM Jr, Hatch KD, Taylor PT, et al.** Perioperative influences on infectious morbidity in radical hysterectomy. *Gynecol Oncol* 1981;11:207–12.

35. **Green T.** Ureteral suspension for prevention of ureteral complications following radical Wertheim hysterectomy. *Obstet Gynecol* 1966;28:1–11.

36. **Lowe J, Mauger G, Carmichael J.** The effect of Wertheim hysterectomy upon bladder and urethral function. *Am J Obstet Gynecol* 1981;139:826–34.

37. **Baltzer J, Lohe K, Kopke W, Zander J.** Histologic criteria for the prognosis of patients with operated squamous cell carcinoma of the cervix. *Gynecol Oncol* 1982;13:184–94.

38. **Chung C, Nahhas W, Stryker J, Curry S.** Analysis of factors contributing to treatment failures in stage IB and IIa carcinoma of the cervix. *Am J Obstet Gynecol* 1980;138:550–6.

39. **Creasman W, Soper J, Clarke-Pearson D.** Radical hysterectomy as therapy for early carcinoma of the cervix. *Am J Obstet Gynecol* 1986;155:964–9.

40. **Van Nagell J, Donaldson E, Parker J.** The prognostic significance of cell type and lesion size in patients with cervical cancer treated by radical surgery. *Gynecol Oncol* 1977;5:142–51.

41. **Inoue T, Okumura M.** Prognostic significance of parametrial extension in patients with cervical carcinoma stage Ib, IIa, and IIIb. *Cancer* 1984;54:1714–9.

42. **Bleker O, Ketting B, Wayjean-eecen B, Kloosterman G.** The significance of microscopic involvement of the parametrium and/or pelvic lymph nodes in cervical cancer stages Ib and IIa. *Gynecol Oncol* 1983;16:56–62.

43. **Gauthier P, Gore I, Shingleton HM.** Identification of histopathologic risk groups in stage Ib squamous cell carcinoma of the cervix. *Obstet Gynecol* 1985;66:569–74.

44. **Van Nagell J, Donaldson E, Wood E, Parker J.** The significance of vascular invasion and lymphocytic infiltration in invasive cervical cancer. *Cancer* 1978;41:228–34.

45. **Nahhas W, Sharkey F, Whitney C.** The prognostic significance of vascular channel involvement in deep stromal penetration in early cervical carcinoma. *Am J Clin Oncol* 1983;6:259–64.

46. **Soisson AP, Soper JT, Clarke-Pearson DL, Berchuck A, Montana G, Creasman WT.** Adjuvant radiotherapy following radical hysterectomy for patients with stage Ib and IIA cervical cancer. *Gynecol Oncol* 1990;37:390–5.

47. **Tinga DJ, Timmer PR, Bouma J, Aalder JG.** Prognostic significance of single versus multiple lymph node metastases in cervical carcinoma stage IB. *Gynecol Oncol* 1990;39:175–80.

48. **Alvarez RD, Soong SJ, Kinney WK, Reid GC, Schray MF, Podratz KC, et al.** Identification of prognostic factors and risk groups in patients found to have nodal metastasis at the time

of radical hysterectomy for early stage squamous carcinoma of the cervix. *Gynecol Oncol* 1989;35:130–35.

49. **Fuller AF, Elliott N, Kosloff C, Hoskins WJ, Lewis JL Jr.** Determinants of increased risk for recurrence in patients undergoing radical hysterectomy for stage IB and IIA carcinoma of the cervix. *Gynecol Oncol* 1989;33:34–9.

50. **Delgado G, Bundy B, Zaino R, Sevin BU, Creasman WT, Major F, et al.** Prospective surgical-pathological study of disease free interval in patients with stage IB squamous cell carcinoma of the cervix: a Gynecologic Oncology Group study. *Gynecol Oncol* 1990;38:352–7.

51. **Gonzalez DG, Ketting BW, Van Bunningen B, Van Duk JDP.** Carcinoma of the uterine cervix stage IB and IIA: results of postoperative irradiation in patients with microscopic infiltration in the parametrium and/or lymph node metastasis. *Int J Radiat Oncol Biol Phys* 1989; 16:389–95.

52. **Martinbeau P, Kjorstad K, Iversen T.** Stage Ib carcinoma of the cervix: the Norwegian Radium Hospital. II. Results when pelvic nodes are involved. *Obstet Gynecol* 1982;60:215–8.

53. **Morrow P.** Panel report: is pelvic irradiation beneficial in the postoperative management of stage Ib squamous cell carcinoma of the cervix with pelvic node metastases treated by radical hysterectomy and pelvic lymphadenectomy? *Gynecol Oncol* 1980;10:105–10.

54. **Inoue T.** Prognostic significance of the depth of invasion relating to nodal metastases, parametrial extension, and cell types. *Cancer* 1984;54:3035–42.

55. **Piver M, Chung W.** Prognostic significance of cervical lesion size and pelvic node metastases in cervical carcinoma. *Obstet Gynecol* 1975;46:507–10.

56. **Hsu CT, Cheng YS, Su SC.** Prognosis of uterine cervical cancer with extensive lymph node metastasis. *Am J Obstet Gynecol* 1972;114:954–62.

57. **Pilleron J, Durand J, Hamelin J.** Prognostic value of node metastasis in cancer of the uterine cervix. *Am J Obstet Gynecol* 1974;119:458–62.

58. **Inoue T, Chihara T, Morita K.** Postoperative extended field irradiation in patients with pelvic and/or common iliac node metastasis from cervical carcinoma stages Ib to IIb. *Gynecol Oncol* 1986;25:234–43.

59. **Larsson G, Alm P, Gullberg B, Grundsell H.** Prognostic factors in early invasive carcinoma of the uterine cervix. *Am J Obstet Gynecol* 1983;146:145–53.

60. **Lohe KJ, Burghardt E, Hillemanns HG, Kaufman C, Ober KG, Zander J.** Early squamous cell carcinoma of the uterine cervix. II. Clinical results of a cooperative study in the management of 419 patients with early stromal invasion and microcarcinoma. *Gynecol Oncol* 1978; 6:31–50.

61. **Burghardt E, Holzer E.** Diagnosis and treatment of microinvasive carcinoma of the cervix uteri. *Obstet Gynecol* 1977;49:641–53.

62. **Van Nagell J Jr, Greenwell N, Powell D, Donaldson E.** Microinvasive carcinoma of the cervix. *Am J Obstet Gynecol* 1983;145:981–91.

63. **Leman M, Benson W, Kurman R, Park R.** Microinvasive carcinoma of the cervix. *Obstet Gynecol* 1976;48:571–8.

64. **Seski JC, Abell MR, Morley GW.** Microinvasive squamous cell carcinoma of the cervix: definition, histologic analysis, late results of treatment. *Obstet Gynecol* 1977;50:410–4.

65. **Roche WO, Norris HC.** Microinvasive carcinoma of the cervix. *Cancer* 1975;36:180–6.

66. **Nahhas WA, Sharkey FE, Whitney CW, Husseinzadeh N, Chung CK, Mortel R.** The prognostic significance of vascular channel involvement and deep stromal invasion in early cervical cancer. *Am J Clin Oncol* 1983;6:259–64.

67. **Shingleton HM, Orr JW Jr.** Primary surgical and combined treatment. In: **Singer A, Jordan J,** eds. *Cancer of the Cervix.* New York: Churchill Livingstone, 1983:76–100.

68. **Barter JF, Soong SJ, Shingleton HM, Hatch KD, Orr JW Jr.** Complications of combined radical hysterectomy: postoperative radiation therapy in women with early stage cervical cancer. *Gynecol Oncol* 1989;32:292–6.

69. **Kinney WK, Alvarez RD, Reid GC, Schray MF, Soong SJ, Morley GW, et al.** Value of adjuvant whole-pelvic irradiation after Wertheim hysterectomy for early-stage squamous carcinoma of the cervix with pelvic nodal metastasis: a matched-control study. *Gynecol Oncol* 1989;34:258–62.

70. **Lai CH, Lin TS, Soong YK, Chen HF.** Adjuvant chemotherapy after radical hysterectomy for cervical carcinoma. *Gynecol Oncol* 1989;35:193–8.

71. **Wertheim MS, Hakes TB, Daghestani AN, Nori D, Smith DH, Lewis JL Jr.** A pilot study of adjuvant therapy in patients with cervical cancer at high risk of recurrence after radical hysterectomy and pelvic lymphadenectomy. *J Clin Oncol* 1985;3:912–16.

72. **Kim DS, Moon H, Kim KT, Hwang YY, Cho SH, Kim SR.** Two-year survival: preoperative adjuvant chemotherapy in the treatment of cervical cancer stages Ib and II with bulky tumor. *Gynecol Oncol* 1989;33:225–30.

73. **Panici PB, Scambia G, Baiocchi G, Greggi S, Ragusa G, Gallo A, et al.** Neoadjuvant chemotherapy and radical surgery in locally advanced cervical cancer: prognostic factors for response and survival. *Cancer* 1991;67:372–9.

74. **Sardi J, Sananes C, Giaroli A, Maya J, di Paola J.** Neoadjuvant chemotherapy in locally advanced carcinoma of the cervix uteri. *Gynecol Oncol* 1990;38:486–93.

75. **Berman M, Keys N, Creasman W, DiSaia P.** Survival and patterns of recurrence in cervical cancer metastatic to paraaortic lymph nodes. *Gynecol Oncol* 1984;19:8–16.

76. **Piver MS, Barlow JJ, Krishnamsetty R.** Five-year survival (with no evidence of disease) in patients with biopsy-confirmed aortic node metastasis from cervical carcinoma. *Am J Obstet Gynecol* 1981;193:575–8.

77. **Wharton JT, Jones HW III, Day TG, Rutledge FN, Fletcher GH.** Preirradiation celiotomy and extended field irradiation for invasive carcinoma of the cervix. *Obstet Gynecol* 1977;49:333–8.

78. **Ballon SC, Berman ML, Lagasse LD, Petrilli ES, Castaldo TW.** Survival after extraperitoneal pelvic and paraaortic lymphadenectomy and radiation therapy in cervical carcinoma. *Obstet Gynecol* 1981;57:90–5.

79. **Twiggs LB, Potish RA, George RJ, Adcock LL.** Pretreatment extraperitoneal surgical staging in primary carcinoma of the cervix uteri. *Surg Gynecol Obstet* 1984;158:243–50.

80. **Weiser EB, Bundy BN, Hoskins WJ, Heller PB, Whittington RR, DiSaia PJ, et al.** Extraperitoneal versus transperitoneal selective paraaortic lymphadenectomy in the pretreatment surgical staging of advanced cervical carcinoma (a Gynecologic Oncology Group study). *Gynecol Oncol* 1989;33:283–9.

81. **Stehman FB, Bundy BN, DiSaia PJ, Keys HM, Larson JE, Fowler WC.** Carcinoma of the cervix treated with radiation therapy. I. A multi-variate analysis of prognostic variables in the Gynecologic Oncology Group. *Cancer* 1991;67:2776–85.

82. **Lovecchio JL, Averette HE, Donato D, Bell J.** 5-year survival of patients with periaortic nodal metastases in clinical stage IB and IIA cervical carcinoma. *Gynecol Oncol* 1990;38:446.

83. **Rubin SC, Brookland R, Mikuta JJ, Mangan C, Sutton G, Danoff B.** Paraaortic nodal metastases in early cervical carcinoma: long-term survival following extended-field radiotherapy. *Gynecol Oncol* 1984;18:213–7.

84. **Stehman FB, Bundy BN, Hanjani P, Fowler WC, Abulhay G, Whitney CW.** Biopsy of the scalene fat pad in carcinoma of the cervix uteri metastatic to the periaortic lymph nodes. *Surg Gynecol Obstet* 1987;165:503–6.

85. **Jampolis S, Andras J, Fletcher GH.** Analysis of sites and causes of failure of irradiation in invasive squamous cell carcinoma of the intact uterine cervix. *Radiology* 1975;115:681–5.

86. **Hreshchyshyn MM, Aron BS, Boronow RC, Franklin EW III, Shingleton HM, Blessing JA.** Hydroxyurea or placebo combined with radiation to treat stage IIIb and IV cervical cancer confined to the pelvis. *Int J Radiat Oncol Biol Phys* 1979;5:317–22.

87. **Piver MS, Barlow JJ, Vongtama V, Blumenson L.** Hydroxyurea: a radiation potentiator in carcinoma of the uterine cervix. *Am J Obstet Gynecol* 1983;147:803–8.

88. **Thomas G, Dembo A, Beale F.** Concurrent radiation, mitomycin-C and 5-fluorouracil in poor prognosis carcinoma of the cervix: preliminary results of a Phase I-II study. *Int J Radiat Oncol Biol Phys* 1984;10:1785–90.

89. **Bonomi P, Blessing JA, Stehman FB.** A randomized trial of three Cisplatinum dose schedules in squamous cell carcinoma of the uterine cervix. *J Clin Oncol* 1985;3:1079–85.

90. **Choo YC, Choy TK, Wong LC, Ma HK.** Potentiation of radiotherapy by cisdichlorodiammine platinum (II) in advanced cervical carcinoma. *Gynecol Oncol* 1986;23:94–100.

91. **Twiggs LB, Potish RA, McIntyre S, Adcock LL, Savage JE, Prem KA.** Concurrent weekly cis-platinum and radiotherapy in advanced cervical cancer: a preliminary dose escalating toxicity study. *Gynecol Oncol* 1986;24:143–8.

92. **Thomas G, Dembo A, Fyles A, Gadalla T, Beale F, Beam H, et al.** Concurrent chemoradiation in advanced cervical cancer. *Gynecol Oncol* 1990;38:446–51.

93. **Kim RY, Levy DS, Brascho DJ, Hatch KD.** Uterine perforation during intracavitary application: prognostic significance in carcinoma of the cervix. *Radiology* 1983;147:249–51.

94. **White AJ, Buchsbaum HJ, Blythe JG, Lifshitz S.** Use of the bulbocavernosus muscle (Martius procedure) for repair of radiation-induced rectovaginal fistulas. *Obstet Gynecol* 1982;60:114–8.

95. **Bricker EM, Johnston WD.** Repair of postirradiation rectovaginal fistula and stricture. *Surg Gynecol Obstet* 1979;148:499–506.

96. **Smith ST, Seski JC, Copeland LJ, Gershenson DM, Edwards CL, Herson J.** Surgical management of irradiation-induced small bowel damage. *Obstet Gynecol* 1985;65:563–7.

97. **Gallousis S.** Isolated lung metastases from pelvic malignancies. *Gynecol Oncol* 1979;7:206–14.

98. **Nordqvist SR, Sevin BU, Nadji M, Greening SE, Ng AB.** Fine-needle aspiration cytology in gynecologic oncology. I. Diagnostic accuracy. *Obstet Gynecol* 1979;54:719–24.

99. **Krebs HB, Helmkamp BF, Sevin B-U, Poliakoff SR, Nadji M, Averette HE.** Recurrent cancer of the cervix following radical hysterectomy and pelvic node dissection. *Obstet Gynecol* 1982;59:422–7.

100. **Shingleton HM, Orr JW Jr.** Posttreatment surveillance. In: **Singer A, Jordan J,** eds. *Cancer of the Cervix*. New York: Churchill Livingstone, 1983:135–22.

101. **Kjorstad KE.** Adenocarcinoma of the uterine cervix. *Gynecol Oncol* 1977;5:219–23.

102. **Berek JS, Hacker NF, Fu YS, Sokale JR, Leuchter RC, Lagasse LD.** Adenocarcinoma of the uterine cervix: histologic variables associated with lymph node metastasis and survival. *Obstet Gynecol* 1985;65:46–52.

103. **Hopkins MP, Morley GW.** A comparison of adenocarcinoma and squamous cell carcinoma of the cervix. *Obstet Gynecol* 1991;77:912–7.

104. **Shingleton HM, Gore H, Bradley DH, Soong SJ.** Adenocarcinoma of the cervix. I. Clinical evaluation and pathologic features. *Am J Obstet Gynecol* 1981;139:799–814.

105. **Kilgore LC, Soong S-J, Gore H, Shingleton HM, Hatch KD, Partridge EE.** Analysis of prognostic features in adenocarcinoma of the cervix. *Gynecol Oncol* 1988;31:137–53.

106. **Berek JS, Castaldo TW, Hacker NF, Petrilli ES, Lagasse LD, Moore JG.** Adenocarcinoma of the uterine cervix. *Cancer* 1981;48:2734–41.

107. **Mayer EG, Galindo J, Davis J, Wurzel J, Aristizabal S.** Adenocarcinoma of the uterine cervix: incidence and the role of radiation therapy. *Radiology* 1976;121:725–9.

108. **Rutledge FN, Galakatos AE, Wharton JT, Smith JP.** Adenocarcinoma of the uterine cervix. *Am J Obstet Gynecol* 1975;122:236–45.

109. **Gallup DG, Abell MR.** Invasive adenocarcinoma of the uterine cervix. *Obstet Gynecol* 1977;49:596–603.

110. **Eifel PJ, Morris M, Oswald MJ, Wharton JT, Delclos L.** Adenocarcinoma of the uterine cervix: prognosis and patterns of failure in 367 cases. *Cancer* 1990;65:2507–14.

111. **Gallup DG, Harper RH, Stock RJ.** Poor prognosis in patients with adenosquamous cell carcinoma of the cervix. *Obstet Gynecol* 1985;65:416–22.

112. **Maier RC, Norris HJ.** Coexistence of cervical intraepithelial neoplasia with primary adenocarcinoma of the endocervix. *Obstet Gynecol* 1980;56:361–4.

113. **Hacker NF, Berek JS, Lagasse LD, Charles EH, Savage EW, Moore JG.** Carcinoma of the cervix associated with pregnancy. *Obstet Gynecol* 1982;59:735–46.

114. **Averette HE, Nasser N, Yankow SL, Little WA.** Cervical conization in pregnancy. *Am J Obstet Gynecol* 1970;106:543–9.

115. **Lee RB, Neglia W, Park RC.** Cervical carcinoma in pregnancy. *Obstet Gynecol* 1981;58:584–9.

116. **Shingleton HM, Orr JW Jr.** Cancer complicating pregnancy. In: **Singer A, Jordan J,** eds. *Cancer of the Cervix*. New York: Churchill Livingstone, 1983:193–209.

117. **Green TH, Morse WJ Jr.** Management of invasive cervical cancer following inadvertent simple hysterectomy. *Obstet Gynecol* 1969;33:763–9.

118. **Orr JW Jr, Ball GC, Soong SJ, Hatch KD, Partridge EE, Austin JM.** Surgical treatment of women found to have invasive cervix cancer at the time of total hysterectomy. *Obstet Gynecol* 1986;68:353–6.

119. **Durrance FY.** Radiotherapy following simple hysterectomy in patients with stage I and II carcinoma of the cervix. *Am J Roentgenol Radium Ther Nucl Med* 1968;102:165–9.

120. **Andras EJ, Fletcher GH, Rutledge F.** Radiotherapy of carcinoma of the cervix following simple hysterectomy. *Am J Obstet Gynecol* 1973;115:647–55.

121. **Heller PB, Barnhill DR, Mayer AR, Fontaine TP, Hoskins WJ, Park RC.** Cervical carcinoma found incidentally in a uterus removed for benign indications. *Obstet Gynecol* 1986;67: 187–90.

122. **Million RR, Rutledge F, Fletcher GH.** Stage IV carcinoma of the cervix with bladder invasion. *Am J Obstet Gynecol* 1972;113:239–46.

123. **Taylor PT, Andersen WA.** Untreated cervical cancer complicated by obstructive uropathy and renal failure. *Gynecol Oncol* 1981;11:162–74.

124. **Fletcher GH, Wharton JT.** Principles of irradiation therapy for gynecologic malignancy. *Curr Probl Obstet Gynecol* 1978;2:2–44.

125. **Gaddis O Jr, Morrow CP, Klement V, Schlaerth JB, Nalick RH.** Treatment of cervical carcinoma employing a template for transperineal interstitial Iridium brachytherapy. *Int J Radiat Oncol Biol Phys* 1983;9:819–27.

126. **O'Quinn AG, Fletcher GH, Wharton JT.** Guidelines for conservative hysterectomy after irradiation. *Gynecol Oncol* 1980;9:68–79.

127. **Homesley HD, Raben M, Blake DD, Ferree CR, Bullock MS, Linton EB, et al.** Relationship of lesion size to survival in patients with stage IB squamous cell carcinoma of the cervix uteri treated by radiation therapy. *Surg Gynecol Obstet* 1980;150:529–31.

128. **Oldham RK, Greco FA.** Small cell lung cancer, a curable disease. *Cancer Chem Pharmacol* 1980;4:173–7.

129. **Sheets EE, Berman ML, Hrountas CK, Liao SY, DiSaia PJ.** Surgically treated early-stage neuroendocrine small-cell cervical carcinoma. *Obstet Gynecol* 1988;71:10–4.

130. **Feder BH, Syed AMN, Neblett D.** Treatment of extensive carcinoma of the cervix with the "transperineal parametrial butterfly"—a preliminary report on the revival of Waterman's approach. *Int J Radiat Oncol Biol Phys* 1978;4:735–42.

131. **Mikuta JJ, Giuntoli RL, Rubin EL, Mangan CE.** The radical hysterectomy. *Am J Obstet Gynecol* 1977;128:119–27.

132. **Symmonds RE, Pratt JH, Welch JS.** Extended Wertheim operation for primary, recurrent, or suspected recurrent carcinoma of the cervix. *Obstet Gynecol* 1964;24:15–27.

133. **Ketcham AS, Chretien PB, Hoye RC, Harrah JD, Deckers PJ, Sugarbaker EU, et al.** Occult metastases to the scalene lymph nodes in patients with clinically operable carcinoma of the cervix. *Cancer* 1973;31:180–3.

134. **Morley GW, Lindenauer SM.** Pelvic exenterative therapy for gynecologic malignancy: an analysis of 70 cases. *Cancer* 1976;38:581–6.

135. **Rutledge FN, Smith JP, Wharton JT, O'Quinn AG.** Pelvic exenteration: an analysis of 296 patients. *Am J Obstet Gynecol* 1977;129:881–92.

136. **Averette HE, Lichtinger M, Sevin BU, Girtanner RE.** Pelvic exenteration: a 150-year experience in a general hospital. *Am J Obstet Gynecol* 1984;150:179–84.

137. **Hatch KD, Shingleton HM, Soong SJ, Baker VV, Gelder MS.** Anterior pelvic exenteration. *Gynecol Oncol* 1988;31:205–16.

138. **Orr JW Jr, Shingleton HM, Hatch KD, Taylor PT, Partridge EE, Soong SJ.** Gastrointestinal complications associated with pelvic exenteration. *Am J Obstet Gynecol* 1983;145: 325–32.

139. **Berek JS, Hacker NF, Lagasse LD.** Rectosigmoid colectomy and reanastomosis to facilitate resection of primary and recurrent gynecologic cancer. *Obstet Gynecol* 1984;64:715–20.

140. **Hatch KD, Shingleton HM, Potter ME, Baker VV.** Low rectal resection and anastomosis at the time of pelvic exenteration. *Gynecol Oncol* 1988;31:262–7.

141. **Kock NG, Nilson AE, Nilsson LO, Norlen LJ, Philipson BM.** Urinary diversion via a continent ileal reservoir: clinical results in 12 patients. *J Urol* 1982;128:469–75.

142. **Penalver MA, Bejany DE, Averette HE, Donato DM, Sevin BU, Suarez G.** Continent urinary diversion in gynecologic oncology. *Gynecol Oncol* 1989;34:274–88.

143. **Mannel RS, Braly PS, Buller RE.** Indiana pouch continent urinary reservoir in patients with previous pelvic irradiation. *Obstet Gynecol* 1990;75:891–3.

144. **Berek JS, Hacker NF, Lagasse LD.** Vaginal reconstruction performed simultaneously with pelvic exenteration. *Obstet Gynecol* 1984;63:318–23.

145. **Thigpen JT.** Single agent chemotherapy in carcinoma of the cervix. In: **Surwit EA, Alberts DS,** eds. *Cervix Cancer.* Boston: Martinus Nijhoff, 1987:119–36.

146. **Barter JF, Soong SJ, Hatch KD, Orr JW, Shingleton HM.** Diagnosis and treatment of pulmonary metastases from cervical carcinoma. *Gynecol Oncol* 1990;38:347–51.

147. **Vermorken JB.** The role of chemotherapy in squamous cell carcinoma of the uterine cervix: a review. *Int J Gynecol Cancer* 1993;3:129.

148. **Rutledge F.** Cancer of the vagina. *Am J Obstet Gynecol* 1967;97:635–55.

149. **Perez CA, Arneson AN, Dehner LP, Galakatos A.** Radiation therapy in carcinoma of the vagina. *Obstet Gynecol* 1974;44:862–72.

150. **Weed JC, Lozier C, Daniel SJ.** Human papillomavirus in multifocal, invasive femal genital tract malignancy. *Obstet Gynecol* 1986;68:333.

151. **Benedet JL, Murphy KJ, Fairey RN, Boyes DA.** Primary invasive carcinoma of the vagina. *Obstet Gynecol* 1983;62:715–9.

152. **Peters WA III, Kuman NB, Morley GW.** Carcinoma of the vagina. *Cancer* 1985;55:892–7.

153. **Rubin SC, Young J, Mikuta JJ.** Squamous carcinoma of the vagina: treatment, complications, and long-term follow up. *Gynecol Oncol* 1985;20:346–53.

154. **Benedet JL, Saunders BH.** Carcinoma *in situ* of the vagina. *Am J Obstet Gynecol* 1984;148:695–700.

155. **Lenehan PM, Meffe F, Lickrish GM.** Vaginal intraepithelial neoplasia: biologic aspects and management. *Obstet Gynecol* 1986;68:333–7.

156. **Cramer DW, Cutler SJ.** Incidence and histopathology of malignancies of the female genital organs in the United States. *Am J Obstet Gynecol* 1974;118:443–60.

157. **Herman JM, Homesley HD, Dignan MB.** Is hysterectomy a risk factor for vaginal cancer? *JAMA* 1986;256:601–3.

158. **Frick HC, Jacox HW, Taylor HC.** Primary carcinoma of the vagina. *Am J Obstet Gynecol* 1986;101:695.

159. **Hoffman MS, DeCesare SL, Roberts WS, et al.** Upper vaginectomy for *in situ* and occult superficially invasive carcinoma of the vagina. *Am J Obstet Gynecol* 1992;166:30–3.

160. **Al-Kurdi M, Monaghan JM.** Thirty-two years experience in management of primary tumors of the vagina. *Br J Obstet Gynecol* 1981;88:1145–50.

161. **Eddy GL, Singh KP, Gansler TS.** Superficially invasive carcinoma of the vagina following treatment for cervical cancer: a report of six cases. *Gynecol Oncol* 1990;36:376–9.

162. **Reddy S, Lee MS, Graham JE, Yordan EL, Phillips R, Saxena VS, et al.** Radiation therapy in primary carcinoma of the vagina. *Gynecol Oncol* 1987;26:19–24.

163. **Kucera H, Langer M, Smekal G, Weyhaupt K.** Radiotherapy of primary carcinoma of the vagina: management and results of different therapy schemes. *Gynecol Oncol* 1985;21:87–93.

164. **Houghton CRS, Iversen T.** Squamous cell carcinoma of the vagina: a clinical study of the location of the tumor. *Gynecol Oncol* 1982;13:365–72.

165. **Eddy GL, Marks RD, Miller MC III, Underwood PB Jr.** Primary invasive vaginal carcinoma. *Am J Obstet Gynecol* 1991;165:292–6.

166. **Pride GL, Schultz AE, Chuprevich TW, Buchler DA.** Primary invasive squamous carcinoma of the vagina. *Obstet Gynecol* 1979;53:218–25.

167. **Ballon SC, Lagasse LD, Chang NH, Stehman FB.** Primary adenocarcinoma of the vagina. *Surg Gynecol Obstet* 1979;149:233–7.

168. **Herbst AL, Scully RE.** Adenocarcinoma of the vagina in adolescence. *Cancer* 1970;25:745–57.

169. **Herbst AL, Ulfelder H, Poskanzer DC.** Adenocarcinoma of the vagina: association of maternal stilbestrol therapy with tumor appearance in young women. *N Engl J Med* 1971;284: 878–81.

170. **Herbst AL, Cole P, Norusis MJ, Welch WR, Scully RE.** Epidemiologic aspects of factors related to survival in 384 Registry cases of clear cell adenocarcinoma of the vagina and cervix. *Am J Obstet Gynecol* 1979;135:876–86.

171. **Reid GC, Schmidt RW, Roberts JA, Hopkins MP, Barrett RJ, Morley GW.** Primary melanoma of the vagina: a clinicopathologic analysis. *Obstet Gynecol* 1989;74:190–9.

172. **Chung AF, Casey MJ, Flannery JT, Woodruff JM, Lewis JL Jr.** Malignant melanoma of the vagina—report of 19 cases. *Obstet Gynecol* 1980;55:720–7.

33

Ovarian Cancer

Jonathan S. Berek
Yao S. Fu
Neville F. Hacker

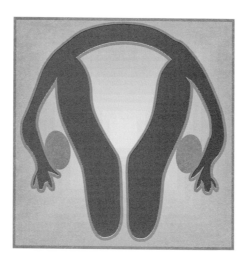

Of all the gynecologic cancers, ovarian malignancies represent the greatest clinical challenge. Epithelial cancers are the most common ovarian malignancies, and because they are usually asymptomatic until they have metastasized, patients present with advanced disease in more than two-thirds of the cases. Ovarian cancer represents a major surgical challenge, requires intensive and often complex therapies, and is extremely demanding of the patient's psychological and physical energy. It has the highest fatality-to-case ratio of all the gynecologic malignancies. There are more than 26,700 new cases annually in the U.S., and 14,800 women can be expected to succumb to their illness (1).

Epithelial Ovarian Cancer

Approximately 90% of ovarian cancers are derived from tissues that come from the coelomic epithelium or "mesothelium" (2). The cells are a product of the primitive mesoderm, which can undergo metaplasia. A classification of the histologic types of Epithelial tumors of the ovary is presented in Table 33.1. Neoplastic transformation can occur when the cells are genetically predisposed to oncogenesis and/or exposed to an oncogenic agent (3).

Pathology

Seventy-five percent of epithelial cancers are of the serous histologic type. Less common types are mucinous (20%), endometrioid (2%), clear cell, Brenner, and undifferentiated carcionomas; each of the last three types represent less than 1% of epithelial lesions (2). Each tumor type has a histologic pattern that reproduces the mucosal features of a section of the lower genital tract (3). For example, the serous or papillary pattern has an appearance similar to that of the glandular epithelium lining and fallopian tube. Mucinous tumors contain cells that resemble the endocervical glands, and the endometrioid tumors resemble the endometrium.

Borderline Tumors

An important group of tumors to distinguish is the *tumor of low malignant potential,* also called the *borderline* tumor. Borderline tumors are lesions that tend to remain confined to

Table 33.1   Epithelial Ovarian Tumors

Histologic Type	*Cellular Type*
I. Serous A. Benign B. Borderline C. Malignant	Endosalpingeal
II. Mucinous A. Benign B. Borderline C. Malignant	Endocervical
III. Endometrioid A. Benign B. Borderline C. Malignant	Endometrial
IV. Clear-Cell "Mesonephroid" A. Benign B. Borderline C. Malignant	Müllerian
V. Brenner A. Benign B. Borderline ("proliferating") C. Malignant	Transitional
VI. Mixed epithelial A. Benign B. Borderline C. Malignant	Mixed
VII. Undifferentiated	Anaplastic
VIII. Unclassified	Mesothelioma, etc.

Adapted with permission from **Seroy SF, Scully RE, Sobin LH.** *International Histological Classification of Tumours no. 9. Histological Typing of Ovarian Tumors.* Geneva: World Health Organization, 1973.

the ovary for long periods, occur predominantly in premenopausal women, and are associated with a very good prognosis (2–6). They are encountered most frequently in women between the ages of 30 and 50 years, whereas invasive carcinomas occur more often in women between the ages of 50 and 70 years (2).

Although uncommon, metastatic implants may occur with borderline tumors. Such implants have been divided into noninvasive and invasive forms. The latter group have a higher likelihood of developing into progressive, proliferative disease in the peritoneal cavity, which can lead to intestinal obstruction and death (2, 6).

The criteria for the diagnosis of borderline tumors (Fig. 33.1) are as follows (7):

1.   Epithelial proliferation with papillary formation and pseudostratification

2.   Nuclear atypia and increased mitotic activity

3.   Absence of true stromal invasion (i.e., without tissue destruction).

It should be emphasized that about 20–25% of borderline malignant tumors spread beyond the ovary. The peritoneal implants may not be distinguished from those secondary to a well-differentiated carcinoma. Thus, the diagnosis of borderline malignant versus malignant ovarian tumor must be based on the histologic features of the primary tumor. In the malignant tumors, stromal invasion is present. Rare examples of microinvasion have been reported in borderline malignant tumors (7).

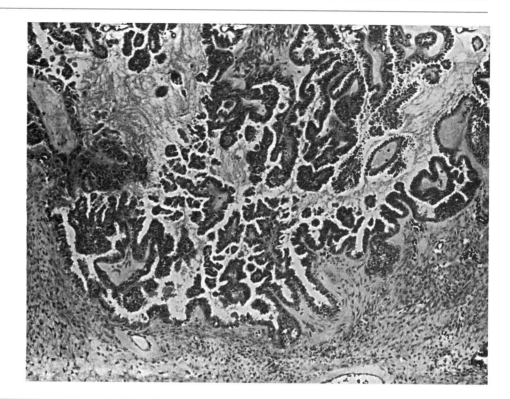

Figure 33.1   Borderline malignant serous tumor of the ovary. Complex papillary fronds are lined with pseudostratified columnar cells. The epithelium and the stroma are clearly separated by a basement membrane, indicating no stromal invasion. (Reproduced with permission from **Berek JS, Hacker NF.** *Practical Gynecologic Oncology.* 2nd ed. Baltimore: Williams & Wilkins, 1994:138.)

Serous Tumors

The serous tumors develop by invagination of the surface ovarian epithelium and are so classified because they secrete serous fluid (as do tubal secretory cells). *Psammoma bodies,* more correctly foci of foreign material, frequently are associated with these invaginations and may be a response to irritative agents that produce adhesion formation and the entrapment of the surface epithelium. In the wall of the mesothelial invaginations, papillary ingrowths are common, representing the early stages of development of a papillary serous cystadenoma. There are may variations in the proliferation of these mesothelial inclusions. Several foci may be lined with flattened inactive epithelium; in adjacent cavities, papillary excrescences are present, often resulting from local irritants.

Borderline Serous Tumors   Approximately 10% of all ovarian serous tumors fall into the category of a "tumor of low malignant potential" or "borderline" tumor, and 50% occur before the age of 40 years. As many as 40% of women with ovarian serous borderline tumors have extraovarian implants, and as many as 40% of these women eventually die of disease (7). Although multiple foci of disease have been documented in the abdominal cavity with secondary deposits in the pelvis, omentum, and adjacent tissues, including lymph nodes, metastases outside the abdominal cavity are exceptional. Death can occur as the result of intestinal obstruction (8).

The implants are divided histologically into invasive and noninvasive groups. In the *noninvasive group,* papillary proliferations of atypical cells involve the peritoneal surface and form smooth invaginations. The degree of nuclear atypia is similar to that of the primary tumor. A desmoplastic stromal reaction, characterized by dense layers of fibroblasts and infiltration with acute and chronic inflammatory cells, can occur in association with some of the implants. Atypical cells, single or in clusters, may be associated with psammoma bodies, necrosis, cholesterol clefts, or hemorrhage (6).

The *invasive implants* resemble well-differentiated serous carcinoma and are characterized by atypical cells forming irregular glands with sharp borders. The interface between the epithelium and stroma is ill-defined and obliterated. Marked cytologic atypia is usually present. Single cells may be found in both invasive and noninvasive implants.

Bell et al. (6) have reported that only three of 50 women with noninvasive implants died, whereas four of six women with invasive implants died. In the series of McCaughey, two of 13 patients with noninvasive implants and all five patients with invasive implants died (9). Others have noted no differences in prognosis (10, 11).

Rare examples of borderline malignant serous tumors with foci of microinvasion have been reported by Bell and Scully (12). These foci can be recognized by single cells, cribiform glands, or papillary clusters extending into the stroma, often with empty spaces between the epithelium and the stroma. Invasion of lymphatic spaces may be seen. Most patients are young, International Federation of Gynecology and Obstetrics (FIGO) stage I, and sometimes pregnant. Only one of 30 such patients died of disease. This patient had stage III disease and died 1 month after surgery (12).

Malignant Serous Carcinomas   The grade of tumor should be identified. In well-differentiated serous adenocarcinoma, papillary and glandular structures predominate. The nuclei are uniformly round to oval with 0–2 mitoses per high-powered field (HPF) (Fig. 33.2). Poorly differentiated neoplasms are characterized by solid sheets of cells, nuclear pleomorphism, and high mitotic activity, usually 2–3 mitoses per HPF. A moderately dif-

Figure 33.2   Well-differentiated serous papillary adenocarcinoma of ovary. Clusters and papillae of malignant cells are in direct contact with fibrous stroma indicative of stromal invasion. (Reproduced with permission from **Berek JS, Hacker NF.** *Practical Gynecologic Oncology.* 2nd ed. Baltimore: Williams & Wilkins, 1994:140.)

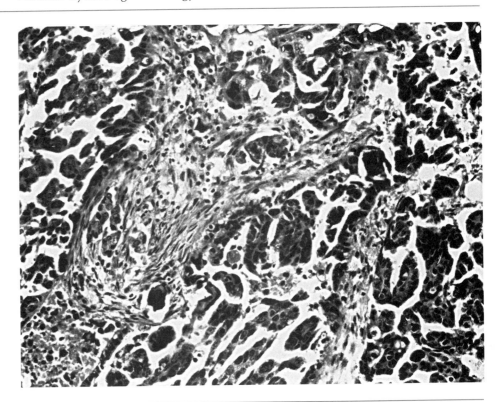

ferentiated tumor is intermediate between the well-differentiated and poorly differentiated groups. Laminated, calcified psammoma bodies are found in 80% of serous carcinomas.

Mucinous Tumors

These cystic tumors with locules lined with mucin-secreting epithelium constitute approximately 8–10% of primary epithelial ovarian tumors. They may reach an enormous size, filling the entire abdominal cavity.

Borderline Mucinous Tumors   The mucinous "tumor of low malignant potential" is an enigma. Mucinous tumors are made up largely of endocervical mucus-secreting cells and may reveal areas in which intestinal, serous, or endometrioid epithelia seem to suggest immaturity. Such foci do not change the prognosis but are simply demonstrations of the multipotentiality of the surface epithelium. Tumors with more than four stratified layers or cytologically malignant cells are best classified as well-differentiated mucinous carcinoma. Although it is common to find a rather uniform pattern from section to section in the borderline malignant serous lesions, this is not true in the mucinous tumors. Frequently, well-differentiated mucinous epithelium may be seen immediately adjacent to a poorly differentiated focus. Therefore, it is important to take multiple sections from many areas in the mucinous tumor to identify the most significant anaplastic alteration.

Malignant Mucinous Carcinomas   Although papillary proliferations are much less common in the mucinous tumors than in the serous tumors, such alterations are basic evidence of atypical proliferation, and it is in these foci that the true mitotic activity of the mucinous carcinoma can be most accurately identified (Fig. 33.3). **Bilateral tumors occur in 8–10% of**

Figure 33.3   Mucinous adenocarcinoma of the ovary. Irregular glandular spaces are lined with a layer of tall columnar cells with abundant mucinous cytoplasm, resembling endocervical cells. The nuclei are mildly atypical. (Reproduced with permission from **Berek JS, Hacker NF.** *Practical Gynecologic Oncology.* 2nd ed. Baltimore: Williams & Wilkins, 1994:142.)

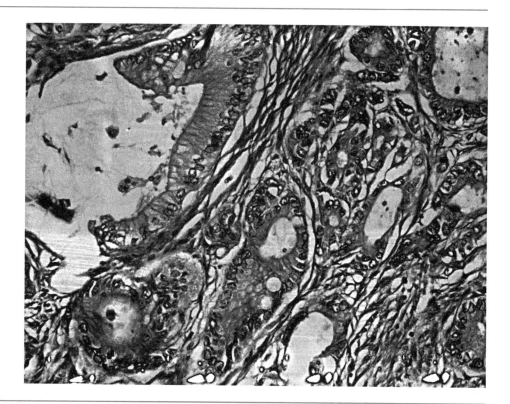

cases. The mucinous lesions are intraovarian in 95–98% of cases. Malignancy develops in 5–10% of benign mucinous cysts. Because most ovarian mucinous carcinomas contain intestinal type cells, they cannot be distinguished from metastatic carcinoma of the gastrointestinal tract on the basis of histology alone. Primary ovarian neoplasms rarely metastasize to the mucosa of the bowel, although they commonly involve the serosa, whereas gastrointestinal lesions frequently involve the ovary by direct extension of vascular lymphatic spread.

Pseudomyxoma Peritonei   In pseudomyxoma peritonei, the neoplastic epithelium secretes large amounts of gelatinous mucinous material. It is most commonly secondary to an ovarian mucinous carcinoma, a mucocele of the appendix, or a well-differentiated colon carcinoma.

Endometrioid Tumors

Endometrioid lesions constitute 6–8% of epithelial tumors. Endometrioid neoplasia includes all the benign demonstrations of endometriosis.

In 1925, Sampson (13) suggested that certain cases of adenocarcinoma of the ovary probably arose in areas of endometriosis. His criteria were so strict that few cases were reported until 1960, because he required that typical benign endometriosis be found in association with adenocarcinoma and that a transition between the two be identified. The adenocarcinomas were similar to those seen in the uterine cavity and approximately 50% contained squamous elements. Tumors that met these criteria were associated with an excellent prognosis.

The malignant potential of endometriosis is very low, although a transition from benign to malignant epithelium may be demonstrated (Fig. 33.4). Malignancies arising in endometriosis may show the hemorrhagic foci characteristic of benign lesions. The neo-

Figure 33.4   Endometrioid cancer arising in adjacent endometriosis. (Reproduced with permission from **Berek JS, Hacker NF.** *Practical Gynecologic Oncology.* 2nd ed. Baltimore: Williams & Wilkins, 1994:143.)

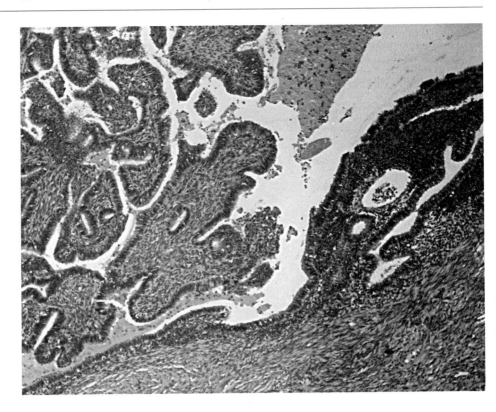

plasms that develop *de novo* from the mesothelium are not distinctive. Most are not as large as the mucinous tumors or as papillary as the serous tumors.

Borderline Endometrioid Tumors   The endometrioid tumor of low malignant potential has a wide morphologic spectrum. Tumors may resemble an endometrial polyp or complex endometrial hyperplasia with crowding of glands. When there are back-to-back glands with no intervening stroma, the tumor is classified as a well-differentiated endometrioid carcinoma. Some borderline malignant tumors have a prominent fibromatous component. In such cases, the word "adenofibroma" is used.

Malignant Endometrioid Carcinomas   Endometrioid tumors are characterized by an adenomatous pattern with all the potential variations of epithelia found in the uterus. Adenocarcinoma with benign-appearing squamous metaplasia has an excellent prognosis. Conversely, patients with mixed adenosquamous carcinomas have a very low survival rate. In poorly differentiated ovarian malignancies, there are frequently "adenoid" foci, but these areas are not sufficient to allow classification of these lesions as "endometrioid."

Multifocal Disease   The "endometrial" or endometrioid tumors afford the greatest opportunity to evaluate "multifocal disease." **Endometrioid tumors of the ovary are often associated with similar lesions in the endometrium.** Identification of multifocal disease is important, because patients with disease metastatic from the uterus to the ovaries have a 30–40% 5-year survival, whereas those with synchronous multifocal disease have a 75–80% 5-year survival (14). When the histologic appearance of endometrial and ovarian tumors is different, the two tumors most likely represent two separate primary lesions. When they appear similar, the endometrial tumor can be considered a separate primary tumor if it is well differentiated and only superficially invasive.

Clear Cell (Mesonephroid) Tumors

The incidence of clear cell carcinoma among all ovarian tumors is difficult to assess, although it is 3% at The Johns Hopkins Hospital. A more accurate figure is lacking because of the high frequency with which clear cells coexist with other cell types. Clinically, these tumors are the most common ovarian neoplasms associated with hypercalcemia or hyperpyrexia, and most such cases are associated with metastatic disease. They are commonly unilateral with a smooth surface unless the malignancy has extended beyond the confines of the ovary. Cystic and solid components are commonly associated.

Malignant Clear Cell Carcinomas   Several basic histologic patterns are present in the clear cell adenocarcinoma (i.e., tubulocystic, papillary, and solid). The tumors are made up of *clear cells* and *hobnail cells*. The tall clear cells have abundant clear or vacuolated cytoplasm, hyperchromatic, irregular nuclei, and nucleoli of various sizes. Hobnail cells project their nuclei to the apical cytoplasm (Fig. 33.5). Other tumor cells have densely eosinophilic cytoplasm. Focal areas of endometriosis and endometrioid carcinoma sometimes occur. The clear cell carcinoma seen in the ovary is histologically identical to that seen in the uterus or vagina of the young patient who has been exposed to diethylstilbestrol (DES) *in utero*.

Brenner Tumors

Borderline Brenner Tumors   Borderline or "proliferating" Brenner tumors have been described. In such cases, the epithelium does not invade the stroma. Some investigators subclassify those tumors that resemble low-grade papillary transitional cell carcinoma of the urinary bladder as proliferating tumors and those with a higher grade of transitional cell carcinoma *in situ* as borderline malignant Brenner tumors (15). Complete surgical removal usually results in cure.

Malignant Brenner Tumors   These are rare and are defined as benign Brenner tumors coexisting with invasive transitional cells or another type of carcinoma. The tumor infiltrates the tissue with associated destruction.

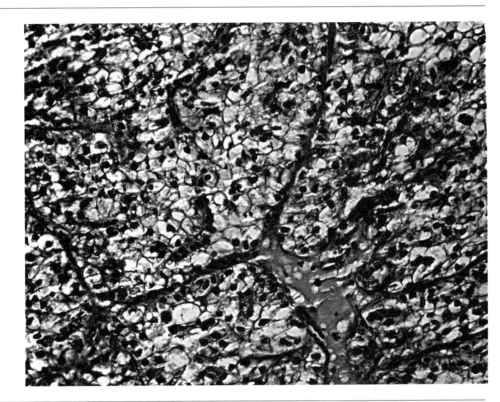

Figure 33.5   Clear-cell "mesonephroid" carcinoma of the ovary. Note the solid variant of clear cell carcinoma with sheets of cells that have clear cytoplasm ("hobnail" cells). (Reproduced with permission from **Berek JS, Hacker NF.** *Practical Gynecologic Oncology.* 2nd ed. Baltimore: Williams & Wilkins, 1994:144.)

Transitional Cell Tumors   The designation transitional cell tumor refers to a primary ovarian carcinoma resembling transitional cell carcinoma of the urinary bladder without a recognizable Brenner tumor. An important finding is that those ovarian carcinomas that contain more than 50% of TCC are more sensitive to chemotherapy and have a more favorable prognosis than other poorly differentiated ovarian carcinomas of comparable stage (16, 17). Transitional cell tumors differ from malignant Brenner tumors in that they are more frequently diagnosed in an advanced stage and, therefore, are associated with a poorer survival rate (18).

Undifferentiated Carcinomas

The undifferentiated carcinomas include large- and small-cell types. In the former, cells with large round to oval nuclei, prominent nucleoli, a moderate amount of cytoplasm, and high mitotic activity are arranged in solid sheets without glandular or squamous differentiation. In small-cell carcinoma, the cells have small, hyperchromatic nuclei, scanty cytoplasm, and high mitotic activity. This neoplasm occurs mainly in young women, who may present with hypercalcemia. Immunohistochemical stains are helpful to differentiate this tumor from a lymphoma, leukemia, or sarcoma.

Mesotheliomas

Peritoneal malignant mesotheliomas fall into four categories (19): 1) fibrosarcomatous, 2) tubopapillary (papillary-alveolar), 3) carcinomatous, and 4) mixed. These lesions appear as multiple intraperitoneal masses and can develop after hysterectomy and bilateral salpingo-oophorectomy for benign disease. Malignant mesotheliomas should be distinguished from ovarian tumor implants and primary peritoneal mullerian neoplasms.

Peritoneal Carcinomas

The primary malignant transformation of the peritoneum has been called *primary peritoneal carcinoma* or *primary peritoneal papillary serous carcinoma*. Peritoneal carcinoma simulates ovarian cancer clinically. In patients for whom exploratory surgery is performed, there may be microscopic or small macroscopic cancer on the surface of the ovary and extensive disease in the upper abdomen, particularly in the omentum. This phenomenon can thus produce a condition in which "ovarian cancer" can arise in a patient whose ovaries were surgically removed many years earlier (20).

Primary peritoneal tumors indistinguishable from primary ovarian serous tumors are well documented. In the case of borderline serous peritoneal tumors and serous peritoneal carcinomas, the ovaries are normal or minimally involved and the tumors affect predominantly the uterosacral ligaments, pelvic peritoneum, or omentum. The overall prognosis for borderline serous peritoneal tumors is excellent and comparable to that of ovarian borderline serous tumors (21–23). In the review of 38 cases of peritoneal borderline serous tumors from the literature, 32 women had no persistent disease, four were well after resection of recurrence, one developed an invasive serous carcinoma, and one died of tumor (21).

Peritoneal serous carcinomas have the appearance of a moderately to poorly differentiated serous ovarian carcinoma. Primary peritoneal endometrioid carcinoma is less common.

Clinical Features

More than 80% of epithelial ovarian cancers are found in postmenopausal women (Fig. 33.6). The peak incidence of this disease occurs at 62 years. Before the age of 45, these cancers are

Figure 33.6   Ovarian Cancer Incidence: Distribution by age. (Reproduced with permission from *J Natl Cancer Inst* 1995;87(17):1280.

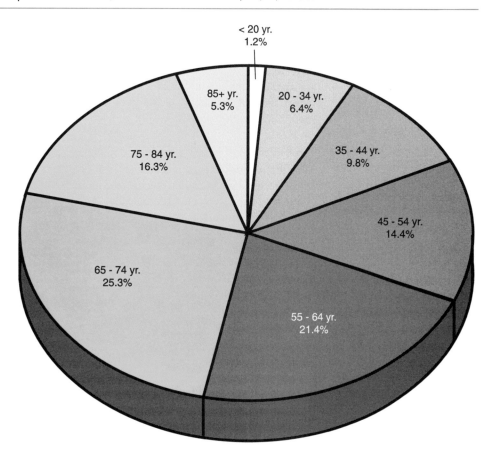

relatively uncommon. Fewer than 1% of epithelial ovarian cancers occur before the age of 21 years, two-thirds of ovarian malignancies in such patients being germ cell tumors (2, 24, 25). About 30% of ovarian neoplasms in postmenopausal women are malignant, whereas only about 7% of ovarian epithelial tumors in premenopausal patients are frankly malignant (2).

Screening

The value of tumor markers and ultrasonography to screen for epithelial ovarian cancer has not been clearly established by prospective studies. Screening results with transabdominal ultrasonography has been encouraging (26), but specificity have been limited. However, recent advances in transvaginal ultrasonography have been shown to have a very high (>95%) sensitivity for the detection of early-stage ovarian cancer, although this test alone might require as many as 10–15 laparotomy procedures for each case of per ovarian cancer detected (27, 28). Routine annual pelvic examinations have had disappointing results in the early detection of ovarian cancer (29). Transvaginal color-flow Doppler to assess the vascularity of the ovarian vessels has been shown to be a useful adjunct to ultrasonography (30, 31), but its role in screening remains to be defined.

CA125 has been shown to contribute to the early diagnosis of epithelial ovarian cancer (32–37). Regarding the sensitivity of the test, CA125 can detect 50% of patients with stage I disease and 60% of patients if those with stage II disease are included (33). Data suggest that the specificity of CA125 is improved when the test is combined with transvaginal ultrasonography (34) or when the CA125 levels are followed over time (35, 36). These data have encouraged the development of prospective screening studies in Sweden and the U.K. (37, 38). In these studies, patients with elevated CA125 levels (>30 U/ml) have undergone abdominal ultrasonography and 14 ovarian cancers have been discovered among 27,000 women screened. About four laparotomies were performed for each case of cancer detected.

Considering the false-positive results for both CA125 and transvaginal ultrasonography, particularly for premenopausal women, these tests are not cost-effective and should not be used routinely to screen for ovarian cancer. In the future, new markers or technologies may improve the specificity of ovarian cancer screening, but proof of their effectiveness will require a large prospective study. A large prospective, randomized mortality trial using serial CA125 and OVX1 blood tests and transvaginal ultrasound is ongoing in the U.K. Screening in women who have a familial risk may have a better yield, but additional study is necessary (39).

Genetic Risk for Epithelial Ovarian Cancer

The lifetime risk of ovarian carcinoma for women in the U.S. is about 1.4% (40). The risk of ovarian cancer is higher in women with certain family histories (39–46). Most epithelial ovarian cancer occurs sporadically; familial or hereditary patterns account for fewer than 5% of all malignancies (46). A patient can have a genetic risk of a *site-specific familial ovarian cancer,* a hereditary *breast/ovarian familial cancer syndrome,* or hereditary nonpolyposis colon cancer syndrome (HNPCC), also known as the *Lynch II syndrome.*

Site-Specific Familial Ovarian Cancer   The risk of developing epithelial ovarian cancer is higher in the presence of a positive family history. The precise risk is difficult to determine but depends on the number of first- or second-degree relatives with a history of epithelial ovarian carcinoma.

1. In families with two first-degree relatives (i.e., mother, sister, or daughter) with documented epithelial ovarian cancer, the risk that a female first-degree relative will have an affected gene could be as high as 50% (43). The pedigree type is consistent with an autosomal dominant mode of inheritance (43, 44).

2. In families with a single first-degree relative and a single second-degree relative (i.e., grandmother, aunt, first cousin, or granddaughter) with epithelial ovarian

cancer, the risk that a woman will have an affected gene also may be increased, but the degree of risk may be difficult to determine precisely unless one performs a full pedigree analysis. The relative risk may be threefold to 10-fold higher (39) than for those without a familial history of the disease.

3. In families with a single first-degree relative with epithelial ovarian carcinoma, a woman has a slightly increased risk of having an affected gene; the relative increase is two- to fourfold (39).

Hereditary ovarian cancers generally occur in women about 10 years younger than those with nonhereditary tumors (44). Based on the median age of about 61 years for development of epithelial ovarian cancer, a woman with a first- or second-degree relative who had ovarian cancer before 50 years of age will have a higher probability of carrying an affected gene.

Breast/Ovarian Familial Cancer Syndrome   Breast/ovarian familial cancer syndrome may exist in a family in which there is a combination of epithelial ovarian and breast cancers, affecting a mixture of first- and second-degree relatives (41, 45). Women with this syndrome tend to have these tumors at a young age, and the breast cancers may be bilateral. If two first-degree relatives are affected, this pedigree is consistent with an autosomal dominant mode of inheritance (41, 43). The relative risk of developing ovarian cancer may be two- to fourfold greater than the general population (40). Women with a primary history of breast cancer have twice the expected incidence of subsequent ovarian cancer (43).

A gene locus on the 17q chromosome, the BRCA1 gene, has been associated with the breast/ovarian syndrome (47). The BRCA1 gene has been cloned, which suggests the prospect of screening of women at risk. The prevalence of BRCA1 mutations is about one in every 800–1000 women. Individuals who have a mutation in the BRCA1 have a cumulative lifetime risk of 85–90% of developing breast cancer and 50% risk of ovarian cancer (48). Women who are of Ashkenazi Jewish extraction have about a 1% risk of carrying a BRCA1 mutation, which is 10-fold greater than the general population.

Lynch II Syndrome   The Lynch II syndrome (hereditary nonpolyposis colon cancer, or HNPCC), which includes multiple adenocarcinomas, involves a combination of familial colon cancer (known as the Lynch I syndrome) and a high rate of ovarian, endometrial, and breast cancers and other malignancies of the gastrointestinal and genitourinary systems (43). The risk that a woman who is a member of one of these families will develop epithelial ovarian cancer depends on the frequency of this disease in first- and second-degree relatives, although these women seem to have at least three times the relative risk of the general population (43). A full pedigree analysis of such families should be performed by a geneticist to more accurately determine the risk.

In all of these syndromes, women at risk benefit from a thorough pedigree analysis. Testing to determine whether there is a mutation in the BRCA1 gene locus is likely to play an important role. A geneticist should evaluate the family pedigree for at least three generations. Decisions about management are best made after careful study and, whenever possible, verification of the histologic diagnosis of the family members' ovarian cancer.

The care of a woman with a strong family history of epithelial ovarian cancer depends on her age, her reproductive plans, and the extent of risk. The plan must be individualized, because the value of screening with transvaginal ultrasonography. CA125 levels, or other procedures has not been clearly established in women at high risk. Bourne et al. (39) have shown that this approach can detect tumors about 10 times more often than in the general population, and thus, they recommend screening for women at high risk. The current recommendations of the Committee on Gynecologic Practice of the American College of Obstetricians and Gynecologists are summarized below (40):

1. Women who wish to preserve their reproductive capacity should undergo periodic screening by transvaginal ultrasonography every 6 months and should consider prophylactic oophorectomy when childbearing has been completed. Oral contraceptives may be given to a young woman before she has children, although the protective effect for women at high risk has not been evaluated.

2. Women with familial ovarian or hereditary breast/ovarian cancer syndrome who do not wish to maintain their fertility should be offered prophylactic bilateral salpingo-oophorectomy. The risk should be clearly documented, preferably established by pedigree analysis, before oophorectomy. These women should be counseled that this operation does not offer absolute protection because peritoneal carcinomas occasionally can occur after bilateral oophorectomy (20). The role of BRCA1 testing in these women is being evaluated.

3. Women with a documented Lynch II syndrome should be treated in the same manner as women with familial breast/ovarian cancer syndrome, but in addition, they should undergo periodic screening mammography, colonoscopy, and endometrial biopsy.

Symptoms

Most women with epithelial ovarian cancer have no symptoms for long periods of time. When symptoms do develop, they are often vague and nonspecific (24). In early-stage disease, the patient may experience irregular menses if she is premenopausal. If a pelvic mass is compressing the bladder or rectum, she may report urinary frequency or constipation. Occasionally, she may perceive lower abdominal distention, pressure, or pain, such as dyspareunia. Acute symptoms, such as pain secondary to rupture or torsion, are unusual.

In advanced-stage disease, patients most often have symptoms related to the presence of ascites, omental metastases, or bowel metastases. The symptoms include abdominal distention, bloating, constipation, nausea, anorexia, or early satiety. Premenopausal women may complain of irregular or heavy menses, whereas vaginal bleeding may occur in postmenopausal women.

Signs

The most important sign of epithelial ovarian cancer is the presence of a pelvic mass on physical examination. A solid, irregular, fixed pelvic mass is highly suggestive of an ovarian malignancy. If, in addition, an upper abdominal mass or ascites is present, the diagnosis of ovarian cancer is almost certain. Because the patient usually complains of abdominal symptoms, she may not have a pelvic examination, and the presence of a tumor may be missed.

In patients who are at least 1 year past menopause, the ovaries should have become atrophic and not palpable. It has been proposed that any palpable pelvic mass in these patients should be considered potentially malignant, a situation that has been referred to as the *postmenopausal palpable ovary syndrome* (49). This concept has been challenged, as subsequent authors have reported that only about 3% of palpable masses measuring <5 cm in postmenopausal women are malignant (29).

Diagnosis

Ovarian epithelial cancers must be differentiated from benign neoplasms and functional cysts of the ovaries. A variety of benign conditions of the reproductive tract, such as pelvic inflammatory disease, endometriosis, and pedunculated uterine leiomyomas, can simulate ovarian cancer. Nongynecologic causes of a pelvic tumor, such as an inflammatory or neoplastic colonic mass, must be excluded (50). A pelvic kidney can simulate ovarian cancer.

Serum CA125 levels have been shown to be useful in distinguishing malignant from benign pelvic masses (51). For postmenopausal patients with an adnexal mass and a very high serum CA125 level (>95 U/ml), there is a 96% positive predictive value for malignancy. For premenopausal patients, however, the specificity of the test is low because the CA125 level tends to be elevated in common benign conditions.

For the premenopausal patient, a period of observation is reasonable, provided the adnexal mass does not have characteristics that suggest malignancy (i.e., it is mobile, mostly cystic, unilateral, and of regular contour). Generally, an interval of no more than 2 months is allowed, during which hormonal suppression with the oral contraceptive may be used. If the lesion is not neoplastic, it should regress, as measured by pelvic examination and pelvic ultrasonography. If the mass does not regress or if it increases in size, it must be presumed to be neoplastic and must be removed surgically.

The size of the lesion is important. If a cystic mass is >8 cm in diameter, the probability is high that the lesion is neoplastic, unless the patient has been taking *clomiphene citrate* or other agents to induce ovulation (26–29). Patients whose lesions are suggestive of malignancy (i.e., predominantly solid, relatively fixed, or irregularly shaped) should undergo laparotomy, as should postmenopausal patients with adnexal masses.

The diagnosis of an ovarian cancer requires an exploratory laparotomy. Before the planned exploration, the patient should undergo routine hematologic and biochemical assessments. A preoperative evaluation in a patient undergoing laparotomy should include an x-ray of the chest and an assessment of the urinary tract with an intravenous pyelography. Abdominal and pelvic computed tomography (CT) or magnetic resonance imaging (MRI) scans are of no value for patients with a definite pelvic mass. A CT or MRI scan should be performed for patients with ascites and no pelvic mass to look for liver or pancreatic tumors. The findings only rarely preclude laparotomy (52). If the hepatic enzymes are normal, the likelihood of liver disease is low. Liver-spleen scans, bone scans, and brain scans are unnecessary unless symptoms or signs suggest metastases to these sites.

The preoperative evaluation should exclude other primary cancers metastatic to the ovary. A barium enema or colonoscopy is indicated in some patients over the 45 years of age to exclude a primary colonic lesion with ovarian metastasis. This study should be performed for any patient who has evidence of occult blood in the stool or evidence of intestinal obstruction. An upper gastrointestinal series or gastroscopy is indicated if symptoms indicate gastric involvement (52, 53). Bilateral mammography is indicated if there is any breast mass, because occasionally breast cancer metastatic to the ovaries can simulate primary ovarian cancer.

Cervical cytologic study should be performed, although its value for the detection of ovarian cancer is very limited. Patients who have irregular menses or postmenopausal vaginal bleeding should have an endometrial biopsy and an endocervical curettage to exclude the presence of uterine or endocervical cancer metastatic to the ovary.

Patterns of Spread

Ovarian epithelial cancers spread primarily by exfoliation of cells into the peritoneal cavity, by lymphatic dissemination, and by hematogenous spread.

Transcoelomic The most common and earliest mode of dissemination of ovarian epithelial cancer is by exfoliation of cells that implant along the surfaces of the peritoneal cavity. The cells tend to follow the circulatory path of the peritoneal fluid. The fluid tends to move with the forces of respiration from the pelvis, up the paracolic gutters, especially on the right, along the intestinal mesenteries, to the right hemidiaphragm. Therefore, metastases are typically seen on the posterior cul-de-sac, paracolic gutters, right hemidiaphragm, liver capsule, the peritoneal surfaces of the intestines and their mesenteries, and the omentum. The disease seldom invades the intestinal lumen but progressively agglutinates loops of bowel, leading to a functional intestinal obstruction. This condition is known as *carcinomatous ileus*.

Lymphatic   Lymphatic dissemination to the pelvic and para-aortic lymph nodes is common, particularly in advanced-stage disease (53–55). Spread through the lymphatic channels of the diaphragm and through the retroperitoneal lymph nodes can lead to dissemination above the diaphragm, especially to the supraclavicular lymph nodes (48). Burghardt et al. (54) reported that 78% of patients with stage III disease have metastases to the pelvic lymph nodes. In another series (55), the rate of positive para-aortic lymph nodes was 18% in stage I, 20% in stage II, 42% in stage III, and 67% in stage IV.

Hematogenous   Hematogenous dissemination at the time of diagnosis is uncommon. Spread to vital organ parenchyma, such as the lungs and liver, occurs in only about 2–3% of patients. Most patients with disease above the diaphragm at the time of presentation have a right pleural effusion (3, 5). Systemic metastases are seen more frequently in patients who have survived for some years. Dauplat et al. (56) reported that distant metastasis consistent with stage IV disease ultimately occurred in 38% of the patients whose disease was originally intraperitoneal.

Prognostic Factors

The outcome of treatment can be evaluated in the context of prognostic factors, which can be grouped into pathologic, biologic, and clinical factors (57).

Pathologic Factors   The morphology and histologic pattern, including the architecture and grade of the lesion, are important prognostic variables (3). Histologic type has not generally been believed to be of prognostic significance, but several papers recently have suggested that clear cell carcinomas are associated with prognosis worse than that of other histologic types (57, 58).

Histologic grade, as determined either by the pattern of differentiation or by the extent of cellular anaplasia and the proportion of undifferentiated cells, seems to be of prognostic significance (59–62). However, studies of the reproducibility of grading ovarian cancers have shown a high degree of intraobserver and interobserver variation (63, 64). Because there is significant heterogeneity of tumors and observational bias, the value of histologic grade as an independent prognostic factor has not been clearly established. Baak et al. (65) have presented a standard grading system based on morphometric analysis, and the system seems to correlate with prognosis, especially in its ability to distinguish low-grade or borderline patterns from other tumors.

Biologic Factors   Several biologic factors have been correlated with prognosis in epithelial ovarian cancer. Using *flow cytometry,* Friedlander et al. (66) showed that ovarian cancers were commonly aneuploid. Furthermore, they and others showed that there was a high correlation between FIGO stage and ploidy; i.e., low-stage cancers tend to be diploid and high-stage tumors tend to be aneuploid (67–73). Patients with diploid tumors have a significantly longer median survival than those with aneuploid tumors: 5 years versus 1 year, respectively (67). Multivariate analyses have demonstrated that ploidy is an independent prognostic variable and one of the most significant predictors of survival (67). *Flow cytometric analysis* also provides data on the cell cycle, and the proliferation fraction (S phase) determined by this technique has correlated with prognosis in some studies (68–77).

More than 60 *proto-oncogenes* have been identified, and studies have focused on the amplification or expression of these genetic loci and their relationship to the development and progression of ovarian cancer. For example, Slamon et al. (78) reported that 30% of epithelial ovarian tumors expressed HER-2/*neu* oncogene and that this group had a poorer prognosis, especially patients with >5 copies of the gene (78). Berchuck et al. (79) reported a similar incidence (32%) of HER-2/*neu* expression. In their series, patients whose tumors expressed the gene had a poorer median survival (15.7 months vs. 32.8 months). Others have not substantiated this finding (80), and a review of the literature by Leary et al. (81) revealed an overall incidence of HER-2/*neu* expression of only 11%. Thus, the prognostic value of HER-2/*neu* expression in ovarian cancer is unclear and further study is required.

The *in vitro clonogenic assay* has been studied in relation to ovarian cancer. A significant inverse correlation has been reported between clonogenic growth *in vitro* and survival (82, 83). Multivariate analysis has found that clonogenic growth in a semisolid culture medium is a significant independent prognostic variable (82), but further study will be needed to evaluate the clinical usefulness of this essay.

Clinical Factors   In addition to stage, the extent of residual disease after primary surgery, the volume of ascites, patient age, and performance status are all independent prognostic variables (84–87). Among patients with stage I disease, Dembo et al. (88) showed, in a multivariate analysis, that tumor grade and "dense adherence" to the pelvic peritoneum had a significant adverse impact on prognosis, whereas intraoperative tumor spillage or rupture did not. Sjövall et al. (89) confirmed that ovarian cancers that undergo intraoperative rupture or spillage do not worsen prognosis whereas tumors found to have already ruptured preoperatively do have a poorer prognosis.

Staging

Ovarian epithelial malignancies are staged according to the FIGO system listed in Table 33.2. The FIGO staging is based on findings at surgical exploration. A preoperative evaluation should exclude the presence of extraperitoneal metastases.

The importance of thorough surgical staging cannot be overemphasized, because subsequent treatment will be determined by the stage of disease. For patients in whom exploratory laparotomy does not reveal any macroscopic evidence of disease on inspection and palpation of the entire intraabdominal space, a careful search for microscopic spread must be undertaken. In earlier series in which patients did not undergo careful surgical staging, the overall 5-year survival for patients with apparent stage I epithelial ovarian cancer was only about 60% (24). Since then, survival rates of 90–100% have been reported for patients who were properly staged and were found to have stage Ia or Ib disease (90, 91).

Technique for Surgical Staging

For patients whose preoperative evaluation suggests a probable malignancy, a midline or paramedian abdominal incision is recommended to allow adequate access to the upper abdomen. When a malignancy is unexpectedly discovered in a patient who has a lower transverse incision, the rectus muscles can be either divided or detached from the symphysis pubis to allow better access to the upper abdomen. If this is not sufficient, the incision can be extended on one side to create a "J" incision.

The ovarian tumor should be removed intact, if possible, and a frozen histologic section should be obtained. If ovarian malignancy is present and the tumor is apparently confined to the ovaries or the pelvis, thorough surgical staging should be performed. Staging involves the following steps:

1. *Any free fluid, especially in the pelvic cul-de-sac, should be submitted for cytologic evaluation.*

2. *If no free fluid is present, peritoneal washings should be performed* by instilling and recovering 50–100 ml of saline from the pelvic cul-de-sac, each paracolic gutter, and beneath each hemidiaphragm. Obtaining the specimens from under

Table 33.2   FIGO Staging for Primary Carcinoma of the Ovary

Stage I		Growth limited to the ovaries.
	Stage Ia	Growth limited to one ovary; no ascites containing malignant cells. No tumor on the external surface; capsule intact.
	Stage Ib	Growth limited to both ovaries; no ascites containing malignant cells. No tumor on the external surfaces; capsules intact.
	Stage Ic*	Tumor either stage Ia or Ib but with tumor on the surface of one or both ovaries; or with capsule ruptured; or with ascites present containing malignant cells or with positive peritoneal washings.
Stage II		Growth involving one or both ovaries with pelvic extension.
	Stage IIa	Extension and/or metastases to the uterus and/or tubes.
	Stage IIb	Extension to other pelvic tissues.
	Stage IIc*	Tumor either stage IIa or IIb but with tumor on the surface of one or both ovaries; or with capsule(s) ruptured; or with ascites present containing malignant cells or with positive peritoneal washings.
Stage III		Tumor involving one or both ovaries with peritoneal implants outside the pelvis and/or positive retroperitoneal or inguinal nodes. Superficial liver metastasis equals stage III. Tumor is limited to the true pelvis, but with histologically proven malignant extension to small bowel or omentum.
	Stage IIIa	Tumor grossly limited to the true pelvis with negative nodes but with histologically confirmed microscopic seeding of abdominal peritoneal surfaces.
	Stage IIIb	Tumor of one or both ovaries with histologically confirmed implants of abdominal peritoneal surfaces, none exceeding 2 cm in diameter. Nodes negative.
	Stage IIIc	Abdominal implants >2 cm in diameter and/or positive retroperitoneal or inguinal nodes.
Stage IV		Growth involving one or both ovaries with distant metastasis. If pleural effusion is present, there must be positive cytologic test results to allot a case to stage IV. Parenchymal liver metastasis equals stage IV.

These categories are based on findings at clinical examination and/or surgical exploration. The histologic characteristics are to be considered in the staging, as are results of cytologic testing as far as effusions are concerned. It is desirable that a biopsy be performed on suspicious areas outside the pelvis.
*In order to evaluate the impact on prognosis of the different criteria for allotting cases to stage Ic or IIc, it would be of value to know if rupture of the capsule was 1) spontaneous or 2) caused by the surgeon and if the source of malignant cells detected was 1) peritoneal washings or 2) ascites.

the diaphragms can be facilitated with the use of a rubber catheter attached to the end of a bulb syringe.

3. *A systematic exploration of all the intra-abdominal surfaces and viscera is performed,* proceeding in a clockwise fashion from the cecum cephalad along the paracolic gutter and the ascending colon to the right kidney, the liver and gallbladder, the right hemidiaphragm, the entrance to the lesser sac at the paraaortic area, across the transverse colon to the left hemidiaphragm, down the left gutter and the descending colon to the rectosigmoid colon. The small intestine and its mesentery from the Trietz ligament to the cecum should be inspected.

4. *Any suspicious areas or adhesions on the peritoneal surfaces should be biopsied. If there is no evidence of disease, multiple intraperitoneal biopsies should be performed.* The peritoneum of the pelvic cul-de-sac, both paracolic gutters, the peritoneum over the bladder, and the intestinal mesenteries should be biopsied.

5. *The diaphragm should be sampled either by biopsy or by scraping with a tongue depressor and obtaining a sample for cytologic assessment.* Biopsies of any irregularities on the surface of the diaphragm can be facilitated by use of the laparoscope and the associated biopsy instrument.

6. *The omentum should be resected from the transverse colon, a procedure called an "infracolic omentectomy."* The procedure is initiated on the underside of the greater omentum, where the peritoneum is incised just a few millimeters away from the transverse colon. The branches of the gastroepiploic vessels are clamped, ligated, and divided, along with all the small branching vessels that feed the infracolic omentum. If the gastrocolic ligament is palpably normal, it does not need to be resected.

7. *The retroperitoneal spaces should be explored to evaluate the pelvic and paraaortic lymph nodes.* The retroperitoneal dissection is performed by incision of the peritoneum over the psoas muscles. This may be performed on the ipsilateral side only for unilateral tumors. Any enlarged lymph nodes should be resected and submitted for frozen section. If no metastases are present, a formal pelvic lymphadenectomy should be performed.

Results

Metastases in apparent stage I and II epithelial ovarian cancer occur in as many as three in 10 patients whose tumor appears to be confined to the pelvis have occult metastatic disease in the upper abdomen or the retroperitoneal lymph nodes (55, 91–100) In a review of the literature (90), occult metastases were found in biopsies of the diaphragm in 7.3% of such patients, biopsies of the omentum in 8.6%, the pelvic lymph nodes in 5.9%, the aortic lymph nodes in 18.1%, and in 26.4% of peritoneal washings.

The importance of careful initial surgical staging is emphasized by the findings of a cooperative national study (91) in which 100 patients with apparent stage I and II disease who were referred for subsequent therapy underwent additional surgical staging. In this series, 28% of the patients initially believed to have stage I disease were "upstaged" and 43% of those believed to have stage II disease had more advanced lesions. A total of 31% of the patients were upstaged as a result of additional surgery, and 77% were reclassified as having stage III disease. Histologic grade was a significant predictor of occult metastasis; i.e., 16% of the patients with grade 1 lesions were upstaged, compared with 34% with grade 2 disease and 46% with grade 3 disease.

Treatment of Epithelial Ovarian Cancer

Stage I

The primary treatment for stage I epithelial ovarian cancer is surgical, i.e., a total abdominal hysterectomy, bilateral salpingo-oophorectomy, and surgical staging (90, 91). In certain circumstances, a unilateral oophorectomy may be performed.

Borderline Tumors

The principal treatment of borderline ovarian tumors is surgical resection of the primary tumor. There is no evidence that either subsequent chemotherapy or radiation therapy improves survival. After a frozen section has determined that the histology is borderline, premenopausal patients who desire preservation of ovarian function may undergo "conservative" operation, i.e., a unilateral oophorectomy (101). In a study of patients who underwent unilateral ovarian cystectomy only for apparent stage I borderline serous tumors, Lim-Tan et al. (102) found that this conservative operation was also safe; only 8% of the patients had recurrences 2–18 years later, all with curable disease confined to the ovaries. Recurrence was associated with "positive margins" of the removed ovarian cyst (102). Thus, hormonal function and fertility can be maintained (5, 101, 102). For patients in whom an oophorectomy or cystectomy has been performed and a borderline tumor is later documented in the permanent pathology, no additional immediate surgery is necessary.

Stages Ia and Ib, Grade 1

For patients who have undergone a thorough staging laparotomy and for whom there is no evidence of spread beyond the ovary, abdominal hysterectomy and bilateral salpingo-oophorectomy are appropriate therapy. *The uterus and the contralateral ovary can be preserved in women with stage Ia, grade 1 disease who desire to preserve fertility.* The conditions of the women should be monitored carefully with routine periodic pelvic examinations and determinations of serum CA125 levels. Generally, the other ovary and the uterus are removed at the completion of childbearing.

Guthrie et al. (100) studied the outcome of 656 patients with early-stage epithelial ovarian cancer. No untreated patients who had stage Ia, grade 1 cancer died of their disease; thus, adjuvant radiation and chemotherapy are unnecessary. Furthermore, the Gynecologic Oncology Group (GOG) carried out a prospective, randomized trial of observation versus *melphalan* for patients with stage Ia and Ib, grade 1 disease (58). Five-year survival for each group was 94% and 96%, respectively, confirming that no further treatment is needed for such patients.

Stages Ia and Ib (Grades 2 and 3) and Stage Ic

For patients whose disease is more poorly differentiated or in whom there are malignant cells either in ascitic fluid or in peritoneal washings, additional therapy is indicated. Although the optimal therapy for these patients is not known, treatment options include chemotherapy or radiation therapy, the latter with intraperitoneal radiocolloids or whole-abdominal radiation. Some comparisons of these modalities have been made, although most are retrospective and therefore inconclusive.

Chemotherapy

Either single-agent or multi-agent chemotherapy can be used to treat patients with stages Ia and Ib, grade 2 or 3, and stage Ic epithelial ovarian cancer. The most frequently used single-agent chemotherapy has been *melphalan* given orally on a "pulse" basis for 5 consecutive days every 28 days (58, 103–105). The advantage of this approach is the relative ease of administration. The principal disadvantage is that about 10% of the patients who receive more than 12 cycles of alkylating agent therapy will develop acute nonlymphocytic leukemia over the next 5–10 years (104). This is an important issue for patients with stage I disease, and *melphalan* should not be given for more than six cycles in such patients.

Because *cisplatin, carboplatin,* and *paclitaxel* (*Taxol*) are active single agents against epithelial ovarian cancer, they may be preferable to *melphalan* for patients with low-stage disease. There are some series in which *cisplatin* and *cyclophosphamide,* with or without *doxorubicin* (*Adriamycin*) (PC or PAC), have been used to treat patients with stage I disease (58, 100–105), but there are no data comparing the use of *cisplatin* combination chemotherapy with either single-agent chemotherapy or radiation therapy (105). The results of a GOG trial of PC versus intraperitoneal ^{32}P in patients with stage Ib and Ic disease is pending. The ongoing GOG trial compares *paclitaxel* for six cycles with carboplatin plus *paclitaxel* for three cycles.

Radiation Therapy

There are two general approaches to the treatment of low-stage epithelial cancers with radiation: intraperitoneal radiocolloids or whole-abdominal radiation therapy. In one retrospective trial of ^{32}P, the 5-year survival for patients thus treated was 85% (108). In a series of patients with stage I disease treated with whole abdominal radiation (109), the 5-year relapse-free survival was only 78%, but many of these patients had high-risk variables (e.g., poor histologic grade).

A prospective trial was conducted by the GOG in patients with stage Ib, grade 3, stage Ic, or stage II with no residual disease. Twelve cycles of *melphalan* were compared with intraperitoneal ^{32}P; there was no difference in survival (Fig. 33.7) (58). In a multicenter Italian trial (107), a randomized comparison of six cycles of *cisplatin* as a single agent versus ^{32}P showed an 84% disease-free survival with *cisplatin* and 61% with ^{32}P (P <0.01). Therefore, it appears that the use of ^{32}P produces results similar to single-agent *melphalan* chemotherapy, although *cisplatin* as a single agent may be preferable (Table 33.4). If further relapses are to be prevented, the use of combination chemotherapy may be indicated, but the data are as yet unavailable to support this. Pelvic radiation alone is not as effective as *melphalan* for these patients and should not be used in ovarian cancer (86).

Current recommendations for treatment of patients with stage Ia and Ib (high-grade) and stage Ic epithelial ovarian cancer depend on the patient's overall health and status. Treatment with *cisplatin, carboplatin,* or combination chemotherapy of one of these drugs plus paclitaxel for three to four cycles seems desirable in young patients, whereas a short course of *melphalan* (four to six cycles) may be preferable for older women. The role of *paclitaxel* for these patients is currently being studied by the GOG.

Figure 33.7   Overall survival of patients with Stage I or II epithelial ovarian cancer treated on two GOG trials. (Reproduced with permission from **Young RC, Walton LA, Ellenberg SS, Homesley HD, Wilbanks GD, Decker DG, et al.** Adjuvant therapy in stage I and stage II epithelial ovarian cancer: results of two prospective randomized trials. *N Engl J Med* 1990:332:1021.

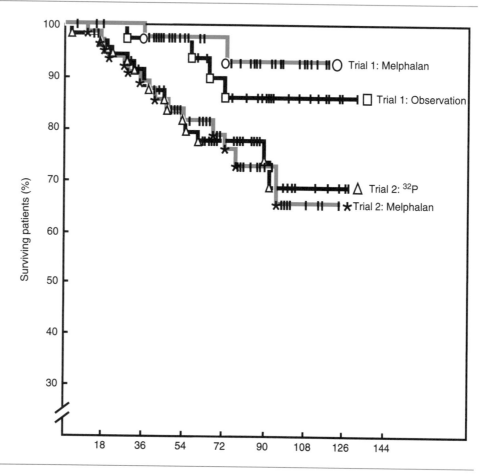

| **Stages II, III, and IV** | The treatment of all patients with advanced-stage disease is approached in a similar manner, with modifications based on the overall status and general health of the patient, as well as the extent of residual disease present at the time treatment is initiated. A treatment scheme is outlined in Figure 33.8. |

An initial exploratory procedure with removal of as much disease as possible should be performed. The operation to remove the primary tumor as well as the associated metastatic disease is referred to as "debulking" or *cytoreductive* surgery. Most patients subsequently receive combination chemotherapy for an empiric number of cycles. For some patients with completely resected disease, whole-abdominal radiation therapy may be used. For patients with no clinical evidence of disease and negative tumor markers at the completion of chemotherapy, a reassessment laparotomy, or "*second-look,*" surgery may be performed. For patients with persistent disease at second-look laparotomy, second-line or "salvage" therapy may be recommended. There are many possible salvage therapies available, but all are of limited effectiveness.

Cytoreductive Surgery

Patients with advanced-stage epithelial ovarian cancer documented at initial exploratory laparotomy should undergo cytoreductive surgery to remove as much of the tumor and its metastases as possible (110–117). The operation typically includes the performance of a total abdominal hysterectomy and bilateral salpingo-oophorectomy, along with a complete omentectomy and resection of any metastatic lesions from the peritoneal surfaces or from the intestines. The pelvic tumor often directly involves the rectosigmoid colon, the terminal ileum, and the cecum (Fig. 33.9). In a minority of patients, most or all of the disease is confined to the pelvic viscera and the omentum, so that removal of these organs will result in extirpation of all gross tumor, a situation that is associated with a reasonable chance of prolonged progression-free survival.

The removal of bulky tumor masses may reduce the volume of ascites present. Often, ascites will completely disappear after removal of the primary tumor and a large omental "cake." Also, removal of the omental cake often alleviates the nausea and early satiety that many patients experience. Removal of intestinal metastases may restore adequate intestinal function and lead to an improvement in the overall nutritional status of the patient, thereby facilitating the patient's ability to tolerate subsequent chemotherapy.

A large, bulky tumor may contain areas that are poorly vascularized, and such areas will be exposed to suboptimal concentrations of chemotherapeutic agents. Similarly, these areas are poorly oxygenated, so that radiation therapy, which requires adequate oxygenation to achieve maximal cell kill, will be less effective. Thus, surgical removal of these bulky tumors may eliminate areas that are most likely to be relatively resistant to treatment.

In addition, larger tumor masses tend to be composed of a higher proportion of cells that are either nondividing or in the "resting" phase (i.e., G_0 cells, which are essentially resistant to the therapy). A low *growth fraction* is characteristic of bulky tumor masses, and cytoreductive surgery can result in smaller residual masses with a relatively higher growth fraction.

The *fractional cell kill hypothesis* of Skipper (117) postulates that a constant proportion of the tumor cells are destroyed with each treatment. This theory suggests that a given dose of a drug will kill a constant fraction of cells as long as the growth fraction and phenotype are

Figure 33.8   Treatment scheme for patients with advanced-stage ovarian cancer. (Modified from **Berek JS, Hacker NF.** *Practical Gynecologic Oncology.* 2nd ed. Baltimore: Williams & Wilkins, 1994:342.)

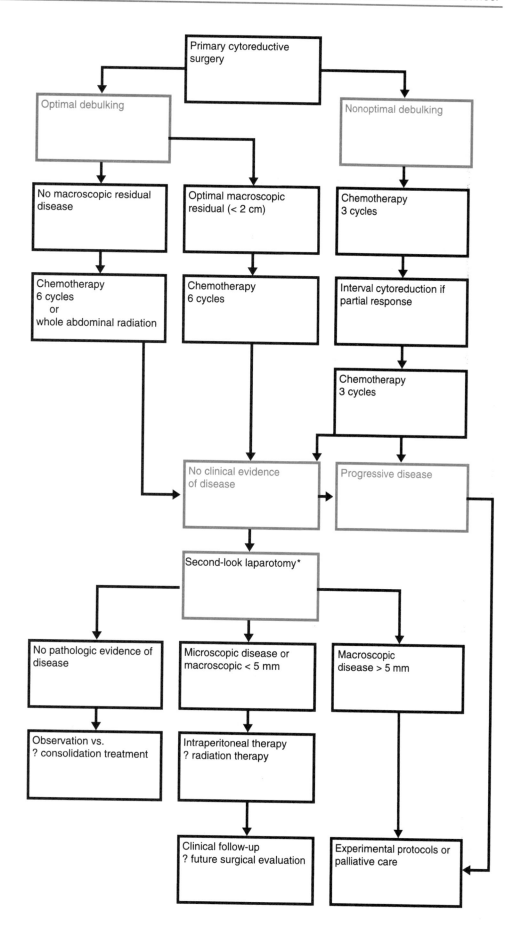

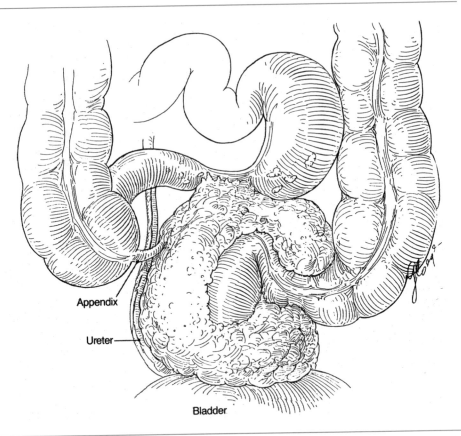

Figure 33.9 Extensive ovarian carcinoma involving the bladder, rectosigmoid, and ileocecal area. (Reproduced with permission from **Heintz APM, Berek JS.** Cytoreductive surgery for ovarian carcinoma. In: Piver MS, ed. *Ovarian Malignancies.* Edinburgh: Churchill Livingstone, 1987:134).

the same. Therefore, treatment that reduces a population of tumor cells from 10^9 to 10^4 cells also would reduce a population of 10^5 cells to a single cell. If the absolute number of tumor cells is lower at the initiation of treatment, fewer cycles of therapy should be necessary to eradicate the cancer, provided that the cells are not inherently resistant to the therapy.

The larger the initial tumor burden, the longer the necessary exposure to the drug and, therefore, the greater the chance of developing *acquired* drug resistance. However, because the spontaneous mutation rate of tumors is an inherent property of the malignancy, the likelihood of developing *phenotypic* drug resistance also increases as the size of the tumor increases. The chance of developing a clone of cells resistant to a specific agent is related to both the tumor size and its mutation frequency (118). This is one of the inherent problems with cytoreductive surgery for large tumor masses: phenotypic drug resistance may have already developed before any surgical intervention. Furthermore, larger tumors are more likely to be immunosuppressive (119).

The ability of cytoreductive surgery to improve the overall outcome of patients with ovarian cancer has been challenged (120). Concern has been expressed that these operations are excessively morbid and that modern chemotherapies are sufficient. Although no randomized prospective study has ever been performed to define the value of primary cytoreductive surgery, a recent prospective trial of "interval" cytoreductive surgery (performed after three cycles of platinum-combination chemotherapy) demonstrated a survival benefit for patients who had an optimal resection of their disease at that time compared with those who did not (121). All retrospective studies indicate that the diameter of the largest residual tumor nodule before the initiation of chemotherapy is significantly related to progression-free survival in patients with advanced ovarian cancer. In addition, quality of life is likely to be significantly enhanced by removal of bulky tumor masses from the pelvis and upper abdomen (122).

Goals of Cytoreductive Surgery

The principal goal of cytoreductive surgery is removal of all of the primary cancer and, if possible, all metastatic disease. If resection of all metastases is not feasible, the goal is to reduce the tumor burden by resection of all individual tumors to an "optimal" status. Griffiths (110) initially proposed that all metastatic nodules should be reduced to <1.5 cm in maximum diameter and showed that survival was significantly longer in patients for whom this was achieved.

Subsequently, Hacker and Berek (111) showed that patients whose largest residual lesions were <5 mm had a superior survival rate, which was substantiated by Van Lindert et al. (114). The median survival of patients in this category was 40 months, compared with 18 months for patients whose lesions were <1.5 cm and 6 months for patients with nodules >1.5 cm (Fig. 33.10).

Figure 33.10   Survival versus diameter of largest residual disease. (Redrawn with permission from **Hacker NF, Berek JS, Lagasse LD, et al.** *Obstet Gynecol* 1983; 61:413).

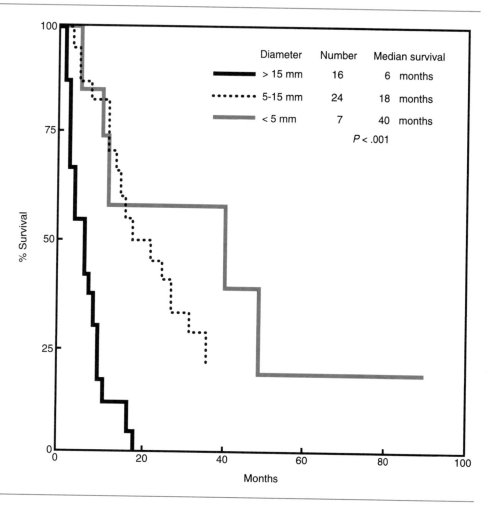

The resectability of the metastatic tumor is usually determined by the location of the disease. Optimal cytoreduction is difficult to achieve in the presence of extensive disease on the diaphragm, in the parenchyma of the liver, along the base of the small-bowel mesentery, in the lesser omentum, or in the porta hepatis.

The ability of cytoreductive surgery to influence survival is limited by the extent of metastases before cytoreduction, presumably because of the presence of phenotypically resistant clones of cells in large metastatic masses. Patients whose metastatic tumor is very large (i.e., >10 cm before cytoreductive surgery) have a shorter survival than those with smaller areas of disease (113). Extensive carcinomatosis, the presence of ascites, the poor tumor grade, even with lesions that measure <5 mm, may also worsen the survival (116).

Exploration

The supine position on the operating table may be sufficient for surgical exploration of most patients. However, for those with extensive pelvic disease for whom a low resection of the colon may be necessary, the low lithotomy position should be used. Debulking operations should be performed through a vertical incision to gain adequate access to the upper abdomen as well as to the pelvis.

After the peritoneal cavity is opened, ascitic fluid, if present, should be evacuated. In some centers, fluid is submitted routinely for appropriate *in vitro* research studies, such as molecular analyses. In cases of massive ascites, careful attention must be given to hemodynamic monitoring, especially for patients with borderline cardiovascular function. For such patients, monitoring of the central venous pressure alone may be inadequate, and a Swan-Ganz catheter may be used.

The peritoneal cavity and retroperitoneum are thoroughly inspected and palpated to assess the extent of the primary tumor and the metastatic disease. All abdominal viscera must be palpated to exclude the possibility that the ovarian disease is metastatic, particularly from the stomach, colon, or pancreas. If optimal status is not considered achievable, extensive bowel and urologic resections are not indicated, except to overcome a bowel obstruction. However, removal of the primary tumor and omental cake is usually both feasible and desirable.

Pelvic Tumor Resection

The essential principle of removal of the pelvic tumor is to use the retroperitoneal approach. To accomplish this, the retroperitoneum is entered laterally, along the surface of the psoas muscles, which avoids the iliac vessels and the ureters. The procedure is initiated by division of the round ligaments bilaterally if the uterus is present. The peritoneal incision is extended cephalad, lateral to the ovarian vessels within the "infundibulopelvic ligament," and caudally toward the bladder. With careful dissection, the retroperitoneal space is explored, and the ureter and pelvic vessels are identified. The pararectal and paravesicle spaces are identified and developed as described in Chapter 32.

The peritoneum overlying the bladder is dissected to connect the peritoneal incisions anteriorly. The vesicouterine plane is identified, and with careful sharp dissection, the bladder is mobilized from the anterior surface of the cervix. The ovarian vessels are isolated, doubly ligated, and divided.

Hysterectomy, which is often not a "simple" operation, is then performed. The ureters must be carefully displayed to avoid injury. During this procedure, the uterine vessels can be identified. The hysterectomy and resection of the contiguous tumor are completed by ligation of the uterine vessels and the remainder of the tissues within the cardinal ligaments.

Because epithelial ovarian cancers tend not to invade the lumina of the colon or bladder, it is usually feasible to resect pelvic tumors without having to resect portions of the lower colon or the urinary tract (123, 124). However, if the disease surrounds the rectosigmoid colon and its mesentery, it may be necessary to remove that portion of the colon to clear the pelvic disease (Fig. 33.11) (123). This is justified if the patient will be left with "optimal" disease at the end of the cytoreduction. After the pararectal space is identified in such patients, the proximal site of colonic involvement is identified, the colon and its mesentery are divided, and the rectosigmoid is removed along with the uterus *en bloc*. A reanastomosis of the colon is performed. It is rarely necessary to resect portions of the lower urinary tract—resection of a small portion of the bladder may be required, and if so, a cystotomy should be performed to assist in resection of the disease (124).

Omentectomy   Advanced epithelial ovarian cancer often completely replaces the omentum, forming an "omental cake." This disease may be adherent to the parietal peritoneum of the anterior abdominal wall, making entry into the abdominal cavity difficult. After freeing the omentum from any adhesions to parietal peritoneum, adherent loops of small intestine are freed by sharp dissection. The omentum is then lifted and pulled gently in the cranial direction, exposing the attachment of the infracolic omentum to the transverse colon. The peritoneum is incised to open the appropriate plane, which is developed by

Figure 33.11   The resection of the pelvic tumor may include removal of the uterus, tubes, and ovaries, as well as portions of the lower intestinal tract. The arrows represent the plane of resection. (Reproduced with permission from **Berek JS, Hacker NF.** *Practical Gynecologic Oncology.* 2nd ed. Baltimore: Williams & Wilkins, 1994:348.)

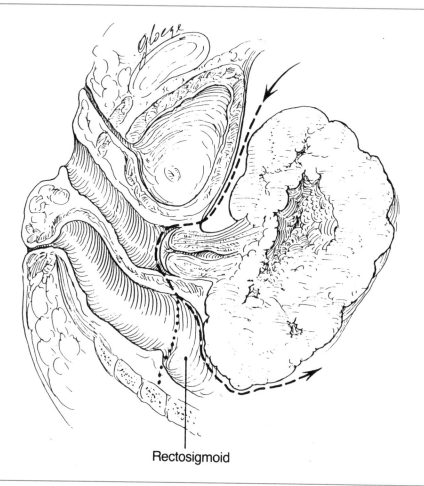

Rectosigmoid

sharp dissection along the serosa of the transverse colon. Small vessels are ligated with hemoclips. The omentum is then separated from the greater curvature of the stomach by ligation of the right and left gastroepiploic arteries and ligation of the short gastric arteries (Fig. 33.12).

The disease in the gastrocolic ligament can extend to the hilus of the spleen and splenic flexure of the colon on the left and to the capsule of the liver and the hepatic flexure of the colon on the right. Usually, the disease does not invade the parenchyma of the liver or spleen, and a plane can be found between the tumor and these organs. However, it will occasionally be necessary to perform splenectomy to remove all the omental disease (125).

Intestinal Resection

The disease may involve focal areas of the small or large intestine, and resection should be performed if it would permit the removal of all or most of the abdominal metastases. Apart from the rectosigmoid colon, the most frequent sites of intestinal metastasis are the terminal ileum, the cecum, and the transverse colon. Resection of one or more of these segments of bowel may be necessary (123, 125).

Resection of Other Metastases

Other large masses of tumor that are located on the parietal peritoneum should be removed, particularly if they are isolated masses, and their removal will permit optimal cytoreduction. Resection of extensive disease from the surfaces of the diaphragm is generally neither practical nor feasible, although solitary metastases may be resected, the diaphragm sutured, and a chest tube placed for a few days (126, 127). The use of the Cavitron Ultrasonic

Figure 33.12   Separation of the omentum from stomach and transverse colon. (Reproduced with permission from **Heintz APM, Berek JS.** Cytoreductive surgery for ovarian carcinoma. In: **Piver MS,** ed. *Ovarian Malignancies.* Edinburgh: Churchill Livingstone, 1987:134).

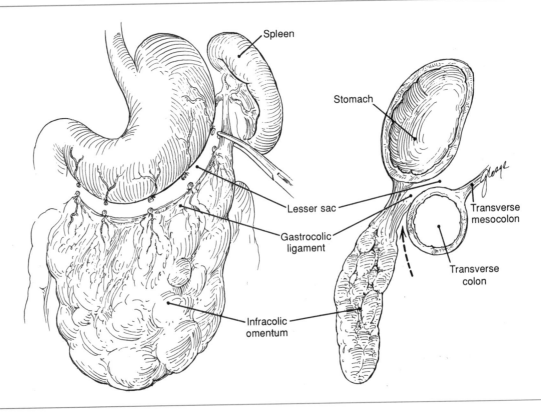

Surgical Aspirator (CUSA) and the argon beam coagulator may help facilitate resection of small tumor nodules, especially those on flat surfaces (128, 129).

Feasibility and Outcome

The only prospective study performed to assess the role of debulking surgery demonstrated a survival advantage in women who underwent successful interval cytodeduction (121). An analysis of the retrospective data available suggests that these operations are feasible for 70–90% of patients when performed by gynecologic oncologists (125, 130). Major morbidity is in the range of 5% and operative mortality is in the range of 1% (125, 131). Intestinal resection in these patients does not appear to increase the overall morbidity of the operation (123, 125). The performance of a pelvic lymphadenectomy in patients with stage III disease has been reported to prolong survival (54), although verification of this awaits a prospective, randomized study.

Chemotherapy

Systemic chemotherapy is the standard treatment for metastatic epithelial ovarian cancer. For many years, oral single-agent alkylating therapy was used (132), but the introduction of *cisplatin* in the latter half of the 1970s changed the therapeutic approach for most patients, and *cisplatin*-based combination chemotherapy has been the most frequently used treatment regimen in the U.S. for the past decade. Recently, *paclitaxel* has become part of the standard primary therapy for advanced ovarian cancer.

Single-Agent Therapy

The standard dose for the single alkylating agent *melphalan,* is 0.2 mg/kg/day given for 5 consecutive days every 28 days. In three separate GOG studies of suboptimal stage III ovarian cancer, 193 patients were treated with this regimen. Sixty-two patients (33%) had a clinical response, with a 16% complete response rate and a 17% partial response rate (133). However, the median duration of response was only 7 months and median survival was 12 months. The results of these prospective studies are comparable to many retrospective studies in the literature.

Other active drugs that have been used as single agents include *cisplatin, carboplatin, paclitaxel, cyclophosphamide, doxorubicin, hexamethylmelamine,* and *5-fluorouracil* (5-FU) (105, 133–141). *Cisplatin, carboplatin,* and *paclitaxel* seem to be more active than alkylating agents, whereas the others are somewhat less active. *Cisplatin, carboplatin,* and *paclitaxel* produce sufficiently high response rates to justify their routine use in primary therapy. The individual activities and their complementary toxicities serve as the rationale for their incorporation into combination regimens.

The use of single-agent chemotherapy for metastatic epithelial ovarian cancer is generally reserved for patients whose overall physical condition precludes the use of more toxic therapy. For elderly or debilitated patients, or for those who refuse intravenous chemotherapy, the use of an oral agent is simple and appealing.

Single-agent drugs, orally administered, are sometimes used for second-line chemotherapy because of their relative ease of administration and low toxicity. Second-line responses to *paclitaxel* (137), *hexamethylmelamine* (139), *carboplatin* (140), and *cisplatin* (141) have been observed in 10–36% of patients who have responded previously to *cisplatin.*

Combination Chemotherapy

Numerous combinations chemotherapeutic regimens have been tested in the treatment of advanced epithelial ovarian cancer. A summary of the most often used regimens is presented in Table 33.3.

Table 33.3   Chemotherapeutic Regimens for Advanced Ovarian Cancer

	Regimen	Interval
PT	*Cisplatin* (75–100 mg/M^2) *Paclitaxel* (175–210 mg/M^2)	Q 3 weeks
CT	*Carboplatin* (starting dose, AUC = 5) *Paclitaxel (135–175 mg/M^2)*	Q 3–4 weeks
PC	*Cisplatin* (75–100 mg/M^2) *Cyclophosphamide* (650–1000 mg/M^2)	Q 3 weeks
CC	*Carboplatin* (AUC = 5–7) *Cyclophosphamide* (600 mg/M^2)	Q 4 weeks
PAC	*Cisplatin* 50 mg/M^2 *Doxorubicin* 50 mg/M^2 *Cyclophosphamide* 500 mg/M^2	Q 3–4 weeks
CHAP	*Hexamethylmelamine* 150 mg/M^2 orally days 1–14 *Cyclophosphamide* 350 mg/M^2 IV day 1 and day 8 *Doxorubicin* 20 mg/M^2 IV day 1 and day 8 *Cisplatin* 60 mg/M^2 IV day 1	Q 3–4 weeks

AUC, area under the curve.

Single-Agent Versus Combination Chemotherapy   Combination chemotherapy has been shown to be superior to single-agent therapy for most patients with advanced epithelial ovarian cancer (142). The era of this testing began in the latter half of the 1970s, when combinations of agents found to have activity against epithelial tumors were compared with single-agent therapy. The first study to show any benefit for combination therapy compared a regimen called Hexa-CAF (*hexamethylmelamine, cyclophosphamide, methotrexate, 5-FU* with *melphalan* (143). This randomized, prospective study showed that the response rate and the median survival with the combination regimen were better than with the single drug. The Hexa-CAF regimen produced a complete response rate of 33% with a median survival of 29 months, compared with 16% and 17 months for *melphalan*.

Cisplatin-Based Combination Chemotherapy   Very soon after these data were published, *cisplatin* became available for the treatment of ovarian cancer, and it was soon recognized as a very active single agent against the disease. In a prospective study in England, it was shown that *cisplatin* was better than an alkylator, *cyclophosphamide*, as a single agent (144). Concurrently, *cisplatin* was tested in a variety of different combinations. One such regimen, CHAP (*cyclophosphamide, hexamethylmelamine, doxorubicin, cisplatin*), was shown to be active and generally tolerable (145). A prospective randomized study (146) comparing CHAP with Hexa-CAF showed a surgically documented complete response rate of 40% for the CHAP regimen, compared with 19% for patients treated with Hexa-CAF. The median survivals were 26 months and 19 months, respectively. Therefore, the *cisplatin*-based combination regimen seemed superior. Because of the toxicity of *hexamethylmelamine*, particularly the depression that some patients experience with the drug, many physicians omitted that agent.

In a meta-analysis performed on studies of patients with advanced-stage disease, patients given *cisplatin*-containing combination chemotherapy were compared with patients treated with regimens that did not include *cisplatin* (142). Survival differences between the groups were seen between 2 and 5 years; the *cisplatin* group had a slight survival advantage, but this difference disappeared by 8 years (Fig. 33.13) (142).

The PAC (*cisplatin, doxorubicin,* and *cyclophosphamide*) regimen has been extensively used for advanced ovarian cancer. Ehrlich et al. (147) reported on 56 patients treated with the PAC regimen every 3 weeks for 12 cycles. The median survival of patients with opti-

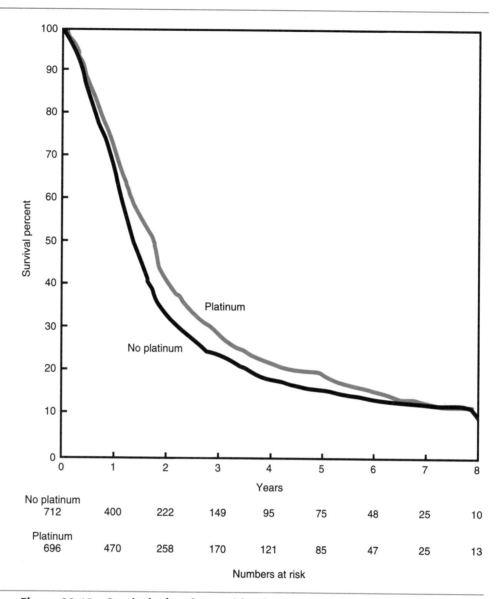

The following numbers at risk appear below the graph:

No platinum								
712	400	222	149	95	75	48	25	10
Platinum								
696	470	258	170	121	85	47	25	13

Numbers at risk

Figure 33.13   Survival of patients with advanced-stage ovarian cancer: a meta-analysis of multiple trials comparing cisplatin-containing combination chemotherapy with regimens without cisplatin. (Reproduced with permission from **Advanced Ovarian Cancer Trialists Group.** Chemotherapy in advanced ovarian cancer: an overview of randomized clinical trials. *BMJ* 1991;303:884).

mal residual disease was 45 months, compared with 23 months for those with suboptimal disease.

Most studies using the PC (*cisplatin* and *cyclophosphamide*) or PAC regimen report response rates and survival times similar to those produced by the CHAP regimen (135, 148). However, updated survival data suggest that the addition of *hexamethylmelamine* may be of benefit in some subsets of patients with advanced disease (149, 150). In the Mayo Clinic study, the initial analysis of a randomized prospective trial of CHAP versus PC for 181 patients with advanced-stage ovarian cancer showed no survival difference (149). An updated analysis showed a small, statistically significant difference in survival for the CHAP regimen for patients with no gross residual or minimal residual disease (149). Therefore, the precise role of *hexamethylmelamine* in the long-term survival of patients with minimal residual disease epithelial ovarian cancer has not been determined and will require additional randomized trials.

Because of the cardiotoxicity of *doxorubicin*, it would be desirable to omit the drug if overall response rates were not significantly changed. A large prospective randomized study of CHAP versus PC in the Netherlands showed that the response rates and median survivals were almost identical (148). Because the toxicity of PC was significantly less than that of the four-drug treatment, it was concluded that PC should be considered the treatment of choice.

There have been several trials comparing PAC with PC (151–154). No study showed a significant difference in survival between treatment arms. The GOG's randomized prospective comparison of equitoxic doses of PAC versus PC showed no benefit to the inclusion of *doxorubicin* in the combination (154). However, a meta-analysis of the combined data from these four trials showed a 7% survival advantage at 6 years for patients treated with the *doxorubicin*-containing regimen (155). The survival curves appear to converge at 8 years. The GOG study used a higher dose of *cyclophosphamide* in the PC arm to produce the same amount of myelosuppression as the PAC arm, but in the other trials, *doxorubicin* was added to the standard doses of PC (151–154).

Dose-Intensification with Cisplatin   With the two-drug regimen PC, higher doses of each drug can be used. This is particularly important for *cisplatin*, because it has a clinically relevant dose-response curve (i.e., the higher the dose, the greater the theoretical probability of response). The principle of *dose-intensity* is discussed more fully in Chapter 30.

The issue of dose-intensification of *cisplatin* was examined in a prospective trial conducted by the GOG (156). In this study, 243 patients with suboptional ovarian cancer were randomized to receive either 50 mg/M^2 or 100 mg/M^2 *cisplatin* plus 500 mg/M^2 *cyclophosphamide*. There was no difference in response rates for patients with measurable disease, and the overall survival times were identical. There was greater toxicity associated with the high-dose regimen. In a study conducted in Scotland, patients who received 100 mg/M^2 *cisplatin* plus 750 mg/M^2 *cyclophosphamide* initially had a significantly longer median survival compared with patients receiving 50 mg/M^2 *cisplatin* plus the same dose of *cyclophosphamide* (157). However, with an almost 5-year follow-up, there are no significant differences in overall survival for the patients with optimal residual disease.

A randomized, prospective trial of intraperitoneal (IP) *cisplatin* versus intravenous (IV) *cisplatin* (100 mg/M^2), each given with 750 mg/M^2 *cyclophosphamide*, has been performed jointly by the Southwest Oncology Group (SWOG), the GOG, and the Eastern Cooperative Oncology Group (ECOG) for patients with minimal residual disease (158). The IP *cisplatin* plus *cyclophosphamide* arm is associated with a longer median survival (49 vs. 41 months) and lower overall morbidity with less ototoxicity and neurotoxicity. **These data suggest that intraperitoneal *cisplatin* has a benefit in patients with minimal residual disease.**

Carboplatin   The second-generation platinum analog, *carboplatin*, was introduced and developed to have less toxicity than its parent compound, *cisplatin*. In toxicity and early efficacy trials, *carboplatin* was shown to have lower toxicity (159–162).; Fewer gastrointestinal side effects, especially nausea and vomiting, were observed than with *cisplatin*, and there was less nephrotoxicity, neurotoxicity, and ototoxicity.

The initial studies showed that *carboplatin* and *cisplatin* have approximately a 4:1 equivalency ratio (159). Thus, a standard single-agent dose of about 400 mg/M^2 has been used in most phase II trials (135). The dose is calculated by using the area under the curve (AUC) and the glomerular filtration rate (GFR) according to the Calvert formula (159), as discussed in Chapter 30. The target AUC is 6–9 (average = 7) for untreated patients with ovarian cancer. Alternatively, a dose of approximately 350–450 mg/M^2 *carboplatin* can be used initially for patients with a normal serum creatinine levels and adjusted based on toxicity. A platelet nadir of approximately 50,000 ml is a suitable target (135). Prospective randomized trials of *carboplatin* plus *cyclophosphamide* (CC) versus PC have been carried out in patients with stage III and IV disease (160, 161). These studies show that the *carboplatin* combination has a better therapeutic index for these patients (i.e., equivalent survival with a lower toxicity). **Thus, both studies conclude that the *carboplatin* combination should be the treatment of choice for patients with suboptimal disease.** A comparison of the two regimens has not been made in a sufficient number of patients with optimal disease, so the question of relative efficacy in this group is unresolved. However, Ozols (135) has argued that *carboplatin* should replace *cisplatin* in the primary treatment of all of these patients on the basis of available comparative efficacy data. Although the combination of *paclitaxel* and *carboplatin* is being compared with *paclitaxel* and *cisplatin,* it is reasonable to use *cisplatin* for patients with optimal disease, unless its use is precluded by toxicity or compromised renal or neurologic function. The gastrointestinal toxicities of *cisplatin* can now be ameliorated reasonably effectively by use of the potent antiemetic, *ondancetron.* In general, older patients (over 65 years of age) or those with significant medical conditions (e.g., diabetes mellitus) tolerate *cisplatin* less well and may do better with *carboplatin.*

Paclitaxel (Taxol)   The introduction of *paclitaxel (Taxol)* as an active agent in ovarian cancer requires the examination of this agent in first-line therapeutic strategies (134–138). *Paclitaxel* is the most active agent because *cisplatin,* with overall response rates in phase II trials of 36% in previously treated patients. This is a higher rate than was seen for *cisplatin* when it was first tested (137).

The randomized trial of the GOG was a two-arm comparison of *paclitaxel* plus *cisplatin* (PT) versus PC in patients with suboptimal stage III disease (138). An analysis of the trial shows a progression-free survival (18 versus 13 months) and overall survival (38 versus 24 months) benefit for the PT arm; therefore, the preferred regimen in patients with suboptimally cytoreduced disease is the combination of *paclitaxel* plus a *platinum* drug (138).

Chemotherapeutic Recommendation in Advanced Ovarian Cancer   Combination chemotherapy with *cisplatin* and *paclitaxel* is the treatment of choice for patients with advanced epithelial ovarian cancer. The recommended doses are *cisplatin* (75 mg/M^2) and *paclitaxel (Taxol)* (135–210 mg/M^2) (PT). For those in whom the toxicity of *cisplatin* is likely to preclude administration, carboplatin (starting dose AUC = 5) plus *paclitaxel (Taxol)* (175 mg/M^2) (CT) can be given. Dose escalations of *paclitaxel* and *carboplatin* that require G-CSF because of the combined myelosuppressive effects are currently undergoing clinical trials. A trial of *paclitaxel* and *cisplatin* versus *paclitaxel* and *carboplatin* is being performed to determine the best combination for optimal patients. The mature results of a completed GOG trial will define whether *paclitaxel* or *cisplatin* alone is better than the combination of the two drugs in suboptimal disease. The role of the intraperitoneal administration of *cisplatin* and *paclitaxel* must be studied to determine if this approach is superior to the intravenous administration of the two drugs.

Administration of Chemotherapy and Amelioration of Toxicity

Cisplatin   *Cisplatin* combination chemotherapy is given every 3–4 weeks by intravenous infusion over 1–1.5 hours. *Cisplatin* requires appropriate hydration and can be administered on either an inpatient or outpatient basis. Hydration is administered with one-half normal saline given intravenously at a rate of 300–500 ml/hour for 2–4 hours until the urinary output is greater than 100 ml/hour. It is preferable to place a Foley catheter to monitor the output. Immediately before chemotherapy, 12.5 g of *mannitol* in 50 ml of normal saline solution is infused. When the urinary output is satisfactory, the *cisplatin* is infused in normal saline; the IV fluid rate is decreased to 150–200 ml/hour for 6 hours and then is discontinued if the patient is stable. The principal toxicities of this regimen are renal, gastrointestinal, hematologic, and neurologic. The renal and neurologic toxicities limit the duration of treatment to no more than six to nine cycles.

The acute gastrointestinal toxicity of *cisplatin* (i.e., nausea and vomiting) can be minimized with a strong antiemetic, *ondancetron,* given as a 32-mg intravenous bolus, followed every 4–6 hours with 10 mg intravenously. Alternative regimens include *diphenhydramine* (25 mg orally) and *lorazepam* (2 mg sublingually) both given 1 hour before the initiation of treatment, followed by *lorazepam* (2 mg sublingually every 3 hours), *metoclopramide* (100 mg intravenously every 3–4 hours), and one dose of *dexamethasone* (20 mg intravenously).

Paclitaxel and Carboplatin   The renal and gastrointestinal toxicities of *carboplatin* are modest compared with those of *cisplatin;* thus, patients being treated with *carboplatin* do not require prehydration, and outpatient administration is more feasible. *Carboplatin* does tend to have appreciable bone marrow toxicity, and growth factors such as G-CSF and GM-CSF have facilitated the administration of drug combinations that have neutropenia as a dose-limiting toxicity. The combination of *carboplatin* with *cisplatin, cyclophosphamide,* or *paclitaxel* can produce considerable neutropenia, and the concomitant administration of 250 μg/M^2 of G-CSF given subcutaneously on days 1–10 of a treatment cycle may be protective (162, 163). The use of growth factors is discussed more fully in Chapter 30.

Radiation Therapy

An alternative to combination chemotherapy for selected patients with metastatic ovarian cancer is the use of whole-abdominal radiation therapy. Although this approach is not often used in the U.S., it is standard treatment in some institutions in Canada for patients with no residual macroscopic tumor in the upper abdomen (109). The treatment involves a radiation field that extends from 1–2 cm above the level of the diaphragm to include the entire pelvis (Chapter 30).

Whole-abdominal radiation seems to be useful for patients with metastatic disease that is microscopic or completely resected. The treatment has not been tested against combination chemotherapy. Radiation therapy has been compared with oral use of *chlorambucil* and seems to be superior (109). The currently available data suggest that whole-abdominal radiation is inappropriate for patients with macroscopic residual disease.

A trial of three cycles of high-dose *cisplatin* and *cyclophosmade* "induction" chemotherapy followed by whole-abdominal radiation therapy to "consolidate" the initial response has been reported (164). No apparent benefit could be shown by adding whole-abdominal radiation after chemotherapy in patients with optimal disease.

Immunotherapy

Although there is currently a great deal of interest in the use of biologic response modifiers in ovarian cancer, none has demonstrated efficacy as primary treatment as yet. The use of cytokines has been treated in a salvage setting, and the activity of α-interferon, γ-interferon, and interleukin-2 has been demonstrated (119). Trials of these and other biologics are developing because they have become increasingly available through recombinant DNA technology.

Hormonal Therapy

There is no evidence that hormonal therapy alone is appropriate primary therapy for advanced ovarian cancer. The use of progestational agents in the treatment of recurrent well-differentiated endometrioid carcinomas is supported by the current data. In a study by Rendina et al. (165), 30 evaluable patients with recurrent epithelial cancers were treated; 17 (57%) had an objective response, and three (10%) of these patients achieved a complete response. All responding patients had well-differentiated, estrogen receptor-positive tumors. A trial of *tamoxifen* in combination with multi-agent chemotherapy is being conducted.

Treatment Assessment

Many patients who undergo optimal cytoreductive surgery and subsequent chemotherapy for epithelial ovarian cancer will have no evidence of disease at the completion of treatment. Tumor markers and radiologic assessments have proven to be too insensitive to exclude the presence of subclinical disease. Therefore, a second-look surgery is often performed to evaluate these patients (90, 166–180). Most often, patients have undergone a formal reassessment laparotomy, although the laparoscope has also been used in this circumstance (178–180). However, there is a 35% false-negative rate if laparoscopy is used for a second-look procedure (90, 179).

Tumor Markers

Tumor markers are not reliable enough to predict accurately which patients with epithelial tumors will experience complete eradication of disease with a particular therapy. Carcinoembronic antigen (CEA) levels are often elevated in patients with ovarian cancer, but it is too nonspecific and insensitive to have much use in the management of patients with ovarian cancer (119).

The level of CA125, a surface glycoprotein associated with müllerian epithelial tissues, is elevated in about 80% of patients with epithelial ovarian cancers, particularly those with nonmucinous tumors. The levels frequently become undetectable after the initial surgical resection and one or two cycles of chemotherapy.

Levels of CA125 have been correlated with findings at second-look operations. Positive levels are useful in predicting the presence of disease, but negative levels are an insensitive determinant of the absence of disease. In a prospective study (181), the predictive value of a positive test was shown to be 100%; i.e., if the level of CA125 was positive (>35 U/ml), disease was always detectable in patients at the second-look procedure. The predictive value of a negative test was only 56%; i.e., if the level was < 35 U/ml, disease was present in 44% of the patients at the time of the second-look surgery. **A review of the literature suggests that an elevated CA125 level predicts persistent disease at second-look surgery in 97% of the cases** (33), **but the CA125 level is not sensitive enough to exclude subclinical disease in many patients.**

Serum CA125 levels can be used during chemotherapy to follow those patients whose levels were positive at the initiation of therapy (33, 182). The change in level generally correlates with response. Those patients with persistently elevated levels after three cycles of treatment most likely have resistant clones. When levels rise after treatment, almost invariably treatment has failed and continuation of the current regimen is futile.

Radiologic Assessment

For patients with stage I to III epithelial ovarian cancer, radiologic tests generally have been of limited value in assessing the response to therapy for subclinical disease. Ascites can be readily detected, but even quite large omental metastases can be missed on CT scan (183). If liver enzymes are abnormal, the liver can be evaluated with a CT scan or ultrasonography. A positive CT scan and fine-needle aspiration (FNA) cytology indicating tumor persistence could obviate the need for second-look surgery, but the false-negative rate of a CT scan is about 45% (183).

Second-Look Operations

A second-look operation is one performed on a patient who has no clinical evidence of disease after a prescribed course of chemotherapy to determine the response to therapy.

Second-Look Laparotomy

The technique of the second-look laparotomy is essentially identical to that for the staging laparotomy (90). The operation should be performed through a vertical abdominal incision. The incision should be initiated below the level of the umbilicus, so that if pelvic disease is detected in the absence of any palpable upper abdominal disease, a smaller incision might suffice. The incision can be extended cranially as needed.

After multiple cytologic specimens have been obtained, biopsies of the peritoneal surfaces should be performed, particularly in any areas of previously documented tumor. These are the most important areas to sample for biopsy because they are most likely to give a positive result. Any adhesions or surface irregularities should be sampled. In addition, biopsy specimens should be taken from the pelvic side walls, the pelvic cul-de-sac, the bladder, the paracolic gutters, the residual omentum, and the diaphragm. A pelvic and para-aortic lymph node dissection should be performed for those patients whose nodal tissues have not been previously removed.

About 30% of patients with no evidence of macroscopic disease will have microscopic metastases (166). Also, for many patients with microscopic disease, it will be detected in only the occasional biopsy or cytologic specimen. Therefore, a large number of specimens (at least 20–30) should be obtained to minimize the "false-negative" rate of the operation. For selected patients in whom gross residual tumor is discovered at second-look surgery, resection of isolated masses may be performed. The removal of all macroscopic areas of disease might facilitate response to salvage therapies (184, 185), and it also permits the collection of tissue for *in vitro* analyses.

Second-look laparotomies have not been shown to influence patient survival (175, 177). **Therefore, they should be performed only in a research setting, in which second-line or "salvage" therapies are undergoing clinical trials.**

The findings at second-look correlate with subsequent outcome and survival (90, 166–177). Patients who have no histologic evidence of disease have a significantly longer survival than those in whom microscopic or macroscopic disease is documented at laparotomy (172, 173).

The attainment of negative findings with second-look surgery is not tantamount to a cure (164, 166). Indeed, the reported probability that a patient will have a recurrence after a negative second-look laparotomy ranges from 30–50% at 5 years (90, 166–177). Clearly, it is not possible to sample every potential site of disease. In addition, disease can become clinically apparent in sites that are occult, such as the liver parenchyma (56). Most recurrences after a negative second-look laparotomy occur in patients with poorly differentiated cancers (177).

Variables associated with the outcome of the second-look laparotomy are: 1) initial stage, 2) tumor grade, 3) the size of the residual tumor and the size of the largest metastatic tumor before treatment, and 4) the type of chemotherapy. No single variable or combination of variables is sufficiently predictive to obviate a planned second-look laparotomy (90).

Second-Look Laparoscopy   The advantage of laparoscopy is that it is less invasive than laparotomy; the disadvantage is that visibility may be limited by the frequent presence of intraperitoneal adhesions (168–172). The development of newer techniques for retroperitoneal lymph node dissection has potentially increased the utility of the endoscopic approach to second-look. The morbidity and role of this technique are currently being studied by the GOG.

One technique that has been used for second-look is "open" laparoscopy. This procedure allows placement of the scope after a "cutdown" to the fascia of the rectus abdominous. The peritoneum is entered under direct vision, thus avoiding the blind insertion that can be associated with intestinal injury (179).

The sensitivity of the laparoscopic technique has been determined by an exploratory laparotomy performed immediately after a negative laparoscopy. Thirty-five percent of those who have a negative findings on laparoscopy have evidence of disease at laparotomy (180), but these patients did not undergo a lymphadenectomy at laparoscopy.

Laparoscopy has been used immediately before a planned laparotomy. If gross disease is detected and secondary resection of the tumor is not possible, a laparotomy may be omitted (179).

Thus, the role of the laparoscope for patients with epithelial ovarian cancer is still being defined. It may be used to stage disease in patients who have undergone a prior laparotomy for a tumor that was incompletely staged. Second-look laparoscopy may also be useful for patients on experimental treatment protocols, especially second-line treatments that require some evaluation of response.

Second-line Therapy

Secondary Cytoreduction   Patients with persistent or recurrent pelvic and abdominal tumors after primary therapy for ovarian cancer may be candidates for surgical excision of their disease. This operation has been referred to as "secondary" cytoreductive surgery (184). Tumor resection, under these circumstances, should be restricted to carefully selected patients for whom resection has a reasonable chance of either prolonging life or resulting in significant palliation of symptoms, because there is no benefit for most patients with persistent or progressive disease after primary therapy. The patient for whom secondary cytoreduction might be appropriate should be in good general medical condition. A suitable patient would be one who has no evidence of ascites, has not yet received *cisplatin* combination chemotherapy, has had at least a partial response to prior alkylating agent therapy, and has had a reasonably long interval since primary diagnosis (longer than 9–12 months). If the patient has previously received *cisplatin,* secondary cytoreduction is justified if there has been a long disease-free survival (>24 months), because such patients are likely to respond again to the primary chemotherapy (185–190).

The goal of secondary debulking is to remove all residual gross tumor, if possible, or to reduce the metastatic tumor burden to <5 mm maximum dimension. Some patients with minimal residual disease will respond to second-line treatment. Those patients in whom the residual disease is completely resected have a significantly longer survival than those who do not (185).

Second-Line Chemotherapy   If disease persists at the time of second-look laparotomy, or if clinically progressive disease develops during primary therapy, patients usually are switched to an alternative treatment, often a second-line chemotherapy. The response rates for second-line chemotherapies have been less than 10–30% for most drugs tested by the oral or intravenous route (105, 133, 135).

Secondary response rates as high as 30% have been reported for high-dose *cisplatin* (100–150 mg/M^2) for patients in whom alkylating agents or low-dose *cisplatin* (50 mg/M^2) have failed (135, 186, 187). Unfortunately, this approach is associated with considerable toxicity, particularly renal and neural. **The *cisplatin* analog, *Carboplatin*, is active as a second-line agent in patients who have responded to prior *cisplatin* treatment, and response rates for these patients have been 20–30%** (163, 188–190). For *cisplatin*-refractory patients, response rates to second-line *carboplatin* are <10% (188, 190).

Depending on the prior chemotherapy, persistent disease can be treated with *cisplatin, carboplatin, paclitaxel, ifosfamide,* or *hexamethylmelamine,* with or without other agents. Although responses occur, this approach is not curative. **For patients treated initially with platinum therapy,** *paclitaxel* **has responses occurring in 20–36% of patients** (134–137). *Hexamethylmelamine* produced second-line complete clinical responses for 15% of the patients (8 of 52) (139) and *ifosfamide* for 20% of the patients (9 of 26) in a GOG trial (191). For patients with minimal residual (<5 mm) or microscopic disease confined to the peritoneal cavity, consideration can be given to intraperitoneal chemotherapy or immuntotherapy (192).

Intraperitoneal Therapy

The failure of second-line intravenous chemotherapy to control residual disease has led to the use of intraperitoneal therapies for small, persistent disease. Cytotoxic chemotherapeutic agents, such as *cisplatin, 5-FU, cytosine arabinoside (Ara-C), Etoposide (VP-16),* and *mitoxantrone,* have been used for patients with persistent epithelial ovarian cancer (192–200), and complete responses have been seen for patients who begin treatment with minimal residual disease. The surgically documented response rates reported with this approach are about 20–40% for carefully selected patients, and the complete response rate is about 10–20%. *Cisplatin* seems to be the best drug, although various combinations of agents (e.g., *cisplatin* plus *etoposide*) have been shown to have significant activity (197, 198). Although it has been suggested that this approach produces a significant subsequent improvement in survival (200), there are no prospective phase III data, and the patients so treated tend to be those with a more favorable prognosis regardless of subsequent therapy.

Another approach is the use of intraperitoneal biologic response modifiers (BRMs) such as interferon (201–207). Interferon has been found to have some activity for patients with minimal residual disease (201, 202). Because of recombinant DNA technology, other BRMs, particularly the cytokines, are becoming increasingly available for clinical testing. Trials of intraperitoneal α-interferon, γ-interferon, tumor necrosis factor, and interleukin-2 have been performed. The response rate for the intraperitoneal cytokines, α-interferon and γ-interferon, is the same as that for the cytotoxic agents, i.e., about 30–50% (201, 202, 205). The intraperitoneal administration of α-interferon has produced a 32% (9 of 28) surgically documented complete response rate, and a 50% (14 of 28) total response rate for patients with minimal residual disease after primary combination chemotherapy with *cisplatin* (201, 202).

The interferons have been combined with cytotoxic agents in an effort to increase the overall response rates. In two trials, the combination of *cisplatin* and α-interferon seemed to produce a 50% complete response rate, which was greater than that produced by either single agent (203, 204). However, in a prospective, single-arm, phase II trial conducted by the GOG, the intraperitoneal administration of *cisplatin* and α-interferon produced only a 7% response rate (207). In this GOG trial, most patients had *cisplatin*-refractory tumors with >5 mm residual disease, generalized carcinomatosis, and ascites. Surgically documented responses to intraperitoneal therapy have been generally limited to patients with minimal residual disease (i.e., <5 mm maximum tumor dimension) and patients whose tumors have been responsive to *cisplatin* chemotherapy.

Intraperitoneal treatment is not suitable for all patients because it can be cumbersome, requiring catheters that remain functional. Neither patients with extensive intraperitoneal adhesions nor patients with extraperitoneal disease are appropriate candidates. On the basis of these issues and the failure to achieve responses in most patients with bulky, platinum-refractory disease, second-line intraperitoneal chemotherapy and immunotherapy should still be considered experimental.

Whole-Abdominal Radiation

Whole-abdominal radiation therapy given as a "salvage" treatment has been shown to be potentially effective in a small subset of selected patients with microscopic disease, but it is associated with a relatively high morbidity. The principal problem associated with this approach is the development of acute and chronic intestinal morbidity. As many as 30% of patients treated with this approach develop intestinal obstruction, which will necessitate potentially morbid exploratory surgery (208).

Experimental Combination Chemotherapy Regimens

In light of the poor responses to second-line drugs in phase II trials, several new combinations of chemotherapy are now being tested in advanced epithelial ovarian cancer. The use of autologous bone marrow transplantation (ABMT) and peripheral stem cell protection is being tested for patients with advanced ovarian cancer (20–211). In one trial of high-dose *carboplatin* with autologous bone marrow transplantation, seven of the 11 patients with extensive refractory disease had an objective response. The maximum tolerated dose of high-dose *carboplatin* was 2 gm/M^2 (209). In a retrospective analysis of 35 patients treated with high-dose *melphalan* and ABMT, nine of 12 patients with residual disease capable of evaluation had a measurable response (210). The morbidity of this approach is high, and its role remains to be determined. The use of peripheral stem cell transplantation as an alternative to autologous bone marrow harvest and transplantation is currently being investigated.

Intestinal Obstruction

Patients with epithelial ovarian cancer often develop intestinal obstruction, either at the time of initial diagnosis or, more frequently, in association with recurrent disease (212–219). Obstruction may be related to a mechanical blockage or to carcinomatous ileus.

The intestinal blockage can be corrected in most patients whose obstruction appears at the time of initial diagnosis (111). However, the decision to perform an exploratory procedure to ease intestinal obstruction in patients with recurrent disease is more difficult. For patients whose life expectancy is very short (e.g., <2 months), surgical relief of the obstruction is not indicated (212). For those whose projected life-span is longer, features that predict a reasonable likelihood of correcting the obstruction include young age, good nutritional status, and the absence of rapidly accumulating ascites (213).

For most patients with recurrent ovarian cancer who present with intestinal obstruction, initial management should include proper radiographic documentation of the obstruction, hydration, correction of any electrolyte disturbances, parenteral alimentation, and intestinal intubation. For some patients, the obstruction may be alleviated by this conservative approach. A preoperative upper gastrointestinal series and a barium enema will define possible sites of obstruction.

If exploratory surgery is deemed appropriate, the type of operation to be performed will depend on the site and the number of obstructions. Multiple sites of obstruction are not uncommon in patients with recurrent epithelial ovarian cancer. More than one-half of the patients have small-bowel obstruction, one-third have colonic obstruction, and one-sixth have both (214–218). If the obstruction is principally contained in one area of the bowel (e.g., the terminal ileum), this area can either be resected or bypassed, depending on whether a concomitant effort at secondary cytoreduction is indicated. If multiple obstructions are present, resection of several segments of intestine in patients with recurrent disease is usually not indicated, and intestinal bypass surgery or colostomy, or both, should be performed.

Intestinal bypass is generally associated with less morbidity than resection (214, 215), and in patients with recurrent, progressive cancer, the survival time after these two operations is the same (214). Most frequently, an enteroenterostomy or an enterocolostomy is performed (215–218). Colostomy may be necessary when there is a distal large-bowel obstruction. Occasionally, the performance of an ileostomy or a jejunostomy is warranted when the large bowel is completely encased in tumor (51). In very advanced cases, a gastrostomy may be used for palliative purposes, and the gastrostomy can be placed percutaneously if there is no carcinomatosis around the stomach (219).

Among 268 patients reported to have undergone operations for intestinal obstruction resulting from ovarian cancer, the operative mortality was 14% and major complications were seen in 34% of the patients (212–215). The need for multiple reanastamoses and prior radiation therapy increased the morbidity, which consisted primarily of sepsis and enterocutaneous fistulas.

The median survival time for patients who have undergone intestinal surgery for obstruction secondary to ovarian cancer ranges from 2.5–7 months, although Castaldo et al. (212) reported that 17% of such patients survived longer than 12 months.

Survival

The prognosis for patients with epithelial ovarian cancer is related to several clinical variables. Including patients in all stages of disease, patients younger than 50 years of age have a 5-year survival rate of about 40%, compared with about 15% for patients older than 50 years of age (1, 59, 84–87, 105). The 5-year survival rate for carefully and properly staged patients with stage I and II tumors is 80–100%, depending on the tumor grade. The 5-year survival rate for stage IIIa is about 30–40%, compared with about 20% for stage IIIb and only 5% for those with stages IIIc and IV (84–87, 90, 142, 155). Including patients of all stages, the overall 5-year survival rate for grade 1 epithelial ovarian cancers is about 40%, compared with about 20% for grade 2 and 5–10% for grade 3 (59–61, 65). The 10- and 20-year survival rates among patients with borderline ovarian tumors is about 95% and 90%, respectively (3, 5, 101, 102). Patients with microscopic residual disease at the start of treatment have a 5-year survival rate of about 40–75%, compared with about 30–40% for those with optimal disease and only 5% for those with suboptimal disease (90, 111–114). Patients without any evidence of disease at second-look laparotomy have a 5-year survival rate of 50% compared with about 35% for those with microscopic disease and about 5% for those with macroscopic disease (90, 166–174, 177). Patients whose Karnofsky's index (KI) is low (<70) have a significantly shorter survival than those with a KI >70 (220).

Nonepithelial Ovarian Cancers

Compared with epithelial ovarian cancers, other malignant tumors of the ovary are uncommon. Nonepithelial malignancies of the ovary account for about 10% of all ovarian cancers (2, 221). Nonepithelial ovarian cancers include malignancies of germ-cell origin, sex cord-stromal cell origin, metastatic carcinomas to the ovary, and a variety of extremely rare ovarian cancers (e.g., sarcomas, lipoid cell tumors). Although there are many similarities in the presentation, evaluation, and management of these patients, these tumors also have many unique qualities that require a special approach.

Germ-Cell Malignancies

Germ-cell tumors are derived from the primordial germ cells of the ovary. Their incidence is only about one-tenth the incidence of malignant germ-cell tumors of the testis, so most of the advances in the management of these tumors have been extrapolations from experience with the corresponding testicular tumors. Although malignant germ-cell tumors can arise in extragonadal sites such as the mediastinum and the retroperitoneum, most germ-cell tumors arise in the gonad from undifferentiated germ cells. The variation in the site of these cancers is explained by the embryonic migration of the germ cells from the caudal part of the yolk sac to the dorsal mesentery before their incorporation into the sex cords of the developing gonads (2, 222).

Classification

A histologic classification of ovarian germ-cell tumors is presented in Table 33.4 (223). Both α-fetoprotein (AFP) and human chorionic gonadotropin (hCG) are secreted by some germ cell malignancies; therefore, the presence of circulating hormones can be clinically useful in the diagnosis of a pelvic mass and in monitoring the course of a patient after surgery. Placental alkaline phosphatase (PLAP) and lactate dehydrogenase (LDH) are commonly produced by dysgerminomas and may be useful for monitoring the disease. α-1-antitrypsin (AAT) can rarely be detected in association with germ-cell tumors. When the histologic and immunohistologic identification of these substances in tumors is correlated, a classification of germ-cell tumors emerges (Fig. 33.14) (224).

In this scheme, embryonal carcinoma, which is a cancer composed of undifferentiated cells, synthesizes both hCG and AFP, and this lesion is the progenitor of several other germ cell tumors (222, 224). More differentiated germ-cell tumors, such as the endodermal sinus tumor, which secretes AFP, and the choriocarcinoma, which secretes hCG, are derived from the extraembryonic tissues; the immature teratomas derived from the embryonic cells have lost the ability to secrete these substances. Pure germinomas do not secrete these markers.

Epidemiology

Although 20–25% of all benign and malignant ovarian neoplasms are of germ-cell origin, only about 3% of these tumors are malignant (202). Germ-cell malignancies account for fewer than 5% of all ovarian cancers in Western countries. Germ-cell malignancies represent up to 15% of ovarian cancers in Asian and African-American socieites, where epithelial ovarian cancers are much less common.

In the first two decades of life, almost 70% of ovarian tumors are of germ-cell origin, and one-third of these are malignant (2, 221). Germ-cell tumors account for two-thirds of the ovarian malignancies in this age group. Germ-cell cancers also are seen in the third decade, but thereafter they become quite rare.

Table 33.4   Histologic Typing of Ovarian Germ Cell Tumors

1. Dysgerminoma

2. Teratoma
   A. Immature
   B. Mature
      1) Solid
      2) Cystic
         a. Dermoid cyst (mature cystic teratoma)
         b. Dermoid cyst with malignant transformation
   C. Monodermal and highly specialized
      1) Struma ovarii
      2) Carcinoid
      3) Struma ovarii and carcinoid
      4) Others

3. Endodermal sinus tumor

4. Embryonal carcinoma

5. Polyembryoma

6. Choriocarcinoma

7. Mixed forms

Reproduced with permission from **Seroy SF, Scully RE, Robin IH.** *Histological Typing of Ovarian Tumors: International Histological Classification of Tumors, No. 9.* Geneva: World Health Organization, 1973.

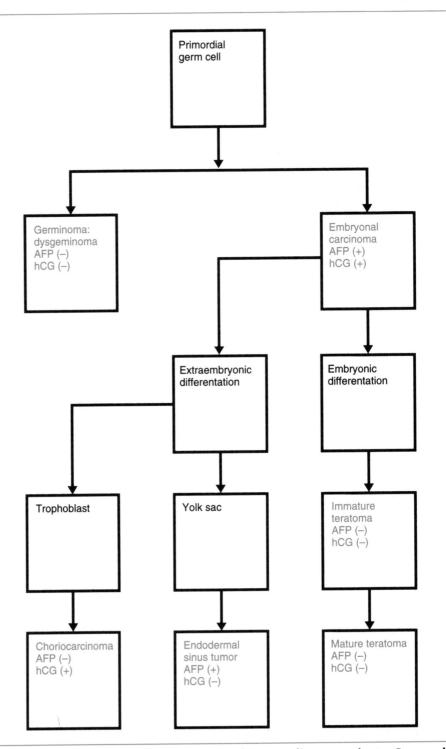

Figure 33.14   Relationship between types of pure malignant patients. Germ cell tumors and their secreted marker substances. (Reproduced with permission from **Berek JS, Hacker NF.** *Practical Gynecologic Oncology.* 2nd ed. Baltimore: Williams & Wilkins, 1994:379.)

Clinical Features

Symptoms

In contrast to the relatively slow-growing epithelial ovarian tumors, germ-cell malignancies grow rapidly and often are characterized by subacute pelvic pain related to capsular distention, hemorrhage, or necrosis. The rapidly enlarging pelvic mass may produce pressure symptoms on the bladder or rectum, and menstrual irregularities also may occur in menarchal patients. Some young patients may misinterpret the early symptoms of a neoplasm as those of pregnancy, and this can lead to a delay in the diagnosis. Acute symptoms associated with torsion or rupture of the adnexa can develop. These symptoms may be confused with acute appendicitis. In more advanced cases, ascites may develop, and the patient can have abdominal distention (222).

Signs

For patients with a palpable adnexal mass, the evaluation can proceed as outlined. Some patients with germ cell tumors will be premenarchal and may require examination under anesthesia. If the lesions are principally solid or a combination of solid and cystic, as might be noted on an ultrasonographic evaluation, a neoplasm is probable and a malignancy is possible (see Fig. 13.11 and Chapter 13). During the remainder of the physical examination, effort should be directed to searching for signs of ascites, pleural effusion, and organomegaly.

Diagnosis

Adnexal masses measuring 2 cm or larger in premenarchal girls or 8 cm or larger in other premenopausal patients will usually require surgical exploration. For young patients, blood tests should include serum hCG and AFP titers, a complete blood count, and liver function tests. An x-ray of the chest is important because germ-cell tumors can metastasize to the lungs or mediastinum. A karyotype should be obtained preoperatively for all premenarcheal girls because of the propensity of these tumors to arise in dysgenetic gonads. A preoperative CT scan or MRI may document the presence and extent of retroperitoneal lymphadenopathy or liver metastases; however, because these patients require surgical exploration, such extensive and time-consuming evaluation is unnecessary. If postmenarcheal patients have predominantly cystic lesions up to 8 cm in diameter, they may be observed or given oral contraceptives for two menstrual cycles (225).

Dysgerminoma

Dysgerminoma is the most common malignant germ-cell tumor, accounting for about 30–40% of all ovarian cancers of germ-cell origin (221, 224). The tumors represent only 1–3% of all ovarian cancers, but they represent as many as 5–10% of ovarian cancers in patients younger than 20 years of age. Seventy-five percent of dysgerminomas occur between the ages of 10 and 30 years, 5% occur before the age of 10 years, and they rarely occur after 50 years of age (2, 222). Because these malignancies occur in young women, 20–30% of ovarian malignancies associated with pregnancy are dysgerminomas.

Dysgerminomas are found in both sexes and may arise in gonadal or extragonadal sites. The latter include the midline structures from the pineal gland to the mediastinum and the retroperitoneum. Histologically, they represent abnormal proliferations of the basic germ cell. In the ovary, the germ cells are encapsulated at birth (the primordial follicle), and the unencapsulated or free cells die. If either of the latter processes fails, it is conceivable that the germ cell could free itself of its normal control and multiply indiscriminately.

The size of dysgerminomas varies widely, but they are usually 5–15 cm in diameter (226). The capsule is slightly bosselated, and the consistency of the cut surface is spongy and gray-brown in color (Fig. 33.15).

The histologic characteristics of the dysgerminoma are very distinctive. The large round, ovoid, or polygonal cells have abundant, clear, very pale-staining cytoplasm, large and ir-

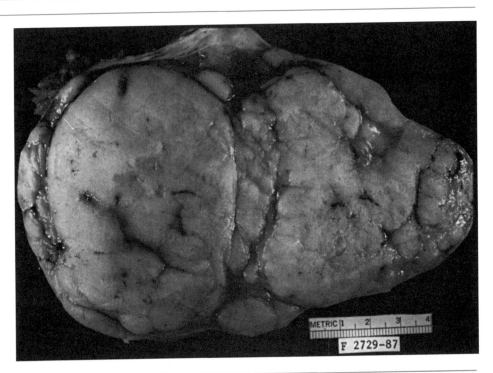

Figure 33.15   Dysgerminoma of the ovary. Note that the lesion is principally solid with some cystic areas. (Reproduced with permission from **Berek JS, Hacker NF.** *Practical Gynecologic Oncology.* 2nd ed. Baltimore: Williams & Wilkins, 1994:380.)

regular nuclei, and prominent nucleoli (Fig. 33.16). Mitotic figures are seen in varying numbers, although they are usually numerous. Another characteristic feature is the arrangement of the elements in lobules and nests separated by fibrous septa, which are often extensively infiltrated with lymphocytes, plasma cells, and granulomas with epitheloid cells and multinucleated giant cells. When necrosis is extensive, the lesion may be confused with tuberculosis. Occasional dysgerminomas may contain syncytiotrophoblastic giant cells and may be associated with precocious puberty or virilization. The presence of these cells does not seem to alter the behavior of the tumor (227).

Because the dysgerminoma is a germ-cell tumor and parthenogenesis (stimulation of the basic germ cell to atypical division) is the most commonly accepted genesis for the more immature teratomas, it is logical that these two tumors may coexist. Choriocarcinoma, endodermal sinus tumor, and other extraembryonal lesions are also commonly associated with the dysgerminoma.

Approximately 5% of dysgerminomas are discovered in phenotypic females with abnormal gonads (2). This malignancy can be associated with patients who have pure gonadal dysgenesis (46XY, bilateral streak gonads), mixed gonadal dysgenesis (45X/46XY, unilateral streak gonad, contralateral testis), and the androgen insensitivity syndrome (46XY, testicular feminization). Therefore, for premenarcheal patients with a pelvic mass, the karyotype should be determined (see Chapter 23.)

For most patients with gonadal dysgenesis, dysgerminomas arise in gonadoblastomas, which are benign ovarian tumors that are composed of germ cells and sex cord stroma. If gonadoblastomas are left *in situ* in patients with gonadal dysgenesis, more than 50% will develop into ovarian malignancies (228).

About 75% of dysgerminomas are stage I (i.e., confined to one or both ovaries) at diagnosis (226, 228–231). About 85–90% of stage I tumors are confined to one ovary; 10–15%

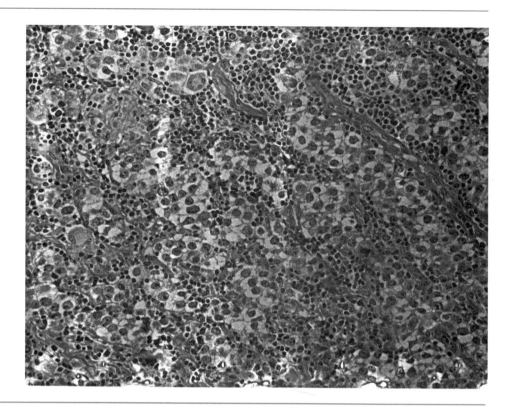

Figure 33.16   Dysgerminoma of ovary. Primitive germ cells are divided into clusters and lobules by fibrous septa rich in lymphocytes. Rare multinucleated giant cells are present in the left upper corner. (Reproduced with permission from **Berek JS, Hacker NF.** *Practical Gynecologic Oncology.* 2nd ed. Baltimore: Williams & Wilkins, 1994:147.)

are bilateral. In fact, dysgerminoma is the only germ-cell malignancy that has this significant rate of bilaterality, othe germ-cell tumors are rarely bilateral.

For patients whose contralateral ovary has been preserved, disease can develop in 5–10% of the retained gonads over the next 2 years (2). This figure includes those not given additional therapy, as well as patients with gonadal dysgenesis.

In the 25% of patients who present with metastatic disease, the tumor most commonly spreads via the lymphatic system. It can also spread hematogenously or by direct extension through the capsule of the ovary with exfoliation and dissemination of cells throughout the peritoneal surfaces. Metastases to the contralateral ovary may be present when there is no other evidence of spread. An uncommon site of metastatic disease is bone; when metastasis to this site occurs, the lesions are seen principally in the lower vertebrae. Metastases to the lungs, liver, and brain are seen most often in patients with long-standing or recurrent disease. Metastasis to the mediastinum and supraclavicular lymph nodes is usually a late manifestation of disease.

Treatment

The treatment of patients with early dysgerminoma is primarily surgical, including resection of the primary lesion and proper surgical staging. Chemotherapy or radiation is administered to patients with metastatic disease. Because the disease principally affects girls and young women, special consideration must be given to the preservation of fertility whenever possible. An algorithm for the management of ovarian dysgerminoma is presented in Figure 33.17.

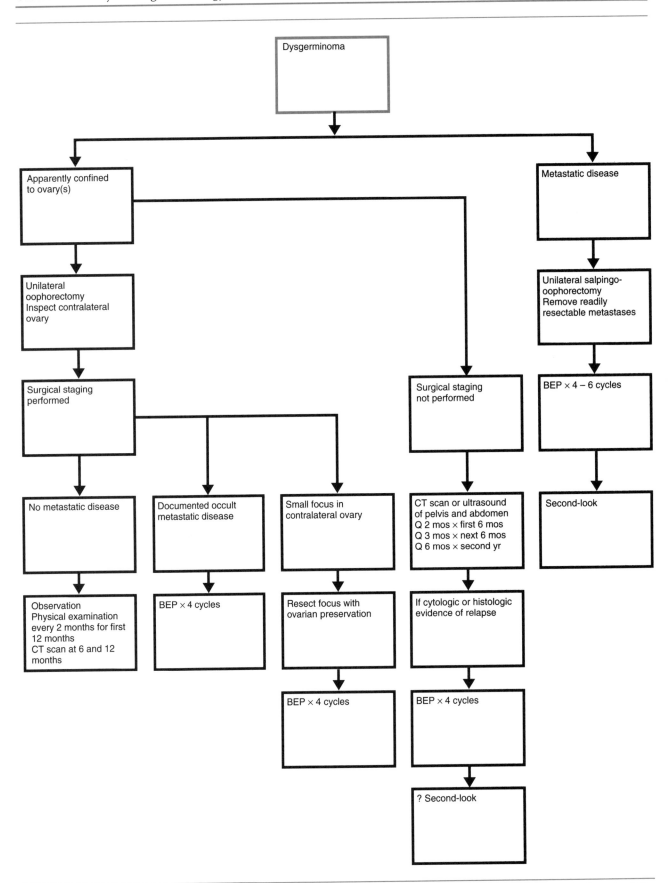

Figure 33.17   Management of dysgerminoma of the ovary. Reproduced from **Berek JS, Hacker NF.** *Practical Gynecologic Oncology.* 2nd ed. Baltimore: Williams & Wilkins. 1994:383.

Surgery

The minimum operation for ovarian dysgerminoma is a unilateral oophorectomy. If there is a desire to preserve fertility, the contralateral ovary, fallopian tube, and uterus should be left *in situ,* even in the presence of metastatic disease, because of the sensitivity of the tumor to chemotherapy. If fertility need not be preserved, it may be appropriate to perform a total abdominal hysterectomy and bilateral salpingo-oophorectomy for patients with advanced disease. For patients whose karyotype analysis reveals a Y chromosome, both ovaries should be removed, although the uterus may be left *in situ* for possible future embryo transfer. Whereas cytoreductive surgery is of unproven value, bulky disease that can be readily resected (e.g., an omental cake) should be removed at the initial operation.

For patients in whom the neoplasm appears on inspection to be confined to the ovary, a careful staging operation should be undertaken to determine the presence of any occult metastatic disease. All peritoneal surfaces should be inspected and palpated, and any suspicious lesions should be biopsied. Unilateral pelvic lymphadenectomy and at least careful palpation and biopsy of enlarged para-aortic nodes are particularly important parts of the staging. These tumors often metastasize to the para-aortic nodes around the renal vessels. Dysgerminoma is the only germ-cell tumor that tends to be bilateral, and not all of the bilateral lesions are associated with obvious ovarian enlargement. Therefore, bisection of the contralateral ovary and excisional biopsy of any suspicious lesion are desirable (229, 230). If a small contralateral tumor is found, it may be possible to resect it and preserve some normal ovary.

Radiation

Dysgerminomas are very sensitive to radiation therapy, and doses of 2500–3500 cGy may be curative, even for gross metastatic disease. Loss of fertility is a problem with radiation therapy, however, so radiation should rarely be used as first-line treatment (232).

Chemotherapy

Many patients with a dysgerminoma will have a tumor that is apparently confined to one ovary and will be referred after unilateral salpingo-oophorectomy without surgical staging. The options for such patients are repeat laparotomy for surgical staging, regular pelvic and abdominal surveillance with CT scans, and adjuvant chemotherapy. As dysgerminomas are rapidly growing tumors, regular CT surveillance is preferable. Tumor markers (AFP and βhCG) should also be monitored in case occult mixed germ-cell elements are present.

There have been numerous reports of successful control of metastatic dysgerminomas with systemic chemotherapy, and this technique should now be regarded as the treatment of choice (232–239). The obvious advantage is the preservation of fertility (235).

The most frequently used chemotherapeutic regimens for germ-cell tumors are BEP (*bleomycin, etoposide,* and *cisplatin*), VBP (*vinblastine, bleomycin,* and *cisplatin*), and VAC (*vincristine, actinomycin,* and *cyclophosphamide*) (234–240) (Table 33.5). The GOG is currently studying three cycles of *carboplatin* (400 mg/M^2 intravenously on day 1 every 4 weeks) and *etoposide* (120 mg/M^2 intravenously on days 1, 2, and 3 every 4 weeks) for patients with completely resected ovarian dysgerminoma, stages Ib, Ic, II, or III (239).

For patients with advanced, incompletely resected germ-cell tumors, the GOG studied *cisplatin*-based chemotherapy on two consecutive protocols. In the first study, patients received four cycles of *vinblastine* (12 mg/M^2 every 3 weeks), *bleomycin* (20 units/M^2 intravenously every week for 12 weeks), and *cisplatin* (20 mg/M^2/day intravenously for 5 days every 3 weeks). Patients with persistent or progressive disease were treated with six cycles of VAC. In the second ongoing trial, patients received three cycles of BEP initially, followed by con-

1199

Table 33.5   Combination Chemotherapy for Germ Cell Tumors of the Ovary

Regimen and Drugs	Dose and Schedule*
BEP	
Bleomycin	15 units/M^2/week × 5; then on day 1 of course 4
Etoposide	100 mg/M^2/day × 5 days every 3 weeks
Cisplatin	20 mg/M^2/day × 5 days, or 100 mg/M^2/day × 1 day every 3 weeks
VBP	
Vinblastine	0.15 mg/kg days 1 and 2 every 3 weeks
Bleomycin	15 units/M^2/week × 5; then on day 1 of course 4
Cisplatin	100 mg/M^2 on day 1 every 3 weeks
VAC	
Vincristine	1–1.5 mg/M^2 on day 1 every 4 weeks
Actinomycin-D	0.5 mg/day × 5 days every 4 weeks
Cyclophosphamide	150 mg/M^2/day × 5 days every 4 weeks

*All doses given intravenously.

---

solidation with VAC, which was later discontinued for patients with dysgerminomas (237). The VAC consolidation after BEP for patients with tumors other than dysgerminoma is still being investigated, but VAC does not seem to improve the outcome of the BEP regimen (240). A total of 20 patients with stage III and IV dysgerminoma were treated in these two protocols, and 19 were alive and free of disease after 6–68 months (median = 26 months) (237). Fourteen of these patients had a second-look laparotomy, and all findings were negative. Another study at M.D. Anderson Hospital (238) used BEP for 14 patients with residual disease, and all patients were free of disease with long-term follow-up. These results suggest that patients with advanced-stage, incompletely resected dysgerminoma have an excellent prognosis when treated with *cisplatin*-based combination chemotherapy. The optimal regimen is unknown, but three to four cycles of BEP seem sufficient.

There seems to be no need to perform a second-look laparotomy for patients with dysgerminoma whose macroscopic disease has all been resected at the primary operation (232). For patients with extensive macroscopic residual disease at the start of chemotherapy, a second-look operation could be used because effective second-line therapy is available, and because the earlier persistent disease is identified, the better the prognosis should be.

Recurrent Disease

About 75% of recurrences occur within the first year after initial treatment (222), the most common sites being the peritoneal cavity and the retroperitoneal lymph nodes. These patients should be treated with either radiation or chemotherapy, depending on their primary treatment. Patients with recurrent disease who have had no therapy other than surgery should be treated with chemotherapy. If prior chemotherapy with BEP has been given, POMB-ACE may be used (Table 33.6), and consideration should be given to the use of high-dose chemotherapy (e.g., with *carboplatin* and *etoposide*) and autologous bone marrow transplantation. Alternatively, radiation therapy is effective for this disease; the major disadvantage is loss of fertility if pelvic and abdominal radiation is required.

Pregnancy

Because dysgerminomas tend to occur in young patients, they may coexist with pregnancy. When a stage Ia cancer is found, the tumor can be removed intact and the pregnancy continued. For patients with more advanced disease, continuation of the pregnancy depends on gestational age. Chemotherapy can be given in the second and third trimesters in the same dosages as given for the nonpregnant patient without apparent detriment to the fetus (234).

Table 33.6   POMB/ACE Chemotherapy For Germ Cell Tumors of the Ovary

POMB

Day 1	*Vincristine* 1 mg/M² intravenously; *methotrexate* 300 mg/M² as a 12-hr infusion
Day 2	*Bleomycin* 15 mg as a 24-hr infusion: *folinic acid* rescue started at 24 hrs after the start of *methotrexate* in a dose of 15 mg every 12 hrs for 4 doses
Day 3	*Bleomycin* infusion 15 mg by 24-hr infusin
Day 4	*Cisplatin* 120 mg/M² as a 12-hr infusion, given together with hydration and 3 g magnesium sulfate supplementation

ACE

Days 1–5	*Etoposide* (VP16-213) 100 mg/M², days 1–5
Days 3, 4, 5	*Actinomycin D* 0.5 mg IV, days 3, 4, and 5
Day 5	*Cyclophosphamide* 500 mg/M² IV, day 5

OMB

Day 1	*Vincristine* 1 mg/M² intravenously; *methotrexate* 300 mg/M² as a 12-hr infusion
Day 2	*Bleomycin* 15 mg by 24-hr infusion; *folinic acid* rescue started at 24 hrs after start of *methotrexate* in a dose of 15 mg every 12 hrs for 4 doses
Day 3	*Bleomycin* 15 mg by 24-hr infusion

The sequence of treatment schedules is two courses of POMB followed by ACE. POMB is then alternated with ACE until patients are in biochemical remission as measured by hCG and AFP, PLAP and LDH. The usual number of courses of POMB is three to five. Following biochemical remission, patients alternate ACE with OMB until remission has been maintained for approximately 12 weeks. The interval between courses of treatment is kept to the minimum (usually 9 to 11 days). If delays are caused by myelosuppression after courses of ACE, the first 2 days of etoposide are omitted from subsequent courses of ACE. Reproduced with permission from **Newlands ES, Southall PJ, Paradinas FJ, Holden L.** Management of ovarian germ cell tumours. In: **Williams CJ, Kaikorian JG, Green MR, Ragharan D,** eds. *Textbook of Uncommon Cancer.* New York: John Wiley & Sons, 1988:47.

Prognosis

For patients whose initial disease is stage Ia (i.e., a unilateral encapsulated dysgerminoma), unilateral oophorectomy alone results in a 5-year disease-free survival rate of greater than 95% (226, 232–234, 239). The features that have been associated with a higher tendency to recurrence include lesions larger than 10–15 cm in diameter, age younger than 20 years, and a microscopic pattern that includes numerous mitoses, anaplasia, and a medullary pattern (221, 226).

Although in the past surgery for advanced disease followed by pelvic and abdominal radiation resulted in a 5-year survival rate of 63–83%, cure rates of 85–90% for this same group of patients are now being reported with the use of VBP or BEP combination chemotherapy (236–240).

Immature Teratomas

Immature teratomas contain elements that resemble tissues derived from the embryo. Immature teratomatous elements may occur in combination with other germ-cell tumors as mixed germ-cell tumors. The pure immature teratoma accounts for fewer than 1% of all ovarian cancers, but it is the second most common germ-cell malignancy. This lesion represents 10–20% of all ovarian malignancies seen in women younger than 20 years of age and 30% of the deaths from ovarian cancer in this age group (2). About 50% of pure immature teratomas of the ovary occur in women between the ages of 10 and 20 years, and they rarely occur in postmenopausal women.

Of fundamental importance in the understanding of the teratoma is a recognition of the maturation of the various elements. If maturation continues along normal lines, the mature or adult teratoma results, and the prognosis is excellent. Conversely, abnormal maturation of these elements produces undisciplined growth that can be fatal. Teratomas containing immature elements, although relative rate, have been recognized more commonly during the past two decades (Fig. 33.18). Among the tumors with embryonal elements, those containing neural tissues demonstrate most clearly the importance of the ability to mature.

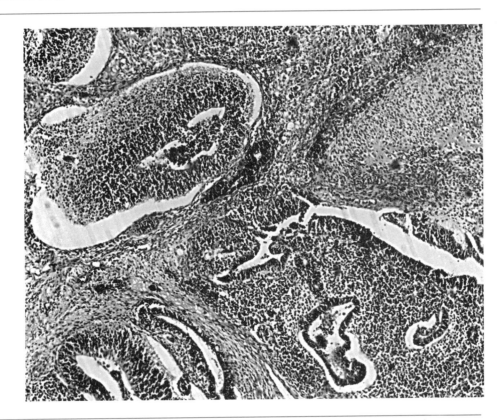

Figure 33.18   Ovarian teratoma. This tumor contains both mature and immature neural elements with a neural tube-like structure near its center. (Reproduced from **Berek JS, Hacker NF.** *Practical Gynecologic Oncology.* 2nd ed. Baltimore: Williams & Wilkins, 1994:150.)

Gliomatosis peritonei is the most dramatic demonstration of the significance of maturation, because most of these patients have survived, even with this disseminated disease.

Immature teratomas are classified according to a grading system (grades 1–3) that is based on the degree of differentiation and the quantity of immature tissue (241). **A determination of the amount of undifferentiated neural tissue is of prognostic importance. A grade 1 tumor is one in which <low-power microscopic field (LPF) contains immature neural elements, a grade 2 tumor has 1–3 LPFs with immature elements, and a grade 3 tumor has >3 LPFs with these elements. The prognosis can be correlated with the grade of these immature neural elements, i.e., with a higher grade, there is a poorer prognosis.**

Previously, most "malignant teratomas" have been classified as secondary neoplasms developing in a primarily benign teratoma. During the last decade, lesions composed primarily of immature embryonal or extraembryonal elements have become more prevalent, and the basic demonstration of malignancy is the inability of the tissue to mature rather than the presence of individual cell anaplasia, i.e., the mitotic activity may be low. This unique aspect is demonstrated by an absence of anueploidy in the few cases that have been studied.

Malignant change in benign cystic teratomas has been recorded as occurring in 1–2% of cases, usually after the 40 years of age (242). The most common malignancy developing in the initially benign teratoma is squamous cell carcinoma. Other neoplasms have been reported (e.g., melanomas, which may arise from the skin or retinal anlage, and sarcomas, including leiomyosarcomas and mixed mesodermal tumors). Carcinomas may arise from any of the epithelial elements.

Diagnosis

The preoperative evaluation and differential diagnosis of immature teratomas are the same as for other germ-cell tumors. Some of these lesions will contain calcifications similar to mature teratomas, which can be detected by an x-ray of the abdomen or by ultrasonography. Rarely, they are associated with the production of steroid hormones and can be accompanied by *sexual pseudoprecosity* (222). Tumor markers are negative unless a mixed germ-cell tumor is present.

Treatment

Surgery

For a premenopausal patient whose lesion appears to be confined to a single ovary, unilateral oophorectomy and surgical staging should be performed. For postmenopausal patients, a total abdominal hysterectomy and bilateral salpingo-oophorectomy may be performed. Contralateral involvement is rare, and routine resection or wedge biopsy of the contralateral ovary is unnecessary (241). Any lesions on the peritoneal surfaces should be sampled and submitted for histologic evaluation. The most frequent site of dissemination is the peritoneum and, much less commonly, the retroperitoneal lymph nodes. Bloodborne metastases to organ parenchyma, such as the lungs, liver, or brain, are uncommon. When present, they are usually seen in patients with late or recurrent disease and most often in tumors that are poorly differentiated (i.e., grade 3) (222).

Chemotherapy

Patients with stage Ia, grade 1, tumors have an excellent prognosis, and no adjuvant therapy is required. For patients whose tumors are stage Ia, grades 2 or 3, adjuvant chemotherapy should be used (222, 242). Chemotherapy is also indicated for patients who have ascites regardless of tumor grade. The most frequently used combination chemotherapeutic regimen in the past has been VAC (234, 239, 243–246). However, in a GOG study, the relapse-free survival rate in patients with incompletely resected disease was only 75% (222, 245). The newer approach has been to incorporate *cisplatin* into the primary treatment of these tumors, and most of the experience has been with the VBP and BEP regimens (236, 239, 240). No direct comparison of these regimens with VAC has been reported, but the BEP combination can save some patients who have persistent or recurrent disease after VAC (240, 246, 247).

The GOG has been prospectively studying three courses of BEP therapy for patients with completely resected stage I, II, and III ovarian germ cell tumors (248). Overall, the toxicity has been acceptable, and all 38 patients with nondysgerminomatous tumors treated (19 immature teratomas, 10 mixed, and 9 endodermal sinus tumors) are clinically free of disease. Thus, the BEP regimen, which is used more extensively for testicular cancer, seems to be superior to the VAC regimen in the treatment of completely resected nondysgerminomatous germ cells tumors of the ovary. Because some patients can progress rapidly, treatment should be initiated as soon as possible after surgery, preferably within 7–10 days (239).

The switch from VBP to BEP has been prompted by the experience in patients with testicular cancer, in which the replacement of vinblastine with etoposide has been associated with a better therapeutic index (i.e., equivalent efficacy and lower morbidity), especially less neurologic and gastrointestinal toxicity. Furthermore, the use of bleomycin seems to be important for this group of patients. In a randomized study of three cycles of *etoposide* plus *cisplatin* with or without *bleomycin* (EP vs. BEP) in 166 patients with germ-cell tumors of the testes, the BEP regimen had a relapse-free survival rate of 84% compared with 69% for the EP regimen (P = 0.03) (249). **In addition, cisplatin**

may be slightly better than carboplatin in the setting of metastatic germ-cell tumors. One hundred ninety-two patients with germ-cell tumors of the testes were entered into a study of four cycles of *etoposide* plus *cisplatin* (EP) versus four cycles of *etoposide* plus *carboplatin* (EC). There have been three relapses with the EP regimen versus seven with the EC regimen, although the overall survival of the two groups is identical thus far (250). **In view of these results, BEP is the preferred treatment regimen for patients with gross residual disease and is replacing the VAC regimen for patients with completely resected disease.**

Immature teratomas with malignant squamous elements seem to have a poorer prognosis than those tumors without these elements (251). The treatment in these patients is identical to that outlined for immature teratomas without these elements (i.e., chemotherapy with BEP regimen).

Radiation

Radiation therapy is generally not used in the primary treatment of patients with immature teratomas. Furthermore, there is no evidence that the combination of chemotherapy and radiation has a higher rate of disease control than chemotherapy alone. Radiation should be reserved for patients with localized persistent disease after chemotherapy (234, 241).

Second-Look Laparotomy

The need for a second-look operation has been questioned (239). It seems not to be jsutified in patients who have received chemotherapy in an adjuvant setting (i.e., stage Ia, grades 2 and 3), because chemotherapy in these patients is so effective. Second-look laparotomy in patients with macroscopic residual disease is of value at the start of chemotherapy, because there are no reliable tumor markers for this disease and such patients are at higher risk of failure (239, 252).

If a second-look operation is performed, sampling of any peritoneal lesions should be performed and the retroperitoneal lymph nodes should be evaluated carefully. If only mature elements are found during the second-look procedure, chemotherapy should be discontinued. If the presence of persistent immature elements is documented, alternative chemotherapy should be employed. An enlarged contralateral ovary may contain a benign cyst or a mature cystic teratoma, which may be managed with an ovarian cystectomy (222).

Prognosis

The most important prognostic feature of the immature teratoma is the grade of the lesion (220, 233, 253). In addition, the stage of disease and the extent of tumor at the initiation of treatment also have an impact on the curability of the lesion. Patients whose tumors have been incompletely resected before treatment have a significantly lower probability of 5-year survival than those whose lesions have been completely resected (i.e., 94% vs. 50%) (222). Overall, the 5-year survival rate for patients with all stages of pure immature teratomas is 70–80%, and it is 90–95% for patients with surgical stage I lesions (239–242).

The degree or grade of immaturity generally predicts the metastatic potential and curability. The 5-year survival rates for all stages combined have been reported to be 82%, 62%, and 30% for patients with grades 1, 2, and 3, respectively (241). Occasionally, these tumors are associated with mature or low-grade glial elements that have implanted throughout the peritoneum, and such patients usually have a favorable long-term survival (222).

Endodermal Sinus Tumor

Endodermal sinus tumors (EST) have also been referred to as "yolk sac carcinomas," because they are derived from the primitive yolk sac (221). These lesions are the third most frequent malignant germ-cell tumors of the ovary. Endodermal sinus tumors have a median age of 16–18 years (222). About one-third of the patients are premenarcheal at the time of initial presentation. Abdominal or pelvic pain is the most frequent presenting symptom, occurring in about 75% of patients, whereas an asymptomatic pelvic mass is documented in 10% of patients (238).

The gross appearance of an EST is soft grayish-brown. Cystic areas caused by degeneration are present in these rapidly growing lesions. The capsule is intact in most cases.

The endodermal sinus tumor is unilateral in 100% of cases; thus, biopsy of the opposite ovary in such young patients is contraindicated. The association of such lesions with gonadal dysgenesis must be appreciated, and chromosomal analysis should be performed preoperatively in premenarchael patients.

Microscopically, the characteristic feature is the endodermal sinus, or *Schiller-Duval body* (Fig. 33.19). The cystic space is lined with a layer of flattened or irregular endothelium into which projects a glomerulus-like tuft with a central vascular core. These structures vary throughout the tumor, and the reticular, myxoid elements represent undifferentiated mesoblast. The lining of the papillary infolding and the cavity is irregular, with an occasional cell containing clear, glassy cytoplasm, simulating the hobnail appearance of the epithelium in clear-cell tumors. The association of EST with dysgerminoma must be emphasized if diagnosis and therapy are to be optimal.

Most EST lesions secrete α-fetoprotein (AFP) and, rarely, they may elaborate detectable α-1-antitrypsin (AAT). Alpha-fetoprotein (AFP) can be demonstrated in the tumor by means of the immunoperoxidase technique. There is a good correlation between the extent of disease and the level of AFP, although discordance also has been observed. The serum

Figure 33.19   Endodermal sinus tumor of the ovary. Note the classic "Schiller-Duval body" with its central vessel and mantle of endoderm (*arrow*). (Reproduced with permission from **Berek JS, Hacker NF.** *Practical Gynecologic Oncology.* 2nd ed. Baltimore: Williams & Wilkins, 1994:151.)

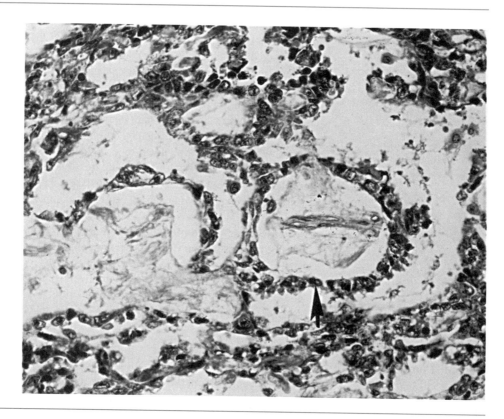

level of these markers, particularly AFP, is useful in monitoring the patient's response to treatment (253, 254).

| **Treatment** | ## Surgery |

The treatment of the EST consists of surgical exploration, unilateral salpingo-oophorectomy, and a frozen section for diagnosis. The addition of a hysterectomy and contralateral salpingo-oophorectomy does not alter outcome (222, 232). Any gross metastases should be removed if possible, but thorough surgical staging is not indicated because all patients need chemotherapy. At surgery, the tumors tend to be solid and large, ranging in size from 7 to 28 cm (median = 15 cm) in the GOG series (222, 246, 252). Because bilaterality is not seen in these lesions, the other ovary is involved with metastatic disease only when there are other metastases in the peritoneal cavity. Most patients have early-stage disease: 71%, stage I; 6%, stage II; and 23%, stage III (243).

Chemotherapy

All patients with endodermal sinus tumors are treated with either adjuvant or therapeutic chemotherapy. Befroe the routine use of combination chemotherapy for this disease, the 2-year survival rate was only about 25%. After the introduction of the VAC regimen, this rate improved to 60–70%, indicating the chemosensitivity of most of these tumors (243, 244). Furthermore, with conservative surgery and adjuvant chemotherapy, fertility can be preserved as with other germ-cell tumors.

VPB is a more effective regimen in the treatment of EST, particularly in the treatment of measurable of incompletely resected tumors (244, 245). In the GOG series, only about 20% of patients with residual metastatic disease responded completely to the VAC regimen, whereas about 60% of those treated with VBP had a complete response (240). In addition, this regimen may save some patients in whom VAC therapy has failed.

Workers at the Charing Cross Hospital in London have developed the POMB-ACE regimen for high-risk germ-cell tumors of any histologic type (255) (Table 33.7). This protocol introduces seven drugs into the initial management, which is intended to minimize the chances of developing drug resistance. Drug resistance, particularly relevant for patients with massive metastatic disease, and the POMB-ACE regimen may be used as primary therapy for such patients as well as for those with liver or brain metastases. The POMB schedule is only moderately myelosuppressive, so the intervals between each course can be kept to a maximum of 14 days (usually 9–11 days), thereby minimizing the time for tumor regrowth between courses. When bleomycin is given by a 48-hour infusion, pulmonary toxicity is reduced. With a maximum of 9 years of follow-up, the Charing Cross group has seen no long-term side effects for patients treated with POMB-ACE. Children have developed normally, menstruation has been physiologic, and several have completed normal pregnancies.

Cisplatin-containing combination chemotherapy, preferably BEP or POMB-ACE, should be used as primary chemotherapy for EST. The optimal number of treatment cycles has not been established. The GOG protocols have used three–four treatment cycles given every 4 weeks (237, 239, 240). Alternatively, three cycles can be given to patients with stage I and completely resected disease and two further cycles can be given after negative tumor marker status for patients with macroscopic residual disease before chemotherapy.

| **Second-Look Laparotomy** | The value of a second-look operation has yet to be established in patients with EST. It seems reasonable to omit the operation for patients with pure low-stage lesions and for patients whose AFP values return to normal and remain normal for the balance of their treat- |

ment (239, 252). There have been reported cases in which the AFP has returned to normal despite persistent measurable disease; some of these cases have been mixed germ-cell tumors (252). For patients whose AFP levels do not return to normal, persistent disease can be assumed and alternative chemotherapy (e.g., POMB-ACE) can be offered.

Embryonal Carcinoma

Embryonal carcinoma of the ovary is an extremely rare tumor that is distinguished from a choriocarcinoma of the ovary by the absence of syncytiotrophoblastic and cytotrophoblastic cells. The patients are very young; ages ranged between 4 and 28 years (median = 14 years) in two series (2, 253). Embryonal carcinomas may secrete estrogens, with the patient exhibiting symptoms and signs of precocious pseudopuberty or irregular bleeding (2). The presentation is otherwise similar to that of the EST. The primary lesions tend to be large, and about two-thirds are confined to one ovary at the time of presentation. These lesions frequently secrete AFP and hCG, which are useful for following the response to subsequent therapy (254). The treatment of embryonal carcinomas is the same as for the EST (i.e., a unilateral oophorectomy followed by combination chemotherapy with BEP) (234, 237–239). Radiation does not seem to be useful for primary treatment.

Choriocarcinoma of the Ovary

Pure nongestational choriocarcinoma of the ovary is an extremely rare tumor. Histologically, it has the same appearance as gestational choriocarcinoma metastatic to the ovaries (2). Most patients with this cancer are younger than 20 years of age. The presence of hCG can be useful in monitoring the patient's response to treatment. In the presence of high hCG levels, isosexual precocity has been seen to occur in about 50% of patients whose lesions appear before menarche.

There are only a few limited reports on the use of chemotherapy for nongestational choriocarcinomas, but complete responses have been reported with the MAC (*methotrexate, actinomycin D,* and *cyclophosphamide*) regimen used in a manner described for gestational trophoblastic disease (256) (see Chapter 35). Alternatively, the BEP regimen can be used (239, 248). The prognosis of ovarian choriocarcinomas has been poor, with most patients have metastases to organ parenchyma at the time of initial diagnosis (2, 257).

Polyembryoma

Polyembryoma of the ovary is another extremely rare tumor, which is composed of "embryoid bodies." This tumor replicates the structures of early embryonic differentiation (i.e., the three somatic layers: endoderm, mesoderm, and ectoderm) (2, 224). The lesion tends to occur in very young, premenarcheal girls with signs of pseudopuberty and elevated AFP and hCG titers. Anecdotally, the VAC chemotherapeutic regimen has been reported to be effective (218).

Mixed Germ-Cell Tumors

Mixed germ-cell malignancies of the ovary contain two or more elements of the lesions described above. In one series (258), the most common component of a mixed malignancy was dysgerminoma, which occurred in 80%, followed by EST in 70%, immature teratoma in 53%, choriocarcinoma in 20%, and embryonal carcinoma in 16%. The most frequent combination was a dysgerminoma and an EST. The mixed lesions may secrete either AFP, hCG, or both or neither of these markers, depending on the components.

These lesions should be managed with combination chemotherapy, preferably BEP. The serum marker, if positive initially, may become negative during chemotherapy, but this finding may reflect regression of only a particular component of the mixed lesion. Therefore, for these patients, a second-look laparotomy may be indicated to determine the precise response to therapy if macroscopic disease was present at initiation of chemotherapy.

The most important prognostic features are the size of the primary tumor and the relative amount of its most malignant component (258). For stage Ia lesions smaller than 10 cm, survival is 100%. Tumors composed of less than one-third EST, choriocarcinoma, or grade

3 immature teratoma also have an excellent prognosis, but it is less favorable when these components constitute most of the mixed lesions.

Sex Cord-Stromal Tumors

Sex cord-stromal tumors of the ovary account for about 5–8% of all ovarian malignancies (2, 221, 255). This group of ovarian neoplasms is derived from the sex cords and the ovarian stroma or mesenchyme. The tumors usually are composed of various combinations of elements, including the "female" cells (i.e., granulosa and theca cells), and "male" cells (i.e., Sertoli and Leydig cells), as well as morphologically indifferent cells. A classification of this group of tumors is presented in Table 33.7.

Granulosa-Stromal Cell Tumors

Granulosa-stromal cell tumors include granulosa cell tumors, thecomas, and fibromas. The granulosa cell tumor is a low-grade malignancy; rarely, thecomas and fibromas have morphologic features of malignancy and then may be referred to as *fibrosarcomas*.

Granulosa-cell tumors, which secrete estrogen, are seen in women of all ages. They are found in prepubertal girls in 5% of cases; the remainder are found in women throughout their reproductive and postmenopausal years (259). Granulosa-cell tumors are bilateral in only 2% of patients.

Granulosa-cell tumors range from a few millimeters to 20 cm or more in diameter. The tumors are rarely bilateral, and they have a smooth, lobulated surface. The solid portions of the tumor are granular, frequently traveculated, and are commonly yellow or gray-yellow in color. The graulosa-theca-cell tumor is probably the most inaccurately diagnosed lesion of the female gonad. Of 477 ovarian tumors from the Emil Novak Ovarian Tumor Registry diagnosed initially as granulosa-theca-cell tumors, almost 15% were reclassified after histologic review. Lesions misdiagnosed as granulosa-cell tumors included metastatic carcinomas, teratoid tumors, and poorly differentiated mesothelial tumors (260).

The classic granulosa cell is round or ovoid with scant cytoplasm. The nucleus contains compact, finely granular cytoplasm suggesting hyperchromatism. "Coffee-bean" grooved nuclei are common, as are mitoses, thus simulating the corresponding elements in the nor-

---

Table 33.7   Sex Cord-Stromal Tumors

1. Granulosa-stromal-cell tumors
    A. Granulosa-cell tumor
    B. Tumors in thecoma-fibroma group
        1) Thecoma
        2) Fibroma
        3) Unclassified

2. Androblastomas; Sertoli-Leydig-cell tumors
    A. Well-differentiated
        1) Sertoli cell tumor
        2) Sertoli-Leydig-cell tumor
        3) Leydig-cell tumor; hilus cell tumor
    B. Moderately differentiated
    C. Poorly differentiated (sarcomatoid)
    D. With heterologous elements

3. Gynandroblastoma

4. Unclassified

Modified and reprinted with permission from **Young RE, Scully RE.** Ovarian sex cord-stromal tumors: recent progress. *Int J Gynecol Pathol* 1980; 1:153.

mal, mature follicle. Conversely, if the "epithelial elements" are bizarre with atypical mitoses, the lesion should not be categorized as a "poorly differentiated granulosa cell tumor" but instead as an undifferentiated mesothelial neoplasm. In the most common variety, the granulosa cells show a tendency to arrange themselves in small clusters or rosettes around a central cavity, so there is a resemblance to primordial follicles (i.e., *Call-Exner bodies*) (Fig. 33.20). The stroma is similar to the theca and may be luteinized. Several histologic patterns have been described: 1) folliculoid, 2) diffuse, 3) cylindroid, 4) pseudoadenomatous, and 5) mixed (261). In children and adolescents, the granular-cell tumors are often cystic, contain luteinized cells, and are associated with precocious puberty.

Diagnosis

Of the rare prepubertal lesions, 75% are associated with sexual pseudoprecocity because of the estrogen secretion (259). For women of reproductive age, most patients have menstrual irregularities or secondary amenorrhea, and cystic hyperplasia of the endometrium is frequently present. For postmenopausal women, abnormal uterine bleeding is frequently the presenting symptom. Indeed, the estrogen secretion in these patients can be sufficient to stimulate the development of endometrial cancer. **Endometrial cancer occurs in association with granulosa-cell tumors in at least 5% of cases and 25%–50% are associated with endometrial hyperplasia** (2, 259, 262, 263).

The other symptoms and signs of granulosa-cell tumors are nonspecific and the same as most ovarian malignancies. Ascites is present in about 10% of cases, and rarely a pleural effusion is present (259, 261–263). Granulosa tumors tend to be hemorrhagic: occasionally, they rupture and produce a hemoperitoneum (263).

Figure 33.20   Granulosa cell tumor of the ovary. Note the classic "Call-Exner bodies" (*arrow*) with a minimal stromal component in this tumor of folliculoid pattern. (Reproduced with permission from **Berek JS, Hacker NF.** *Practical Gynecologic Oncology.* 2nd ed. Baltimore: Williams & Wilkins, 1994:153.)

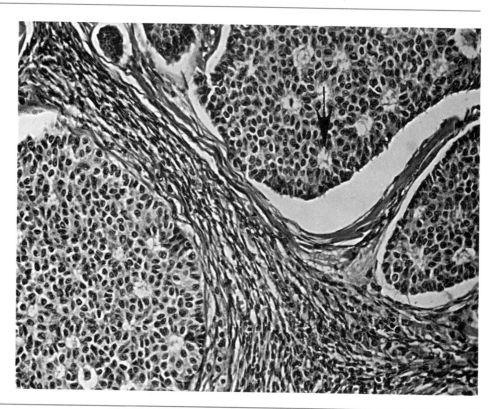

Granulosa-cell tumors are usually stage I at diagnosis but may recur 5–30 years after initial diagnosis (262). The tumors may also spread hematogenously, and metastases can develop in the lungs, liver, and brain years after initial diagnosis. When granulosa-cell tumors do recur, they can progress quite rapidly. Malignant thecomas are extremely rare, and their presentation, management, and outcome are similar to those of the granulosa-cell tumors (259, 262–265). Inhibin has been reported to be secreted by some granulosa-cell tumors and may be a useful marker for the disease (266).

Treatment

The treatment of granulosa-cell tumors depends on the age of the patient and the extent of disease. For most patients, surgery alone is sufficient primary therapy; radiation and chemotherapy are reserved for the treatment of recurrent or metastatic disease (263–265).

Surgery

Because granulosa-cell tumors are bilateral in only about 2% of patients, a unilateral salpingo-oophorectomy is appropriate therapy for stage Ia tumors in children or in women of reproductive age (262). At the time of laparotomy, if a granulosa-cell tumor is identified by frozen section, a staging operation is performed, including an assessment of the contralateral ovary. If the opposite ovary appears enlarged, it should be biopsied. For perimenopausal and postmenopausal women for whom ovarian preservation is not important, a hysterectomy and bilateral salpingo-oophorectomy should be performed. For premenopsual patients in whom the uterus is left *in situ,* a dilatation and curettage of the uterus should be performed, because of the possibility of a coexistent adenocarcinoma of the endometrium (258).

Radiation

There is no evidence to support the use of adjuvant radiation therapy for granulosa cell tumors (259), although pelvic radiation may help to palliate isolated pelvic recurrences (262).

Chemotherapy

There is no evidence that adjuvant chemotherapy will prevent recurrence of disease. Metastatic lesions and recurrences have been treated with a variety of antineoplastic drugs. There has been no consistently effective regimen for these patients, although complete responses have been reported anecdotally for patients treated with a single agent, *cyclophosphamide* or *melphalan,* as well as in those treated with the combinations VAC (*vincristine, doxorubicin, cyclophosphamide*) and PAC (*cisplatin, doxorubicin, cyclophosphamide*) (207). The AcFuCy regimen (*actinomycin D, 5-FU,* and *cyclophosphamide*) was used by the GOG and produced only a 20% partial response rate (222, 264). The use of hormonal agents such as progestins or antiestrogens has been suggested, but there are no data available to suggest effectiveness (262).

Prognosis

Granulosa-cell tumors have a prolonged natural history and a tendency toward late relapse, reflecting their low-grade biology. As such, 10-year survival rates of about 90% have been reported, with 20-year survival rates dropping to 75% (262). Most histologic types have the same prognosis, but the more poorly differentiated diffuse or sarcomatoid type tends to do worse (259).

The DNA ploidy of the tumors has recently been correlated with survival. Holland and colleagues (267) reported DNA aneuploidy in 13 of 37 patients (35%) with primary granulosa-cell tumors. The presence of residual disease was found to be the most important predictor of progression-free survival, but DNA ploidy was an independent prognostic factor.

Patients with residual-negative DNA diploid tumors had a 10-year progression-free survival of 96%.

Sertoli-Leydig Tumors

Sertoli-Leydig tumors occur most frequently in the third and fourth decades of life; 75% of the lesions are seen in women younger than 40 years. These lesions are extremely rare and account for less than 0.2% of ovarian cancers (2). Sertoli-Leydig-cell tumors are most frequently low-grade malignancies, although occasionally a poorly differentiated variety may behave more aggressively.

The tumors typically produce androgens, and clinical virilization is noted in 70–85% of patients (222). Signs of virilization include oligomenorrhea followed by amenorrhea, breast atrophy, acne, hirsutism, clitoromegaly, deepening of the voice, and a receding hairline. Measurement of plasma androgens may reveal elevated testosterone and androstenedione, with normal or slightly elevated dehydroepiandrosterone sulphate (222). Rarely, the Sertoli-Leydig tumor can be associated with manifestations of estrogenization (i.e., isosexual precocity, irregular or postmenopausal bleeding).

Treatment

Because these low-grade lesions are only rarely bilateral (<1%), the usual treatment is unilateral salpingo-oophorectomy and evaluation of the contralateral ovary for patients who are in their reproductive years (268). For older patients, hysterectomy and bilateral salpingo-oophorectomy are appropriate.

Data are insufficient to document the utility of radiation or chemotherapy for patients with persistent disease, but some responses in patients with measurable disease have been reported with pelvic radiation and the VAC chemotherapy regimen (222, 252).

Prognosis

The 5-year survival rate is 70–90%, and recurrences thereafter are uncommon (222, 256). Most fatalities occur in the presence of poorly differentiated lesions.

Uncommon Ovarian Cancers

There are several varieties of malignant ovarian tumors that together constitute only 0.1% of ovarian malignancies (2). Two of these lesions are the lipoid (or lipid) cell tumors and the primary ovarian sarcomas.

Lipoid-Cell Tumors

Lipoid-cell tumors are believed to arise in adrenal cortical rests that reside in the vicinity of the ovary. More than 100 cases have been reported, and bilaterally has been noted in only a few (2). Most are associated with virilization and, occasionally, with obesity, hypertension, and glucose intolerance reflecting glucocorticoid secretion. Rare cases of estrogen secretion and isosexual precocity have been reported.

Most of these tumors have benign or low-grade behavior, but about 20%, most of which are initially larger than 8 cm in diameter, develop metastatic lesions. Metastases are usually in the peritoneal cavity but rarely occur at distant sites (224). The primary treatment is surgical extirpation of the primary lesion. There are no data regarding the effectiveness of radiation or chemotherapy for this disease.

Sarcomas

Malignant mixed mesodermal sarcomas of the ovary are extremely rare; only about 100 cases have been reported. Most lesions are heterologous, and 80% occur in postmenopausal women. The presentation is similar to that of most ovarian malignancies. These lesions are biologically aggressive, and most patients have evidence of metastases.

There is no effective treatment for ovarian sarcomas, and most patients die within 2 years. *Doxorubicin,* with or without *cyclophosphamide,* has produced an occasional partial response, and cisplatin is currently undergoing clinical trials (269). For patients in whom all macroscopic disease can be resected, we have observed disease-free survival of more than 3 years in two patients treated with six cycles of *cisplatin* and *epirubicin.*

Metastatic Tumors

About 5–6% of ovarian tumors are metastatic from other organs, most frequently from the female genital tract, the breast, or the gastrointestinal tract (270). The metastases may occur from direct extension of another pelvic neoplasm, by hematogenous spread, lymphatic spread, or transcoelomic dissemination, with surface implantation of tumors that spread in the peritoneal cavity.

Gynecologic

Nonovarian cancers of the genital tract can spread by direct extension or they may metastasize to the ovaries. Tubal carcinoma involves the ovaries secondarily in 13% of cases (271), usually by direct extension. Under some circumstances, it is difficult to know whether the tumor originates in the tube or in the ovary when both are involved. Cervical cancer spreads to the ovary only in rare cases (<1%), and most of these are of an advanced clinical stage or are adenocarcinomas (272). Although adenocarcinoma of the endometrium can spread and implant directly onto the surface of the ovaries in as many as 5% of cases, two synchronous primary tumors probably occur with greater frequency. In these cases, an endometrioid carcinoma of the ovary is usually associated with the adenocarcinoma of the endometrium.

Nongynecologic

The frequency of metastatic breast carcinoma to the ovaries varies according to the method of determination, but the phenomenon is common (Fig. 33.21). **Autopsy data of women who die of metastatic breast cancer show that the ovaries are involved in 24% of cases and 80% of the involvement is bilateral** (273, 274). Similarly, when ovaries are removed to palliate advanced breast cancer, about 20–30% of the cases reveal ovarian involvement (60% bilaterally) (274). The involvement of ovaries in early-stage breast cancer seems to be considerably lower, but precise figures are not available. In almost all cases, either ovarian involvement is occult or a pelvic mass is discovered after other metastatic disease becomes apparent.

Krukenberg Tumor

The Krukenberg tumor, which can account for 30–40% of metastatic cancers to the ovaries, arises in the ovarian stroma and has characteristic mucin-filled, signet-ring cells (275) (Fig. 33.22). The primary tumor is most frequently located in the stomach and less commonly in the colon, breast, or biliary tract. Rarely, the cervix or the bladder may be the primary site (2). Krukenberg tumors can account for about 2% of ovarian cancers at some institutions, and they are usually bilateral. The lesions are usually not discovered until the primary disease is advanced, and therefore, most patients die of their disease within 1 year (275). In some cases, a primary tumor is not found.

Other Gastrointestinal

In other cases of metastasis from the gastrointestinal tract to the ovary, the tumor does not have the classic histologic appearance of a Krukenburg tumor; most of these are from the colon and, less commonly, the small intestine. As many as 1–2% of women with intestinal carcinomas will develop metastases to the ovaries during the course of their disease (276). Before exploration for an adnexal tumor in a woman older than 40 years of age, a barium enema is indicated to exclude a primary gastrointestinal carcinoma with metastases to the ovaries, particularly if there are any gastrointestinal symptoms. Metastatic colon cancer can mimic a mucinous cystadenocarcinoma of the ovary histologically (275, 276).

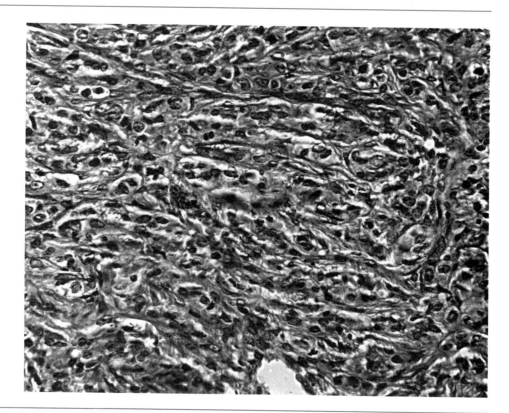

Figure 33.21 Metastatic carcinoma in the ovary. Note the "Indian file" pattern found in this metastatic breast carcinoma. (Reproduced with permission from **Berek JS, Hacker NF.** *Practical Gynecologic Oncology.* 2nd ed. Baltimore: Williams & Wilkins, 1994:157.)

Carcinoid

Metastatic carcinoid tumors represent fewer than 2% of metastatic lesions to the ovaries (277). Conversely, only about 2% of primary carcinoids have evidence of ovarian metastasis, and only 40% of these patients have the carcinoid syndrome at the time of discovery of the metastatic carcinoid. However, in perimenopausal and postmenopausal women explored for an intestinal carcinoid, it is reasonable to remove the ovaries to prevent subsequent ovarian metastasis. Furthermore, the discovery of an ovarian carcinoid should prompt a careful search for a primary intestinal lesion (277).

Lymphoma and Leukemia

Lymphomas and leukemia can involve the ovary. When they do, the involvement is usually bilateral (272, 278). About 5% of patients with Hodgkin's disease will have lymphomatous involvement of the ovaries, but this involvement occurs typically with advanced-stage disease. **With Burkitt's lymphoma, ovarian involvement is very common (279). Other types of lymphoma involve the ovaries much less frequently, and leukemic infiltration of the ovaries is uncommon.** Sometimes the ovaries can be the only apparent site of involvement of the abdominal or pelvic viscera with a lymphoma; if this circumstance is found, a careful surgical exploration may be necessary. Intraoperatively, a hematologist-oncologist should be consulted to determine the need for these procedures if frozen section of a solid ovarian mass reveals a lymphoma. In general, most lymphomas no longer require extensive surgical staging, although enlarged lymph nodes should generally be biopsied. In some cases of Hodgkin's disease, a more extensive evaluation may be necessary. Treatment involves that of the lymphoma or leukemia in general. Removal of a large ovarian mass may improve patient comfort and facilitate a response to subsequent radiation or chemotherapy.

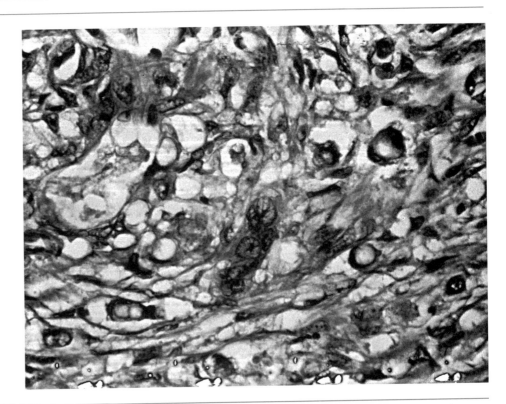

Figure 33.22   Krukenberg tumor of the ovary metastatic from a gastric carcinoma. Malignant cells have discrete vacuoles that push nuclei eccentrically, giving a signet-ring appearance. Nucicarmine stain demonstrates the cytoplasmic vacuoles to be mucin. (Reproduced with permission from **Berek JS, Hacker NF.** *Practical Gynecologic Oncology.* 2nd ed. Baltimore: Williams & Wilkins, 1994:158.)

Fallopian Tube Cancer

Carcinoma of the fallopian tube accounts for 0.3% of all cancers of the female genital tract (221, 271, 279). In histologic features and behavior, fallopian tube carcinoma is similar to ovarian cancer; thus, the evaluation and treatment are also essentially the same (Fig. 33.23). The fallopian tubes are frequently involved secondarily from other primary sites, most often the ovaries, endometrium, gastrointestinal tract, or breast. They may also be involved in primary peritoneal carcinomatosis. Almost all cancers are of "epithelial" origin, most frequently of serous histology. Rarely, sarcomas have also been reported.

Clinical Features

Tubal cancers are seen most frequently in the fifth and sixth decades, with a mean age of 55–60 years (221, 271). There are no known predisposing factors.

Symptoms and Signs

The classic triad of symptoms and signs associated with fallopian tube cancer is 1) a prominent watery vaginal discharge (i.e., *hydrops tubae profluens*); 2) *pelvic pain;* and 3) *a pelvic mass. However, this triad is noted in fewer than 15% of patients* (271).

Either vaginal discharge or bleeding is the most common symptom reported by patients with tubal carcinoma and is documented in more than 50% of patients (271, 280). Lower abdominal or pelvic pressure and pain also are noted in many patients. However, the presentation may be rather vague and nonspecific. For perimenopausal and postmenopausal women with an unusual, unexplained, or persistent vaginal discharge, even in the absence of bleeding, the clinician should be concerned about the possibility of an occult tubal cancer. Fallopian tube cancer is often found incidentally in asymptomatic women at the time of abdominal hysterectomy and bilateral salpingo-oophorectomy.

On examination, a pelvic mass is present in about 60% of patients, and ascites may be present if advanced disease exists. For patients with tubal carcinoma, the results of dilation and curettage will be negative (280), although abnormal or adenocarcinomatous cells may be seen in cytologic specimens obtained from the cervix in 10% of patients.

Tubal cancers spread in much the same manner as epithelial ovarian malignancies, principally by the transcoelomic exfoliation of cells that implant throughout the peritoneal cavity. In about 80% of the patients with advanced disease, metastases are confined to the peritoneal cavity at the time of diagnosis (281).

The fallopian tube is richly permeated with lymphatic channels, and spread to the para-aortic and pelvic lymph nodes is common. Metastases to the para-aortic lymph nodes have been documented in at least 33% of the patients with all stages of disease (282).

Staging

Although there is no official FIGO staging for tubal cancer, the ovarian staging system has been adapted to apply to fallopian tube disease (283). Thus, staging is based on the surgical findings at laparotomy (Table 33.8). According to this system, about 20–25% of patients have stage I disease, 20–25% have stage II disease, 40–50% have stage III disease, and 5–10% have stage IV disease (283). A somewhat lower incidence of advanced disease is seen in these patients than in patients with epithelial ovarian carcinomas, presumably because of the earlier occurrence of symptoms, particularly vaginal bleeding or unusual vaginal discharge.

Treatment

The treatment of this disease is similar to that of epithelial ovarian cancer (280–283). Exploratory laparotomy is necessary to remove the primary tumor, to stage the disease, and to resect metastases. After surgery, the most frequently employed treatment is combination chemotherapy, although radiation is also used in selected cases.

Surgery

Patients with tubal carcinoma should undergo total abdominal hysterectomy and bilateral salpingo-oophorectomy (221). If there is no evidence of gross tumor spread, a staging op-

Table 33.8   Surgical Stage of Fallopian Tube Cancer

Stage I	Carcinoma confined to fallopian tube(s)	
	Stage Ia	Unilateral disease; no ascites
	Stage Ib	Bilateral disease; no ascites
	Stage Ic	Either *a* or *b* with ascites and/or neoplastic cells in peritoneal washings
Stage II	Carcinoma extends beyond fallopian tube(s) but confined to pelvis	
	Stage IIa	Extension to uterus and/or ovary
	Stage IIb	Extension to other pelvic organs
	Stage IIc	Either *a* or *b* with ascites and/or neoplastic cells in peritoneal washings
Stage III	Carcinoma extends beyond pelvis but confined to abdominal cavity	
	Stage IIIa	Tumor microscopic only
	Stage IIIb	Tumor metastasis ≤2 cm
	Stage IIIc	Tumor metastasis >2 cm
Stage IV	Carcinoma extends beyond abdominal cavity	

Modified with permission from **Podratz KC, Podczaski ES, Gaffey TA, O'Brien PC, Schray MF, Malkasian GD Jr.** Primary carcinoma of the fallopian tube. *Am J Obstet Gynecol* 1986; 154:1319–26.

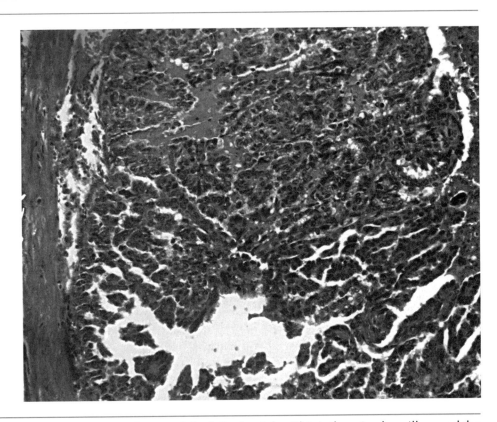

Figure 33.23   Carcinoma of the fallopian tube. This is the mixed papillary and the papillary alveolar pattern. (Reproduced with permission from **Berek JS, Hacker NF.** *Practical Gynecologic Oncology.* 2nd ed. Baltimore: Williams & Wilkins, 1994:159.)

eration is performed. The retroperitoneal lymph nodes should be adequately evaluated, and peritoneal cytologic studies and biopsies should be performed, along with an infracolic omentectomy.

In patients with metastatic disease, an effort should be made to remove as much tumor bulk as possible. The role of cytoreductive surgery in this disease is unclear, but extrapolation from the experience with epithelial ovarian cancer indicates that significant benefit might be expected, particularly if all macroscopic disease can be resected.

Chemotherapy

The most active single agents seem to be alkylating agents and *cisplatin*. Recent experience with *cisplatin* given in combination with *cyclophosphamide* (PC) or *doxorubicin* and *cyclophosphamide* (PAC) indicates that complete responses can be obtained (283). It seems justifiable, therefore, to use the same protocols that are used for epithelial ovarian cancer in patients with epithelial tubal malignancies, i.e., *paclitaxel* and *cisplatin*.

Data on well-staged lesions are scarce. Therefore, it is unclear whether patients with disease confined to the fallopian tube (i.e., a stage Ia, grade 1 or 2 carcinoma), benefit from additional therapy.

Radiation

Although most patients with tubal cancers have been treated with radiation in the past, the role of radiation in the management of the disease remains unclear because patients have not been treated in any consistent manner and the small numbers treated preclude any meaningful conclusions (280). Pelvic radiation alone was once popular, but this approach seems inappropriate when the pattern of spread of this disease to the upper abdomen is considered (279, 281, 282). Intarperitoneal ^{32}P has also been used, but these data are limited. More recently, whole-abdominal radiation with a pelvic boost has been used in patients with no evidence of gross disease in the abdomen (i.e., completely resected disease or microscopic metastases only). As with epithelial ovarian cancer, there may be a role in properly selected patients (281).

Prognosis

The overall 5-year survival for patients with epithelial tubal carcinomas is about 40%. This number is higher than for patients with ovarian cancer and reflects the somewhat higher proportion of patients with early-stage disease. The outlook is clearly related to the stage of disease, but the available data relate to patients who have not been surgically staged. Thus, the reported 5-year survival rate for patients with stage I disease is only about 65%. The 5-year survival rate for patients with stage II disease is 50–60%, but it is only 10–20% for patients with stages III and IV (271, 280, 281).

Tubal Sarcomas

Tubal sarcomas, particularly malignant mixed mesodermal tumors, have been described but are rare. They occur mainly in the sixth decade and are typically advanced at the time of diagnosis. If all gross disease can be resected, *cisplatin*-based combination chemotherapy should be tried. However, survival is generally poor, and most patients die of their disease within 2 years (269).

References

1. **Parker SL, Tong T, Bolden S, Wingo PA.** Cancer statistics, 1996. *CA–Cancer J Clin* 1996; 65:5–27.

2. **Scully RE.** *Tumors of the Ovary and Maldeveloped Gonads.* Fascicle 16. Washington, DC: Armed Forces Institute of Pathology, 1979.

3. **Julian CG, Goss J, Blanchard K, Woodruff JD.** Biologic behavior of primary ovarian malignancy. *Gynecol Oncol* 1974;44:873–84.

4. **Julian CG, Woodruff JD.** The biologic behavior of low-grade papillary serous carcinoma of the ovary. *Obstet Gynecol* 1972;40:860–7.

5. **Genadry R, Poliakoff S, Rotmensch J, Rosenshein NB, Parmley TH, Woodruff JD.** Primary, papillary peritoneal neoplasia. *Obstet Gynecol* 1981;58:730–4.

6. **Bell DA, Weinstock MA, Scully RE.** Peritoneal implants of ovarian serous borderline tumors: histologic features and prognosis. *Cancer* 1988;62:2212–22.

7. **Bell DA.** Ovarian surface epithelial-stromal tumors. *Hum Pathol* 1991;22:750–62.

8. **Bell DA, Scully RE.** Clinical perspectives on borderline tumors of the ovary. In: **Greer BE, Berek JS,** eds. *Gynecologic Oncology: Treatment Rationale and Techniques.* New York: Elsevier, 1991:119–34.

9. **McCaughey WT, Kirk ME, Lester W, Dardick I.** Peritoneal epithelial lesions associated with proliferative serous tumours of the ovary. *Histopathology* 1984;8:195–208.

10. **Michael H, Roth LM.** Invasive and noninvasive implants in ovarian serous tumors of low malignant potential. *Cancer* 1986;57:1240–7.

11. **Gershenson DM, Silva EG.** Serous ovarian tumors of low malignant potential with peritoneal implants. *Cancer* 1990;65:578–85.

12. **Bell DA, Scully RE.** Ovarian serous borderline tumors with stromal microinvasion: a report of 21 cases. *Hum Pathol* 1990;21:397–403.

13. **Sampson JA.** Endometrial carcinoma of the ovary. *Arch Surg* 1925;10:1.

14. **Kurman RJ, Craig JM.** Endometrioid and clear cell carcinomas of the ovary. *Cancer* 1972;29: 1653–64.

15. **Roth LM, Dallenbach-Hellweg G, Czernobilsky B.** Ovarian Brenner tumors. I. Metaplastic proliferating and of low grade potential. *Cancer* 1985;56:582–91.

16. **Robey SS, Silva EG, Gershenson DM, McLemore D, el-Naggar A, Ordonez NG.** Transitional cell carcinoma in high-grade stage ovarian carcinoma: an indicator of favorable response to chemotherapy. *Cancer* 1989;63:839–47.

17. **Silva EG, Robey-Cafferty SS, Smith TL, Gershenson DM.** Ovarian carcinomas with transitional cell carcinoma pattern. *Am J Clin Pathol* 1990;93:457–62.

18. **Austin RM, Norris HJ.** Malignant Brenner tumor and transitional cell carcinoma of the ovary: a comparison. *Int J Gynaecol Pathol* 1987;6:29–34.

19. **Thor AD, Young RH, Celement PB.** Pathology of the fallopian tube, broad ligament, peritoneum, and pelvic soft tissue. *Hum Pathol* 1991;22:856–67.

20. **Tobachman JK, Greene MH, Tucker MA, Costa J, Kase R, Fraumeri JF Jr.** Intraabdominal carcinomatosis after prophylactic oophorectomy in ovarian cancer-prone families. *Lancet* 1982;2:795–7.

21. **Bell DA, Scully RE.** Serous borderline tumors of the peritoneum. *Am J Surg Pathol* 1990;14:230–9.

22. **Fromm GL, Gershenson DM, Silva EG.** Papillary serous carcinoma of the peritoneum. *Obstet Gynecol* 1990;75:89–95.

23. **Truong LD, Maccato ML, Awalt H, Cagle PT, Schwartz MR, Kaplan AL.** Serous surface carcinoma of the peritoneum: a clinicopathology study of 22 cases. *Hum Pathol* 1990;21:99–110.

24. **Aure JC, Hoeg K, Kolstad P.** Clinical and histologic studies of ovarian carcinoma: long-term follow-up of 950 cases. *Obstet Gynecol* 1971;37:1.

25. **Norris HJ, Jensen RD.** Relative frequency of ovarian neoplasms in children and adolescents. *Cancer* 1972;30:713–9.

26. **Campbell S, Bhan V, Royston P, Whitehead MI, Collins WP.** Transabdominal ultrasound screening for early ovarian cancer. *BMJ* 1989;299:1363–7.

27. **Higgins RV, van Nagell JR Jr, Donaldson ES, Gallion HH, Pavlik EJ, Endicott B, et al.** Transvaginal sonography as a screening method for ovarian cancer. *Gynecol Oncol* 1989;34:402–6.

28. **van Nagell JR Jr, DePriest PD, Puls LE, Donaldson ES, Gallion HH, Pavlik EJ, et al.** Ovarian cancer screening in asymptomatic postmenopausal women by transvaginal sonography. *Cancer* 1991;68:458–62.

29. **Rulin MC, Preston AL.** Adnexal masses in postmenopausal women. *Obstet Gynecol* 1987;70:578–81.

30. **Kurjak A, Zalud I, Jurkovic D, Alfirevic Z, Miljan M.** Transvaginal color flow Doppler for the assessment of pelvic circulation. *Acta Obstet Gynecol Scand* 1989;68:131–5.

31. **Kurjak A, Zalud I, Alfirevic Z.** Evaluation of adnexal masses with transvaginal color ultrasound. *J Ultrasound Med* 1991;10:295–7.

32. **Zurawski VR, Broderick SF, Pickens P, Knapp RC, Bast RC Jr.** Serum CA125 levels in a group of nonhospitalized women: relevance for the early detection of ovarian cancer. *Obstet Gynecol* 1987;69:606–11.

33. **Jacobs I, Bast RC Jr.** The CA125 tumour associated antigen: a review of the literature. *Hum Reprod* 1989;4:1–12.

34. **Jacobs I, Stabile I, Bridges J, Kemsley P, Reynolds C, Grndzinskas J, et al.** Multimodal approach to screening for ovarian cancer. *Lancet* 1988;2:268–71.

35. **Zurawski VR Jr, Orjaseter H, Andersen A, Jellum E.** Elevated serum CA125 prior to diagnosis of ovarian neoplasia: relevance for early detection of ovarian cancer. *Int J Cancer* 1988;42:677–80.

36. **Zurawski VR Jr, Sjövall K, Schoenfeld DA, Broderick SF, Hall P, Bast RC Jr, et al.** Prospective evaluation of serum CA125 levels in a normal population, phase I: the specification of single and serial determinations in testing for ovarian cancer. *Gynecol Oncol* 1990;36:299–305.

37. **Einhorn N, Sjovall K, Knapp RC, Hall P, Scully RE, Bast RC Jr, et al.** A prospective evaluation of serum CA125 levels for early detection of ovarian cancer. *Obstet Gynecol* 1992;80:14–8.

38. **Jacobs I, Prys Davies A, Oram D.** Role of CA125 in screening for ovarian cancer. In: **Sharp F, Mason WP, Creasman W,** eds. *Ovarian Cancer. 2 Biology, Diangosis and Management.* London: Chapman and Hall Medical, 1992:265–75.

39. **Bourne TH, Whitehead MI, Campbell S, Royston P, Bhan V, Collins WP.** Ultrasound screening for familial ovarian cancer. *Gynecol Oncol* 1991;43:92–7.

40. **American College of Obstetricians and Gynecologists.** Genetic risk and screening techniques for epithelial ovarian cancer. ACOG Committee Opinion 117. Washington, DC: ACOG, 1992.

41. **Lynch HT, Harris RE, Guirgis HA, Maloney K, Carmody LL, Lynch JF.** Familial association of breast/ovarian carcinoma. *Cancer* 1978;41:1543–9.

42. **Lynch HT, Lynch PM.** Tumor variation in the cancer family syndrome: ovarian cancer. *Am J Surg* 1979;138:439–42.

43. **Lynch HT, Conway T, Lynch J.** Hereditary ovarian cancer. In: **Sharp F, Mason WP, Leake RE,** eds. *Ovarian Cancer: Biological and Therapeutic Challenges*. Cambridge: Chapman and Hall Medical, 1990:719–.

44. **Lynch HT, Watson P, Bewtra TA, Conway TA, Hipper CR, Kaur P, et al.** Hereditary ovarian cancer: heterogeneity in age at diagnosis. *Cancer* 1991;61:1460–6.

45. **Schildkraut JM, Thompson WD.** Familial ovarian cancer: a population-based case-control study. *Am J Epidemiol* 1988;128:456–66.

46. **Ponder BAJ, Easton DF, Peto J.** Risk of ovarian cancer associated with a family history: preliminary report of the OPCS study. In: **Sharp F, Mason WP, Leake RE,** eds. *Ovarian Cancer: Biological and Therapeutic Challenges*. Cambridge: Chapman and Hall Medical, 1990:3.

47. **Miki Y, Swensen J, Shattuck-Eidens D, Futreal A, Harshman K, Tautigian S, et al.** A strong candidate for the breast and ovarian cancer susceptibility gene BRCA1. *Science* 1994;266:66–71.

48. **Easton DF, Ford D, Bishop DT, and the Breast Cancer Linkage Consortium.** Breast and ovarian cancer incidence in BRCA 1-mutation carriers. *Am J Hum Genet* 1995;56:265–71.

49. **Barber HK, Graber EA.** The PMPO syndrome (postmenopausal palpable ovary syndrome). *Obstet Gynecol* 1971;38:921–3.

50. **Lewis E, Wallace S.** Radiologic diagnosis of ovarian cancer. In: **Piver MS,** ed. *Ovarian Malignancies*. Edinburgh: Churchill Livingstone, 1987:59–80.

51. **Hacker NF, Berek JS, Lagasse LD.** Gastrointestinal operations in gynecologic oncology. In: **Knapp RE, Berkowitz RS,** eds. *Gynecologic Oncology*. 2nd ed. New York: McGraw-Hill, 1993:361–75.

52. **Malkasian GD, Knapp RC, Lavin PT, Zurawski UR Jr, Podratz KC, Stanhope CR, et al.** Preoperative evaluation of serum CA125 levels in premenopausal and postmenopausal patients with pelvic masses: discrimination of benign from malignant disease. *Am J Obstet Gynecol* 1988;159:341–6.

53. **Plentl AM, Friedman EA.** *Lymphatic System of the Female Genitalia*. Philadelphia: WB Saunders; 1971.

54. **Burghardt E, Hellmuth P, Lahousen M, Stettner H.** Pelvic lymphadenectomy in operative treatment of ovarian cancer. *Am J Obstet Gynecol* 1986;155:315–9.

55. **Chen SS, Lee L.** Incidence of paraaortic and pelvic lymph node metastasis in epithelial ovarian cancer. *Gynecol Oncol* 1983;16:95–100.

56. **Dauplat J, Hacker NF, Neiberg RK, Berek JS, Rose TP, Sagae S.** Distant metastasis in epithelial ovarian carcinoma. *Cancer* 1987;60:1561–6.

57. **Krag KJ, Canellos GP, Griffiths CT, Knapp RC, Parker LM, Welch WR, et al.** Predictive factors for long term survival in patients with advanced ovarian cancer. *Gynecol Oncol* 1989;34:88–93.

58. **Young RC, Walton LA, Ellenberg SS, Homesley HD, Wilbanks GD, Decker DG, et al.** Adjuvant therapy in stage I and stage II epithelial ovarian cancer: results of two prospective randomized trials. *N Engl J Med* 1990;322:1021–7.

59. **Bjorkholm E, Pettersson F, Einhorn N, Krebs I, Nilsson B, Tjernberg B.** Long term follow-up and prognostic factors in ovarian carcinoma. The Radiumhemmet series 1958 to 1973. *Acta Radiol Oncol* 1982;21:413–9.

60. **Malkasian GD, Decker DG, Webb MJ.** Histology of epithelial tumours of the ovary: clinical usefulness and prognostic significance of histologic classification and grading. *Semin Oncol* 1975;2:191–201.

61. **Silverberg SG.** Prognostic significance of pathologic features of ovarian carcinoma. *Curr Top Pathol* 1989;78:85–109.

62. **Jacobs AJ, Deligdisch L, Deppe G, Cohen CJ.** Histologic correlations of virulence in ovarian adenocarcinoma. 1. Effects of differentiation. *Am J Obstet Gynecol* 1982;143:574–80.

63. **Baak JP, Langley FA, Talerman A, Delemarre JF.** Interpathologist and intrapathologist disagreement in ovarian tumor grading and typing. *Anal Quant Cytol Histol* 1986;8:354–7.

64. **Hernandez E, Bhagavan BS, Parmley TH, Rosenshein NB.** Interobserver variability in the interpretation of epithelial ovarian cancer. *Gynecol Oncol* 1984;17:117–23.

65. **Baak JP, Chan KK, Stolk JG, Kenemans P.** Prognostic factors in borderline and invasive ovarian tumours of the common epithelial type. *Pathol Res Pract* 1987;182:755–74.

66. **Friedlander ML, Heldey DW, Swanson C, Russell P.** Prediction of long term survivals by flow cytometric analysis of cellular DNA content in patients with advanced ovarian cancer. *J Clin Oncol* 1988;6:282–90.

67. **Friedlander ML, Taylor IW, Russell P, Musgrove EA, Hedley DW, Tattersall MH.** Ploidy as a prognostic factor in ovarian cancer. *Int J Gynaecol Pathol* 1983;1:55–63.

68. **Punnonen R, Kallioniemi OP, Mattila J, Koivula T.** Prognostic assessment in stage I ovarian cancer using a discriminant analysis with clinicopathological and DNA flow cytometric data. *Gynecol Obstet Invest* 1989;27:213–6.

69. **Murray K, Hopwood L, Volk D, Wilson JF.** Cytofluorometric analysis of the DNA content in ovarian cancer and its relation to patient survival. *Cancer* 1989;63:2456–60.

70. **Volm M, Bruggemann A, Gunther M, Kleine W, Pfleiderer A, Vogt-Schader M.** Prognostic relevance of ploidy, proliferation and resistance predictive tests in ovarian carcinoma. *Cancer Res* 1985;45:5180–5.

71. **Friedlander ML, Russell P, Taylor IN, Hedley DW, Tattersall MH.** Flow cytometric analysis of cellular DNA content as an adjunct to the diagnosis of ovarian tumours of borderline malignancy. *Pathology* 1984;16:301–6.

72. **Blumenfeld D, Braly PS, Ben-Ezra J, Klevecz RR.** Tumor DNA content as a prognostic feature in advanced epithelial ovarian carcinoma. *Gynecol Oncol* 1987;27:389–402.

73. **Khoo SK, Hurst T, Kearsley J, Dickie G, Free K, Parsons PG, et al.** Prognostic significance of tumor ploidy in patients with advanced ovarian carcinoma. *Gynecol Oncol* 1990;39:284–8.

74. **Kallioniemi OP, Punnonen R, Mattila J, Lehtinen M, Koivula T.** Prognostic significance of DNA index, multiploidy and S-phase fraction in ovarian cancer. *Cancer* 1988;61:334–9.

75. **Wils J, van Guens H, Baak J.** Proposal for therapeutic approach based on prognostic factors including morphometric and flow-cytometric features in stage III–IV ovarian cancer. *Cancer* 1988;61:1920–5.

76. **Conte PF, Alama A, Rubagotti A, Chiara S, Nicolin A, Nicolo R, et al.** Cell kinetics in ovarian cancer: relationship to clinicopathologic features, responsiveness to chemotherapy and survival. *Cancer* 1989;64:1188–91.

77. **Kuhn W, Kaufmann M, Feichter GE, Rummell HH, Schmid H, Heberling D.** DNA flow cytometry, clinical and morphological pararmeters as prognostic factors for advanced malignant and borderline tumors. *Gynecol Oncol* 1989;33:360–7.

78. **Slamon DJ, Godolphin W, Jones LA, Hoh JA, Wong SG, Keith DE, et al.** Studies of the HER-2/*neu* protooncogene in human breast and ovarian cancer. *Science* 1989;244:707–12.

79. **Berchuck A, Kamel A, Whitakeer R, Kerns B, Olt G, Kinney R, et al.** Overexpression of HER-2/*neu* is assocaited with poor survival in advanced epithelial ovarian cancer. *Cancer Res* 1990;50:4087–9.

80. **Rubin SC, Finstad CL, Wong GY, Aldadrones L, Plante M, Lloyd KO.** Prognostic significance of HER-2/*neu* expression in advanced epithelial ovarian cancer: a multivariate analysis. *Am J Obstet Gynecol* 1993;168:162–9.

81. **Leary JA, Edwards BG, Houghton CRS.** Amplification of HER-2/*neu* oncogene in human ovarian cancer. *Int J Gynaecol Oncol* 1993;2:293–98.

82. **Dittrich C, Dittrich E, Sevelda P, Huder M, Salzer H, Grunt T.** Clonogenic growth in vitro: an independent biologic prognostic factor in ovarian carcinoma. *J Clin Oncol* 1991;9:381–8.

83. **Bertoncello I, Bradley TR, Campbell JJ, Day AJ, McDonald IA, McLeish GR, et al.** Limitations of the clonal agar assay for the assessment of primary human ovarian tumour biopsies. *Br J Cancer* 1982;45:803–11.

84. **Voest EE, van Houwelingen JC, Neijt JP.** A meta-analysis of prognostic factors in advanced ovarian cancer with median survival and overall survival measured with log (relative risk) as main objectives. *Eur J Cancer Clin Oncol* 1989;25:711–20.

85. **Swenerton KD, Hislop TG, Spinelli J, LeRiche JC, Yang N, Boyes DA.** Ovarian carcinoma: a multivariate analysis of prognostic factors. *Obstet Gynecol* 1985;65:264–70.

86. **van Houwelingen JC, ten Bokkel Huinink W, van der Burg ATM, van Oosterom AT, Neijt JP.** Predictability of the survival of patients with ovarian cancer. *J Clin Oncol* 1989;7:769–73.

87. **Omura GA, Brady MF, Homesley HD, Yordan E, Major FJ, Buchsbaum HJ, et al.** Long-term follow-up and prognostic factor analysis in advanced ovarian carcinoma: the Gynecologic Oncology Group experience. *J Clin Oncol* 1991;9:1138–50.

88. **Dembo AJ, Davy M, Stenwig AE, Behle EJ, Bush RS, Kjorstad K.** Prognostic factors in patients with stage I epithelial ovarian cancer. *Obstet Gynecol* 1990;75:263–73.

89. **Sjövall K, Nilsson B, Einhorn N.** Different types of rupture of the tumor capsule and the impact on survival in early ovarian cancer. *Int J Gynecol Cancer* 1994;4:333–6.

90. **Berek JS, Hacker NF.** Staging and second-look operations in ovarian cancer. In: **Alberts DS, Surwit EA,** eds. *Ovarian Cancer.* Boston: Martinus Nijhoff, 1985:109–27.

91. **Young RC, Decker DG, Wharton JT, Piver MS, Sindelar WF, Edwards BK, et al.** Staging laparotomy in early ovarian cancer. *JAMA* 1983;250:3072–6.

92. **Buchsbaum HJ, Lifshitz S.** Staging and surgical evaluation of ovarian cancer. *Semin Oncol* 1984;11:227–37.

93. **Yoshimuna S, Scully RE, Bell DA, Taft PD.** Correlation of ascitic fluid cytology with histologic findings before and after treatment of ovarian cancer. *Am J Obstet Gynecol* 1984;148:716–21.

94. **Piver MS, Barlow JJ, Lele SB.** Incidence of subclinical metastasis in stage I and II ovarian carcinoma. *Obstet Gynecol* 1978;52:100–4.

95. **Delgado G, Chun B, Caglar H.** Paraaortic lymphadenectomy in gynecologic malignancies confined to the pelvis. *Obstet Gynecol* 1977;50:418–23.

96. **Rosenoff SH, Young RC, Anderson T, Bagley C, Chabner B, Schein PS, et al.** Peritoneoscopy: a valuable staging tool in ovarian carcinoma. *Ann Intern Med* 1975;83:37–41.

97. **Knapp RC, Friedman EA.** Aortic lymph node metastases in early ovarian cancer. *Am J Obstet Gynecol* 1974;119:1013–7.

98. **Keetel WC, Pixley EL, Buchsbaum HJ.** Experience with peritoneal cytology in the management of gynecologic malignancies. *Am J Obstet Gynecol* 1974;120:174–82.

99. **Creasman WT, Rutledge F.** The prognostic value of peritoneal cytology in gynecologic malignant disease. *Am J Obstet Gynecol* 1971;110:773–81.

100. **Guthrie D, Davy MLJ, Phillips PR.** Study of 656 patients with "early" ovarian cancer. *Gynecol Oncol* 1984;17:363–9.

101. **Bostwick DG, Tazelaar HD, Ballon SC, Hendrickson MR, Kempson RL.** Ovarian epithelial tumors of borderline malignancy: a cliniical and pathologic study of 109 cases. *Cancer* 1986;58:2052–65.

102. **Lim-Tan SK, Cajigas HE, Scully RE.** Ovarian cystectomy for serous borderline tumors: a follow-up study of 35 cases. *Obstet Gynecol* 1988;72:775–81.

103. **Hreshchyshyn MM, Park RC, Blessing JA, Norris HJ, Levy D, Lagasse LD, et al.** The role of adjuvant therapy in Stage I ovarian cancer. *Am J Obstet Gynecol* 1980;138:139–45.

104. **Greene MH, Boice JD, Greer BE, Blessing JA, Dembo AJ.** Acute nonlymphocytic leukemia after therapy with alkylating agents for ovarian cancer. *N Engl J Med* 1982;307:1416–21.

105. **Young RC, Knapp RC, Di Saia PJ, Fuks Z.** Cancer of the ovary. In: **DeVita VT, Hellman S, Rosenberg SA,** eds. *Principles and Practices of Oncology.* Philadelphia: JB Lippincott, 1985:1083–117.

106. **Dembo AJ, Bush RS, DeBoer G.** Therapy in stage I ovarian cancer. *Am J Obstet Gynecol* 1981;14:231–3.

107. **Bolis G, Marsoni S, Chiari N, Colombo M, Franchi F, Landoni, W. et al.** Cooperative randomized clinical trial for stage I ovarian carcinoma. In: **Conte PF, Ragni N, Rosso R, Vermorken JB,** eds. *Multimodal Treatment of Ovarian Cancer.* New York: Raven Press, 1989;20:81–86.

108. **Piver MS, Barlow JJ, Lele SB, Bakshi S, Parthasarathy KL, Bender MA.** Intraperitoneal chromic phosphate in peritoneoscopically confirmed Stage I ovarian adenocarcinoma. *Am J Obstet Gynecol* 1982;144:836–40.

109. **Dembo AJ, Bush RS, Beale FA, Pringle JF, Sturgeon JF.** The Princess Margaret Hospital study of ovarian cancer: stages I, II and asymptomatic III presentations. *Cancer Treat Rep* 1979;63:249–54.

110. **Griffiths CT.** Surgical resection of tumor bulk in the primary treatment of ovarian carcinoma. *Natl Cancer Inst Monogr* 1975;42:101–4.

111. **Hacker NF, Berek JS.** Cytoreductive surgery in ovarian cancer. In: **Albert PS, Surwit EA,** eds. *Ovarian Cancer.* Boston: Martinus Nijhoff, 1986:53–67.

112. **Heintz APM, Berek JS.** Cytoreductive surgery in ovarian cancer. In: **Piver MS,** eds. *Ovarian Cancer.* Edinburgh: Churchill Livingstone, 1987:129–43.

113. **Hacker NF, Berek JS, Lagasse LD, Nieberg RK, Elashoff RM.** Primary cytoreductive surgery for epithelial ovarian cancer. *Obstet Gynecol* 1983;61:413–20.

114. **Van Lindert AM, Alsbach GJ, Barents JW, Heintz APM, Kooyman C.** The role of the abdominal radical tumor reduction procedure (ARTR) in the treatment of ovarian cancer. In: **Heintz APM, Griffiths CT, Trimbos JB,** eds. *Surgery in Gynecologic Oncology.* The Hague, Netherlands: Martinus Nijhoff, 1984:275–87.

115. **Hoskins WJ, Bundy BN, Thigpen TJ, Omura GA.** The influence of cytoreductive surgery on recurrence-free interval and survival in small volume stage III epithelial ovarian cancer: a Gynecologic Oncology Group study. *Gynecol Oncol* 1992;47:159–66.

116. **Farias-Eisner R, Teng F, Oliveira M, Leuchter R, Karlan B, Lagasse LD, Berek JS.** The influence of tumor grade, distribution and extent of carcinomatosis in minimal residual stage III epithelial ovarian cancer after optimal primary cytoreductive surgery. *Gynecol Oncol* 1995;5:108–10.

117. **Skipper HE.** Adjuvant chemotherapy. *Cancer* 1978;41:936–40.

118. **Goldie JH, Coldman AJ.** A mathematical model for relating the drug sensitivity of tumors to their spontaneous mutation rate. *Cancer Treat Rep* 1979;63:1727–33.

119. **Bookman M, Berek JS.** Biologic and immunologic therapy of ovarian cancer. *Hematol Oncol Clin North Am* 1992;6:941–65.

120. **Hunter RW, Alexander NDE, Soutter WP.** Meta-analysis of surgery in advanced ovarian carcinoma: is maximum cytoreductive surgery an independent determinant of prognosis. *Am J Obstet Gynecol* 1992;166:504–11.

121. **van der Burg MEL, van Lent M, Buyse M, Kobierska A, Colombo N, Favalli G, et al.** The effect of debulking surgery after induction chemotherapy on the prognosis in advanced epithelial ovarian cancer: an EROTC Gynecologic Cancer Cooperative Group study. *N Engl J Med* 1995;332:629–34.

122. **Berek JS.** Interval debulking of epithelial ovarian cancer: an interim measure. *N Engl J Med* 1995;332:675–7.

123. **Berek JS, Hacker NF, Lagasse LD.** Rectosigmoid colectomy and reanastamosis to facilitate resection of primary and recurrent gynecologic cancer. *Obstet Gynecol* 1984;64:715–20.

124. **Berek JS, Hacker NF, Lagasse LD, Leuchter RS.** Lower urinary tract resection as part of cytoreductive surgery for ovarian cancer. *Gynecol Oncol* 1982;13:87–92.

125. **Heintz AM, Hacker NF, Berek JS, Rose TP, Munoz AK, Lagasse LD.** Cytoreductive surgery in ovarian carcinoma: feasibility and morbidity. *Obstet Gynecol* 1986;67:783–8.

126. **Deppe G, Malviya VK, Boike G, Hampton A.** Surgical approach to diaphragmatic metastases from ovarian cancer. *Gynecol Oncol* 1986;24:258–60.

127. **Montz FJ, Schlaerth J, Berek JS.** Resection of diaphragmatic peritoneum and muscle: role in cytoreductive surgery for ovarian carcinoma. *Gynecol Oncol* 1989;35:338–40.

128. **Brand E, Pearlman N.** Electrosurgical debulking of ovarian cancer: a new technique using the argon beam coagulator. *Gynecol Oncol* 1990;39:115–8.

129. **Deppe G, Malviya VK, Boike G, Malone JM Jr.** use of Cavitron surgical aspirator for debulking of diaphragmatic metastases in patients with advanced carcinoma of the ovaries. *Surg Gynecol Obstet* 1989;168:455–6.

130. **Chen SS, Bochner R.** Assessment of morbidity and mortality in primary cytoreductive surgery for advanced ovarian cancer. *Gynecol Oncol* 1985;20:190–5.

131. **Venesmaa P, Ylikorkala O.** Morbidity and mortality associated with primary and repeat operations for ovarian cancer. *Obstet Gynecol* 1992;79:168–72.

132. **Smith JP, Day TG.** Review of ovarian cancer at the University of Texas Systems Cancer Center, M.D. Anderson Hospital and Tumor Institute. *Am J Obstet Gynecol* 1979;135:984–93.

133. **Thigpen JT.** Single agent chemotherapy in the management of ovarian carcinoma. In: **Alberts DS, Surwit EA,** eds. *Ovarian Cancer.* Boston: Martinus Nijhoff, 1985:115–46.

134. **Rowinsky EK, Czaenave LA, Donehower RC.** Taxol: a novel investigational antimicrotubule agent. *J Natl Cancer Inst* 1990;82:1247–59.

135. **Ozols RF.** Chemotherapy for advanced epithelial ovarian cancer. *Hematol Oncol Clin North Am* 1992;6:879–94.

136. **McGuire WP, Rowinsky EK, Rosensheim NE, Grumbine FC, Ettinger DS, Armstrong DK, et al.** Taxol: a unique antineoplastic agent with signficant activity in advanced ovarian epithelial neoplasms. *Ann Intern Med* 1989;111:273–9.

137. **Thigpen T, Blessing J, Ball H, Hummel S, Barrett R.** Phase II trial of Taxol as a second-line therapy for ovarian carcinoma: a Gynecologic Oncology Group study. *Proc Am Soc Clin Oncol* 1990;9:156.

138. **McGuire WP, Hoskins WJ, Brady MF, Kucera PR, Partridge EE, Look KY, et al.** Cyclophosphamide and cisplatin compared with paclitaxel and cisplatin in patients with stage III and stage IV ovarian cancer. *N Engl J Med* 1996;334:1–6.

139. **Manetta A, MacNeill C, Lyter JA, Scheffler B, Podczaski ES, Larson JE, et al.** Hexamethylmelamine as a second-line agent in ovarian cancer. *Gynecol Oncol* 1990;36:93–6.

140. **Ozols RF, Ostchega Y, Curt G, Young RC.** High-dose carboplatin in refractory ovarian cancer patients. *J Clin Oncol* 1987;5:197–201.

141. **Markman M, Rothman R, Hakes T, Reichman B, Hoskins W, Rubin S, et al.** Second-line platinum therapy in patients with ovarian cancer previously treated with cisplatin. *J Clin Oncol* 1991;9:389–93.

142. **Advanced Ovarian Cancer Trialists Group.** Chemotherapy in advanced ovarian cancer: an overview of randomized clinical trials. *BMJ* 1991;303:884–93.

143. **Young RC, Chabner BA, Hubbard SP, Fisher RI, Bender RA, Anderson T, et al.** Advanced ovarian adenocarcinoma: a prospective clinical trial of melphalan (L-PAM) versus combination chemotherapy. *N Engl J Med* 1978;299:1261–6.

144. **Lambert HE, Berry RJ.** High dose cisplatin compared with high dose cyclophosphamide in the management of advanced epithelial ovarian cancer (FIGO Stages III and IV): report from the North Thames Cooperative Group. *BMJ* 1985;290:889–93.

145. **Greco FA, Julian CG, Richardson RL.** Advanced ovarian cancer: brief intensive combination chemotherapy and second-look laparotomy. *Obstet Gynecol* 1981;58:202–35.

146. **Neijt JP, ten Bokkel Huinink WW, van der Burg ME, van Oosterom AT, Vriesendorp R, Kooyman CD et al.** Randomised trial comparing two combination chemotherapy regimens (Hexa-CAF vs. CHAP-5) in advanced ovarian carcinoma. *Lancet* 1984;2:594–600.

147. **Ehrlich EC, Einhorn L, Williams SD, Morgan J.** Chemotherapy for stage III–IV epithelial ovarian cancer with cis-dichlorodiamineplatinum (II), Adriamycin, and cyclophosphamide: a preliminary report. *Cancer Treat Rep* 1979;63:281–8.

148. **Neijt JP, ten Bokkel Huinink WW, van der Burg MET, van Oosterman AT, Willemse PH, Heintz AP, et al.** Randomized trial comparing two combination chemotherapy regimens (CHAP-5 versus CP) in advanced ovarian carcinoma: a randomized trial of the Netherlands joint study group for ovarian cancer. *J Clin Oncol* 1987;5:1157–68.

149. **Edmonson JH, McCormack GW, Weiand HS.** Late emerging survival differences in a comparative study of HCAP versus CP in stage III–IV ovarian carcinoma. In: **Salmon S,** ed. *Adjuvant Therapy of Cancer.* Philadelphia: WB Saunders, 1990:512–21.

150. Hainsworth JD, Grosh WW, Burnett LS, Jones HW, Wolff SN, Greco FA, et al. Advanced ovarian cancer: long term results of treatment with intensive cisplatin based chemotherapy of brief duration. *Ann Intern Med* 1988;108:165–70.

151. Omura G, Bundy B, Berek JS, Curry S, Delgado G, Mortel R. Randomized trial of cyclophosphamide plus cisplatin with or without doxorubicin in ovarian carcinoma: a Gynecologic Oncology Group study. *J Clin Oncol* 1989;7:457–65.

152. Bertelsen K, Jacobsen A, Andersen JE, Ahrons S, Pedersen PH, Kiaer H, et al. A randomized study of cyclophosphamide and cisplatin with or without doxorubicin in advanced ovarian cancer. *Gynecol Oncol* 1987;28:161–9.

153. Conte PF, Bruzzone M, Chiara S, Sertoli MR, Daga MG, Rubagotti A, et al. A randomized trial comparing cisplatin plus cyclophosphamide versus cisplatin, doxorubicin and cyclophosphamide in advanced ovarian cancer. *J Clin Oncol* 1986;4:965–71.

154. Gruppo Interegionale Cooperativo Oncologico Ginecologia. Randomized comparison of cisplatin with cyclophosphamide/cisplatin with cyclophosphamide/doxorubicin/cisplatin in advanced ovarian cancer. *Lancet* 1987;2:353–9.

155. Ovarian Cancer Meta-Analysis Project. Cyclophosphamide plus cisplatin versus cyclophosphamide, doxorubicin, and cisplatin chemotherapy of ovarian carcinoma: a meta-analysis. *J Clin Oncol* 1991;9:1668–74.

156. McGuire WP, Hoskins WJ, Brady MS, Homesley HD, Creasman WT, Berman ML, et al. Assessment of dose-intensive therapy in suboptimally debulked ovarian cancer: a Gynecologic Oncology Group Study. *J Clin Oncol* 1995;13:1589–99.

157. Kaye SB, Lewis CR, Paul J, Duncan ID, Gordon HK, Kitchener HC, et al. Randomized study of two doses of cisplatin with cyclophosphamide in epithelial ovarian cancer. *Lancet* 1992;340:329–33.

158. Alberts DS, Liu PY, Hannigan EV, O'Toole R, Williams SD, Young J, et al. Phase II study of intraperitoneal cisplatin/IV cyclophosphamide versus IV cisplatin/IV cyclophosphamide in patients with optimal disease stage III ovarian cancer: A SWOG-GOG-ECOG Intergroup Study (INT 0051). *Proc Am Soc Clin Oncol* 1995;Abstract 760.

159. Calvert AH, Newall DR, Gumbrell LA, O'Reilly S, Burnell M, Boxall FE, et al. Carboplatin dosage: prospective evaluation of a simple formula based on renal function. *J Clin Oncol* 1989;7:1748–56.

160. Alberts DS, Green S, Hannigan EV, O'Toole R, Stock-Novack D, Anderson P, et al. Improved therapeutic index of carboplatin plus cyclophosphamide versus cisplatin plus cyclophosphamide: final report by the Southwest Oncology Group of a phase III randomized trial in stages III (suboptimal) and IV ovarian cancer. *J Clin Oncol* 1992;10:706–17.

161. Swenerton K, Jeffrey J, Stuart G, Roy M, Krepart G, Carmichael J, et al. Cisplatin-cyclophosphamide versus carboplatin-cyclophosphamide in advanced ovarian cancer: a randomized phase III study of the Natioinal Cancer Institute of Canada Clinical Trials Group. *J Clin Oncol* 1992;10:718–26.

162. Sarosy G, Kohn E, Stone DA, Rothenberg M, Jacob J, Adamo DO, et al. Phase I study of Taxol and granulocyte colony-stimulating factor in patients with refractory ovarian cancer. *J Clin Oncol* 1992;10:1165–70.

163. Reed E, Janik J, Bookman MA, Rothenberg M, Smith J, Young RC, et al. High-dose carboplatin and recombinant granulocyte-macrophage colony-stimulating factor in advanced-stage recurrent ovarian cancer. *J Clin Oncol* 1993;11:2118–26.

164. Rothenberg ML, Ozols RF, Glatstein E, Steinberg SM, Reed E, Young RC. Dose-intensive induction therapy with cyclophosphamide, cisplatin and consolidative abdominal radiation in advanced stage epithelial cancer. *J Clin Oncol* 1992;10:727–34.

165. Rendina GM, Donadio C, Giovanni M. Steroid receptors and progestinic therapy in ovarian endometrioid carcinoma. *Eur J Gynaecol Oncol* 1982;3:241–6.

166. Berek JS, Hacker NF, Lagasse LD, Poth T, Resnick B, Nieberg RK, et al. Second-look laparotomy in stage III epithelial ovarian cancer: clinical variables associated with disease status. *Obstet Gynecol* 1984;64:207–12.

167. Schwartz PE, Smith JP. Second-look operation in ovarian cancer. *Am J Obstet Gynecol* 1980;138:1124–30.

168. Webb MJ, Snyder JA, Williams TJ, Decker DG. Second-look laparotomy in ovarian cancer. *Gynecol Oncol* 1982;14:285–93.

169. **Cohen CJ, Goldberg JD, Holland JF, Bruckner HW, Deppe G, Gusberg SB.** Improved therapy with cisplatin regimens for patients with ovarian carcinoma (FIGO stages III and IV) as measured by surgical end-staging (second-look operation). *Am J Obstet Gynecol* 1983; 145:955–67.

170. **Barnhill DR, Hoskins JW, Heller PB, Park RC.** The second-look surgical reassessment for epithelial ovarian carcinoma. *Gynecol Oncol* 1984;19:148–54.

171. **Podratz KC, Malkasian GD, Hilton JF, Harris EA, Gaffey TA.** Second-look laparotomy in ovarian cancer: evaluation of pathologic variables. *Am J Obstet Gynecol* 1985;152:230–8.

172. **Copeland LJ, Gershenson DM, Wharton JT, Atkinson EN, Sneige N, Edwards CL, et al.** Microscopic disease at second-look laparotomy in advanced ovarian cancer. *Cancer* 1985;55:472–8.

173. **Gershenson DM, Copeland LJ, Wharton JT, Atkinson EN, Sneige N, Edwards CL, et al.** Prognosis of surgically determined complete responders in advanced ovarian cancer. *Cancer* 1985;55:1129–35.

174. **Smira LR, Stehman FB, Ulbright TM, Sutton GP, Ehrlich CE.** Second-look laparotomy after chemotherapy in the management of ovarian malignancy. *Am J Obstet Gynecol* 1985; 152:661–8.

175. **Freidman JB, Weiss NS.** Second thoughts about second-look laparotomy in advanced ovarian cancer. *N Engl J Med* 1990;322:1079–82.

176. **Berek JS.** Second-look versus second-nature. *Gynecol Oncol* 1992;44:1–2.

177. **Rubin SC, Hoskins WJ, Hakes TB, Markman M, Cain JM, Lewis JL Jr.** Recurrence after negative second-look laparotomy for ovarian cancer: analysis of risk factors. *Am J Obstet Gynecol* 1988;159:1094–8.

178. **Berek JS, Griffith CT, Leventhal JM.** Laparoscopy for second-look evaluation in ovarian cancer. *Obstet Gynecol* 1981;58:192–8.

179. **Berek JS, Hacker NF.** Laparoscopy in the management of patients with ovarian carcinoma. In: **DiSaia P,** ed. *The Treatment of Ovarian Cancer.* Philadelphia: WB Saunders, 1983: 213–22.

180. **Lele S, Piver MS.** Interval laparoscopy prior to second-look laparotomy in ovarian cancer. *Obstet Gynecol* 1986;68:345–7.

181. **Berek JS, Knapp RC, Malkasian GD, Lavin PT, Whitney C, Niloff JM, et al.** CA125 serum levels correlated with second-look operations among ovarian cancer patients. *Obstet Gynecol* 1986;67:685–9.

182. **Lavin PT, Knapp RC, Malkasian GD, Whitney CW, Berek JS, Bast RC Jr.** CA125 for the monitoring of ovarian carcinoma during primary therapy. *Obstet Gynecol* 1987;69:223–7.

183. **Brenner DE, Shaft MI, Jones HW, Grosh WW, Greco FA, Burnett LS.** Abdominopelvic computed tomography: evaluation in patients undergoing second-look laparotomy for ovarian carcinoma. *Obstet Gynecol* 1985;65:715–9.

184. **Berek JS, Hacker NF, Lagasse LD, Nieberg RK, Elashoff RM.** Survival of patients following secondary cytoreductive surgery in ovarian cancer. *Obstet Gynecol* 1983;61:189–93.

185. **Hoskins WJ, Rubin SC, Dulaney E, Chapman D, Almadrones L, Saigo P, et al.** Influence of secondary cytoreduction at the time of second-look laparotomy on the survival of patients with epithelial ovarian carcinoma. *Gynecol Oncol* 1989;34:365–71.

186. **Ozols RF, Ostchega Y, Myers CE, Young RC.** High dose cisplatin in hypertonic saline in refractory ovarian cancer. *J Clin Oncol* 1985;3:1246–50.

187. **Gershenson DM, Kavanagh JJ, Copeland LJ, Stringer CA, Morris M, Wharton JT.** Retreatment of patients with recurrent epithelial ovarian cancer with cisplatin-based chemotherapy. *Obstet Gynecol* 1989;73:798–802.

188. **Ozols RF, Ostchega Y, Curt G, Young RC.** High dose carboplatin in refractory ovarian cancer patients. *J Clin Oncol* 1987;5:197–201.

189. **Markman M, Rothman R, Hakes T, Reichman B, Hoskins W, Rubin S, et al.** Second-line platinum therapy in patients with ovarian cancer previously treated with cisplatin. *J Clin Oncol* 1991;9:389–93.

190. **Gore ME, Fryatt I, Wiltshaw E, Dawson T.** Treatment of relapsed carcinoma of the ovary with cisplatin or carboplatin following initial treatment with these compounds. *Gynecol Oncol* 1990;36:207–11.

191. **Sutton GP, Blessing JA, Homesley HD, Berman ML, Malfetano J.** Phase II trial of ifosfamide and mesna in advanced ovarian carcinoma: a Gynecologic Oncology Group study. *J Clin Oncol* 1989;7:1672–6.

192. **Markman M, Howell SB.** Intraperitoneal chemotherapy for ovarian cancer. In: **Alberts DS, Surwit EA,** eds. *Ovarian Cancer.* Boston: Martinus Nijhoff, 1985:179–212.

193. **Hacker NF, Berek JS, Pretorius G, Zuckerman J, Eisenkop S, Lagasse LD.** Intraperitoneal cisplatin as salvage therapy in persistent epithelial ovarian cancer. *Obstet Gynecol* 1987;70:759–64.

194. **Markman M, Howell SB, Lucas WE, Pfeifle CE, Green MR.** Combination intraperitoneal chemotherapy with cisplatin, cytarabine, and doxorubicin for refractory ovarian carcinoma and other malignancies principally confined to the peritoneal cavity. *J Clin Oncol* 1984;2:13–6.

195. **King ME, Pfeiffe CE, Howell SB.** Intraperitoneal cytosine arabinoside therapy in ovarian carcinoma. *J Clin Oncol* 1984;2:662–9.

196. **Howell SB, Pfeiffe CE, Wung WE, Olshen RA, Lucas WE, Yon JL, et al.** Intraperitoneal cisplatin with systemic thiosulfate protection. *Ann Intern Med* 1982;97:845–51.

197. **Howell SB, Kirmani S, Lucas WE, Zimm S, Goel R, Kim S, et al.** A phase II trial of intraperitoneal cisplatin and etoposide for primary treatment of ovarian epithelial cancer. *J Clin Oncol* 1990;8:137–45.

198. **Kirmani S, Lucas WE, Kim S, Goel R, McVey L, Morris J.** A phase II trial of intraperitoneal cisplatin and etoposide as salvage treatment for minimal residual ovarian carcinoma. *J Clin Oncol* 1991;9:649–57.

199. **Markman M, Hakes T, Reichman B, Lewis JL Jr, Rubin S, Jones W, et al.** Phase II trial of weekly or biweekly intraperitoneal mitoxantrone in epithelial ovarian cancer. *J Clin Oncol* 1991;9:978–82.

200. **Howell SB, Zimm S, Markman M, Abramson IS, Cleary S, Lucas WE, et al.** Long-term survival of advanced refractory ovarian carcinoma patients with small-volume disease treated with intraperitoneal chemotherapy. *J Clin Oncol* 1987;5:1607–12.

201. **Berek JS, Hacker NF, Lichtenstein A, Jung T, Spina C, Knox RM, et al.** Intraperitoneal recombinant alpha₂ interferon for "salvage" immunotherapy in stage III epithelial ovarian cancer immunotherapy in Stage III: a Gynecologic Oncology Group study. *Cancer Res* 1985; 45:4447–53.

202. **Willemse PHB, De Vries EGE, Mulder NH, Aalders JG, Bouma J, Sleijfer DT.** Intraperitoneal human recombinant interferon alpha-2b in minimal residual ovarian cancer. *Eur J Cancer* 1990;26:353–8.

203. **Nardi M, Lognetti F, Pallera F, Giulia MD, Lombardi A, Atlante GI, et al.** Intraperitoneal alpha-2-interferon alternating with cisplatin as salvage therapy for minimal residual disease ovarian cancer: a phase II study. *J Clin Oncol* 1990;6:1036–41.

204. **Bezwoda WR, Golombick T, Dansey R, Keeping J.** Treatment of malignant ascites due to recurrent/refractory ovarian cancer: the use of interferon-alpha or interferon-alpha plus chemotherapy. In vivo and in vitro observations. *Eur J Cancer* 1991;27:1423–9.

205. **Pujade-Lauraine E, Guastella JP, Colombo N, Naner N, Fumoleau P, Monnier A, et al.** Intraperitoneal recombinant human interferon gamma (IFNg) in residual ovarian cancer: efficacy is independent of previous response to chemotherapy. *Proc Am Soc Clin Oncol* 1991;713:225.

206. **Steis RG, Urba WJ, Vandermolen LA, Bookman MA, Smith JW 2d, Clark JW, eet al.** Intraperitoneal lymphokine-activated killer cell and interleukin 2 therapy for malignancies limited to the peritoneal cavity. *J Clin Oncol* 1990;10:1618–29.

207. **Markman M, Berek JS, Blessing JA, McGuire WP, Bell J, Homesley HD, et al.** Characteristics of patients with small-volume residual ovarian cancer unresponsive to cisplatin-based ip chemotherapy: lessons learned from a Gynecologic Oncology Group phase II trial of ip cisplatin and recombinant α-interferon. *Gynecol Oncol* 1992;45:3–8.

208. **Hacker NF, Berek JS, Burnison CM, Heintz PM, Juillard GJ, Lagasse LD.** Whole abdominal radiation as salvage therapy for epithelial ovarian cancer. *Obstet Gynecol* 1985;65: 60–6.

209. **Shea TC, Flaherty M, Elias A, Eder JP, Antman K, Begg C et al.** A phase I clinical pharmacokinetic study of carboplatin and autologous bone marrow support. *J Clin Oncol* 1989; 7:651–61.

210. **Stoppa A, Maraninchi D, Viens P.** High doses of melphalan and autologous marrow rescue in advanced common epithelial ovarian carcinomas: a retrospective analysis in 35 patients. In: **Nicke K, Spitzer G, Zander A,** eds. *Autologous Bone Marrow Transplantation: Proceedings of the Fourth International Symposium.* Houston: University of Texas Cancer Center, MD Anderson Hospital, 1989:125–134.

211. **Shpall EJ, Clarke-Pearson D, Soper JT, Berchuck A, Jones RB, Bast RC Jr, et al.** High-dose alkylating agent chemotherapy with autologous bone marrow support in patients with stage III/IV epithelial ovarian cancer. *Gynecol Oncol* 1990;38:386–391.

212. **Castaldo TW, Petrilli ES, Ballon SC, Lagasse LD.** Intestinal operations in patients with ovarian carcinoma. *Am J Obstet Gynecol* 1981;139:80–84.

213. **Krebs HB, Goplerud DR.** Surgical management of bowel obstruction in advanced ovarian cancer. *Obstet Gynecol* 1983;61:327–330.

214. **Tunca JC, Buchler DA, Mack EA, Ruzicka FF, Crowley JJ, Carr WF.** The management of ovarian cancer caused bowel obstruction. *Gynecol Oncol* 1981;12:186–192.

215. **Piver MS, Barlow JJ, Lele SB, Frank A.** Survival after ovarian cancer induced intestinal obstruction. *Gynecol Oncol* 1982;13:44–49.

216. **Clarke-Pearson DL, DeLong ER, Chin N, Rice R, Creasman WT.** Intestinal obstruction in patients with ovarian cancer: variables assocaited with surgical complications and survival. *Arch Surg* 1988;123:42–45.

217. **Fernandes JR, Seymour RJ, Suissa S.** Bowel obstruction in patients with ovarian cancer: a search for prognostic factors. *Am J Obstet Gynecol* 1988;158:244–9.

218. **Rubin SC, Hoskins WJ, Benjamin I, Lewis JL Jr.** Palliative surgery for intestinal obstruction in advanced ovarian cancer. *Gynecol Oncol* 1989;34:16–9.

219. **Malone JM Jr, Koonce T, Larson DM, Freedman RS, Carrasco CH, Saul PB.** Palliation of small bowel obstruction by percutaneous gastrostomy in patients with progressive ovarian carcinoma. *Obstet Gynecol* 1986;68:431–3.

220. **Gruppo Interegionale Cooperativo Oncologico Ginecologia.** Randomized comparison of cisplatin with cyclophosphamide/cisplatin and with cyclophosphamide/doxorubicin/cisplatin in advanced ovarian cancer. *Lancet* 1987;8555:353–359.

221. **Berek JS, Hacker NF.** Ovarian and fallopian tubes. In: Haskell CM, ed. *Cancer Treatment.* 4th ed. Philadelphia: WB Saunders, 1995.

222. **Slayton RE.** Management of germ cell and stromal tumors of the ovary. *Semin Oncol* 1984; 11:299–313.

223. **Serov SF, Scully RE, Robin IH.** histological typing of ovarian tumors. In: *International Histological Classification of Tumors.* No. 9. Geneva: World Health Organization, 1973.

224. **Kurman RJ, Scardino PT, Waldmann TA, McIntire KK, Javadpour N, Norris HJ, et al.** Malignant germ cell tumors of the ovary and testis: an immunologic study of 69 cases. *Ann Clin Lab Sci* 1979;9:462–6.

225. **Spanos WJ.** Preoperative hormonal therapy of cystic adnexal masses. *Am J Obstet Gynecol* 1973;116:551–6.

226. **Gordon A, Lipton D, Woodruff JD.** Dysgerminoma: a review of 158 cases from the Emil Novak Ovarian Tumor Registry. *Obstet Gynecol* 1981;58:497–504.

227. **Zaloudek CJ, Tavassoli FA, Norris HJ.** Dysgerminoma with syncytiotrophoblastic giant cells: a histologically and clinically distinctive subtype of dysterminoma. *Am J Surg Pathol* 1981;5:361–7.

228. **Kurman RJ, Norris HJ.** Germ cell tumors of the ovary. *Hum Pathol* 1978;1:291–325.

229. **Asadourian L, Taylor H.** Dysgerminoma. *Obstet Gynecol* 1969;33:370–9.

230. **Malkasian G, Symmonds R.** Treatment of the unilateral encapsulated ovarian dysgerminoma. *Am J Obstet Gynecol* 1964;90:379–82.

231. **Freel JH, Cassir JF, Pierce VK, Woodruff JD, Lewis JL Jr.** Dysgerminoma of the ovary. *Cancer* 1979;43:798–805.

232. **Thomas GM, Dembo AJ, Hacker NF, DePetrillo AD.** Current therapy for dysgerminoma of the ovary. *Obstet Gynecol* 1987;70:268–75.

233. **Gershenson DM, Wharton JT, Kline RC, Larson DM, Kavanaugh JJ, Rutledge FN.** Chemotherapeutic complete remission in patients with metastatic ovarian dysgerminoma. Potential for cure and preservation of reproductive capacity. *Cancer* 1986;58:2594–9.

234. **Gershenson DM, Wharton JT.** Malignant germ cell tumors of the ovary. In: **Albert DS, Surwit EA,** eds. *Ovarian Cancer.* Boston: Bartinus Nijhoff, 1985;227–269.

235. **Gershenson DM.** Menstrual and reproductive function after treatment with combination chemotherapy for malignant ovarian germ cell tumors. *J Clin Oncol* 1988;6:270–5.

236. **Williams SD, Birch R, Einhorn LH, Irwin L, Greco FA, Loehrer PJ.** Disseminated germ cell tumors: chemotherapy with cisplatin plus bleomycin plus either vinblastine or etoposide. *N Engl J Med* 1987;316:1435–40.

237. **Williams SD, Blessing JA, Hatch K, Homesley HD.** Chemotherapy of advanced ovarian dysgerminoma: trials of the Gynecologic Oncology Group. *J Clin Oncol* 1991;9:1950–5.

238. **Gershenson DM, Morris M, Cangir A, Kavanaugh JJ, Stringer CA, Edwards CL, et al.** Treatment of malignant germ cell tumors of the ovary with bleomycin, etoposide, and cisplatin. *J Clin Oncol* 1990;8:715–20.

239. **Williams SD.** Germ cell tumors. In: **Ozols RF,** ed. *Ovarian Cancer.* Philadelphia: WB Saunders, 1992:967–74.

240. **Williams SD, Blessing JA, Moore DH, Homesley HD, Adcock L.** Cisplatin, vinblastine, and bleomycin in advanced and recurrent ovarian germ-cell tumors. A trial of the Gynecologic Oncology Group. *Ann Intern Med* 1989;111:22–7.

241. **Norris HJ, Zirken HJ, Benson WL.** Immature (malignant) teratoma of the ovary: a clinical and pathologic study of 58 cases. *Cancer* 1976;37:2359–72.

242. **Curry SL, Smith JP, Gallagher HS.** Malignant teratoma of the ovary: prognostic factors and treatment. *Am J Obstet Gynecol* 1978;131:845–9.

243. **Cangir A, Smith J, Van Eys J.** Improved prognosis in children with ovarian cancers following modified VAC (vincristine sulfate, dactinomycin, and cyclophosphamide) chemotherapy. *Cancer* 1978;42:1234–8.

244. **Slayton RE, Hreshchyshyn MM, Silverberg SC, Shingleton HM, Park RC, DiSaia PJ, et al.** Treatment of malignant ovarian germ cell tumors: response to vincristine, dactinomycin and cyclophosphamide. *Cancer* 1978;42:390–8.

245. **Slayton RE, Park RC, Silverberg SC, Shingleton H, Creasman WT, Blessing JA.** Vincristine, dactinomycin, and cyclophosphamide (VAC) in the treatment of malignant germ cell tumors of the ovary: a Gynecologic Oncology Group study (a final report). *Cancer* 1985; 56:243–8.

246. **Creasman WJ, Soper JT.** Assessment of the contemporary management of germ cell malignancies of the ovary. *Am J Obstet Gynecol* 1985;153:828–34.

247. **Taylor MH, DePetrillo AD, Turner AR.** Vinblastine, bleomycin and cisplatinum in malignant germ cell tumors of the ovary. *Cancer* 1985;56:1341–9.

248. **Williams SD, Blessing JA, Liao SY, Ball H, Hanjani P.** Adjuvant therapy of ovarian germ cell tumors with cisplatin, etoposide, and bleomycin: an adjuvant trial of the Gynecologic Oncology Group. *J Clin Oncol* 1994;12:701–6.

249. **Loehrer PJ, Elson P, Johnson DH, Williams SD, Trump DL, Einhorn LH.** A randomized trial of cisplatin plus etoposide with or without bleomycin in favorable prognosis disseminated germ cell tumors: an ECOG study. *Proc Am Soc Clin Oncol* 1991;10:540.

250. **Bajorin DF, Sarosdy MF, Pfister DG, Mazumdar M, Motzer RJ, Scher HI, et al.** A randomized trial of etoposide plus carboplatin versus etoposide plus cisplatin in patients with metastatic germ cell tumors. *J Clin Oncol* 1993;11:598–606.

251. **Loehrer PJ Sr, Hui S, Clark S, Seal M, Einhorn LH, Williams SD, et al.** Teratoma following cisplatin-based combination chemotherapy for nonseminomatous germ cell tumors: a clincopathological correlation. *J Urol* 1986;135:1183–9.

252. **Gershenson DM, Copeland JL, Del Junco G, Edwards LL, Wharton JT, Rutledge FN.** Second-look laparotomy in the management of malignant germ cell tumors of the ovary. *Obstet Gynecol* 1986;67:789–93.

253. **Kurman RJ, Norris HJ.** Endodermal sinus tumor of the ovary: a clinical and pathological analysis of 71 cases. *Cancer* 1976;38:2404–19.

254. **Talerman A, Haije WG, Baggerman L.** Serum alpha-fetoprotein (AFP) in patients with germ cell tumors of the gonads and extragonadal sites: correlation between endodermal sinus (yolk sac) tumors and raised serum AFP. *Cancer* 1980;46:380–5.

255. **Newlands ES, Southall PJ, Paradinas FJ, Holden L.** Management of ovarian germ cell tumours. In: **Williams CJ, Krikorian JG, Green MR, Ragavan D,** eds. *Textbook of Uncommon Cancer.* New York: John Wiley & Sons Ltd., 1988:37–53.

256. **Kurman RJ, Norris HJ.** Embryonal carcinoma of the ovary: a clinicopathologic entity distinct from endodermal sinus tumor resembling embryonal carcinoma of the adult testis. *Cancer* 1976;38:2420–33.

257. **Gerbie MV, Brewer JI, Tamimi H.** Primary choriocarcinoma of the ovary. *Obstet Gynecol* 1975;46:720–3.

258. **Kurman RJ, Norris HJ.** Malignant mixed germ cell tumors of the ovary: a clinical and pathologic analysis of 30 cases. *Obstet Gynecol* 1976;48:579–89.

259. **Young RH, Scully RE.** Ovarian sex cord-stromal tumors: recent progress. *Int J Gynaecol Pathol* 1982;1:101–23.

260. **Thor AD, Young RH, Clement PB.** Pathology of the fallopian tube, broad ligament, peritoneum, and pelvic soft tissue. *Hum Pathol* 1991;9:856–67.

261. **Novak ER, Kutchmeshgi J, Mupas RS, Woodruff JD.** Feminizing gonadal stromal tumors: analysis of the granulosa-theca cell tumors of the ovarian tumor registry. *Obstet Gynecol* 1971;38:701–13.

262. **Bjorkholm E, Pettersson F.** Granulosa-cell and theca cell tumors: the clinical picture and long-term outcome for the Radiumhemmet series. *Acta Obstet Gynecol Scand* 1980;59:361–5.

263. **Fox H, Agarawal K, Langley FA.** A clinicopathologic study of 92 cases of granulosa cell tumors of the ovary with special reference to the factors influencing prognosis. *Cancer* 1975;35:231–41.

264. **Slayton RE, Johnson G, Brady L, Blessing J.** Radiotherapy and chemotherapy in malignant tumors of the ovarian stroma: a Gynecologic Oncology Group study. *Proc Am Soc Clin Oncol* 1980;C444.

265. **Norris HJ, Taylor HB.** Prognosis of granulosa-theca tumors of the ovary. *Cancer* 1968; 21:255–63.

266. **Lappohn RE, Burger HG, Bouma J, Bangah M, Kraus M, de Bruijn HW.** Inhibin as a marker for granulosa-cell tumors. *N Engl J Med* 1989;321:790–3.

267. **Holland DR, LeRiche J, Swenerton KD, Elit L, Spinelli J.** Flow cytometric assessment of DNA ploidy is a useful prognostic factor for patients with granulosa cell ovarian tumors. *Int J Gynaecol Cancer* 1991;1:227–32.

268. **Roth LM, Anderson MC, Govan AD, Langley FA, Growing NF, Woodcock AS.** Sertoli-Leydig cell tumors: a clinicopathologic study of 34 cases. *Cancer* 1981;48:187–97.

269. **Berek JS, Hacker NF.** Sarcomas of the female genital tract. In: **Eilber FR, Morton DL, Sondak VK, Economou JS,** eds. *The Soft Tissue Sarcomas.* Orlando: Grune & Stratton, 1987: 229–38.

270. **Fox H, Langley FA.** *Tumors of the Ovary.* Chicago: Mosby Year Book, 1976.

271. **Sedlis A.** Carcinoma of the fallopian tube. *Surg Clin North Am* 1978;58:121–9.

272. **Woodruff JD, Murthy YS, Bhaskar TN, Bordbar F, Tseng SS.** Metastatic ovarian tumors. *Am J Obstet Gynecol* 1970;107:202–9.

273. **Kasilag FB, Rutledge FN.** Metastatic breast carcinoma to the ovary. *Am J Obstet Gynecol* 1957;74:989–92.

274. **Lee YN, Hori JM.** Significance of ovarian metastasis in therapeutic oophorectomy for advanced breast cancer. *Cancer* 1971;27:1374–8.

275. **Woodruff JD, Novak ER.** The Krukenberg tumor: study of 48 cases from the Emil Novak Ovarian Tumor Registry. *Obstet Gynecol* 1960;15:351–60.

276. **Webb MJ, Decker DG, Mussey E.** Cancer metastatic to the ovary: factors influencing survival. *Obstet Gynecol* 1975;45:391–6.

277. **Robboy SJ, Scully RE, Norris HJ.** Carcinoid metastatic to the ovary: a clinicopathologic analysis 35 cases. *Cancer* 1974;33:798–811.

278. Freeman C, Berg JW, Cutler SJ. Occurrence and prognosis of extranodal lymphomas. *Cancer* 1972;29:252–60.

279. Arseneau JC, Canellos GP, Banks DM, Berard CW, Gralnick HR, De Vita VT Jr. American Burkitt's lymphoma: a clinicopathologic study of 30 cases. I. Clinical factors relating to prolonged survival. *Am J Med* 1975;58:314–21.

280. Podczaski E, Herbst Al. Cancer of the vagina and fallopian tube. In: Knapp RC, Berkowitz RS, eds. *Gynecologic Oncology.* New York: MacMillan, 1986:394–424.

281. Podratz KC, Podczaski ES, Gaffey TA, O'Brien PC, Schray MR, Malksian GD Jr. Primary carcinoma of the fallopian tube. *Am J Obstet Gynecol* 1986;254:1319–26.

282. Tamimi HK, Figge DC. Adenocarcinoma of the uterine tube: potential for lymph node metastases. *Am J Obstet Gynecol* 1981;141:132–7.

283. Deppe G, Bruckner HW, Cohen CJ. Combination chemotherapy for advanced carcinoma of the fallopian tube. *Obstet Gynecol* 1980;56:530–2.

Modified from Berek JS, Hacker NF. *Practical Gynecologic Oncology.* 2nd ed. Baltimore: Williams & Wilkins. 1994:136–59, 327–401.

34 Vulvar Cancer

Neville F. Hacker

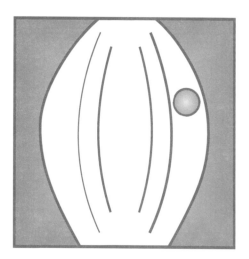

Vulvar cancer is uncommon, representing about 4% of malignancies of the female genital tract. Squamous cell carcinomas account for about 90% of the cases, whereas melanomas, adenocarcinomas, basal cell carcinomas, and sarcomas are much less common. **The incidence of** *in situ* **vulvar cancer nearly doubled between the mid-1970s and the mid-1980s, whereas the rate of invasive squamous cell carcinoma has remained stable (1).**

Since the reports of Taussig (2) in the United States and Way (3) in Great Britain, radical vulvectomy and *en bloc* groin dissection, with or without pelvic lymphadenectomy, has been considered standard treatment for all operable patients. During the past 15 years, however, a number of significant advances have been made in the management of vulvar cancer. These changes have not improved the survival for the disease, but have markedly decreased the physical and psychological morbidity associated with the treatment. These changes include the following:

1. Individualization of treatment for all patients with invasive disease (4, 5)

2. Vulvar conservation for patients with unifocal tumors and an otherwise normal vulva (4–8)

3. Omission of the groin dissection for patients with T_1 tumors and ≤ 1 mm of stromal invasion (4, 5)

4. Elimination of routine pelvic lymphadenectomy (9–13)

5. The use of separate groin incisions for the groin dissection to improve wound healing (14, 15)

6. Omission of the contralateral groin dissection in patients with lateral T_1 lesions and negative ipsilateral nodes (5, 16)

1231

7. The use of preoperative radiation therapy to obviate the need for exenteration in patients with advanced disease (17, 18)

8. The use of postoperative radiation to decrease the incidence of groin recurrence in patients with multiple positive groin nodes (13)

Etiology

No specific etiologic factor has been identified for vulvar cancer, and the relationship of the invasive disease to vulvar dystrophy and to vulvar intraepithelial neoplasia remains unclear. Chronic pruritus is usually an important antecedent phenomenon in patients with invasive vulvar cancer (19). Vulvar cancer has been reported to be more common in patients who are obese, hypertensive, diabetic, or nulliparous (20, 21), but a recent case-control study of vulvar cancer was unable to confirm any of these as risk factors (22).

A second primary malignancy, usually invasive or preinvasive cervical cancer, has been reported in as many as 22% of cases (16, 23). The common association between cervical, vaginal, and vulvar cancer suggests a common pathogen, and the case-control study by Brinton et al. found a significantly increased risk in association with multiple sexual partners, a history of genital warts, and smoking (22). Human papillomavirus (HPV) DNA has been reported in 20–60% of patients with invasive vulvar cancer (24). The HPV-positive group has been characterized by a younger mean age, more tobacco use, and the presence of vulvar intraepithelial neoplasia (VIN) in association with the invasive component (25–27).

Vulvar cancer is occasionally associated with syphilis and nonluetic granulomatous venereal disease, particularly lymphogranuloma venereum and granuloma inguinale (*donovanosis*). In approximately 5% of patients with vulvar cancer, a serologic test for syphilis is positive; these patients develop the disease at an earlier age and have more poorly differentiated lesions (20, 21). Antecedent chronic granulomatous disease has been reported in 66% of black patients with vulvar cancer in Jamaica (28), but such diseases are not seen commonly in Western countries.

Types of Invasive Vulvar Cancer

The varieties of invasive vulvar cancer are shown in Table 34.1.

Squamous Cell Carcinoma

Approximately 90–92% of all invasive vulvar cancers are of the squamous cell type. In these malignancies, mitoses are noted, but atypical keratinization is the histologic hallmark of invasive vulvar cancer (29). Most vulvar squamous carcinomas reveal keratinization (Fig. 34.1). *Anaplastic carcinoma* may consist of large immature cells, spindle sarco-

Table 34.1   Types of Vulvar Cancer

Type	Percent
Squamous	92
Melanoma	2–4
Basal cell	2–3
Bartholin gland (adenocarcinoma, squamous cell, transitional cell, adenoid cystic)	1
Metastatic	1
Verrucous	<1
Sarcoma	<1
Appendage (e.g., hidradenocarcinoma)	rare

matoid cells, or small cells. The latter may simulate small-cell anaplastic carcinoma of the lung or *Merkel's cell tumor*. Histologic features that correlate with the occurrence of inguinal lymph node metastasis, in the order of importance, are vascular invasion, tumor thickness, depth of stromal invasion, and increased amount of keratin (30–36).

Microinvasive Squamous Carcinoma

Microinvasive carcinoma of the vulva has been characterized as lesions ≤2 cm with <1 mm stromal invasion (37). In the past, attempts had been made to use the same criteria as those used to define microinvasive carcinoma of the cervix (i.e., identifying the depth of invasion from the adjacent basement membrane), but this was difficult and confusing (29). For example, when measured from the adjacent basement membrane, an elongated rete peg of 6 mm may be misconstrued as invasive cancer. Consequently, the term "microinvasive carcinoma of the vulva" should be used with caution. Although the cervix routinely shows the presence of *in situ* changes adjacent to invasive cancer, the same is not true for the vulva. On the vulva, the transition from normal tissue to invasive cancer may be abrupt without intervening histopathologic abnormalities. The International Society of Gynecologic Pathologists recommended that the depth of stromal invasion be measured vertically from the most superficial basement membrane to the deepest tumor (32) (Fig. 34.2). Tumor thickness is the distance between the granular layer of epidermis and the deepest tumor. **When the tumor is <1 mm in depth or thickness, metastasis to the inguinal lymph nodes is extremely rare** among reported series, as discussed below. However, **when invasion is >1 mm, there is a significant risk of inguinal lymph node metastasis.**

Clinical Features

Squamous cell carcinoma of the vulva is predominantly a disease of postmenopausal women; the mean age at diagnosis is about 65 years. Most patients present with a vulvar

Figure 34.1   Squamous cell carcinoma of the vulva, keratinizing type. The multiple pearl formations consist of laminated keratin. (Figures 34.1–34.9 Reproduced from **Berek JS, Hacker NF.** *Practical Gynecologic Oncology.* 2nd ed. Baltimore: Williams & Wilkins, 1994.

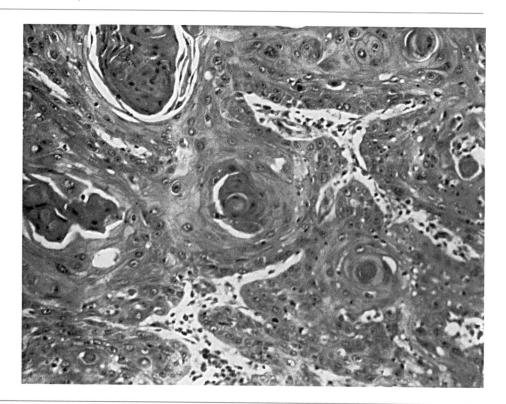

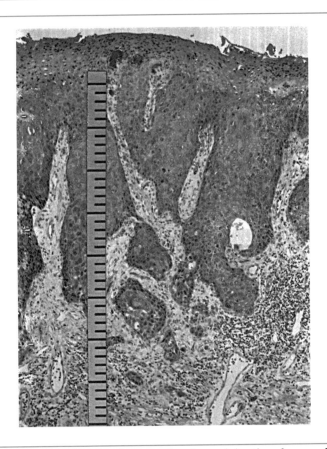

Figure 34.2   Early invasive carcinoma of vulva originating from vulvar intraep-ithelial neoplasia. Multiple irregular nests of malignant cells extend from the base of rete pegs. Desmoplastic stromal reaction and chronic inflammation are useful diag-nostic signs of stromal invasion. The depth of stromal invasion is measured from the base of the most superficial dermal papilla vertically to the deepest tumor cells. In this tumor, it is 3.6 mm in depth.

lump or mass, although there is often a long history of pruritus, which may be caused by an associated vulvar dystrophy. Less common presenting symptoms include vulvar bleed-ing, discharge, or dysuria. Occasionally, a large metastatic mass in the groin may be the initial presenting symptom.

On physical examination, the lesion is usually raised and may be fleshy, ulcerated, leuko-plakic, or warty in appearance. There is an increasing incidence of warty carcinoma of the vulva, and such lesions account for about 20% of all cases (38).

Most squamous carcinomas of the vulva occur on the labia majora, but the labia minora, clitoris, and perineum also may be primary sites. Approximately 10% of the cases are too extensive to determine a site of origin, and about 5% of the cases are multifocal.

As part of the clinical assessment, the groin lymph nodes should be evaluated carefully and a complete pelvic examination should be performed. A Papanicolaou (Pap) smear should be taken from the cervix, and colposcopy of the cervix and vagina should be performed be-cause of the common association with other squamous intraepithelial neoplasms of the lower genital tract.

Diagnosis

Diagnosis requires a wedge biopsy specimen, which usually can be taken in the office with the patient under local anesthesia. If the lesion is only about 1 cm in diameter, excisional biopsy is preferable.

Physician delay is a common problem in the diagnosis of vulvar cancer, particularly if the lesion has a warty appearance. Although isolated condylomas do not require histologic confirmation for diagnosis, any confluent warty lesion should be biopsied before medical or ablative therapy is initiated.

Routes of Spread

Vulvar cancer spreads by the following routes:

1. Direct extension, to involve adjacent structures such as the vagina, urethra, and anus

2. Lymphatic embolization to regional lymph nodes

3. Hematogenous spread to distant sites, including the lungs, liver, and bone

Lymphatic metastases may occur early in the disease. Initially, spread is usually to the inguinal lymph nodes, which are located between Camper's fascia and the fascia lata (6). From these superficial groin nodes, the disease will spread to the femoral nodes, which are located along the femoral vessels (Fig. 34.3). *Cloquet's node,* situated beneath the inguinal ligament, is the most cephalad of the femoral node group. **Metastases to the femoral nodes without involvement of the inguinal nodes have been reported (39–42).**

From the inguinal-femoral nodes, the cancer spreads to the pelvic nodes, particularly the external iliac group. Although direct lymphatic pathways from the clitoris and Bartholin gland to the pelvic nodes have been described, these channels seem to be of minimal clin-

Figure 34.3   Inguinal-femoral lymph nodes.

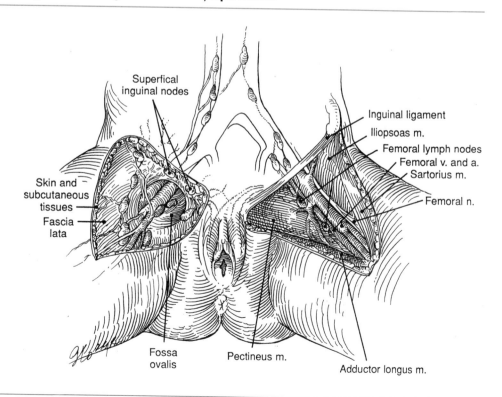

gland to the pelvic nodes have been described, these channels seem to be of minimal clinical significance (9, 43, 44).

Since 1978, the overall incidence of lymph node metastases is reported to be about 30% (9, 10, 45–51) (Table 34.2). The incidence in relation to depth of invasion is shown in Table 34.3 (4, 5, 40, 52–58).

Metastases to pelvic nodes occur in about 9% of cases (59). Pelvic nodal metastases are rare in the absence of clinically suspicious (N_2) groin nodes (10) and three or more positive groin nodes (9, 10, 50). About 20% of patients with positive groin nodes have positive pelvic nodes (59).

Hematogenous spread usually occurs late in the course of vulvar cancer and is rare in the absence of lymph node metastases.

Staging

A clinical staging system based on the TNM classification was adopted by the International Federation of Gynecology and Obstetrics (FIGO) in 1969 (Table 34.4). The staging was based on a clinical evaluation of the primary tumor and regional lymph nodes and a limited search for distant metastases. Microscopic metastases may be present in nodes that are not clinically suspicious, and suspicious nodes may be enlarged because of inflammation only. **When compared with surgical staging of vulvar cancer, the percentage of error in clinical staging increases from 18% for stage I disease to 44% for stage IV disease** (51).

These factors led the Cancer Committee of FIGO to introduce a surgical staging for vulvar cancer in 1988, which was revised in 1995 (Table 34.5). There are two major problems with this staging system. First, patients with negative lymph nodes have a very good prognosis,

Table 34.2   Incidence of Lymph Node Metastases in Operable Vulvar Cancer

Author	*No. of Cases*	*Positive Nodes*	*Percent*
Green, 1978 (47)	142	54	38.0
Krupp and Bohm, 1978 (48)	195	40	20.5
Benedet et al., 1979 (49)	120	34	28.3
Curry et al., 1980 (9)	191	57	29.8
Iversen et al., 1980 (50)	268	86	32.1
Hacker et al., 1983 (10)	113	31	27.4
Podratz et al., 1983 (51)	175	59	33.7
Homesley et al., 1993 (46)	588	203	34.5
Paladini et al., 1994 (45)	350	75	21.2
Total	2142	639	29.8

Table 34.3   Nodal Status in T₁ Squamous Cell Carcinoma of the Vulva Versus Depth of Stromal Invasion

Depth of Invasion	*No.*	*Positive Nodes*	*Nodes*
<1 mm	163	0	0
1.1–2 mm	145	11	7.7
2.1–3 mm	131	11	8.3
3.1–5 mm	101	27	26.7
>5 mm	38	13	34.2
Total	578	62	10.7

Data compiled from Parker, 1975 (40); Magrina, 1979 (53); Iversen, 1981 (4); Wilkinson, 1982 (54); Hoffman, 1983 (52); Hacker, 1984 (5); Boice, 1984 (55); Ross, 1987 (56); Rowley, 1988 (57); Struyk, 1989 (58).

Table 34.4   Clinical Staging of Carcinoma of the Vulva

FIGO Stage	TNM	Clinical Findings
Stage 0		Carcinoma *in situ,* e.g., VIN 3, noninvasive Paget's disease.
Stage I	$T_1N_0M_0$ $T_1N_1M_0$	Tumor confined to the vulva, 2 cm or less in largest diameter, and no suspicious groin nodes.
Stage II	$T_2N_0M_0$ $T_2N_1M_0$	Tumor confined to the vulva more than 2 cm in diameter, and no supicious groin nodes.
Stage III	$T_3N_0M_0$ $T_3N_1M_0$ $T_3N_2M_0$ $T_1N_2M_0$ $T_2N_2M_0$	Tumor of any size with: (1) adjacent spread to the urethra and/or the vagina, the perineum, and the anus, and/or (2) clinically suspicious lymph nodes in either groin.
Stage IV	$T_xN_3M_0$ $T_4N_0M_0$ $T_4N_1M_0$ $T_4N_2M_0$ $T_xN_xM_{1a}$ $T_xN_xM_{1b}$	Tumor of any size: (1) infiltrating the bladder mucosa, or the rectal mucosa, or both, including the upper part of the urethral mucosa, and/or (2) fixed to the bone and/or (3) other distant metastases.

TNM Classification

T: Primary Tumor

T_1 Tumor confined to the vulva, 2 cm in largest diameter.

T_2 Tumor confined to the vulva, >2 cm in diameter.

T_3 Tumor of any size with adjacent spread to the urethra and/or vagina and/or perineum and/or anus.

T_4 Tumor of any size infiltrating the bladder mucosa and/or the rectal mucosa or including the upper part of the urethral mucosa and/or fixed to the bone.

N: Regional Lymph Nodes

N_0 No nodes palpable.

N_1 Nodes palpable in either groin, not enlarged, mobile (not clinically suspicious for neoplasm).

N_2 Nodes palpable in either or both groins, enlarged, firm and mobile (clinically suspicious for neoplasm).

N_3 Fixed or ulcerated nodes.

M: Distant Metastases

M_0 No clinical metastases.

M_{1a} Palpable deep pelvic lymph nodes.

M_{1b} Other distant metastases.

x = any T or N category; VIN, vulvar intraepithelial neoplasia.

regardless of the size of the primary tumor (10, 60), so survival for both stages I and II should be better than 80%. Second, survival is dependent on the number of positive lymph nodes (9, 10, 51, 60). Therefore, stage III represents a very heterogeneous group of patients, ranging from those with negative nodes and involvement of the distal urethra or vagina, who should have an excellent prognosis, to those with multiple positive groin nodes, who have a very poor prognosis.

Treatment

After the pioneering work of Taussig (2) in the United States and Way (3) in Great Britain, *en bloc* radical vulvectomy and bilateral dissection of the groin and pelvic nodes became the standard treatment for most patients with operable vulvar cancer. If the disease involved the anus, rectovaginal septum, or proximal urethra, some type of pelvic exenteration was combined with the above dissection.

Although the survival improved markedly with this aggressive surgical approach, several factors have led to modifications of this "standard" treatment plan during the past 15 years. These factors may be summarized as follows:

1.   An increasing proportion of patients with early-stage disease—up to 50% of patients in many centers have T_1 tumors.

Table 34.5   Revised FIGO Staging for Vulvar Cancer

1988 FIGO Stage	*TNM*	*Clinical/Pathological Findings*
Stage 0	T_{IS}	Carcinoma *in situ*, intraepithelial carcinoma.
Stage I	$T_1N_0M_0$	Tumor confined to the vulva or perineum, <2 cm in greatest dimension, nodes are negative
Ia		Stromal invasion <1 mm
Ib		Stromal invasion ≥1 mm
Stage II	$T_2N_0M_0$	Tumor confined to the vulva and/or perineum, >2 cm in greatest dimension, nodes are negative.
Stage III	$T_3N_0M_0$ $T_3N_1M_0$ $T_1N_1M_0$ $T_2N_1M_0$	Tumor of any size with 1. Adjacent spread to the lower urethra or the anus 2. Unilateral regional lymph-node metastasis.
Stage IVA	$T_1N_2M_0$ $T_2N_2M_0$	Tumor invades any of the following: Upper urethra, bladder mucosa, rectal mucosa, pelvic bone or bilateral regional node metastasis.
	$T_3N_2M_0$ T_4 any N M_0	
Stage IVB	Any T, any N M_1	Any distant metastasis including pelvic lymph nodes

TNM Classification

T: **Primary Tumor**

T_x Primary tumor cannot be assessed

T_0 No evidence of primary tumor

T_{IS} Carcinoma *in situ* (preinvasive carcinoma)

T_1 Tumor confined to the vulva and/or perineum 2 cm or less in greatest dimension

T_2 Tumor confined to the vulva and/or perineum more than 2 cm in greatest dimension

T_3 Tumor involves any of the following: lower urethra, vagina, anus

T_4 Tumor involves any of the following: bladder mucosa, rectal mucosa, upper urethra, pelvic bone

N: **Regional Lymph Nodes**
Regional lymph nodes are the femoral and inguinal nodes

N_x Regional lymph nodes cannot be assessed

N_0 No lymph node metastasis

N_1 Unilteral regional lymph node metastasis

N_2 Bilateral regional lymph node metastasis

M: **Distant Metastasis**

M   Presence of distant metastasis cannot be assessed

M_0 No distant metastasis

M_1 Distant metastasis (pelvic lymph node metastasis is M_1)

2. Concern about the postoperative morbidity and associated long-term hospitalization common with the *en bloc* radical dissection.

3. Increasing awareness of the psychosexual consequences of radical vulvectomy.

Management of Early Vulvar Cancer (T_1N_{0-1})

The modern approach to the management of patients with T1 carcinoma of the vulva should be individualized (4, 5). There is no "standard" operation applicable to every patient, and emphasis is on performing the most conservative operation that is consistent with cure of the disease.

In considering the appropriate operation, it is necessary to determine independently the appropriate management of the following:

1. The primary lesion

2. The groin lymph nodes.

Before any surgery, all patients should have colposcopy of the cervix, vagina, and vulva, because preinvasive (and rarely invasive) lesions may be present at other sites along the lower genital tract.

Management of the Primary Lesion   Although radical vulvectomy has been regarded as the standard treatment for the primary vulvar lesion, this operation is associated with significant disturbances of sexual function and body image. DiSaia et al. (6) regarded the psychosexual disturbances as the major long-term morbidity associated with the treatment of vulvar cancer. Andersen and Hacker (61) reported that sexual arousal was reduced to the eighth percentile and body image was reduced to the fourth percentile for women who had undergone vulvectomy when compared with healthy adult women.

During the past 15 years, several investigators have advocated a radical local excision rather than a radical vulvectomy for the primary lesion for patients with T_1 tumors (4–7). Traditionally, vulvar cancer has been considered to be a "diffuse disease involving the entire vulva" (21). Anything less than radical vulvectomy has been considered inadequate local treatment that is likely to result in local recurrence. In addition, there has been concern that without an *en bloc* resection, intervening tissue left between the primary tumor and the regional lymph nodes may contain microscopic tumor foci in draining lymphatics. However, experience with a separate incision technique for node dissection has confirmed that metastases rarely occur in the skin bridge in patients without clinically suspicious (N_2) nodes in the groin (15).

Regardless of whether a radical vulvectomy or a radical local excision is performed, the surgical margins adjacent to the tumor will be the same, and an analysis of the available literature indicates that the incidence of local invasive recurrence after radical local excision is not higher than that after radical vulvectomy (59). This suggests that in the presence of an otherwise normal-appearing vulva, radical local excision is a safe surgical option, regardless of the depth of invasion.

There has been uncertainty regarding the surgical margins that must be obtained to prevent local recurrence, but a recent review of 135 patients from the UCLA with all stages of disease revealed that a 1-cm tumor-free surgical margin on the vulva resulted in a very high rate of local control (62). Neither clinical tumor size nor the presence of coexisting benign vulvar pathology correlated with local recurrence.

When vulvar cancer arises in the presence of VIN or some nonneoplastic epithelial disorder, treatment will be influenced by the patient's age. Elderly patients who often have had many years of chronic itching are usually not disturbed by the prospect of a radical vulvectomy. In younger women, it will be desirable to conserve as much of the vulva as possible; thus, radical local excision should be performed for the invasive disease and the associated disease should be treated in the most appropriate manner. For example, topical steroids may be required for squamous hyperplasia, whereas VIN may require superficial local excision and primary closure.

Radical local excision is most appropriate for lesions on the lateral or posterior aspects of the vulva (Fig. 34.4), **where preservation of the clitoris is feasible.** For anterior lesions that involve the clitoris or that are in proximity to it, any type of surgical excision will have psychosexual consequences, particularly for younger patients. In addition, marked edema of the posterior vulva may occur. For young patients with periclitoral lesions, consideration should be given to treating the primary lesion with a small field of radiation therapy. Small vulvar lesions will respond very well to about 5000 cGy external radiation, and biopsy can be performed after therapy to confirm the absence of any residual disease.

After radical local excision, some type of vulvar reconstruction may be preferable to primary closure. For posterior defects, the rhomboid flap is ideal (63), whereas for lateral defects, a mons pubis pedicle flap has been advocated (64).

Management of the Groin Lymph Nodes   Groin dissection is associated with postoperative wound infection and breakdown and chronic leg edema. Although the incidence of

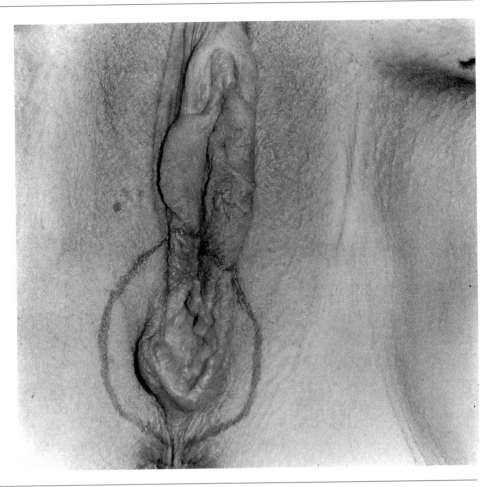

Figure 34.4   Small (T_1) vulvar carcinoma at the posterior fourchette.

wound breakdown is reduced significantly when separate incisions are used for the groin dissection (15), chronic leg edema remains a major problem.

The early papers on early vulvar cancer suggested that it was reasonable to omit the groin dissection for most patients with clinical stage I disease, provided that the depth of stromal invasion was <5 mm (40, 65). On the basis of these reports, the groin dissection was omitted in many such patients. However, with an increasing number of reports in the literature, two facts have become clear:

1. **The only patients with virtually no risk of lymph node metastases are those whose tumor invades the stroma to ≤1 mm.**

2. **Patients who develop recurrent disease in an undissected groin have a very high mortality** (5, 11, 52, 53, 66).

In 1984, the International Society for the Study of Vulvar Diseases (ISSVD) recommended (67) that the term "stage Ia carcinoma of the vulva" be adopted for a single lesion 2 cm or less in diameter, with 1 mm or less of stromal invasion. The recommendation has been adopted by FIGO in 1995 (37). **Appropriate groin dissection is the single most important factor in decreasing the mortality for early vulvar cancer. All patients with more than 1 mm of stromal invasion require inguinal-femoral lymphadenectomy.** A wedge biopsy specimen of the primary tumor should be obtained, and the depth of invasion should be determined. If it is smaller than 1 mm on the wedge biopsy specimen, the entire lesion should be locally excised and analyzed histologically to determine the depth of invasion. If there is still no invasive focus larger than 1 mm, groin dissection may be omitted. Although an occasional patient with less than 1 mm of stromal invasion has had documented groin node metastases (68), the incidence is so low that it is of no practical significance. In frail, elderly patients with up to 3 mm of invasion, it may be reasonable to omit groin dissection, provided that there is no vascular space invasion, the tumor is not poorly differentiated, and the tumor does not have a "spray" pattern of infiltration.

If groin dissection is indicated in patients with early vulvar cancer, it should be a thorough inguinal-femoral lymphadenectomy. The Gynecologic Oncology Group (GOG) recently reported six groin recurrences among 121 patients with T_1N_{0-1} tumors after a superficial (inguinal) dissection, even though the inguinal nodes were negative (69). Whether all of these recurrences were in the femoral nodes is unclear, but this large multi-institutional study does indicate that modification of the groin dissection will increase groin recurrences and, therefore, mortality.

From the accumulated experience now available in the literature, it is clear that it is not necessary to perform a bilateral groin dissection if the primary lesion is unilateral although lesions involving the anterior labia minora should have bilateral dissection because of the more frequent contralateral lymph flow from this region (70).

Measurement of Depth of Invasion   The Nomenclature Committee of the International Society of Gynecological Pathologists has recommended that depth of invasion should be measured from the most superficial dermal papilla adjacent to the tumor to the deepest focus of invasion. This method was originally proposed by Wilkinson et al. (54). Tumor thickness is also commonly measured (53, 71), and Fu and Reagan (72) estimated that the average difference between tumor thickness and depth of invasion as determined by the Wilkinson method was 0.3 mm.

Management of a Patient with Positive Groin Nodes   No additional treatment is recommended if one microscopically positive groin node is found. The prognosis for this group of patients is excellent (10), and only careful observation is required. Even if a unilateral groin dissection has been performed for a lateral lesion, there seems to be no indication for dissection of the other groin, because contralateral lymph node involvement is likely only if there are multiple ipsilateral inguinal node metastases (13, 73).

If two or more positive groin nodes are found, which is unusual in patients with T_1 vulvar cancer, the patient is at increased risk of groin and pelvic recurrence and should receive postoperative groin and pelvic radiation (13).

Management of Patients with T_2 and Early T_3 Tumors and N_{0-1} Nodes

In general, the management of patients with T_2 and early T_3 tumors consists of radical vulvectomy and bilateral inguinal-femoral lymphadenectomy. If the disease involves the distal urethra or vagina, partial resection of these organs will be required. Alternatively, it may be preferable to give preoperative radiation therapy to allow a less radical resection.

There are two basic surgical approaches that can be used:

1. The *en bloc* approach through a trapezoid or butterfly incision (74, 75).

2. The separate-incision approach, involving three separate incisions, one for the radical vulvectomy and one for each groin dissection (14, 15) (Fig. 34.5).

In general, there is a greater likelihood of primary healing with the separate-incision technique, and it is being used increasingly.

1241

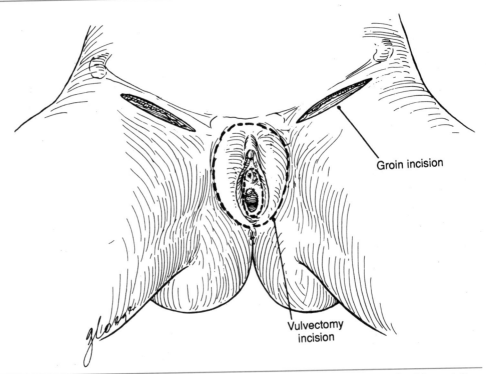

Groin incision

Vulvectomy
incision

Figure 34.5   Skin incision for groin dissection through a separate incision. A line is drawn 1 cm below and parallel to the groin crease, and a narrow ellipse of skin is removed.

Closure of Large Defects   It is usually possible to close the vulvar defect without tension. However, if a more extensive dissection has been required because of a large primary lesion, a number of options are available to repair the defect. These include the following:

1. An area may be left open to granulate, which it will usually do over a period of 6 to 8 weeks (76).

2. Full-thickness skin flaps may be devised (64, 77, 78). An example is the rhomboid flap, which is best suited for covering large defects of the posterior vulva (63).

3. Unilateral or bilateral gracilis myocutaneous grafts may be developed. These are most useful when an extensive area from the mons pubis to the perianal area has been resected. Because the graft brings a new blood supply to the area, it is particularly applicable if the vulva is poorly vascularized from prior surgical resection or radiation (79).

4. If extensive defects exist in the groin and vulva, the tensor fascia lata myocutaneous graft is applicable (80).

Vulvar Conservation for T_2 and Early T_3 Tumors   In recent years, the indications for vulvar conservation have been extended by some surgeons to selected patients with T_2 and early T_3 tumors. Although the reported experience is limited (7, 8, 81, 82), a recent study at UCLA suggests that the local recurrence rate for patients with conservatively treated stage II tumors is identical to that for patients with stage I tumors (83) as long as surgical margins of at least 1 cm are obtained. The tumor-free margin should be the same, whether or not a radical vulvectomy or a radical local excision is performed, so it would seem to be both feasible and desirable to extend the indications for vulvar conservation, particularly for younger patients. Tumors that are most suitable for a more conservative resection are those involving the posterior half of the vulva, where preservation of the clitoris and mon pubis is feasible.

Management of the Pelvic Lymph Nodes   In the past, pelvic lymphadenectomy has been considered to be part of the routine surgery for invasive vulvar cancer. However, the incidence of pelvic node metastases is <10%, so a more selective approach is justified. A more critical examination of pelvic lymph node metastases indicates that they are rare in the absence of clinically suspicious groin nodes or three or more positive groin nodes (9, 10, 12, 51).

Most authors (16, 74) suggest that pelvic lymphadenectomy should be reserved for patients with positive groin nodes, unless the primary tumor involves the clitoris or Bartholin gland. It has been demonstrated that even with clitoral (9, 50) and Bartholin gland carcinomas (43), pelvic node metastases are rare in the absence of inguinal-femoral metastases, so there is no reason to make an exception for these tumors.

In 1977, the GOG initiated a prospective trial in which patients with positive groin nodes were randomized to either ipsilateral pelvic node dissection or bilateral pelvic plus groin irradiation (3). Radiation therapy consisted of 4500–5000 cGy to the midplane of the pelvis at a rate of 180–200 cGy per day. Survival for the radiation group (68% at 2 years) was significantly better than the survival for the pelvic lymphadenectomy group (54% at 2 years) (P=0.03). The survival advantage was limited to patients with clinically evident groin nodes or more than one positive groin node. Groin recurrence occurred in three of 59 patients (5%) treated with radiation, compared with 13 of 55 (23.6%) patients treated with lymphadenectomy (P=0.02). Four patients who received radiation had a pelvic recurrence, compared with one who had lymphadenectomy. These data indicate no benefit from pelvic irradiation compared with pelvic lymphadenectomy for the prevention of pelvic recurrence, but they do highlight the value of prophylactic groin irradiation in preventing groin recurrence in patients with multiple positive groin nodes.

From the above observations, it would seem that patients with one microscopically positive groin node require no further therapy. Patients with two or more positive groin nodes are best treated with pelvic and groin irradiation.

Postoperative Management   Despite the age and general medical condition of most patients with vulvar cancer, surgery is usually remarkably well tolerated. However, a postoperative mortality rate of about 2% can be expected, usually as a result of pulmonary embolism or myocardial infarction. Patients should be able to commence a low-residue diet on the first postoperative day. Bedrest is advisable for 3–5 days to allow immobilization of the wounds to foster healing. Pneumatic calf compression or subcutaneous heparin should be given to help prevent deep venous thrombosis, and active, nonweight-bearing leg movements are to be encouraged. Frequent wound dressings and perineal swabs are given. Suction drainage of each groin is continued for about 10 days to help decrease the incidence of groin seromas. A Foley catheter is left in the bladder until the patient is walking around. When the patient is fully mobilized, Sitz baths or whirlpool therapy is helpful, followed by drying of the perineum with a hair dryer.

Early Postoperative Complications   The major immediate morbidity is related to groin wound infection, necrosis, and breakdown, and this has been reported in as many as 85% of patients having an *en bloc* operation (51). With the separate-incision approach, the incidence of wound breakdown can be reduced to about 44%; major breakdown occurs in about 14% of patients (15). With debridement and wound dressings, the area will granulate and reepithelialize over the next few weeks and may be managed with home nursing. Whirlpool therapy is effective for areas of extensive breakdown.

Other early postoperative complications include urinary tract infection, seromas in the femoral triangle, deep venous thrombosis, pulmonary embolism, myocardial infarction, hemorrhage, and, rarely, osteitis pubis. Seromas occur in about 10–15% of cases and should be managed by periodic sterile aspiration. Anesthesia of the anterior thigh from femoral nerve injury is common and usually resolves slowly.

Late Complications   The major late complication is chronic leg edema, which has been reported in as many as 69% of patients (51). Recurrent lymphangitis or cellulitis of the leg occurs in about 10% of patients and usually responds to erythromycin tablets. Urinary stress incontinence, with or without genital prolapse, occurs in about 10% of patients and may require corrective surgery. Introital stenosis can lead to dyspareunia and may require a vertical relaxing incision, which is sutured transversely. An uncommon late complication is femoral hernia, which can usually be prevented intraoperatively by closure of the femoral canal with a suture from the inguinal ligament to Cooper's ligament. Pubic osteomyelitis and rectovaginal or rectoperineal fistulas are rare late complications.

Advanced Disease

Vulvar cancer may be considered to be advanced on the basis of a large T_3 or T_4 primary tumor or the presence of bulky, positive groin nodes. As with early vulvar cancer, management must be individualized.

Management of Patients with a Large T_3 or T_4 Primary Tumor   When the primary disease involves the anus, rectum, rectovaginal septum, or proximal urethra, adequate surgical clearance of the primary tumor is possible, only by pelvic exenteration combined with radical vulvectomy and bilateral groin dissection. Such radical surgery is often inappropriate for these elderly patients, and even in suitable surgical candidates, psychological morbidity is high (61, 84). In addition, operative mortality is about 10%, and the postoperative physical morbidity is significant. Nevertheless, a 5-year survival rate of about 50% can be expected with this approach (85–88). Surgery alone is rarely curative for patients with fixed or ulcerated (N_3) groin nodes.

Radiation therapy traditionally has been considered to have a limited role in the management of patients with vulvar cancer. In the orthovoltage era, local tissue tolerance was poor and vulvar necrosis was common, but with megavoltage therapy, tolerance has improved significantly.

Boronow (17) was the first to suggest a combined radiosurgical approach as an alternative to pelvic exenteration for patients with advanced vulvar cancer. In his initial report, he recommended intracavitary radium, with or without external irradiation, to eliminate the internal genital disease and subsequent surgery, usually radical vulvectomy and bilateral groin dissection, to treat the external genital disease.

In 1984, Hacker et al. (18) reported the use of preoperative teletherapy for patients with advanced vulvar cancer; brachytherapy was reserved for patients with persistent disease that would otherwise necessitate exenteration. Rather than radical vulvectomy for all patients, only the tumor bed was resected, on the assumption that any microscopic foci originally present in the vulva would have been sterilized by the radiation. In specimens from one-half of the patients, there was no residual disease. Long-term morbidity was low with the predominant use of teletherapy, and no patient developed a fistula. Two patients whose primary tumor was fixed to bone were long-term survivors (18). Backstrom et al. (89) from the Radiumhemmet reported cure of only four of 19 patients (21%) with advanced vulvar cancer when external radiation alone was used, emphasizing the need for a combined radiosurgical approach.

In 1987, Boronow et al. (90) updated their experience with preoperative radiation for locally advanced vulvovaginal cancer, reporting 37 primary cases and 11 cases of recurrent disease. The 5-year survival rate for the primary cases was 75.6%, whereas the recurrent cases had a 5-year survival rate of 62.6%. Seventeen of 40 vulvectomy specimens (42.5%) contained no residual disease. Local recurrence occurred in eight patients (17%), and a fistula developed in five patients (10.4%).

As the experience of these investigators has evolved, their approach has been refined. They now recommend external beam therapy for all cases, with more selective use of brachytherapy. The radicality of the surgery has also been significantly modified. A more limited vulvar resection is now advocated, and bulky N_2 and N_3 nodes are resected without full groin dissection to avoid the leg edema associated with groin dissection and radiation.

In 1989, Thomas et al. (91) reported on the use of radiation with concurrent infusional *5-fluorouracil,* with or without *mitomycin C,* for 33 patients with vulvar cancer. Median follow-up was 16 months. Of nine patients who received primary chemoradiation, six had an initial complete response in the vulva, but three of the six subsequently had a local recurrence. This suggests that chemoradiation should always be combined with excision of the tumor bed. Berek et al. (92) treated 12 patients with preoperative chemoradiation using *cisplatin* and *5-fluorouracil* as the radiation sensitizers. The 3-year survival rate was 83%. Using preoperative radiation alone, Rotmensch et al. (93) reported a 45% survival rate for 13 patients with advanced vulvar cancer.

With the experience now accrued, preoperative radiation, with or without concurrent chemotherapy, should be regarded as the treatment of first choice for patients with advanced vulvar cancer who would otherwise require some type of pelvic exenteration.

Management of Patients with Bulky Positive Groin Nodes   In the past, such patients would have undergone a pelvic lymphadenectomy after full groin dissection. The GOG study showed the advantage of postoperative pelvic and groin irradiation in decreasing the incidence of groin recurrence and improving survival for patients with bulky, positive groin nodes (13). However, the incidence of pelvic recurrence was higher in the group receiving pelvic radiation, presumably because of the inability of external beam therapy to sterilize bulky positive pelvic nodes. In addition, our experience is that full groin dissection, combined with groin irradiation, often produces quite severe leg edema.

In view of these considerations, our current approach to patients with N_2 or N_3 groin nodes is as follows:

1. A preoperative computed tomography (CT) scan or ultrasonogram of the pelvis is obtained to determine whether there are any enlarged pelvic nodes.

2. All enlarged groin nodes are removed through a separate-incision approach and sent for frozen-section diagnosis. If metastatic disease is confirmed, full lymphadenectomy is not performed.

3. Any enlarged pelvic nodes seen on CT scan or ultrasonogram are removed via an extraperitoneal approach.

4. Full pelvic and groin irradiation is given as soon as the groin incisions are healed.

5. If the frozen section reveals no metastatic disease in the removed nodes, full groin dissection is performed.

Role of Radiation

Radiation therapy, with or without the addition of concurrent chemotherapy, is likely to have an increasingly important role in the management of patients with vulvar

cancer. The indications for radiation therapy for patients with this disease are still evolving. At present, radiation seems to be clearly indicated in the following situations:

1. Preoperatively, in patients with advanced disease who would otherwise require pelvic exenteration (17, 18).

2. Postoperatively, to treat the pelvic lymph nodes and groin of patients with two or more positive groin nodes (13).

Possible roles for radiation therapy include the following:

1. Postoperatively, to help prevent local recurrences in patients with involved or close surgical margins (<5 mm) (94, 95).

2. As primary therapy for patients with small primary tumors, particularly clitoral or periclitoral lesions in young and middle-aged women, for whom surgical resection would have significant psychological consequences.

Groin irradiation has been proposed as an alternative to groin dissection in patients with N_0 lymph nodes. However, the GOG recently reported the results of a phase III trial in which patients with T_1, T_2, or T_3 tumors and N_{0-1} groin nodes were randomized between surgical resection (and postoperative irradiation for patients with positive groin nodes) and primary groin irradiation (96). Patients with N_1 nodes were allowed fine-needle aspiration cytology of the nodes and exclusion from the trial if findings were positive. The study was closed prematurely because five of 26 patients in the groin-irradiation arm of the study had recurrences in the groin. Of 23 patients undergoing groin dissection, five showed groin node metastases, but no groin recurrences occurred after postoperative irradiation. The dose of radiation was 5000 cGy given in daily 200-cGy fractions to a depth of 3 cm below the anterior skin surface.

Recurrent Vulvar Cancer

Recurrence of vulvar cancer correlates most closely with the number of positive groin nodes (10). **Patients with fewer than three positive nodes, particularly if the nodes are only microscopically involved, have a low incidence of recurrence at any site, whereas patients with three or more positive nodes have a high incidence of local, regional, and systemic recurrences** (10, 13).

Local vulvar recurrences are most likely in patients with primary lesions larger than 4 cm in diameter (94) and are usually amenable to further surgical excision, often with a gracilis myocutaneous graft to cover the defect. If this is the only site of recurrence, most patients can be cured (15, 97). Radiation therapy, particularly a combination of external beam therapy plus interstitial needles, has also been used to treat vulvar recurrences. Hoffman et al. (98) recently reported on 10 patients treated in this manner, and nine were still alive with a mean follow-up of 28 months. However, six of the 10 patients developed severe radionecrosis at a median of 8.5 months after radiation, and the authors concluded that, although this treatment was highly effective, it was also highly morbid.

Regional and distant recurrences are difficult to manage (94). Radiation therapy may be used in conjunction with surgery for groin recurrence, whereas chemotherapeutic agents that have activity against squamous carcinomas may be offered for distant metastases. The most active agents are *cisplatin, methotrexate, cyclophosphamide, bleomycin,* and *mitomycin C,* but response rates are low and the duration of response is usually disappointing. Long-term survival is very uncommon with regional or distant recurrence (94).

Prognosis

With appropriate management, the prognosis for vulvar cancer is generally good; the overall 5-year survival rate in operable cases is about 70%.

The number of positive groin nodes is the single most important prognostic variable (10, 12, 13, 51). Patients with one microscopically positive node have a good prognosis, regardless of the stage of disease (10, 12), but patients with three or more positive nodes have a poor prognosis. Because the number of positive nodes correlates with the clinical status of the groin nodes (10), survival also correlates significantly with this variable. In the GOG study, patients with N_0 or N_1 nodes had a 2-year survival rate of 78%, compared with 52% for patients with N_2 nodes and 33% for patients with N_3 nodes (P=0.01) (13). The survival rate for patients with positive pelvic nodes is about 11% (59).

As discussed earlier, the FIGO surgical staging is flawed, and it is hoped that it will be revised. However, the GOG staged 588 patients with vulvar cancer by the new criteria and reported 5-year survival rates of 98%, 85%, 74%, and 31% for stages I, II, III, and IV, respectively (60).

Workers at the Norwegian Radium Hospital evaluated DNA ploidy for its prognostic significance in 118 squamous cell carcinomas of the vulva (99). The 5-year crude survival rate was 62% for the diploid and 23% for the aneuploid tumors (P<0.001). Aneuploid tumors without lymph node metastases had a 5-year cancer-related survival rate of 44% as compared with 58% for the diploid tumors with lymph node metastases. In a multivariate Cox regression analysis, the most important independent prognostic parameters were as follows:

1. Lymph node involvement (P<0.0001)

2. Tumor ploidy (P=0.0001)

3. Tumor size (P=0.0039)

Melanoma

Vulvar melanomas are rare, although they are the second most common vulvar malignancy. Most arise *de novo* (100), but they may arise from a preexisting junctional nevus. They occur predominantly in postmenopausal white women, most commonly on the labia minora or the clitoris (Fig. 34.6). The incidence of cutaneous melanomas worldwide is increasing significantly.

Most patients with a vulvar melanoma have no symptoms except for the presence of a pigmented lesion that may be enlarging. Some patients have itching or bleeding, and a few present with a groin mass.

There are three basic histologic types. The most common is the *superficial spreading melanoma,* which tends to remain relatively superficial early in its development (Fig. 34.7). The *lentigo maligna melanoma* is a flat freckle, which may become quite extensive but also tends to remain superficial. The most aggressive lesion is the *nodular melanoma,* which is a raised lesion that penetrates deeply and may metastasize widely. Amelanotic varieties occasionally occur. Any pigmented lesion on the vulva should be excised or biopsied, unless it is known to have been present and unchanged for some years.

Staging

The FIGO staging used for squamous lesions is not applicable for melanomas, because these lesions are usually much smaller and the prognosis is related to the depth of penetration rather than to the diameter of the lesion (101–103). The leveling system established by Clark et al. (104) for cutaneous melanomas is less readily applicable to vulvar lesions because of the different skin morphology. Chung et al. (101) proposed a modified system that retained Clark's definitions for levels I and V but arbitrarily defined levels II, III, and IV, using measurements in millimeters. Breslow (105) measured the thickest portion of the melanoma from the surface of intact epithelium to the deepest point of invasion. A comparison of these systems is shown in Table 34.6.

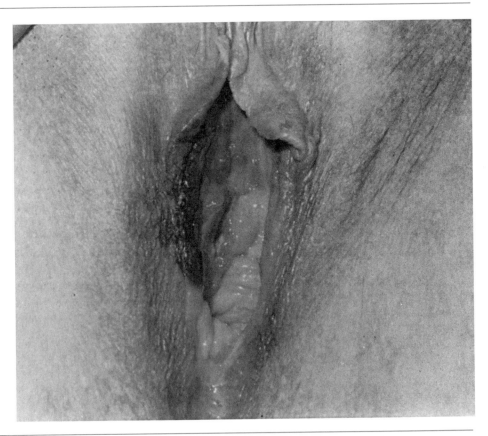

Figure 34.6   Melanoma of the vulva involving the right labium minus.

Treatment

With better understanding of the prognostic significance of the microstage, some individualization of treatment has developed. **Lesions with less than 1 mm of invasion may be treated with radical local excision alone** (101, 102). With more invasive lesions, *en bloc* resection of the primary tumor and regional groin nodes is required. In line with trends toward more conservative surgery for cutaneous melanomas (106, 107), there is a trend toward more conservative resection for vulvar melanomas (108–110). Radical vulvectomy is being performed less frequently, and survival does not seem to be compromised. Davidson et al. (109) reported on 32 patients with vulvar melanoma who underwent local excision (N=14), simple vulvectomy (N=7), or radical resection (N=11). No group had a superior survival, although the overall survival rate at 5 years was only 25%. More recently, Trimble et al. (110) reported on 59 patients who underwent radical vulvectomy and 19 who underwent more conservative resections. Survival was not improved by the more radical approach, and they recommended radical local excision for the primary tumor, with groin dissection for tumors with a thickness of more than 1 mm.

As melanomas commonly involve the clitoris and labia minora, the vaginourethral margin of resection is a common site of failure, and care should be taken to obtain an adequate "inner" resection margin (111). Podratz et al. (103) demonstrated a 10-year survival rate of 61% for lateral lesions, compared with 37% for medial lesions (P=0.027).

Pelvic node metastases do not occur in the absence of groin node metastases (111–113). In addition, the prognosis for patients with positive pelvic nodes is so poor that there seems to be no value in performing pelvic lymphadenectomy for this disease.

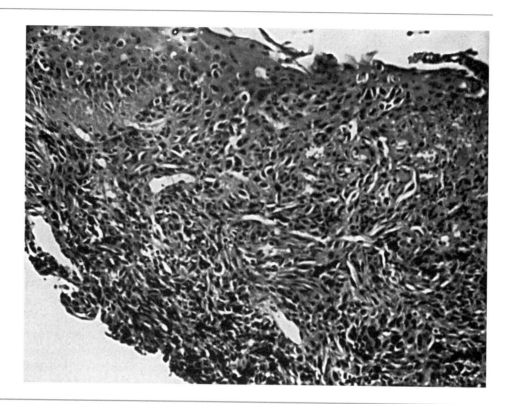

Figure 34.7   Vulvar melanoma. Spindle-shaped melanoma cells form interlacing bundles, and some contain melanin pigment (left lower corner). Epidermal invasion is evident in the form of Pagetoid migration (left upper corner).

Table 34.6   Microstaging of Vulvar Melanomas

	Clark's Levels	*Chung*	*Breslow*
I	Intraepithelial	Intraepithelial	<0.76 mm
II	Into papillary dermis	≤1 mm from granular layer	0.76–1.50 mm
III	Filling dermal papillae	1.1–2 mm from granular layer	1.51–2.25 mm
IV	Into reticular dermis	>2 mm from granular layer	2.26–3.0 mm
V	Into subcutaneous fat	Into subcutaneous fat	>3 mm

Chemotherapy and immunotherapy for vulvar melanoma are disappointing. Estrogen receptors have been demonstrated in human melanomas (114), and responses to tamoxifen have been reported (115, 116).

Prognosis

The behavior of melanomas can be quite unpredictable, but the overall prognosis is poor. The mean 5-year survival rate for reported cases of vulvar melanoma ranges from 21.7% (100) to 54% (103). Patients with lesions invading to 1 mm or less have an excellent prognosis, but as depth of invasion increases, prognosis worsens. Chung et al. (101) reported a corrected 5-year survival rate of 100% for patients with level II lesions, 40% for level III or IV lesions, and 20% for level V lesions. Tumor volume has been reported to correlate with prognosis; patients whose lesions have a volume under 100 mm³ have an excellent prognosis (113).

Bartholin Gland Carcinoma

Primary carcinoma of the Bartholin gland accounts for about 5% of vulvar malignancies. Because of its rarity, individual experience with the tumor is limited, and recommendations for management must be based on literature reviews. To date, about 280 cases have been reported (43, 117).

The bilateral Bartholin glands are greater vestibular glands situated posterolaterally in the vulva. Their main duct is lined with stratified squamous epithelium, which changes to transitional epithelium as the terminal ducts are reached. As tumors may arise from the gland or the duct, a variety of histologic types may occur, including adenocarcinomas, squamous carcinomas, and, rarely, transitional cell, adenosquamous, and adenoid cystic carcinomas.

Classification of a vulvar tumor as a Bartholin gland carcinoma has typically required that it fulfill *Honan's criteria,* which are as follows:

1. The tumor is in the correct anatomic position.

2. The tumor is located deep in the labium majus.

3. The overlying skin is intact.

4. There is some recognizable normal gland present.

Strict adherence to these criteria will result in underdiagnosis of some cases. Large tumors may ulcerate through the overlying skin and obliterate the residual normal gland. Although transition between normal and malignant tissue is the best criterion, some cases will be diagnosed on the basis of their histologic characteristics and anatomic location.

A history of preceding inflammation of the Bartholin gland may be obtained for about 10% of patients, and malignancies may be mistaken for benign cysts or abscesses. Therefore, delay of diagnosis is common, particularly for premenopausal patients. The differential diagnosis of any pararectovaginal neoplasm should include cloacogenic carcinoma and secondary neoplasm (117).

Treatment

Traditionally, treatment has been by radical vulvectomy, with bilateral groin and pelvic node dissection (118). However, there seems to be no indication for dissection of the pelvic nodes in the absence of positive groin nodes, and Copeland et al. (117) at the M.D. Anderson Hospital have reported good results with hemivulvectomy or radical local excision for the primary tumor. Because these lesions are deep in the vulva, extensive dissection is required in the ischiorectal fossa, and even then, surgical margins are often close. Postoperative radiation to the vulva decreased the likelihood of local recurrence in Copeland's series from 27% (six of 22 patients) to 7% (one of 14 patients). If the ipsilateral groin nodes are positive, bilateral groin and pelvic radiation may decrease regional recurrence. If the tumor is fixed to the inferior pubic ramus or involving adjacent structures, such as the anal sphincter or rectum, preoperative radiation is preferable to avoid exenterative surgery and permanent colostomy.

Prognosis

Because of the deep location of the gland, cases tend to be more advanced than squamous carcinomas at the time of diagnosis, but stage for stage, the prognosis is similar.

The *adenoid cystic* variety is less likely to metastasize to lymph nodes and carries a somewhat better prognosis (Fig 34.8). Local recurrences are common, however, and they may metastasize, particularly to the lungs. The slowly progressive nature of these tumors is reflected in the disparity between progression-free interval and survival curves (119).

Other Adenocarcinomas

Adenocarcinomas of the vulva usually arise in a Bartholin gland or occur in association with Paget's disease. They may rarely arise from the skin appendages, paraurethral glands,

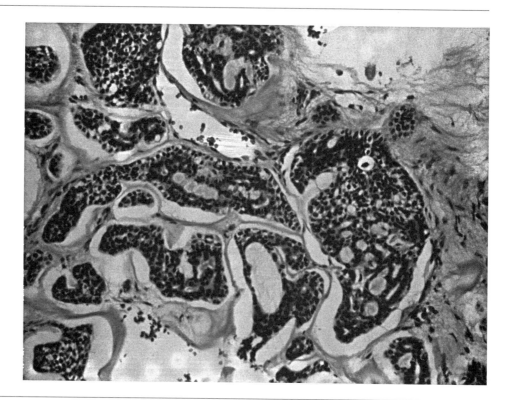

Figure 34.8   Adenoid cystic tumor of the Bartholin gland. Basaloid cells form cribiform, sieve-like spaces containing mucinous material. The hyaline stroma is another distinct feature of this tumor.

minor vestibular glands, aberrant breast tissue, endometriosis, or a misplaced cloacal remnant (72).

A particularly aggressive type is the *adenosquamous carcinoma*. This tumor has a number of synonyms, including cylindroma, pseudoglandular squamous cell carcinoma, and adenoacanthoma of the sweat gland of Lever. The tumor has a propensity for perineural invasion, early lymph node metastasis, and local recurrence. Underwood et al. (120) reported a crude 5-year survival rate of 5.5% (one of 18) for adenosquamous carcinoma of the vulva, compared with 62.3% (48 of 77) for patients with squamous cell carcinoma. Treatment should be by radical vulvectomy and bilateral groin dissection, and postoperative radiation may be appropriate.

Basal Cell Carcinoma

Basal cell carcinomas represent about 2% of vulvar cancers. As with other basal cell carcinomas, vulvar lesions commonly appear as a "rodent ulcer" with rolled edges, although nodules and macules are other morphologic varieties. Most lesions are smaller than 2 cm in diameter and are usually situated on the anterior labia majora. Giant lesions occasionally occur (121). They usually affect postmenopausal white women and are locally aggressive. Radical local excision is generally adequate treatment. Metastasis to regional lymph nodes has been reported but is rare (122–124). The local recurrence rate is about 20% (125).

About 3–5% of basal cell carcinomas contain a malignant squamous component, the socalled *basosquamous carcinoma*. These lesions are more aggressive and should be treated as squamous carcinomas (124). Another subtype of basal cell carcinoma is the *adenoid basal cell carcinoma,* which must be differentiated from the more aggressive adenoid cystic carcinoma arising in a Bartholin gland or the skin (124).

1251

Verrucous Carcinoma

Verrucous carcinoma is a variant of squamous cell carcinoma and has distinctive clinical and pathologic characteristics (126). Although most commonly found in the oral cavity, verrucous lesions may be found on any moist membrane composed of squamous epithelium (127).

Grossly, the tumors have a "cauliflower-like" appearance; microscopically, they contain multiple papillary fronds that lack the central connective tissue core that characterizes condylomata acuminata (Fig. 34.9). The gross and microscopic features of a verrucous carcinoma are very similar to those of the *giant condyloma of Buschke-Loewenstein,* and they probably represent the same disease entity (72). Adequate biopsy from the base of the lesion is required to differentiate a verrucous carcinoma from a benign condyloma acuminatum or a squamous cell carcinoma with a verrucous growth pattern.

Clinically, verrucous carcinomas usually occur in postmenopausal women, and they are slowly growing but locally destructive lesions. Even bone may be invaded. Metastasis to regional lymph nodes is rare but has been reported (128). Radical local excision is the basic treatment, although if there are palpably suspicious groin nodes, these should be evaluated with fine-needle aspiration cytology or excisional biopsy. Usually, enlarged nodes will be caused by inflammatory hypertrophy (129). If the nodes contain metastases, radical vulvectomy and bilateral inguinal-femoral lymphadenectomy are indicated.

Radiation therapy is contraindicated, because it may induce anaplastic transformation with subsequent regional and distant metastasis (130). Japaze et al. (129) reported a corrected 5-year survival rate of 94% for 17 patients treated with surgery alone, compared with 42% for 7 patients treated with surgery and radiation. If there is a recurrence, further surgical excision is the treatment of choice. This may occasionally necessitate some type of exenteration.

Figure 34.9   Verrucous carcinoma of the vulva. Note the exophytic hyperkeratotic papillary fronds and endophytic bulky rete pegs with smooth borders.

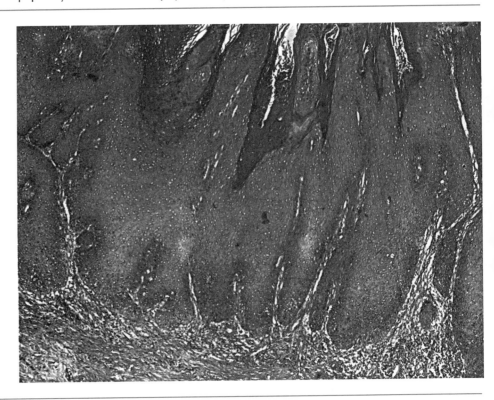

Vulvar Sarcomas

Sarcomas represent 1–2% of vulvar malignancies and constitute a heterogenous group of tumors. Leiomyosarcomas are the most common, and other histologic types include fibrosarcomas, neurofibrosarcomas, liposarcomas, rhabdomyosarcomas, angiosarcomas, epithelioid sarcomas, and malignant schwannomas (72).

Leiomyosarcomas usually appear as enlarging, often painful masses, usually in the labium majus. In a review of 32 smooth muscle tumors of the vulva, Tavassoli and Norris (131) reported that recurrence was associated with three main determinants: diameter larger than 5 cm, infiltrating margins, 5 or more mitotic figures per 10 high-power fields. Neoplasms with these three features should be regarded as sarcomas. The absence of one, or even all, of these features does not guarantee that recurrence will not occur (131). Lymphatic metastases are uncommon, and radical local excision is the usual treatment.

Epithelioid sarcomas characteristically develop in the soft tissues of the extremities of young adults but may rarely occur on the vulva. Ulbright et al. (132) described two cases and reviewed three other reports. They concluded that these tumors may mimic a Bartholin cyst, thus leading to inadequate initial treatment. They also believed that vulvar epithelioid sarcomas behave more aggressively than their extragenital counterparts, with four of the five patients dying of metastatic disease. They suggested that early recognition and wide excision should improve the prognosis.

Rhabdomyosarcomas are the most common soft tissue sarcomas in childhood, and 20% involve the pelvis or genitourinary tract (133). Dramatic gains have been made in the treatment of these tumors during the past 20 years. Previously, radical pelvic surgery was the standard approach, but results were poor. More recently, a multimodality approach has evolved and survival rates have improved significantly, with a corresponding decrease in morbidity.

Hays et al. (134) reported the experience of the Intergroup Rhabdomyosarcoma Study I and II (1972–1984) with primary tumors of the female genital tract. Nine patients aged 1 to 19 years had primary vulvar tumors, and these were often regarded as a form of Bartholin gland infection before biopsy. They were all managed with chemotherapy (*vincristine, actinomycin D/cyclophosphamide/doxorubicin*), with or without radiotherapy. Wide local excision of the tumor, with or without inguinal-femoral lymphadenectomy, was carried out before or after the chemotherapy. Seven of the nine patients were free of disease 4 or more years from diagnosis, one patient was free of disease when lost to follow-up at 5 years, and one patient was alive with disease.

Rare Vulvar Malignancies

Other than the tumors mentioned above, a number of malignancies more commonly seen in other areas of the body may rarely present as isolated vulvar tumors. These include the following.

Lymphomas   The genital tract may be involved primarily by malignant lymphomas, but more commonly, involvement is a manifestation of systemic disease. In the lower genital tract, the cervix is most commonly involved, followed by the vulva and the vagina (72). Most patients are in their third to sixth decade of life, and about three-fourths of the cases involve diffuse large-cell or histiocytic non-Hodgkin's lymphomas. The remainder are nodular or Burkitt's lymphomas (135). Treatment is by surgical excision followed by chemotherapy and/or radiation, and the overall 5-year survival rate is about 70% (135).

Endodermal Sinus Tumor   There have been four case reports of endodermal sinus tumor of the vulva, and three of the four patients died of distant metastases (72, 136). All patients were in their third decade of life, but none were treated with modern chemotherapy.

Merkel Cell Carcinoma   Merkel cell carcinomas are primary small-cell carcinomas of the skin, which resemble oat cell carcinomas of the lung. They metastasize widely and have a very poor prognosis (137, 138). They should be locally excised and treated with cis-platinum-based chemotherapy.

Dermatofibrosarcoma Protuberans   This is a rare, low-grade cutaneous malignancy that occasionally involves the vulva. It has a marked tendency for local recurrence but a low risk of systemic spread (139). Radical local excision should be sufficient treatment.

Malignant Schwannoma   Five cases of malignant schwannoma in the vulvar region have been reported. The patients ranged in age from 25 to 45 years. Four of the five were free of tumor from 1–9 years after radical surgery, and the fifth patient died of multiple pulmonary metastases (72).

Secondary Vulvar Tumors

Eight percent of vulvar tumors are metastatic (72). The most common primary site is the cervix, followed by the endometrium, kidney, and urethra. Most patients in whom vulvar metastases develop have advanced primary tumors at presentation, and in about one-fourth of the patients, the primary lesion and the vulvar metastasis are diagnosed simultaneously (140).

References

1. **Sturgeon SR, Brinton LA, Devesa SS, Kurman RJ.** In situ and invasive vulvar cancer incidence trends (1973 to 1987). *Am J Obstet Gynecol* 1992;166:1482–5.

2. **Taussig FJ.** Cancer of the vulva: an analysis of 155 cases. *Am J Obstet Gynecol* 1940;40:764–78.

3. **Way S.** Carcinoma of the vulva. *Am J Obstet Gynecol* 1960;79:692–7.

4. **Iversen T, Abeler V, Aalders J.** Individualized treatment of stage I carcinoma of the vulva. *Obstet Gynecol* 1981;57:85–9.

5. **Hacker NF, Berek JS, Lagasse LD, Nieberg RK, Leuchter RS.** Individualization of treatment for stage I squamous cell vulvar carcinoma. *Obstet Gynecol* 1984;63:155–62.

6. **DiSaia PJ, Creasman WT, Rich WM.** An alternative approach to early cancer of the vulva. *Am J Obstet Gynecol* 1979;133:825–32.

7. **Burke TW, Stringer CA, Gershenson DM, Edwards CL, Morris M, Wharton JT.** Radical wide excision and selective inguinal node dissection for squamous cell carcinoma of the vulva. *Gynecol Oncol* 1990;38:328–32.

8. **Burrell MO, Franklin EW III, Campion MJ, Crozier MA, Stacey DW.** The modified radical vulvectomy with groin dissection. An eight-year experience. *Am J Obstet Gynecol* 1988;159:715–22.

9. **Curry SL, Wharton JT, Rutledge F.** Positive lymph nodes in vulvar squamous carcinoma. *Gynecol Oncol* 1980;9:63–7.

10. **Hacker NF, Berek JS, Lagasse LD, Leuchter RS, Moore JG.** Management of regional lymph nodes and their prognostic influence in vulvar cancer. *Obstet Gynecol* 1983;61:408–12.

11. **Monaghan JM, Hammond IG.** Pelvic node dissection in the treatment of vulval carcinoma—is it necessary? *Br J Obstet Gynaecol* 1984;91:270–4.

12. **Hoffman JS, Kumar NB, Morley GW.** Prognostic significance of groin lymph node metastases in squamous carcinoma of the vulva. *Obstet Gynecol* 1985;66:402–5.

13. **Homesley HD, Bundy BN, Sedlis A, Adcock L.** Radiation therapy versus pelvic node resection for carcinoma of the vulva with positive groin nodes. *Obstet Gynecol* 1986;68:733–40.

14. **Byron RL, Mishell DR, Yonemoto RH.** The surgical treatment of invasive carcinoma of the vulva. *Surg Gynecol Obstet* 1965;121:1243–51.

15. **Hacker NF, Leuchter RS, Berek JS, Castaldo TW, Lagasse LD.** Radical vulvectomy and bilateral inguinal lymphadenectomy through separate groin incisions. *Obstet Gynecol* 1981;58:574–9.

16. **Figge DC, Gaudenz R.** Invasive carcinoma of the vulva. *Am J Obstet Gynecol* 1974;119:382–95.

17. **Boronow RC.** Therapeutic alternative to primary exenteration for advanced vulvo-vaginal cancer. *Gynecol Oncol* 1973;1:223–30.

18. **Hacker NF, Berek JS, Juillard GJF, Lagasse LD.** Preoperative radiation therapy for locally advanced vulvar cancer. *Cancer* 1984;54:2056–61.

19. **Zacur H, Genadry R, Woodruff JD.** The patient-at-risk for development of vulvar cancer. *Gynecol Oncol* 1980;9:199–208.

20. **Franklin EW, Rutledge FD.** Epidemiology of epidermoid carcinoma of the vulva. *Obstet Gynecol* 1972;39:165–72.

21. **Green TH Jr, Ulfelder H, Meigs JV.** Epidermoid carcinoma of the vulva: an analysis of 238 cases. Parts I and II. *Am J Obstet Gynecol* 1958;73:834–64.

22. **Brinton LA, Nasca PC, Mallin K, Baptiste MS, Wilbanks GD, Richart RM.** Case control study of cancer of the vulva. *Obstet Gynecol* 1990;75:859–66.

23. **Collins CG, Lee FY, Roman-Lopez JJ.** Invasive carcinoma of the vulva with lymph node metastases. *Am J Obstet Gynecol* 1971;109:446–52.

24. **Rusk D, Sutton GP, Look KY, Roman A.** Analysis of invasive squamous cell carcinoma of the vulva and vulvar intraepithelial neoplasia for the presence of human papillomavirus DNA. *Obstet Gynecol* 1991;77:918–22.

25. **Bloss JD, Liao SY, Wilczynski SP, Macri C, Walker J, Peake M, et al.** Clinical and histologic features of vulvar carcinomas analysed for human papillomavirus status: evidence that squamous cell carcinoma of the vulva has more than one etiology. *Hum Pathol* 1991;22:711–8.

26. **Toki T, Kurman RJ, Park JS, Kessis T, Daniel RW, Shah KV.** Probable nonpapillomavirus etiology of squamous cell carcinoma of the vulva in older women: a clinicopathologic study using *in situ* hybridization and polymerase chain reaction. *Int J Gynecol Pathol* 1991;10:107–25.

27. **Nuovo GJ, Delvenne P, MacConnell P, Chalas E, Neto C, Mann WJ.** Correlation of histology and detection of human papillomavirus DNA in vulvar cancers. *Gynecol Oncol* 1991;43:275–80.

28. **Hay DM, Cole FM.** Primary invasive carcinoma of the vulva in Jamaica. *J Obstet Gynaecol Br Commonw* 1969;76:821–30.

29. **Woodruff JD.** Early invasive carcinoma of the vulva. *Clin Oncol* 1982;1:349.

30. **Binder SW, Huang I, Fu YS, Hacker NF, Berek JS.** Risk factors for the development of lymph node metastasis in vulvar squamous cell carcinoma. *Gynecol Oncol* 1990;37:9–16.

31. **Committee on Terminology, International Society for the Study of Vulvar Disease.** New nomenclature for vulvar disease. *Int J Gynecol Pathol* 1989;8:83.

32. **Buscema J, Woodruff JD.** Progressive histobiologic alterations in the development of vulvar cancer. *Am J Obstet Gynecol* 1980;138:146–50.

33. **Collins CG, Lee FY, Roman-Lopez JJ.** Invasive carcinoma of the vulva with lymph node metastases. *Am J Obstet Gynecol* 1971;109:446–52.

34. **Krupp PJ, Lee FY, Batson HWK, Allen PM, Collins JH.** Carcinoma of the vulva. *Gynecol Oncol* 1973;1:345–362.

35. **Donaldson ES, Powell DE, Hanson MB, Van Nagell JR Jr.** Prognostic parameters in invasive vulvar cancer. *Gynecol Oncol* 1981;11:184–90.

36. **Chou CY.** Double primary epidermoid carcinoma of the vulva and cervix. *Gynecol Oncol* 1980;9:124–33.

37. **Creasman WT.** New gynecologic cancer staging. *Gynecol Oncol* 1995;58:157–8.

38. **Rastkar G, Okagaka T, Twiggs LB, Clark BA.** Early invasive and in situ warty carcinoma of the vulva: clinical, histologic, and electron microscopic study with particular reference to viral association. *Am J Obstet Gynecol* 1982;143:814–20.

39. **Hacker NF, Nieberg RK, Berek JS, Leuchter RS, Lucas WE, Tamimi HK, et al.** Superficially invasive vulvar cancer with nodal metastases. *Gynecol Oncol* 1983;15:65–77.

40. **Parker RT, Duncan I, Rampone J, Creasman W.** Operative management of early invasive epidermoid carcinoma of the vulva. *Am J Obstet Gynecol* 1975;123:349–55.

41. **Chu J, Tamimi HK, Figge DC.** Femoral node metastases with negative superficial inguinal nodes in early vulvar cancer. *Am J Obstet Gynecol* 1981;140:337–9.

42. **Podczaski E, Sexton M, Kaminski P, Singapuri K, Sorosky J, Larson J, et al.** Recurrent carcinoma of the vulva after conservative treatment for "microinvasive" disease. *Gynecol Oncol* 1990;39:65–8.

43. **Leuchter RS, Hacker NF, Voet RL, Berek JS, Townsend DE, Lagasse LD.** Primary carcinoma of the Bartholin gland: a report of 14 cases and a review of the literature. *Obstet Gynecol* 1982;60:361–8.

44. **Piver MS, Xynos FP.** Pelvic lymphadenectomy in women with carcinoma of the clitoris. *Obstet Gynecol* 1977;49:592–5.

45. **Paladini D, Cross P, Lopes A, Monaghan JM.** Prognostic significance of lymph node variables in squamous cell carcinoma of the vulva. *Cancer* 1994;74:2491–6.

46. **Homesley HD, Bundy BN, Sedlis A, Yordan E, Berek JS, Jahshan A, et al.** Prognostic factors for groin node metastasis in squamous cell carcinoma of the vulva (A Gynecologic Oncology Group Study). *Gynecol Oncol* 1993;49:279–83.

47. **Green TH Jr.** Carcinoma of the vulva: a reassessment. *Obstet Gynecol* 1978;52:462–9.

48. **Krupp PJ, Bohm JW.** Lymph gland metastases in invasive squamous cell cancer of the vulva. *Am J Obstet Gynecol* 1978;130:943–52.

49. **Benedet JL, Turko M, Fairey RN, Boyes DA.** Squamous carcinoma of the vulva: results of treatment, 1938 to 1976. *Am J Obstet Gynecol* 1979;134:201–7.

50. **Iversen T, Aalders JG, Christensen A, Kolstad P.** Squamous cell carcinoma of the vulva: a review of 424 patients, 1956–1974. *Gynecol Oncol* 1980;9:271–9.

51. **Podratz KC, Symmonds RE, Taylor WF, Williams TJ.** Carcinoma of the vulva: analysis of treatment and survival. *Obstet Gynecol* 1983;61:63–74.

52. **Hoffman JS, Kumar NB, Morley GW.** Microinvasive squamous carcinoma of the vulva: search for a definition. *Obstet Gynecol* 1983;61:615–8.

53. **Magrina JF, Webb MJ, Gaffey TA, Symmonds RE.** Stage I squamous cell cancer of the vulva. *Am J Obstet Gynecol* 1979;134:453–9.

54. **Wilkinson EJ, Rico MJ, Pierson KK.** Microinvasive carcinoma of the vulva. *Int J Gynaecol Pathol* 1982;1:29–39.

55. **Boice CR, Seraj IM, Thrasher T, King A.** Microinvasive squamous carcinoma of the vulva: present status and reassessment. *Gynecol Oncol* 1984;18:71–6.

56. **Ross M, Ehrmann RL.** Histologic prognosticators in stage I squamous cell carcinoma of the vulva. *Obstet Gynecol* 1987;70:774–84.

57. **Rowley KC, Gallion HH, Donaldson ES, van Nagell JR, Higgins RV, Powell DE, et al.** Prognostic factors in early vulvar cancer. *Gynecol Oncol* 1988;31:43–9.

58. **Struyk APHB, Bouma JJ, van Lindert ACM.** Early stage cancer of the vulva: a pilot investigation on cancer of the vulva in gynecologic oncology centers in the Netherlands. *Proc Int Gynecol Cancer Soc* 1989;2:303.

59. **van der Velden J, Hacker NF.** Update on vulvar carcinoma. In: **Rothenberg ML,** ed. *Gynecologic Oncology. Controversies and New Developments.* Boston: Kluwer Academic Publishers, 1994:101–19.

60. **Homesley HD, Bundy BN, Sedlis A, Yordan E, Berek JS, Jahshan A, et al.** Assessment of current International Federation of Gynecology and Obstetrics staging of vulvar carcinoma relative to prognostic factors for survival (a Gynecologic Oncology Group study). *Am J Obstet Gynecol* 1991;164:997–1003.

61. **Andersen BL, Hacker NF.** Psychological adjustment after vulvar surgery. *Obstet Gynecol* 1983;62:457–62.

62. **Heaps JM, Fu YS, Montz FJ, Hacker NF, Berek JS.** Surgical-pathologic variables predictive of local recurrence in squamous cell carcinoma of the vulva. *Gynecol Oncol* 1990;38:309–14.

63. **Barnhill DR, Hoskins WJ, Metz P.** Use of the rhomboid flap after partial vulvectomy. *Obstet Gynecol* 1983;62:444–7.

64. **Potkul RK, Barnes WA, Barter JF, Delgado G, Spear SL.** Vulvar reconstruction using a mons pubis pedicle flap. *Gynecol Oncol* 1994;55:21–4.

65. **Wharton JT, Gallager S, Rutledge RN.** Microinvasive carcinoma of the vulva. *Am J Obstet Gynecol* 1974;118:159–62.

66. **Lingard D, Free K, Wright RG, Battistutta D.** Invasive squamous cell carcinoma of the vulva: behaviour and results in the light of changing management regimes. *Aust N Z J Obstet Gynaecol* 1992;32:137–45.

67. **ISSVD Task Force.** Microinvasive cancer of the vulva. *J Reprod Med* 1984;29:454–5.

68. **Atamdede F, Hoogerland D.** Regional lymph node recurrence following local excision for microinvasive vulvar carcinoma. *Gynecol Oncol* 1989;34:125–8.

69. **Stehman FB, Bundy BN, Droretsky PM, Creasman WT.** Early stage I carcinoma of the vulva treated with ipsilateral superficial inguinal lymphadenectomy and modified radical hemivulvectomy: a prospective study of the Gynecologic Oncology Group. *Obstet Gynecol* 1992;79:490–7.

70. **Iversen T, Aas M.** Lymph drainage from the vulva. *Gynecol Oncol* 1983;16:179–89.

71. **Sedlis A, Homesley H, Bundy BN, Marshall R, Yordan E, Hacker N, et al.** Positive groin lymph nodes in superficial squamous cell vulvar cancer. A Gynecologic Oncology Group Study. *Am J Obstet Gynecol* 1987;156:1159–64.

72. **Fu YS, Reagan JW.** Benign and malignant epithelial tumors of the vulva. In: **Fu YS, Reagan JW,** eds. *Pathology of the Uterine Cervix, Vagina, and Vulva.* Philadelphia: WB Saunders, 1989:138–92.

73. **Dvoretsky PM, Bonfiglio TA, Helmkamp F, Ramsey G, Chuang C, Beecham JB.** The pathology of superficially invasive thin vulvar squamous cell carcinoma. *Int J Gynecol Pathol* 1984;3:331–42.

74. **Morley GW.** Infiltrative carcinoma of the vulva: results of surgical treatment. *Am J Obstet Gynecol* 1976;124:874–88.

75. **Abitbol MM.** Carcinoma of the vulva: improvements in the surgical approach. *Am J Obstet Gynecol* 1973;117:483–9.

76. **Simonsen E, Johnsson JE, Tropé C.** Radical vulvectomy with warm-knife and open-wound techniques in vulvar malignancies. *Gynecol Oncol* 1984;17:22–31.

77. **Trelford JD, Deer DA, Ordorica E, Franti CE, Trelford-Sander M.** Ten-year prospective study in a management change of vulvar carcinoma. *Am J Obstet Gynecol* 1984;150:288–96.

78. **Julian CG, Callison J, Woodruff JD.** Plastic management of extensive vulvar defects. *Obstet Gynecol* 1971;38:193–8.

79. **Ballon SC, Donaldson RC, Roberts JA.** Reconstruction of the vulva using a myocutaneous graft. *Gynecol Oncol* 1979;7:123–7.

80. **Chafe W, Fowler WC, Walton LA, Currie JL.** Radical vulvectomy with use of tensor fascia lata myocutaneous flap. *Am J Obstet Gynecol* 1983;145:207–13.

81. **Hacker NF.** Surgery for malignant tumors of the vulva. In: **Gershenson DM, Curry S,** eds. *Operative Gynecology.* Philadelphia: WB Saunders, 1993.

82. **Andrews SJ, Williams BT, De Priest PD, Gallion HH, Hunter JE, Buckley SL, et al.** Therapeutic implications of lymph node spread in lateral T1 and T2 squamous cell carcinoma of the vulva. *Gynecol Oncol* 1994;55:41–6.

83. **Farias-Eisner R, Cirisano FD, Grouse D, Leuchter RS, Karlan BY, Lagasse CD, Berek JS.** Conservative and individualized surgery for early squamous carcinoma of the vulva: the treatment of choice for stages I and II (T_{1-2}, N_{0-1}, M_0) disease. *Gynecol Oncol* 1994;53:33–8.

84. **Andersen BL, Hacker NF.** Psychosexual adjustment following pelvic exenteration. *Obstet Gynecol* 1983;61:457–62.

85. **Kaplan AL, Kaufman RH.** Management of advanced carcinoma of the vulva. *Gynecol Oncol* 1975;3:220–32.

86. **Phillips B, Buchsbaum HJ, Lifshitz S.** Pelvic exenteration for vulvovaginal carcinoma. *Am J Obstet Gynecol* 1981;141:1038–44.

87. **Cavanagh D, Shepherd JH.** The place of pelvic exenteration in the primary management of advanced carcinoma of the vulva. *Gynecol Oncol* 1982;13:318–22.

88. **Grimshaw RN, Aswad SG, Monaghan JM.** The role of anovulvectomy in locally advanced carcinoma of the vulva. *Int J Gynecol Cancer* 1991;1:15.

89. **Backstrom A, Edsmyr F, Wicklund H.** Radiotherapy of carcinoma of the vulva. *Acta Obstet Gynecol* 1972;51:109–15.

90. **Boronow RC, Hickman BT, Reagan MT, Smith RA, Steadham RE.** Combined therapy as an alternative to exenteration for locally advanced vulvovaginal cancer. II. Results, complications and dosimetric and surgical considerations. *Am J Clin Oncol* 1987;10:171–81.

91. **Thomas G, Dembo A, DePetrillo A, Pringle J, Ackerman I, Bryson P, et al.** Concurrent radiation and chemotherapy in vulvar carcinoma. *Gynecol Oncol* 1989;34:263–7.

92. **Berek JS, Heaps JM, Fu YS, Juillard GJ, Hacker NF.** Concurrent cisplatin and 5-fluorouracil chemotherapy and radiotherapy for advanced stage squamous carcinoma of the vulva. *Gynecol Oncol* 1991;42:197–207.

93. **Rotmensch J, Rubin SJ, Sutton HG, Javaheri G, Halpern HJ, Schwartz JL, et al.** Preoperative radiotherapy followed by radical vulvectomy with inguinal lymphadenectomy for advanced vulvar carcinomas. *Gynecol Oncol* 1990;36:181–4.

94. **Podratz KC, Symmonds RE, Taylor WF.** Carcinoma of the vulva: analysis of treatment failures. *Am J Obstet Gynecol* 1982;143:340–51.

95. **Malfetano J, Piver MS, Tsukada Y.** Stage III and IV squamous cell carcinoma of the vulva. *Gynecol Oncol* 1986;23:192–8.

96. **Stehman FB, Bundy BN, Thomas G, Varia M, Okagaki T, Roberts J, et al.** Groin dissection versus groin radiation in carcinoma of the vulva: a Gynecologic Oncology Group study. *Int J Radiat Oncol Biol Phys* 1992;24:389–96.

97. **Hopkins MP, Reid GC, Morley GW.** The surgical management of recurrent squamous cell carcinoma of the vulva. *Obstet Gynecol* 1990;75:1001–5.

98. **Hoffman M, Greenberg S, Greenberg H, Fiorica JV, Roberts WS, LaPolla JP, et al.** Interstitial radiotherapy for the treatment of advanced or recurrent vulvar and distal vaginal malignancy. *Am J Obstet Gynecol* 1990;162:1278–82.

99. **Kaern J, Iversen T, Tropé C, Petterson EO, Nesland JM.** Flow cytometric DNA measurements in squamous cell carcinoma of the vulva: an important prognostic method. *Int J Gynecol Cancer* 1992;2:169–74.

100. **Blessing K, Kernohan NM, Miller ID, Al Nafussi AI.** Malignant melanoma of the vulva: clinicopathological features. *Int J Gynecol Oncol* 1991;1:81–7.

101. **Chung AF, Woodruff JM, Lewis JL Jr.** Malignant melanoma of the vulva: a report of 44 cases. *Obstet Gynecol* 1975;45:638–46.

102. **Phillips GL, Twiggs LB, Okagaki T.** Vulvar melanoma: a microstaging study. *Gynecol Oncol* 1982;14:80–8.

103. **Podratz KC, Gaffey TA, Symmonds RE, Johansen KL, O'Brien PC.** Melanoma of the vulva: an update. *Gynecol Oncol* 1983;16:153–68.

104. **Clark WH, From L, Bernardino EA, Mihm MC.** The histogenesis and biologic behavior of primary human malignant melanomas of the skin. *Cancer Res* 1969;29:705–27.

105. **Breslow A.** Thickness, cross-sectional area and depth of invasion in the prognosis of cutaneous melanoma. *Ann Surg* 1970;172:902–8.

106. **Aitken DR, Clausen K, Klein JP, James AG.** The extent of primary melanoma excision—a re-evaluation. How wide is wide? *Ann Surg* 1983;198:634–41.

107. **Day CL, Mihm MC Jr, Sober AJ, Fitzpatrick TB, Malt RA.** Narrower margins for clinical stage I malignant melanoma. *N Engl J Med* 1982;306:479–82.

108. **Rose PG, Piver MS, Tsukada Y, Lau T.** Conservative therapy for melanoma of the vulva. *Am J Obstet Gynecol* 1988;159:52–5.

109. **Davidson T, Kissin M, Wesbury G.** Vulvovaginal melanoma—should radical surgery be abandoned? *Br J Obstet Gynaecol* 1987;94:473–6.

110. **Trimble EL, Lewis JL Jr, Williams LL, Curtin JP, Chapman D, Woodruff JM, et al.** Management of vulvar melanoma. *Gynecol Oncol* 1992;45:254–8.

111. **Morrow CP, Rutledge FN.** Melanoma of the vulva. *Obstet Gynecol* 1972;39:745–52.

112. **Jaramillo BA, Ganjei P, Averette HE, Sevin BU, Lovecchio JL.** Malignant melanoma of the vulva. *Obstet Gynecol* 1985;66:398–401.

113. **Beller U, Demopoulos RI, Beckman EM.** Vulvovaginal melanoma: a clinicopathologic study. *J Reprod Med* 1986;31:315–9.

114. **Fisher RI, Neifeld JP, Lippman ME.** Oestrogen receptors in human malignant melanoma. *Lancet* 1976;2:337–9.

115. **Masiel A, Buttrick P, Bitran J.** Tamoxifen in the treatment of malignant melanoma. *Cancer Treat Rep* 1981;65:531–2.

116. **Nesbit RA, Woods RL, Tattersall MH, Fox RM, Forbes JF, Mackay IR, et al.** Tamoxifen in malignant melanoma. *N Engl J Med* 1979;301:1241–2.

117. **Copeland LJ, Sneige N, Gershenson DM, McGuffee VB, Abdul-Karim F, Rutledge FN.** Bartholin gland carcinoma. *Obstet Gynecol* 1986;67:794–801.

118. **Barclay DL, Collins CG, Macey HB.** Cancer of the Bartholin gland: a review and report of 8 cases. *Obstet Gynecol* 1964;24:329–36.

119. **Copeland LJ, Sneige N, Gershenson DM, Saul PB, Stringer CA, Seski JB.** Adenoid cystic carcinoma of Bartholin gland. *Obstet Gynecol* 1986;67:115–20.

120. **Underwood JW, Adcock LL, Okagaki T.** Adenosquamous carcinoma of skin appendages (adenoid squamous cell carcinoma, pseudoglandular squamous cell carcinoma, adenoacanthoma of sweat gland of Lever) of the vulva: a clinical and ultrastructural study. *Cancer* 1978; 42:1851–8.

121. **Dudzinski MR, Askin FB, Fowler WC.** Giant basal cell carcinoma of the vulva. *Obstet Gynecol* 1984;63:57S–60S.

122. **Jimenez HT, Fenoglio CM, Richart RM.** Vulvar basal cell carcinoma with metastasis: a case report. *Am J Obstet Gynecol* 1975;121:285–6.

123. **Sworn MJ, Hammond GT, Buchanan R.** Metastatic basal cell carcinoma of the vulva: a case report. *Br J Obstet Gynaecol* 1979;86:332–4.

124. **Hoffman MS, Roberts WS, Ruffolo EH.** Basal cell carcinoma of the vulva with inguinal lymph node metastases. *Gynecol Oncol* 1988;29:113–9.

125. **Palladino VS, Duffy JL, Bures GJ.** Basal cell carcinoma of the vulva. *Cancer* 1969;24: 460–70.

126. **Isaacs JH.** Verrucous carcinoma of the female genital tract. *Gynecol Oncol* 1976;4:259–69.

127. **Partridge EE, Murad R, Shingleton HM, Austin JM, Hatck KD.** Verrucous lesions of the female genitalia. II. Verrucous carcinoma *Am J Obstet Gynecol* 1980;137:419–24.

128. **Gallousis S.** Verrucous carcinoma: report of three vulvar cases and a review of the literature. *Obstet Gynecol* 1972;40:502–7.

129. **Japaze H, Van Dinh TV, Woodruff JD.** Verrucous carcinoma of the vulva: study of 24 cases. *Obstet Gynecol* 1982;60:462–6.

130. **Demian SDE, Bushkin FL, Echevarria RA.** Perineural invasion and anaplastic transformation of verrucous carcinoma. *Cancer* 1973;32:395–401.

131. **Tavassoli FA, Norris HJ.** Smooth muscle tumors of the vulva. *Obstet Gynecol* 1979;53: 213–7.

132. **Ulbright TM, Brokaw SA, Stehman FB, Roth LM.** Epithelioid sarcoma of the vulva. *Cancer* 1983;52:1462–9.

133. **Bell J, Averette H, Davis J, Toledano S.** Genital rhabdomyosarcoma: current management and review of the literature. *Obstet Gynecol Surv* 1986;41:257–63.

134. **Hays DM, Shimada H, Raney RB Jr, Tefft M, Newton W, Crist WM, et al.** Clinical staging and treatment results in rhabdomyosarcoma of the female genital tract among children and adolescents. *Cancer* 1988;61:1893–903.

135. **Harris NL, Scully RE.** Malignant lymphoma and granulocytic sarcoma of the uterus and vagina. *Cancer* 1984;53:2530–45.

136. **Dudley AG, Young RH, Lawrence WD, Scully RE.** Endodermal sinus tumor of the vulva in an infant. *Obstet Gynecol* 1983;61:76S–9S.

137. **Bottles K, Lacy CG, Goldberg J, Lanner-Cusin K, Hom J, Miller TR.** Merkel cell carcinoma of the vulva. *Obstet Gynecol* 1984;63:61S–5S.

138. **Husseinzadeh N, Wesseler T, Newman N, Shbaro I, Ho P.** Neuroendocrine (Merkel cell) carcinoma of the vulva. *Gynecol Oncol* 1988;29:105–12.

139. **Bock JE, Andreasson B, Thorn A, Holck S.** Dermatofibromasarcoma protuberans of the vulva. *Gynecol Oncol* 1985;20:129–35.

140. **Dehner LP.** Metastatic and secondary tumors of the vulva. *Obstet Gynecol* 1973;42:47–57.

Modified from **Berek JS, Hacker WF.** *Practical Gynecologic Oncology.* 2nd ed. Baltimore: Williams & Wilkins, 1994:1–73.

35 Gestational Trophoblastic Disease

Ross S. Berkowitz
Donald P. Goldstein

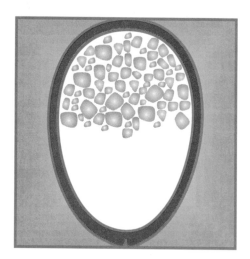

Gestational trophoblastic disease (GTD) is among the rare human tumors that can be cured even in the presence of widespread dissemination (1, 2). GTD includes a spectrum of interrelated tumors, including complete and partial hydatidiform mole, placental-site trophoblastic tumor, and choriocarcinoma, which have varying propensities for local invasion and metastasis. Although persistent gestational trophoblastic tumor (GTT) most commonly follows a molar pregnancy, it may ensue after any gestational event, including therapeutic or spontaneous abortion, ectopic or term pregnancy. Advances in the understanding of the pathogenesis, natural history and treatment of GTD and the current approach to management are reviewed.

Hydatidiform Mole

Epidemiology

Estimates of the incidence of GTD vary dramatically in different regions of the world. For example, the incidence of molar pregnancy in Japan (2.0 per 1000 pregnancies) has been reported to be about threefold higher than the incidence in Europe or North America (about 0.6–1.1 per 1000 pregnancies) (3). The variation in the incidence rates of molar pregnancy may in part result from differences between reporting population-based versus hospital-based data. The incidence of both complete and partial mole has been investigated in Ireland by reviewing all products of conception from first- and second-trimester abortions (4). Based on a complete pathologic review, the incidence of complete and partial mole was found to be 1:1945 and 1:695 pregnancies, respectively.

Careful case-control studies have been undertaken to identify risk factors for both complete and partial molar pregnancy. The high incidence of molar pregnancy in some populations has been attributed to nutritional and socioeconomic factors. **Case-control studies** from both Italy and the United States have shown that low dietary intake of carotene may be associated with an increased risk of complete molar pregnancy (5, 6). **Areas with a high incidence of molar pregnancy also have a high frequency of vitamin A deficiency. Dietary factors may, therefore, partly explain regional variations in the incidence of complete mole.**

Maternal age older than 35 years has consistently been shown to be a risk factor for complete mole. Ova from older women may be more susceptible to abnormal fertilization. In one study, the risk for complete mole was increased twofold for women older than 35 years of age and 7.5-fold for women older than 40 years of age (7).

Limited information is available concerning risk factors for partial molar pregnancy. However, the epidemiologic characteristics of complete and partial mole may differ. There is no association between maternal age and the risk for partial mole (7).

Complete versus Partial Hydatidiform Mole

Hydatidiform moles may be categorized as either complete or partial moles on the basis of gross morphology, histopathology, and karyotype (Table 35.1).

Complete Hydatidiform Mole

Pathology **Complete moles lack identifiable embryonic or fetal tissues, and the chorionic villi exhibit generalized hydatidiform swelling and diffuse trophoblastic hyperplasia** (Fig. 35.1).

Chromosomes **Cytogenetic studies have demonstrated that complete hydatidiform moles usually have a 46XX karyotype, and the molar chromosomes are entirely of paternal origin** (Fig. 35.2) (8). **Complete moles appear to usually arise from an ovum that has been fertilized by a haploid sperm, which then duplicates its own chromosomes. The ovum nucleus may be either absent or inactivated** (9). **Although most complete moles have a 46XX chromosomal pattern, about 10% have a 46XY karyotype** (10). Chromosomes in a 46XY complete mole also appear to be entirely of paternal origin. Although chromosomes of complete moles are entirely of paternal origin, mitochondrial DNA is of maternal origin (11).

Partial Hydatidiform Mole

Pathology   Partial hydatidiform moles are characterized by the following pathologic features (12) (Fig. 35.3):

1. Chorionic villi of varying size with focal hydatidiform swelling, cavitation, and trophoblastic hyperplasia

2. Marked villous scalloping

3. Prominent stromal trophoblastic inclusions

4. Identifiable embryonic or fetal tissues.

Table 35.1   Features of Complete and Partial Hydatidiform Moles

	Complete Mole	*Partial Mole*
Fetal or embryonic tissue	Absent	Present
Hydatidiform swelling of chorionic villi	Diffuse	Focal
Trophoblastic hyperplasia	Diffuse	Focal
Scalloping of chorionic villi	Absent	Present
Trophoblastic stromal inclusions	Absent	Present
Karyotype	46XX (90%); 46XY	Triploid (90%)

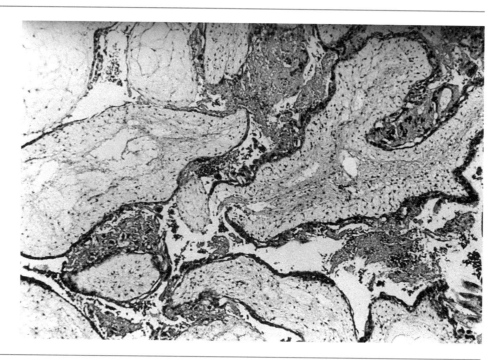

Figure 35.1   Photomicrograph of complete mole demonstrating diffusely hydropic chorionic villi and diffuse trophoblastic hyperplasia.

Figure 35.2   The karyotype of complete hydatidiform mole.

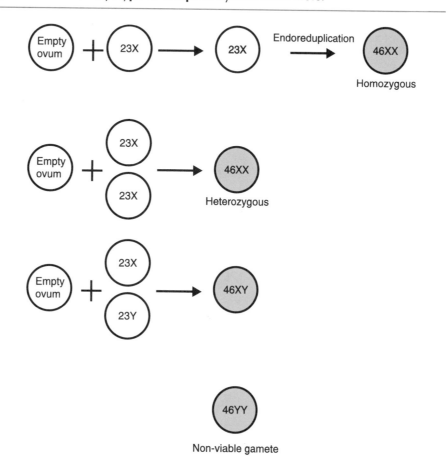

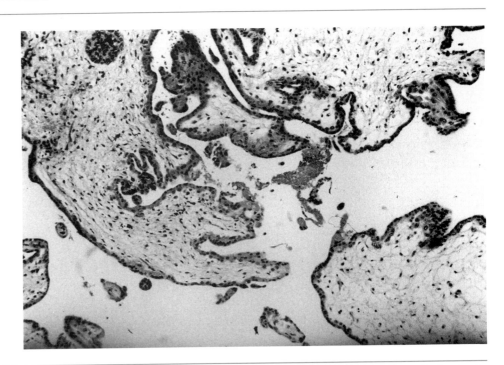

Figure 35.3 Photomicrograph of partial mole showing varying-sized chorionic villi with focal trophoblastic hyperplasia, stroma trophoblastic inclusions, and villous scalloping. (Reproduced with permission from **Berkowitz RS, Goldstein OP.** Gestational trophoblastic diseases. In: **Ryan KJ, Berkowitz R, Barbieri R,** eds. *Kistner's Gynecology Principles and Practice.* 5th ed. Chicago: Year Book Medical Publishers, 1990:433.)

Chromosomes **Partial moles generally have a triploid karyotype (69 chromosomes); the extra haploid set of chromosomes usually is derived from the father** (Fig. 35.4) (13). Lawler et al. and Lage et al. reported that 93 and 90%, respectively, of partial moles were triploid (13, 14). When a fetus is present in conjunction with a partial mole, it generally exhibits the stigmata of triploidy, including growth retardation and multiple congenital malformations such as syndactyly and hydrocephaly (Fig. 35.5).

Clinical Features	Increasingly, patients with complete molar pregnancy are being treated before they develop the classic clinical signs and symptoms. This may be due to changes in clinical practice, such as the frequent use of vaginal probe ultrasound in early pregnancy in women with vaginal staining and even asymptomatic women. The following description of the clinical features of complete mole represents the classic presentation.
Complete Hydatidiform Mole	***Vaginal Bleeding*** **Vaginal bleeding is the most common presenting symptom in patients with complete molar pregnancy and occurs in 97% of cases** (15). Molar tissues may separate from the decidua and disrupt maternal vessels, and large volumes of retained blood may distend the endometrial cavity. Because vaginal bleeding may be considerable and prolonged, half of these patients may have anemia (hemoglobin <10 g/100 ml). ***Excessive Uterine Size*** **Excessive uterine enlargement relative to gestational age is one of the classic signs of a complete mole, although it is present in only about half of the patients.** The endometrial cavity may be expanded by both chorionic tissue and retained blood. Excessive uterine size is generally associated with markedly elevated levels of human chorionic gonadotropin (hCG), because uterine enlargement results in part from trophoblastic overgrowth.

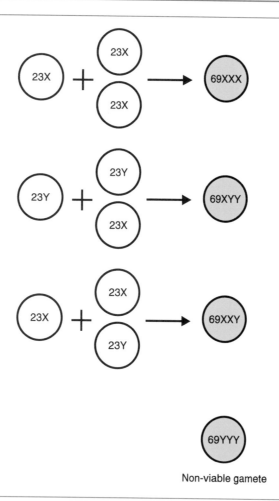

Figure 35.4   The karyotype of partial hydatidiform mole.

Figure 35.5   Photomicrograph of a fetal hand demonstrating syndactyly. The fetus had a triploid karyotype and the chorionic tissues were a partial mole.

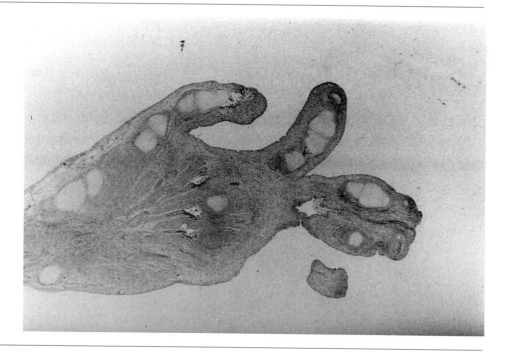

Preeclampsia   **Preeclampsia is observed in 27% of patients with a complete hydatidiform mole.** Although preeclampsia is associated with hypertension, proteinuria, and hyperreflexia, eclamptic convulsions rarely occur. Preeclampsia develops almost exclusively in patients with excessive uterine size and markedly elevated hCG levels. Curry et al. observed that 81% of patients with molar pregnancy and preeclampsia had excessive uterine enlargement (16). The diagnosis of hydatidiform mole should be considered whenever preeclampsia develops early in pregnancy.

Hyperemesis Gravidarum   **Hyperemesis requiring antiemetic or intravenous replacement therapy occurs in one-fourth of women with a complete mole, particularly those with excessive uterine size and markedly elevated hCG levels.** Severe electrolyte disturbances may develop and require treatment with parenteral fluids.

Hyperthyroidism   **Clinically evident hyperthyroidism may be observed in 7% of patients with a complete molar gestation.** These women may present with tachycardia, warm skin, and tremor, and the diagnosis can be confirmed by detection of elevated serum levels of free thyroxine (T_4) and triiodothyronine (T_3).

If hyperthyroidism is suspected before the induction of anesthesia for molar evacuation, β-adrenergic blocking agents should be administered because anesthesia or surgery may precipitate thyroid storm. Thyroid storms may be manifest by hyperthermia, delirium, convulsions, tachyrhythmia, high-output heart failure, or cardiovascular collapse. Administration of β-adrenergic blocking agents prevents or rapidly reverses many of the metabolic and cardiovascular complications of thyroid storm. After molar evacuation, thyroid function tests return rapidly to normal.

Hyperthyroidism develops almost exclusively in patients with very high hCG levels (17). Some investigators have suggested that hCG is the thyroid stimulator in women with GTD because positive correlations between serum hCG and total T_4 or T_3 concentrations have been observed. However, Amir et al. (18) measured thyroid function in 47 patients with a complete mole and reported no significant correlation between serum hCG levels and serum values of free T_4 index or free T_3 index. Although some investigators have speculated about a separate chorionic thyrotropin, this substance has not yet been isolated.

Trophoblastic Embolization   **Respiratory distress develops in 2% of patients with a complete mole.** Respiratory distress is usually diagnosed in patients with excessive uterine size and markedly elevated hCG levels. Twiggs et al. observed respiratory complications in 12 (27%) of 44 patients with a molar pregnancy of at least 16 weeks' size (19). These patients may have chest pain, dyspnea, tachypnea, and tachycardia and may experience severe respiratory distress during and after molar evacuation. Auscultation of the chest usually reveals diffuse rales, and the chest x-ray may demonstrate bilateral pulmonary infiltrates. Respiratory distress usually resolves within 72 hours with cardiopulmonary support. In some circumstances, patients may require mechanical ventilation. Respiratory insufficiency may result from trophoblastic embolization or from the cardiopulmonary complications of thyroid storm, preeclampsia, and massive fluid replacement.

Theca Lutein Ovarian Cysts   **Prominent theca lutein ovarian cysts (>6 cm in diameter) develop in about half the patients with a complete mole** (17). Theca lutein ovarian cysts result from high serum hCG levels, which cause ovarian hyperstimulation (20). Because the uterus also may be excessively enlarged, theca lutein cysts may be difficult to palpate during physical examination; however, ultrasonography can accurately document their presence and size. After molar evacuation, theca lutein cysts normally regress spontaneously within 2–4 months.

Prominent theca lutein cysts may cause symptoms of marked pelvic pressure, and they may be decompressed by laparoscopic or ultrasound-directed aspiration. If acute pelvic pain develops, laparoscopy should be performed to assess possible cystic torsion or rupture. Incomplete ovarian torsion or cystic rupture may be managed successfully with laparoscopic manipulation (21).

Partial Hydatidiform Mole

Patients with a partial hydatidiform mole usually do not present with the dramatic clinical features characteristic of complete molar pregnancy. **In general, these patients present with the signs and symptoms of incomplete or missed abortion, and the diagnosis of partial mole may be made only after histologic review of the curettings (22).**

In a survey of 81 patients with a partial mole, the main presenting sign was vaginal bleeding, which occurred in 59 patients (72.8%) (23). Excessive uterine enlargement and preeclampsia were present in only three patients (3.7%) and two (2.5%) patients, respectively. No patients presented with theca lutein ovarian cysts, hyperemesis, or hyperthyroidism. The presenting clinical diagnosis was an incomplete or missed abortion in 74 patients (91.3%) and hydatidiform mole in only five patients (6.2%). Preevacuation hCG levels were measured in 30 patients and were higher than 100,000 mIU/ml in only two patients (6.6%).

Natural History

Complete Hydatidiform Mole

Complete moles have a potential for local invasion and dissemination. **After molar evacuation, local uterine invasion occurs in 15% of patients and metastases occurs in 4% (17).**

A review of 858 patients with complete hydatidiform mole revealed that two-fifths of the patients had the following signs of marked trophoblastic proliferation at the time of presentation (17):

1. hCG level >100,000 mIU/ml

2. Excessive uterine enlargement

3. Theca lutein cysts >6 cm in diameter

Patients with any one of these signs were considered at high risk. After molar evacuation, local uterine invasion occurred in 31% and metastases developed in 8.8% of the 352 high-risk patients. For the 506 low-risk patients, local invasion was found in only 3.4% and metastases developed in 0.6%.

Older patients are also at increased risk of developing postmolar gestational trophoblastic tumor. Tow and Tsukamoto et al. reported that persistent tumor developed after a complete molar pregnancy in 37% of women older than 40 years of age and 56% of women older than 50 years of age (24, 25).

Partial Hydatidiform Mole

Persistent tumor, usually nonmetastatic, develops in approximately 4% of patients with a partial mole, and chemotherapy is required to achieve remission (26). Patients who develop persistent disease have no distinguishing clinical or pathologic characteristics (27). Additionally, Lage et al. reported that 11 (85%) of 13 partial moles that developed persistent tumor had a triploid karyotype (28).

Diagnosis

Ultrasonography is a reliable and sensitive technique for the diagnosis of complete molar pregnancy. Because the chorionic villi exhibit diffuse hydropic swelling, complete moles produce a characteristic vesicular sonographic pattern.

Ultrasonography may also contribute to the diagnosis of partial molar pregnancy by demonstrating focal cystic spaces in the placental tissues and an increase in the transverse diameter of the gestational sac (29). When both of these criteria are present, the positive predictive value for partial mole is 90%.

Treatment

After molar pregnancy is diagnosed, the patient should be evaluated carefully for the presence of associated medical complications, including preeclampsia, hyperthyroidism, electrolyte imbalance, and anemia. After the patient's condition has been stabilized, a decision must be made concerning the most appropriate method of evacuation.

Hysterectomy

If the patient desires surgical sterilization, a hysterectomy may be performed with the mole *in situ*. The ovaries may be preserved at the time of surgery, even though prominent theca lutein cysts are present. Large ovarian cysts may be decompressed by aspiration. Hysterectomy does not prevent metastasis; therefore, patients still require follow-up with assessment of hCG levels.

Suction Curettage

Suction curettage is the preferred method of evacuation, regardless of uterine size, for patients who desire to preserve fertility. It involves the following steps:

1. *Oxytocin infusion*—This is begun in the operating room before the induction of anesthesia.

2. *Cervical dilation*—As the cervix is being dilated, the surgeon frequently encounters increased uterine bleeding. Retained blood in the endometrial cavity may be expelled during cervical dilation. However, active uterine bleeding should not deter the prompt completion of cervical dilation.

3. *Suction curettage*—Within a few minutes of commencing suction curettage, the uterus may decrease dramatically in size and the bleeding is generally well controlled. The use of a 12-mm cannula is strongly advised to facilitate evacuation. If the uterus is larger than 14 weeks of gestation in size, one hand should be placed on top of the fundus and the uterus should be massaged to stimulate uterine contraction and reduce the risk of perforation.

4. *Sharp curettage*—When suction evacuation is believed to be complete, gentle sharp curettage is performed to remove any residual molar tissue.

Because trophoblast cells express Rh D factor, patients who are Rh negative should receive Rh immune globulin at the time of evacuation.

Prophylactic Chemotherapy

The use of prophylactic chemotherapy at the time of molar evacuation is controversial (30). The debate concerns the wisdom of exposing all patients to potentially toxic treatment when only about 20% are at risk of developing persistent tumor.

In a study of 247 patients with complete molar pregnancy who prophylactically received a single course of actinomycin D at the time of evacuation, local uterine invasion subsequently developed in only 10 patients (4%) and no patients developed metastases (31). Furthermore, all 10 patients with local invasion achieved remission after only one additional course of chemotherapy. Prophylactic chemotherapy, therefore, not only prevented metastases but also reduced the incidence and morbidity of local uterine invasion.

In a prospective randomized study of prophylactic chemotherapy in patients with a complete mole, a significant decrease in persistent tumor was detected in patients with high-risk mole who received prophylactic chemotherapy (47 vs. 14%) (32). **Prophylaxis may be particularly useful in the management of high-risk complete molar pregnancy, especially when hormonal follow-up is unavailable or unreliable.**

Follow-Up

Human Chorionic Gonadotropin

After molar evacuation, patients should be monitored with weekly determinations of β-subunit hCG levels until these are normal for 3 consecutive weeks, followed by monthly determinations until the levels are normal for 6 consecutive months. The average time to achieve the first normal hCG level after evacuation is about 9 weeks (33). **At the completion of follow-up, pregnancy may be undertaken.**

Contraception

Patients are encouraged to use effective contraception during the entire interval of gonadotropin follow-up. Because of the potential risk of uterine perforation, intrauterine devices should not be inserted until the patient achieves a normal hCG level. If the patient does not desire surgical sterilization, the choice is to use either oral contraceptives or barrier methods.

The incidence of postmolar persistent tumor has been reported to be increased among patients who used oral contraceptives before gonadotropin remission (34). However, more recent data indicate that oral contraceptives do not increase the risk of postmolar trophoblastic disease (35, 36). In addition, the method of contraception used does not influence the mean hCG regression time. **It appears that oral contraceptives may be used safely after molar evacuation during the entire interval of hormonal follow-up.**

Persistent Gestational Trophoblastic Tumor

Nonmetastatic Disease

Locally invasive gestational trophoblastic tumor (GTT) develops in about 15% of patients after molar evacuation and infrequently after other gestations (1). These patients usually present clinically with the following symptoms:

1. Irregular vaginal bleeding

2. Theca lutein cysts

3. Uterine subinvolution or asymmetric enlargement

4. Persistently elevated serum hCG levels.

The trophoblastic tumor may perforate through the myometrium, causing intraperitoneal bleeding, or erode into uterine vessels, causing vaginal hemorrhage. Bulky, necrotic tumor may involve the uterine wall and serve as a nidus for infection. Patients with uterine sepsis may have a purulent vaginal discharge and acute pelvic pain.

After molar evacuation, persistent GTT may exhibit the histologic features of either hydatidiform mole or choriocarcinoma. After a nonmolar pregnancy, however, persistent GTT always has the histologic pattern of choriocarcinoma. Histologically, choriocarcinoma is characterized by sheets of anaplastic syncytiotrophoblast and cytotrophoblast without chorionic villi.

Placental-Site Trophoblastic Tumor   Placental-site trophoblastic tumor is an uncommon but important variant of choriocarcinoma that consists predominantly of intermediate trophoblast (37). Relative to their mass, these tumors produce small amounts of hCG and human placental lactogen, and they tend to remain confined to the uterus, metastasizing late in their course. **In contrast to other trophoblastic tumors, placental-site tumors are relatively insensitive to chemotherapy.**

Metastatic Disease

Metastatic GTT occurs in about 4% of patients after molar evacuation but is seen more commonly when GTT develops after other pregnancies (1). Metastasis is usually associated with choriocarcinoma, which has a tendency toward early vascular invasion with widespread dissemination. Because trophoblastic tumors are often perfused by fragile vessels, they are frequently hemorrhagic. Symptoms of metastases may result from spontaneous bleeding at metastatic foci. The most common sites of metastases are lung (80%), vagina (30%), pelvis (20%), liver (10%), and brain (10%).

Pulmonary   **At the time of presentation, lung involvement is shown on chest x-rays of 80% of patients with metastatic GTT.** Patients with pulmonary metastases may have chest pain, cough, hemoptysis, dyspnea, or an asymptomatic lesion on chest x-ray. Respiratory symptoms may be acute or chronic, persisting over many months.

GTT may produce four principal pulmonary radiographic patterns:

1. An alveolar or "snowstorm" pattern

2. Discrete rounded densities

3. Pleural effusion

4. An embolic pattern caused by pulmonary arterial occlusion

Because respiratory symptoms and radiographic findings may be dramatic, the patient may be thought to have primary pulmonary disease. Some patients with extensive pulmonary involvement have minimal if any gynecologic symptoms because the reproductive organs may be free of trophoblastic tumor. Unfortunately, the diagnosis of GTT may be confirmed only after thoracotomy has been performed, particularly in patients with a nonmolar antecedent pregnancy.

Pulmonary hypertension may develop in patients with GTT secondary to pulmonary arterial occlusion by trophoblastic emboli. The development of early respiratory failure requiring intubation is associated with a dismal clinical outcome (38, 39).

Vaginal   **Vaginal metastases are present in 30% of the patients with metastatic tumor. These lesions are usually highly vascular and may bleed vigorously if biopsied.** Metastases to the vagina may occur in the fornices or suburethrally and may produce irregular bleeding or a purulent discharge.

Hepatic   **Liver metastases occur in 10% of patients with disseminated trophoblastic tumor.** Hepatic involvement is encountered almost exclusively in patients with protracted delays in diagnosis and extensive tumor burdens. Epigastric or right upper quadrant pain may develop if metastases stretch the hepatic capsule. Hepatic lesions may be hemorrhagic, causing hepatic rupture and exsanguinating intraperitoneal bleeding.

Central Nervous System   **Metastatic trophoblastic disease involves the brain in 10% of patients.** Cerebral involvement is generally seen in patients with far-advanced disease; virtually all patients with brain metastases have concurrent pulmonary or vaginal involvement or both. Because cerebral lesions may spontaneously hemorrhage, patients may develop acute focal neurologic deficits.

Staging

An anatomic staging system for GTT has been adopted by the International Federation of Gynecology and Obstetrics (FIGO) (Table 35.2). It is hoped that this staging system will encourage the objective comparison of data among various centers.

Table 35.2   Staging of Gestational Trophoblastic Tumors

Stage I	**Disease confined to uterus**
Stage Ia	Disease confined to uterus with no risk factors
Stage Ib	Disease confined to uterus with one risk factor
Stage Ic	Disease confined to uterus with two risk factors
Stage II	**Gestational trophoblastic tumor extending outside uterus but limited to genital structures (adnexa, vagina, broad ligament)**
Stage IIa	Gestational trophoblastic tumor involving genital structures without risk factors
Stage IIb	Gestational trophoblastic tumor extending outside uterus but limited to genital structures with one risk factor
Stage IIc	Gestational trophoblastic tumor extending outside uterus but limited to genital structures with two risk factors
Stage III	**Gestational trophoblastic disease extending to lungs with or without known genital tract involvement**
Stage IIIa	Gestational trophoblastic tumor extending to lungs with or without genital tract involvement and with no risk factors
Stage IIIb	Gestational trophoblastic tumor extending to lungs with or without genital tract involvement and with one risk factor
Stage IIIc	Gestational trophoblastic tumor extending to lungs with or without genital tract involvement and with two risk factors
Stage IV	**All other metastatic sites**
Stage IVa	All other metastatic sites without risk factors
Stage IVb	All other metastatic sites with one risk factor
Stage IVc	All other metastatic sites with two risk factors

Risk factors affecting staging include the following: 1) human chorionic gonadotropin > 100,000 MIU/ml and 2) duration of disease longer than 6 months from termination of antecedent pregnancy.
The following factors should be considered and noted in reporting: 1) prior chemotherapy has been given for known gestational trophoblastic tumor; 2) placental site tumors should be reported separately; 3) histologic verification of disease is not required.

Stage I   **Patients with persistently elevated hCG levels and tumor confined to the uterine corpus.**

Stage II   **Patients with metastases to the vagina and/or pelvis.**

Stage III   **Patients with pulmonary metastases with or without uterine, vaginal, or pelvic involvement.** The diagnosis is based on a rising hCG level in the presence of pulmonary lesions on chest x-ray.

Stage IV   **Patients with advanced disease and involvement of the brain, liver, kidneys, or gastrointestinal tract.** These patients are in the highest risk category, because they are most likely to be resistant to chemotherapy. The histologic pattern of choriocarcinoma is usually present, and disease commonly follows a nonmolar pregnancy.

Prognostic Scoring System

In addition to anatomic staging, it is important to consider other variables to predict the likelihood of drug resistance and to assist in selecting appropriate chemotherapy (2). **A prognostic scoring system has been proposed by the World Health Organization and reliably predicts the potential for resistance to chemotherapy (Table 35.3).**

When the prognostic score is ≥8, the patient is categorized as high-risk and requires intensive combination chemotherapy to achieve remission. Patients with stage I disease usually have a low-risk score, and those with stage IV disease have a high-risk score. The distinction between low and high risk applies mainly to patients with Stage II or III disease.

Table 35.3 Scoring System Based on Prognostic Factors

	Score			
	0	**1**	**2**	**4**
Age (years)	≤39	>39		
Antecedent pregnancy	Hydatidiform mole	Abortion	Term	
Interval between end of antecedent pregnancy and start of chemotherapy (months)	<4	4–6	7–12	>12
Human chorionic gonadotropin (IU/liter)	$<10^3$	$10^3–10^4$	$10^4–10^5$	$>10^5$
ABO groups		O or A	B or AB	
Largest tumor, including uterine (cm)	<3	3–5	>5	
Site of metastases		Spleen, kidney	Gastrointestinal treat, liver	Brain
Number of metastases		1–3	4–8	>8
Prior chemotherapy			1 drug	≥2 drugs

The total score for a patient is obtained by adding the individual scores for each prognostic factor. Total score: <4 = low-risk; 5–7 = middle risk; ≥8 = high risk.

Diagnostic Evaluation

Optimal management of persistent GTT requires a thorough assessment of the extent of the disease prior to the initiation of treatment. **All patients with persistent GTT should undergo a careful pretreatment evaluation, including the following:**

1. Complete history and physical examination

2. Measurement of the serum hCG value

3. Hepatic, thyroid, and renal function tests

4. Determination of base line peripheral white blood cell and platelet counts.

The metastatic workup should include the following:

1. Chest x-ray or computed tomography (CT) scan

2. Ultrasonogram or CT scan of the abdomen and pelvis

3. CT scan of the head

4. Selective angiography of abdominal and pelvic organs, if indicated.

If the pelvic examination and chest x-ray are negative, it is very uncommon to have metastatic involvement of other sites.

Liver ultrasonography and CT scanning will document most hepatic metastases in patients with abnormal liver function tests. CT scan of the head has facilitated the early diagnosis of asymptomatic cerebral lesions (40). Chest CT scans may demonstrate micrometastases in the presence of a normal chest x-ray.

In patients with choriocarcinoma or metastatic disease, hCG levels may be measured in the cerebrospinal fluid (CSF) to exclude cerebral involvement if the CT scan of the brain is normal. The plasma/CSF hCG ratio tends to be lower than 60 in the presence of cerebral metastases (41). However, a single plasma/CSF hCG ratio may be misleading, because rapid changes in plasma hCG levels may not be reflected promptly in the CSF (42).

Pelvic ultrasonography appears to be useful in detecting extensive trophoblastic uterine involvement and may also aid in identifying sites of resistant uterine tumor (43). Because ultrasonography can accurately and noninvasively detect extensive uterine tumor, it may help select patients who would benefit from hysterectomy.

Management of Persistent GTT

A protocol for the management of GTT is presented in Table 35.4.

Stage I

In patients with stage I disease, the selection of treatment is based primarily on whether the patient desires to retain fertility.

Hysterectomy Plus Chemotherapy

If the patient does not wish to preserve fertility, hysterectomy with adjuvant single-agent chemotherapy may be performed as primary treatment. Adjuvant chemotherapy is administered for three reasons:

1. To reduce the likelihood of disseminating viable tumor cells at surgery.

2. To maintain a cytotoxic level of chemotherapy in the bloodstream and tissues in case viable tumor cells are disseminated at surgery.

3. To treat any occult metastases that may already be present at the time of surgery.

Chemotherapy can be administered safely at the time of hysterectomy without increasing the risk of bleeding or sepsis. In a series of 29 patients treated at our institution with primary hysterectomy and a single course of adjuvant chemotherapy, all have achieved complete remission with no additional therapy.

Hysterectomy is also performed in all patients with stage I *placental-site trophoblastic tumor*. Because placental-site tumors are resistant to chemotherapy, hysterectomy for presumed nonmetastatic disease is the only curative treatment. To date, only a small number of patients with metastatic placental-site tumor have been reported to be in sustained re-

Table 35.4   Protocol for Treatment of GTT

Stage I	
Initial	Single-agent chemotherapy or hysterectomy with adjunctive chemotherapy
Resistant	Combination chemotherapy
	Hysterectomy with adjunctive chemotherapy
	Local resection
	Pelvic infusion
Stage II and III	
Low Risk*	
Initial	Single-agent chemotherapy
Resistant	Combination chemotherapy
High Risk*	
Initial	Combination chemotherapy
Resistant	Second-line combination chemotherapy
Stage IV	
Initial	Combination chemotherapy
Brain	Whole-heat irradiation (3000 cGy)
	Craniotomy to manage complications
Liver	Resection to manage complications
Resistant*	Second-line combination chemotherapy
	Hepatic arterial infusion

*Local resection optional.

of patients with metastatic placental-site tumor have been reported to be in sustained remission as a result of chemotherapy (44).

Chemotherapy Alone

Single-agent chemotherapy is the preferred treatment in patients with stage I disease who desire to retain fertility. When primary single-agent chemotherapy was administered at our institution to 399 patients with stage I GTT, 373 patients (93.5%) attained complete remission. The remaining 26 resistant patients subsequently achieved remission after combination chemotherapy or surgical intervention.

When patients are resistant to single-agent chemotherapy and desire to preserve fertility, combination chemotherapy should be administered. If the patient is resistant to both single-agent and combination chemotherapy and wants to retain fertility, local uterine resection may be considered. When local resection is planned, a preoperative ultrasonogram, magnetic resonance imaging (MRI), or arteriogram may help define the site of the resistant tumor.

Stages II and III

Low-risk patients are treated with primary single-agent chemotherapy, and high-risk patients are managed with primary intensive combination chemotherapy.

Vaginal and Pelvic Metastasis

All 26 patients with Stage II disease treated at our institution achieved remission. Single-agent chemotherapy induced complete remission in 16 (88.9%) of 18 low-risk patients. In contrast, only two of eight high-risk patients achieved remission with single-agent treatment; the others required combination chemotherapy.

Vaginal metastases may bleed profusely because they are highly vascular and friable. When bleeding is substantial, it may be controlled by packing the vagina or by wide local excision. Infrequently, arteriographic embolization of the hypogastric arteries may be required to control hemorrhage from vaginal metastases.

Pulmonary Metastasis

Of 130 patients with stage III disease treated at our institution, 129 (99%) attained complete remission. Gonadotropin remission was induced with single-agent chemotherapy in 71 of 85 (83.5%) patients with low-risk disease. All patients who were resistant to single-agent treatment subsequently achieved remission with combination chemotherapy.

Thoracotomy Thoracotomy has a limited role in the management of stage III disease. **If a patient has a persistent viable pulmonary metastasis despite intensive chemotherapy, however, thoracotomy may be attempted to excise the resistant focus.** A thorough metastatic workup should be performed before surgery to exclude other sites of persistent disease. Evidence of fibrotic pulmonary nodules may persist indefinitely on chest x-rays, even after complete gonadotropin remission has been attained. In patients undergoing thoracotomy for resistant disease, chemotherapy should be administered postoperatively to treat potential occult sites of micrometastases.

Hysterectomy

Hysterectomy may be required in patients with metastatic disease to control uterine hemorrhage or sepsis. Furthermore, in patients with extensive uterine tumor, hysterectomy may substantially reduce the trophoblastic tumor burden and thereby limit the need for multiple courses of chemotherapy (45).

Follow-Up

All patients with stage I through stage III disease should receive follow-up with:

1. Weekly measurement of hCG levels until they are normal for 3 consecutive weeks

2. Monthly measurement of hCG values until levels are normal for 12 consecutive months

3. Effective contraception during the entire interval of hormonal follow-up

Stage IV

Patients with stage IV disease are at greatest risk of developing rapidly progressive and unresponsive tumors despite intensive multimodal therapy. **They should preferably be referred to centers with special expertise in the management of trophoblastic disease.**

All patients with stage IV disease should be treated with primary intensive combination chemotherapy and the selective use of radiation therapy and surgery. Before 1975, only six of 20 patients (30%) with stage IV disease treated at our institution attained complete remission, whereas after that time, 14 of 18 patients (77.8%) achieved remission. This improvement in survival has resulted from the use of primary combination chemotherapy in conjunction with radiation and surgical treatment.

Hepatic Metastasis

The management of hepatic metastases is particularly difficult. If a patient is resistant to systemic chemotherapy, hepatic arterial infusion of chemotherapy may induce complete remission in selected cases. Hepatic resection may also be required to control acute bleeding or to excise a focus of resistant tumor. New techniques of arterial embolization may reduce the need for surgical intervention.

Cerebral Metastasis

If cerebral metastases are diagnosed, whole-brain irradiation (3000 cGy in 10 fractions) is instituted promptly in our institution. The risk of spontaneous cerebral hemorrhage may be lessened by the concurrent use of combination chemotherapy and brain irradiation because irradiation may be both hemostatic and tumoricidal. However, excellent remission rates (86%) have been reported in patients with cranial metastases treated with intensive intravenous combination chemotherapy and intrathecal methotrexate (46).

Craniotomy Craniotomy may be required to provide acute decompression or to control bleeding and should be performed to manage life-threatening complications in the hope that the patient ultimately will be cured with chemotherapy. Weed et al. (47) reported the use of craniotomy to control bleeding in six patients, three of whom subsequently achieved complete remission. Infrequently, cerebral metastases that are resistant to chemotherapy may be amenable to local resection. Fortunately, patients with cerebral metastases who achieve sustained remission generally have no residual neurologic deficits.

Follow-Up

Patients with stage IV disease should receive follow-up with:

1. Weekly determination of hCG levels until they are normal for 3 consecutive weeks.

2. Monthly determination of hCG levels until they are normal for 24 consecutive months.

These patients require prolonged gonadotropin follow-up because they are at increased risk of late recurrence.

An algorithm for the management of persistent gestational trophoblastic tumor is presented in Figure 35.6.

Chemotherapy

Single-Agent Chemotherapy

Single-agent chemotherapy with either *actinomycin D (Act-D)* or *methotrexate (MTX)* has achieved comparable and excellent remission rates in both nonmetastatic and low-risk metastatic GTT (48). Several protocols using these agents are available. *Act-D* can be given every other week as a 5-day regimen or in a pulsatile fashion; similarly, *MTX* can be given either in a 5-day regimen or pulsatile weekly. No study has compared all of these protocols with regard to success. An optimal regimen should maximize the response rate while minimizing morbidity and cost.

The administration of *methotrexate* with *folinic acid (MTX-FA)* in GTT to limit systemic toxicity was first reported in 1964 (49). Subsequently, it has been confirmed that *MTX-FA* is both effective and safe in the management of GTT (50).

MTX-FA has been the preferred single-agent regimen in the treatment of GTT in our institution since 1974. An evaluation of 185 patients treated in this manner between 1974 and 1984 revealed that complete remission was achieved in 162 patients (87.6%); and 132 of these patients (81.5%) required only one course of *MTX-FA* to attain remission (50). *MTX-FA* induced remission in 147 of 163 patients (90.2%) with stage I GTT and in 15 of 22 patients (68.2%) with low-risk stages II and III GTT. Resistance to therapy was more common in patients with choriocarcinoma, metastases, and pretreatment serum hCG levels higher than 50,000 mIU/ml. After treatment with *MTX-FA*, thrombocytopenia, granulocytopenia, and hepatotoxicity developed in only three (1.6%), 11 (5.9%) and 26 (14.1%) patients, respectively. Thus, *MTX-FA* achieved an excellent therapeutic outcome with minimal toxicity and attained this goal with limited exposure to chemotherapy.

Rustin et al. (51) investigated the incidence of second tumors after cytotoxic chemotherapy in 457 long-term survivors treated for GTT. MTX was administered to all but two patients, and 261 (57%) also received other cytotoxic drugs. There was no increase in second tumors after cytotoxic chemotherapy for GTT.

Technique of Single-Agent Treatment

The serum hCG level is measured weekly after each course of chemotherapy, and the hCG regression curve serves as the primary basis for determining the need for additional treatment.

After the first treatment:

1. Further chemotherapy is withheld as long as the hCG level is falling progressively.

2. Additional single-agent chemotherapy is not administered at any predetermined or fixed time interval.

1276

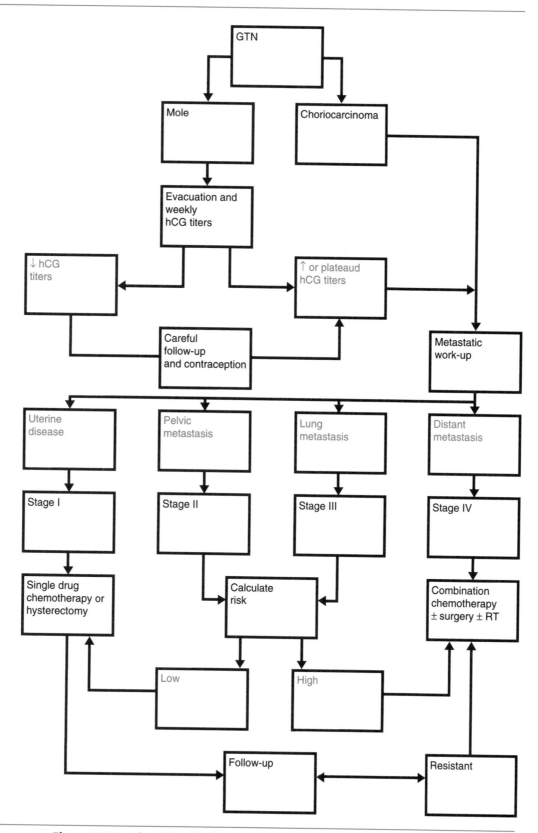

Figure 35.6   Algorithm for the management of persistent gestational trophoblastic tumor. (Reproduced with permission from **Berek JS, Hacker NF,** eds. *Practical Gynecologic Oncology.* 2nd ed. Baltimore: Williams & Wilkins, 1994:473.)

A second course of chemotherapy is administered under the following conditions:

1. If the hCG level plateaus for more than 3 consecutive weeks or begins to rise again.

2. If the hCG level does not decline by 1 log within 18 days after completion of the first treatment.

If a second course of *MTX-FA* is required, the dosage of *MTX* is unaltered if the patient's response to the first treatment was adequate. An adequate response is defined as a fall in the hCG level by 1 log after a course of chemotherapy.

If the response to the first treatment is inadequate, the dosage of *MTX* is increased from 1.0 mg/kg/day to 1.5 mg/kg/day for each of the four treatment days. If the response to two consecutive courses of *MTX-FA* is inadequate, the patient is considered to be resistant to *MTX* and *Act-D* is promptly substituted. If the hCG levels do not decline by 1 log after treatment with *Act-D*, the patient is also considered resistant to *Act-D* as a single agent. She must then be treated intensively with combination chemotherapy to achieve remission.

Combination Chemotherapy

Triple Therapy

Triple therapy with *MTX*, *Act-D*, and *cyclophosphamide* is inadequate as an initial treatment in patients with metastases and a high-risk prognostic score. Collectively, data from various centers indicate that triple therapy induced remission in only 21 (49%) of 43 patients with metastases and high-risk score (score $\geq$8) (52–54).

EMA-CO

Etoposide has been reported to induce complete remission in 56 (95%) of 60 patients with nonmetastatic and low-risk metastatic GTT (55). In 1984, Bagshawe first described a new combination regimen that included *etoposide, MTX, Act-D, cyclophosphamide,* and *vincristine* (EMA-CO) and reported an 83% remission in patients with metastases and a high-risk score (56). Importantly, Bolis et al. (57) confirmed that primary EMA-CO induced complete remission in 76% of the patients with metastatic GTT and a high-risk score. Similarly, Quinn et al. reported that EMA-CO induced complete sustained remission in 61 (94%) of 65 patients with high-risk (score $\leq$5) GTT (58). Furthermore, Rustin et al. (46) reported remission with EMA-CO in 13 (86%) of 15 patients with brain metastases.

The EMA-CO regimen is generally well tolerated, and treatment seldom has to be suspended because of toxicity. The EMA-CO regimen may now be the preferred primary treatment in patients with metastases and a high-risk prognostic score. However, the optimal combination drug protocol in GTT has not yet been clearly defined. Surwit and Childers have proposed a modification of the EMA-CO regimen by substituting *cisplatin* and *etoposide* on day 8 (59). The optimal combination drug protocol will most likely include *etoposide, MTX,* and *Act-D* and perhaps other agents, administered in the most dose-intensive manner.

Duration of Therapy

Patients who require combination chemotherapy must be treated intensively to attain remission. Combination chemotherapy should be given as often as toxicity permits until the patient achieves three consecutive normal hCG levels. After normal hCG levels are attained, at least two additional courses of chemotherapy are administered to reduce the risk of relapse.

1278

Subsequent Pregnancies

Pregnancies After Hydatidiform Mole

Patients with hydatidiform moles can anticipate normal reproduction in the future (60). From 1965 until 1992, patients who were treated at our institution for complete mole had 1205 subsequent pregnancies that resulted in 826 full-term live births (68.5%), 90 premature deliveries (7.5%), 11 ectopic pregnancies (0.9%), seven stillbirths (0.5%), and 17 repeat molar pregnancies (1.5%). First- and second-trimester spontaneous abortions occurred in 198 (16.4%) and 18 (1.5%) pregnancies, respectively. Major and minor congenital malformations were detected in 38 infants (4.1%), and primary cesarean section was performed in 56 of 318 (17.6%) term or premature births from 1979 until 1992.

While data regarding later pregnancies after partial mole are limited (149 subsequent pregnancies), the information is reassuring (60). **Patients with both complete and partial mole should be reassured that they are at no increased risk of complications in later gestations.**

When a patient has had a molar pregnancy, she is at an increased risk of having a molar gestation in subsequent conceptions (60). **After one molar pregnancy, the risk of having molar disease in a future gestation is about 1%.** Of 24 patients with at least two documented molar pregnancies, every possible combination of repeat molar pregnancy was observed. After two molar gestations, these 24 patients had 20 later conceptions resulting in 13 full-term deliveries, four complete moles, two spontaneous abortions, and one ectopic pregnancy. In five cases, the medical records indicated that the patient had a different partner at the time of different molar pregnancies.

Therefore, for any subsequent pregnancy, it seems prudent to:

1. Obtain a pelvic ultrasonogram during the first trimester to confirm normal gestational development.

2. Obtain a thorough histologic review of the placenta or products of conception.

3. Obtain an hCG measurement 6 weeks after completion of the pregnancy to exclude occult trophoblastic neoplasia.

Pregnancies After Persistent GTT

Patients with GTT who are treated successfully with chemotherapy can expect normal reproduction in the future. Patients who were treated with chemotherapy at our institution from 1965 until 1992 had 420 subsequent pregnancies that resulted in 295 term live births (70.2%), 18 premature deliveries (4.3%), 4 ectopic pregnancies (1.0%), seven stillbirths (1.6%), and two repeat molar pregnancies (0.6%) (60). First- and second-trimester spontaneous abortions occurred in 65 (15.5%) and seven (1.6%) pregnancies, respectively. Major and minor congenital malformations were detected in only seven infants (2.2%). Primary cesarean section was performed in 32 (15%) of 214 subsequent term and premature births from 1979 until 1992. It is particularly reassuring that the frequency of congenital anomalies is not increased, although chemotherapeutic agents are known to have teratogenic and mutagenic potential.

References

1. **Berkowitz RS, Goldstein DP.** The management of molar pregnancy and gestational trophoblastic tumors. In: **Knapp RC, Berkowitz RS,** eds. *Gynecologic Oncology.* 2nd ed. New York: McGraw-Hill, 1993:328–38.

2. **Bagshawe KD.** Risks and prognostic factors in trophoblastic neoplasia. *Cancer* 1976;38:1373–85.

3. **Palmer JR.** Advances in the epidemiology of gestational trophoblastic disease. *J Reprod Med* 1994;39:155–62.

4. **Jeffers MD, O'Dwyer P, Curran B, Leader M, Gillan JE.** Partial hydatidiform mole: a common but underdiagnosed condition. *Int J Gynecol Pathol* 1993;12:315–23.

5. **Parazzini F, La Vecchia C, Mangili G, Caminiti C, Negri E, Cecchetti G, et al.** Dietary factors and risk of trophoblastic disease. *Am J Obstet Gynecol* 1988;158:93–9.

6. **Berkowitz RS, Cramer DW, Bernstein MR, Cassells S, Driscoll SG, Goldstein DP.** Risk factors for complete molar pregnancy from a case-control study. *Am J Obstet Gynecol* 1985; 152:1016–20.

7. **Parazzini F, La Vecchia C, Pampallona S.** Parental age and risk of complete and partial hydatidiform mole. *Br J Obstet Gynaecol* 1986;93:582–5.

8. **Kajii T, Ohama K.** Androgenetic origin of hydatidiform mole. *Nature* 1977;268:633–4.

9. **Yamashita K, Wake N, Araki T, Ichinoe K, Makoto K.** Human lymphocyte antigen expression in hydatidiform mole: androgenesis following fertilization by a haploid sperm. *Am J Obstet Gynecol* 1979;135:597–600.

10. **Pattillo RA, Sasaki S, Katayama KP, Roesler M, Mattingly RF.** Genesis of 46XY hydatidiform mole. *Am J Obstet Gynecol* 1981;141:104–5.

11. **Azuma C, Saji F, Tokugawa Y, Kimura T, Nobunaga T, Takemura M, et al.** Application of gene amplification by polymerase chain reaction to genetic analysis of molar mitochondrial DNA: the detection of anuclear empty ovum as the cause of complete mole. *Gynecol Oncol* 1991;40:29–33.

12. **Szulman AE, Surti U.** The syndromes of hydatidiform mole. I. Cytogenetic and morphologic correlations. *Am J Obstet Gynecol* 1978;131:665–71.

13. **Lawler SD, Fisher RA, Dent J.** A prospective genetic study of complete and partial hydatidiform moles. *Am J Obstet Gynecol* 1991;164:1270–7.

14. **Lage JM, Mark SD, Roberts DJ, Goldstein DP, Bernstein MR, Berkowitz RS, et al.** A flow cytometric study of 137 fresh hydropic placentas: correlation between types of hydatidiform moles and nuclear DNA ploidy. *Obstet Gynecol* 1992;79:403–10.

15. **Goldstein DP, Berkowitz RS.** Current management of complete and partial molar pregnancy. *J Reprod Med* 1994;39:139–46.

16. **Curry SL, Hammond CB, Tyrey L, Creasman WT, Parker RT, et al.** Hydatidiform mole: diagnosis, management and long-term follow-up of 347 patients. *Obstet Gynecol* 1975;45:1–8.

17. **Berkowitz RS, Goldstein DP.** Pathogenesis of gestational trophoblastic neoplasms. *Pathobiol Annu* 1981;11:391–411.

18. **Amir SM, Osathanondh R, Berkowitz RS, Goldstein DP.** Human chorionic gonadotropin and thyroid function in patients with hydatidiform mole. *Am J Obstet Gynecol* 1984;150:723–8.

19. **Twiggs LB, Morrow CP, Schlaerth JB.** Acute pulmonary complications of molar pregnancy. *Am J Obstet Gynecol* 1979;135:189–94.

20. **Osathanondh R, Berkowitz RS, de Cholnoky C, Smith BS, Goldstein DP, Tyson JE.** Hormonal measurements in patients with theca lutein cysts and gestational trophoblastic disease. *J Reprod Med* 1986;31:179–83.

21. **Berkowitz RS, Goldstein DP, Bernstein MR.** Laparoscopy in the management of gestational trophoblastic neoplasms. *J Reprod Med* 1980;24:261–4.

22. **Szulman AE, Surti U.** The clinicopathologic profile of the partial hydatidiform mole. *Obstet Gynecol* 1982;59:597–602.

23. **Berkowitz RS, Goldstein DP, Bernstein MR.** Natural history of partial molar pregnancy. *Obstet Gynecol* 1985;66:677–81.

24. **Tow WSH.** The influence of the primary treatment of the hydatidiform mole on its subsequent course. *J Obstet Gynaecol Br Commonw* 1966;73:545–52.

25. **Tsukamoto N, Iwasaka T, Kashimura Y, Uchino H, Kashimura M, Matsuyama T.** Gestational trophoblastic disease in women aged 50 or more. *Gynecol Oncol* 1985;20:53–61.

26. **Berkowitz RS, Goldstein DP, Bernstein MR.** Advances in management of partial molar pregnancy. *Contemp Obstet Gynecol* 1991;36:33–44.

27. **Rice LW, Berkowitz RS, Lage JM, Goldstein DP, Bernstein MR.** Persistent gestational trophoblastic tumor after partial hydatidiform mole. *Gynecol Oncol* 1990;36:358–62.

28. **Lage JM, Berkowitz RS, Rice LW, Goldstein DP, Bernstein MR, Weinberg DS.** Flow cytometric analysis of DNA content in partial hydatidiform moles with persistent gestational trophoblastic tumor. *Obstet Gynecol* 1991;77:111–5.

29. **Fine C, Bundy AL, Berkowitz RS, Boswell SB, Berezin AF, Doubilet PM.** Sonographic diagnosis of partial hydatidiform mole. *Obstet Gynecol* 1989;73:414–8.

30. **Goldstein DP.** Prevention of gestational trophoblastic disease by use of actinomycin-D in molar pregnancies. *Obstet Gynecol* 1974;43:475–9.

31. **Berkowitz RS, Goldstein DP, DuBeshter B, Bernstein MR.** Management of complete molar pregnancy. *J Reprod Med* 1987;32:634–9.

32. **Kim DS, Moon H, Kim KT, Moon YJ, Hwang YY.** Effects of prophylactic chemotherapy for persistent trophoblastic disease in patients with complete hydatidiform mole. *Obstet Gynecol* 1986;67:690–4.

33. **Genest DR, LaBorde O, Berkowitz RS, Goldstein DP, Bernstein MR, Lage J.** A clinicopathologic study of 153 cases of complete hydatidiform mole (1980–1990): histologic grade lacks prognostic significance. *Obstet Gynecol* 1991;78:402–9.

34. **Stone M, Dent J, Kardana A, Bagshawe KD.** Relationship of oral contraception to development of trophoblastic tumour after evacuation of a hydatidiform mole. *Br J Obstet Gynaecol* 1976;83:913–6.

35. **Berkowitz RS, Goldstein DP, Marean AR, Bernstein MR.** Oral contraceptives and postmolar trophoblastic disease. *Obstet Gynecol* 1981;58:474–7.

36. **Curry SL, Schlaerth JB, Kohorn EI, Boyce JB, Gore H, Twiggs LB, et al.** Hormonal contraception and trophoblastic sequelae after hydatidiform mole (a Gynecologic Oncology Group study). *Am J Obstet Gynecol* 1989;160:805–9.

37. **Finkler NJ, Berkowitz RS, Driscoll SG, Goldstein DP, Bernstein MR.** Clinical experience with placental site trophoblastic tumors at the New England Trophoblastic Disease Center. *Obstet Gynecol* 1988;71:854–7.

38. **Kelly MP, Rustin GJ, Ivory C, Phillips P, Bagshawe KD.** Respiratory failure due to choriocarcinoma: a study of 103 dyspneic patients. *Gynecol Oncol* 1990;38:149–54.

39. **Bakri YN, Berkowitz RS, Khan J, Goldstein DP, von Sinner W, Jabbar FA.** Pulmonary metastases of gestational trophoblastic tumor—risk factors for early respiratory failure. *J Reprod Med* 1994;39:175–8.

40. **Athanassiou A, Begent RHJ, Newlands ES, Parker D, Rustin GJ, Bagshawe KD.** Central nervous system metastases of choriocarcinoma: 23 years' experience at Charing Cross Hospital. *Cancer* 1983;52:1728–35.

41. **Bagshawe KD, Harland S.** Immunodiagnosis and monitoring of gonadotropin-producing metastases in the central nervous system. *Cancer* 1976;38:112–8.

42. **Bakri Y, Berkowitz RS, Goldstein DP, Subhi J, Senoussi M, von Sinner W, et al.** Brain metastases of gestational trophoblastic tumor. *J Reprod Med* 1994;39:179–84.

43. **Berkowitz RS, Birnholz J, Goldstein DP, Bernstein MR.** Pelvic ultrasonography and the management of gestational trophoblastic disease. *Gynecol Oncol* 1983;15:403–12.

44. **Dessau R, Rustin GJ, Dent J, Paradinas FJ, Bagshawe KD.** Surgery and chemotherapy in the management of placental site tumor. *Gynecol Oncol* 1990;39:56–9.

45. **Soper JT.** Surgical therapy for gestational trophoblastic disease. *J Reprod Med* 1994;39:168–74.

46. **Rustin GJ, Newlands ES, Begent RHJ, Dent J, Bagshawe KD.** Weekly alternating etoposide, methotrexate, actinomycin D/vincristine and cyclophosphamide chemotherapy for the treatment of CNS metastases of choriocarcinoma. *J Clin Oncol* 1989;7:900–3.

47. **Weed JC Jr, Hammond CB.** Cerebral metastatic choriocarcinoma: intensive therapy and prognosis. *Obstet Gynecol* 1980;55:89–94.

48. **Homesley HD.** Development of single-agent chemotherapy regimens for gestational trophoblastic disease. *J Reprod Med* 1994;39:185–92.

49. **Bagshawe KD, Wilde CE.** Infusion therapy for pelvic trophoblastic tumors. *J Obstet Gynaecol Br Commonw* 1964;71:565–70.

50. **Berkowitz RS, Goldstein DP, Bernstein MR.** Ten years' experience with methotrexate and folinic acid as primary therapy for gestational trophoblastic disease. *Gynecol Oncol* 1986;23: 111–8.

51. **Rustin GJ, Rustin F, Dent J, Booth M, Salt S, Bagshawe KD.** No increase in second tumors after cytotoxic chemotherapy for gestational trophoblastic tumors. *N Engl J Med* 1983;308: 473–6.

52. **Curry SL, Blessing JA, DiSaia PJ, Soper JT, Twiggs LB.** A prospective randomized comparison of methotrexate, dactinomycin and chlorambucil versus methotrexate, dactinomycin, cyclophosphamide, doxorubicin, melphalan, hydroxyurea and vincristine in "poor prognosis" metastatic gestational trophoblastic disease: a Gynecologic Oncology Group study. *Obstet Gynecol* 1989;73:357–62.

53. **Gordon AN, Gershenson DM, Copeland LJ, Stringer CA, Morris M, Wharton JT.** High-risk metastatic gestational trophoblastic disease: further stratification into clinical entities. *Gynecol Oncol* 1989;34:54–6.

54. **DuBeshter B, Berkowitz RS, Goldstein DP, Cramer DW, Bernstein MR.** Metastatic gestational trophoblastic disease: experience at the New England Trophoblastic Disease Center, 1965–1985. *Obstet Gynecol* 1987;69:390–5.

55. **Wong LC, Choo YC, Ma HK.** Primary oral etoposide therapy in gestational trophoblastic disease: an update. *Cancer* 1986;58:14–7.

56. **Bagshawe KD.** Treatment of high-risk choriocarcinoma. *J Reprod Med* 1984;29:813–20.

57. **Bolis G, Bonazzi C, Landoni F, Mangili G, Vergadoro F, Zanaboni F, et al.** EMA-CO regimen in high-risk gestational trophoblastic tumor (GTT). *Gynecol Oncol* 1988;31:439–44.

58. **Quinn M, Murray J, Friedlander M, Steigrad S, Khoo S, Marsden D, et al.** EMACO in high risk gestational trophoblastic disease—the Australian experience. *Aust N Z J Obstet Gynecol* 1994;34:90–2.

59. **Surwit EA, Childers JM.** High-risk metastatic gestational trophoblastic disease: a new dose-intensive, multiagent chemotherapeutic regimen. *J Reprod Med* 1991;36:45–8.

60. **Berkowitz RS, Bernstein MR, LaBorde O, Goldstein DP.** Subsequent pregnancy experience in patients with gestational trophoblastic disease: New England Trophoblastic Disease Center, 1965–1992. *J Reprod Med* 1994;39:228–32.

36 Breast Cancer

Armando E. Giuliano

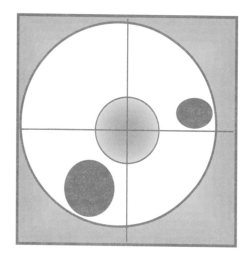

Breast cancer accounts for approximately one-third of all cancers in women and is second only to lung cancer as the leading cause of cancer deaths in women. According to estimates from the American Cancer Society, in the U.S. during 1996, there will be 184,300 new cases of breast cancer and 44,300 deaths from this disease (1). During the past 50 years, the incidence of breast cancer in this country has increased significantly; nearly one in every eight American women will develop breast cancer. On the bright side, the mortality rate has remained stable, implying an increased rate of cure.

Predisposing Factors

Age

Less than 1% of all breast cancers occur in women under 25 years of age. After 30 years of age, however, there is a sharp increase in the incidence of breast cancer; except for a short plateau between the ages of 45 and 50 years (2), this incidence increases steadily with age.

Family History

Any family history of breast cancer increases the overall relative risk of breast cancer (3). However, the risk is not increased significantly in women whose mothers or sisters had breast cancer after menopause, whereas women whose mothers or sisters had bilateral premenopausal breast cancer have at least a 40–50% lifetime risk. If the patient's mother or sister had unilateral premenopausal breast cancer, her lifetime risk of developing breast cancer is approximately 30%.

Diet, Obesity, and Alcohol

Marked geographic differences in the incidence of breast cancer may be related to diet, particularly variations in fat intake (4). It is not clear, however, that a high-fat diet is a specific risk factor because most studies have not clearly separated obesity from other known risk factors (5). Alcohol consumption may increase the risk of breast cancer (6), but again this relationship is not clear.

Reproductive and Hormonal Factors

The longer a women's reproductive phase, the higher her risk of breast cancer (7). Thus, the median age at menarche is lower for women who develop breast cancer (5), and either natural or artificial early menopause protects against the development of breast cancer (8). Artificial menopause as a result of oophorectomy lowers the risk of breast cancer farther than early natural menopause. There is no clear association between the risk of breast cancer and menstrual irregularity or duration of menses. There is some evidence that these reproductive factors, although decreasing the risk of developing breast cancer, may adversely affect a patient's prognosis (9).

Lactation does not affect the incidence of breast cancer, but women who have never been pregnant have a higher risk of breast cancer than those who are multiparous. Also, women bearing their first child later in life have a higher incidence of breast cancer than younger primigravida females (10).

A well-controlled study from the Centers for Disease Control and Prevention showed that oral contraceptive use does not increase the risk of breast cancer, regardless of duration of use, family history, or coexistence of benign breast disease (11).

Although estrogen treatment for menopausal symptoms probably does not increase the risk of breast cancer, prolonged estrogen use (longer than 10 years) or higher doses of estrogen may increase the risk. A meta-analysis suggests that postmenopausal estrogen administration is a risk factor (12). The current consensus is that, postmenopausally, estrogen should be given in a relatively low dose either cyclically or in combination with progestins. Although estrogens may slightly increase the incidence of breast cancer, their judicious use is justified by decreased mortality from osteoporosis and heart disease.

History of Cancer

Women with a history of breast cancer have an approximately 50% risk of developing microscopic breast cancer in the contralateral breast (13). Lobular carcinoma has a higher incidence of bilaterality than does ductal carcinoma. A history of endometrial carcinoma, ovarian carcinoma, or colon cancer has also been associated with an increased risk of breast cancer (8).

Diagnosis

Breast cancer most commonly arises in the upper outer quadrant, where there is more breast tissue. Breast masses are most often discovered by the patient and less frequently by the physician during routine breast examination. The increasing use of screening mammography has increased the detection of nonpalpable abnormalities. An axillary mass without obvious malignancy in the breast is a rare presentation of metastatic breast cancer.

Masses are easier to palpate in older women with fatty breasts than in younger women with dense, often nodular breasts. An area of thickening amid normal nodularity may be the only clue to an underlying malignancy. Skin dimpling, nipple retraction, or skin erosion is usually obvious, but these are later-stage disease signs. Algorithms for the evaluation of breast masses in premenopausal and postmenopausal women are presented in Chapter 18.

A dominant breast mass must be considered a possible carcinoma, and biopsy is essential for diagnosis. **About 30–40% of lesions believed clinically to be malignant will be benign on histologic examination** (14). **Conversely, 20–25% of clinically benign lesions will be proven malignant by biopsy** (15).

Biopsy Techniques

For patients with obvious malignancy, it is reasonable to obtain a biopsy specimen and a frozen section immediately before mastectomy or other definitive treatment. Because it is psychologically preferable for the patient to be involved in the planning of her therapy, initial biopsy may be followed by subsequent definitive treatment in the two-step approach. When biopsy and treatment procedures are separated, patients who do not have a malignancy do not need to be admitted to the hospital. This approach also allows the physician to discuss alternative forms of therapy with the patient who has a malignancy, and it gives the patient an opportunity to obtain a second opinion before undergoing definitive treatment.

Fine-Needle Aspiration Cytology

Fine-needle aspiration (FNA) cytology is performed with a 20-or 22-gauge needle. The technique has a high level of diagnostic accuracy, with a 10–15% false-negative rate and rare but persistent false-positive results (16). If a mass appears to be malignant on physical examination or mammography or both, FNA cytology results can be useful in discussing alternatives with the patient. Negative FNA cytologic results do not exclude malignancy and usually are followed by excisional biopsy. In young women, it is prudent to follow a benign-appearing mass for one or two menstrual cycles. In a young woman, confirmation of a clinically apparent fibroadenoma with FNA can serve as the basis for observational follow-up.

Open Biopsy

Open biopsy may be performed if FNA cytology has not been performed or if the results are negative or equivocal. **An unequivocal histologic diagnosis of cancer should be obtained before treatment of breast cancer is undertaken.** Cytologic diagnosis may be relied on if the mass is clinically malignant. A partial mastectomy can be performed and a frozen section can be obtained to confirm the diagnosis of cancer before the axillary dissection is started. An alternative to open biopsy is removal of a core of tissue through a Vim-Silverman-type cutting needle. These procedures must also be followed by open biopsy if cancer is not diagnosed.

Open biopsy can usually be performed in an outpatient operating room with local anesthesia in the following manner:

1. The patient is positioned and the location of the mass confirmed.

2. Local anesthesia is used to infiltrate the skin and subcutaneous tissue surrounding the palpable mass.

3. An incision is made directly over the mass. It should be planned to allow an ellipse of skin to be either excised with the mastectomy or placed cosmetically so that partial mastectomy can be performed through the same incision. Para-areolar incisions should be avoided, particularly if the tumor is far from the areola and would result in dragging malignant cells through a large segment of breast.

4. After the skin and underlying tissue are incised, the mass is gently grasped with Allis forceps or with a stay suture and moved into the operative field.

5. The mass should be completely excised whenever possible. Large masses that are difficult to excise totally with local anesthesia can be incised. When an incisional biopsy is used, a frozen section should be obtained to confirm that malignant tissue has been obtained. Such masses are usually biopsied with FNA or core biopsy.

6. Once the mass is excised, adequate hemostasis is achieved and the incision is closed. A cosmetically superior result will be achieved if the breast parenchyma is not reapproximated deeply. The most superficial subcutaneous fat can be reapproximated with fine, absorbable sutures. The skin should be closed with a subcuticular suture and adhesive strips to achieve the most cosmetically pleasing result. Usually a drain is not necessary.

Mammographic Localization Biopsy

Biopsy of nonpalpable lesions is a potentially difficult procedure that requires close cooperation between the surgeon and the mammographer. The mammographer places a needle or specialized wire into the breast parenchyma at or near the site of the suspected abnormality. Many mammographers will also inject a biologic dye to assist localization further. The surgeon then reviews the films with the mammographer and localizes the abnormality with respect to the tip of the wire or needle. An incision is made directly over this area, and a small portion of the breast that is suspected of containing the abnormality is excised. A mammogram of the surgical specimen is obtained to ensure that the abnormality has been excised. Often, the mammographer can place a needle in the specimen at the site of the abnormality to facilitate histologic evaluation and ensure that the pathologist examines the site of the abnormality.

Stereotactic Core Biopsy

Mammographic units with computerized stereotactic modifications can be used to localize abnormalities and perform needle biopsy without surgery. Under mammographic guidance, a biopsy needle is inserted into the lesion and a core of tissue is removed for histologic examination. **Because it is less invasive and less expensive than mammographic localization biopsy, core biopsy is preferred for accessible lesions.**

Pathology and Natural History

Breast cancer may arise in the intermediate-sized ducts or terminal ducts and lobules. In most cases, the diagnosis of lobular and intraductal carcinoma is based more on histologic appearance than site of origin. The cancer may be either invasive (infiltrating ductal carcinoma, infiltrating lobular carcinoma) or *in situ* (ductal carcinoma *in situ* or lobular carcinoma *in situ*). Morphologic subtypes of infiltrating ductal carcinoma can be described as scirrhous, tubular, medullary, and mucinous.

Infiltrating ductal carcinoma of nonspecified type accounts for 60–70% of the breast cancers in the U.S. (17). Mammographically, it is characterized by a stellate density or by microcalcifications. Macroscopically, there are gritty, chalky streaks within the tumor that most likely represent a desmoplastic response; microscopically, there is invasion of the surrounding stroma and fat. There is often a fibrotic response surrounding the invasive carcinoma.

Other types of infiltration ductal carcinoma are far less common. Medullary carcinoma, which accounts for approximately 5–8% of breast carcinomas, arises from larger ducts within the breast and has a dense lymphocytic infiltrate. The tumor appears to be a slow-growing, less aggressive malignancy than the infiltrating ductal carcinoma. Mucinous (colloid) carcinoma accounts for <5% of all breast cancers. Grossly, the tumor may have areas that appear mucinous or gelatinous. Infiltrating comedo carcinoma accounts for <1% of breast malignancies. It is an invasive cancer characterized by foci of necrosis that exude a comedo, necrosis-like substance when biopsied. Usually, comedo carcinomas are *in situ* malignancies. Papillary carcinoma is predominantly a noninvasive ductal carcinoma; when invasive components are present, it should be specified as invasive papillary carcinoma. Tubular carcinoma is a well-differentiated breast cancer that accounts for <1% of all breast malignancies. Adenoid cystic carcinomas are extremely rare and are similar histologically to those seen in the salivary glands. They tend to be well differentiated and slow to metastasize (17).

Growth Patterns

The growth potential of breast cancer and the patient's resistance to malignancy vary widely with the individual and the stage of disease. The doubling time of breast cancer can range from several weeks for rapidly growing tumors to months or years for slowly growing ones. If the doubling time of a breast tumor was constant and a tumor originated from one cell, a doubling time of 100 days would result in a 1-cm tumor in about 8 years (Fig. 36.1) (18). During the preclinical phase, tumor cells may be circulating throughout the body.

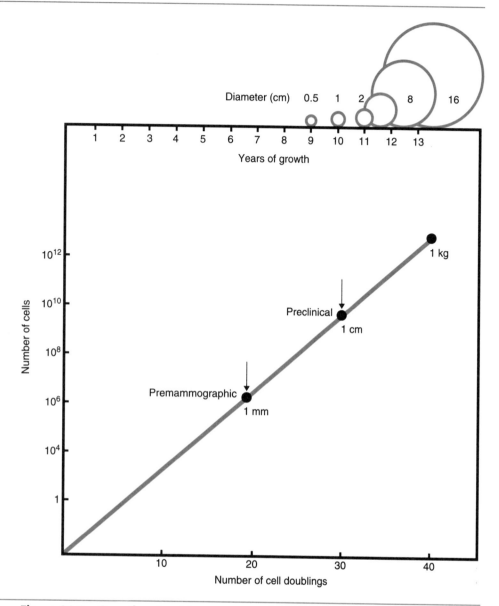

Figure 36.1   Growth rate of breast cancer indicating long preclinical phase. (Redrawn with permission from **Gullino PM.** Natural history of breast cancer: progression from hyperplasia to neoplasia as predicted by angiogenesis. *Cancer* 1977;39:2697.)

Because of the long preclinical tumor growth phase and the tendency of infiltrating lesions to metastasize early, many clinicians view breast cancer as a systemic disease at the time of diagnosis. Although cancer cells may be released from the tumor prior to diagnosis, variations in the tumor's ability to grow in other organs and the host's response to the tumor may inhibit dissemination of the disease. Indeed, many women can be treated successfully with surgery alone for breast cancer, and some women have been cured even in the presence of palpable axillary disease. Thus, a pessimistic attitude that breast cancer is systemic and incurable at the time of diagnosis is unwarranted. A more realistic approach may be to view breast cancer as a two-component disease: one is the primary tumor in the breast, with all the inherent problems of local and regional extension and primary tumor control, and the other consists of the systemic metastases with their life-threatening consequences.

Although the natural history of breast cancer can involve metastases to any organ, involvement of bone, lungs, or liver occurs in 85% of women with metastatic breast cancer (19–21).

If any of these sites is involved, metastases in other organs is highly likely. The use of systemic chemotherapy affects the sites of metastases, and more unusual metastatic sites are occurring with greater frequency.

Staging

After the diagnosis of breast cancer has been established either cytologically or histologically, the clinical stage of disease should be determined. The Columbia Clinical Staging System was widely used for many years (22) but has been replaced largely by the tumor-nodes-metastases (TNM) system recommended by the International Union Against Cancer (IUCC) and the American Joint Committee on Cancer (23). This system allows both preoperative clinical staging and postoperative pathologic staging (Tables 36.1 and 36.2).

Table 36.1   Tumor–Nodes–Metastasis (TNM) Classification

Primary Tumor (T)

TX	Primary tumor cannot be assessed
TO	No evidence of primary tumor
Tis	Carcinoma *in situ*: intraductal carcinoma, lobular carcinoma *in situ*, or Paget's disease of the nipple with no tumor
T1	Tumor 2 cm or less in greatest dimension
T1a	0.5 cm or less in greatest dimension
T1b	More than 0.5 cm but not more than 1 cm in greatest dimension
T1c	More than 1 cm but not more than 2 cm in greatest dimension
T2	Tumor more than 2 cm but not more than 5 cm in greatest dimension
T3	Tumor more than 5 cm in greatest dimension
T4	Tumor of any size with direct extension to chest wall or skin
T4a	Extension to chest wall
T4b	Edema (including peau d'orange) or ulceration of the skin of breast or satellite skin nodules confined to same breast
T4c	Both T4a and T4b
T4d	Inflammatory carcinoma

Lymph Node (N)

NX	Regional lymph nodes cannot be assessed (e.g., previously removed)
N0	No regional lymph node metastasis
N1	Metastasis to movable ipsilateral axillary lymph node(s)
N2	Metastasis to ipsilateral axillary lymph node(s) fixed to one another or to other structures
N3	Metastasis to ipsilateral internal mammary lymph node(s)

Pathologic Classification (pN)

pNX	Regional lymph nodes cannot be assessed (e.g., previously removed or not removed for pathologic study)
pN0	No regional lymph node metastasis
pN1	Metastasis to movable ipsilateral axillary lymph node(s)
pN1a	Only micrometastasis (none larger than 0.2 cm)
pN1b	Metastasis to lymph nodes, any larger than 0.2 cm
pN1bi	Metastasis in one to three lymph nodes, any more than 0.2 cm and all less than 2 cm in greatest dimension
pN1bii	Metastasis to four or more lymph nodes, any more than 0.2 cm and all less than 2 cm in greatest dimension
pN1biii	Extension of tumor beyond the capsule of a lymph node metastasis less than 2 cm in greatest dimension
pN1biv	Metastasis to a lymph node 2 cm or more in greatest dimension
pN2	Metastasis to ipsilateral axillary lymph nodes that are fixed to one another or to other structures
pN3	Metastasis to ipsilateral internal mammary lymph node(s)

Distant Metastasis (M)

MX	Presence of distant metastasis cannot be assessed
M0	No distant metastasis
M1	Distant metastasis (includes metastasis to ipsilateral supraclavicular lymph node(s))

Reproduced with permission from **Beahrs OH, Henson DE, Hutter RVP, Kennedy BJ.** *American Joint Committee on Cancer: Manual for Staging of Cancer.* 4th ed. Philadelphia: JB Lippincott, 1992:153.

Table 36.2   Staging of Breast Carcinoma

| Stage | TNM Classification* | | |
	Tumor	Node	Metastasis
Stage 0	Tis	N0	M0
Stage I	T1	N0	M0
Stage IIA	T0	N1†	M0
	T1	N1*	M0
	T2	N0	M0
Stage IIB	T2	N1	M0
	T3	N0	M0
Stage IIIA	T0	N2	M0
	T1	N2	M0
	T2	N2	M0
	T3	N1	M0
	T3	N2	M0
Stage IIIB	T4	Any N	M0
	Any T	N3	M0
Stage IV	Any T	Any N	M1

*See Table 36.1.

†*Note:* The prognosis of patients with N1a is similar to that of patients with pN0.

Reproduced with permission from **Beahrs OH, Henson DE, Hutter RVP, Kennedy BJ.** *American Joint Committee on Cancer: Manual for Staging of Cancer.* 4th ed. Philadelphia: JB Lippincott, 1992:152.

Preoperative Evaluation

The extent of preoperative workup varies with the initial stage of the disease (24). For most patients with small tumors, no palpable lymph nodes (TMN stage I), and no symptoms of metastases, the preoperative evaluation should consist of bilateral mammography, chest x-ray, complete blood count, and screening blood chemistry tests. A bone scan and computed tomography (CT) scan are not necessary unless symptoms or abnormal blood chemistry suggest bone or liver metastases. For patients with clinical stage II disease, a bone scan should be obtained, but a CT scan of the liver is not necessary unless symptoms or liver function tests suggest liver metastasis. Patients with clinical stage III or IV disease should undergo both a bone scan and a liver scan. A bone marrow biopsy should be performed if there is obvious bone marrow dysfunction but metastases are not evident on bone scan.

Treatment

Mastectomy

Traditionally, treatment of breast cancer has been surgical, but the type of operation employed has remained a controversial and highly emotional issue. In the 19th century, surgical treatment of breast cancer was haphazard, varying from local excision alone to total mastectomy. Halsted devised the radical mastectomy in an attempt to treat carcinoma of the breast as a local infiltrative process (25). Thus, radical mastectomy removes the entire breast, the underlying pectoral muscles, and the axillary lymph nodes in continuity (26) (Fig. 36.2A). Haagensen and Bodian reported a 51-year experience with radical mastectomy. Their data, which included 1036 patients with a follow-up of 47 years, remain unequalled in evaluating any single method of treating breast cancer (27).

During the 20th century, extensions and modifications of the radial mastectomy procedure were devised that involved removal of more local and regional tissue. Supraclavicular node dissections were added to the radial mastectomy (28). In addition, supraclavicular, mediastinal, and internal mammary lymph node dissections were performed (29).

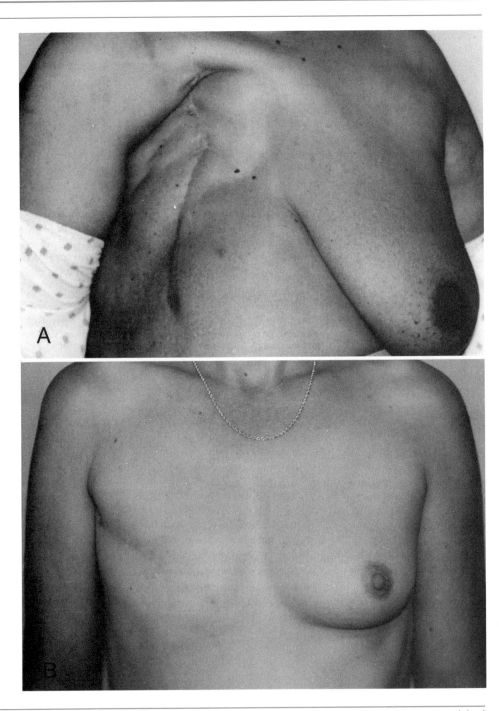

Figure 36.2   Appearance of breast after radical mastectomy (*A*) versus modified mastectomy (*B*). (Reproduced with permission from **Berek JS, Hacker NF,** eds. *Practical Gynecologic Oncology*. 2nd ed. Baltimore: Williams & Wilkins, 1994:500.)

Urban (30) added *en bloc* internal mammary lymph node dissection to the standard radical mastectomy. This technique became popular and is the operation commonly referred to as the "extended radical mastectomy ." The extended radical mastectomy did not enhance overall survival rates (31). About 10% of patients in whom axillary lymph nodes are not involved will have involvement of internal mammary nodes. Locally destructive surgery is not justified, however, based on current understanding of the biologic behavior of breast cancer.

Modified Radical Mastectomy

Modified radical mastectomy preserves the pectoralis major muscle (Fig. 36.2B) (32, 33). The breast is removed in a manner similar to that of the radical mastectomy; however, removal of the skin and the axillary lymph node dissection are not as extensive, and there is no need for skin grafting. There is no difference in survival rates between radical mastectomy and modified radical mastectomy (34), but the latter procedure has a better functional and cosmetic result. **Modified radical mastectomy has replaced radical mastectomy and is the procedure Most often performed for breast cancer.**

Total (Simple) Mastectomy

Total mastectomy is the removal of the entire breast, nipple, and areolar complex without the underlying muscles or axillary lymph nodes. There is generally no need for skin grafts, and axillary nodes are not removed intentionally. However, low-lying lymph nodes in the upper outer portion of the breast and low axilla usually are included in the specimen. Total mastectomy has local control rates comparable to those of radical or modified radical mastectomy. Because the axillary lymph nodes are not examined microscopically, allowing the addition of adjuvant systemic chemotherapy in survival rates in certain patients, this operation generally is less desirable than radical procedures. Regional recurrence will occur in at least 15–20% of patients treated with total mastectomy alone.

Adjuvant Radiation Therapy

The combination of total mastectomy with radiation therapy was developed by McWhirter (35). Many have advocated adjuvant radiation therapy in combination with various operative procedures. Studies claiming improvements in overall survival usually are flawed by the use of historical controls and inaccurate preoperative staging. Most trials, both prospective randomized studies and historical control studies, show that adjuvant radiation therapy improves local control but not survival rates (36–39).

In a prospective randomized trial performed by the National Surgical Adjuvant Breast Project (NSABP), the role of postoperative radiation therapy was examined (41). Patients were randomly assigned to therapy consisting either of total mastectomy, radical mastectomy, or total mastectomy with radiation therapy. This trial showed no difference in survival rates among the three groups of patients, whereas radiation therapy improved local control in patients treated with total mastectomy.

Conservative Surgery With or Without Radiation Therapy

Radiation therapy alone without excision of the tumor is associated with a high local failure rate (41–44). Veronesi et al. (45, 46) reported the first major prospective randomized trial comparing radical surgery with a combination of conservative surgery and modern radiotherapeutic techniques. Patients were randomly assigned to treatment with either standard Halsted radical mastectomy or a combination of quadrantectomy, axillary lymph node dissection, and postoperative radiation. Only patients in whom tumors were <2 cm and not centrally located and who had no clinical evidence of axillary lymph node disease ($T_1N_0M_0$) were considered for this trial. All 701 women in the study were comparable in age, tumor size, menopausal status, and histologic involvement of the axillary lymph nodes (46). After more than 12 years of follow-up, there has been no statistically significant difference between the two groups in either local control or overall survival rates.

The NSABP conducted a trial that extended these observations and provided further information (47). Eligible patients could have a primary tumor ≤4 cm, with or without palpable axillary lymph nodes, provided that the lymph nodes were not fixed (i.e., stage I or stage II, T_1 or T_2 and N_0 or N_1). Patients were assigned randomly to one of three groups: 1) modified radical mastectomy; 2) segmental mastectomy (lumpectomy) and axillary lymph node dissection; or 3) segmental mastectomy, axillary lymph node dissection, and postoperative radiation therapy. Unlike the quadrantectomy, segmental mastectomy or "lumpectomy" consists of removing only the tumor and a small rim of normal surrounding tissue (Fig. 36.3). Patients were considered ineligible if they were found to have microscopic involvement of the margins. A total of 1843 women were randomized among the

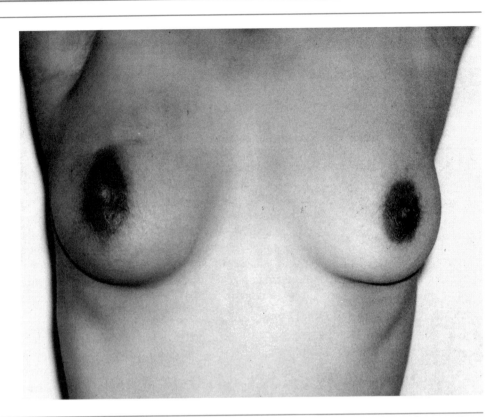

Figure 36.3   Appearance of breast after lmnpectomy, axillary dissection, and radiation therapy. (Reproduced with permission from **Berek JS, Hacker NF,** eds. *Practical Gynecologic Oncology.* 2nd ed. Baltimore: Williams & Wilkins, 1994:503.)

three treatment arms, and the groups were comparable. The lowest local recurrence rate was seen among patients treated with segmental mastectomy and postoperative radiation therapy. Of these patients, 90% were free of local recurrence after 8 years of observation, whereas 39% of the patients undergoing segmental mastectomy without radiation therapy had a local recurrence. Although the addition of radiation therapy clearly improved the local control rate, no significant difference in overall survival rates or disease-free survival could be seen among the three treatment arms; there was a trend, however, in favor of patients who received radiation. This NSABP study clearly shows that segmental mastectomy, axillary lymph node dissection, and postoperative radiation therapy were as effective as modified radical mastectomy for the management of patients with stage I and II breast cancer. The high local recurrence rate without radiation therapy makes limited surgery alone generally unacceptable, except in unusual circumstances.

Adjuvant Systemic Therapy

For most patients, local-regional control of breast cancer is achieved readily with surgery and radiation therapy. More than 90% of patients will never experience a local recurrence; however, patients may still develop metastatic disease. The 10-year survival rate for women with palpable metastatic axillary lymph nodes is only about 40–50%. Even when it is not clinically palpable, lymph node metastases portend an unfavorable course. The goal of adjuvant systemic therapy is to eliminate occult metastases in the early postoperative period while theoretically they are most vulnerable to anticancer agents (48).

Chemotherapy

Initial trials involved a single perioperative course of chemotherapy in an attempt to eradicate circulating tumor cells. The Nissen-Meyer study from Norway (49) showed that a single course of *cyclophosphamide* improved overall survival rates. Subsequently, numerous trials have shown the benefit of adjuvant chemotherapy for certain subgroups of patients (50). In the initial NSABP adjuvant trial, a 2-year course of melphalan was shown to be superior to no treatment (51). Subsequent trials have shown the beneficial effect of multiple drugs and a combination of hormonal manipulation with chemotherapy in the adjuvant setting (52).

The most frequently used adjuvant combination chemotherapy has been *CMF: cyclophosphamide, methotrexate,* and *5-fluorouracil (5-FU)*. In the original study by Bonadonna and Valagussa (55), patients with positive axillary lymph nodes were randomized to receive either 12 monthly cycles of *CMF* or no therapy after radical mastectomy. A statistically significant benefit was found with *CMF* for premenopausal patients, especially those with 1–3 positive nodes. A subsequent study (54) showed six cycles of *CMF* to be as effective as 12 cycles. However, no significant effect was seen for postmenopausal women. This was believed to be because postmenopausal women were less likely to tolerate the full course of *CMF* (55). The value of adjuvant chemotherapy in postmenopausal women has been controversial, and other studies have shown beneficial results (53, 56, 57). Most recent trials confirm a beneficial effect of adjuvant therapy in postmenopausal as well as premenopausal women (58).

Until recently, adjuvant systemic therapy was generally reserved for patients with involved lymph nodes. In 1988, the National Cancer Institute alerted clinicians to the value of adjuvant chemotherapy in patients without axillary lymph node involvement (58). In several cooperative group trials (59–64), lymph node-negative patients were randomly assigned to receive either a systemic treatment or observation. Treatment was initiated 2–6 weeks after primary therapy. With a median follow-up of 3–4 years, these studies have shown a significant improvement in disease-free survival for patients with node-negative breast cancers who received systemic chemotherapy.

In another NSABP study (81), patients with estrogen-receptor (ER)-negative tumors were randomly assigned to receive either no further treatment or chemotherapy with *methotrexate* (100 mg/m^2 intravenously) followed 1 hour later by *5-FU* (600 mg/m^2 intravenously) and *citrovorum factor* (10 mg/m^2 every 6 hours for six doses commencing 24 hours after *methotrexate* administration). The treatments were given on days 1 and 8 of each 24-day cycle for 13 3-week cycles. With a total of 741 patients entered and a median follow-up of 4 years, 80% of the group receiving chemotherapy were alive and free of disease, compared with 71% of the untreated controls (P=0.003). The disease-free survival was longer for both premenopausal and postmenopausal women.

In the Intergroup Study (INT-0011) (64), a trial of adjuvant *CMF plus prednisone (CMFP)* versus observation alone was undertaken in patients with negative axillary nodes, ER-negative tumors of any size, and ER-positive tumors larger than 3 cm. The *CMFP* regimen consisted of *cyclophosphamide* (100 mg/m^2 orally on days 1 through 14), *methotrexate* (40 mg/m^2; 5-FU 600 mg/m^2 intravenously on days 1 and 8), and *prednisone* (40 mg/m^2 orally on days 1 through 14). The chemotherapy was given every 28 days for six cycles. With a median follow-up of 3 years, the disease-free survival rate for the patients treated with *CMFP* was 84% compared with 67% for the control group (P=0. 0001). This benefit was demonstrated for patients with both ER-positive and ER-negative tumors, as well as for both premenopausal and postmenopausal patients.

In NSABP study B-14 (61), 2644 patients with ER-positive tumors and no axillary metastases were randomized, double-blind, to either *tamoxifen* (10 mg orally twice daily for 5 years) or a placebo control. With a 4-year median follow-up, the disease-free survival rate for the 1318 patients treated with *tamoxifen* was 82% compared with 77% for the 1326 patients treated with placebo (P=0.00001). An advantage existed for both premenopausal and postmenopausal women.

Adjuvant cytotoxic chemotherapy appears to affect the natural history of patients with axillary node-negative breast cancer. A 1990 consensus statement from the National Institutes of Health on early-stage breast cancer (65) advised that all patients be considered for clinical trials and offered the opportunity to participate and that node-negative patients who are not candidates for clinical trials should be made aware of the benefits and potential risks of adjuvant systemic therapy. Most high-risk node-negative patients are now being treated with adjuvant systemic chemotherapy.

Hormonal Therapy

Hormonal manipulation may improve the results of adjuvant systemic therapy. *Tamoxifen* has been shown to enhance the effects of *melphalan* and *5-FU* in women with ER-positive tumors. In one NSABP study (66), significant improvement in disease-free survival rates was seen only in postmenopausal women. Patients with ER-negative tumors may have a higher recurrence rate than patients with ER-positive tumors, even in the absence of axillary lymph node metastases. In NSABP study B-14 (61), both premenopausal and postmenopausal patients who had ER-positive, node-negative disease benefitted from the adjuvant use of *tamoxifen*. Clinical studies currently are under way to investigate the value of adjuvant hormonal therapy in women with ER-negative tumors and negative lymph nodes. The possibility of substituting *tamoxifen* for radiotherapy in patients with small <1 cm) tumors is also being studied prospectively.

The relative merits of *tamoxifen* plus cytotoxic chemotherapy compared with *tamoxifen* alone for postmenopausal patients with positive axillary lymph nodes and positive hormonal receptors are not clear and are the subject of current investigation. Survival benefit has yet to be established in premenopausal patients with positive axillary lymph nodes when *tamoxifen* is used in combination with cytotoxic chemotherapy. The Early Breast Cancer Trialists' Collaborative Group performed a meta-analysis of adjuvant systemic therapy for breast cancer (90). They analyzed randomized trials involving adjuvant systemic hormonal, cytotoxic, or immune therapy administered to more than 75,000 women with stage I or II carcinoma. The investigators concluded that, for postmenopausal women with ER-positive tumors, *tamoxifen* in a dose of 20 mg daily for at least 2 years had a significant beneficial effect on disease-free survival rates. This beneficial effect lasted up to 10 years. *Tamoxifen* appeared to have some effect even in patients with ER-negative tumors. Data demonstrated a decreased incidence of carcinoma in the contralateral breast and a decreased death rate from heart disease. Cytotoxic chemotherapy decreased recurrences and increased survival for both pre- and postmenopausal women.

Metastatic disease may respond to drugs that block hormonal receptor sites or drugs that block synthesis of hormones (67, 68). Hormonal manipulation should not be attempted in women with ER-negative tumors. Such patients should receive cytotoxic chemotherapy.

In premenopausal patients, *tamoxifen* therapy has replaced bilateral oophorectomy as the primary method of hormonal manipulation because of its ease of administration and lack of morbidity. About 60% of premenopausal patients with ER-positive tumors respond to either *tamoxifen* or bilateral oophorectomy. Patients who respond to *tamoxifen* should be treated with *Megace* if they experience subsequent tumor progression. Some oncologists advocate the use of *aminoglutethimide*, an inhibitor of adrenal hormone synthesis, but its use is more complicated and offers no therapeutic advantage over *tamoxifen*. Currently, oophorectomy is rarely performed for treatment of metastatic breast cancer.

Primary hormonal manipulation in postmenopausal women should be undertaken with *tamoxifen*. *Tamoxifen* has fewer side effects than *diethylstilbestrol (DES)*, which was formerly the therapy of choice and appears to be just as effective. Women whose tumors respond to *tamoxifen* initially and then progress are given *DES* or, more often, *Megace*. Patients with tumors that do not respond to *tamoxifen* should be treated with cytotoxic chemotherapy. Further endocrine manipulation is probably best performed with *Megace* or *aminoglutethimide*.

General Recommendations

Adjuvant systemic therapy, either with *tamoxifen* or polychemotherapy, lowers the incidence of recurrence by about 25%. Caution should be exercised when using these agents. Patients in whom the risk of recurrence is low are likely to derive little overall benefit from the use of adjuvant systemic therapy, whereas those whose overall risk of recurrence is high are likely to receive the greatest benefit. When the risk of recurrence is extremely low, as would be expected for tumors <1 cm with no lymph node metastases, the reduction in recurrence may not justify the side effects of the drugs.

In practice, systemic adjuvant therapy is used for most patients with early-stage breast cancer. In addition to lymph node status, other prognostic factors are being considered in decisions regarding the institution of adjuvant systemic therapy. The factors that determine the patient's risk of recurrence are tumor size, estrogen and progesterone receptor status, nuclear grade, histologic type, proliferative rate, and oncogene expression (65). Table 36.3 summarizes these prognostic factors and their effects on recurrence. The assumption is made that patients with high-risk prognostic factors are more likely to benefit from adjuvant therapy and, thus, these patients are generally given such therapy. Current studies are under way to investigate whether this assumption is true, and it remains to be seen whether these patients constitute the subgroup most likely to benefit from adjuvant systemic therapy. On the basis of these new data, the current recommendations for adjuvant systemic therapy in breast cancer can be summarized as follows:

1. Premenopausal women with lymph node involvement should be treated with adjuvant combination chemotherapy. *Tamoxifen* may be added to the regimen for patients with ER-positive tumors.

2. Premenopausal women without evidence of axillary lymph node involvement but with risk factors such as large, aneuploid, or ER-negative tumors should be treated with combination chemotherapy.

3. Postmenopausal patients who have negative lymph nodes and positive hormone receptor levels should receive adjuvant *tamoxifen* therapy. Those with positive lymph nodes may receive *tamoxifen* or combination chemotherapy.

4. Postmenopausal women who have lymph node metastasis and negative hormone receptor levels may be treated with adjuvant chemotherapy.

5. Adjuvant systemic therapy is not recommended for patients with small nonpalpable tumors or palpable tumors <1 cm. The hazards of chemotherapy and its

Table 36.3   Prognostic Factors in Node-Negative Breast Carcinoma

Factor	Increased Risk of Recurrence
Size	Larger tumors
Histologic grade	High-grade tumors
DNA ploidy	Aneuploid tumors
Labeling index	High index (>3%)
S phase fraction	High fraction (>5%)
Lymphatic/vascular invasion	Present
Cathepsin D	High levels
HER-2/*neu* oncogene expression	High expression
Epidermal growth factor	High levels

Reproduced with permission from **Tierney LM, McPhee SJ, Papadakis MA.** *Current Medical Diagnosis and Treatment.* Lange, 1995.

effect on quality of life must be carefully evaluated, especially in older post-menopausal women. Such a patient, even with axillary node involvement, may be better treated with adjuvant *tamoxifen,* which has relatively few side effects.

Special Breast Cancers

Paget's Disease

Sir James Paget described a nipple lesion similar to eczema and recognized that this nipple change was associated with an underlying breast malignancy (69). The erosion results from invasion of the nipple and surrounding areola by characteristic large cells with irregular nuclei, which are now called Paget's cells. The origin of these cells has been much debated by pathologists. However, they are probably extensions of an underlying carcinoma into the major ducts of the nipple-areolar complex. There may be no visible changes associated with the initial invasion of the nipple. Often, the patient will notice a nipple discharge, which is actually a combination of serum and blood from the involved ducts.

The overall prognosis for patients with Paget's disease depends on the underlying malignancy. In patients who have an intraductal carcinoma alone, the prognosis is favorable, whereas in those with infiltrating ductal carcinoma metastatic to the regional lymph nodes, the prognosis is poor. Traditionally, treatment has almost always been total mastectomy and lymph node dissection, although radiotherapy with resection of the tumor and nipple areolar complex is being performed (70).

Inflammatory Carcinoma

Inflammatory carcinoma of the breast initially appears to be an acute inflammation with redness and edema. Inflammatory cancer rather than infiltrating ductal carcinoma should be diagnosed when more than one-third of the breast is involved by erythema and edema and when biopsy of this area shows metastatic cancer in the subdermal lymphatics. There may be no distinct palpable mass, because the tumor infiltrates through the breast with ill-defined margins or there may be a dominant mass. There may even be satellite nodules within the parenchyma. Most of the tumors are poorly differentiated, and mammographically the breast shows skin thickening with an infiltrative process.

Except for biopsy of the lesion, surgery usually should not be used in the initial management of inflammatory carcinoma. Mastectomy in the face of inflammatory carcinoma usually fails locally and does not improve survival rates. The best results are achieved with a combination of chemotherapy and radiation therapy. Mastectomy may be indicated for patients who remain free of distant metastatic disease after initial chemotherapy and radiation (71, 72).

***In Situ* Carcinomas**

Both lobular carcinoma and ductal carcinoma may be confined by the basement membrane of the ducts. These carcinomas do not invade the surrounding tissue and, theoretically, lack the ability to spread. Because of their unusual natural history, they represent a special form of breast cancer.

Lobular Carcinoma *In Situ*

If treated by biopsy alone, 25–30% of patients with lobular carcinoma *in situ* (LCIS), also known as lobular neoplasia, will subsequently develop invasive cancer. In women with lobular neoplasia, cancer can occur in either breast (73).

Most women with lobular neoplasia are premenopausal. The tumor typically is not a discrete mass, but it is a multifocal lesion within one or both breasts found incidentally at biopsy of a mass or mammographic assessment of an abnormality not related to the LCIS. Lobular neoplasia is usually managed with excisional biopsy followed by careful observation and mammography. It should not be considered a malignancy but rather a risk factor.

Patients should be informed that they have a higher risk of developing invasive breast cancer. Occasionally, a patient may request bilateral prophylactic mastectomy.

Ductal Carcinoma *In Situ*

Ductal carcinoma *in situ* (DCIS) typically occurs in postmenopausal women. It may present as a palpable mass with features typical of an invasive ductal carcinoma but usually is detected mammographically as a cluster of branched or Y-shaped microcalcifications. By definition, the intraductal disease does not invade beyond the basement membrane. Unlike patients with LCIS, however, at least 30–50% of patients with DCIS will develop invasive cancer within the same breast when treated by excisional biopsy alone (74).

Although modified radical mastectomy has been standard treatment for intraductal carcinoma, more conservative surgery with or without radiation therapy can yield good results (75). In NSAPB trial B17, 818 patients were randomly assigned to treatment with excision alone or excision followed by radiation therapy (76). The mean extent of DCIS lesions was 13 mm, and 88% were ≤20 mm. All lesions were completely resected with negative margins. After a median follow-up of 43 months, the actuarial 5-year local recurrence rate was 10.4% without radiation versus 7.5% with radiation (P=0.055) for noninvasive cancers, and 10.5% without radiation versus 2.9% with irradiation (P<0.001) for invasive cancers. Of 83 recurrences, only nine (11%) were not in the index quadrant. A recent analysis with a median follow-up of 57 months confirmed these 5-year results (77). These data suggest that segmental mastectomy offers excellent local control.

Axillary metastases occur in fewer than 5% of patients, indicating that an invasive component has been missed during biopsy. For small true DCIS, axillary dissection is not indicated. About 5% of patients whose initial biopsy results show intraductal carcinoma will be found to have infiltrating ductal carcinoma when treated with mastectomy. The incidence of contralateral breast cancer in women with intraductal carcinoma is the same as in those with invasive ductal carcinoma (i.e., 5–8%) (78).

Breast Cancer in Pregnancy

Breast cancer complicates approximately one in 3000 pregnancies (79–81). Initial studies suggested a significantly worse prognosis for patients with breast cancer diagnosed during pregnancy, but more recent data indicate that the hormonal changes associated with pregnancy seem to have little if any influence on prognosis (82). **When pregnant patients are stage-matched with nonpregnant patients, survival rates seem equivalent** (83).

The treatment of breast cancer in pregnant women must be highly individualized. Considerations include the patient's age and desire to have the child. The overall prognosis should be considered, especially when axillary lymph nodes are involved, because adjuvant chemotherapy can be teratogenic or lethal, particularly in the first trimester. It is not known whether interruption of pregnancy improves the prognosis for patients with potentially curable breast cancer.

The following are recommendations for treatment of pregnant women with breast cancer:

1. Localized disease found during the first or second trimester of pregnancy is probably best treated with definitive surgery and radiation therapy similar to nonpregnant patients. Although adjuvant chemotherapy theoretically can be given after the first trimester, most oncologists prefer not to give it to pregnant women.

2. Localized tumors found in the third trimester of pregnancy must be managed on an individual basis. Initially, tumors should be excised using local anesthesia. Early in the third trimester, definitive treatment should be initiated. If delivery is imminent, standard therapy can be performed immediately postpartum.

3. If the breast cancer is diagnosed during lactation, lactation should be suppressed and the cancer should be treated definitively.

4. Advanced, incurable cancer should be treated with palliative therapy and the pregnancy may be continued or interrupted depending on the therapy necessary and the desires of the mother.

Counseling regarding future childbearing is important for women who have had carcinoma of the breast. Although it generally has been assumed that subsequent pregnancies are detrimental because of the high levels of circulating estrogens, **there is no clear difference in survival for women who become pregnant after the diagnosis of breast cancer** (72, 82). Theoretically, it may be that only women with ER-positive or progesterone-positive tumors would be affected deleteriously by subsequent pregnancy, but this possibility has not been studied. Because recurrences are most frequent within the first 2–3 years after diagnosis, patients with receptor-positive tumors probably should wait before becoming pregnant again (if ever).

Prognosis

The most reliable predictor of survival is the stage of breast cancer at the time of diagnosis. The overall 5-year survival rate for patients with breast cancer is 70–75% (Table 36.4). Patients with stage I disease and small tumors and no evidence of regional spread after careful examination of the dissected lymph nodes ($T_1N_0M_0$) have an 80–90% 5-year disease-free survival rate. When the axillary lymph nodes are involved with tumor (stage II), the survival rate drops to 22–63% at 5 years. The number of involved axillary lymph nodes is inversely related to the rate of survival. Large lesions (T_3) or lesions with skin involvement or fixation to the underlying fascia have a 5-year survival rate of only about 20–30% (84).

Estrogen receptor status may also predict survival, with ER-positive tumors appearing to be less aggressive than ER-negative tumors. Patients with T_1N_0 lesions that are ER-positive have a 5-year survival rate $\geq$90%. In general, breast cancer appears to be somewhat more malignant in younger women than in older women; however, this may be because fewer younger women have ER-positive tumors. Other prognostic parameters—tumor grade, histologic type, and lymphatic or blood vessel involvement—have been proposed as important variables, but most microscopic findings other than lymph node involvement have correlated poorly with prognosis (85). Other biochemical and biologic factors such as ploidy, S-phase fraction, HER-2/*neu* oncogene amplification, and cathepsin D levels appear to have some prognostic significance, especially in node-negative patients (86–89), but these findings also are of limited value. Tumor size and lymph node involvement remain the main predictors of survival.

Table 36.4   Year Survival According to Stage of Breast Cancer

AJCC Stage	Breast Cancer Cases (%)	5-Year Survival (%)
0	9.4	99
I	40.9	82
II	36.6	73
III	8.9	55
IV	4.2	23

AJCC, American Joint Committee on Cancer.
Data from **Osteen RT, Karnell LH.** Breast cancer. In: **Steele GD Jr, Winchester DP, Menck HR, Murphy GP,** eds. *National Cancer Data Base Annual Review of Patient Care,* 1993. Atlanta: American Cancer Society, 1993:10–9.

References

1. **Parker SL, Tong T, Bolden S, Wingo PA.** Cancer Statistics, 1996. *CA Cancer J Clin* 1996;46:5–27.

2. **Brian DD, Melton LJ, Goellner JR, Williams RL, O'Fallon WM.** Breast cancer incidence, prevalence, mortality, and survivorship in Rochester, Minnesota. *Mayo Clin Proc* 1980;55:355–9.

3. **Mesko TW, Dunlap JN, Sutherland CM.** Risk factors for breast cancer. *Compr Ther* 1990;16:3–9.

4. **Van't Veer P, Van Leer EM, Rietdijk A, Kok FJ, Schouten EG, Hermus RJ, Sturmans F.** Combination of dietary factors in relation to breast cancer occurrence. *Int J Cancer* 1991;47:649–53.

5. **Hsieh CC, Trichopoulos D, Katsouyanni K, Yuasa S.** Age at menarche, age at menopause, height and obesity as risk factors for breast cancer: associations and interactions in an international case-control study. *Int J Cancer* 1990; 46: 796–80.

6. **Schatzkin A, Jones Y, Hoover RN, Taylor PR, Brinton LA, Ziegler RG, et al.** Alcohol consumption and breast cancer in the epidemiologic follow up: study of the first national health and nutrition examination survey. *N Engl J Med* 1987;316:1169–73.

7. **Pike MC, Krailo MD, Henderson BE, Casagrande JT, Hoel DG.** "Hormonal" risk factors, "breast tissue age" and the age-incidence of breast cancer. *Nature* 1983;303:767–70.

8. **Brinton LA, Hoover R, Fraumeni JF Jr.** Reproductive factors in the etiology of breast cancer. *Br J Cancer* 1983;47:757–62.

9. **Korzeniowski S, Dyba T.** Reproductive history and prognosis in patients with operable breast cancer. *Cancer* 1994;14:1591–4.

10. **Trapido EJ.** Age at first birth, parity, and breast cancer risks. *Cancer* 1983;51:946–8.

11. **The Cancer and Steroid Hormone Study of the Centers for Disease Control and the National Institute of Child Health and Human Development.** Oral-contraceptive use and the risk of breast cancer. *N Engl J Med* 1986;315:405–11.

12. **Kaufmann DW, Miller DR, Rosenberg L, Hellmrich SP, Stolley P, Schottenfeld D, Shapiro S.** Noncontraceptive estrogen use and the risk of breast cancer. *JAMA* 1984;252:63–7.

13. **Nielsen M, Christensen L, Andersen J.** Contralateral cancerous breast lesions in women with clinical invasive breast carcinoma. *Cancer* 1986;57:897–903.

14. **Bassett LW, Liu TH, Giuliano AE, Gold RH.** The prevalence of carcinoma in palpable vs non-palpable mammographically detected lesions. *Am J Roentgenol* 1991;157:21–4.

15. **Miller AB, Bulbrook RD.** Screening, detection and diagnosis of breast cancer. *Lancet* 1982;1:1109–11.

16. **Frable WJ.** Fine-needle aspiration biopsy: a review. *Hum Pathol* 1983;14:9–28.

17. **McDivitt RW, Stewart FW, Bert JW.** *Atlas of Tumor Pathology Tumors of the Breast.* Second series, fascicle 2. Washington DC: Armed Forces Institute of Pathology, 1968.

18. **Tubiana M, Pejovic JM, Renaud A, Contesso G, Chauaudra N, Gioanni J, Malaise EP.** Kinetic parameters and the course of the disease in breast cancer. *Cancer* 1981;47:937–43.

19. **Lee YT.** Breast carcinoma: pattern of metastasis at autopsy. *J Surg Oncol* 1983;23:175–80.

20. **Giuliano A.** The pattern of recurrence of early stage breast cancer. *J Surg Oncol* 1989;31:152–8.

21. **Bloom HJG, Richardson MB, Harris EJ.** Natural history of untreated breast cancer (1805–1933). *BMJ* 1962;47:937.

22. **Haagensen CD.** *Diseases of the Breast.* 3rd ed. Philadelphia: WB Sounders, 1986.

23. **American Joint Conunittee on Cancer.** In: **Beahrs OH, Hensen DE, Hutter RVP, Kennedy BJ,** eds. *Manuel for Staging of Cancer.* 4th ed. Philadelphia: JB Lippincott CO, 1992;149–54.

24. **Bassett LW, Giuliano AE, Gold RH.** Staging for breast carcinoma. *Am J Surg* 1989;157:250–5.

25. **Halsted WS.** The results of radical operation for cure of carcinoma of the breast. *Ann Surg* 1907;46:1–19.

26. **Meyer W.** Carcinoma of the breast; ten years experience with my method of radical operation. *JAMA 1905;45:297–313.*

27. **Haagensen CD, Bodian C.** A personal experience with Halsted's radical mastectomy. *Ann Surg* 1984;199:143–50.

28. **Dahl-Iversen E, Tobiassen T.** Radical mastectomy with parasternal and supraclavicular dissection for mammary carcinoma. *Ann Surg* 1963;157:170–3.

29. **Lewis FJ.** Extended or super radical mastectomy for cancer of the breast. *Minn Med* 1953; 36:763–6.

30. **Urban JA.** Extended radical mastectomy for breast cancer. *Ann Surg* 1963;106:399.

31. **Veronesi U, Valagussa P.** Inefficacy of internal mammary node dissection in breast cancer surgery. *Cancer* 1981;47:170–3.

32. **Handley RS.** The conservative radical mastectomy of Patey: 10-year results in 425 patients. *Breast* 1976;2:16–9.

33. **Maier WP, Leber D, Rosemond GP, Goldman LI, Tyson RR.** The technique of modified radical mastectomy. *Surg Gynecol Obstet* 1977;145:68–74.

34. **Robinson GN, Van Heerden JA, Payne SW, Taylor WF, Gaffey TA.** The primary surgical treatment of carcinoma of the breast: a changing trend toward modified radical mastectomy. *Mayo Clin Proc* 1976;51:433–42.

35. **McWhirter R.** Should more radical treatment be attempted in breast cancer? *Am J Roentgenol* 1964;92:3–13.

36. **Montague ED.** Radiation therapy and breast cancer. Past, present and future. *Am J Clin Oncol* 1985;8:455–62.

37. **Montague ED, Fletcher GH.** The curative value of irradiation in the treatment of nondisseminated breast cancer. *Cancer* 1980;46:995–8.

38. **Wallgren A, Arner O, Bergstrom J, Blomstedt B, Granberg PO, Karnstrom L, et al.** The value of preoperative radiotherapy in operable mammary carcinoma. *Int J Radiat Oncol Biot Phys* 1980;6:287–90.

39. **Nevin JE, Baggerly JT, Laird TK.** Radiotherapy as an adjuvant in the treatment of cancer of the breast. *Cancer* 1982;49:1194–200.

40. **Fisher B, Redmond C, Fisher ER, Bauer M, Wolmark N, Wickerham DL, et al.** Ten-year results of a randomized clinical trial comparing radical mastectomy and total mastectomy with or without radiation. *N Engl J Med* 1985;312:674–81.

41. **Keynes G.** Conservative treatment of cancer of the breast. *BMJ* 1937;2:643–47.

42. **Calle R, Pilleron JP, Schlienger P, Vilcoq JR.** Conservative management of operable breast cancer: ten years' experience at the Foundation Curie. *Cancer* 1978;42:2045–53.

43. **Prosnitz LR, Goldenberg IS, Packard RA, Levene MB, Harris J, Hellman S, et al.** Radiation therapy as initial treatment for early stage cancer of the breast without mastectomy. *Cancer* 1977;39:917–23.

44. **Harris JR, Helllman S, Silen W.** *Conservative Management of Breast Cancer.* Philadelphia: JB Lippincott, 1983.

45. **Veronesi U, Saccozzi R, Del Veccio M, Saccozzi R, Clemente C, Greco M, et al.** Comparing radical mastectomy with quadrantectomy, axillary dissection and radiotherapy in patients with small cancers of the breast. *N Engl J Med* 1985;312:665.

46. **Veronesi U, Zucali R, Luini A.** Local control and survival in early breast cancer: the Milan trial. *Int J Radiat Oncol Biol Phys* 1986;12:717–20.

47. **Fisher B, Bauer M, Margolese R, Poisson R, Pilch Y, Redmond C, et al.** Five-year results of a randomized clinical trial comparing total mastectomy and segmental mastectomy with or without radiation in the treatment of cancer. *N Engl J Med* 1989;320:822–8.

48. **Schabel FM Jr.** Rationale for adjuvant chemotherapy. *Cancer* 1977;39:2875–82.

49. **Nissen-Meyer R.** The Scandanavian clinical trials. *Experientia Suppl* 1982;41:571–9.

50. **Bonadonna G, Valagussa P.** Adjuvant systemic therapy for resectable breast cancer. *J Clin Oncol* 1985;3:259–75.

51. **Fisher B, Carbone P, Economou SG, Frelick R, Glass A, Lerner H, et al.** L-phenylalanine mustard in the management of primary breast cancer. A report of early findings. *N Engl J Med* 1975;292:117–22.

52. **Mueller CB, Lesperance ML.** NSABP trials of adjuvant chemotherapy for breast cancer. A further look at the evidence. *Ann Surg* 1991;214:206–11.

53. **Bonadonna G, Rossi A, Valagussa P.** Adjuvant CMF chemotherapy in operable breast cancer: ten years later. *World J Surg* 1985;9:707–13.

54. **Tancine G, Bonadonna G, Valagussa P, Marchini S, Veronesi U.** Adjuvant CMF in breast cancer: comparative 5-year results of 12 versus 6 cycles. *J Clin Oncol* 1983;1:2–10.

55. **Bonadonna G, Valagussa P.** Dose-response effect of adjuvant chemotherapy in breast cancer. *N Engl J Med* 1981;304:10–15.

56. **Castiglione M, Gelber RD, Goldhirsch A.** Adjuvant systemic therapy for breast cancer in the elderly: competing causes of mortality. International Breast Cancer Study Group. *J Clin Oncol* 1990;8:519–26.

57. **Henderson IC.** Adjuvant systemic therapy for early breast cancer: current problems. *Cancer* 1987;11:125–207.

58. **Abeloff MD, Beveridge RA.** Adjuvant chemotherapy of breast cancer. The Consensus Development Conference revisited. *Oncology (Huntingt)* 1988;2:21–26,29–33.

59. **Fisher B, Redmond C, Dimitrov NV, Bowman D, Legault-Poisson S, Wickerham DL, et al.** A randomized clinical trial evaluating sequential methotrexate and fluorouracil in the treatment of patients with node-negative breast cancer who have estrogen-receptor-negative tumors. *N Engl J Med* 1989;320:473–8.

60. **Mansour EG, Gray R, Shatila AH, Osborne CK, Tormey DC, Gilchrist KW, et al.** Efficacy of adjuvant chemotherapy in high-risk node-negative breast cancer. An intergroup study. *N Engl J Med* 1989;320:485–90.

61. **Fisher B, Costantino A, Redmond C, Poisson R, Bowman D, Couture J, et al.** A randomized clinical trial evaluating tamoxifen in the treatment of patients with node-negative breast cancer who have estrogen-receptor-positive tumors. *N Engl J Med* 1989;320:479–84.

62. **Baum MB, Brinkley DM, Dosset JA, McPherson IM, Jackson RD, Rubens FG, et al.** Controlled trial of tamoxifen as a single adjuvent agent in the management of early breast cancer: analysis at eight years by Nolvadex adjuvant trial organization. *Br J Cancer* 1988;57:608–11.

63. **Breast Cancer Trials Committee.** Scottish Cancer Trials Office (MRC) Edinburgh. Adjuvant tamoxifen in the management of operable breast cancer: The Scottish trial. *Lancet* 1987;2:171–5.

64. **Breast Cancer Study Group.** Prolonged disease-free survival after one course of perioperative adjuvant chemotherapy for node-negative breast cancer. *N Engl Med* 1989;320:491–6.

65. **National Institutes of Health Consensus Statement.** NIH consensus development conference: adjuvant chemotherapy for breast cancer. Washington, DC: National Institutes of Health, 1990;8:16.

66. **Fisher B, Redmond C, Brown A, Wolmack N, Wittliff J, Fisher ER, et al.** Treatment of primary breast cancer with chemotherapy and tamoxifen. *N Engl J Med* 1981;305:1–6.

67. **Buzdar AU.** Current status of endocrine treatment of carcinoma of the breast. *Semin Surg Oncol* 1990;6:77–82.

68. **Henderson IC, Garber JE, Breitmeyer JB, Hayes DF, Harris JR.** Comprehensive management of disseminated breast cancer. *Cancer* 1990;66:1439–48.

69. **Paget J.** Disease of the mammary areola preceding cancer of the mammary gland. *St Bart Host Rep* 1874;10:89.

70. **Bulens P, Vanuytsel L, Rijnders A, van der Schueren E.** Breast conserving treatment of Paget's disease. *Radiother Oncol* 1990;17:305–9.

71. **Droulias CA, Sewell CW, McSweeney MB, Powell RW.** Inflammatory carcinoma of the breast: a correlation of clinical, radiologic and pathologic findings. *Ann Surg* 1976;184:217–22.

72. **Donegan WL, Padrta B.** Combined therapy for inflammatory breast cancer. *Arch Surg* 1990;125:578–82.

73. **Sunshine JA, Moseley HS, Fletcher WS, Krippaehne WW.** Breast carcinoma *in situ:* a retrospective review of 112 cases with a minimum 10-year follow up. *Am J Surg* 1985;150:44–51.

74. **Barth A, Brenner RJ, Giuliano AE.** Current management of ductal carcinoma in situ. *West J Surg.* 1995;163:360–6.

75. **Stotter AT, McNeese M, Oswald MJ, Ames FC, Romsdahl MM.** The role of limited surgery with irradiation in primary treatment of ductal in situ breast cancer. *Int J Radial Ther Oncol Biol Phys* 1990;18:283–7.

76. **Fisher B, Constantino J, Redmond C, Fisher E, Margolese R, Dixnitrov N, et al.** Lumpectomy compared with lumpectomy and radiation therapy for the treatment of intraductal breast cancer. *N Engl J Med* 1993;328:1581–6.

77. **Recht A, van Dongen JA, Peterse JL.** Ductal carcinoma in situ. *Lancet* 1994;343:969.

78. **Kinne DW, Petrek JA, Osborne MP, Fracchia AA, DePalo AA, Rosen PP.** Breast carcinoma in situ. *Arch Surg* 1989;124:33–6.

79. **Donegan WL.** Cancer and pregnancy. *CA Cancer J Clin* 1983;33:194–214.

80. **Hornstein E, Skornick Y, Rozin R. The management of breast carcinoma in pregnancy and lactation.** *J Surg Oncol* 1982;21:179–82.

81. **Hoover HC Jr.** Breast cancer during pregnancy and lactation. *Surg Clin North Am* 1990;70:1151–63.

82. **Yon Schoultz E, Johansson H, Wilking N, Rutqvist LE.** Influence of prior and subsequent pregnancy on breast cancer prognosis. *J Clin Oncol* 1995;13:430–4.

83. **Petrek JA.** Breast cancer and pregnancy. *Monogr Natl Cancer Inst* 1994;16:113–21.

84. **Steele GD, Winchester DP, Menck HR, Murphy GP.** National cancer data base. *Anno Rev Patient Care* 1992.

85. **Fisher ER, Redmond C, Fisher B, Bass G.** Pathologic findings from the National Surgical Adjuvant Breast and Bowel Projects (NSABP). Prognostic discriminants for 8-year survival for node-negative invasive breast cancer patients. *Cancer* 1990;65:2121–8.

86. **Merkel DE, Osborne CK.** Prognostic factors in breast cancer. *Hematol Oncol Clin North Am* 1989;3:641–52.

87. **McGuire WL, Clark GM.** Prognostic factors and treatment decisions in axillary node-negative breast cancer. *N Engl J Med* 1992;326:1756–61.

88. **Tandon AK, Clark GM, Chamness GC, Chirgwin JM, MCGuire WL.** Cathepsin D and prognosis in breast cancer. *N Engl J Med* 1990;322:297–302.

89. **Lewis WE.** Prognostic significance of flow cytometric DNA analysis in node-negative breast cancer patients. *Cancer* 1990;65:2315–20.

Recent references that confirm the findings of prior randomized trials:

90. **Early Breast Cancer Trialists' Collaborative Group.** Systemic treatment of early breast cancer of hormonal, cytotoxic, or immune therapy. 133 randomized trials involving 31,000 recurrences and 24,000 deaths among 75,000 women. *Lancet* 1992;339(8785):71–85.

91. **Early Breast Cancer Trialists' Collaborative Group.** Effects of radiotherapy and surgery in early breast cancer. *N Engl J Med* 1995;333:1444–55.

92. **Fisher B, Anderson S, Redmond CK, Wolmark N, Wickerham DL, Cronin WM.** Reanalysis and results after 12 years of follow-up in a randomized clinical trial comparing total mastectomy with lumpectomy with or without irradiation in the treatment of breast cancer. *N Engl J Med* 1995;333:1456–61.

93. **Christian MC, McCabe MS, Korn EL, Abrams JS, Kaplan RS, Friedman MA.** The National Cancer Institute audit of the National Surgical Adjuvant Breast and Bowel Project protocol B-06. *N Engl J Med* 1995;333:1469–74.

37 Palliative Care and Pain Management

J. Norelle Lickiss
Jennifer Wiltshire

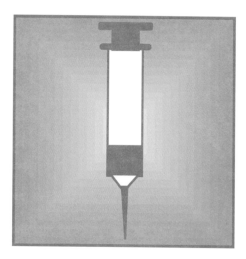

There are no circumstances that justify a gynecologist's ever telling a patient or her family that "nothing more can be done." A patient with advanced, progressive gynecological cancer, even if anticancer therapy is still ongoing, needs and has a right to good palliative care.

The World Health Organization, in a recent statement, offers a definition embodying these elements (1):

Palliative care is the active total care of patients whose disease is not responsive to curative treatment. Control of pain, of other symptoms, and of psychological, social, and spiritual problems is paramount. The goal of palliative care is achievement of the best possible quality of life for patients and their families. Many aspects of palliative care are also applicable earlier in the course of the illness, in conjunction with anticancer treatment. Palliative care:

- *affirms life and regards dying as a normal process*
- *neither hastens nor postpones death*
- *provides relief from pain and other distressing symptoms*
- *integrates the psychological and spiritual aspects of patient care*
- *offers a support system to help patients live as actively as possible until death*
- *offers a support system to help the family during the patient's illness and in their bereavement.*

Radiotherapy, chemotherapy, and surgery have a place in palliative care if the symptomatic benefits of treatment clearly outweigh the disadvantages. Investigative procedures are kept to a minimum.

In general, effective cancer therapy offers the best chance of good symptom relief if the patient is a "responder," but the quality of life of a "nonresponder" to therapy may be worse than that of an untreated patient. When the patient's condition is clearly deteriorating and a plateau in therapy has been reached, with a high price being paid for very small gains, a revision of management is essential. It is crucial for the bond between the patient and her physicians to be strengthened at this time. One of the skills required of the palliative care practitioner is to be nonintrusive whenever possible. Indeed, the patient's own primary care physician becomes central, assisted when necessary by specialist palliative medical and nursing staff, preferably those who are already known by the patient. **Continuity of as many professional relationships as possible is beneficial. As the patient moves from a chronic phase into a deteriorating late phase, a total change of personnel is undesirable, but advice should be readily sought from colleagues versed in palliative medicine and care.**

Overall Approach to Palliative Care

The care of a woman with advanced gynecologic cancer involves several components:

1. diagnosis

2. delineation of therapeutic possibilities

3. implementation of treatment

4. evaluation of outcome

Step 1

Make a comprehensive diagnosis—this involves at least the following:

1. Ascertainment of the patient's symptoms and other problems, in her order of priority

2. Clarification of the nature and the extent of the neoplastic process, with careful consideration of other diseases that may be contributing to the present problems

3. Delineation of the personal and social contexts within which the patient is living and from which she may draw support

4. Elucidation of her personal objectives

The pursuit of an adequate diagnosis involves not only careful listening to the patient but also, if the patient gives consent, interaction with family members and close friends.

Step 2

Delineate the therapeutic possibilities now. On the basis of a comprehensive diagnosis, with or without further investigations to elucidate the mechanisms of troublesome symptoms, it is possible to delineate the therapeutic possibilities. If the symptoms are not adequately ascertained, the mechanisms are not adequately understood, and the patient's priorities are not appreciated, then therapeutic endeavors are likely to be ineffective.

Step 3

Make decisions concerning treatment and implementation. Palliative care is concerned with quality of life and the facilitation of freedom. The therapeutic options should reflect this.

In general, the least restrictive alternative involving the least dependence on medical facilities and the least use of the patient's time, resources, and personal energy should be selected. Careful consideration of other relevant antitumor measures (i.e., surgery, radiotherapy, or chemotherapy) is mandatory, because control of the neoplastic process usually offers the best chance of alleviating symptoms. Decision-making in this area requires genuine clinical wisdom, going far beyond the consideration of known statistics with respect to specific outcomes.

Decisions concerning treatment should normally involve the patient, who should be adequately informed about the foreseeable advantages and disadvantages of the various options. Although the patient should share in decision-making insofar as she wishes, her physician should, on the whole, clearly indicate the course of action he or she favors and ultimately take the responsibility for an intervention. This is not necessarily true for an omission, if the patient clearly prefers not to have an advised intervention. The burden of decision-making is considerable, and ways of reaching decisions vary according to social, cultural, economic, and medical contexts. However, the physician has the duty of bearing a part of the burden, so that a distressing outcome should not engender guilt in the patient and her family. However, the physician should not compromise his or her better judgment or conscience in the face of patient or family pressure (2).

Step 4

Evaluation of palliative interventions is best performed by the informed patient, although the observations of the medical and nursing staff are also important. Some form of monitoring is essential, because time, often the patient's most precious possession, should not be wasted by ineffective intervention if further treatment options are available or if modifications are possible. The more restricted the life expectancy, the more grave the misuse of time. Formal outcome measures based on subjective criteria ideally should be introduced into routine clinical practice.

The clinical process also involves the recognition of a patient who is clearly dying. There are many indicators of this phase, and these are well known to clinicians, nurses, and family members. There may be a change in the tempo of the disease, a change in the function of the critical organs with no possibility for reversibility, or a rapid deterioration in strength or physical performance in the absence of reversible factors, such as anemia, septicemia, hypercalcemia, or drug interactions. What is medically possible at this stage, such as treatment of septicemia or hypercalcemia, may not necessarily be medically wise.

Some word is necessary concerning prognosis, because the matter ultimately will arise. In the face of a question concerning prognosis, there is a strong case for a response offering some time boundaries within which death may eventually occur. Such boundaries are useful for thinking and planning and certainly reinforce the fact that, as in the case of all mortals, time is finite and the "horizon is in view." These boundaries do not give a patient or her family an agonizing date around which to focus, nor do they suggest that what is still quite uncertain can be predicted precisely. The end of life is too serious a matter to be diverted by such a false focus.

Management of Major Gynecologic Symptoms

Symptoms are subjective, even though the person with severe symptoms may have objective manifestations, such as vomiting. A patient in severe pain may or may not show signs of distress. Her behavior will be influenced by cultural and environmental factors, as well as by personal and interpersonal relationships. **Accurate assessment of symptoms requires skill, patience, active listening, and unconditional regard for the patient. The patient is always right about symptoms because of their intrinsic subjectivity** (3–7).

Symptoms vary in their significance. Certain symptoms may cause much emotional distress, whereas other symptoms that are more serious in the physiologic consequences (e.g., severe constipation) may not evoke the same fear. It is important to give the patient a chance to express her fears and to offer some simple explanation for the symptom, because this will at least reduce her anxiety. Whatever the cause, symptom relief is essential and usually possible with relatively simple measures.

Pain Management

Pain has been defined by the International Association for Management for the Study of Pain as "an unpleasant sensory and emotional experience associated with actual or potential tissue damage or described in terms of such damage." Pain is a subjective phenomenon, an experience. It is not surprising, therefore, that there are difficulties both in measuring pain and in pain management. Because of its subjective nature, the patient is always correct in her appraisal of the severity of the pain.

The advances of the last decade in pain management should be readily available to all patients with advanced gynecological cancer. Improvements have been based on a more adequate understanding of pain physiology and classification, as well as on precise research with respect to drug management (7–9). Conolly (10) stated, "What is needed now is not a stunning new understanding of pain pharmacology, but the consistent and rational application of what is already known." Cancer pain assessment and treatment guidelines have recently been developed by the American Society of Clinical Oncology (11).

The following simple scheme may provide some guidelines in the face of the complexity of recent research and practice. Pain management may be considered as having four steps (Fig. 37.1).

Step One—Reduce the Noxious Stimulus at the Periphery

This step demands an adequate understanding of the mechanisms of the pain stimulus in the individual patient, on the basis of a carefully focused history, physical examination, and if necessary, other investigations. A precise history, including the mode of onset, characteristics, distribution, aggravating factors, trends over time, and response to therapeutic endeavors, provides the fundamental guide to the likely mechanism. Pain caused by treatment requires as close attention as that resulting directly from tumor. The noxious stimulus may arise from soft-tissue distortion or infiltration, bone involvement, neural involvement, muscle spasm, infection within or near tumor masses, intestinal colic, or sheer pressure. Therapeutic approaches vary according to the mechanism that is operative. Consideration should be given to specific therapeutic measures (e.g., radiotherapy, chemotherapy, antibiotics, regional neural blockade, or occasionally, surgical approaches).

Bone metastases frequently cause inflammatory changes with release of prostaglandins that may sensitize the tissues to other noxious stimuli. When the pain is clearly arising from bone

Figure 37.1   Four-step approach to cancer pain.

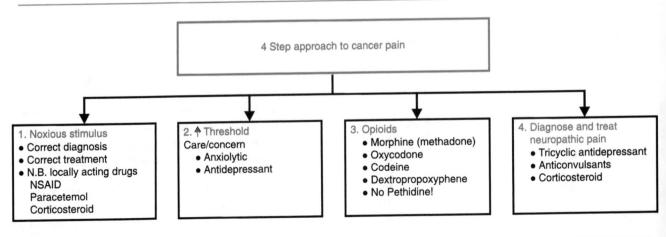

metastases and has the characteristics of bone pain, the use of drugs that interfere in some way with prostaglandin synthesis, e.g., nonsteroidal anti-inflammatory drugs (*NSAIDS*), is logical. These drugs should be avoided or used with caution for patients who have a history of peptic ulceration, excessive alcohol consumption, bleeding diatheses, or known idiosyncratic reaction to aspirin or related drugs. When the use of *NSAIDS* is precluded, acetaminophen is useful, although the mechanism of action of this drug is obscure. It may have central effects as well as some peripheral action. Whereas *acetaminophen* is fairly well tolerated and safe, it should be used in reduced dosage for patients with extensive liver damage, especially alcoholic cirrhosis.

Peripherally acting drugs such as *acetaminophen* and *NSAIDS* are also useful for pain arising in nonosseous sites and for postoperative pain. They should rarely be omitted from drug analgesic regimens, even for moribund patients. Rectal preparations may prove useful as an adjunct to rectal opioids for patients who are unable to take oral drugs.

Step Two—Raise the Pain Threshold

The concept of threshold is useful, and it is clear that the threshold for pain perception is varied by many factors. The threshold for pain may well be raised significantly by comfort, care, concern, diversion, and various forms of relaxation; the threshold is lowered by depression, anxiety, loneliness, and isolation.

A wide range of strategies exist to raise the threshold and to facilitate coping with pain, and simple nonpharmacologic measures should be tried initially. The diagnosis of "extreme anguish" as a major component of unrelieved pain is difficult and may not be clear until an empiric approach to pain therapy has been initiated. Anguish is aggravated by unrelieved pain more often than anguish is the factor that makes the relief of pain more difficult.

Step Three—Reduce Pain Perception by the Careful and Precise Use of Opioid Drugs

There is abundant literature on opioid use, and a range of opioids are available (7–12). In practice, weak opioids, such as *codeine* or *dextropropoxyphene,* or stronger opioids, typically *morphine,* are combined with drugs such as *acetaminophen* or *aspirin,* with regard for contraindications. **It is now widely recognized that opioids should be given regularly, at precisely determined doses and at fixed intervals in accordance with the half-life of the drug concerned, rather than haphazardly in response to a severe pain stimulus** (Table 37.1).

Morphine

1. The most commonly used *morphine* preparation, *morphine sulfate* solution, is best given every 4 hours, with a double dose (or 1.5 times the standard dose in the frail) at bedtime and a break of approximately 8 hours overnight to permit sleep for both the patient and caregivers. Many find the following schedule to be useful: 6 AM, 10 AM, 2 PM, 6 PM, and 10 PM.

2. A reasonable starting dose of oral *morphine* for a patient not already on an opioid drug would be 5–10 mg for a patient of average size and 3–5 mg for a frail or elderly patient, with repetition of the original dose in 1–2 hours if there has been no relief from pain.

3. During the next 24–48 hours, dose finding is undertaken by prescription of regular doses given every 4 hours, together with the provision of one or two "breakthrough" doses equal to the standard dose. The correct dose may range from 2 mg to more than 100 mg every 4 hours, but most patients will need less than 50 mg every 4 hours.

Table 37.1   Equivalency of Various Narcotic Analgesics to 10 mg of Intramuscular Morphine

Drug	Route*	Dose (mg)	Duration (hr)	Plasma (half-life)	Comments
Morphine	SQ/IM	10	4–6	2–3.5	Also available in a slow-release form and as rectal suppositories
	PO	30–60			
Codeine	SQ/IM	130	4–6	3	Metabolized to morphine
	PO	200			
Oxycodone	SQ/IM	15	3–4	—	Often, 5 mg combined with ASA and acetaminophen
	PO	30			
Levorphanol	IM	2	4–6	12–16	May accumulate and result in delayed toxities
	PO	4			
Hydromorphone	SQ/IM	1.5	4–5	2–3	Available up to 10 mg/ml for injection and as rectal suppositories
	PO	7.5			
Oxymorphone	SQ/IM	1	4–6	2–3	No oral preparation
	PR	10			
Meperidine	SQ/IM	75	2–3	3–4	Toxic metabolite causes CNS excitation; avoid in renal failure
	PO	300			
Methadone	SQ/IM	10	4–6	15–30	May accumulate and result in delayed toxicities
	PO	20			
Fentanyl	IV	0.1	0.5–1	3–12	Transdermal delivery requires days to reach steady state
	Patch	0.5	72		

Reproduced with permission from **Grossman SA.** Is pain undertreated in cancer patients? *Advances Oncol* 1993;9:11.
IM, intramuscular; IV, intravenous; PO, oral; SQ, subcutaneous; ASA, acetylsalicylic acid (aspirin); PR, rectally, CNS, central nervous system.
*Subcutaneous route is preferable to intramuscular in most situations.

4. Controlled-release *morphine* tablets offer a convenience of administration, with the proviso that dose findings should be initially undertaken with the use of morphine sulfate solution. After the correct dose has been determined, the total 24-hour dose can be given in two fractions every 12 hours. It is essential that the tablets not be crushed. Controlled-release *morphine* should not be used for patients with uncontrolled or unstable pain or for patients with extensive upper abdominal disease that is likely to interfere with drug absorption or gastrointestinal motility. Aqueous *morphine* or subcutaneous *morphine* is a wiser choice in such circumstances.

5. Occasionally, the oral route cannot be used and calibration can then be undertaken by the subcutaneous route; the conversion ratio of oral to subcutaneous is 3:1. Occasionally, the rectal route may be a useful alternative to oral or subcutaneous *morphine* (4).

6. There is usually no need for the intramuscular route, and intravenous pulses give only short-lived analgesia. The intravenous route, although often useful, can be hazardous. One risk is the development of acute tolerance, which may not always be overcome by the addition of more *morphine* (13). Cessation of the infusion and resumption of appropriate subcutaneous doses every 4 hours is often helpful, and advice must be sought if a patient has rapidly escalating pain not controlled by rapidly increasing doses of *morphine*, especially given as an intravenous infusion. No patient should be left in such a state.

If significant drowsiness or other *morphine* toxicity occurs after the first 24 hours, the *morphine* level is probably above the therapeutic range for that patient. Other causes of drowsiness should be excluded, such as sedative drugs or hypercalcemia, but the *morphine* dose should not be raised further. In such circumstances, the pain therapy usually requires another approach. Some types of pain are relatively unresponsive to opioids, including pain caused by bone metastases, nerve irritation, or extreme muscle spasm. In such circumstances, other drugs are essential, not optional, as adjuncts to *morphine*.

The efficacy of the regular dosing approach to *morphine* administration may be dependent on the contribution of an active metabolite (*morphine 6-glucuronide*), which is a more powerful analgesic than *morphine*. Hepatic impairment, if severe, interferes with *morphine* metabolism to glucuronides (12). Renal impairment, even if only moderate, interferes with excretion of these metabolites, and in both of these circumstances, dose reduction is essential.

The side effects of opioid drugs are avoidable largely by precise prescribing. Predictable side effects such as constipation can usually be prevented with concomitant use of a laxative that combines softening and stimulant properties. Care should be taken to avoid laxatives that increase the bulk of the stool in patients liable to bowel obstruction. Nausea is uncommon unless the patient is very anxious, inadequately counselled, or already constipated. It can also occur if *morphine* is introduced in such a manner that serum levels rise rapidly.

Morphine Myths

Morphine (if correctly used) does not hasten death or lead to addiction in most cases, but some physicians continue to harbor misconceptions about its use. When morphine is to be commenced, counselling is usually necessary, and the following issues should be stressed to counteract widely held fears.

1. The use of *morphine* with careful dose-finding and monitoring does not, in most patients, lead to addiction (although physical dependence occurs).

2. The introduction of *morphine* does not mean that the patient is actually dying but rather that morphine is the most appropriate opioid at that time. It is the type of pain and its severity, not the prognosis for the patient, that dictate whether an opioid should be introduced.

3. Patients and their families may need to be reassured that the introduction of *morphine* will not mean that there will be no adequate analgesic available at a later stage in the illness when the situation may be worse.

4. Tolerance to *morphine* may be a major clinical problem if the *morphine* is not introduced and calibrated correctly. When the drug is used correctly, increased requirements during the course of an illness usually signify an increase in the noxious stimulus, rather than a reduction in the effectiveness of *morphine*.

Other Strong Opioids

Although *morphine* is currently the most useful opioid, other strong opioids are occasionally preferable. Availability varies, but gynecologists should become familiar with a narrow range of opioids, e.g., *morphine, oxycodone, codeine,* and other relevant available drugs.

Oxycodone is approximately equianalgesic with morphine and is most often used in a dose of 5–15 mg every 4–6 hours. Some patients tolerate *oxycodone* better than *morphine* at the same dose and vice versa.

Meperidine (pethidine) is of very little value in palliative care. At high doses, the drug is clearly neurotoxic and can add much to the distress of dying patients (4).

Heroin offers no advantage over *morphine* except higher solubility, and its efficiency depends on metabolism to morphine.

Methadone is occasionally useful, but its long half-life is sometimes disadvantageous and its sedative action outlasts its analgesic activity, making the drug difficult to use. Transdermal preparations of opioids such as *fentanyl* may prove to be very convenient if used correctly. Opioids such as *codeine*, often combined with *aspirin, acetaminophen,* or *dextropropoxyphene*, are useful for mild pain, but these opioids should not be combined with *morphine*. Care should be taken to use only one opioid at a time; a combination of two opioids is unwise, unnecessary, and hazardous. A change from one opioid to another, however, is frequently justified.

If fecal impaction has occurred as a result of opioids given without a laxative, pelvic and abdominal pain may occur and nausea may increase. Such patients are in preventable misery, and the diagnosis should always be suspected in a patient with diarrhea, nausea, abdominal distension, abdominal pain, or in the case of an elderly patient, confusion.

Step Four—Recognize Neuropathic Pain and Treat Correctly

Neuropathic pain may result from irritation or destruction of peripheral nerves secondary to disease or its therapy. The quality of neuropathic pain varies but can be described as burning, lancinating, anesthetic, or hyperesthetic in nature.

When the pain is neuropathic in origin, an opioid and a peripherally acting drug should be supplemented by low doses of other drugs, such as tricyclic antidepressants, anticonvulsants, corticosteroids, or oral anesthetic agents. In general, the management of neuropathic pain is difficult. The drugs used have significant side effects, and assistance of a specialist will be necessary. Anesthetists with special interests in pain management may be most helpful. Regional blockade with local anesthetic techniques may be worthy of consideration. Epidural *morphine* with *marcaine* is useful for carefully selected patients.

Difficult Pain Problems

Lumbosacral Plexopathy

The lumbosacral plexus lies in the retroperitoneal space medial to the iliopsoas muscle and lateral to the cervix. This plexus can be compressed or invaded by locally advanced pelvic tumors, particularly cervical tumors, or it may be compressed by a pelvic abscess or hematoma. Fibrosis of the lumbosacral plexus, especially when patients are treated with combinations of external and intracavitary radiation, has also been documented (14). The lumbar portion of the plexus (L1–4) forms the femoral nerve and receives its blood supply from branches of the abdominal aorta. The sacral portion of the plexus (L5–S3) forms the sciatic nerve and receives its blood supply from branches of the internal iliac artery (14).

Assessment

Pain is normally the first sign of lumbosacral plexopathy and often precedes the weakness and sensory dysfunction by weeks to months. The pain may be confined to the lumbosacral region or radiate down the leg along the sensory distribution of the nerve roots. It may be sharp, shooting, lancinating pain or a continuous burning dysesthesia. Occasionally, there may be an incident component with extension of the hip or weight bearing.

Signs vary depending on which part of the plexus is compressed. When the lower part of the plexus is involved (L5–S3 nerve roots), there may be signs of foot-drop, a pelvic tilt, and sensory loss in the thigh, sole, and perineum. Compression of the upper plexus (L1–4) results in hip flexor weakness and difficulty climbing steps, together with paraesthesia in the anterior thigh (4).

Investigations to assist diagnosis include a computed tomography (CT) scan or magnetic resonance imaging (MRI) of the pelvis to diagnose tumor, abscess, or hematoma and a CT myelogram or MRI of the lumbosacral spine to rule out epidural metastasis compressing the cord or nerve roots. Specialist assistance will normally be needed to clarify the etiology and the treatment options.

Management

Management of these symptoms is aimed at reversing the underlying cause, including specific antitumor therapy (i.e., radiotherapy, surgery, or chemotherapy) when appropriate; for example, antibiotics for an abscess, and drainage of a hematoma. Specific symptom management includes *dexamethasone, acetaminophen,* or *NSAIDS* to help reduce edema. Opioids should be given as per Step Three (Fig. 37.1), anticonvulsants should be given for lancinating neuropathic pain, and antidepressants should be given for continuous or burning dysesthesias. Nonpharmacological measures such as transcutaneous electronic nerve stimulation (TENS) may also be useful.

Psoas Muscle Spasm

The psoas muscle forms the posterior abdominal wall. The lumbar part of the lumbosacral plexus lies in the substance of the muscle. Spasm of this muscle can occur when infiltrated by tumor or compressed by nodal disease or a benign space-occupying lesion.

The main symptom is severe pain. This occurs in the abdomen, iliac, or inguinal region with radiation to the hip or posterior thigh. If the lumbosacral plexus is involved, neuropathic pain will occur in the areas corresponding to the affected lumbar nerve roots. The hip is often held in a fixed flexed position, and extension or internal rotation of the hip is very painful and may not be possible. Management is aimed at reversing any aggravating factors, such as antitumor treatment (i.e., radiotherapy, chemotherapy, or surgery when appropriate). Concomitant and early symptom management is essential and will reduce the risk of myopathy and chronic pain problems. Such measures include the following:

1. Reducing local noxious stimuli as per Step One above with *acetaminophen* or *NSAIDS*

2. Adding carefully calibrated opioids

3. Reducing muscle spasm with a muscle relaxant, e.g., *diazepam* 2–5 mg every 6–8 hours

4. Reducing tumor edema with *dexamethasone* if it is not contraindicated

5. Treating lumbosacral plexopathy if it is involved

The goal of medicine is concerned with the relief of suffering, which Cassell defines as a sense of disintegration of the self (15): in common parlance, a sense of "going to pieces." It is essential to recognize that although pain is a subjective experience (and therefore the patient is always the arbiter of its severity), it is usually possible to differentiate pain from suffering. Occasionally, anxiety and depression are so clearly pathological that the patient is being impeded in her attempts to relate to her loved ones and to come to terms with her disease. In such a circumstance, a formal psychiatric consultation may be of assistance and, occasionally, anxiolytics or antidepressants may be used in the usual fashion. However, threshold issues, including extreme anguish, futility, loss of sense of meaning, personal guilt, and other forms of spiritual pain, require a different approach. With the help of skilled counsellors, pastors, and above all, those persons who are close to the patient, the patient must be allowed to have her private space for suffering.

Other Symptoms

Gastrointestinal Symptoms

Pain remains the most common symptom in patients with advanced gynecological cancer, but gastrointestinal symptoms are also a major source of distress and may arise from the cancer or its treatment. Each symptom requires precise diagnosis and competent management (16).

Oral

Mouth symptoms can be most distressing, and mouth care is crucial in very ill patients. Discomfort arising from oral candidiasis responds to antifungal agents such as *nystatin* mouthwashes (every 2–3 hours), *amphotericin* lozenges, or *ketoconazole* tablets. Pain from mucositis caused by radiotherapy may be relieved by *sucralfate* suspension and by *acetaminophen*, with *morphine* (orally or subcutaneously) if necessary. Vitamins may assist stomatitis and glossitis in seriously malnourished patients.

Anorexia

Anorexia is a common and significant symptom with a multitude of causes and serious nutritional consequences, which often are not appreciated. The best initial approach includes careful preparation of small meals, good mouth care, emotional support, and direct nutritional supplements. Progestins may increase appetite and weight without undue side effects. Attention to reversible factors, such as gastric stasis and nutritional supplements, should be considered.

Nausea

Nausea and vomiting are common in advanced gynecological cancer. These symptoms require precise diagnosis so that rational therapy may be applied.

Nausea with or without vomiting is mediated finally by the vomiting center situated in the reticular formation of the medulla oblongata, an area rich in histamine receptors. The vomiting center is influenced by several connections, each of which can be the causal pathway for nausea. These include the following:

1. Cerebral cortex (e.g., anxiety-conditioned responses)

2. Vestibular center, which is rich in histamine receptors (H1) (e.g., some forms of morphine induce nausea, occasionally cerebral metastases)

3. Chemosensitive trigger zone (CTZ), which is rich in dopamine receptors (D) (e.g., nausea induced by some drugs, including chemotherapeutic agents, hypercalcemia, uremia)

4. Gastrointestinal tract (e.g., gastric stasis, intestinal obstruction, fecal impaction, abnormalities of gut motility)

After the likely mechanism has been determined by means of a careful history, clinical examination, and investigations (if indicated), the appropriate antinauseant can be prescribed (Table 37.2).

When anxiety dominates the scene, anxiolytics may be crucial in reducing the nausea. When vestibular mechanisms are suspected or when no specific pathway can be identified, relatively nonsedating antihistamines (e.g., *cyclizine* and *meclozine*), that act directly on the vomiting center and the vestibular center, may be useful. Drugs such as *prochlorperazine* have some affinity for both muscarinic and histaminic receptors and are moderately useful although less specific.

Table 37.2   Commonly Used Antinauseant Drugs

Drug	Dose	Comment
Metoclopramide	10–20 mg every 4 hours (oral or subcutaneous)	Avoid if patient has bowel colic
Haloperidol	1–3 mg bid or tid (oral)	Lower doses required than when used as a sedative
Prochlorperazine	5–25 mg bid or tid (oral or rectal)	May be useful if vomiting mechanism is unknown
Meclozine	10–75 mg per day in divided doses (oral)	Antihistamine with doses that produce minimal sedation
Cyclizine	10–75 mg per day in divided doses (oral, rectal, or subcutaneous)	Useful if patient has bowel obstruction
Hyoscine	0.1–0.4 mg every 6–8 hours (subcutaneous)	CNS side effects can occur, particularly drowsiness and confusion
Ondansetron	0.15 mg/kg every 4 hours for 3 doses IV 4–8 mg tid (oral)	Main use is for chemotherapy-related nausea Constipation can be troublesome

See text and manufacturers' information before prescribing; watch for side effects; review frequently; cease ineffective drugs.

Nausea clearly related to the CTZ requires a drug with high affinity for dopamine receptors, such as *haloperidol*. A dose of 3 mg or less at night (orally or subcutaneously) may be sufficient. Nausea related to chemotherapy has become less of a problem for many patients with the introduction of new drugs such as *ondansetron*, a 5-HT (serotonin) receptor agonist (which has central and peripheral effects), but care must be taken with respect to side effects, which can include constipation.

Nausea arising from stimuli in the gastrointestinal tract associated with slowing of the gut should respond to gastrokinetic antinauseants such as *metaclopramide* or *domperidone*, which promote gastric emptying and increase gut motility. These actions will be counterproductive in a patient with a very high gastrointestinal obstruction, and vomiting will be aggravated.

Clearly, drugs available by more than one route—especially oral, subcutaneous, and rectal routes—are advantageous. Both *metaclopramide* and *haloperidol* may be used subcutaneously as well as orally, but other useful drugs (notably *prochlorperazine*) cannot be used subcutaneously. Many other drugs have useful antinauseant activity through various mechanisms, including *amitriptyline*, which has a central action.

In addition to the established antinauseant drugs, *dexamethasone*, which acts by an unknown mechanism, is also useful in suppressing nausea, and the drug is used in some premedication programs before chemotherapy. It is also useful in some patients with advanced disease, but it should be used in the lowest possible dose and as an adjunct to other therapy. Small doses (e.g., 2 mg *dexamethasone*) may reduce nausea associated with tumors involving the gastrointestinal tract, especially hepatic metastases or motility disturbances. If benefit is not obvious within 1 week, it could be discontinued (17). Caution must be exercised if the patient has a history of active peptic ulceration, tuberculosis, or diabetes mellitus.

Constipation

Constipation, a common symptom, may result from a change of diet, inactivity, opioids used without laxatives, or from varying degrees of tumor-induced intestinal obstruction. Opioid-induced fecal impaction is almost always avoidable. When present, vigorous local treatment is required, such as glycerine or stimulant suppositories, careful enemas, or occasionally, manual removal with analgesia. Laxatives including large bowel stimulants, softeners, and occasionally small bowel flushers are also essential.

Constipation resulting from intestinal obstruction as a direct effect of tumor or adhesions requires either relief of the obstruction by medical or surgical means or acceptance as an end-stage manifestation.

Bowel Obstruction

Gynecological malignancies are frequently complicated by the development of bowel obstruction. This is most common in ovarian cancer, in which the incidence varies from 14.6%

(18) to 42% of patients with advanced disease developing partial or complete bowel obstruction (19, 20). Obstruction may occur at any level of the gastrointestinal tract and frequently involves several separate sites.

The management of patients with recurrent cancer and those with progressive disease on chemotherapy includes the recognition that definitive surgical treatment is not always associated with acceptable results. Although surgery must be considered for all of these patients, an attempt to define those who will not benefit must be made. These poor prognostic factors include hypoalbuminemia, raised blood urea nitrogen, raised serum alkaline phosphatase, obstruction associated with a normal abdominal x-ray or the presence of massive ascites or palpable abdominal masses (20, 21).

In a patient with end-stage obstruction, the totally symptomatic approach developed at St. Christopher's Hospice may be helpful (22). In brief, this approach avoids the use of both a nasogastric tube and intravenous fluids. It relies on careful mouth care, with a little food and drink as desired. The patient remains mildly dehydrated, but this is beneficial in reducing gastrointestinal secretions and, hence, the amount of vomiting. Medications are used with care.

For a practical point of view, bowel obstructions can be divided into three groups: complete bowel obstruction, partial bowel obstruction, and motility disorders. It is important to note that fecal impaction may mimic a bowel obstruction.

Complete Bowel Obstruction

The surgical correction or bypass for complete bowel obstruction depends on the location of the obstruction or obstructions, the extent of the cancer, and the estimated time of survival. If surgery is not indicated, medical management should be undertaken. Steps that can be taken are as follows:

1. Consider a trial of steroids to reduce pain and tumor edema, if not contraindicated, thereby determining whether any reversibility exists

2. If irreversible, the aim is
   - to decrease volumes of gastrointestinal secretions by reducing or ceasing parenteral fluids.
   - to decrease spasmodic pain and increase bowel capacity by judicial use of anticholinergic agents such as *hyoscine hydrobromide* (10–20 mg subcutaneously every 4 hours). *Hyoscine hydrobromide* has similar effects but crosses the blood-brain barrier and may cause drowsiness. Subcutaneous *morphine* may also be needed for pain control.
   - to decrease nausea with appropriate antiemetics such as *haloperidol,* 0.5 mg at bedtime increasing to 1.5 mg or 3 mg subcutaneously divided into two daily doses. *Metaclopramide* must be used with care in bowel obstruction. If the obstruction is high, it may induce worsening of vomiting and colic. However, with a low obstruction, it may assist by enhancing gastric emptying and therefore keeping the upper gut empty.

3. If obstruction is high with large-volume vomiting, gastric and intestinal secretions can be reduced further by *somatostatin,* 300–600 mg subcutaneously over 24 hours.

4. With the above approach, most patients' pain and symptoms can be controlled, enabling them to continue to drink and tolerate small amounts of food without nausea, vomiting only once every 24–72 hours.

5. If vomiting of large volumes persists despite the above measures, a skinny nasogastric tube may be considered or a venting gastrostomy may be performed to enable decompression.

Partial Obstruction

Partial bowel obstruction may be difficult to differentiate from a motility disorder, but it tends to be associated with more vomiting, more pain, and characteristic bowel sounds.

1. Surgery should be considered, especially if there is single-level bowel obstruction.

2. If surgery is not appropriate and the partial obstruction is caused by tumor, then the following measures should be tried:
   - steroids (if not contraindicated)
   - *metoclopramide* to empty the stomach (cease if vomiting is exacerbated)
   - antiemetics, antispasmodics, and analgesia (as for complete bowel obstruction)
   - gentle enemas to empty the rectum and lower bowel.

Motility Disorders

Gastrointestinal motility disorders behave like bowel obstructions and are diagnosed by a history of progressive, worsening constipation out of proportion with the effects of opioids or other medications. The situation is characterized clinically by little or no vomiting and is usually painless, with only minimal abdominal distension and diminished or absent bowel sounds.

Motility disorders may result from direct tumor invasion of the myenteric plexus or bowel wall, from radiotherapy, or secondary to autonomic neuropathy from chemotherapy. It can involve the entire length of the bowel or cause a single loop of atonic bowel.

The management is aimed at stimulating the bowel as much as possible with prokinetic agents such as *cisapride* and stimulants such as *senna*. The rectum and lower colon are emptied using enemas. If a single loop of bowel is involved, surgical resection may be appropriate.

Diarrhea, Fistula, and Tenesmus

Diarrhea in a patient with advanced gynecological cancer is probably best considered as a sign of fecal impaction until proven otherwise. True irritative diarrhea can occur when tumor involves the bowel wall. *Loperamide* is useful in the management of such patients. When diarrhea is associated with a rectovaginal fistula and surgical diversion is not possible, the emphasis is on nursing procedures calculated to keep the vagina clean and comfortable and to support the patient in her quite extreme distress.

Fistulas between bowel and bowel, bowel and skin, and/or involving pelvic viscera are serious causes of major distress for some patients. Obviously, surgical options are considered, especially when the etiology is not tumor recurrence but radiation damage. When surgical approaches are not feasible, other measures must be taken.

Measures that may benefit the patient include the following:

1. Maintenance of soft, formed stools by judicious use of bulking agents

2. Reduction of bowel secretions by trial of *somatostatin* in some circumstances

3. Antibiotics, especially *metronidazole,* locally as well as systemically, may be valuable in reducing some of the distressing odor when necrosis has occurred

4. Local measures to reduce soiling: for example, correctly selected and placed catheters or other appliances

5. Skin care involving stoma therapists when possible

6. Constant emotional support

Tenesmus can often be problematic and may require the advice of a specialist. The approach to management of tenesmus should follow guidelines as outlined in Figure 37.1. The use of antispasmodics, including anticholinergic agents, calcium channel blockers, and occasionally drugs used for neuropathic pain, may be helpful.

Abdominal Distension and Ascites

This symptom may have many causes, including simple tumor bulk, obstructed bowel, or ascites. Abdominal distension resulting from intractable ascites can be a major cause of distress. Recurrent paracentesis has a limited but definite place, whereas shunting procedures have severe limitations. Diuretics, especially *spironolactone* 50–150 mg per day, may prove helpful initially. Occasionally, corticosteroids in very low doses may reduce production and are worthy of trial. The actual discomfort is readily controlled with a combination of a drug such as *acetaminophen* and a low dose of an opioid. Cytotoxics (systemic or intraperitoneal) may be worthy of consideration, but in practice, their potential is limited in a late-stage patient, and care must be taken not to waste the patient's time and energy or increase her distress.

Respiratory Symptoms

Dyspnea is common, and the dominant cause can usually be clarified by a clinical history, physical examination, and a chest x-ray. It should be possible to differentiate between a pleural effusion, bronchial obstruction, diffuse lung involvement, reduced excursion caused by massive ascites, bronchial asthma, chronic obstructive airway disease, cardiac failure, and respiratory infection.

When the dyspnea is not reversible and medical management is required, the careful use of *morphine* may improve the symptoms considerably (23). Oral *morphine* should be commenced at doses of 2–5 mg every 4 hours and increased until no further benefit is gained. In practice, this usually means doses of around 10 mg every 4 hours, with or without corticosteroids in low dosage. *Morphine* may improve dyspnea not only through central mechanisms but possibly also through peripheral effects. If a patient is already receiving morphine calibrated correctly for pain relief but becomes dyspneic because of tumor progression, *morphine* may be increased by an additional 30–50% to give relief (4). If medical management of dyspnea is optimal, oxygen is rarely necessary or truly advantageous, even with widespread pulmonary metastases. Anxiolytics, however, may be valuable in modest doses. Benzodiazepines (for example, 2 mg *diazepam* orally or 0.5 mg *lorazepam* sublingually) may have significant benefit for the anxious patient.

Urinary Tract Symptoms

Urinary tract symptoms are common in women with far-advanced gynecological cancer. Hydronephrosis, with subsequent infection, pain, and obstructive nephropathy, may justify mechanical measures such as nephrostomy or stent insertion if the prognosis, on other grounds, is for at least several good-quality months of life. Although some patients clearly benefit, complications are frequent and the personal and financial costs can be considerable. Fine judgment is required for the individual case.

In the short term, patency of ureters, with a significant reduction in serum creatinine level and improved quality of life, may be achieved by short courses of modest doses of corticosteroids (e.g., oral *dexamethasone*, 4 mg daily for 3–5 days). Bladder symptoms may yield to the use of *NSAIDS* to reduce detrusor irritability or drugs with an anticholinergic action to reduce bladder contractility. Catheterization may be unavoidable in some circumstances and may increase comfort. Renal failure of even minor degree may mandate the need for dose reduction with respect to several drugs, including *morphine*.

Edema

Leg swelling caused by venous or lymphatic obstruction can be distressing and may respond either to small doses of diuretics or to careful massage toward the trunk, beginning at the top of the leg. Systematic bandaging of the legs by experienced personnel when the edema is minimal may improve the patient's comfort. Compression bandages or support hosiery should not be applied to grossly edematous legs, because venous circulation may be further compromised.

Weakness

Weakness can be a dominant symptom when there is a large tumor load, but there are also many reversible causes for weakness. These include nutritional deficiencies, hypotension, hypokalemia or hyperglycemia, hypoadrenalism, hypercalcemia, renal failure, infection, and anemia.

At least some of these may be either easily excluded or readily treated in appropriate circumstances. Nutritional deficiencies may aggravate the debility associated with advanced cancer, and some of these problems may be readily reversible. Anemia is not necessarily an indication for transfusion, as benefit may be short-lived and not proportionate to the expenditure of resources. If the hemoglobin is very low and weakness is a dominant symptom, transfusion may be justified.

Hypercalcemia

Hypercalcemia (raised ionized plasma calcium level) is a recognized complication of malignancy, which is often, but not always, associated with bony metastases. Hypercalcemia is a potent cause of symptoms, ranging from aggravation of bone pain, lethargy, weakness, and constipation to severe nausea, vomiting, and confusion. In general, such distressing symptoms should be reversed if possible. Assistance of a specialist may be wise both to clarify the diagnosis (because each of the symptoms above can have complex causes) and to supervise the treatment.

Treatment may not be justified for a patient who is clearly dying, but in most instances, treatment is justified at least once after due consideration of the ethical principles involved. Treatment involves the use of preparations such as *pamidronate,* 30–60 mg by intravenous infusion in 250 ml of crystalloid over 4–8 hours.

Improvement of symptoms with these measures can be expected within 2–3 days, with continuation of the effect for 2–3 weeks, when repetition of *pamidronate* infusion can be performed. The rate of relapse of hypercalcemia is partially dependent on the availability of effective therapy for the underlying tumor, as well as on the biologic characteristics and tempo of the neoplastic process.

Care of the Patient Close to Death

No person should die in despair. The physician should assist the patient to center hope not on what will fail in the end (e.g., chemotherapy, radiotherapy, surgery) but on what will not fail—such as the physician's commitment to care, the control of pain and other symptoms, and the intrinsic value of the patient as a unique individual. No patient should die with hope focused on the next course of chemotherapy or on another surgical intervention. Unrealistic expectations may increase, not relieve, suffering (15).

After it is clear that the patient is dying, the goal is dignity and peace, which are best served by precise control of major symptoms. This usually involves continuing indicated drugs in correct dosage, by either the subcutaneous or the rectal route. Sometimes one is justified in offering direct sedation when, despite adequate pain control, distress is extreme and opportunities for verbal communication no longer exist. Phenothiazines such as *chlorpromazine* may cause distressing dissociation, and anxiolytics of the *benzodiazepine* group are preferable. In such circumstances, sublingual *lorazepam,* 0.5–2.5 mg every 4–6 hours, may be valuable. Alternatively, parenteral *midazolam* (e.g., 2–5 mg subcutaneously or intramuscularly) or *clonazepam* (subcutaneously or sublingual) may assist in achieving appropriate sedation, whereas a subcutaneous infusion of 30–50 mg every 24 hours may be helpful if the situation is protracted. Large doses of opioids are not appropriate for sedation of dying patients.

Complex equipment should be avoided if possible. It is consoling to both the patient and the family to avoid tubes of all sorts wherever possible, to facilitate maximum physical contact with loved ones.

The process of dying is fraught with uncertainties. Space, time, privacy, and peacefulness are the essence of good care, and these are facilitated by the presentation of a clear therapeutic plan. In the face of imminent death, respect for individual religious and cultural customs is mandatory. It is essential that medical and nursing staff accept and understand the value and personal significance of the final phase of life, even the last days.

Ethical issues abound in relation to gynecological oncology, as in all areas of clinical practice. Such issues include the rights of the patient, the responsibilities of the clinical staff and of society, and the requirements to ensure at least good symptomatic relief and basic care in accord with human dignity throughout the course of the illness. It is crucial to recognize when the time has come to allow a patient to die, but deliberate acceleration of death is not necessary nor the wisest course to ensure dignity in most circumstances if skilled palliative care is available.

It is the physician's responsibility and privilege to provide care, support, and concern, no matter what ensues, with as much attention to the palliation of symptoms as has been given to diagnosis and anticancer treatment. The patient should be encouraged in every effort she exerts to combat her disease but also to accept her personal reality profoundly.

Nothing should be said or done by doctors to induce despair, either by encouraging false hope or by failure to offer skilled care. Instead, all should be said and done to facilitate the emergence of a final integrity and wholeness, no matter what the preceding shape of the patient's life has been. This is real hope rooted in reality, which is abiding. Good palliative care is concerned with enrichment of life, even when facing death, the human task that is common to all.

References

1. **World Health Organization.** *Cancer Pain Relief and Palliative Care.* WHO: Geneva, 1991.

2. **Feinstein AR.** *Clinical Judgement.* Baltimore: Williams & Wilkins, 1967:91–7.

3. **Twycross RG, Lack SA.** Therapeutics in terminal cancer. In: *Pain Relief.* 2nd ed. London: Churchill Livingstone, 1990.

4. **Doyle D, Hanks GW, MacDonald N** *Oxford Textbook of Palliative Medicine.* Oxford: Oxford University Press, 1993.

5. **Billings JA.** *Outpatient Management of Advanced Cancer.* Philadelphia: JB Lippincott, 1985.

6. **Walsh TD.** *Symptom Control.* Oxford: Blackwell Scientific, 1989.

7. **Hanks GW, Justin DM.** Cancer pain management. *Lancet* 1992;339:1031–9.

8. **Foley KM.** Controversies in cancer pain: medical perspectives. *Cancer* 1989;63:2257–65.

9. **Matthiessen HV.** Pain treatment in gynecological cancer. *Postgrad Med J* 1991;67(Suppl 2):26–30.

10. **Conolly ME.** Recent advances in the control of pain. In: **Bates TD,** ed. *Contemporary Palliative of Difficult Symptoms. In: Bailliere's Clinical Oncology.* Vol 1. London: Bailliere Tindall, 1987:417–41.

11. **Ad Hoc Committee on Cancer Pain of the American Society of Clinical Oncology: ASCO Cancer.** Pain assessment and treatment curriculum guidelines. *J Clin Oncol* 1992;10:1976–82.

12. **Glare PA, Walsh TD.** Clinical pharmacokinetics of morphine. *Ther Drug Monit* 1991;13:1–23.

13. **Portenoy RK, Moulin DE, Rogers A, Inturrisi CE, Foley KM.** IV infusion of opioids for cancer pain: clinical review and guidelines for use. *Cancer Treat Rep* 1986;70:575–81.

14. **Creed Pettigrew L, Glass JP, Maor M, Zornoza J.** Diagnosis and treatment of lumbosacral plexopthies in patients with cancer. *Arch Neurol* 1984;41:1282–5.

15. **Cassell EJ.** The nature of suffering and the goals of medicine. *N Engl J Med* 1982;306(11): 639–45.

16. **Twycross RG, Lack SA.** *Control of Alimentary Symptoms in Far Advanced Cancer*. London: Churchill Livingstone, 1986.

17. **Twycross RG.** *Cancer Pain*. London: Churchill Livingstone, 1993.

18. **Granei MD.** Ovarian cancer: unrealistic expectations. *N Engl J Med* 1992;327:197–200.

19. **Solomon HJ, Atkinson KH, Coppleson JV, Elliot PM, Houghton CR.** Bowel complications in the management of ovarian cancer. *Aust N Z J Obstet Gynaecol* 1983;23:65–8.

20. **Krebs HB, Goplerud DR.** Surgical management of bowel obstruction in advanced ovarian carcinoma. *Obstet Gynecol* 1983;61(3):327–30.

21. **Fernandes JR, Seymour RJ, Suissa S.** Bowel obstruction in patients with ovarian cancer: a search for prognostic factors. *Am J Obstet Gynecol* 1988;158:344–9.

22. **Baines M, Oliver DJ, Carter RL.** Medical management of intestinal obstruction in patients with advanced malignant disease. *Lancet* 1985;2:990–3.

23. **Cowcher KC, Hanks GW.** Long term management of respiratory symptoms in advanced cancer. *J Pain Symptom Manage* 1990;5:320–30.

Appendix: Reference Values

Measure	SI	Conventional (C)	Conversion Factor (CF) $C \times CF = SI$
Acetoacetate, plasma	<100 μmol/l	<1.0 mg/dl	97.95
Adrenal steroids, plasma			
Aldosterone, supine, saline suppression	<220 pmol/l	<8 ng/dl	27.74
Cortisol			
8:00 AM	220–660 nmol/l	8–24 μg/dl	27.59
4:00 PM	50–410 nmol/l	2–15 μg/dl	27.59
Overnight dexamethasone suppression	<140 nmol/l	<5 μg/dl	27.59
Dehydroepiandrosterone (DHEA)	0.6–70 nmol/l	0.2–20 μg/l	3.467
Dehydroepiandrosterone sulfate (DHEAS)	5.4–9.2 μmol/l	820–3380 ng/ml	0.002714
11-Deoxycortisol (compound S)	<60 nmol/l	<2 μg/dl	28.86
17α-Hydroxyprogesterone, women	1–13 nmol/l	0.3–4.2 μg/l	3.026
Adrenal steroids, urinary excretion			
Aldosterone	15–70 nmol/d	5–26 μg/d	2.774
Cortisol, free	30–300 nmol/d	10–100 μg/d	2.759
17-Hydroxycorticosteroids	5.5–28 μmol/d	2–10 mg/d	2.759
17-Ketosteroids, women	14–52 μmol/d	4–15 mg/d	3.467
Ammonia (as NH_3), venous whole blood	6–45 μmol/l	10–80 μg/dl	0.5872
Angiotensin II, plasma, 8 AM	10–30 ng/l	10–30 pg/ml	1.0
Arginine vasopressin (AVP), plasma, random fluid intake	2.3–7.4 pmol/l	2.5–8 ng/l	0.92
Bicarbonate, serum	18–23 mmol/l	18–23 meq/l	1.0
Calciferols (see vitamin D)			
Calcitonin, serum	<50 ng/l	<50 pg/ml	1.0
Calcium			
Ionized serum	1–1.5 mmol/l	4–4.6 mg/dl	0.2495
Total serum	2.2–2.6 mmol/l	9–10.5 mg/dl	0.2495
β-Carotene, serum	0.9–4.6 μmol/l	50–250 μg/dl	0.01863
Catecholamines, plasma			
Epinephrine, basal supine	170–520 pmol/l	30–95 pg/ml	5.458
Norepinephrine, basal supine	0.3–2.8 nmol/l	15–475 pg/ml	0.005911
Catecholamines, urinary			
Epinephrine	<275 nmol/d	<50 μg/d	5.458
Normetanephrine	0–11 μmol/d	0–2.0 mg/d	5.458
Total catecholamines (as norepinephrine)	<675 nmol/d	<120 μg/d	5.911
Vanillylmandelic acid (VMA)	<35 μmol/d	<68 mg/d	5.046
Chloride, serum	98–106 mmol/l	98–106 meq/l	1.0
Cholesterol, plasma			
Total cholesterol			
Desirable	<5.20 mmol/l	<200 mg/dl	0.02586
Borderline high	5.2–6.18 mmol/l	200–239 mg/dl	0.02586
High	≥6.21 mmol/l	≥240 mg/dl	0.02586
High-density lipoprotein (HDL) cholesterol			
Desirable	≥1.29 mmol/l	≥50 mg/dl	0.02586
Borderline high	0.9–1.27 mmol/l	36–49 mg/dl	0.02586
High	≤0.91 mmol/l	≤35 mg/dl	0.02586
Low-density lipoprotein (LDL) cholesterol			
Desirable	<3.36 mmol/l	<130 mg/dl	0.02586
Borderline high	3.39–4.11 mmol/l	131–159 mg/dl	0.02586
High	≥4.14 mmol/l	≥160 mg/dl	0.02586
Corticotropin (ACTH), plasma	4–22 pmol/l	20–100 pg/ml	0.2202
C peptide, plasma	0.5–2 μg/l	0.5–2 ng/ml	1.0
Creatinine, serum	<133 μmol/l	<1.5 mg/dl	88.40
Fatty acids, nonesterified or free (FFA), plasma	<0.7 mmol/l	<18 mg/dl	0.03906
Gastrin, serum	<120 ng/l	<120 pg/ml	1.0
Glucagon, plasma	50–100 ng/l	50–100 pg/ml	1.0
Glucose, plasma			
Overnight fast, normal	4.2–6.4 mmol/l	75–115 mg/dl	0.05551
Overnight fast, diabetes mellitus	7.8 mmol/l	>140 mg/dl	0.05551
72-hour fast, normal women	>2.2 mmol/l	>40 mg/dl	0.05551
Glucose tolerance test, 2-hour postprandial plasma glucose			
Normal	<7.8 mmol/l	<140 mg/dl	0.05551
Imparied glucose tolerance	7.8–11.1 mmol/l	140–200 mg/dl	0.05551
Diabetes mellitus	>11.1 mmol/l	>200 mg/dl	0.05551

Measure	SI	Conventional (C)	Conversion Factor (CF) $C \times CF = SI$
Gonadal steroids, plasma			
Androstenedione, women	3.5–7.0 nmol/l	1–2 ng/ml	3.492
Estradiol, women			
Basal	70–220 pmol/l	20–60 pg/ml	3.671
Ovulatory surge	>740 pmol/l	>200 pg/ml	3.671
Dihydrotestosterone, women	0.17–1.0 nmol/l	0.05–3 ng/ml	3.467
Progesterone, women			
Luteal phase	6–64 nmol/l	2–20 ng/ml	3.180
Follicular phase	<6 nmol/l	<2 ng/ml	3.180
Testosterone			
Women	<3.5 nmol/l	<1 ng/ml	3.467
Prepubertal boys and girls	0.2–0.7 nmol/l	0.05–0.2 ng/ml	3.467
Gonadotropins, plasma			
Women, basal			
Follicle-stimulating hormone	5–20 IU/l	5–20 mIU/ml	1.0
Luteinizing hormone	5–25 IU/l	5–25 mIU/ml	1.0
Women, ovulatory peak			
Follicle-stimulating hormone	12–30 IU/l	12–30 mIU/ml	1.0
Luteinizing hormone	25–100 IU/l	25–100 mIU/ml	1.0
Prepubertal boys and girls			
Follicle-stimulating hormone	<5 IU/l	<5 mIU/ml	1.0
Luteinizing hormone	<5 IU/l	<5 mIU/ml	1.0
Growth hormone, plasma			
After 100 g glucose orally	<5 μg/l	<5 ng/ml	1.0
After insulin-induced hypoglycemia	>9 μg/l	>9 ng/ml	1.0
Human chorionic gonadotropin, beta subunit, plasma; nonpregnant women	<3 IU/l	<3 mIU/ml	1.0
β-Hydroxybutyrate, plasma	<300 nmol/l	<3.0 mg/dl	96.05
Insulin, plasma			
Fasting	35–145 pmol/l	5–20 μU/ml	7.175
During hypoglycemia (plasma glucose <2.8 nmol/l [<50 mg/dl])	<35 pmol/l	<5 μU/ml	7.175
Insulin-like growth factor I (IGF I, somatomedin-C), women	0.45–2.2 kU/l	0.45–2.2 U/ml	1.0
Lactate, plasma	0.56–2.2 mmol/l	5–20 mg/dl	0.111
Magnesium, serum	0.8–1.20 mmol/l	1.8–3.0 mg/dl	0.4114
Osmolality, plasma	285–295 mmol/kg	285–295 mosm/kg	1.0
Oxytocin, plasma			
Random	1–4 pmol/l	1.25–5 ng/l	0.80
Ovulatory peak in women	408 pmol/l	5–10 ng/l	0.80
Parathyroid hormone, serum (intact PTH using immunoradiometric assay [IRMA])	10–65 ng/l	10–65 pg/ml	1.0
Phosphorus, inorganic, serum	1–1.5 mmol/l	3.0–4.5 mg/dl	0.3229
Potassium, serum	3.5–5.0 mmol/l	3.5–5.0 meq/l	1.0
Prolactin, serum	2–15 μg/l	2–15 ng/ml	1.0
Pyruvate, blood	39–102 μmol/l	0.3–0.9 mg/dl	0.01129
Renin activity, plasma, normal-sodium diet			
Supine	3.2 ± 1 μg/l/h	3.2 ± 1.1 ng/ml/h	1.0
Standing	9.3 ± 4.3 μg/l/h	9.3 ± 4.3 ng/ml/h	1.0
Sodium, serum	136–145 mmol/l	136–145 meq/l	1.0
Thyroid function tests			
Radioactive iodine uptake, 24 hours	0.05–0.30	5–30%	—
Reverse triiodothyronine (rT_3), serum	0.15–0.61 nmol/l	10–4 ng/dl	0.01536
Thyrotropin (TSH), highly sensitive assay, serum	0.6–4.6 mU/l	0.6–4.6 μU/ml	1.0
Thyroxine (T_4), serum	51–42 nmol/l	4–11 μg/dl	12.87
Thyroxine-binding globulin, serum (as thyroxine)	150–360 nmol/l	12–28 μg/ml	12.87
Triiodothyronine (T_3), serum	1.2–3.4 nmol/l	75–220 ng/dl	0.01536
Triiodothyronine resin uptake, serum	0.25–0.35	25–35%	—
Triglycerides, plasma (as Triolein)	<1.80 mmol/l	<160 mg/dl	0.01129
Uric acid, serum	120–420 μmol/l	2–7 mg/dl	59.48
Vitamin D (as vitamin D_3, cholecalciferol), plasma			
1,25-Dihydroxycholecalciferol (1,25$(OH)_2$D)	36–144 pmol/l	15–60 pg/ml	2.400
25-Hydroxycholecalciferol (25-OHD)	20–100 nmol/l	8–40 ng/ml	2.496

Modified with permission from **Wilson JD, Foster DW.** *Williams Textbook of Endocrinology,* 8th ed. Philadelphia: WB Saunders, 1991.

Index

Page numbers in *italics* denote figures; those followed by "t" denote tables.